de Swiet's Medical Disorders in Obstetric Practice

Dedication

The name Michael de Swiet is synonymous with obstetric medicine. He has generously inspired generations of obstetric physicians throughout the world. Through his education, his writing and his practice, Professor de Swiet has imparted his wisdom to obstetricians, physicians and other clinicians, so raising the profile and understanding of maternal medicine. This has improved the safety of women with medical disorders in pregnancy and of their babies. A gentle, but great, man to whom we and all our patients owe an enormous debt, Professor de Swiet's contribution to the practice, teaching and research in the field has influenced maternal medicine around the world. We grew up with *Medical Disorders in Obstetric Practice* as our bible and we are delighted that the 5th edition has been aptly renamed *"de Swiet's Medical Disorders in Obstetric Practice"*.

Catherine Nelson-Piercy
Consultant Obstetric Physician
Guy's & St Thomas' Foundation Trust and
Queen Charlotte's & Chelsea Hospital
London, UK

Robyn A. North
Professor of Maternal and Fetal Medicine
Division of Reproduction and Endocrinology
King's College London
London, UK

Karen Rosene-Montella
Professor of Medicine and Obstetrics-Gynecology
Warren Alpert Medical School of Brown University
Chief of Medicine, Women & Infants' Hospital of Rhode Island
Providence, RI, USA

de Swiet's Medical Disorders in Obstetric Practice

Edited by

Raymond O. Powrie MD FRCP FACP
Professor of Medicine and Obstetrics and Gynecology
Warren Alpert Medical School of Brown University
Senior Vice President Quality and Clinical Effectiveness
Women & Infants' Hospital of Rhode Island
Providence, RI, USA

Michael F. Greene MD
Professor of Obstetrics, Gynecology and Reproductive Biology, Harvard Medical School;
Chief of Obstetrics, Massachusetts General Hospital, Boston, MA, USA

William Camann MD
Associate Professor of Anaesthesia, Harvard Medical School
Director of Obstetric Anesthesiology
Brigham and Women's Hospital, Harvard Medical School
Boston, MA, USA

FIFTH EDITION

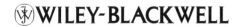

WILEY-BLACKWELL

A John Wiley & Sons, Ltd., Publication

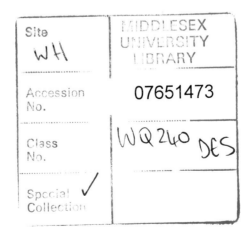

Contents

List of contributors

Brenna Anderson
Department of Obstetrics and Gynecology, Warren Alpert Medical School of Brown University, Providence, RI, USA

Teresa Baker
Department of Obstetrics and Gynecology, Texas Tech University of Medicine, Amarillo, TX, USA

Mrinalini Balki
Department of Anesthesia, Mount Sinai Hospital, Toronto, Ontario, Canada

Emma Barber
Department of Obstetrics, Gynecology and Reproductive Sciences, Yale University School of Medicine, New Haven, CT, USA

Marianne Berwick
Department of Internal Medicine and the Cancer Research and Treatment Center, University of New Mexico Health Sciences Center, Albuquerque, NM, USA

David Birnbach
Department of Anesthesia, University of Miami and Jackson Memorial Hospital, Miami, FL, USA

Ghada Bourjeily
Department of Medicine, Warren Alpert Medical School of Brown University, Women & Infants' Hospital of Rhode Island, Providence, RI, USA

Brian Brost
Department of Obstetrics and Gynecology, Mayo Clinic, Rochester, MN, USA

Mark A. Brown
Department of Renal Medicine, St George Hospital and University of New South Wales, Sydney, Australia

Brenda Bucklin
Department of Anesthesiology, University of Colorado Health Sciences Center, Denver, CO, USA

William Camann
Department of Anesthesiology, Perioperative and Pain Medicine, Brigham and Women's Hospital, Boston, MA, USA

Michael P. Carson
UMDNJ-Robert Wood Johnson Medical Scholl, Departments of Medicine and Obstetrics/Gynecology, Jersey Shore University Medical Center, Neptune, NJ, USA

Brian M. Casey
Department of Obstetrics and Gynecology, Division of Maternal-Fetal Medicine, University of Texas Southwestern Medical Center, Dallas, TX, USA

Eliana Castillo
Department of Medicine, University of British Columbia; Women's Health Research Institute, British Columbia Women's Hospital, Vancouver, BC, Canada

Wee Shian Chan
Department of Medicine, University of Toronto, Sunnybrooke and Women's Health Sciences Center, Toronto, Canada

Kenneth K. Chen
Department of Medicine, Warren Alpert Medical School of Brown University, Women & Infants' Hospital of Rhode Island, Providence, RI, USA

Edward K.S. Chien
Department of Obstetrics and Gynecology, Warren Alpert Medical School of Brown University, Women & Infants' Hospital of Rhode Island, Providence, RI, USA

Kue Chung Choi
Department of Anesthesiology, Women & Infants' Hospital of Rhode Island, Providence, RI, USA

Megan E. B. Clowse
Division of Rheumatology and Immunology, Duke University Medical Center, Durham, NC, USA

Anne-Marie Côté
Department of Medicine, Université de Sherbrooke, Sherbrooke, Quebec, Canada

Ilana B. Crome
Academic Psychiatry Unit, Keele University Medical School, St George's Hospital, Stafford, UK

Judith S. Currier
Division of Infectious Diseases, Center for Clinical AIDS Research and Education, David Geffen School of Medicine at UCLA, Los Angeles, CA, USA

Peter von Dadelszen
Department of Obstetrics and Gynecology, University of British Columbia, British Columbia Women's Hospital, Vancouver, BC, Canada

Mark Davis
Department of Dermatology, Mayo Clinic, Rochester, MN, USA

Joanne Douglas
Department of Anesthesia, British Columbia Women's Hospital, Vancouver, BC, Canada

Hugh M. Ehrenberg
Division of Maternal Fetal Medicine, Ohio State University Medical Center, Columbus, OH, USA

Chris Elton
Department of Anaesthesia, Leicester Royal Infirmary, Leicester, UK

Silvia Degli Esposti
Department of Medicine, Warren Alpert Medical School of Brown University, Women & Infants' Hospital of Rhode Island, Providence, RI, USA

Roshan Fernando
Department of Anaesthesia, Royal Free Hospital, London, UK

Véronique Filippi
Department of Epidemiology and Population Health, London School of Hygiene and Tropical Medicine, London, UK

Melissa Gaitanis
Department of Medicine/Infectious Diseases, Warren Alpert Medical School of Brown University, Providence, RI, USA

Stephen Gatt
Division of Anaesthesia and Intensive Care, Prince of Wales and Sydney Children's Hospitals and Royal Hospital for Women, Randwick, New South Wales, Australia

Paul S. Gibson
Departments of Medicine and Obstetrics and Gynecology, University of Calgary, Foothills Medical Centre, Calgary, Alberta, Canada

T. Murphy Goodwin
Department of Medicine, Keck School of Medicine, University of Southern California, Los Angeles, CA, USA

Dorothy Graham
Obstetric Medicine, University of Western Australia and King Edward Memorial Hospital, Perth, Australia

Michael F. Greene
Vincent Memorial Obstetrics and Gynecology Department, Massachusetts General Hospital, Boston, MA, USA

Ian Greer
Faculty of Health and Life Sciences, University of Liverpool, Liverpool, UK

Kalpalatha K. Guntupalli
Pulmonary, Critical Care and Sleep Medicine, Baylor College of Medicine, Houston, TX, USA

Thomas W. Hale
Department of Pediatrics, Texas Tech University of Medicine, Amarillo, TX, USA

Dominic C. Heaney
UCL Institute of Neurology, University College London and UCL Hospitals NHS Foundation Trust, London, UK

Linda Heffner
Department of Obstetrics and Gynecology, Boston University School of Medicine, Boston, MA, USA

Timothy Hurley
Department of Obstetrics and Gynecology, University of New Mexico Health Sciences Center, Albuquerque, NM, USA

Jessica Illuzzi
Department of Obstetrics, Gynecology and Reproductive Sciences, Yale University School of Medicine, New Haven, CT, USA

Khaled M.K. Ismail
Keele University Medical School and The Maternity Centre, University Hospital of North Staffordshire, Stoke-on-Trent, UK

Sig-Linda Jacobson
Department of Obstetrics and Gynecology, Oregon Health and Science University, Division of Maternal-Fetal Medicine, Portland, OR, USA

Andra H. James
Division of Maternal-Fetal Medicine, Department of Obstetrics and Gynecology, Duke University Medical Center, Durham, NC, USA

Dilip R. Karnad
Seth G S Medical College and Medical Intensive Care Unit, KEM Hospital, Mumbai, India, and Baylor College of Medicine, Houston, TX, USA

Warwick D. Ngan Kee
Department of Anesthesia and Intensive Care, Chinese University of Hong Kong, Prince of Wales Hospital, Hong Kong, China

Erin Keely
Department of Endocrinology and Metabolism, The Ottawa Hospital, Ottawa, Ontario, Canada

Hanan Khalil
Department of Diagnostic Imaging, Warren Alpert Medical School of Brown University, Providence, RI, USA

Rshmi Khurana
Departments of Medicine and Obstetrics and Gynecology, University of Alberta, Royal Alexandra Hospital, Edmonton, Alberta, Canada

Sailesh Kumar
Centre for Fetal and Maternal Medicine, Queen Charlotte's and Chelsea Hospital, Imperial College London, London, UK

Sandra L. Kweder
Department of Medicine, Uniformed Services University, Bethesda, MD, USA

Lucia Larson
Department of Obstetrics and Gynecology, Warren Alpert Medical School of Brown University, Women & Infants' Hospital of Rhode Island, Providence, RI, USA

Men-Jean Lee
Department of Obstetrics, Gynecology and Reproductive Science, Mount Sinai School of Medicine, NY, USA

Stephanie L. Lee
Section of Endocrinology, Diabetes, and Nutrition, Boston Medical Center, Boston, MA, USA

Kimberly K. Leslie
Department of Obstetrics and Gynecology, and the Cancer Research and Treatment Center, University of New Mexico Health Sciences Center, Albuquerque, NM, USA

Sandra A. Lowe
Department of Medicine, Royal Hospital For Women and School of Women's and Children's Health, University of New South Wales, Sydney, Australia

Cynthia Maxwell
Obstetrics and Maternal Fetal Medicine, Mount Sinai Hospital, Toronto, Ontario, Canada

Elizabeth McGrady
Department of Anesthesia, Princess Royal Maternity Unit, Glasgow Royal Infirmary, Glasgow, Scotland, UK

Claire McLintock
National Women's Health, Auckland City Hospital, Auckland, New Zealand

Laura A. Magee
Department of Medicine, University of British Columbia, British Columbia Women's Hospital , Vancouver, BC, Canada

Moke Magoma
Department of Epidemiology and Population Health, London School of Hygiene and Tropical Medicine, London, UK

George J. Mangos
Department of Renal Medicine, St George Hospital and University of New South Wales, Sydney, Australia

Niharika Mehta
Department of Medicine, Warren Alpert Medical School of Brown University, Women & Infants' Hospital of Rhode Island, Providence, RI, USA

Margaret A. Miller
Department of Medicine, Warren Alpert Medical School of Brown University, Women & Infants' Hospital of Rhode Island, Providence, RI, USA

Mark E. Molitch
Division of Endocrinology, Metabolism and Molecular Medicine, Northwestern University Feinberg School of Medicine, Chicago, IL, USA

Deborah M. Money
Department of Obstetrics and Gynecology, University of British Columbia; Women's Health Research Institute, British Columbia Women's Hospital, Vancouver, BC, Canada

Martin N. Montoro
Department of Obstetrics and Gynecology, Keck School of Medicine, University of Southern California, Los Angeles, CA, USA

Carolyn Muller
Department of Obstetrics and Gynecology, University of New Mexico Health Sciences Center, Albuquerque, NM, USA

Uma Munnur
Department of Anesthesiology, Baylor College of Medicine, Houston, TX, USA

Catherine Nelson-Piercy
Guy's & St Thomas' Foundation Trust and Queen Charlotte's & Chelsea Hospital, London, UK

James A. O'Brien
Department of Obstetrics and Gynecology, Warren Alpert Medical School of Brown University, Women & Infants' Hospital of Rhode Island, Providence, RI, USA

Patrick O'Brien
UCL Institute of Women's Health, University College London and UCL Hospitals NHS Foundation Trust, London, UK

Nollag O'Rourke
Department of Anesthesia, Perioperative and Pain Medicine, Brigham and Women's Hospital, Harvard Medical School, Boston, MA, USA

Medge D. Owen
Department of Anesthesia, Wake Forest University, Winston-Salem, NC, USA

Elvis R. Pagan
Virginia Tech Carilion School of Medicine, Department of Medicine, Carilion Clinic, Roanoke, VA, USA

Michael J. Paglia
Department of Obstetrics and Gynecology, Warren Alpert Medical School of Brown University, Women & Infants' Hospital of Rhode Island, Providence, RI, USA

Michael Paidas
Department of Obstetrics, Gynecology and Reproductive Sciences, Yale Women and Children's Center for Blood Disorders, Yale-New Haven Hospital, New Haven, CT, USA

Alan Peaceman
Division of Maternal-Fetal Medicine, Department of Obstetrics and Gynecology, Northwestern University Feinberg School of Medicine, Chicago, IL, USA

Teri Pearlstein
Department of Psychiatry and Human Behavior, Warren Alpert Medical School of Brown University and Women's Behavioral Health Program, Women & Infants' Hospital of Rhode Island, Providence, RI, USA

Michael Peek
Department of Obstetrics and Gynaecology, University of Sydney and Nepean Hospital, Sydney, Australia

Robert A. Peterfreund
Harvard Medical School and Massachusetts General Hospital, Boston, MA, USA

Michelle Petri
Division of Rheumatology, Johns Hopkins University School of Medicine, Baltimore, MD, USA

Rudiger Pittrof
Department of Epidemiology and Population Health, London School of Hygiene and Tropical Medicine, London, UK

Felicity Plaat
Department of Anaesthesia, Queen Charlotte's and Hammersmith Hospitals, London, UK

Athena Poppas
Division of Cardiology, Department of Medicine, Warren Alpert Medical School of Brown University and Echocardiography Laboratory, Rhode Island Hospital, Providence, RI, USA

Raymond O. Powrie
Department of Medicine, Warren Alpert Medical School of Brown University, Women & Infants' Hospital of Rhode Island, Providence, RI, USA

Christopher W.G. Redman
Nuffield Department of Obstetrics and Gynaecology, University of Oxford, Oxford, UK

John T. Repke
Penn State Milton S. Hershey Medical Center, MSHMC Maternal Fetal Medicine, Hershey, PA, USA

Marc A. Rodger
Division of Hematology, The Ottawa Hospital, University of Ottawa; Clinical Epeidemiology Program, Ottawa Health Research Institute, Ottawa, Ontario, Canada

Robin Russell
Nuffield Department of Anaesthetics, John Radcliffe Hospital, Oxford, UK

Sunanda Sadanandan
Department of Obstetrics and Gynecology, University of New Mexico Health Sciences Center, Albuquerque, NM, USA

Sumona Saha
Department of Medicine, Warren Alpert Medical School of Brown University, Women & Infants' Hospital of Rhode Island, Providence, RI, USA

Scott Segal
Department of Anesthesia, Harvard Medical School, Brigham and Women's Hospital, Boston, MA, USA

Mathew Sermer
Department of Obstetrics and Gynecology, University of Toronto, and Obstetrics and Maternal Fetal Medicine, Mount Sinai Hospital, Toronto, Ontario, Canada

Daniel I. Sessler
Department of Outcomes Research, Cleveland Clinic, Cleveland, OH, USA

Winnie W. Sia
Departments of Medicine and Obstetrics and Gynecology, University of Alberta, Royal Alexandra Hospital, Edmonton, Alberta, Canada

Caren G. Solomon
Department of Medicine, Brigham and Women's Hospital, Boston, MA, USA

Jami Star
Department of Obstetrics and Gynecology, University of Massachusetts Medical School, University of Massachusetts Memorial Medical Center, Worcester, MA, USA

Iris Tong
Department of Medicine, Warren Alpert Medical School of Brown University, Women & Infants' Hospital of Rhode Island, Providence, RI, USA

Lawrence Tsen
Department of Anesthesiology, Center for Reproductive Medicine, Perioperative and Pain Medicine, Brigham and Women's Hospital, Boston, MA, USA

Ruth E. Tuomala
Department of Obstetrics, Gynecology, and Reproductive Biology, Harvard Medical School and Brigham and Women's Hospital, Boston, MA, USA

Susan Cu-Uvin
Departments of Medicine and Obstetrics and Gynecology, Brown University; The Immunology Center, The Miriam Hospital, Providence, RI, USA

Claire Verschraegen
Department of Internal Medicine and the Cancer Research and Treatment Center, University of New Mexico Health Sciences Center, Albuquerque, NM, USA

Mark C. Walker
Ottawa Health Research Institute and Department of Obstetrics and Gynecology, University of Ottawa, Ontario, Canada

Charles L. Wiggins
Department of Internal Medicine and the Cancer Research and Treatment Center, University of New Mexico Health Sciences Center, Albuquerque, NM, USA

David J. Williams
UCL Institute of Women's Health, University College London and UCL Hospitals NHS Foundation Trust, London, UK

Catherine Williamson
Institute of Reproductive and Developmental Biology, Imperial College London, London, UK

Richard N. Wissler
Department of Anesthesiology, Obstetrics and Gynecology, University of Rochester, School of Medicine and Dentistry, Rochester, NY, USA

David Wlody
Department of Anesthesiology, State University of New York Downstate Medical Center, Brooklyn, NY, USA

Edward R. Yeomans
Department of Obstetrics and Gynecology, University of Texas Medical School at Houston and Texas Tech University Health Sciences Center, Lubbock, TX, USA

Preface

Professor Michael de Swiet's ground breaking first edition of *Medical Disorders in Obstetric Practice* was published more than 35 years ago and was one of the first international textbooks to focus exclusively on providing expert guidance to obstetricians, medical specialists and anesthesiologists for the care of medical illness during pregnancy. It has remained one of the foremost books in the field with each subsequent edition. We have been privileged to serve as the new multidisciplinary editorial team for this fifth edition. We have entirely revised and updated the last edition while striving to maintain Professor de Swiet's high standards of scholarship. This edition introduces several innovations that we hope will assist care providers in ensuring that women with medical disorders have the best possible outcomes for themselves and their pregnancies.

• Each chapter is now co-written and co-edited by an expert team of practicing clinicians including a high-risk obstetrician, a medical subspecialist and, where appropriate, an obstetric anesthesiologist. This team approach provides a uniquely broad interdisciplinary, practical perspective to the care of medical illness in pregnancy that expertly addresses the entire period from preconception through to postpartum follow up.

• An entirely new section has been added that provides brief, practical, evidence-based advice from highly experienced clinicians about how to properly investigate and safely manage many of the most common medical problems that present to obstetricians. Topics covered include syncope, palpitations, headaches and abnormal liver function tests.

• Additional chapters have been added on a wide range of topics including cancer, critical care, obesity, advanced maternal age and prescribing in pregnancy and lactation.

• The text makes much greater use of tables, algorithms, text boxes and figures to summarize and illustrate key points for busy clinicians.

• A special section of each major chapter now addresses issues related to the provision of anesthesia care to obstetric patients with medical illness to help obstetricians and medical specialists understand the concerns of their obstetric anesthesiology colleagues.

As doctors caring for medical illness in pregnancy, and building on the foundation of the four prior editions of his textbook, each of the editors feels much in debt to Professor de Swiet. We also gratefully acknowledge our debts to our wonderful partners and families (Harvey Makadon, Laurie, Jonathan and Rebecca Greene and Rhonda, Zac and Andy Camann for the time and attention that was taken from each of them while we worked on this book); our expert authors (for taking time they likely did not have to provide their excellent contributions); and the critical daily assistance from Linda J. Hunt, Lynne Mottola-Doherty and our remarkable publishing team at Wiley-Blackwell.

Raymond O. Powrie
Michael F. Greene
William Camann

Foreword

Obstetric medicine has never been more important. Every minute somewhere in the world a woman dies of complications arising from pregnancy or childbirth. More than six million newborns and 600,000 women die needlessly each year. In the developed world indirect deaths and other "medical" causes such as thromboembolism are the major causes of women dying in pregnancy. This is not so in the developing world where sepsis and obstructed labour are still major worries, but medical problems such as eclampsia are still very important. Therefore, it is essential that all who care for pregnant women have insight into medical disorders and they way that these are influenced by pregnancy.

Traditional teaching in obstetrics and midwifery in the past concentrated on obstetric matters. Internists have been so unfamiliar with obstetrics that they have ignored the influence of pregnancy on their diseases in most of their teaching and writing. These issues have emphasized the need for a comprehensive textbook on medical disorders in pregnancy and have underwritten the success of previous editions of *Medical Disorders in Obstetric Practice*.

In this 5th edition, the new editors, Dr. Powrie, Dr. Greene and Dr. Camann, have made radical and welcome changes. Every chapter has been rewritten by new authors who are world leaders in their subjects. Most chapters are now a collaborative effort of clinicians from different specialties: maternal-fetal medicine, medical subspecialists, obstetric anesthetists and obstetric internists. This approach emphasizes the importance of multidisciplinary care for women with medical illness in pregnancy in order to achieve the best possible outcomes throughout their reproductive years.

There are new chapters on difficult subjects such as cancer in pregnancy, prescribing in pregnancy and during lactation and on diagnostic imaging. The coverage has also been expanded by including a new section on specific problems such as how to manage chest pain and new onset seizures in pregnancy. These sections will be particularly useful for practitioners new to the field and, I suspect, will also be stimulating to those who are more experienced.

I am delighted that Raymond Powrie, and his colleagues have taken on the task of editing *Medical Disorders in Obstetric Practice*; I congratulate them on their magnificent achievement in editing this book and cannot recommend it too highly.

Michael de Swiet
Emeritus Professor of Obstetric Medicine,
Imperial College, London.

Pulmonary disease in pregnancy

Lucia Larson[1], Niharika Mehta[2], Michael J. Paglia[1], Ghada Bourjeily[2] with Warwick D. Ngan Kee[3]

[1]Department of Obstetrics and Gynecology, Warren Alpert Medical School of Brown University, Women & Infants' Hospital of Rhode Island, Providence, RI, USA
[2]Department of Medicine, Warren Alpert Medical School of Brown University, Women & Infants' Hospital of Rhode Island, Providence, RI, USA
[3]Department of Anesthesia and Intensive Care, Chinese University of Hong Kong, Prince of Wales Hospital, Hong Kong, China

Introduction

The respiratory system undergoes a number of changes during pregnancy so that the gravid woman can meet the metabolic needs of both the mother and the fetus. The implications of these changes for the diagnosis and management of specific pulmonary diseases as well as for pregnancy will be considered in this chapter.

Physiologic adapations to pregnancy

Anatomic changes

Many anatomic changes occur in and around the respiratory system. In the upper airway, hyperemia and glandular hyperactivity are observed in pregnancy and are associated with edema and friability. These changes are likely the result of the expansion of plasma volume that starts early in pregnancy and progresses with increasing gestational age. Also contributing to this is the indirect effect of the elevated levels of estrogens. Consequently, up to 30% of pregnant women suffer from nasal congestion and epistaxis. This condition is known as gestational rhinitis and it usually resolves very quickly after delivery. Other consequences of mucosal edema of the upper airway include difficulties in airway management and failed endotracheal intubations as well as problems with the introduction of nasogastric tubes, necessitating liberal lubrication and extreme care. The higher propensity to snoring in pregnancy as compared to the nonpregnant population is also related to these changes.

Changes also occur in the chest wall. The lower ribcage widens, leading to an increase in the anteroposterior and transverse diameters of the chest, resulting in an overall increase of 5–7 cm in the chest wall circumference and a widening of the costal angle by about 50%. However, impaired chest wall compliance related to the enlarging uterus can occur late in pregnancy, causing decreased total lung compliance.

Physiologic measurements in pregnancy

Flow rates are relatively unchanged in pregnancy. Forced expiratory volume in 1 second (FEV_1), a helpful measurement in obstructive lung diseases, is not affected by pregnancy. In addition, peak expiratory flow rates are unchanged. Therefore, the interpretation and monitoring value of these tests in patients with asthma, for instance, are unchanged in pregnancy. The major effect of pregnancy on lung physiology occurs on volumes. There is an increase in tidal volume (TV) and a reduction in functional residual capacity (FRC) secondary to a decreased residual volume and expiratory reserve volume. FRC is further reduced in the supine position late in gestation. The inspiratory capacity is increased so that total lung capacity remains the same in the pregnant and nonpregnant state (Figure 1.1).

Ventilation

Minute ventilation, a product of tidal volume and respiratory rate, is increased by about 40% in pregnancy. This increase is achieved mainly by a proportional increase in tidal volume from 500 mL to 700 mL (about 40%). There is minimal change in the respiratory rate in pregnancy and any change should be interpreted as pathologic rather than physiologic.

This increase in ventilation leads to a reduction in $PaCO_2$ levels from 35–40 mmHg in the pre-pregnant state to an average of 30 mmHg during pregnancy. The drop in $PaCO_2$ is matched by an increased renal excretion of bicarbonate, leading to lower plasma bicarbonate levels. The end result is a plasma pH that is not significantly changed but there may be less buffering capacity in the face of an acidosis.

More profound changes occur in pregnancy at high altitude. Ventilation usually increases at high altitudes to compensate

de Swiet's Medical Disorders in Obstetric Practice, 5th edition. Edited by R. O. Powrie, M. F. Greene, W. Camann. © 2010 Blackwell Publishing.

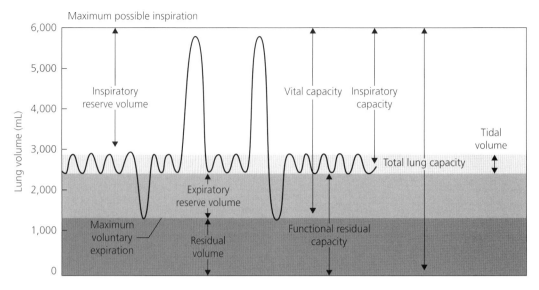

Figure 1.1 Lung volumes and capacities. Reproduced with permission of Anaesthesia UK Image Library.

for the drop in ambient oxygen. This response in pregnancy further accentuates the drop in $PaCO_2$ and levels of 24–28 mmHg have been reported at high altitude. Although residence at high altitude is associated with decreased maternal PaO_2, intrauterine growth restriction and pre-eclampsia, modern aircraft are pressurized to about 2500 m (8200 ft) and at these pressures Huch found no evidence of ill effects on mother or fetus in 10 pregnancies studied during commercial flights [1].

The increase in ventilation and associated fall in $PaCO_2$ occurring in pregnancy are probably due to progesterone, which may act via a number of mechanisms. Progesterone lowers the threshold and increases the sensitivity of the respiratory center to CO_2. It is also possible that progesterone acts as a primary stimulant to the respiratory center independently of any change in CO_2 sensitivity or threshold. Not only does progesterone stimulate ventilation, but it also increases the level of carbonic anhydrase B in the red blood cell. An increase in carbonic anhydrase will facilitate CO_2 transfer, and also tends to decrease $PaCO_2$ independently of any change in ventilation.

Oxygenation

Maternal PaO_2 increases in pregnancy to 100–105 mmHg at sea level. This increase is in part secondary to an increment in cardiac output leading to an improvement in ventilation/perfusion matching in the upper lobes. The alveolar–arterial gradient (the difference between PO_2 in the alveoli and that measured in the arterial blood) has been reported to increase slightly in the late stages of pregnancy from 15 to about 20. Position can also have an important effect on maternal arterial blood gases late in pregnancy. PaO_2 has been shown to decrease and the alveolo-arterial gradient to increase in the supine position in pregnancy. This has been attributed to a

reduction in functional residual capacity and earlier airway closing during normal tidal breathing. Alterations in cardiac output between the sitting and the supine position may also contribute to that reduction in arterial oxygen tension. Therefore, arterial blood gases are ideally obtained while pregnant women are in the sitting position.

Oxygen consumption is increased in pregnancy by about 20% and increases further during labor and delivery. About one-third of the increased oxygen consumption is necessary for the metabolism of the fetus and placenta. The remainder is supplied for the extra metabolism of the mother, in particular the extra work of increased secretion and reabsorption by the kidney.

Breathlessness in pregnancy

Approximately 50% of normal pregnant women will note dyspnea before 19 weeks gestation and 76% by 31 weeks [2]. Reasons for experiencing the sensation during normal pregnancy may be related to the effect of progesterone on the respiratory center, mechanical changes associated with weight gain or decreased venous return, and/or the demands of the fetus. Women often describe their symptoms as "needing to take a deep breath." Since these women are otherwise normal, there should be no suggestion of cardiopulmonary disease on history or physical exam such as sudden onset of symptoms, cough, chest pain or wheezing and patients should be able to perform activities of daily living. Likewise, physical exam is normal and oxygen saturation is normal at rest and with exertion. The presence of an anemia should be sought as this is common in pregnancy. If there is no underlying disease as a cause of dyspnea, the patient can be reassured that there is no increased risk for complications during pregnancy or labor and delivery.

Specific conditions

The remainder of this chapter discusses the most common and the most serious respiratory problems that may complicate a pregnancy. Although each requires specific management, a general approach to the care of the pulmonary patient can be found at the end of this chapter in Table 1.12.

Asthma

Asthma is characterized by heightened airway responsiveness to triggers and reversible airway obstruction. According to the National Asthma Education and Prevention Program, it is defined as "a chronic inflammatory disorder of the airways in which many cells and cellular elements play a role. . ." In susceptible individuals, this inflammation causes recurrent coughing (particularly at night or early in the morning), wheezing, breathlessness, and chest tightness. These episodes are usually associated with widespread but variable airflow obstruction that is often reversible either spontaneously or with treatment [3].

Epidemiology

Asthma affects 3.7–8.4% of all pregnancies and is one of the most common serious medical complications encountered in pregnancy in the United States [4]. Other estimates from both the United Kingdom and Australia show rates close to 12–13% in pregnancy [5]. It is estimated that 10% of the population has airway hyper-responsiveness. The prevalence of asthma has significantly increased since the 1980s and cannot be solely explained by an increased awareness of the disease since the rate of death from asthma has also increased. Asthma has become the leading cause of hospitalization of children under 15 and is emerging as the most common chronic and potentially life-threatening disease of childhood, affecting one in seven children in Great Britain. Pregnant women and their children are also more likely to experience asthma than any other chronic disease.

Physiology

Asthma is a chronic inflammatory disease characterized by a reversible airway obstruction and airway hyper-reactivity. Reversible airway obstruction is defined as an obstruction on spirometry which is documented during acute attacks with normal physiology between attacks. Reversibility may also be documented by complete resolution of obstruction following the administration of a short-acting bronchodilator. Airway hyper-responsiveness, an exaggerated bronchospastic response to nonspecific agents such as methacholine and histamine or specific antigens, is the physiologic cornerstone of this disorder. Multiple factors lead to narrowing of the airway, resulting in reduced air flow, such as smooth muscle contraction, thickening of the airway wall and the presence of secretions within the airway lumen.

Pathophysiology

The predominant causes of airway obstruction in asthma include airway inflammation, cellular infiltration, and subsequent cytokine production.

Airway inflammation has many components involving cellular infiltration with Th2 lymphocytes as well as eosinophils, the former playing an important role in initiating and perpetuating inflammation through cytokine release as well as by affecting IgE production. When Th2 lymphocytes are stimulated by the appropriate antigens, they release interleukins (IL) such as IL-3, IL-4 and IL-5 as well as granulocyte macrophage-colony stimulating factor (GM-CSF). Airway cells such as smooth muscle cells and secretory cells undergo hypertrophic and hyperplastic changes whereas mast cells become sensitized with IgE and secrete tumor necrosis factor alpha (TNF-alpha), a pleiotropic inflammatory cytokine that plays a role in airway hyper-responsivess. Remodeling of the airway structure occurs as a result of collagen deposition in the basement membrane and thickening of the subepithelial connective tissue.

Clinical manifestations

Typically, patients with asthma present with periodic symptoms of shortness of breath, wheezing or chest tightness that occur in response to various stimuli. Common stimuli include exercise, cold temperatures, allergens or irritants. Common allergens could be indoor or outdoor allergens and include grass, pollen, pet dander, cockroaches, mice, dust mites and mold. A careful history should be taken regarding possible triggers and the history needs to include questioning about the home, work or even school environment.

During attacks, patients usually have expiratory wheezing which typically resolves once the symptoms improve. Depending on the severity of the attack, patients may use their accessory respiratory muscles (the parasternal, scalene, sternocleidomastoid, trapezius, and pectoralis muscles that do not normally contract with respiration) and even have paradoxic breathing (normally the abdomen should expand with inspiration but in paradoxic breathing, the abdomen may retract with inspiration, indicating marked respiratory muscle fatigue). In severe attacks leading to hyperinflation, there may be some compromise to the venous return and subsequent hypotension.

Diagnosis

The diagnosis of asthma is usually suggested by the history of episodic symptoms that follow specific triggers. The physical exam is suggestive during attacks but not when the attacks have resolved. The diagnosis is usually established by the documentation of a reversible obstruction on spirometry. Obstruction is defined on spirometry by a reduced FEV_1 forced vital capacity (FVC) (normally the ratio of FEV_1 to FVC should be about 75%, meaning that 75% of the total volume of a breath can be exhaled within 1 second) with variable degrees of FEV_1 reduction. Normalization of FEV_1 following administration of bronchodilators determines reversibility.

Spirometry is often normal in patients with asthma outside an acute attack. Establishing a diagnosis may be difficult in that case and an airway challenge may be performed to trigger an obstructive physiology. The most commonly used challenge in making the diagnosis of asthma is performed with methacholine chloride but other challenges can be used such as cold air and allergen challenges. Methacholine is a quaternary ammonium compound and likely does not cross the placenta. There are no human studies looking at the safety of methacholine in pregnancy. Advantages obtained from testing during the pregnancy should be weighed against the potential risks.

Effect of pregnancy on asthma

The course of asthma is usually unpredictable in pregnancy and numerous studies have suggested that one-third of patients improve, one-third remain the same and the last third worsen [6]. Factors contributing to improvement may be the pregnancy-associated rise in serum cortisol, an anti-inflammatory hormone, or the increase in progesterone which acts as a potent smooth muscle relaxant. However, more is known in terms of factors that predispose to worsening of asthma during pregnancy. There is clear evidence linking upper airway and nasal symptoms and asthma control. The course of asthma seems to parallel that of gestational rhinitis and those patients who have an improvement in their symptoms of rhinitis during pregnancy also have improvements in their asthma symptoms [7]. These findings suggest that the same systemic factors may be affecting both upper and lower airways. In addition, the rate of bacterial sinusitis is 5–6 times higher in pregnant women and may contribute to worsening of asthma symptoms. Gastroesophageal reflux disease (GERD), common in pregnancy, may also play a role in worsening asthma control during pregnancy both through reflux of gastric acid into the airway and through a reflex bronchoconstriction that can occur following acidification of the lower esophagus.

How hormonal factors related to pregnancy affect asthma control is not as well understood. There are many studies of premenstrual asthma that suggest changes in beta-agonist receptor density in the airways that occur during the menstrual cycle. Declines in FEV_1 have been shown to occur in the luteal phase in women with premenstrual exacerbations of their symptoms. Emergency room visits were more frequent in the premenstrual period than in the pre-, peri- or postovulatory periods of the menstrual cycle but these findings were not consistent in other studies that showed more visits in the preovulatory phase of the cycle. Unfortunately, however, this information does not translate directly into pregnancy and the presence of premenstrual asthma does not necessarily suggest that asthma will worsen during pregnancy.

Epidemiologic studies done in both the US and Finland suggest that asthma exacerbations are most common between gestation weeks 17–24 [8] and symptoms worsen mostly between 29 and 32 weeks [9]. There is usually an improvement in symptoms after 36 weeks. It is possible that this improvement late in the pregnancy is related to cortisol levels at term reaching four times pre-pregnancy levels.

Of those patients who have worsening of their asthma during pregnancy, close to 60% improve in the postpartum period, whereas worsening was seen in 87% of women whose asthma had improved during pregnancy [10]. When women were followed during successive pregnancies, only 60% followed the same course in the second pregnancy as in the first. Thus, it is difficult to predict with certainty the course asthma will take in an individual pregnancy.

Effect of asthma on pregnancy

Case–control studies have shown that well-controlled pregnant asthmatics do not have a significantly higher rate of adverse outcomes than women without asthma [11,12]. Pregnancy outcomes are not as favorable in women with severe or poorly controlled disease. Of 37,000 women with asthma and 2495 exacerbations, those with exacerbations were more likely to have miscarriage or therapeutic abortions than those without [13]. Suboptimal control appears to be associated with low birthweight, intrauterine growth restriction, and cesarean section. Other adverse pregnancy outcomes thought to be associated with asthma include preterm delivery and maternal hypertension but these risks have not been shown consistently and systemic steroid use may have a confounding effect.

Pre-eclampsia has also been associated with severe asthma in some studies, but it is unclear whether it is the underlying disease or the concomitant use of systemic steroids and co-morbidities that is the culprit [14].

The manner by which poorly controlled asthma affects obstetric outcomes remains unclear. While maternal hypoxia is often offered as an explanation, the majority of pregnant women with even poorly controlled asthma are unlikely to have chronic hypoxia to the degree that would explain these obstetric outcomes. A relationship between obstetric outcomes and chronic inflammatory mediators associated with poorly controlled asthma is therefore speculated although it remains unproven.

Classification of asthma severity

The National Asthma Expert Panel Report (EPR 3) [15] classifies asthma into severity according to two domains – impairment and risk. The term "mild intermittent" has been eliminated and the classification now falls into the following four categories: intermittent, mild persistent, moderate persistent, and severe persistent. Patients within each category can be classified as well controlled, not well controlled or poorly controlled (Tables 1.1 and 1.2). These same categories should be used in evaluating pregnant women with asthma and are useful in directing appropriate management with step therapy.

The advantage of the new guidelines compared to the previous guidelines is the fact that risk is now an important feature of the disease severity classification. Need for emergency room visits, frequency of exacerbations and steroid tapers are now taken into account when assessing disease severity. Furthermore, the more recent guidelines reinforce the need to monitor quality of life by using validated measures and emphasize the need for objective measurements with spirometry as part of the initial evaluation and follow-up care.

Management

The first step in management is establishing the diagnosis of asthma. Many patients are misdiagnosed with asthma for many years before they are correctly diagnosed with asthma mimics such as chronic obstructive lung disease, sinus disease or vocal cord dysfunction. Review of medical records and

Table 1.1 Severity assessment and initial treatment

Assessing severity and initiating treatment for patients who are not currently taking long-term control medications

Components of Severity		Classification of Asthma Severity ≥12 years of age			
				Persistent	
		Intermittent	Mild	Moderate	Severe
Impairment	Symptoms	≤2 days/week	>2 days/week but not daily	Daily	Throughout the day
	Nighttime awakenings	≤2x/month	3–4x/month	>1x/week but not nightly	Often 7x/week
	Short-acting β_2-agonist use for symptom control (not prevention of EIB)	≤2 days/week	>2 days/week but not daily, and not more than 1x on any day	Daily	Several times per day
Normal FEV_1/FVC: 8–19 y 85% 20–39 y 80% 40–59 y 75% 60–80 y 70%	Interference with normal activity	None	Minor lmitation	Some limitation	Extremely limited
	Lung function	• Normal FEV_1 between exacerbations • $FEV_1 > 80\%$ predicted • FEV_1/FVC normal	• $FEV_1 > 80\%$ predicted • FEV_1/FVC normal	• $FEV_1 > 60\%$ but 80% predicted • FEV_1/FVC reduced $> 5\%$	• $FEV_1 < 60\%$ predicted • FEV_1/FVC reduced $> 5\%$
Risk	Exacerbations requiring oral systemic corticosteroids	0–1/year (see note)	≥2/year (see note)		
		Consider severity and interval since last exacerbation. Frequency and severity may fluctuate over time for patients in any severity category. Relative annual risk of exacerbations may be related to FEV_1.			
Recommended Step for Initiating Treatment (See "Stepwise Approach for Managing Asthma" for treatment steps.)		Step 1	Step 2	Step 3 and consider short course of oral systemic corticosteroids	Step 4 or 5
		In 2–6 weeks, evaluate level of asthma control that is achieved and adjust therapy accordingly.			

*Notes:
- The stepwise approach is meant to assist, not replace, the clinical decision-making to meet individual patient needs.
- Level of severity is determined by assessment of both impairment and risk. Assess impairment domain by patient's/caregiver's recall of previous 2–4 wk and spirometry. Assign severity to the most severe category in which any feature occurs.
- Currently there are inadequate date to correspond frequencies of exacerbations with deferent levels of asthma severity. In general, more frequent and intense exacerbations (eg. requiring urgent, unscheduled care, hospitalization, or ICU admission) indicate greater underlying disease severity. For treatment purposes, patients who had ≥2 exacerbations requiring oral systemic corticosteroids in the past year may be considered the same as patients who have persistent asthma, even in the absence of impairment levels consistent with persistent asthma.

EIB, exercise-induced bronchospasm; FEV, forced expiratory volume; FVC, forced vital capacity; ICU, intensive care unit.
Reproduced with permission from the National Asthma Education and Prevention Program [15].

Table 1.2 Control classification

Components of Control		Classification of Asthma Control (≥12 years of age)		
		Well Controlled	Not Well Controlled	Very Poorly Controlled
Impairment	Symptoms	≤2 days/week	>2 days/week	Throughout the day
	Nighttime awakenings	≤2x/month	1–3x/week	≥4x/week
	Interference with normal activity	None	Some lmitation	Extremely limited
	Short-acting β₂-agonist use for symptom control (not prevention of EIB)	≤2 days/week	> 2 days/week	Several times per day
	FEV₁ or peak flow	>80% predicted/ personal best	60–80% predicted/ personal best	<60% predicted/ personal best
	Validated questionnaires	0	1–2	3–4
	ATAQ	≤0.75*	≥1.5	N/A
	ACQ	≥20	16–19	≤15
	ACT			
Risk	Exacerbations requiring oral systemic corticosteroids	0–1/year	≥2/year (see notes)	
		Consider severity and interval since last exacerbation		
	Progressive loss of lung function	Evaluation requires long-term follow-up care.		
	Treatment-related adverse effects	Medication side effects can vary in intensity from none to very troublesome and worrisome. The level of intensity does not correlate to specific levels of control but should be considered in the overall assessment of risk.		
Recommended Action for Treatment (See "Stepwise Approach for Managing Asthma" for treatment steps.)		• Maintain current step. • Regular follow-up at every 1–6 months to maintain control. • Consider step down if well controlled for at least 3 months.	• Step up 1 step. • Re-evaluate in 2–6 weeks. • For side effects, consider alternative treatment options.	• Consider short course of oral systemic corticosteroids. • Step up 1–2 steps. • Re-evaluate in 2 weeks. • For side effects, consider alternative treatment options.

*ACQ values of 0.76–1.4 are indeterminate regarding well controlled asthma.

†Notes:
• The stepwise approach is meant to assist, not replace, the clinical decision-making required to meet individual patient needs.
• The level of control is based on the most severe impairment or risk category. Assess impairment domain by patient's recall of previous 2–4 wk and by spirometry/or peak flow measures. Symptom assessment for longer periods should reflect a global assessment, such as inquiring whether the patient's asthma is better or worse since the last visit.
• Currently there are inadequate date to correspond frequencies of exacerbations with different levels of asthma control. In general, more frequent and intense exacerbations (eg. requiring urgent, unscheduled care, hospitalization, or ICU admission) indicate poorer disease control. For treatment purposes, patients who had ≥2 exacerbations requiring oral systemic corticosteroids in the past year may be considered the same as patients who have not-well controlled asthma, even in the absence of impairment levels consistent with not-well controlled asthma.
• Validated questionnaires for the impairment domain (the questionnaires do not assess lung function or the risk domain).
• Minimal important difference: 1.0 for the ATAQ: 0.5 for the ACQ; not determined for the ACT.
• **Before step up in therapy:**
    — Review adherence to medication, inhaler technique, environmental control, and comorbid conditions.
    — If an alternative treatment option was used in a step, discontinue and use the preferred treatment for that step.

ACQ, asthma control questionaire; ACT, asthma control test; ATAQ, asthma therapy assessment questionaire; ICU, intensive care unit.
Reproduced with permission from the National Asthma Education and Prevention Program [15].

ensuring that the diagnosis is accurate and the history is suggestive are crucial steps.

Another important step is the identification of triggers. Once those have been recognized, every effort should be made to avoid exposure to known triggers. Frequent vacuuming of carpeted areas, avoiding contact with stuffed toys, and using a mattress cover to avoid exposure to dust mites should be encouraged.

According to the US national health interview survey in 2005, 21% of women of childbearing age in the US smoke. Many of those patients are likely to be asthmatic and it is paramount to address smoking habits with every patient. All smokers should be encouraged to quit especially since smoking is the most modifiable risk factor for adverse pregnancy outcomes. Counseling regarding the ill effects of smoking on asthma and fetal health should be done periodically. Strong statements such as: "As your clinician, I need you to know that quitting smoking is the most important thing you can do to protect your baby and your own health" help send a clear message to the pregnant smoker (see section on smoking cessation below).

In addition, pregnant asthmatic patients should be asked about sulfite (additives to prepared foods that preserve freshness) and aspirin sensitivity, rhinitis and sinusitis, GERD, exercise- or cold-induced asthma, and nocturnal asthma. Many pregnant women have GERD so that counseling about lifestyle modifications, including elevating the head of the bed, eating smaller meals, and eating earlier in the evening, can be helpful. Identification and treatment of sinus disease or nasal congestion secondary to allergic rhinitis or gestational rhinitis may also help control symptoms.

Compliance and proper use of medications is another major issue in patients with asthma as poor asthma control results in many cases from inadequate use of the drugs. Pregnancy poses an additional challenge since patients may not be compliant with their medications because of fear of fetal harm. This fear may be propagated by family members, friends, or even other healthcare providers who are less familiar with treating pregnant women. Counseling regarding the safety of the drugs should be done with all asthma patients and it is important to clarify that the benefits of asthma control far outweigh the risks of medications. Reviewing inhaler techniques with all patients should be done not only on their first visit but also periodically on follow-up visits. It should never be assumed that patients who have had asthma for many years know how to properly use their drugs. In our experience, many of those patients use their inhalers incorrectly (Box 1.1).

The National Asthma Education and Prevention Program (NAEPP) has placed substantial emphasis on patient education to help with disease monitoring. In essence, asthma patients need to be educated about their disease, the triggers, ways to avoid them, identifying signs of an attack, monitoring of peak flows and understanding the implications of different stages of obstruction suggested by peak flow meters. In our practice, a written asthma management plan is provided to every patient with asthma after proper education.

Drugs

General principles regarding drug prescription in pregnancy include:

- finding out whether the condition is self-limited and how necessary the medications are;
- evaluating the possible outcomes to the mother and fetus of the untreated condition
- assessing safety data of the drug to be administered and whether other drugs with a better safety profile and similar efficacy could be used instead
- understanding how the patient's value system and cultural beliefs affect decision making with regard to taking medications during pregnancy.

Box 1.1 Instructions for proper inhaler use

- Inhalers come as metered dose inhalers (MDI), MDI with a spacer, and dry powder inhalers. The latter two have the advantage that hand–breath co-ordination is not critical. The disadvantage of dry powder inhalers, which is not a problem with MDI, is that they do require patients to be able to take a deep, fast breath to get the medication and that an accidental exhalation will blow medication away.
- To use an MDI (e.g. albuterol or salbutamol), shake the inhaler 5–6 times. Remove the mouthpiece cover and place the spacer over the mouthpiece if a spacer is being used. If you are using a spacer, place the lips and teeth over the spacer. If a spacer is not being used, hold the inhaler mouthpiece just outside your open mouth. Breathe in slowly while giving a single squeeze to the top of the canister. Continue to inhale slowly and deeply even after the squeeze has been completed. When you have completely inhaled, hold the breath for 10 seconds. Repeat this procedure in a minute to administer a second "puff."
- To use a dry powder inhaler (e.g. Pulmicort®), there is no need shake the inhaler. Twist the cover off. "Load" the medication by twisting the base grip to the right as far as it will go and then twist it back to the left. A click should be heard, meaning the medication is loaded. Place the inhaler between your lips in a horizontal position and take a fast, deep breath through your mouth and not your nose, continuing to inhale deeply. Repeat this procedure in a minute to administer a second "puff."
- To use a dry powder disk inhaler (e.g. Advair®), there is no need to shake the inhaler. Hold the disk level in one hand. With the other hand, put the thumb in the appropriate notch and push it away from you as far as it will go to expose the mouthpiece and the lever for "loading" the medication. Move the lever as far as it will go. A click should be heard, meaning the medication is loaded. Place the mouthpiece between your lips and take a fast, deep breath through your mouth (not your nose) and continue to inhale deeply. Repeat this procedure to administer a second "puff."

In a patient with asthma, the answer to the first two questions is clear: the attacks should not be assumed to be self-limited and the disease can be life threatening. Therefore the need for therapy is obvious. Below, we will review safety data regarding all the medications used in asthma. Individual counseling should be undertaken in patients with different beliefs and cultural influences to explain the need for therapy and the downside of withholding therapy. The NAEPP published guidelines on pharmacologic management of pregnant patients with asthma in 2004 after reviewing data on fetal safety of the drugs [16].

Short-acting beta-agonists

Short-acting beta-agonists, also called rescue inhalers, are the most potent and rapidly acting bronchodilators currently available for clinical use. Beta-agonists interact with beta-receptors on the surface of a variety of cells implicated in asthma pathogenesis. Among other things, beta-agonists have the potential to relax bronchial smooth muscle and affect vascular tone and edema formation. These drugs have not been shown to affect the maternal circulation even at high doses and are thought to be safe to use in pregnancy.

Long-acting beta-agonists

Formoterol and salmeterol are available in the US. Their safety profile and toxicologic data are similar to those of short-acting beta-agonists. Animal data were suggestive of possible teratogenic effect in one animal species, later labeled as "sensitive rabbits," when salmeterol was used intravenously at very high doses. However, inhaled use of the drug results in minimal absorption. Further animal studies have not shown such effects even at doses 1600 times higher than the human dose. The use of long-acting beta-agonists is certainly justifiable in pregnancy in patients who are poorly controlled on inhaled corticosteroids alone.

Anticholinergics

Anticholinergic drugs such as ipratropium bromide lead to parasympathetic blockade and further accentuate the bronchodilating effect of beta-agonists. Anticholinergic drugs can be of use in acute exacerbations in the emergency room or hospital (and are often given in combination with beta-agonists in this setting) but have not been shown to have any benefit in long-term therapy of asthma. Although the published data about the safety of these agents in pregnancy are scarce, the systemic absorption is minimal and their use for exacerbations leading to hospital visits is readily justifiable.

Inhaled corticosteroids

Inhaled corticosteroids (ICS) should be the first alternative in patients with poorly controlled symptoms on beta-agonists. Corticosteroids have been shown to inhibit multiple cell types such as mast cells, eosinophils and basophils as well as mediator production and secretion (e.g. histamine and cytokines) involved in asthma pathogenesis. Beclomethasone and budesonide are the most studied inhaled corticosteroids in pregnancy and are thought to be safe for use. However, patients who have been well controlled on a different inhaled steroid prior to conception may be maintained on their drugs since the goal in asthma therapy is optimal control and especially since ICS should be the first-line controller medication.

Leukotriene inhibitors

Leukotrienes are substances that induce numerous biologic activities including augmentation of neutrophil and eosinophil migration, neutrophil and monocyte aggregation as well as increasing capillary permeability and smooth muscle contraction. All these effects contribute to the inflammation, edema, bronchoconstriction, and mucus secretion seen in asthma. Leukotriene inhibitors block the physiologic effects of leukotrienes.

Animal data regarding these drugs suggest that they are likely to be safe for use in pregnancy; however, human data are lacking. Therefore, the risks and benefits need to be balanced in an individual patient. For instance, those patients who required a leukotriene inhibitor in addition to their steroid inhaler and long-acting beta-agonist for optimal symptom control would need to remain on all their drugs during the pregnancy, including leukotriene inhibitors. Patients who are on a leukotriene inhibitor without adequate inhaled steroids may be switched to steroids since more data regarding those are available in pregnancy.

Other drugs

In the most recent report from the National Institutes of Health (NIH) on asthma management in pregnancy, the NAEPP guidelines [16] suggest using low-dose inhaled corticosteroids as a preferred agent in patients with mild persistent asthma, with accepted alternatives listed alphabetically: cromolyn, leukotriene receptor antagonists or theophylline (Figure 1.2). In our experience and in many studies, use of inhaled steroids is certainly superior to the use of any of these agents in the general population. In addition, a study comparing a low-potency steroid (beclomethasone) with theophylline in pregnancy has shown comparable benefit but the steroids were much better tolerated [17]. We believe that inhaled steroids should certainly be used first especially because a superior benefit may be expected from higher potency inhaled steroids compared to beclomethasone, making them a better choice than theophylline.

Other studies have suggested that the use of systemic steroids in pregnant asthmatics increases the risk of orofacial clefts (a 2–7-fold increase in risk to 2–14 per 1000 births with use in the first trimester), pre-eclampsia, premature rupture of the membranes and the delivery of both preterm

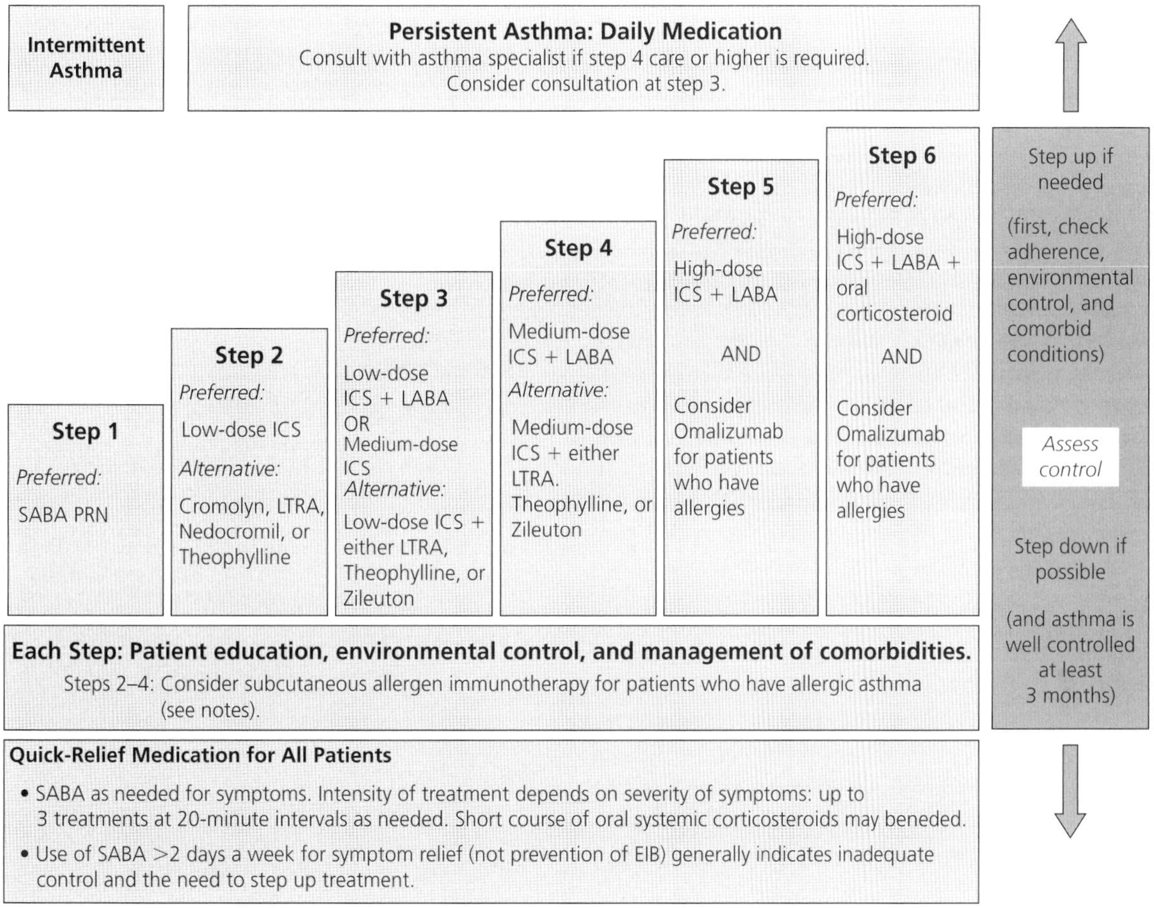

Intermittent Asthma	**Persistent Asthma: Daily Medication** Consult with asthma specialist if step 4 care or higher is required. Consider consultation at step 3.

Step 1

Preferred:

SABA PRN

Step 2

Preferred:

Low-dose ICS

Alternative:

Cromolyn, LTRA, Nedocromil, or Theophylline

Step 3

Preferred:

Low-dose ICS + LABA OR Medium-dose ICS

Alternative:

Low-dose ICS + either LTRA, Theophylline, or Zileuton

Step 4

Preferred:

Medium-dose ICS + LABA

Alternative:

Medium-dose ICS + either LTRA. Theophylline, or Zileuton

Step 5

Preferred:

High-dose ICS + LABA

AND

Consider Omalizumab for patients who have allergies

Step 6

Preferred:

High-dose ICS + LABA + oral corticosteroid

AND

Consider Omalizumab for patients who have allergies

Step up if needed

(first, check adherence, environmental control, and comorbid conditions)

Assess control

Step down if possible

(and asthma is well controlled at least 3 months)

Each Step: Patient education, environmental control, and management of comorbidities.

Steps 2–4: Consider subcutaneous allergen immunotherapy for patients who have allergic asthma (see notes).

Quick-Relief Medication for All Patients

- SABA as needed for symptoms. Intensity of treatment depends on severity of symptoms: up to 3 treatments at 20-minute intervals as needed. Short course of oral systemic corticosteroids may beneded.

- Use of SABA >2 days a week for symptom relief (not prevention of EIB) generally indicates inadequate control and the need to step up treatment.

'Notes:

- The stepwise approach is meant to assist, not replace, the clinical decision-making required to meet individual patient needs.

- If alternative treatment is used and response is inadequate, discontinue it and use the preferred treatment before stepping up.

- Zileuton is a less desirable alternative because of limited studies as adjunctive therapy and the need to monitor liver function. Theophylline requires monitoring of serum concentration levels.

- In step 6, before oral corticosteroids are introduced, a trial of high-dose ICS + LABA + LTRA, theophylline, or zileuton may be considered, although this approach has not been studied in clinical trials.

- Step 1, 2, and 3 preferred therapies are based on Evidence A: step 3 alternative therapy is based on Evidence A for LTRA, Evidence B for theophylline, and Evidence D for zileuton. Step 4 preferred therapy is based on Evidence B, and alternative therapy is based on Evidence B for LTRA and theophylline and Evidence D for zileuton. Step 5 preferred therapy is based on Evidence B. Step 6 preferred therapy is based on (EPR-2 1997) and Evidence B for omalizumab.

- Immunotherapy for steps 2–4 is based on Evidence B for house dust mites, animal danders, and pollens; evidence is weak or lacking for molds and cockroaches. Evidence is strongest for immunotherapy with single allergens. The role of allergy in asthma is greater in children than in adults.

- Clinicians who administer immunotherapy or omalizumab should be prepared and equipped to identify and treat anaphylaxis that may occur.

- Alphabetical order is used when more than 1 treatment option is listed within either preferred or alternative therapy.

Figure 1.2 Step therapy for asthma. Reproduced with permission from the National Asthma Education and Prevention Program [15]. EIB, exercise induced bronchospasm; ICS, inhaled corticosteroid; LABA, long-acting beta agonist; LTRA, leukotriene receptor antagonist; PRN, as needed; SABA, short-acting beta agonist.

and low birthweight children [14], despite the fact that 87% of prednisone is metabolized by the placenta before it reaches the fetus. Systemic steroids may also contribute to the development of gestational diabetes. However, if indicated, the benefit of systemic steroids to treat inadequately controlled asthma certainly outweighs these risks.

The monoclonal antibody omalizumab blocks the binding of IgE to the IgE receptors and is now being used in moderate to severe asthmatics who are not well controlled on the usual regimen and have significant allergic triggers to their disease. Animal data do not seem to show significant teratogenicity but there have been no safety data in human studies since the initial trials have excluded pregnant patients. Postmarketing data are also limited given that the drug was only recently introduced to the market. For those reasons, the use of omalizumab cannot yet be recommended in pregnancy.

Cimetidine, ranitidine, and metoclopramide can all be used safely in pregnant women with GERD who need pharmacologic treatment. Rhinitis in the pregnant woman can be treated with nasal ipratropium and inhaled nasal steroids. See Table 1.3 for an overview of the drugs used to treat asthma in pregnancy. It is also recommended that all pregnant women receive immunization for influenza regardless of gestation and this is particularly important in asthmatics (see influenza section below).

Management of acute exacerbations

Patients presenting with an acute exacerbation should be assessed promptly. Those with a clear history of asthma and an exam suggesting an acute exacerbation should receive bronchodilators without delay. Peak flow measurements help determine the severity of the attack, guide therapy, and monitor for a response to interventions (Box 1.2). On physical exam, patients should be assessed for the use of accessory muscles since this suggests a severe exacerbation. Arterial blood gases should be obtained if patients are not improving with initial treatment or if a severe exacerbation is suspected. It is important to recognize that normal $PaCO_2$ in pregnancy is 30–35 mmHg. Therefore, a tachypneic patient with a $PaCO_2$ above that range should prompt the suspicion of impending respiratory failure.

The NAEPP guidelines published in 2004 have clear advice on the management of acute exacerbations of asthma in pregnancy and are shown in Figure 1.3. It should be noted that this is essentially unchanged from treatment in nonpregnant patients.

Fetal surveillance during pregnancy

The primary affect on the fetus from asthma, or any other pulmonary disease, is chronic hypoxia. The impact of hypoxia can manifest in several ways, including growth restriction or, more significantly, fetal death. Shortly after a woman with asthma becomes pregnant, she should have an early ultrasound to confirm her pregnancy dating. Women should be instructed to monitor fetal activity during the course of the pregnancy. A third-trimester ultrasound can be considered in a woman with well-controlled asthma who has appropriate growth in the fundal height. The NAEPP Working Group recommends serial ultrasounds starting at 32 weeks gestation in women with suboptimally controlled asthma and women with moderate-to-severe asthma [16]. If the growth is not appropriate or the woman has an acute exacerbation, fetal testing should be started. Testing may include umbilical artery Doppler flow velocity studies, nonstress testing (NST) or biophysical profiles (BPP). The frequency of such testing would depend on the severity of the patient's asthma or the degree of growth restriction.

Labor and delivery

Asthma exacerbations are rare in labor and delivery. This is thought to be related to the increase in serum cortisol that occurs during that period. Despite that, it is advisable to administer stress doses of steroids to patients who have been on prolonged systemic steroids during the pregnancy (see Chapter 47). Asthma medications should not be discontinued through labor and delivery.

Prostaglandin E2 is safe for cervical ripening, as is oxytocin. The agent 15-methyl prostaglandin F2-alpha should be avoided because it may cause severe bronchospasm. Although methylergonovine may cause dyspnea, asthma is not an absolute contraindication, and therefore it can be used when appropriate in the management of postpartum hemorrhage. Fentanyl is preferred to morphine and meperidine, which can release histamine. Epidural anesthesia is usually advised because it decreases oxygen consumption and minute ventilation. Epidural anesthesia also decreases the possibility of requiring general anesthesia if an emergency cesarean becomes indicated during labor. However, if cesarean delivery is required, a high level of sensory block may produce some degree of patient anxiety in the intraoperative period.

Several published articles in recent years have suggested that the increase in cesarean delivery rates over past years may be linked to the increasing incdence in asthma in the general population [18,19]. The "hygiene hypothesis" is put forward as a possible explanation as the establishment of GI flora in neonates born by cesarean section is delayed and this could have implications for the development of the neonatal immune system which ultimately leads to atopy and asthma. However, the existence of a relationship between asthma and mode of delivery requires further exploration in prospective studies that are controlled for confounding variables at the time of this writing.

Postpartum period

During the postpartum period, women should initially continue the same asthma medications they required during pregnancy. Close peak flow monitoring is indicated, particularly in those with poorly controlled or moderate-to-severe asthma.

Table 1.3 Drugs for treating common pulmonary conditions in pregnancy

Indication for treatment	Pregnancy			Breastfeeding		
	Use justifiable when indicated	Use may be justifiable in rare circumstances	Use almost never justifiable	Use acceptable in breastfeeding	Can be used safely in breastfeeding but may be second choice to column left	Should not be used with breastfeeding
Asthma						
Beta-agonists	–	–	–	–	–	
albuterol$_C$ (*ventolin*™, *Proventil*™)	Yes	–	–	Yes	–	–
formeterol $_C$ (*Foradil*™)	Yes	–	–	–	Yes	–
flunisolide $_C$ (*Aerobid*™)	–	–	–	–	Yes	–
fluticasone $_C$ (*Flovent*™)	–	–	–	–	Yes	–
metaproterenol$_C$ (*Alupent*™)	Yes	–	–	Yes	–	–
montelukast $_B$ *singulair*™	–	Yes	–	–	Yes	–
omalizumab $_B$ (*Xolair*™)	–	Yes	–	–	–	–
pirbuterol $_C$ (*Maxair*™)	Yes		–	Yes	–	–
salmeterol$_C$ (*Serevent*™)	Yes		–	Yes		–
terbutaline$_C$ (*Brethaire*™)	Yes	–	–	Yes	–	–
theophylline $_C$					Yes	
triamcinolone $_C$ (*Azmacort*™)			–		Yes	
zafirlukast$_B$ (*accolate*™)	–	Yes	–	–	Yes	
zileuton $_B$ (*zyflo*™)	–	–	Yes	–	–	–
Inhaled steroids						
beclomethasone $_C$ (*Beclovent*™ *Vanceril*™)	Yes	–	–	Yes	–	–
flunisolide $_C$ (*Aerobid*™)	Yes	–	–	–	–	–
fluticasone $_C$ (*Flovent*™)	Yes	–	–	–	–	–
triamcinolone $_C$ (*Azmacort*™)	Yes	–	–	–	–	–
budesonide $_B$ (*Pulmicort*)	Yes			Yes		
Other	*Other*					
systemic steroids $_C$	Yes			Yes		
ipatropium $_B$ (*Atrovent*™)	Yes			Yes		
cromolyn $_B$ (*Intal*™)	Yes			Yes		
theophylline $_C$	Yes					
minophylline	Yes					
Nasal congestion						
pseudoephedrine$_C$ (*Sudafed*™)	Yes	–	–	–	Yes (*if used short term*)	Yes (*if used long term*)
nasal steroids (*Beconase*™$_C$, *Rhinocort*™$_C$, *Flonase*™$_C$, *Nasacort*™$_C$)	nasal steroids (*Beconase*™$_C$, *Rhinocort*™$_C$, *Flonase*™$_C$, *Nasacort*™$_C$)	–	–	nasal steroids (*Beconase*™$_C$, *Rhinocort*™$_C$, *Flonase*™$_C$)	–	–
oxymetazoline$_C$ (*Afrin*™)	Yes	–	–	Yes	–	–
nasal ipratropium $_B$ (*Atrovent nasal*™)	Yes	–	–	Yes	–	–
Cough						
guaifenesin $_C$ (*Robitussin*™)	Yes	–	–	Yes	–	–
dextromethorphan$_C$ (*Benylin DM*™)	Yes	–	–	Yes	–	–
albuterol $_C$	Yes	–	–	Yes	–	–
codeine $_C$	Yes	–	–	–	Yes	–

Adapted with permission from Powrie RO. Drugs in pregnancy. Respiratory disease. Best Pract Res Clin Obstet Gynaecol 2001;15(6):913–36.

Box 1.2 Use of the peak flow meter

- Peak flow meters are inexpensive portable, hand-held devices that measure the patient's ability to push air out of her lungs and are used as a convenient standardized way for a patient and her provider to monitor the course of her asthma on a daily basis. Peak flow meters also help identify worsening asthma before the patient may be aware of an exacerbation and thereby allow early intervention.
- Patients should measure their peak flow rate around the same time each day, often first thing in the morning and early in the evening. Normal peak flow rates can be obtained in standardized charts and vary with height, gender and race. A 30-year-old white woman with a height of 5′ 5″ will typically have a peak flow rate of 400 L/min. Most experts, however, will have their patients measure themselves against their own "personal best," i.e. the best peak flow rate that they have obtained under stable conditions. Patients can be taught to consider peak flow rates within 80% of their personal best as "normal" (the "green zone"), flow rates that are within 50–80% of normal as cause for concern or caution (the "yellow zone") and flow rates less than 50% of normal as being potentially dangerous (the "red zone"). Patients should be given explicit instructions as to what they should do with results in each zone.

Most drugs used for asthma treatment can be safely used in breastfeeding women (see Table 1.3). In fact, breastfeeding should be encouraged given the many well-recognized benefits for both mother and baby. Whether breastfeeding decreases the likelihood of the development of asthma in offspring is as yet controversial but it does appear to decrease atopy. The need for medication compliance should be reinforced as some mothers will find it more difficult to tend to their own needs when they have a newborn. Women who have quit smoking during their pregnancy are at increased risk for returning to their old habit so a discussion focused on maintaining abstinence may be useful. (See smoking cessation section below.)

Smoking cessation in pregnancy

The health risks of cigarette smoking outside pregnancy are well established and include atherosclerotic cardiovascular disease, cancers of the lung, cervix, pancreas, kidneys, lower urinary tract, and upper digestive tract, as well as respiratory illness including chronic obstructive pulmonary disease and worsening of asthma. It is also associated with diseases such as osteoporosis and peptic ulcer disease. As the leading preventable cause of death worldwide, it is responsible for approximately 1 in 10 deaths in adults and costs billions of dollars in annual health-related economic losses. For the smoking pregnant woman and her fetus, the risks are more immediate and include low birthweight, spontaneous pregnancy loss, stillbirth, premature rupture of membranes, placental abruption, placenta previa, and preterm delivery.

Epidemiology

According to studies from the 1990s, between 1 in 3 and 1 in 5 women living in developed countries reported smoking

during pregnancy [20]. However, the prevalence may be even higher as smoking is notoriously under-reported by gravid women, probably because of the lack of social acceptability of cigarette use in pregnancy. Smoking is particularly common in those who are socially disadvantaged and have low income but poor social support, depression, work stress, and exposure to intimate partner violence are also associated factors. Women with concern about weight gain during pregnancy may use continued smoking as a method of weight control.

Pathophysiology

Smoking is the most important modifiable risk factor for adverse pregnancy outcome. It is estimated that in a population with a high smoking prevalence, smoking cessation could prevent up to 10% of perinatal deaths, 35% of low birthweight babies, and 15% of preterm deliveries [21]. Mechanisms by which these adverse outcomes may occur include impaired oxygen delivery to the fetoplacental unit, exposure to carboxyhemoglobin, direct fetal genetic damage or other toxicities from the multiple substances present in cigarettes and cigarette smoke. In the postpartum period, cigarette smoking is associated with further risks for babies including an increased risk of neonatal death and sudden infant death syndrome, respiratory infections, asthma, otitis media, colic, childhood obesity, and possibly type 2 diabetes mellitus (Box 1.3).

Management

Antepartum

The benefit of smoking cessation both within and outside pregnancy is clear but successful abstinence is difficult.

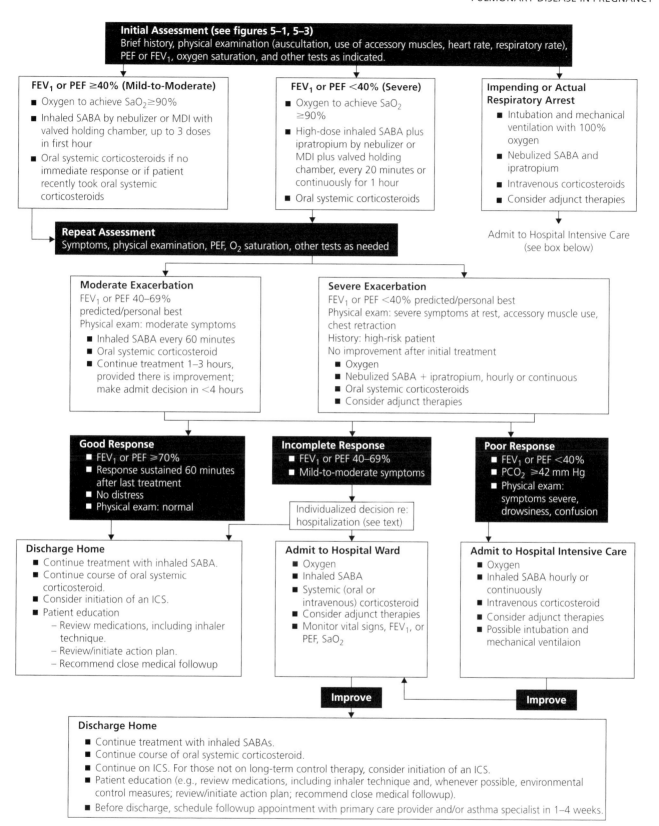

Figure 1.3 Management of asthma exacerbations: emergency department and hospital-based care. Reproduced with permission from The National Asthma Education and Prevention Program [15]. FEV$_1$, forced expiratory volume in 1 seconds; ICS, inhaled corticosteroid; MDI, metered dose inhaler; PCO$_2$, partial pressure carbon dioxide; PEF, peak expiratory flow; SABA, short-acting beta-agonist; SaO$_2$, oxygen saturation.

Box 1.3 Adverse pregnancy outcomes associated with smoking

- Infertility
- Low birthweight
- Spontaneous pregnancy loss
- Stillbirth
- Premature rupture of membranes
- Placental abruption
- Placenta previa
- Preterm delivery
- Possibly congenital malformations

Adverse effects on neonates and infants of mothers who smoke

- Increased risk of neonatal death and sudden infant death syndrome
- Increased respiratory infections (including otitis media)
- Increased asthma
- Increased colic
- Possible increased childhood obesity
- Possible increased type 2 diabetes mellitus

However, factors which may help motivate pregnant women include the desire to have a healthy pregnancy and newborn and the frequent contact with healthcare providers who can provide tobacco abstinence encouragement and support. Complete smoking cessation is only accomplished by approximately 20–40% of smoking pregnant women. Of those who do stop, most have already quit by their first prenatal visit. Risk factors for continued smoking include lower education status, those smoking less than 10 cigarettes per day, having a partner who smokes, and those who have other psychosocial issues. A study looking at a group of women who continued to smoke during pregnancy cited the following reasons for continued smoking: skepticism about smoking-related harms, addiction to nicotine, smoking among partners/family members, doubt about the safety of nicotine patch, and that the provider stopped asking about smoking status [22].

The 5As (Ask, Advise, Assess, Assist, Arrange) remain the cornerstone in approaching smoking pregnant women just as for nonpregnant patients (see Box 1.3, Tables 1.4 and 1.5). Inquiries about smoking status should be made on each visit and appropriate reinforcement given. If a patient is considering smoking cessation, a discussion centered on her continued need for stopping and recommendations for possible cessation strategies should be provided. Once a patient has actually stopped, continued positive reinforcement of useful strategies will be helpful for ongoing success. Additional resources for specific strategies for smoking cessation in pregnancy will be found at the following websites: www.modimes.org, www.helppregnantsmokersquit.com, and www.acog.org.

Drugs

In nonpregnant women, pharmacotherapy is strongly encouraged but because of concerns regarding drug use in pregnancy, medication is often not considered as a tool for use in smoking cessation in pregnancy. However, the considerable risks of ongoing tobacco use in a gravida unable to stop smoking without pharmacotherapy must be balanced against the risks of medication use. In particular, nicotine has known adverse fetal effects for which it has earned an US Food and Drug Administration (FDA) pregnancy safety category D ("studies have demonstrated a risk to the fetus"). However, with continued smoking, a fetus is exposed not only to nicotine but also to many other substances with adverse effects. Interestingly, several recent studies have suggested no worsened and even

Table 1.4 The 5 As for pregnant women

The 5 As	Action	Length of time spent
ASK about smoking status	Ask the pregnant woman to describe herself as one of the following: (a) I have NEVER smoked or have smoked LESS THAN 100 cigarettes in my lifetime (b) I stopped smoking BEFORE I found out I was pregnant, and I am not smoking now (c) I stopped smoking AFTER I found out I was pregnant, and I am not smoking now (d) I smoke some now, but I cut down on the number of cigarettes SINCE I found out I was pregnant (e) I smoke regularly now, about the same as BEFORE I found out I was pregnant	1 minute
ADVISE quitting	Give the patient strong, clear advice to quit smoking describing the impact of smoking and the benefits of quitting on the mother and fetus (see Table 1.5)	1 minute
ASSESS willingness to quit	Discuss whether the patient is willing to quit smoking in the next 30 days	1 minute
ASSIST in helping patient to quit	Discuss problem-solving methods and skills for cessation. Provide pregnancy-specific self-help materials. Encourage social support in the smoker's environment	3 minutes +
ARRANGE follow-up	Periodically assess smoking status and encourage cessation if continued smoking	1 minute

Adapted with permission from the National Partnership to Help Pregnant Smokers Quit: www.helppregnantsmokersquit.org.

Table 1.5 Benefits of smoking cessation in general over time

Time period	Result
Within 20 minutes	Blood pressure drops to near that of before the last cigarette. Temperature of hands and feet increases to normal
Within 12 hours	Carbon monoxide level drops to normal
Within 24 hours	The risk of myocardial infarction decreases
Within 2–3 weeks	Circulation improves and lung function increases
Within 1–9 months	Coughing, sinus congestion, fatigue, and shortness of breath decrease
Within 1 year	The excess risk of heart disease is half that of a smoker's
Within 5 years	The risk of stroke reduces to that of a nonsmoker's
Within 10 years	The risk of many cancers decreases, including lung, mouth, and throat cancer
Within 15 years:	The risk of heart disease reduces to that of a nonsmoker

Adapted with permission from the National Partnership to Help Pregnant Smokers Quit: www.helppregnantsmokersquit.org.

Box 1.4 Specific benefits of smoking cessation to tell pregnant patients

- After you stop smoking more nutrition will go to your baby to help him/her grow.
- After you stop smoking, your chances of having a healthy baby increase, and the baby is more likely to have a healthy childhood.
- After you stop smoking you will have more energy and may feel less stressed.
- After you stop smoking you'll breathe easier and you will be better able to keep up with your active, healthy baby.
- After you stop smoking, you'll reduce your risk for cancer, cardiovascular, and other diseases so you can be around a long time to be a good mother.

Adapted with permission from *You and your baby*, American Lung Association: www.lungusa.org.

improved fetal outcome associated with nicotine replacement therapy. One study looking at the rate of stillbirth in pregnant women using nicotine gum, patch or inhaler did not show an increase in stillbirth in nicotine replacement users [23]. The use of 2 mg nicotine gum in a study by Oncken *et al.* did not show increased quit rates but did show increased birthweight and a lower risk of preterm delivery as compared with placebo [24]. Ideally a pregnant woman would stop smoking without any pharmacologic aids but in the practical world, the likelihood is lower. Therefore, many would consider the benefit of nicotine replacement therapy and the higher likelihood of smoking cessation to be greater than the risk of continued smoking, especially in women who are at high risk for continued smoking.

Though bupropion is more effective for smoking cessation than nicotine replacement therapy outside pregnancy, there are limited data on its use in pregnancy for either smoking cessation or depression. Therefore, nicotine replacement is preferable for use in pregnancy. Both nicotine replacement and bupropion are acceptable for breastfeeding but nicotine replacement is preferable. Likewise, the safety of varenicline in pregnancy and lactation is even less clear and it should be avoided in pregnant and breastfeeding women until more data are available.

Post partum

Among those women who do stop smoking during pregnancy, 90% will relapse in the first postpartum year and most often within the first 6 weeks after delivery. Therefore, cessation programs should target this time period to minimize recidivism. Discussions addressing postpartum relapse should begin in the third trimester (Box 1.4). Risk factors for relapse include women with depressed mood, women who have family members or friends who are continued smokers, those with less social support, and those with less confidence in their ability to remain smoke free. Women who smoke in the postpartum period are also less likely to breastfeed.

Respiratory tract infection

Rhinitis and sinusitis

Up to 30% of women develop symptoms of rhinitis or sinusitis during pregnancy and the risk dramatically increases in smokers [25]. The effects of increased blood volume and vascular congestion on the nasal mucosa are thought to be responsible for gestational rhinitis. In addition, women with underlying allergic rhinitis or nasal polyps may develop worsening of their baseline symptoms with pregnancy.

Rhinitis may be categorized as allergic or nonallergic, both presenting with similar symptoms of rhinorrhea and nasal obstruction but with varied underlying causes. Allergic rhinitis may not be life threatening but its negative impact on quality of life of pregnant women is significant. Allergic rhinitis often co-exists with asthma and up to 40% of rhinitis patients become asthmatics [26]. Furthermore, clinically diagnosed allergic rhinitis is associated with worse asthma control. Of note, rhinitis in pregnancy may be associated with snoring.

Reassurance may be the only intervention necessary for rhinitis but women with particularly bothersome symptoms can try saline nasal spray or intranasal preparations of beclomethasone

Table 1.6 Differential diagnosis of rhinitis in pregnancy and some treatment options

Diagnosis	Clinical features	Treatment
Rhinitis medicamentosa	A condition of rebound nasal congestion brought on by extended use of topical decongestants (e.g. oxymetazoline, phenylephrine, and xylometazoline nasal sprays) that work by constricting blood vessels in the lining of the nose	Discontinue topical vasoconstrictors
Pregnancy rhinitis	Runny nose and nasal congestion presenting at any time in pregnancy caused by mucosal and vascular changes in nasopharynx	Buffered saline nose spray or nasal lavage, external nasal dilator (e.g. Breath-Rite strips)
Infectious rhinosinusitis	Usually a bacterial infection complicating the common cold with symptoms worsening after 5 days or not improving after 10 days and nasal congestion, fever and sinus pain predominating	Antibiotics (usually amoxicillin or azithromycin in penicillin-allergic patients) if no co-morbid conditions and no recent prior antibiotic use), nasal lavage, limited use of oxymetazoline nasal spray or pseudoephedrine after first trimester
Vasomotor rhinitis	Itch, sneeze, cough, nasal congestion, rhinorrhea in response to specific allergens (e.g. hay fever)	No specific therapy. Nasal ipratropium or pseudoephedrine after first trimester for limited period
Allergic rhinitis	Nasal congestion and rhinorrhea in response to nonallergenic environmental stimuli (e.g. cold, heat, alcohol, emotion, spicy food)	Intranasal cromolyn +/− nasal oxymetazoline or pseudoephedrine, topical beclomethasone or fluticasone, oral antihistamines (chlorpheniramine maleate, diphenhydramine)

and/or cromolyn [27]. First-generation antihistamines such as chlorpheniramine or diphenhydramine are reasonably used to treat allergy-related symptoms. Warning against overuse of topical decongestants which can cause rhinitis medicamentosa is important as many women may try these to avoid systemic medications. Table 1.6 outlines the differential diagnosis of rhinitis in pregnancy with recommended treatment options.

Sinusitis is increased sixfold in pregnancy as compared with nonpregnant patients. Complicating its diagnosis is the fact that 50% of pregnant women with documented purulent sinusitis do not have classic sinusitis symptoms (sinus tenderness, purulent discharge, fever). Therefore, despite the common rhinitis symptoms of pregnancy, clinicians should have a high index of suspicion for sinusitis in gravid women. The organisms causing sinusitis in pregnancy are the same as in the general population so antibiotics should be geared towards covering *Haemophilus influenzae*, *Mycoplasma. catarrhalis*, and *Streptococcus pneumoniae*. Assuming antibiotic resistance patterns do not dictate otherwise, reasonable antibiotic choices for use in pregnancy include amoxicillin/clauvulanate, cefuroxime axetil, and azithromycin. However, ciprofloxacin, doxycycline and tetracycline should be avoided.

Acute bronchitis

Acute bronchitis usually refers to a self-limited respiratory illness characterized by the predominance of a productive cough in a patient with no history of chronic obstructive pulmonary disease and no evidence of pneumonia. It affects approximately 5% of adults in the US annually [28].

Most cases of acute bronchitis seem to have a viral etiology; however, atypical bacteria including *Bordetella pertussis*, *Chlamydia pneumoniae* and *Mycoplasma pneumoniae* are important causes [29]. The etiologic pathogen is isolated from the sputum in only a minority of patients.

During the first few days of infection, the illness is indistinguishable from other acute upper respiratory infections. However, with acute bronchitis, coughing persists for more than 5 days, and during this period the results of pulmonary function testing may become abnormal [30]. Reduction in FEV_1 or bronchial hyper-reactivity may be noted, with improvement in the following 5–6 weeks. Typically, cough persists for 3 weeks following acute bronchitis, but may last 4 weeks or more.

Differential diagnosis includes asthma, bronchiolitis, bronchiectasis or acute exacerbation of chronic bronchitis. Chronic bronchitis by definition is the presence of cough and sputum production on most days of the month for at least 3 months of the year during 2 consecutive years.

No studies have looked specifically at the course of acute bronchitis in pregnancy. One retrospective cohort study found an association between placental abruption and acute respiratory illnesses, including acute bronchitis among white women [31].

Most patients with acute cough syndromes require no more than reassurance and symptomatic treatment. A chest X-ray would only be indicated if pneumonia was suspected on clinical exam. Diagnostic testing for a particular pathogen can only be justified when the organism is treatable and a community outbreak is suspected.

Antimicrobial agents are not recommended in most cases of acute bronchitis. Multiple studies indicate that patients with acute bronchitis do not benefit from these drugs. Antimicrobial therapy may be considered in patients when a treatable pathogen is identified or in epidemic settings to limit transmission. Table 1.7 includes suggested treatment regimens for pregnant patients.

Table 1.7 Recognized causes of acute bronchitis and treatment options

Pathogen	Comments	Treatment options in pregnancy	Treatment options with lactation
Influenza virus	Precipitous onset with fever, chills, headache, cough and myalgias	Supportive treatment with acetaminophen, fluids, rest. Antiviral agents recommended for treatment of influenza have either very little or concerning pregnancy safety data (see influenza section)	Supportive treatment with acetaminophen, fluids, and rest (see influenza section)
Parainfluenza virus	Epidemic may occur in fall. Croup in a child at home suggests its presence	Supportive treatment with acetaminophen, fluids, rest	Supportive treatment with acetaminophen, fluids, rest
Respiratory syncytial virus	Outbreaks occur in winter or spring. Approximately 45% of adults exposed to an infant with bronchiolitis become infected	Supportive treatment with acetaminophen, fluids, rest	Supportive treatment with acetaminophen, fluids, rest
Coronavirus	Severe respiratory symptoms may occur	Supportive treatment with acetaminophen, fluids, rest	Supportive treatment with acetaminophen, fluids, rest
Adenovirus	Infection is clinically similar to influenza, with abrupt onset of fever	Supportive treatment with acetaminophen, fluids, rest	Supportive treatment with acetaminophen, fluids, rest
Rhinovirus	Fever is uncommon, infection is generally mild	Supportive treatment with acetaminophen, fluids, rest	Supportive treatment with acetaminophen, fluids, rest
Bordetella pertussis	Incubation period is 1–3 weeks. Post-tussive vomiting may be present. Fever is uncommon	Azithromycin for 5 days (500 mg on day 1, 250 mg days 2–5)*or* Erythromycin for 14 days (500 mg 4 times daily) *or* Trimethoprim/Sulfamethoxazole for 14 days (160/800 mg twice daily)	Acceptable for use in lactation: Erythromycin$_B$ Azithromycin$_B$ Acceptable as second choice: Trimethoprim/sulfamethoxazole$_C$
Mycoplasma pneumoniae	Gradual onset over 2–3 days of headache, fever, malaise and cough. Wheezing may occur. Dyspnea is uncommon	Azithromycin for 5 days (500 mg on day 1, 250 mg days 2–5) or no therapy*	Acceptable for use in lactation: Erythromycin$_B$ Azithromycin$_B$
Chlamydia pneumoniae	Gradual onset of cough with preceding hoarseness	Azithromycin for 5 days (500 mg on day 1, 250 mg days 2–5) or no therapy*	Acceptable for use in lactation: Erythromycin$_B$ Azithromycin$_B$

Adapted with permission from Wenzel RP, Fowler AA 3rd. Clinical practice. Acute bronchitis. N Engl J Med 2006;355(20):2125–30.

Pneumonia

Pneumonia and influenza combined are the seventh leading cause of mortality in the United States and the most common cause of death from an infectious disease [32]. The incidence of pneumonia requiring hospitalization in pregnancy is between 2.6 and 15.1 per 10,000 deliveries, a rate comparable to that seen in nonpregnant women of a similar age [33]. Although historically pneumonia has been cited as the third most frequent cause of indirect obstetric death in North America, several recent studies have reported no or rare maternal deaths, with mortality rates similar to young hospitalized nonpregnant patients [34]. Despite this, pregnancy is associated with reduction in cell-mediated immunity and this may explain the increased risk of severe pneumonia and disseminated disease from atypical pathogens such as herpes virus, influenza, varicella, and coccidioidomycosis in pregnant women. Other anatomic and physiologic changes of pregnancy that may add to the vulnerability of the lung to injury during infection include an increase in thoracic circumference, elevation of the diaphragm (resulting in interference with clearance of secretions), decreased functional residual capacity, and increased oxygen consumption. This section will discuss the various types of pneumonia (Table 1.8).

Bacterial and atypical pneumonia

Although rigorous investigation into specific causes of pneumonia in pregnancy is lacking, the etiology is likely similar to the nonpregnant population, with *Streptococcus pneumoniae* being the most commonly isolated organism. Other causes of pneumonia include *Staphylococcus aureus, Haemophilus influenzae, Legionella* spp, *Mycoplasma pneumoniae, Chlamydia* and viruses. Among patients requiring admission to intensive care units, *Pseudomonas aeruginosa* and Enterobacteriaceae also play an important role. However, even with extensive diagnostic testing, the etiologic agent cannot be identified in at least 50% of cases.

Clinical presentation

Signs and symptoms of pneumonia in pregnancy are similar to those in nonpregnant individuals. Symptoms usually include cough, sputum production, chills, rigors, dyspnea and pleuritic

Table 1.8 Types of pneumonia and their treatment

Type of pneumonia	Recommended antibiotics acceptable for use in pregnancy	Lactation	Other comments
Community-acquired pneumonia Organisms: S. pneumoniae Respiratory viruses M. pneumoniae H. influenza C. pneumoniae Legionella Unknown	Ceftriaxone (2 g IV daily) or cefotaxime or ampicillin/sulbactam (3 g IV q 6 h) PLUS macrolide (azithromycin, erythromycin) If concern for MRSA, add vancomycin (15 mg/kg q 12 h)	All these agents can be used safely in breastfeeding mothers	Avoid tetracycline and doxycycline in pregnant or breastfeeding mothers Antipneumococcal fluoroquinolone may be used in nonpregnant patients but generally avoided in pregnancy or breastfeeding mothers
Hospital-acquired pneumonia/healthcare-associated pneumonia/ventilator-associated pneumonia Organisms: Aerobic gram-negatives (P. aeruginosa, E.coli, Klebsiella pneumoniae, Acinetobacter sp.) Gram-positive cocci (Staph. aureus, esp. methicillin resistant (MRSA) Oropharyngeal commensals (viridans group strep, coagulase-negative staph, Neisseria sp, Corynebacterium sp) Multidrug-resistant organisms (MDR) (as per local patterns)	Ceftriaxone (2 g IV daily) or ampicillin/sulbactam (3 g IV q 6h) If concern for MDR: Ceftazidime (2 g IV q 8 h) or cefepime (2 g IV q 8 h) or imipenem 500 mg q 6 h) or piperacillin/tazobactam (4.5 g q 6 h) or aztreonam (2 g q 6–8 h) PLUS Gentamycin or tobramycin PLUS Vancomycin (15 mg/kg q 12 h)	All these agents can be used safely in breastfeeding mothers	Antipneumococcal fluoroquinolone may be used in nonpregnant patients but generally avoided in pregnancy or breastfeeding mothers Avoid tetracycline and doxycycline in pregnant or breastfeeding mothers
Aspiration pneumonia Organisms: Oropharyngeal commensals (viridans group strep, coagulase-negative staph, Neisseria sp, Corynebacterium sp)	Clindamycin or penicillin	All these agents can be used safely in breastfeeding mothers	
Varicella pneumonia	Acyclovir IV 10 mg/kg q 8 h	Can be used safely in breastfeeding	

chest pain, although nonrespiratory symptoms such as vomiting, abdominal pain and fever may also occur. Physical exam may reveal fever, tachypnea, hypoxia, abnormal breath sounds, including a pleural friction rub, egophony (consolidation causing the patient's spoken "a" to sound like an "e" on auscultation) or tactile fremitus (consolidation causing the spoken words "99" to cause a palpable vibration on the chest wall). Hemodynamic instability may be present in cases of severe illness. Mothers who develop pneumonia are more likely to have co-existing medical problems including asthma, drug abuse, anemia and HIV infection. The use of corticosteroids for enhancement of fetal lung maturity and tocolytic agents has also been associated with antepartum pneumonia [35].

Diagnosis

Information obtained from the history or physical examination cannot rule in or rule out the diagnosis of pneumonia with adequate accuracy. Therefore, to confirm the diagnosis and to assess severity of illness and presence of complications such as pleural effusion or multilobar disease, a chest radiograph should be performed in all patients suspected to have pneumonia.

Laboratory data should include a complete blood count, serum chemistries for hepatic, renal and glucose evaluation, assessment of oxygenation and two sets of blood cultures; however, blood cultures may be positive only 7–15% of the time. The American Thoracic Society (ATS) does not recommend routine performance of sputum culture and gram stain. However, if a drug-resistant pathogen or an organism not covered by usual empiric therapy is suspected, sputum culture should be obtained. HIV status should be reviewed for all pregnant women with pneumonia and testing should be offered if it has not previously been done. Testing for Pneumocystis jiroveci infection should occur in all HIV-positive women who present with pneumonia.

The differential diagnosis for a pregnant woman presenting with symptoms of pneumonia is varied. Pulmonary embolism can present identically to an acute pneumonia with dyspnea, cough, chest pain, low-grade fever and chest X-ray infiltrates and remains the leading direct cause of maternal mortality in the US and the UK. Aspiration chemical pneumonitis, amniotic fluid embolism and pulmonary edema related to sepsis, tocolysis or pre-eclampsia can also present in a similar fashion. Other infectious illnesses, including cholecystitis, appendicitis and pyelonephritis, should also be considered.

Management

Preconception counseling

Pneumonia does not generally prompt preconception counseling because it is an acute infectious illness. There are a few issues worth consideration, however. Women who are HIV infected with low CD4 cell counts should continue prophylaxis for *Pneumocystis jiroveci* (see Chapter 18). Immunizations to prevent pneumonia and its complications are also indicated. The Centers for Disease Control and the American College of Obstetricians and Gynecologists advise that women should routinely receive influenza vaccination (see section on influenza below). Women with diabetes mellitus, asthma, chronic cardiac or pulmonary disease, chronic hypertension or immune compromise disease should receive the pneumococcal vaccine. It is also recommended post splenectomy and in women with functional hyposplenism, such as with sickle cell disease, and for women living in prisons or long-term care facilities. All nonpregnant women of childbearing age who are not immune to varicella should be vaccinated but it is a live vaccine and should not be given during pregnancy.

Potential maternal and fetal complications

Pregnancy increases the risk of maternal complications from pneumonia, including the need for mechanical ventilation. Respiratory failure due to pneumonia is the third leading indication for intubation in pregnancy [36]. Other maternal complications include pulmonary edema, bacteremia, empyema and pneumothorax. Pregnancies complicated by acute respiratory illnesses, including viral and bacterial pneumonia, have been shown to be associated with placental abruption [31]. Increased rates of preterm labor and delivery before 34 weeks of gestation have also been described [37], resulting in significantly lower average birthweight at delivery. The neonatal mortality rate due to antepartum pneumonia ranges from 1.9% to 12%, with most mortality attributable to complications of preterm birth [38]. Although most cases of pneumonia in pregnancy are caused by organisms which do not affect the fetus except through their effects on maternal status, some organisms, such as varicella, may present specific risks to the fetus. The fetus may also be at risk from maternal conditions which predispose to pneumonia, such as anemia or HIV infection.

Treatment

Although several guidelines to assess severity and need for hospitalization have been developed for pneumonia in the nonpregnant population, discriminatory features that identify those pregnant women who can be successfully managed as outpatients have not been determined. Pregnant women with pneumonia should generally be admitted for initial therapy, fetal evaluation and to ensure adequate oxygenation (oxygen saturation $\geq 95\%$ or $pO_2 \geq 70$ mmHg).

Several recommendations for the empiric treatment of community-acquired pneumonia exist. These support the use of a macrolide (erythromycin in any form except estolate ester, or azithromycin) in conjunction with a beta-lactam (cefotaxime, ceftriaxone or ampicillin-sulbactam) for most inpatients with pneumonia. Although levofloxacin and doxycycline are often recommended in the treatment of pneumonia in the nonpregnant population, these drugs should be avoided in pregnancy. Clarithromycin has shown adverse effects in animal trials at doses equivalent to 2–17 times the maximum recommended human dose. It is therefore best avoided in pregnancy, with use limited to those cases where no alternative therapy is appropriate. Monotherapy with high-dose amoxicillin (3–4 g a day) is supported in some European recommendations for nonpregnant patients, but ATS guidelines suggest addition of azithromycin for adequate coverage of *H. influenzae* (see Table 1.8).

With appropriate antibiotic therapy, some improvement in the patient's clinical course should be seen within 72 hours. Patients initially treated with intravenous antibiotics can be switched to oral agents (erythromycin/azithromycin with cefprozil or cefpodoxime) once the patient is afebrile for 24–48 hours. Continuation of therapy for a total of 10–14 days is recommended for all agents except azithromycin which can be given for only a 5-day course because of its extended half-life. Clinicians should ensure that a follow-up chest X-ray is done to confirm that there is no other underlying pathology complicating the pneumonia.

Aspiration pneumonia

Due to significant progress in modern obstetric and anesthetic management, acute aspiration pneumonitis has become a very uncommon cause of pneumonia in pregnancy. Although aspiration usually occurs in association with a difficult intubation or during the postanesthetic period when the gag reflex may be depressed, it may also develop *de novo* in pregnant women. Gastric juice in the lungs leads to intense pulmonary inflammation over 8–24 hours. The patient becomes tachypneic, hypoxic and febrile and the chest X-ray can show a complete "white out." Despite this rapidly deteriorating course, the picture resolves without antibiotics within 48–72 hours unless bacterial superinfection intervenes.

Bacterial aspiration pneumonia usually has a more insidious onset. Clinical manifestations typically begin 48–72 hours after aspiration, with persistent fever, sputum and leukocytosis. In this syndrome, chest X-ray findings are typically localized to the basilar segments (if the patient aspirated while upright) or to the posterior segment of the upper lobe or the superior segment of the lower lobe (if the patient aspirated while supine). The bacterial infection is generally polymicrobial with mouth anaerobes predominating and antibiotic treatment with penicillin or clindamycin is recommended.

Viral pneumonia

Varicella and influenza are the most common pathogens associated with viral pneumonia in pregnancy; however, cases with pneumonia resulting from rubella, hantavirus and SARS have also been reported in pregnancy. Viral pneumonia is often complicated by acute respiratory failure, secondary bacterial infections and acute respiratory distress syndrome (ARDS). This chapter will cover influenza, severe acute respiratory syndrome (SARS), and varicella pneumonia.

Influenza in pregnancy (see also Chapter 17)

Outbreaks or epidemics of influenza generally occur in the fall and winter but can occur year round in the tropics. The viruses causing influenza are of two types, A and B. The A virus is further classified by the hemagglutinin (H) and neuramidase (N) surface antigens and antibodies against these antigens decrease the likelihood of infection. However, antibodies to one subtype do not necessarily confer immunity to another or a variant of a subtype, such as occurs with antigenic drift. This is an important consideration in determining the influenza strains against which the annual vaccines are targeted. A major change in the antigens resulting in essentially a novel influenza virus, termed antigenic shift, has the potential to cause pandemics.

Children have the highest rate of influenza infection but anyone in the general population may become infected. Between the years 1990 and 1999, the average annual number of deaths related to influenza infection in the US was 36,000 [39]. Those who are at the greatest risk for serious infection or death include people ≥65 years old, children <2 years old, those with chronic cardiac and pulmonary disorders, those with chronic metabolic conditions (such as diabetes mellitus), those with chronic medical conditions (such as renal insufficiency, hemoglobinopathies, and immunodeficiencies such as HIV), as well as pregnant women. Complications of influenza include severe primary viral infection as well as secondary bacterial infections causing pneumonia, sinusitis, and otitis media. Further complications are secondary to decompensation of underlying diseases, particularly cardiopulmonary disease.

The influenza virus is spread via respiratory droplets from person to person. The incubation period is approximately 1–4 days and virus may be shed from several days before obvious infection to 5–10 days after. Symptoms include the abrupt onset of fever, headache, myalgia and respiratory symptoms such as cough and sore throat. Uncomplicated infection resolves after 3–7 days but some patients may have persistent malaise for more than 2 weeks.

Influenza is a relatively common infection in pregnancy. One study in 2000 found that of 1659 pregnant women in the United Kingdom, 11% had serologic evidence of a new influenza infection during the pregnancy [40]. Influenza is also associated with increased morbidity and mortality in pregnant women. The mortality for all infected pregnant women in the 1918 flu epidemic was 27% but when women were infected in the last month of pregnancy, the mortality was over 60%. Of the pregnant women who developed pneumonia, over 50% died as compared with 30% of nonpregnant patients who developed pneumonia. During the 1957 Asian flu epidemic in New York City, over half the young women who died with pneumonia were pregnant. Since that time, improved healthcare with wider immunization practices (and possibly the specific antigenic strains of influenza circulating) have been associated with lower mortality rates. Despite this, pregnant women with influenza are still at increased risk for serious complications requiring hospitalization [41]. Neuzil et al. estimated from their data in 1998 that in the average flu season, 25 out of 10,000 pregnant women in the third trimester will require hospitalization for influenza-related morbidity [42]. Pregnant women with influenza and associated co-morbidities such as asthma, diabetes, cardiac disease, cigarette smoking or other high-risk medical diseases are at increased risk for hospitalization with influenza. The likelihood of requiring hospitalization also increases with each trimester. Physiologic changes in pregnancy which may explain the increase of influenza complications in gravid women include changes in immune function, predisposition to the development of pulmonary edema, higher baseline oxygen consumption and a higher cardiac output.

It appears that the effects of influenza on the fetus are primarily related to the severity of maternal illness. Though there are reports of increased congenital anomalies, stillbirths, and prematurity with pandemics, a Tennessee Medicaid population study conducted from 1985 to 1993 did not reveal an increase in adverse perinatal outcomes with respiratory hospitalizations during the influenza season [43]. A few cases of the influenza virus infecting the placenta and fetus have been reported but others have found no increase in obstetric complications, congenital malformations or other evidence of transplacental transmission.

The management of pregnant women with influenza rests primarily on supportive care and aggressive treatment of superinfection. Fevers should be controlled with acetaminophen and adequate hydration provided. Pneumonia, sinusitis, and otitis media require appropriate antibiotics. These patients should be followed closely for any deterioration as those with worsening shortness of breath, hypoxia or abnormal chest exams are at risk for requiring mechanical ventilation. Amantadine and rimantadine are not effective against influenza B and there is emerging resistance in influenza A such that they have not been recommended for use in the United States in recent years. Both agents are teratogenic and embryotoxic in rodents so their use is not recommended in pregnancy anyway. There is only limited information about the neuramidase inhibitors zanamivir and oseltamivir in pregnancy. Use of these agents requires careful consideration of the potential benefits against their unknown risks.

Table 1.9 Use of antiviral drugs for influenza in pregnancy

Antivirals	Use in pregnancy	Use in breastfeeding
Adamantanes: amantadine, rimantadine	Teratogenic and embryotoxic in rodents	Amantadine not reviewed by American Academy of Pediatrics (AAP) but may suppress milk production Rimantadine not reviewed by AAP but concentrated in rodent milk. It is used in pediatric patients over 1 year old, however
Neuramidase inhibitors: zanamivir, oseltamivir	The potential benefits of use in pregnancy must be weighed against the unknown risks. However, during the early 2009 H1N1 epidemic, the use of these agents in pregnant women was recommended by the US CDC	Zanamivir and oseltamivir are not reviewed by AAP but given limited efficacy should probably not be used routinely in breastfeeding patients. However, during the early 2009 H1N1 epidemic, the use of these agents in pregnant women was recommended by the US CDC
	Zanamivir crosses the placenta in rats and rabbits. Congenital abnormalities were not found in rats and rabbits exposed to zanamivir *in utero* In rats, dose-dependent minor skeletal changes were noted in the offspring of mothers given oseltamivir	

Prevention of influenza infection is unequivocally the most important measure in the fight against influenza. Hygiene, such as handwashing measures, is recommended but cannot replace immunization. In one study of more than 2000 pregnant women immunized for influenza, no adverse fetal effects were associated with the vaccination [44]. Further, immunization of pregnant mothers in Bangladesh against influenza reduced influenza illness by 63% in infants up to 6 months of age and reduced by one-third all febrile respiratory illness in both mothers and infants [45]. Universal vaccination of pregnant (regardless of trimester) and breastfeeding women is recommended by the American College of Obstetricians and Gynecologists (ACOG) and the Centers for Disease Control and Prevention (CDC) [46].

Severe acute respiratory syndrome (see also Chapter 17)
Severe acute respiratory syndrome is a new viral illness that was first described in 2002. Prior to its containment in July 2003, the global outbreak of SARS affected more than 8000 people and caused more than 800 deaths worldwide. SARS is caused by a novel coronavirus and results in an atypical pneumonia which can rapidly progress to respiratory failure. Symptoms usually develop 2–7 days after exposure and include fever, chills, malaise, myalgia and headache. A nonproductive cough, dyspnea and diarrhea develop over 3–7 days and respiratory failure may develop in up to 20%. Patients are most infectious in the second week of illness. Laboratory abnormalities include lymphopenia, thrombocytopenia, prolonged partial thrombin time (PTT) and electrolyte abnormalities. Chest radiograph findings include generalized, patchy, interstitial infiltrates. Diagnosis can be confirmed by viral culture, polymerase chain reaction (PCR), ELISA and immunofluorescence assay. Since the clinical presentation of SARS is nonspecific, the differential diagnosis is wide and includes influenza virus, parainfluenza viruses, respiratory syncytial virus, *Haemophilus influenzae*, *Mycoplasma pneumoniae*, *Legionella* spp. and *Chlamydia* spp.

Although there were reports of pregnant women with SARS from several countries, the number of reported cases is too small to permit any definitive conclusions as to whether SARS was more or less severe among pregnant women as compared with nonpregnant women. The largest case series which included 12 pregnant patients with SARS showed high rates of morbidity and mortality [47], with a case fatality rate of 25%. Among the seven women who were infected in the first trimester, four had spontaneous abortions, and two had induced abortions. Of the five women who were infected later in pregnancy, three underwent preterm cesarean delivery (26–32 weeks of gestation) for worsening maternal hypoxemia; two of the three women who underwent cesarean delivery subsequently died. No cases of vertical transmission have been reported. Treatment with ribavirin, oseltamivir, steroids or combination steroids and antiviral medications has demonstrated reduction in mortality in the nonpregnant population [48]. However, ribavirin is teratogenic in animals and its use in pregnancy for this indication is evolving.

Varicella pneumonia (see also Chapter 17)
Although primary varicella infection is a childhood illness, 5–10% of cases occur after age 15 years. Acute VZV infection affects 5–7 of 10,000 pregnancies [49]. Ten to 20% of women with primary varicella infection in pregnancy can develop fulminant pneumonia. Before the availability of antiviral therapy, maternal mortality in cases of VZV pneumonia was as high as 40%. With the advent of antiviral agents, the mortality has decreased but still remains substantial. Risk factors for varicella pneumonia include later gestational age, history of or current smoking and skin involvement with >100 vesicles. Signs and symptoms of pneumonia may become manifest approximately 3–5 days after onset of rash and include dyspnea, tachypnea, cough with blood-tinged sputum, malaise and pleurisy. Chest X-ray may reveal a diffuse interstitial

nodular pattern ("ground-glass" appearance) or focal infiltrates. Mechanical ventilation may be required in up to half the patients. Treatment is parenteral acyclovir.

Management of maternal exposure to varicella during pregnancy is based on maternal immune status to varicella. Previous known varicella infection, previous vaccination or presence of serum IgG against varicella confers immunity and there is no risk from exposure. If exposure to varicella occurs in a gravid woman without immunity, VZ IG should be administered within 96 hours in an attempt to prevent maternal infection. The ability to prevent congenital varicella syndrome with VZ IG is unknown. Oral acyclovir (800 mg five times a day) is recommended for pregnant women with primary varicella infection to prevent serious complications such as pneumonia, but is most effective if given within 24 hours of development of rash. Parenteral acyclovir (10 mg/kg every 8 hours) should also be given to all varicella nonimmune patients who develop respiratory symptoms within 10 days of exposure to varicella.

Fungal pneumonia

Pneumonia caused by fungal organisms is rare in pregnancy. Histoplasmosis and blastomycosis (most commonly acquired in the Ohio or Mississippi River valleys in the southeast US but found throughout the world) have been most commonly associated with fungal pneumonia in pregnancy and cause a mild, self-limiting illness. Cryptococcosis (found worldwide in soil contaminated with bird droppings) also may present in pregnancy, though meningitis is more common than pneumonia. Coccidioidomycosis pneumonia (most commonly acquired in the desert south west of the US) has been associated with disseminated disease, particularly with infection in the third trimester. Disseminated fungal infection in a gravid woman is associated with increased risk of preterm delivery, perinatal and maternal mortality.

Fungal pneumonia may present with slow onset of cough and dyspnea or an acute onset of pleuritic chest pain and hypoxemia. Chest X-rays tend to show nodular disease with adenopathy. Diagnosis may be confirmed by sputum gram stain and culture for fungal organisms or by detection of serum fungal antigens. Severe pneumonia or disseminated disease is treated with amphotericin B. Ketoconazole or itraconazole is an option, although safety data for long-term use in pregnancy are limited and some concerning data exist for ketoconazole that suggest it may be teratogenic.

Pneumocystis jiroveci pneumonia

Pneumocystis jiroveci pneumonia (PJP) is the most common cause of AIDS-related death among pregnant patients. Symptoms include dry cough, tachypnea and dyspnea. Chest radiographs demonstrate diffuse interstitial infiltrates. In most cases, the diagnosis can be made by histologic staining of sputum, although bronchoscopy may be necessary in

some cases. In a review of 22 cases of PJP in pregnancy, high rates of respiratory failure, maternal and fetal mortality were found [50]. However, these numbers may not necessarily reflect the true incidence of complications, because none of the patients in this series were on antiretroviral therapy and the diagnosis of HIV/AIDS was made only after the PJP was detected. Treatment is with trimethoprim-sulfamethoxazole (TMP/SMX) or pentamidine. For patients without hypoxemia (PaO$_2$ >70 mmHg), oral TMP/SMX 2 double-strength tablets or intravenous 15 mg/kg/day of TMP component every 8 hours for 21 days is recommended. For severe cases, oral or intravenous steroids are initiated before addition of TMP/SMX. HIV-infected patients with CD4 counts less than 200/μL, a history of oropharyngeal candidiasis or an AIDS-defining illness should receive prophylaxis with TMP/SMX, one double-strength tablet daily (see Chapter 18).

Tuberculosis in pregnancy

Tuberculosis (TB) is an age-old disease that is still very relevant to the worldwide community, causing 8 million new cases and 2 million deaths annually. Pregnant women are not spared its effects. Of all the TB deaths in women, 80% occur during the childbearing years. Because of its significant impact on pregnant women and their children, TB is targeted in Millennium Development Goals 4 and 5 to reduce childhood mortality and improve maternal health [51] (Box 1.5). In developed nations TB appears to be decreasing in incidence overall but even in the US, inner-city dwellers and immigrants from countries with a high prevalence represent significant populations with untreated TB. Women from these populations may seek healthcare only in the context of pregnancy

---

Box 1.5 Millennium Development Goals

Goal 4 – Reduce child mortality

Certain diseases . . . (including) TB . . . when they occur in pregnancy can lead to underweight and premature babies whose chances of survival are diminished. It follows, then, that treating these diseases in pregnant women will also help reduce under-five mortality.

Goal 5 – Improve maternal health

Target 6: Reduce by three-quarters, between 1990 and 2015, the maternal mortality ratio. Certain diseases . . . possibly including TB . . . when experienced during pregnancy, can be especially hard-hitting, and contribute to maternal mortality.

such that pregnancy presents a public health opportunity to identify and treat infected individuals.

Pathophysiology

Tuberculosis is caused by the acid-fast tubercle bacillus, *Mycobacterium tuberculosis*. It is spread via respiratory droplets from person to person. The inhaled organism is ingested by macrophages and disseminated tuberculosis occurs if the organism is not contained in the local lymph nodes. Granulomas develop secondary to the host's immune response to the mycobacterium. The infected primary lesion may heal and those individuals will not go on to have subsequent evidence of disease. Others may develop reactivation TB years later, particularly in circumstances of physiologic stress or depressed immunity (such as with HIV infection).

Clinical manifestations

Primary infection with TB is typically asymptomatic unless it disseminates. Reactivation TB presents with low-grade fevers, weight loss, and drenching night sweats. Respiratory symptoms may not be prominent even with pulmonary TB but cough and hemoptysis can occur. Symptoms of extrapulmonary TB are referable to the organ system involved.

Diagnosis

The diagnosis of a TB infection is established when the organism is identified in sputum, urine, body tissue or body fluid. Acid-fast bacilli may be seen on stained slides initially but culture can take up to 4–8 weeks to grow on classic culture media. Ideally, 2–3 sputum specimens obtained at least 8 hours apart (with at least one being an early morning specimen) should be sent for evaluation. If patients are unable to produce sputum, a nebulizer of hypertonic saline may be helpful in inducing some. Auramine-rhodamine or auramine O fluorescence staining (ideally used in combination with confirmatory nucleic acid amplification testing or NAAT) is more sensitive and now more commonly used than the classic Ziehl–Neelson stain but definitive diagnosis or exclusion of tuberculosis still requires culture. Positive cultures are typically subjected to confirmatory (DNA/RNA probe or high-pressure liquid chromatography or biochemical methods) and drug susceptibility testing. A rapid detection assay under development, called the microscopic-observation drug-susceptibility (MODS) assay, offers a combined rapid (7 days) tentative detection method and drug susceptibility testing for *M. tuberculosis* in resource-limited settings.

Chest X-ray findings suggestive of tuberculosis include multinodular infiltrates of the upper lobes and superior segments of the lower lobes. Cavitary lesions may also develop. The classic Gohn complex represents a healed primary lesion with a calcified hilar node and calcified peripheral nodule.

However, it is important to be aware that up to 10% of patients with early culture-positive tuberculosis will have normal chest radiographs.

Screening

The CDC and the ATS recommend targeted testing for TB to identify persons with either latent tuberculosis or TB disease who would benefit from treatment [52]. They do not recommend screening for those who are not at high risk for TB exposure and since pregnancy itself does not represent a risk for exposure, pregnant women should be screened as in non-pregnant patients. Indications for tuberculin testing in and out of pregnancy are listed in Box 1.6. The common practice of universal tuberculin testing of pregnant women in hospital-based prenatal clinics is best justified in settings with a large proportion of socio-economically disadvantaged women, immigrants from high-risk areas or women with recent or active substance abuse or malnutrition.

Screening recommendations are established with the Mantoux tuberculin skin test and consist of an intradermal injection of 0.1 mL of purified protein derivative (PPD) containing 5 tuberculin units just beneath the skin surface on the forearm. A trained healthcare worker measures the area of induration (NOT erythema) in millimeters 48–72 hours later to determine the test result. The classification of a positive result depends on the presence of known risk factors (Box 1.7). For instance, a woman who has recently immigrated from a high-risk area has a positive Mantoux or PPD if the area of induration measures 10 mm or more. However, a woman with HIV has a positive test if the area of induration is 5 mm or more. Pregnancy does not impact on the interpretation of the test.

The QuantiFERON-TB Gold test was approved by the US FDA in 2005 for use in diagnosing both TB infection and latent TB infection. The test measures the white blood cell response to two synthetic peptides representing *M. tuberculosis* proteins. Though it is designed to be used in the same circumstances as the Mantoux test, there are limited data on its use in immunocompromised persons as well as in pregnancy. Therefore, until more data are available in these populations, the Mantoux test is preferable. Advantages to the QuantiFERON-TB Gold test are that it only requires a single blood draw, results are available within 24 hours and are not affected by prior BCG vaccination or subject to reader bias, and it is not affected by boost responses. Disadvantages are the need to collect, transport, and process blood samples in a specific manner within 12 hours and the uncertainties about its use in certain populations, as noted.

Course in pregnancy

Before antituberculous drugs were available, the outcome of pregnancy complicated by tuberculosis was poor for both

Box 1.6 Who should receive tuberculin testing outside pregnancy?

Patients who should have annual tuberculin testing

- Persons with HIV infection.
- Presence of a medical condition that increases the risk of active TB (diabetes, end-stage renal disease, alcoholism, solid organ transplant recipients, rapid weight loss or chronic malnutrition, anticipated long-term therapy with glucocorticoids or other immunosuppressive medications, hemodialysis, gastrectomy, jejunoileal bypass, silicosis, hematologic or reticuloendothelial malignancies).
- Ongoing potential close contact with cases of active TB including laboratory personnel handling potentially infected specimens, prison guards, healthcare workers in high-risk settings.
- New immigrants from areas where TB is common (Asia, Africa, Latin America, Eastern Europe, Russia).
- Residents of long-term care facilities (nursing homes, mental and correctional institutions).
- Medically underserved, low-income populations (including migrant farm workers, injection drug users and homeless persons).
- Children exposed to adults in high-risk categories.

Patients who should have a single tuberculin test

- Close exposure to a case of TB.
- Individuals born in Latin America, Asia or Africa or other locations with a high prevalence of TB who have relocated to a low-incidence country in the past 5 years.
- Individuals returning from work in a refugee, relief or healthcare setting in a TB-endemic area.
- Patients with an incidentally discovered fibrotic lung lesion on a CXR.

Adapted with permission from *Core curriculum on tuberculosis: what the clinician should know*. Department of Health and Human Services, Centers for Disease Control and Prevention, 2000. www.cdc.gov/tb

Box 1.7 Classification of tuberculin reactivity

≥ 5 mm induration is positive	≥ 10 mm induration is positive	≥ 15 mm induration is positive
HIV–positive patient	Recent immigration from high-prevalence area	Person with no known risk factors for TB*
Recent contact with person with TB		
Patient with changes on CXR consistent with TB	Injection drug users	
Patient with organ transplant and other immunosuppressed conditions	Residents and employees of high-risk congregate settings	
	Laboratory personnel in mycobacteriology labs	
	Persons with clinical conditions that place them at high risk†	
	Children less than 4 years old or older children exposed to adults in high-risk categories	

*Skin testing programs should only be done among high-risk groups.

†High-risk conditions include: substance abuse, diabetes mellitus, silicosis, prolonged corticosteroid therapy, other immunosuppressive therapy, cancer of the head and neck, hematologic and reticuloendothelial disease (e.g. leukemia, Hodgkin's disease), end-stage renal disease, intestinal bypass or gastrectomy, chronic malabsorption syndromes, low bodyweight (10% or more below ideal bodyweight).

Adapted with permission from *Core curriculum on tuberculosis: what the clinician should know*. Department of Health and Human Services, Centers for Disease Control and Prevention, 2000. www.cdc.gov/tb

mother and fetus and it appeared that there was a tendency for worsening in the postpartum period. In the early 20th century it was even recommended that pregnant women with TB terminate their pregnancies. However, it now appears that the course of tuberculosis is not affected by pregnancy but rather is more related to other risk factors, such as HIV and immune status. Interestingly, active tuberculosis may be more likely to be asymptomatic in pregnancy [53].

Treated tuberculosis in pregnancy does not appear to be associated with adverse maternal or fetal outcome. Untreated and extrapulmonary disease (with the exception of TB lymphadenitis), however, is associated with low birth-weight, intrauterine growth restriction, and lower APGAR scores [54]. Extrapulmonary TB has a high prevalence in pregnancy of up to 50%. Reports of extrapulmonary TB in pregnancy include tuberculous peritonitis associated with a temporary Addisonian state, colonic tuberculosis, pericardial tuberculosis, renal tuberculosis, and tuberculous meningitis. The more common presentation for TB in pregnancy is positive screening by PPD or a suspicious chest X-ray done for other reasons such as cough, purulent sputum, hemoptysis, fever, weight loss, night sweats or chest pain.

Tuberculosis only rarely affects the fetus by transplacental passage but cases of fetal infection have been well documented. Infection may occur via the fetus swallowing infected amniotic fluid or be blood borne via the umbilical vein. Granulomas have been identified in the placenta and the bacillus itself has been found in the decidua, amnion, and chorionic villi. This occurs primarily with endometrial or miliary TB. Pulmonary and lymphadenitis TB generally pose little risk to the fetus assuming oxygenation and maternal well-being is not seriously jeopardized. More commonly, a neonate becomes infected after birth from exposure to an infected mother or family member. Therefore aggressive identification of an infected mother is important. Isolation of a neonate from the mother is only required if the mother is "smear positive" (mycobacteria identified on staining of sputum). Because modern antituberculous agents render the sputum sterile within 2 weeks and markedly reduce the number of organisms within 24 hours, this should not occur frequently. The neonate will require appropriate treatment if the mother is found to have positive sputum.

Management

Pregnancy

Untreated active TB is a greater risk to the fetus than treatment itself. The main fetal concern is the effect of the antituberculous drugs. In general, the recommended initial drug regimen for pregnant women with TB is at least isoniazid (INH), rifampin (RIF), and ethambutol (EMB) (Table 1.10). Pyrazinamide (PZA) is recommended by the World Health Organization [55] and the International Unit

Against Tuberculosis and Lung Disease as a fourth agent [56]. Though INH, RIF, and EMB cross the placenta, teratogenic effects have not been demonstrated. An increased incidence of hepatic toxicity of INH appears to be associated with pregnancy and the first 6 postpartum months so that baseline and monthly liver tests are recommended. In particular, Hispanic and black women seem to be especially prone. Pyridoxine (50 mg) should also be administered to pregnant women taking INH to minimize the risk of neuropathy as they have increased nutritional needs. While there is no disagreement that PZA is necessary when there is concern about drug resistance or co-infection with HIV, some reserve its use for such indications as there are limited data about its effects in pregnancy. However, since multidrug resistance and co-infection with HIV are increasingly common, data about its use are accumulating and it is being recommended more often for initial use in the US.

The emergence of drug-resistant tuberculosis is problematic as some second-line agents such as the quinolones have known risks while others have an as yet unestablished safety profile in pregnancy. Treatment of these pregnant patients requires careful consideration by a multidisciplinary team including an expert in multidrug-resistant TB.

Latent TB infection (LTBI) requires treatment to decrease the likelihood of developing active TB in the future. Isoniazid is considered the safest, most effective drug of choice for use in pregnancy [57]. In general, it is recommended that treatment not be delayed until after delivery as this is associated with fewer recurrences [58]. It is unclear whether this is related to the higher noncompliance rate post partum (which has been shown to be up to 80%) and results in reduced effectiveness of isoniazid from 93–98% to 50% [59]. Certainly if the decision is made to treat LTBI post partum, every effort should be made to ensure compliance. Complicating the treatment of women antepartum is the reluctance of women to take medications during pregnancy, particularly when they otherwise feel well and medication is needed for a prolonged period. If there is a language barrier or transportation issues with obtaining medication for directly observed therapy, success is even more difficult.

Post partum (Box 1.8)

Women should not be discouraged from breastfeeding when taking isoniazid, rifampin, ethambutol or pyrazinamide. These agents do pass into the breast milk but only to a small degree and levels are inadequate to provide any treatment or protection from TB.

Acute respiratory distress syndrome and acute lung injury in pregnancy

Acute respiratory distress syndrome, previously known as adult respiratory distress syndrome, was first described as a

Table 1.10 Antituberculous medication

Medication/dose	Pregnancy data	Adverse effects	Breastfeeding	Other comments
Isoniazid (INH) 5 mg/kg up to a maximum of 300 mg daily Dispensed in the US as 50, 100 and 300 mg tablets and 50 m/5 mL syrup	FDA pregnancy classification C Considerable reassuring pregnancy safety data make this an excellent choice in pregnancy	Hepatotoxicity (risk increased in pregnant and Hispanic patients – recommend screening baseline liver function tests and checking monthly during pregnancy) Peripheral neuritis (risk obviated somewhat by supplementation with pyridoxine 25–50 mg PO daily) Other: GI upset, seizures, rash, and multiple drug interactions	AAP deems compatible with breastfeeding Thomas Hale classifies as L3*	Consider supplementation with vitamin K 10 mg PO daily from 36 weeks gestation on to decrease the risk of postpartum hemorrhage and hemorrhagic disease of the newborn
Rifampin 10 mg/kg up to a maximum of 600 mg daily Dispensed in the US as 150 and 300 mg tablets	FDA pregnancy classification C No evidence of adverse fetal effects	Hepatitis, nausea, fever, anemia, headache, diarrhea, orange secretions, pseudomembranous colitis, multiple drug interactions, flu-like symptoms at high doses, purpura	AAP deems compatible with breastfeeding Thomas Hale classifies as L3*	Consider supplementation with vitamin K 10 mg PO daily from 36 weeks gestation on to decrease the risk of postpartum hemorrhage and hemorrhagic disease of the newborn
Ethambutol 15–25 mg/kg up to a maximum of 2500 mg daily Dispensed in the US as 100 and 400 mg tablets	FDA pregnancy classification B	Optic neuritis in 1% of patients Other: peripheral neuropathy, rash, dizziness, confusion, nausea, vomiting	AAP deems compatible with breastfeeding Thomas Hale classifies as L2*	Screen patient monthly for optic neuritis by asking about blurred vision or scotomata and performing visual acuity and color discrimination testing
Pyrazinamide (PZA) 15–30 mg/kg PO daily up to a maximum of 3000 mg daily	FDA pregnancy classification C Published human data are limited despite broad international experience	Thrombocytopenia, hepatotoxicity, interstitial nephritis, nausea and vomiting, rashes, arthralgia	Not reviewed by the AAP Thomas Hale classifies as L3* No reported neonatal adverse effects	When possible, best to be started after the first trimester
Streptomycin Dose varies	FDA pregnancy classification D Reports of fetal ototoxicity	Deafness, anemia, renal toxicity	AAP deems compatible with breastfeeding Thomas Hale classifies as L3* No neonatal concerns via milk but observe for changes in GI flora	Use in pregnancy to be avoided unless no alternatives identified

AAP, American Academy of Pediatrics.

The Food and Drug Administration (FDA) classifies the safety of medications during pregnancy as category A, B, C, D and X. This classification system is reviewed in Chapter 30

*Thomas Hale in his classic breastfeeding reference *Medications and mothers' milk* (Pharmasoft, 2008), classifies medication safety in breastfeeding as follows: L1, safest; L2, safer; L3, moderately safe; L4, possibly hazardous; L5, contraindicated. See Chapter 31 for details.

clinical entity in 1967. It is characterized by an acute onset of noncardiogenic pulmonary edema resulting in severely impaired oxygenation. The current definition of ARDS was proposed in 1994 in the American-European Consensus Conference [60]. The panel recognized that severity of lung injury varies: patients with less severe hypoxia are considered to have acute lung injury (ALI) and patients with more severe hypoxia are considered to have ARDS. This definition characterizes the illness as having acute onset, bilateral chest infiltrates, pulmonary artery wedge pressure of less than 18 mmHg or absence of clinical evidence of left atrial hypertension, and PaO_2/FiO_2 ratio of 200–300 for ALI and $\geq$200 for ARDS.

The frequency of ARDS in the general population is estimated at 1.5 per 100,000 per year, with a fatality rate of 35–50%. Although no studies clearly elucidate the frequency of ARDS in the obstetric population, the incidence is felt to be similar to the general population. Noncardiogenic pulmonary edema or ALI, on the other hand, is known to occur more frequently in pregnant women, with an estimated

Box 1.8 Management of TB-infected mother and newborn baby

1. Mother with latent TB infection (LBTI + PPD, normal CXR and physical exam, no pulmonary symptoms, negative sputum culture)
   a. No respiratory precautions necessary
   b. Mother and baby do not need separation
   c. Begin or continue treatment for LTBI in women at high risk for progression to active disease and encourage breastfeeding
   d. Contact appropriate agency to evaluate family and contacts, if not already done
   e. Depending on findings for contacts, neonate may or may not need future skin testing
2. Mother has contagious (active pulmonary) TB (+PPD, + sputum smear or culture)
   a. Separate mother and neonate
   b. Respiratory precautions in negative pressure ventilation room
   c. Begin multidrug therapy
   d. Mother can pump breast milk until she is not contagious and can breastfeed
   e. Contact appropriate agency to evaluate family and contacts
   f. Contact pediatrician/neonatologist for neonate evaluation for TB
   g. Neonate can be reunited with mother once she is noncontagious (negative sputum smear or culture). It generally takes 2 weeks with therapy to be noncontagious as long as the TB organism is not resistant to therapy and the mother is compliant with therapy
3. Mother with +PPD and suspicion for active TB but incomplete evaluation
   a. Separate mother and baby until evaluation (CXR, sputum smear and culture) is complete
   b. Place mother on respiratory precautions in negative pressure ventilation room (wearing proper respirator when patient is not in room) until she is determined to not be contagious with 2–3 negative sputums
   c. Mother can pump breast milk for infant

Box 1.9 Causes of ARDS unique to/more common in pregnancy

1. Tocolytic (beta sympathomimetic) induced pulmonary edema
2. Pre-eclampsia
3. Acute fatty liver of pregnancy
4. Septic abortion
5. Amniotic fluid embolism
6. Placental abruption
7. Obstetric hemorrhage
8. Chorioamnionitis
9. Endometritis
10. Pyelonephritis
11. Gastric aspiration

incidence of 80–500 cases per 100,000, and is responsible for 25% of transfers of obstetric patients to intensive care units. Both the normal decrease in serum oncotic pressure that occurs in pregnancy due to a physiologic dilutional hypoalbuminemia and changes in maternal endothelium may explain this pregnancy-related propensity to pulmonary edema.

Causes of ARDS

Eighty-five percent of all ARDS cases result from one of the following four causes, with sepsis being the most common:
- sepsis from pulmonary or nonpulmonary sources
- major trauma
- multiple transfusions
- aspiration of gastric contents.

In the obstetric patient, several causes unique to pregnancy have to be considered. These are listed in Box 1.9. In all cases, the presence of excessive crystalloid administration, anemia and/or multiple gestations can significantly increase the risk that a particular precipitating factor will lead to pulmonary edema.

Pathophysiology

Acute respiratory distress syndrome results from inflammation-induced injury to the alveolar–capillary barrier. In the acute or exudative phase, this leads to flooding of the alveoli with high-protein fluid and subsequent surfactant abnormalities which lead to alveolar collapse and consolidation. Some cases resolve from this phase, which typically lasts 4–7 days, while others progress to fibrosing alveolitis with persistent hypoxemia, increased alveolar dead space, and a further decrease in pulmonary compliance. Pulmonary hypertension, owing to obliteration of the pulmonary–capillary bed, may be severe and may lead to right ventricular failure. After 1–2 weeks, those cases that progressed may begin to resolve with clearance of pulmonary edema and inflammatory cells and reconstitution of the alveolar–capillary barrier.

Prognosis

Most studies of ALI and ARDS report high case fatality rates, though recent reports suggest that mortality from this disease may be decreasing. In most patients who survive, pulmonary function returns to near-normal levels within 6–12 months, despite the severe injury to the lung. Residual impairment of pulmonary mechanics may include mild restriction, obstruction, impairment of the diffusing capacity for carbon monoxide or gas exchange abnormalities with exercise, but these abnormalities are usually asymptomatic. Persistent pulmonary function disability is more likely in patients who required prolonged mechanical ventilation.

Clinical features

Patients with noncardiogenic pulmonary edema resulting in ALI or ARDS experience acute hypoxemic respiratory failure with evidence of dyspnea, orthopnea, tachypnea and tachycardia. Arterial hypoxemia that is refractory to treatment with supplemental oxygen is a characteristic feature of ARDS. The chest may initially be clear to auscultation, but eventually diffuse crackles and/or wheezing develop. Arterial blood gases in patients with pulmonary edema typically show an initial decrease in both PaO_2 and $PaCO_2$. As the condition worsens, PaO_2 will decrease further but $PaCO_2$ may increase if the patient is no longer able to maintain adequate ventilation. The chest radiograph is usually significant for bilateral diffuse alveolar and interstitial infiltrates. As patients move into the resolution phase, there is gradual improvement in oxygenation and most radiographic abnormalities resolve completely.

Fetal considerations

The effect of maternal ARDS on neonatal outcomes is not well studied, but high rates of fetal death, spontaneous preterm labor and fetal heart rate abnormalities are reported. In one series of 13 patients with ARDS [61] who reached gestational age compatible with viability, the perinatal death rate was 23%. Catanzarite et al. [62] reported 10 cases of ARDS in mothers with living fetuses at the time of intubation. Six infants were delivered for fetal heart rate (FHR) abnormalities while four were delivered for maternal reasons. One perinatal death and at least three cases of perinatal asphyxia occurred in the six infants who were delivered for FHR abnormality.

Differential diagnosis

It is important to consider pulmonary edema in the differential diagnosis of ARDS. Pulmonary edema can occur due to cardiac causes such as peripartum cardiomyopathy, ischemic heart disease or occult valvular heart disease and fluid overload. It can also occur in pregnancy due to noncardiogenic causes such as infection, pre-eclampsia or beta-sympathomimetic tocolysis. Unsuspected cardiac abnormalities are not unusual in cases of pulmonary edema even in the setting of pre-eclampsia or tocolytic therapy. Other conditions such as interstitial pneumonia, acute eosinophilic pneumonia, acute bronchiolitis obliterans pneumonia, acute hypersensitivity pneumonitis and diffuse alveolar hemorrhage may have a clinical and radiologic picture similar to ARDS.

Diagnosis

The usual investigations for acute respiratory compromise are summarized in Box 1.10. A chest X-ray is an important initial evaluation but often further investigation is necessary. To clarify possible cardiac causes, a cardiac echo should be considered in any patient with pulmonary edema. An inquiry should be made into any history suggestive of aspiration such as an episode of choking occurring in the setting of altered mental status. A review of the patient's risk factors for thromboembolic disease should also occur and if the onset of the patient's dyspnea was acute and the chest X-ray is not typical for pulmonary edema, a computed tomography (CT) angiogram or

---

Box 1.10 Usual investigations for acute respiratory compromise

Diagnostic tests indicated in the obstetric patient with ALI

1. Complete blood count (CBC) with differential white blood cell count: Rule out anemia as a contributing factor and look for bandemia suggesting infection
2. Creatinine and blood urea nitrogen (BUN): Rule out renal failure
3. PTT, Fibrinogen and fibrinogen degradation products (FDP): Look for evidence of amniotic fluid embolism
4. AST, uric acid and urine protein creatinine ratio (in addition to above mentioned CBC and Creatinine): Look for evidence of preeclampsia
5. Blood and urine cultures in all patients with fever or bandemia
6. Urine drug screen: Look for evidence of cocaine or narcotics as a cause
7. Echocardiogram: Rule out underlying cardiac cause for pulmonary edema or evidence of cardiac compromise in preeclampsia

ventilation/perfusion scan should be considered. A review of the patient's history for any recent transfusions or drug use should also be carried out. Presence of fever, a history of any infectious exposures (particularly influenza and varicella) and any infectious prodrome may suggest the need for empiric antibiotics.

Management

Pulmonary edema in pregnancy is a medical emergency. Its treatment is summarized in Box 1.11. The first and immediate goal is to maintain adequate maternal oxygenation ($PaO_2 \geq 70$ mmHg equivalent to oxygen saturation 95%) through the use of oxygen supplementation to avoid hypoxia in the fetus. Mechanical ventilation may be needed in severe cases to ensure adequate oxygenation.

For tocolytic-induced pulmonary edema, management consists of immediate discontinuation of tocolytic therapy, initiation of IV loop diuretic and administration of supplemental oxygen. Invasive hemodynamic monitoring is rarely necessary for tocolytic-induced pulmonary edema.

When pulmonary edema is suspected to be related to pre-eclampsia, initial management consists of oxygen supplementation, fluid restriction, and blood pressure control while plans are made for delivery. Judicious use of intravenous furosemide is recommended since many pre-eclamptic

patients are relatively volume contracted intravascularly despite having massive amounts of peripheral edema and pulmonary edema. Excessive diuresis of a pre-eclamptic patient can impair maternal renal perfusion, cardiac output, and uteroplacental perfusion, leading to fetal compromise. It is our experience that most patients with pulmonary edema in pregnancy will respond favorably to doses of furosemide as low as 10 mg IV, especially if renal function is normal. Despite the need for careful fluid restriction and gentle diuresis, there is little evidence that central hemodynamic monitoring in these patients improves outcomes and the vast majority of these women can be successfully managed without central or pulmonary artery catherization.

Pulmonary edema in some cases of pre-eclampsia may be cardiogenic. A stiff left ventricle with significant diastolic dysfunction working against a high systemic vascular resistance may contribute. In others, pre-eclampsia-related vasospasm and endothelial effects may induce a transiently stunned myocardium that manifests as ventricular systolic dysfunction. In these cases afterload reduction is appropriate and hydralazine or nitroprusside (or angiotensin-converting enzyme inhibitors or angiotensin receptor blockers in postpartum patients) may be used.

Whether delivery has a positive impact on maternal condition in patients with ARDS is unclear. While there are numerous case reports in which the fetus remained undelivered despite maternal respiratory failure and intubation, most case series in the literature suggest that mothers with ARDS in the third trimester rarely stay pregnant for more than a few days. In general, patients with ARDS secondary to chorio-amnionitis, placental abruption, amniotic fluid embolism and pre-eclampsia need immediate delivery, while those with pyelonephritis or varicella pneumonia can often recover without delivery. The high rates of adverse fetal outcomes do support expeditious delivery for maternal ARDS after 28 weeks gestation.

Box 1.11 Treatment of pulmonary edema

Salient features in management of ARDS in pregnancy

1. Supplemental oxygen to maintain maternal oxygen saturation above 95%
2. Consider intubation for $PaO_2 < 70$ mmHg or $PaCO_2 > 45$ mmHg on 100% oxygen
3. Look for precipitating causes listed in textbox 1 in addition to sepsis, massive transfusion, aspiration of gastric contents or trauma
4. Appropriate diagnostic testing as listed in textbox 2
5. Immediate discontinuation of tocolytic therapy where applicable
6. Fluid restriction
7. IV furosemide 10–20 mg
8. IV antibiotics if infection suspected
9. Echocardiogram to rule out cardiac cause for pulmonary edema
10. Consider afterload reduction with sodium nitroprusside or hydralazine if patient pregnant and angiotensin converting enzyme inhibitors or angiotensin-receptor blockers (ARBs) in the postpartum patient

---

Ventilatory support in pregnancy

Causes of respiratory failure in the pregnant patient include pre-eclampsia, amniotic fluid embolism, massive obstetric hemorrhage/transfusion, and peripartum cardiomyopathy in addition to all the other causes of respiratory failure that occur outside pregnancy such as pneumonia, aspiration, asthma and ARDS. As discussed earlier in this chapter, $PaCO_2$ is decreased and PaO_2 increased in normal pregnancy. General measures to consider for patients requiring assisted ventilation include noninvasive ventilation (NIV) and endotracheal intubation with ventilation.

Noninvasive ventilation

Noninvasive ventilation refers to ventilation delivered to a patient without the need for endotracheal intubation.

It is often used in nonpregnant patients with acute hypoxic respiratory failure. Its use requires that the patient is able to co-operate, clear secretions and protect her airway and is not appropriate in the setting of other organ failure or when a need for prolonged ventilation is expected. The following are general comments about the typical management of noninvasive ventilation but the reader is cautioned that there are many variables to be considered and its use is best undertaken by individuals with specialized training and ongoing experience with noninvasive ventilation.

Positive pressure ventilation is usually delivered by a full facemask in acute settings but nasal masks and plugs can be used. Ventilation can be assisted through several modalities similar to those used for invasive ventilation. Biphasic positive airway pressure (BiPAP) is a modality unique to NIV and involves both pressure support for inspiration and positive airway pressure during expiration. Patients are typically in a bed or chair at a 30° angle. The mask is selected and fit to allow one or two fingers to fit under the strap. The mask is then connected to the ventilator with the appropriate settings for the modality. Continuous positive airway pressure (CPAP) is typically started at 3–5 cmH_2O and increased in steps of 3–5 cmH_2O as needed and tolerated to 10–15 cmH_2O. BiPAP is typically started at an inspiratory pressure of 8–12 cmH_2O and an expiratory pressure of 3–5 cmH_2O. The inspiratory pressure is gradually increased by 1–2 cmH_2O to alleviate dyspnea and achieve adequate oxygenation. Occasional monitoring of blood gases is important for maximizing the success of therapy. Adjusting the patient's mask straps, checking for air leaks and encouraging and reassuring the patient are also important aspects of successful implementation of NIV.

The use of NIV has not been well studied in an obstetric population. Because of the airway edema and the risk of aspiration in pregnancy, NIV may be a suboptimal mode of ventilation. However, given the lack of reports of adverse events in the literature concerning the risk of aspiration, short trials of NIV may be attempted in pregnancy prior to endotracheal intubation, especially in patients who may not require assisted ventilation for prolonged periods of time. If there are contraindications to NIV or if noninvasive measures fail to provide adequate oxygenation and ventilation, endotracheal intubation must be performed.

Endotracheal intubation

Indications for airway intubation in pregnancy are unchanged compared to the nonpregnant state:
• inadequate oxygenation using less invasive methods (often a $PaO_2 < 70$ on 100% oxygen by nonrebreather mask or NIV)
• airway protection in patients with altered levels of consciousness, inability to clear their secretions or impending airway obstruction
• hyperventilation in the setting of increased intracranial pressure.

The possible need for intubation should always be considered early in patients with acute respiratory difficulties and an anesthesiologist should be notified early to assess a patient's airway. The failure rate for intubations is one in 280 compared to one in 2330 in the general surgical population, with a potential higher risk for cardiac arrest and aspiration [63].

A number of factors may contribute to the difficulties with endotracheal intubation in pregnancy, including anatomic changes such as weight, increased breast size and airway edema. Airway edema may be further exaggerated in patients with a prolonged second stage of labor, excessive intravenous fluids and, particularly, in patients with pre-eclampsia. Morbid obesity also increases the risk of failed intubation and gastric aspiration during procedures requiring general anesthesia. Intubation is further complicated by the fact that pregnant women are more predisposed to aspiration and their lower oxygen reserve leads to a tendency to experience more rapid arterial oxygen desaturation and carbon dioxide retention. Therefore, preoxygenation with 100% oxygen with minimal manual ventilation (to avoid the risk of aspiration) is necessary in this patient population.

Because of the increased risk of serious morbidity and mortality associated with airway intubation in pregnancy, it is important that intubation is performed by the provider with the most extensive experience available. Box 1.12 lists the main points for successful intubation in pregnancy.

Mechanical ventilation

Indications for mechanical ventilation are the same as those listed above as indications for endotracheal intubation and are unchanged in pregnancy. These include status asthmaticus, ARDS, pneumonia and shock but also include situations that are specific to the pregnant population such as amniotic fluid embolism. The following are general comments about the typical use of mechanical ventilation but the reader is cautioned that given the many variables that should be considered in individual patients, clinicians with specialized training and experience with mechanical ventilation should be involved when caring for pregnant women requiring mechanical ventilation.

Mechanical ventilation can be performed in a wide range of modalities including assist control (A/C) and pressure support (PSV), and synchronized intermittent mandatory ventilation (SIMV). Choices among these modalities are often based more on institutional preferences and familiarity rather than distinct advantages of one over the other. Mechanical ventilation is a complicated and potentially dangerous intervention and is best undertaken by individuals who routinely manage ventilated patients. For many patients the initial settings might include:
• the amount of air delivered with each breath (tidal volume) of 6–8 mL per kg of ideal body weight
• a rate of 12–16 breaths per minute

Box 1.12 Key points in airway intubation of the pregnant woman

- Assess airway even in urgent intubations
- Position patient in the left lateral decubitus or left-sided tilt to avoid hypotension from compression of inferior vena cava by gravid uterus
- Avoid aspiration (e.g. do not feed patients who may require emergency intubation, have suction ready). Smaller endotracheal tube size may be necessary
- Use a lower dose of sedatives/anesthetics
- Preoxygenate patient prior to attempting intubation but use minimal manual ventilation when possible to decrease risk of aspiration
- Keep each attempt at intubation brief and separated by brief periods of bag-mask ventilation. Hypoxemia and hypercapnia develop rapidly during periods of apnea in pregnancy due to a physiologic decrease in end-respiratory volumes and increased oxygen consumption
- Be prepared for "next step" if intubation fails by having alternative equipment for the difficult airway readily available (all obstetric centers should have an easily accessible standardized "difficult airway cart" or the equivalent)
- Intubation should be performed by the most experienced provider available
- Obtain a measure of end-tidal CO_2 and CXR to verify correct endotracheal tube placement after intubation. Auscultation is not a reliable method of affirming appropriate placement

- a peak end-expiratory pressure (PEEP, used to keep alveoli open between breaths) of 5–10 cmH_2O
- the lowest fraction of inspired oxygen (FiO_2) to achieve the desired level of oxygenation.

Patients with ARDS, ALI or severe obstructive physiology are managed using the smaller tidal volumes of 6 mL per kg of ideal body weight to avoid ventilator-associated lung injury from alveolar distension.

Mechanical ventilation in pregnancy is managed in a similar manner as in nonpregnant patients but is complicated by the fact that the ventilator parameters need to consider not only maternal hemodynamics and oxygen requirements but also fetal well-being. In the nonpregnant patient, institution of positive pressure ventilation may lead to an increase in intrathoracic pressure and a drop in venous return, leading to a reduction in cardiac output and hypotension. Therefore, careful attention should be paid to the intravascular volume status when a patient is placed on positive pressure mechanical ventilation. All of the above is true for the nonpregnant population, but a reduction in venous return in pregnancy may be even more pronounced in late gestation as the uterine size may impair venous return. Placing the pregnant patient in the left lateral decubitus position or tilting her to the left with a wedge under her right hip may displace the uterus off the inferior vena cava, thereby improving venous flow.

Maintaining fetal oxygenation is clearly a significant concern in mothers with acute respiratory failure requiring mechanical ventilation. Data from chronically hypoxic high-altitude residents suggest that growth restriction and pre-eclampsia are potential complications. It is important to recognize that data on the fetal effects of short periods of desaturations in humans are lacking. Fetal oxygenation is more dependent on PaO_2 than it is on oxygen saturations and therefore, more frequent blood gases would be required in the pregnant patient. Although human data on this issue are lacking and most of the evidence is extrapolated from animal models, it would be reasonable to keep maternal PaO_2 above 70 mmHg to avoid fetal compromise. However, it should be noted that supranormal maternal PaO_2 does not carry any benefit since the maternal–fetal gradient of O_2 increases substantially as maternal PaO_2 increases. Continuous fetal monitoring should be initiated when there is an acute change in maternal respiratory status, especially upon initiation of mechanical ventilation. Once the pregnant gravida is appropriately oxygenated, intermittent monitoring (3–4 times/day) may be performed.

Managing mechanical ventilation in the pregnant patient should also consider the adverse effects of hypercapnia and hypocapnia on the fetus and the uteroplacental circulation. A gradient of 10 mmHg exists between the mother and the fetus (the fetus being 10 mm higher). Fetal hypercapnia may be associated with fetal acidosis, an increase in intracranial pressure and levels above 70 mmHg may adversely affect the uterine and placental circulation. In addition, hypercapnia in the first 72 hours of life may lead to retinopathy of prematurity. On the other hand, maternal hypocapnia is not harmless either, as it may lead to uterine artery vasoconstriction. In addition, $PaCO_2$ changes may lead to a "shift" in the oxygen hemoglobin dissociation curve. Increases in $PaCO_2$ will shift this curve to the right, meaning an elevated $PaCO_2$ is associated with a decrease in affinity of hemoglobin for oxygen (decreasing oxygen uptake by blood but facilitating the delivery of oxygen by blood to tissue). Decreases in $PaCO_2$ will shift this curve to the left, meaning a decrease in $PaCO_2$ is associated with an increase in affinity of hemoglobin for oxygen (increasing oxygen uptake by blood but potentially decreasing the delivery of oxygen by blood to tissue). When possible, the maternal $PaCO_2$ in ventilated patients should likely be kept in the range 28–32 mmHg seen in healthy pregnancies.

These goals can represent a challenge when caring for pregnant patients with ARDS. As mentioned above, when ventilating a patient with ARDS, the preponderance of evidence suggests clear mortality and other clinical benefits to using the low tidal volume method [64]. However, the low tidal volume method is frequently associated with hypercapnia (called permissive hypercapnia) and respiratory acidosis, which may be problematic for the fetus. Although bicarbonate infusions have been used to correct acidemia in the nonpregnant patient subjected to permissive hypercapnia, it is not clear whether the rate of transfer of bicarbonate is adequate to protect the fetus from the deleterious effects of maternal hypercapnia. Decisions regarding where to strike the best balance between the risk of maternal ventilator-related lung damage and the desire to maintain normal blood gases during pregnancy need to be individualized but should be guided by the principle that fetal well-being is first and foremost dependent on maternal well-being.

Amniotic fluid embolism

First described in 1941 by Steiner & Lushbaugh [65], amniotic fluid embolism (AFE) has potentially devastating consequences. It is rare, with an estimated incidence of 1.25 (England) to 7.7 (US) per 100,000 births and a case fatality rate of 22%. It remains one of the leading causes of maternal mortality in the developed world, accounting for 6.4% of maternal deaths in Wales [66,67]. Patients who survive may suffer some degree of hypoxic encephalopathy.

Oft-cited risk factors include advanced maternal age, eclampsia, fetal distress, grand multiparity, cesarean or operative delivery, placenta previa, placental abruption, medical induction of labor, and tumultuous or precipitate labor. However, evidence to support any of these as definitive risk factors for AFE is inconclusive.

A classic clinical presentation is the sudden onset of acute respiratory distress associated with hemodynamic collapse (due to cardiac dysfunction that may be complicated by arrhythmias) and disseminated intravascular coagulation (DIC) occurring at the time of labor and delivery and often resulting in death. Cases have been reported in the first trimester, with amniocentesis, and up to 48 hours post partum. Nonspecific symptoms such as nausea, vomiting, chills, and agitation may presage the sudden cardiovascular collapse.

How the amniotic fluid gains access to the maternal vasculature to initiate this cascade of events is unclear but it has been conjectured that the site of entry involves the placenta or cervical tears. Steiner & Lushbaugh suggested that forceful uterine contractions against membranes that may remain partially intact over the cervical os and/or particularly against an applied fetal head could then force amniotic fluid into the maternal circulation. However, cases of AFE have been reported to occur at the time of amniocentesis. At autopsy, fetal material including squamous cells, vernix or fat globules, and lanugo hairs have been found in the maternal pulmonary vasculature. However, the presence of these factors is frequent in the maternal circulation even in patients who have not suffered a clinical picture consistent with AFE. Thus, it has been suggested that AFE may actually represent an anaphylactoid reaction to pregnancy, with a mechanism unrelated to physical presence of fetal materials in the maternal circulation. Gross findings at autopsy have been dilation of the right heart with right-sided vascular congestion, suggesting acute obstruction of the pulmonary vasculature, but also consistent with acute, severe right ventricular failure. Further complicating the clinical picture is hemorrhage and DIC. It has been postulated that ABO incompatibility between the fetal and maternal blood groups could also contribute to the severity of this clinical picture.

Treatment is supportive, with early ventilatory and hemodynamic support. Patients often require extensive blood product support. Although the condition is rare enough that there is no clearly proven course of action to take in caring for these patients, all of the following are commonly recommended:
- cardiac rhythm, pulse oximeter and blood pressure monitoring
- consideration of pulmonary artery catheterization
- intubation and mechanical ventilation
- consideration of fluid, norepinephrine and/or dopamine to maintain blood pressure
- delivery of the fetus if this has not already occurred.

Those patients who do survive often follow a course more consistent with anaphylaxis or pulmonary edema and do not tend to run a protracted course as is seen with ARDS.

Pulmonary hypertension

Pulmonary hypertension (PAH) is a life-threatening disease characterized by elevated pulmonary arterial pressures. Previously described as primary or secondary, pulmonary hypertension now has a clinical classification with five distinct categories, listed in Box 1.13. This section will deal with pulmonary arterial hypertension (Group 1) in pregnancy.

Pulmonary hypertension is defined as pulmonary artery pressure greater than 25 mmHg at rest or 30 mmHg with exercise, when measured by right heart catheterization, in the presence of normal pulmonary capillary wedge pressure. PAH occurs more commonly in women in their third or fourth

Box 1.13 Revised clinical classification of pulmonary hypertension (Venice 2003)

1. Pulmonary arterial hypertension (PAH)
   1.1   Idiopathic (IPAH)
   1.2   Familial (FPAH)
   1.3   Associated with (APAH):
        1.3.1   Collagen vascular disease
        1.3.2   Congenital systemic-to-pulmonary shunts
        1.3.3   Portal hypertension
        1.3.4   HIV infections
        1.3.5   Drugs and toxins
        1.3.6   Other (thyroid disorders, glycogen storage disease, Gaucher's disease, hereditary hemorrhagic telangiectasia, hemoglobinopathies, myeloproliferative disorderes, splenectomy)
   1.4   Associated with significant venous or capillary involvement
        1.4.1   Pulmonary veno-occlusive disease (PVOD)
        1.4.2   Pulmonary capillary hemangiomatosis (PCH)
   1.5   Persistant pulmonary hypertension of the newborn
2. Pulmonary hypertension with left heart disease
   1.1   Left-sided atrial or ventricular heart disease
   1.2   Left-sided valvular heart disease
3. Pulmonary hypertension associated with lung diseases and/or hypoxemia
   3.1   Chronic obstructive pulmonary disease
   3.2   Interstitial lung disease
   3.3   Sleep-disordered breathing
   3.4   Alveolar hypoventilation disorders
   3.5   Chronic exposure to high altitude
   3.6   Developmental abnormalities
4. Pulmonary hypertension due to chronic thrombotic and/or embolic disease
   4.1   Thromboembolic obstruction of proximal pulmonary arteries
   4.2   Thromboembolic obstruction of distal pulmonary arteries
   4.3   Nonthrombotic pulmonary embolism (tumor, parasites, foreign material)
5. Miscellaneous
Sarcoidosis, histiocytosis X, lymphangiomatosis, compression of pulmonary vessels (adenopathy, tumor, fibrosing mediastinitis)

Reproduced with permission from: Simonneau G, Galie N, Rubin LJ, *et al*. Clinical classification of pulmonary hypertension. J Am Coll Cardiol 2004;43:10S. Copyright © 2004 American College of Cardiology Foundation.

decade. It is a progressive disease which is usually fatal. There are numerous causes of PAH including idiopathic PAH (both sporadic and familial), collagen vascular disease, left-to-right intracardiac shunts, anorectic drugs, stimulants (e.g. cocaine, methamphetamine), HIV, and portal hypertension. The presence of medial hypertrophy, intimal fibrosis or fibrinoid necrosis, arteritis and plexiform lesions in the pulmonary vasculature may be evident on histology.

Due to an inability to increase cardiac output with exercise, most patients with PAH initially experience exertional dyspnea, lethargy, and fatigue. As the PAH progresses and right ventricular failure develops, exertional chest pain, exertional syncope, and peripheral edema may develop. Passive hepatic congestion may cause anorexia and abdominal pain in the right upper quadrant. Cough and hemoptysis occur less often.

The initial physical finding is usually increased intensity of the pulmonic component of the second heart sound, which may even become palpable. Signs of right heart failure such as elevated jugular venous pressure, third heart sound, hepatomegaly, a pulsatile liver, peripheral edema, and ascites may occur as PAH worsens and RV failure occurs. Patients with idiopathic PAH (IPAH) have a survival of only 3 years without treatment and less than 1 year if the pulmonary hypertension is severe.

Treatment may include any of the following, depending on the type of PAH that the patient has: diuretics, home oxygen, anticoagulation, digoxin, exercise, and advanced therapy with calcium channel blockers (typically nifedipine and helpful in only a small proportion of patients), prostanoids (e.g. epoprostenol, trepostinil, iloprost), endothelin receptor antagonists (e.g. ambrisentan, bosentan) or phosphodiesterase-5 inhibitors (e.g. sildenafil). Creation of a right-to-left shunt with an atrial septostomy and lung transplantation are options for patients unresponsive to these medical options.

Pregnancy is poorly tolerated in women with significant PAH. In a normal pregnancy, the pulmonary vascular resistance decreases. However, in pregnant women with PAH, the increase in cardiac output coupled with an inability to decrease pulmonary vascular resistance can lead to increased pulmonary artery pressure. In addition, the hypercoagulable state in pregnancy predisposes these women to thromboses in the pulmonary vascular bed which may further worsen pulmonary hypertension.

Maternal mortality in PAH is as high as 30% [68]. In a review of published reports, most of the deaths occurred in the third trimester, with the highest risk in the first 10 days post partum. In view of the high maternal mortality, preconception counseling is of vital importance. Such counseling should emphasize the reduced life expectancy of the patient herself, as well as the significant risk of mortality with pregnancy and poorer fetal outcomes. If a woman does become pregnant and chooses not to proceed with pregnancy, it should be understood that some women with significant pulmonary hypertension may also have difficulty tolerating some termination of pregnancy procedures.

Management of pregnant women with PAH requires close monitoring. Limited data suggest that pregnant patients with pulmonary hypertension who are admitted to hospital early have a better prognosis. Heparin use throughout the pregnancy is recommended because these patients are at increased risk for venous thromboembolism as well as for *in situ* thrombosis. Given the life-threatening nature of this condition, use of any agent effective for treating PAH in nonpregnant patients seems justifiable even in the absence of extensive pregnancy data. Other measures that should be considered in pregnant patients with PAH include work-up and treatment of obstructive sleep apnea (see below) to limit nocturnal arterial oxygen desaturations that may worsen pulmonary artery pressures further.

In patients with PAH, labor and delivery are best performed in a controlled setting with a multidisciplinary team including an obstetrician, maternal-fetal medicine specialist, a pulmonologist and/or a cardiologist experienced in the care of PAH, obstetric anesthesiologist and obstetric internist. Full resuscitation facilities and access to an intensive care unit should be readily available. Some experts recommend right heart catheterization in the intrapartum and postpartum period. Early epidural anesthesia is advisable to control oxygen consumption and minimize the catecholamine surge. Slow administration of the epidural to minimize hypotension is preferred. Supplemental oxygen should be administered. Vasodilator therapy with epoprostenol or nitric oxide should be considered during labor and delivery. Fluid overload should be strictly avoided during labor and in the postpartum period. However, early and aggressive management of postpartum hemorrhage and hypotension is also essential. Patients with severe pulmonary hypertension are encouraged to use nonestrogen-containing contraceptive methods.

Obstructive sleep apnea

Obstructive sleep apnea (OSA) is defined as a combination of disturbed sleep with more than five episodes of apnea/hypopnea per hour at night and daytime symptoms of sleepiness, poor concentration or fatigue. Snoring is a prominent feature of the disease. It is a common condition affecting 9–12% of women and is more common with age, obesity and in African Americans. Untreated OSA can lead to hypertension, pulmonary hypertension, arrhythmias and right-sided heart failure caused by the effects of chronic intermittent hypoxia during the night. Cases suggestive of sleep apnea are confirmed using a sleep study (polysomnography). Treatment includes weight loss, avoidance of alcohol, and the use of positive pressure airway devices or surgery.

The significance of OSA in pregnancy is as yet unclear but there are case reports and reasons for concern. Physiologically, the increased minute ventilation of pregnancy, increased upper airway dilator muscle activity, and decreased REM sleep could potentially decrease the likelihood of OSA. However, other competing factors favoring the development of OSA include increased mucosal edema and hyperemia, decreased oropharyngeal junction (even smaller in pre-eclamptics) and decreased functional residual capacity. Snoring, a marker for OSA, is common in pregnancy, occurring in up to 44% of pregnant women [69]. Further, there is evidence suggesting an association between adverse pregnancy outcomes and OSA. In a case series of 502 women, snoring was found to be an independent risk factor for hypertension and pre-eclampsia even when adjusted for age and weight [70]. Snoring has also been found to be associated with fetal growth restriction [71]. Sleep-disordered breathing, including arterial oxygen desaturations, occurs more in patients with pre-eclampsia than in controls. Interestingly, both pre-eclampsia and OSA are associated with increased inflammatory markers, endothelial dysfunction, obesity and hypertension.

While the prevalence and significance of OSA are not known, screening should be considered in pregnant women in the appropriate setting such as obesity, excessive weight gain, hypertension, snoring, excessive daytime somnolence, and headaches. Once diagnosed in pregnancy, OSA should be treated with CPAP. There are available data in small numbers of patients to suggest that OSA may improve in the postpartum period, even in patients on no therapy. The experience of these authors supports these findings. However, some women will continue to require longer term treatment, suggesting that their sleep apnea was not recognized prior to pregnancy.

Cystic fibrosis

Over the past three decades, the survival of patients with cystic fibrosis (CF) has dramatically improved, resulting in more women with CF reaching reproductive age. Currently about 140 pregnancies in CF women are reported annually to the US Cystic Fibrosis Foundation Registry, with approximately 100 resulting in livebirths.

Pathophysiology

Cystic fibrosis is an autosomal recessive disorder that results from a defect in the CF transmembrane conductance regulator (CFTR) gene. Abnormal production or function of the CFTR protein leads to a dysfunctional chloride channel and subsequent impaired sodium and water transfer across glands in many organ systems. Glandular secretions become thick and tenacious, predisposing to organ failure. While any organ with a significant exocrine component may be affected, most clinically significant disease arises in the lungs, gastrointestinal tract and pancreas. Sweat chloride remains the primary diagnostic test for this disorder and is abnormal if >60 mmol/L.

In the respiratory system, bacterial colonization and recurrent airway infections result in permanent dilation of bronchi (bronchiectasis) and an obstructive physiology. Respiratory failure is the leading cause of death in the vast majority of patients with CF. Pancreatic insufficiency is another common manifestation of CF. Both the male and female reproductive tracts are affected by mutations in CFTR, leading to infertility. Life expectancy for patients with CF has risen steadily since the middle of the last century and the median predicted survival now sits at 35 years of age.

Treatment of CF is reviewed in Box 1.14 and applies equally to both nonpregnant and pregnant patients (see below). Lung transplantation is offered to patients with progressive or severe pulmonary functional impairment (e.g. FEV_1 <30% of predicted, hypoxemia, hypercapnia) or major life-threatening pulmonary complications (e.g. recurrent massive hemoptysis).

Pregnancy

Obstructive azoospermia is the most common cause of infertility in men; however, nonobstructive causes including reduced spermatogenesis, reduced semen volume and low semen pH have also been recognized. Unlike men with CF, women with CF usually have anatomically normal reproductive tracts but infertility remains a significant problem in up to 20% of patients. Amenorrhea (likely caused by patients being anovulatory due to being underweight) and tenacious cervical mucus are two contributing factors.

With improved survival and health outcomes in women with CF, the number of pregnancies in these women has also increased. Although earlier reports of pregnancy in CF were

Box 1.14 Management of cystic fibrosis

1. Respiratory
   a. Antibiotics for treatment and prevention of bacterial infection and colonization
   b. Clearance of thick pulmonary secretions using chest PT, postural drainage, mucolytics (DNase I)
   c. Treatment of bronchospasm and airway inflammation with beta-agonists and steroids
2. Gastrointestinal
   a. Ensure adequate calorie intake
   b. Pancreatic enzyme supplementation
   c. Supplementation of fat-soluble vitamins A, D, E and K
3. Metabolic
   a. Treatment of CF-related diabetes mellitus and impaired glucose tolerance

discouraging, recent publications have attested to the safety of pregnancy in CF women with good lung function.

Long-term survival is not negatively affected by pregnancy in women with CF. In a cohort study of 680 women with CF, followed between 1985 and 1997, 10-year survival rate was higher for women who had been pregnant when compared to never-pregnant controls [72]. Pregnancy was not harmful even in those patients whose FEV_1 was <40% predicted at baseline or those with insulin-dependent diabetes, pancreatic insufficiency or *Pseudomonas aeruginosa* colonization. However, whether the women with CF who became pregnant were somehow healthier than those who did not is not clear.

Cystic fibrosis patients have more outpatient visits and hospitalizations during pregnancy than their baseline and when compared with never-pregnant CF women. Pregnant women may also need more intravenous antibiotics and supplemental nutrition

Pulmonary function may decline in pregnancy but significant irreversible loss of lung function does not occur. CF patients have a tendency to develop gallstones; this risk likely increases somewhat during pregnancy. Pancreatic dysfunction in CF is associated with decreased insulin production which has also been noted in pregnancy. Furthermore, pregnancy in CF is also associated with decreased insulin sensitivity, increased protein turnover and less response to insulin's anticatabolic effect. These changes predispose pregnant CF women to early development of diabetes and poor weight gain. CF patients have higher caloric requirements at baseline secondary to increased work of breathing, poor intestinal absorption and increased metabolic rate related to the inflammatory effects of the disease. Those metabolic demands rise even further during pregnancy.

The ACOG Committee on Genetics recommends that prenatal and preconception carrier screening for CF should be available to all couples regardless of race or ethnicity [73]. All children of a mother with CF will be obligate CF carriers. If the biologic father is of European descent, approximately 2% of children born to a CF mother would be expected to have the disease. Paternal screening for CF should be recommended prior to conception. For postconception diagnosis of CF in the fetus, amniocentesis with genetic analysis can be performed.

The offspring of women with CF may be at increased risk for prematurity and low birthweight [74]. However, other studies have shown a median gestational age of over 40 weeks and a median birthweight of 3.2 kg. Neither the rate of abortions nor that of congenital anomalies is increased in CF women. The overall perinatal mortality rate (7.9–11%) seems to be increased and is directly related to the severity of CF [75] but reports of perinatal mortality vary significantly among available registries. The difference in these reports of neonatal outcomes, including mortality, is likely explained by variations in the access to care and the application of standard of care to these patients. Severity of the disease at the time of conception likely plays an important role in predicting outcomes as well. Risk factors for poor obstetric outcome include severe pulmonary dysfunction, pulmonary hypertension, hypoxemia and poor maternal nutrition. In addition, the likelihood of suffering the loss of the affected parent prior to achieving adulthood is high for children born to CF women [76].

Management

Clinical management of CF involves a multidisciplinary team with medical, nursing, nutrition, physical therapy, social work and sometimes psychotherapy staff. Box 1.14 lists salient features in CF management. Special considerations may apply additionally during pregnancy.

Routine management of CF should be continued throughout gestation as needed. As with any medical issue in pregnancy, the safest possible therapeutic agent should be chosen.

Chest physical therapy should be continued aggressively. Antibiotics, including quinolones, should be used when necessary. Parenteral therapy with aminoglycosides is considered safe in pregnancy. Inhaled tobramycin and colistin have little systemic absorption and can also be safely used. Inhaled beta-agonists and inhaled steroids can be used to improve respiratory function during pregnancy. Short-term use of oral or parenteral steroids may be necessary in some patients. Chronic inhalation therapy with DNAse-I has been shown to reduce the viscosity of sputum and improve lung function. Limited data are available on its use in pregnancy. However, given that systemic absorption from inhaled therapy is minimal, cautious use may be justified under certain circumstances. Supplemental oxygen may be necessary if there is evidence of hypoxia, particularly in late gestation.

Nutritional supplementation may be necessary if normal weight gain is not sustained. Regular assessment of fetal growth should be undertaken and if the growth rate slows then more intensive surveillance for fetal well-being and timely delivery are indicated. The mother may need admission for nutritional supplementation and supplemental oxygen. Maternal weight gain and nutritional status should be monitored closely throughout gestation with greater calorie and protein intake than recommended for normal pregnancy. The 1998 CF Foundation Consortium recommends that all pregnant CF patients have an oral glucose tolerance test (OGTT) to screen for diabetes before pregnancy and at the end of each trimester or until diabetes develops [77]. In patients with pre-existing diabetes, insulin requirements may increase.

Delivery and postpartum issues

Vaginal delivery with optimal pain control and supplemental oxygenation is recommended for all women with CF, with cesarean section being reserved for obstetric indications. Mothers who have CF should be closely monitored for disease exacerbation in the postpartum period, especially because decreased adherence to a medical regimen is common in new mothers. Successful breastfeeding in CF mothers is possible. Breast milk from women who have CF has normal sodium and protein levels, with lipid levels sufficient for the nursing needs of the infant.

Chronic obstructive pulmonary disease

Chronic obstructive pulmonary disease (COPD) is characterized by an irreversible or partially reversible airway obstruction with mucus hypersecretion and ciliary dysfunction on pathologic examination. Though COPD is the fourth leading cause of mortality in the USA and Europe, it is not common during the childbearing years unless there are significant predisposing factors present. The most common risk factor for COPD is cigarette smoking. Other risk factors include chronic exposure to certain environmental factors, airway hyper-responsiveness, recurrent childhood infections and genetic predisposition such as alpha-1 antitrypsin deficiency. Women are more predisposed to developing COPD than men, because of their smaller airway size and an apparently greater susceptibility to smoking [78].

A Th1-dominated response is prominent in COPD and leads to interferon-gamma and tumor necrosis factor (TNF) production. TNF is thought to be responsible for systemic manifestations such as cachexia and peripheral muscle wasting.

The main manifestation of COPD in women is dyspnea on exertion that worsens with disease progression. Sputum production is more common in men. Systemic manifestations of the disease include cachexia and peripheral muscle wasting. COPD may also predispose to osteoporosis and cardiovascular disease. Signs on physical examination include tachypnea, a prolonged expiratory phase, wheezing and rhonchi. Signs of right-sided heart failure may be seen in patients with more advanced disease. COPD is usually diagnosed later in women, and after more prominent symptoms than it is in men. This is in part secondary to physician bias against the diagnosis of the disease in women.

Pulmonary function tests usually help establish the diagnosis. According to the GOLD criteria [79], a postbronchodilator $FEV_1/FVC < 70$ is diagnostic of COPD.

Pregnancy

Chronic obstructive lung disease is rare in women of childbearing age. One case report [80] described a woman with bullous emphysema secondary to alpha-1 antitrypsin deficiency who delivered a healthy baby despite a spontaneous pneumothorax that required a chest tube at 21 weeks of gestation. A pregnant patient was treated at our institution for two episodes of spontaneous pneumothoraces that were secondary to extensive bullous emphysema. The patient had a chest tube placed on both occasions and delivered a healthy baby. No information was available at the time of her pregnancy regarding her lung function.

It is not known whether pregnancy may affect the course of COPD since the reported cases are minimal and the disease is rare in the childbearing years. Patients should continue to use their prescribed inhaled medications and their treatment in pregnancy should not be different from the treatment outside pregnancy. Smoking should be strongly discouraged and clear directions given to help with quitting. Ipratropium has no reported teratogenic effects in pregnant rats and rabbits and has no reported cases of teratogenicity in humans. Ipratropium is preferred to tiotropium as the latter is less well studied in pregnancy. Both short-acting and long-acting beta-agonists are thought to be safe in pregnancy. Oxygen home therapy is given to nonpregnant COPD patients with a $PaO_2 \leq 59$ mmHg or a oxygen saturation of $\leq 88\%$ but should be considered in pregnancy if there is a $PaO_2 \leq 70$ mmHg or oxygen saturation of $\leq 95\%$ at sea level.

Kyphoscoliosis

Kyphoscoliosis is a spinal deformity characterized by abnormal curvature of the spine. It is uncommon, with reported incidence in pregnancy varying from 0.02% to 0.7%. The primary concern with kyphoscoliosis is that there may be cardiopulmonary compromise due to the mechanical restriction caused by the spinal deformity and this may be further exacerbated by pregnancy-related respiratory changes. However, with aggressive treatment of kyphoscoliosis early in life, marked restriction of pulmonary function can be prevented and current literature

suggests that most women with kyphoscoliosis experience normal pregnancy and delivery. In a cohort study, most women who had prior surgical or brace treatments for scoliosis experienced normal pregnancies, with rates of cesarean section and back pain similar to the general population [81]. As in cystic fibrosis, the limiting factors are hypoxemia, pulmonary hypertension and mechanical issues. In patients with severe kyphoscoliosis and hypoventilation, noninvasive ventilatory support can be an option. Epidural or spinal anesthesia may be technically challenging because of the spinal deformity and may lead to an incomplete or unilateral block. These patients are more likely to require cesarean section, because of associated abnormalities of the bony pelvis and abnormal presentation of the fetus. Patients with achondroplasia and other chondrodystrophies may have similar though less severe respiratory and pelvic problems.

Erythema nodosum

Eyrthema nodosum (EN) [82] is a rare disorder, characterized by the presence of inflammatory, tender, nodular lesions, usually located on the anterior aspects of the lower extremities. It is seen most often in women of reproductive age. The process may be associated with a wide variety of diseases, including infections, rheumatologic and autoimmune diseases, inflammatory bowel disease, medications, pregnancy, and malignancies.

Box 1.15 lists some of the conditions associated with EN. Most patients with EN have either an antecedent streptococcal infection or no identifiable cause. Although its pathogenesis is unclear, it is presumed to be a delayed hypersensitivity reaction to antigens associated with the various conditions mentioned above.

The typical eruption is quite characteristic and consists of a sudden onset of symmetric, tender, erythematous, warm nodules and raised plaques usually located on the shins, ankles and knees. Lesions are usually bilateral and may rarely extend to the thighs, anterior aspect of arms and even the face. Within a few days, the nodules evolve into bruise-like lesions which resolve without scarring over 6–8 weeks. Ulceration is never seen with EN.

Diagnosis is mostly clinical, with biopsy reserved for atypical cases and in areas where tuberculosis is endemic. Recommended diagnostic testing is aimed at trying to establish probable cause and includes complete blood count (CBC) with differential, liver function tests, creatinine and urinalysis, antistreptolysin-O titer at diagnosis and 2–4 weeks later (to assess for antecedent streptococcal infection), plain chest radiograph (to assess for hilar adenopathy or other evidence of pulmonary sarcoidosis, tuberculosis or fungal infection) and skin testing for tuberculosis.

Erythema nodosum is self-limited and treatment should be directed at the underlying disorder, if identified. Nonsteroidal

Box 1.15 Conditions associated with EN

- Bacterial infections
  - Streptococcal infections
  - Tuberculosis
  - Syphilis
  - Mycoplasma and Chlamydia infections
- Viral infections
  - CMV
  - Hepatitis B and C
  - HIV
- Fungal infections
- Parasitic infections
- Medications
  - Oral contraceptives
  - Certain antibiotics (including amoxicillin, sulfamethoxazole, nitrofurantoin)
- Malignancy
- Pregnancy
- Sarcoidosis
- Inflammatory bowel disease
- Behçet's disease
- Chronic active hepatitis
- Rheumatoid arthritis
- Reiter's syndrome
- SLE
- Wegener's granulomatosis

anti-inflammatory drugs and potassium iodide, which are used for symptomatic relief in the nonpregnant population, are best avoided in pregnancy. Oral steroids, starting at 40 mg/day and tapered over a few days, may be an option but should be used with caution, keeping in mind the possibility that an underlying neoplastic, inflammatory or infectious condition may be masked.

Sarcoidosis

Sarcoidosis is a multisystem disease of unclear etiology that is characterized by the presence of noncaseating granulomas in the affected organs, which mainly include lungs, lymph nodes, eyes and skin. It can affect individuals between the ages of 20 and 40 years and therefore women of childbearing age represent a group at risk for the disease. The prevalence of the disease is estimated to be 10–20 per 100,000 with a lifetime incidence of 0.85% among whites and 2.4% among blacks in the US.

Sarcoidosis most commonly affects the lung, and cough, dyspnea, and chest pain are common manifestations. However, most cases are detected incidentally on routine chest radiographs before symptoms of sarcoidosis develop. Chest X-ray findings can vary and may be normal or show evidence of hilar lymphadenopathy and/or reticular opacities. Pulmonary function tests may show restrictive or obstructive disease with variable degrees of reduction in the diffusion capacity.

Other common manifestations of sarcoidosis include hypercalciuria and hypercalcemia rashes (erythema nodosum, skin nodules, and maculopapular eruptions), lymphadenopathy, inflammation of the eye (iridocyclitis, chorioretinitis, and keratoconjunctivitis) and hepatic infiltration. Less commonly, sarcoidosis can affect the spleen, neurologic system, bone marrow, heart, kidney, bones, joints, salivary glands, the ear, nose and throat, and muscles.

Although reproductive organs may be affected by the disease, there is no evidence that sarcoidosis affects fertility. No data suggest that patients with sarcoidosis have a higher risk of maternal, fetal or neonatal complications.

There is no single standard way to monitor patients with sarcoidosis. Frequency and type of evaluation will be determined by severity of disease, organs affected and whether treatment has been initiated. Typically patients should have a review of symptoms, physical examination, spirometry and a diffusing capacity (DLCO, a measurement of gas exchange that is very sensitive to the presence of interstitial lung disease) every 3–4 months and a CBC, creatinine, calcium, liver function tests, EKG and ophthalmologic exam yearly or more often if symptomatic or previous abnormalities of these tests have been identified.

Systemic steroids are the mainstay of treatment for sarcoidosis but their use is generally reserved for those with significant symptoms such as ocular disease or pulmonary compromise. It is not clear if steroids affect the long-term course of the disease in more mild cases. A variety of agents are used to treat the minority of cases unresponsive to steroids and include chloroquine, hydroxychloroquine, methotrexate, azathioprine, cyclophosphamide, cyclosoporine and infliximab.

Pregnancy usually has no effect on the course of the disease, but it may result in a temporary improvement. Women with a normal chest radiograph or those without active disease tend to remain stable during pregnancy and the postpartum period. Active disease that is present before pregnancy may show partial or complete resolution during pregnancy, but may relapse 3–6 months post partum.

Pregnancy in a woman with sarcoidosis does not merit a change in frequency of monitoring, which should be dictated by the patient's clinical status. Indications for steroid therapy are unchanged in pregnancy although potential complications of hyperglycemia and infections should be watched for. Stress-dose steroids should be considered at the time of labor in women who have required daily doses of 5 mg or more of prednisone for 3 or more weeks in the year preceding delivery (see Chapter 47). Pre-existing hypoxia, severe restrictive lung disease and secondary pulmonary hypertension increase the risk of maternal and fetal complications.

Management of labor and delivery should be directed by obstetric indications, with general goals aimed at decreasing pain and oxygen consumption. Maternal hypercalcemia can lead to neonatal hypocalcemic tetany and seizures, therefore calcium levels should perhaps be monitored more closely in pregnancy – we would typically do so once a trimester. Fortunately, the hypercalcemia in sarcoidosis is rarely severe and is not likely to lead to neonatal complications. Vitamin supplements with calcium and vitamin D may exacerbate hypercalcemia and should probably be avoided in pregnant patients with sarcoidosis.

Wegener's granulomatosis

Wegener's granulomatosis (WG) is a rare form of systemic vasculitis in which necrotizing granulomatous lesions affect the upper respiratory tract (particularly the nose – causing perforation of the septum), lungs and kidneys. It presents with nasal symptoms, hemoptysis, general malaise or renal failure often accompanied by systemic symptoms of night sweats, fever, weight loss and anorexia. Up to a third of patients will also have cranial or peripheral neuropathies. Diagnosis is confirmed by blood testing for circulating antineutrophil cytoplasmic antibodies (ANCA, both c-ANCA (cytoplasmic) and p-ANCA (plasma)) and biopsy of affected tissue. Patients with WG are at an increased risk of venous thromboembolism that may be as high as 7 per 100 person-years. Untreated, WG is rapidly fatal, with up to 90% of patients dying within 2 years. Treatment with a combination of cyclophosphamide and glucocorticoids, however, has improved survival to 80%, with 75% of patients achieving complete remission. Once remission has been achieved (usually in 3–6 months), patients are typically placed on azathioprine or methotrexate for maintenance therapy. Cyclophosphamide is discontinued and steroid therapy tapered and stopped.

Patients with WG are typically followed on the basis of their symptoms, laboratory parameters (including serial creatinine, BUN, microscopic urine examination, quantification of urinary protein, liver function tests, complete blood count and chest X-ray) and their titer of ANCA. The frequency of testing will depend on symptoms, disease activity and treatment.

The condition is now being diagnosed more frequently in or before pregnancy as less severe cases are recognized and treated earlier with prednisone and cyclophosphamide. There is insufficient experience to comment whether the course of WG is affected by pregnancy. On balance, most reports suggest that pregnancy is associated with exacerbation of the disease but this may just represent selective reporting. It is not likely that the course of WG has direct effects on the fetus aside from the risks associated with maternal organ dysfunction and treatment.

While prednisone may be used throughout pregnancy (see Chapter 47), cyclophosphamide is potentially teratogenic;

normal and malformed offspring have been reported following first-trimester use. Patients who have WG should therefore ideally wait until they are in remission so that cyclophosphamide can be stopped before pregnancy and introduction of maintenance therapy with azathioprine has been accomplished. Patients should be informed, however, that cyclophosphamide may affect their subsequent fertility by causing premature ovarian failure. Patients who have conceived while taking cyclophosphamide should be offered the option of termination because of the risks of both the disease and its treatment. The use of azathioprine in pregnancy is discussed in Chapters 8 and 10 but its use in pregnancy is readily justifiable for the treatment of WG. Methotrexate use in pregnancy is contraindicated, however.

For patients who present with new-onset or a relapse of WG in pregnancy, cyclophosphamide has been used in the latter half of pregnancy with good outcomes. Although transient leukopenia and intrauterine growth restriction have been reported (and there is always the concern about the potential for alkylating agents to induce leukemia), the very serious nature of this disease makes its use in pregnancy for this indication readily justifiable.

Monitoring of patients with Wegener's disease should not be significantly altered in pregnancy from what is described above. Establishment of "baseline" values prior to 20 weeks may be helpful if features of pre-eclampsia arise later in the pregnancy.

Pulmonary lymphangioleiomyomatosis

Pulmonary lymphangioleiomyomatosis (LAM) is a rare disease that primarily affects women, particularly in their childbearing years. It is characterized by non-neoplastic proliferation of atypical smooth muscle cells in the lung parenchyma and cyst formation. It presents similarly to asthma or COPD rather than as an interstitial lung disease. It results in progressive loss of lung function and eventually death. It may occur sporadically or in association with tuberous sclerosis. A variety of intra- and extrathoracic complications have been associated with pulmonary LAM, including spontaneous pneumothorax, chylothorax and chyloperitoneum (chylous lymphatic fluid and free fatty acids in the pleural or abdominal space). Renal angiomyolipomas and meningiomas also occur frequently. Patients present with breathlessness or with symptoms from pneumothorax or chylothorax. In general, the diagnosis should be strongly suspected in any young woman who presents with emphysema, recurrent pneumothorax or a chylous pleural effusion.

Chest radiology may be normal initially or show interstitial thickening, pneumothorax or pleural effusion. High-resolution CT (HRCT) scanning may be necessary to show the typical small cystic changes. Lung function tests show air flow obstruction and characteristically low gas transfer factor. HRCT can often confirm the diagnosis, and tissue confirmation may not always be necessary, especially if a diagnosis of tuberous sclerosis has already been established.

Early reports suggested that most patients died within 10 years of diagnosis. More recent studies, possibly in patients diagnosed earlier in the course of the disease, are more optimistic. Taylor *et al.* [83] found that 78% of patients were alive 8 years after diagnosis. Evidence from case series of close to 70 patients suggest that the risk of complications is higher during pregnancy than at any other time in a woman's life. In another series that described six out of 50 patients who became pregnant and continued their pregnancies, five had very complicated pregnancies with recurrent pneumothoraces and three lung surgeries were required during the pregnancies. Hormonal manipulation and oophorectomy have been used as treatment with limited or no benefit. Lung transplantation may improve survival and overall quality of life, but disease-related complications are frequent.

Pre-pregnancy counseling and decisions about termination of pregnancy can only be based on a frank discussion of the uncertainty about the natural history of this condition. Women contemplating pregnancy should be made aware of their own mortality with or without the pregnancy so that they can make a more informed decision that would include the possibility of the patient not being alive through the adolescent years of their children's lives.

Idiopathic pulmonary fibrosis

Idiopathic pulmonary fibrosis (IPF) is an interstitial lung disease with a progressive and typically fatal outcome, often within 3 years of diagnosis. IPF is a disease of the elderly, with most cases occurring in the sixth or seventh decades of life, making its presentation in a woman of childbearing age extremely unlikely. Very few case reports of pregnancy in a woman with IPF exist in the literature. Consequently little is known about its course during pregnancy or its effects on pregnancy outcomes. A woman with IPF contemplating pregnancy must be advised to consider her own prognosis for survival outside pregnancy. Patients with severe disease may be unable to tolerate the increased oxygen demands of pregnancy. IPF has been treated with steroids and immunomodulatory agents with limited response. Decisions to continue therapy during pregnancy will need to be individualized. Single lung transplant has demonstrated improved survival in these patients and successful pregnancy after lung transplant has been reported.

Churg–Strauss syndrome

Churg–Strauss syndrome (CSS, also known as allergic granulomatous and angiitis) is a rare allergic granulomatosis characterized by asthma, allergic rhinitis, and systemic vasculitis. Manifestations can include eosinophilia, rash, pericarditis, cardiovascular disease, glomerulonephritis, peripheral neuropathies and an eosinophilic gastroenteritis. It is often misdiagnosed as steroid-dependent asthma with other clinical features becoming apparent with attempts at steroid tapering. Diagnosis is made with biopsy of affected tissue. Treatment is with systemic steroids which have greatly improved prognosis in this previously frequently fatal condition.

The literature on CSS in pregnancy is very limited. Although single case reports suggest that Churg–Strauss improves in pregnancy [84], it may also become more obvious in pregnancy because of efforts to withdraw steroid therapy by patients or their physicians.

Lung cancer

Lung cancer in pregnancy is rare. However, with delayed childbearing and increasing incidence of smoking among reproductive age women, its incidence can be expected to rise. Because of the paucity of data in the literature, no specific recommendations with regard to screening and management in pregnancy can be made. In general, when malignancy is suspected in a pregnant woman, diagnostic radiologic testing should not be withheld for fear of fetal radiation exposure, which is usually minimal for most diagnostic tests for lung cancer. Staging involves a thorough history and physical exam, CBC, liver function tests, bone enzymes, a chest X-ray and a CT scan of the chest to determine resectability but may also necessitate additional imaging procedures.

Treatment can be carried out in pregnancy in many cases, but the management depends upon gestational age at diagnosis, clinical staging and histologic type of cancer and whether the tumor is operable (see Chapter 22 for a complete discussion of treatment of the more common causes of cancer in pregnancy). Based upon the few case reports in the literature, prognosis for lung cancer diagnosed in pregnancy is poor. In the largest case series of 19 patients of lung cancer during pregnancy [85], the maternal mortality was 68% within 9 months of diagnosis, but the neonatal outcome of all cases was favorable. Data remain insufficient to opine whether pregnancy affects the natural history of lung cancer.

Pneumothorax and pneumomediastinum

Pneumothorax and pneumediastinum refer to the presence of air in the pleural space or mediastinum respectively. Both these conditions occur infrequently in pregnancy, but probably more commonly than in the nonpregnant state. They most commonly occur in susceptible individuals due to the expulsive efforts of labor [86,87]. However, pneumomediastinum in particular may occur at other times such as in association with bronchial asthma or following vomiting. Pneumothorax may occur in association with other chest conditions, such as emphysema, pulmonary tuberculosis or cystic fibrosis. In most cases of pneumomediastinum, which is more common in pregnancy than pneumothorax, a false passage is created between the airways and the mediastinal tissues. The condition usually, although not invariably, follows a strenuous labor. Air tracks through the mediastinum to the neck or pericardium (pneumopericardium), and there may be subcutaneous emphysema over the thorax or even the whole body. This produces a characteristic crackling sound and sensation on palpation, which does not occur in any other condition. In addition, there may be a crunching noise (Hamman's sign) synchronous with the heartbeat at the left sternal edge due to air. Although most cases of pneumomediastinum in pregnancy will be due to the mechanism just described, the differential diagnosis includes the much more serious esophageal rupture in patients who have undergone trauma, instrumentation or severe retching/vomiting (Boerhaave syndrome). These patients usually have severe chest and abdominal pain and proceed to manifestations of sepsis and septic shock in a short time frame. CT scan of the chest is usually diagnostic.

In pneumothorax there is a false passage between the airways and the pleural cavity. Pneumothorax accompanies about one-third of the cases of pneumomediastinum that occur in pregnancy but may also occur independently [88]. In both conditions, the patient complains of sudden-onset chest pain and breathlessness, and the diagnosis is confirmed by chest radiography. In tension pneumothorax the patient will become cyanosed and hypotensive due to the reduction in venous return. A similar variant of pneumomediastinum, "malignant mediastinum," also occurs but is much rarer.

Pneumomediastinum normally clears spontaneously and the treatment is therefore usually conservative, with oxygen and analgesics. Malignant mediastinum requires urgent relief either by multiple incisions over the subcutaneous tissue where air is trapped or by splitting the sternum. Pneumothorax should be drained via an underwater seal if the lung is more than 25% collapsed. Tension pneumothorax requires immediate relief by a large-bore needle inserted through the chest wall overlying the pneumothorax. If pneumothorax or pneumomediastinum has occurred in pregnancy, an operative vaginal delivery should be considered to minimize the chance of recurrence, caused by raised intrapulmonary pressure due to maternal straining.

Pleural effusion

Pleural effusions can be caused by a variety of conditions as listed in Table 1.11 along with some characteristic findings on pleural fluid analysis. Physiologic changes of pregnancy, including an increased blood volume and decreased colloid osmotic pressure, may promote transudation of fluid into the pleural space. Benign small postpartum pleural effusions have been noted on chest radiographs and ultrasound studies after normal vaginal delivery [89,90] with an incidence of about 25%. In addition, pre-eclampsia and other conditions associated with pulmonary edema in pregnancy may result in pleural effusion.

Signs and symptoms vary according to underlying condition but mainly include dyspnea, cough and pleuritic chest pain. Hypoxia may be present, particularly when the effusion is very large or when the underlying cause involves lung parenchyma or the pulmonary vasculature. Decreased breath sounds, dullness to percussion, decreased tactile and vocal fremitus may be noted on physical exam.

Diagnostic approach is largely guided by findings on history and physical exam and conditions being considered in the differential. While chest radiographs can usually confirm presence of fluid in the pleural space, ultrasound or CT scan may sometimes be necessary to further characterize the effusion and to narrow the differential. A diagnostic thoracocentesis should always be considered for an unexplained pleural fluid collection but especially in the presence of fever, hemoptysis, and weight loss or when hemothorax or empyema is suspected.

Management usually involves treatment of the underlying condition. Rarely, a therapeutic thoracocentesis may be necessary, particularly in case of a large (e.g. TB) or rapidly accumulating (e.g. malignancy) effusion. Presence of blood, pus or chylous effusion warrants placement of a thoracostomy tube. While performing these procedures in pregnancy, it is important to remember that the diaphragm is about 4–5 cm elevated and a higher approach may be needed than in nonpregnant patients and that ultrasound guidance may be desirable.

Anesthetic considerations

Many factors should be considered when administering anesthesia to the parturient with pulmonary disease. Early recognition and assessment of respiratory conditions, both as independent entities as well as complications of other primary conditions, are essential and facilitate disease assessment and optimization, early planning of anesthetic care, and joint discussion with the patient and parent team. Therefore early anesthetic referral during pregnancy should be performed as part of interdisciplinary care.

Labor and delivery

During labor and delivery, pain causes hyperventilation, increased respiratory work and increased oxygen consumption which combine to increase the risk of acute respiratory deterioration. Thus, it is extremely important to provide effective analgesia. This is best achieved using regional anesthesia.

Table 1.11 Some causes of pleural effusion and some characteristic findings on pleural fluid analysis

Etiology	Findings on pleural fluid analysis
Exudative pleural effusions*	
Parapneumonic: a sterile effusion occurring in proximity to an infectious pneumonitis	pH >7.2, glucose >40 mg/dL (2.2 mmol/L) Gram stain and culture negative
Empyema: an infected pleural effusion	Appearance of frank pus, pH <7.3, glucose <40 mg/dL (2.2 mmol/L) Positive gram stain and/or culture
Pulmonary embolism	Bloody appearance (blood may also be caused by malignancy)
Pancreatitis	Elevated amylase (pleural fluid level greater than serum level)
Tuberculosis	Positive stain for acid-fast bacilli (AFB) Glucose <60 mg/dL (3.3 mmol/L)
Esophageal rupture	pH <6.0 Elevated amylase (pleural fluid level greater than serum level)
Malignancy: metastatic or primary mesothelioma	Abnormal cytology Glucose <60 mg/dL Elevated amylase (pleural fluid level greater than serum level)
Chylothorax	High triglycerides (>110 mg/dL or 1.24 mmol/L)
Rheumatoid arthritis	Glucose <60 mg/dL
Ovarian hyperstimulation syndrome (OHSS)	Usually happens in the context of ascites, but OHSS has been reported as an isolated cause of pleural effusion in pregnancy
Transudative pleural effusions*	
Congestive heart failure	Underlying diagnosis usually apparent from other systemic manifestations
Cirrhosis	Underlying diagnosis usually apparent from other systemic manifestations
Nephrotic syndrome	Underlying diagnosis usually apparent from other systemic manifestations
Exudative or transudative pleural effusions*	
Idiopathic	Diagnosis may not be apparent in up to 25% of patients after initial evaluation

Pleural fluid is typically sent for cell count, pH, protein, LDH, glucose, cholesterol, gram stain, culture and cytology. In some circumstances, an amylase, triglyceride should be sent.

*Transudative effusions are caused by disturbances in hydrostatic pressure or oncotic pressure (e.g. congestive heart failure, cirrhosis or nephritic syndrome). Exudative effusions are caused by damage of the pleural membranes and/or vasculature (e.g. cancer, infection, collagen vascular disease). Transudates have none of (and exudates have one of) the following characteristics: (1) pleural fluid protein to serum protein ratio of >0.5; (2) a pleural fluid LDH to serum LDH ratio of >0.6 (or a pleural fluid LDH that is greater than two-thirds the upper limit of normal for the serum level). A pleural fluid cholesterol >45 mg/dL (1.17 mmol/L) is also suggestive, but not diagnostic, of an exudate.

Both epidural analgesia and paracervical block have been shown to reduce oxygen consumption, tidal volume and minute ventilation in labor [91,92]. However, in modern practice, carefully titrated epidural and combined spinal-epidural analgesia are the modalities most commonly used. In addition, placement of an epidural catheter provides the option of rapid extension of the block and avoidance of general anesthesia in the event that cesarean delivery is required. Ideally, epidural analgesia should be commenced early in labor and maintained through the first and second stages.

The main adverse effect of epidural anesthesia is the possibility of diminished respiratory muscle function, especially if a dense or high (thoracic) block occurs [93]. This potentially may reduce breathing effort as well as the ability to cough. The risk is minimized by the use of incremental doses of low concentrations of local anesthetic (e.g. bupivacaine or ropivacaine). Addition of small doses of a lipophilic opioid (e.g. fentanyl or sufentanil) enhances analgesia without additional motor block. Provided that extensive block is avoided, epidural analgesia using low concentrations of local anesthetic has been shown not to decrease spirometric values in

healthy patients during labor and may even improve them slightly [94]. However, all patients should be closely monitored and supplementary oxygen should be administered according to clinical assessment.

Systemic methods of analgesia (e.g. opioids, nitrous oxide) are not as effective as regional anesthesia but may be considered in patients in whom regional anesthesia is contraindicated. However, opioids reduce respiratory drive and cause sedation which may increase the risks of respiratory failure and pulmonary aspiration in some patients. Some opioids (e.g. morphine) stimulate histamine release which theoretically may induce or exacerbate bronchospasm in asthmatics and other susceptible patients, thus fentanyl may be a preferred systemic opioid. Nitrous oxide should be avoided in patients with pulmonary bullae or pneumothorax because of its propensity to expand air-filled cavities.

Cesarean delivery

Regional anesthesia has a number of advantages for cesarean delivery. Importantly, it avoids the risks of airway manipulation which include pulmonary aspiration and hypoxia secondary to difficult or failed tracheal intubation (see previous section in this chapter on ventilatory assistance in pregnancy). Furthermore, airway manipulation and light general anesthesia may stimulate bronchospasm, particularly in asthmatic patients. Epidural anesthesia, spinal anesthesia or combined spinal-epidural anesthesia can be used, the choice depending on the clinical urgency and the preferences and experience of the attending anesthesiologist.

However, because a more dense and more extensive block is required for cesarean delivery compared with vaginal delivery, the potential for motor block to adversely affect respiratory function is greater when regional anesthesia is administered for cesarean delivery compared with labor. Studies of the effect of spinal anesthesia on spirometric pulmonary function during cesarean delivery in normal parturients have shown that most parameters are decreased, including FVC, FEV_1, peak expiratory flow rate (PEFR) and forced expiratory flow (FEF) [95,96]. These changes were shown to be greatest when the abdomen was open [95] and lasted for several hours after induction of anesthesia [96]. The effects of spinal anesthesia on respiratory function are even greater in obese parturients [97]. Studies of epidural anesthesia have shown small or no differences in respiratory function [98]. Peak expiratory pressure (PEP) was shown to be better preserved with the use of bupivacaine 0.5% versus lidocaine

2% with epinephrine [99]. Although the respiratory changes associated with regional anesthesia usually are not clinically important in normal parturients, patients with severe respiratory disease who have diminished reserve may become compromised intraoperatively. Therefore the decision to use regional anesthesia in these patients should be individualized with this consideration in mind.

General anesthesia is required in patients in whom regional anesthesia is contraindicated or in patients with poor respiratory function who are considered unable to tolerate regional anesthesia. In these patients, general anesthesia with mechanical ventilation facilitates adequate gas exchange which may be particularly important in patients with acute deterioration, for example from exhaustion or sepsis. Additionally, endotracheal intubation ensures a secure and protected airway for these patients. However, it is known that regional anesthesia is associated with a lower risk of postoperative pulmonary complications in nonpregnant patients with chronic stable lung undergoing abdominal surgery. Although it is not known whether similar benefits exist for pregnant patients with lung disease undergoing cesarean deliveries, it is likely that regional anesthesia when possible is generally preferable in this setting as well.

Agents chosen for general anesthesia should be those least likely to provoke bronchospasm. In this respect, ketamine is a useful induction agent because of its bronchodilating properties,

Table 1.12 Summary of general recommendations for management of pregnant patients with pulmonary disease

Recommendation	Comments
Assess baseline pulmonary status and confirm diagnosis (ideally done both during pre-pregnancy counseling and at first antenatal visit)	1. Perform indicted genetic testing such as paternal testing for cystic fibrosis 2. Document baseline signs and symptoms. Document baseline respiratory rate and physical exam. Obtain baseline CBC 3. Check oxygen saturation at rest and with ambulation 4. The goal of oxygen saturation for fetal well-being in pregnancy is $\geq 95\%$ or $pO_2 \geq 70$ mmHg. Provide supplemental oxygen to obtain this if necessary 5. Obtain baseline blood gas if abnormal oxygenation or there is concern about possible CO_2 retention 6. Obtain pulmonary function tests (including DLCO if patient has interstitial lung disease) if not recently done 7. Review previous testing such as CXR, chest CT, etc. 8. Consider echocardiogram if there is concern about secondary pulmonary hypertension or if history not typical for pulmonary disease, or concern for concomitant heart disease 9. Consider cardiopulmonary stress testing if there is doubt about the patient's pulmonary reserve for meeting pregnancy needs
Assess and optimize disease control and review medication use for pregnancy	Review the need for medication in light of underlying disease and adjust as necessary. Address effect of the untreated disease as well as the effect of the medicine on the unborn fetus
Reassess pulmonary status at each visit	1. Assess for any changes in signs and symptoms and investigate as indicated 2. Address respiratory rate and any other changes in physical exam and investigate as indicated 3. Check oxygen saturation at rest, and with ambulation, if indicated 4. Evaluate the need for repeat testing, such as repeat pulmonary function testing or repeat imaging as indicated

(Continued on p. 44)

Table 1.12 (Continued)

Recommendation	Comments
Make labor and delivery plan as end of pregnancy nears. (This often requires involvement of anesthesia, obstetric medicine, pulmonary, labor and delivery room nursing, respiratory therapy, in collaboration with maternal-fetal medicine and/or generalist obstetrician)	1. Determine mode and timing of delivery 2. Determine appropriate anesthesia 3. Determine whether second stage should be assisted 4. Determine appropriate maternal monitoring during labor such as continuous pulse oximetry and cardiac monitoring 5. Determine which staff need to be available 6. Determine appropriate management of medication during labor and delivery and make arrangements if special medication should be administered or readily available. (Does the patient need stress-dose steroids? Are there specific medications that should be avoided?) 7. Determine reassuring fetal status prior to beginning an induction of labor 8. Determine when continuous fetal monitoring will be initiated 9. Determine best setting for patient to recover postpartum (such as routine postpartum floor or respiratory care unit, etc.)
Immediate postpartum management	1. Reassess pulmonary status by signs and symptoms, physical exam, and objective findings such as pulse oximetry, peak flow meter 2. Take special note of volume status, given postpartum volume shifts 3. Reassess medication needs (including any special management of pain medication). 4. Consider and discuss safety of medication with lactation
Longer term postpartum management	1. Clarify medications to be taken at discharge 2. Determine whether further testing is indicated postpartum, such as repeat PFT, CT scans, etc. 3. Confirm follow-up appointments with appropriate providers (such as obstetric medicine, pulmonary, obstetrics)

BPP, fetal biophysical profile; CBC, complete blood count; CT, computed tomography; CXR, chest X-ray; DLCO, diffusion lung capacity for carbon dioxide; NST, fetal non stress test; PFT, pulmonary function test.

although both propofol and sodium pentothal are acceptable general anesthetic induction agents. Muscle relaxants with minimal histamine-releasing properties should be used (e.g. rocuronium, vecuronium or cisatracurium). Volatile anesthetics all promote bronchodilation but there is no evidence to support choice of any particular agent. Unnecessary light anesthesia should be avoided and inspired gases should be humidified.

Gas exchange should be closely monitored intraoperatively. Use of pulse oximetry and capnography is standard and in selected patients insertion of an arterial catheter should be considered for repeated blood gas analysis. Intraoperative spirometry is standard and display of continuous flow-volume and pressure-volume loops is particularly useful for monitoring changes in respiratory resistance and compliance [99].

Postpartum care

Postpartum or postoperative care in a high-dependency or intensive care unit should be considered and in some patients postoperative ventilation may be required. Adequate analgesia after cesarean section is important and can be effectively provided using epidural or intrathecal opioids without the risks of decreasing respiratory drive that may be seen with systemic opioids.

References

1. Huch R, Baumann H, Fallenstein F, et al. Physiologic changes in pregnant women and their fetuses during jet travel. Am J Obstet Gynecol 1986;154:996–1000.
2. Milne JA, Howie AD, Pack AI, et al. Dyspnoea during normal pregnancy. Br J Obstet Gynaecol 1978;84:448.
3. National Asthma Education and Prevention Program. Expert Panel Report 3. Guidelines for the diagnosis and management of asthma. NIH Publication Number 08-5846. US Department of Health and Human Services, Washington, DC, 2007.
4. Kwon HL, Belanger K, Bracken MB. Asthma prevalence among pregnant and child-bearing age women in the United States: estimates from national health surveys. Ann Epidemiol 2003;13:317–24.
5. Kurincsuk JJ, Parsons DE, Dawes V, Burton PR. The relationship between asthma and smoking during pregnancy. Women Health 1999;29(3):31–47.
6. Gluck JC, Gluck P. The effects of pregnancy on asthma: a prospective study. Ann Allergy 1976;37:164.
7. Kircher S, Shatz M, Long L. Variables affecting asthma course during pregnancy. Ann Allergy Asthma Immunol 2002;89:463–6.
8. Stenius-Aarniala B, Riikonen S, Teramo K. Asthma and pregnancy: a prospective study of 198 pregnancies. Thorax 1988;43:12–18.
9. Schatz M, Zeigler RS. Asthma and allergy in pregnancy. Clin Perinatol 1997;24:407–32.

10. Schatz M, Harden K, Forsythe A, *et al.* The course of asthma during pregnancy, post partum, and with successive pregnancies: a prospective analysis. J Allergy Clin Immunol 1988;81(3):509–17.

11. Schatz M, Zeiger RS, Hoffman CP, *et al.* Perinatal outcomes in the pregnancies of asthmatic women: a prospective controlled analysis. Am J Respir Crit Care Med 1995;151:1170–4.

12. Mabie WC, Barton JR, Wasserstrum N, Sibai BM. Clinical observations on asthma in pregnancy. J Mat Fet Med 1992;1:45–50.

13. Tata LJ, Lewis SA, McKeever TM, *et al.* A comprehensive analysis of adverse obstetric and pediatric complications in women with asthma. Am J Respir Crit Care Med 2007;175(10):991–7.

14. Perlow JH, Montgomrey D, Morgan MA, Towers CV, Porto M. Severity of asthma and perinatal outcome. Am J Obstet Gynecol 1992;167 (4 Pt 1):963–7.

15. National Asthma Education and Prevention Program. Expert Panel Report 3. Guidelines for the diagnosis and management of asthma. US Department of Health and Human Services, Washington, DC, 2007.

16. NAEPP Working Group. Report on managing asthma during pregnancy: recommendations for pharmacologic treatment – update 2004. NIH Publication No. 05-3279. US Department of Health and Human Services, Washington, DC, 2004.

17. Dombrowski MP, Schatz M, Wise R, *et al.*, National Institute of Child Health and Human Development Maternal-Fetal Medicine Units Network, National Heart, Lung, and Blood Institute. Randomized trial of inhaled beclomethasone dipropionate versus theophylline for moderate asthma during pregnancy. Am J Obstet Gynecol 2004;190(3):737–44.

18. Thavagnanam S, Fleming J, Bromley A, Shields MD, Cardwell CR. A meta-analysis of the association between caesarean section and childhood asthma. Clin Exper Allergy 2007;38:629–33.

19. Tollanes MC, Moster D, Daltveit AK, Irgens LM. Cesarean section and risk of severe childhood asthma: a population-based cohort study. J Pediatr 2008;153(1):112–116.

20. Lumley J, Oliver SS, Chamberlain C, Oakley L. Interventions for promoting smoking cessation during pregnancy. Cochrane Database of Systematic Reviews, 2004;4:CD001055.

21. US Department of Health and Human Services, Public Health Service, Centers for Disease Control, Center for Chronic Disease Prevention and Health Promotion, Office on Smoking Health. The benefits of smoking cessation. US Department of Health and Human Services, Washington, DC, 1990.

22. Hotham ED, Atkinson ER, Gilbert AL, *et al.* Focus groups with pregnant smokers: barriers to cessation, attitudes to nicotine patch use and perceptions of cessation counseling by care providers. Drug Alcohol Rev 2002;21:163.

23. Strandberg-Larsen K, Tinggaard M, Anderson AM, Olsen J, Gronbaek M. Use of nicotine replacement therapy during pregnancy and stillbirth:a cohort study. Br J Obstet Gynaecol 2008;115:1405–10.

24. Oncken C, Dornelas E, Green J, *et al.* Nicotine gum for pregnant smokers. Obstet Gynecol 2008;112(4):859–67.

25. Ellegard E, Hellgren M, Toren K, Karlsson G. The incidence of pregnancy rhinitis. Gynecol Obstet Invest 2000;49(2):98–101.

26. Evans R, Mullally DI, Wilson RW, *et al.* National trends in morbidity and mortality in the US. Chest 1987;91:65–74.

27. Incaudo GA, Takach P. The diagnosis and treatment of allergic rhinitis during pregnancy and lactation. Immunol Allergy Clin North Am 2006;26:137–54.

28. Adams PF, Hendershot GE, Marano MA, *et al.* Current estimates from the National Health Interview Survey 1996. Vital Health Stat 10, 1999;200:1–203.

29. Macfarlane J, Holmes W, Gard P, *et al.* Prospective study of the incidence, aetiology and outcome of adult lower respiratory tract illness in the community. Thorax 2001;56:109–14.

30. Wenzler RP, Fowler AA 3rd. Clincal practice. Acute bronchitis. N Engl J Med 2006;355(20)2125–30.

31. Getahun D, Ananth CV, Peltier MR, *et al.* Acute and chronic respiratory diseases in pregnancy: associations with placental abruption. Am J Obstet Gynecol 2006;195(4):1180–4.

32. Anderson RN, Smith BL. Deaths: leading causes for 2002, Nat Vital Stat Rep 2005;53(17)1–89.

33. Jin Y, Carriere K, Marrie T, *et al.* The effects of community-acquired pneumonia during pregnancy ending with a live birth. Am J Obstet Gynecol 2003;188:800–6.

34. Simpson JC, Macfarlane JT, Watson J, Woodhead MA. A national confidential enquiry into community acquired pneumonia deaths in young adults in England and Wales. Thorax 2000;55:1040–5.

35. Lim WS, Macfarlane JT, Colthorpe CL. Treatment of community-acquired lower respiratory tract infections during pregnancy. Am J Respir Med 2003;2:22.

36. Jenkins TM, Troiano NH, Graves CR, *et al.* Mechanical ventilation in an obstetric population: characteristics and delivery rates. Am J Obstet Gynecol 2003;188:549–52.

37. Munn MB, Groome LJ, Atterbury JL, *et al.* Pneumonia as a complication of pregnancy. J Maternal Fetal Med 1999; 8:151–4.

38. Goodnight WH, Soper DE. Pneumonia in pregnancy. Crit Care Med 2005;33(10S):S390–S397.

39. Fiore AE, Shay DK, Broder K, *et al.* Prevention and control of influenza: recommendations of the Advisory Committee on Immunization Practices (ACIP). MMWR 2008;57:1–60.

40. Laibl V, Sheffield J, *et al.* Presentation of influenza A in pregnancy during the 2003–2004 influenza season. Am J Obstet Gynecol 2004;191(6, suppl 1):528.

41. Bridges CB, Harper SA, et al. Prevention and control of influenza: recommendations of the Advisory Committee on Immunization Practices (ACIP). MMWR Recomm Rep 2002;52(RR-8):1–34. (Erratum in MMWR 2003;52(22):526.)

42. Neuzil KM, Reed GW, Mitchel F, Simonsen L, Griffin MR. Impact of influenza on acute cardiopulmonary hospitalizations in pregnant women. Am J Epidemiol 1998;148:1094–102.

43. Hartert TV, Neuzil KM, Shintani AK, *et al.* Maternal morbidity and perinatal outcomes among pregnant women with respiratory hospitalizations during influenza season. Am J Obstet Gynecol 2003;189:1705–12.

44. Heinonen OP, Shapiro S, Monson RR, *et al.* Immunization during pregnancy against poliomyelitis and influenza in relation to childhood malignancy. Int J Epidemiol 1973;2:229–35.

45. Zaman K, Roy E, Arifeen SE, *et al.* Effectiveness of maternal influenza immunization in mothers and infants. N Engl J Med 2008;359:1–10.

46. Centers for Disease Control and Prevention. Prevention and control of influenza: recommendations of the Advisory Committee on Immunization Practices (ACIP). MMWR 2004;53(RR–6):1–32.

47. Wong SF, Chow KM, Leung TN, *et al.* Pregnancy and perinatal outcomes of women with severe acute respiratory syndrome. Am J Obstet Gynecol 2004;191:292–7.

48. Cheng VCC, Tang BSF, Wu AKL, *et al.* Medical treatment of viral pneumonia including SARS in the immunocompetent adult. J Infect 2004;49:262–73.

49. Chapman SJ. Varicella in pregnancy. Semin Perinatol 1998; 114:426–31.

50. Ahmad H, Mehta NJ, Manikol VM, *et al.* Pneumocystis carinii pneumonia in pregnancy. Chest 2001;120:666–71.

51. United Nations Millennium Development Goals. www.un.org/millenium goals (accessed 2009).

52. Department of Health and Human Services, Centers for Disease Control and Prevention. Core curriculum on tuberculosis: what the clinician should know, 4th edn. 2000. www.cdc.gov/tb.

53. Carter EJ, Mates S. Tuberculosis during pregnancy. The Rhode Island Experience 1987 to 1991. Chest 1994;106:1466–70.

54. Jana N, Vasishta K, Jindal SK, Khunnu B, Ghosh K. Perinatal outcome in pregnancies complicated by pulmonary tuberculosis. Int J Gynaecol Obstet 1994;44:119–24.

55. World Health Organization. Treatment of tuberculosis: guidelines for national programmes, 2nd edn. World Health Organization, Geneva, 1997. www.who.int/gtb/publications/ttgnp/PDF/tb97_220.pdf.

56. Enarson DA, Rieder HL, Arnadottir T, Trebucq A. Management of tuberculosis: a guide for low income countries, 4th edn. International Union against Tuberculosis and Lung Diseases, Paris, 1996.

57. Centers for Disease Control and Prevention. Update: adverse event data and revised Thoracic Society/CDC recommendations against the use of rifampin and pyrazinamide for treatment of latent tuberculosis infection. MMWR 2003;52:735–8.

58. Boggess KA, Myers ER, Hamilton CD. Antepartum or postpartum isoniazide treatment of latent tuberculosis infection. Obstet Gynecol 2000;96(5 Pt 1):757–62.

59. McCarthy FP, Rowlands S, Giles M. Tuberculosis in pregnancy – case studies and a review of Australia's screening process. Aust NZ J Obstet Gynaecol 2006;46:451–5.

60. Bernard GR, Artigas A, Brigham KL, et al. The American-European Consensus Conference on ARDS: definitions, mechanisms, relevant outcomes and clinical trial coordination. Am J Respir Crit Care Med 1994;149(3 Pt 1):818–24.

61. Mabie WC, Barton JR, Sibai BM. Adult respiratory distress syndrome in pregnancy. Am J Obstet Gynecol 1992;167(4 Pt 1):950–7.

62. Catanzarite V, Willms D, Wong G, et al. Acute respiratory distress in pregnancy and the peurperium: auses, courses and outcomes. Obstet Gynecol 2001;97(5 Pt 1):760–4.

63. Hawthorne L, Wilson R, Lyons G, et al. Failed intubation revisited: 17-yr experience in a teaching maternity unit. Br J Anaesth 1996;76(5):680–4.

64. Acute Respiratory Distress Syndrome Network. Ventilation with lower tidal volumes as compared with traditional tidal volumes for acute lung injury and the acute respiratory distress syndrome. N Engl J Med 2000;342(18):1301–8.

65. Steiner PE, Lushbugh CC. Maternal pulmonary embolism by amniotic fluid as a cause of obstetric shock and unexpected deaths in obstetrics. JAMA 1941;117;1340.

66. DHSS. Report on Confidential Enquiries into Maternal Deaths in England and Wales, 1973–75. HMSO, London, 1979: 93–7.

67. Abenhaim HA, Azoulay L, Kramer MS, Leduc L. Incidence and risk factors of amniotic fluid embolism: a population based study on 3 million births in the United States. Am J Obstet Gynecol 2008;199(1):49.

68. Weiss BM, Zemp L, Seifert B, Hess OM. Outcome of pulmonary vascular disease in pregnancy: a systematic overview from 1978 through 1996. J Am Coll Cardiol 1998;31:1650–7.

69. Calaora-Tournadre D, Ragot S, et al. Obstructive sleep apnea syndrome during pregnancy prevalence of main symptoms and relationship with pregnancy-induced hypertension and intra-uterine growth retardation [French]. Revue de Medecine Interne 2006;27(4):291–5.

70. Yinon D, Lowenstein L, Suraya S, et al. Pre-eclampsia is associated with sleep-disordered breathing and endothelial dysfunction. Eur Respir J 2006;27(2):328–33.

71. Franklin KA, Holmgren PA, et al. Snoring, pregnancy-induced hypertension, and growth retardation of the fetus. Chest 2000; 117(1):137–41.

72. Goss CH, Rubenfeld GD, Otto K, Aitken ML. The effect of pregnancy on survival in women with cystic fibrosis. Chest 2003;124:1460–8.

73. American College of Obstetricians and Gynecologists. Update on carrier screening for cystic fibrosis. ACOG Committee Opinion No. 325. Obstet Gynecol 2005;106:465–8.

74. Cheng EY, Goss CH, McKone EF, et al. Aggressive prenatal care results in successful fetal outcomes in CF women. J Cyst Fibros 2006;5:85–91.

75. Hilman BC, Aitken ML, Constantinescu M. Pregnancy in patients with cystic fibrosis. Clin Obstet Gynecol 1996;39:70–86.

76. Tonelli MR, Aitken ML. Pregnancy in cystic fibrosis. Curr Opin Pulm Med 2007;13(6):537–40.

77. Hardin DS. The diagnosis and managment of cystic fibrosis related diabetes. Endocrinologist 1998;8:265–72.

78. Kirkpatrick P, Dransfield MT. Racial and sex differences in chronic obstructive pulmonary disease susceptibility, diagnosis, and treatment. Curr Opin Pulm Med 2009;15(2):100–4.

79. Pauwels RA, Buist AS, Calverley PM, Jenkins CR, Hurd SS. Global strategy for the diagnosis, management, and prevention of chronic obstructive pulmonary disease. NHLBI/WHO Global Initiative for the Chronic Obstructive Lung Disease (GOLD) Workshop summary. Am J Respir Crit Care Med 2001;163:1256–76.

80. Atkinson AR. Pregnancy and alpha-1 antitrypsin deficiency. Postgrad Med J 1987;63:817–20.

81. Danielsson AJ, Nachemson AL. Childbearing, curve progression and sexual function in women 22 years after treatment for adolescent idiopathic scoliosis: a case control study. Spine 2001;26:1449–56.

82. Requena L, Requena C. Erythema nodosum. Dermatol Online J 2002;8(1):4.

83. Taylor RJ, Tym J, Colby TV, Raffin TA. Lymphangiomyomatosis-clinical course in 32 patients. N Engl J Med 1990;323:1254–84.

84. Zeilonka TM, Dabrowski A, Droszcz W. Efficacite de la betamethazone-retard dans le syndrome de Churg et Strauss. A propos d'une cas. (Efficacy of slow release betamethasone in Churg–Strauss Syndrome. Report of a case.) Rev Pneumol Clin 1994;50(2):77–9.

85. Mujaibel K, Benjamin A, Delisle MF, Williams K. Lung cancer in pregnancy: case reports and review of the literature. J Maternal-Fetal Med 2001;10:426–32.

86. Burgener L, Solmes JG. Spontaneous pneumothorax and pregnancy. Can Med Assoc J 1979;120:19.

87. Spellacy WN, Prem KA. Subcutaneous emphysema in pregnancy. Report of 3 cases. Obstet Gynecol 1963;22:521–3.

88. Farrell SJ. Spontaneous pneumothorax in pregnancy: a case report and review of the literature. Obstet Gynecol 1983;62:43S–45S.

89. Hughson WG, Friedman PJ, Feigin DS, et al. Postpartum pleural effusion: a common radiologic finding. Ann Int Med 1982;97:856–8.

90. Gourgoulianis KI, Karantanas AH, Diminikou G, et al. Benign postpartum pleural effusion. Eur Respir J 1995;8:1748–50.

91. Sangoul F, Fox GS, Houle GL. Effect of regional analgesia on maternal oxygen consumption during the first stage of labor. Am J Obstet Gynecol 1975;121:1080–3.

92. Hagerdal M, Morgan CW, Sumner AE, Gutsche BB. Minute ventilation and oxygen consumption during labor with epidural analgesia. Anesthesiology 1983;59:425–7.

93. Von Ungern-Sternberg BS, Regli A, Bucher E, Reber A, Schneider MC. The effect of epidural analgesia in labour on maternal respiratory function. Anaesthesia 2004;59:350–3.

94. Conn DA, Moffat AC, McCallum GD, Thorburn J. Changes in pulmonary function tests during spinal anaesthesia for caesarean section. Int J Obstet Anesth 1993;2:12–14.

95. Kelly MC, Fitzpatrick KT, Hill DA. Respiratory effects of spinal anaesthesia for caesarean section. Anaesthesia 1996;51:1120–2.

96. Von Ungern-Sternberg BS, Regli A, Bucher E, Reber A, Schneider MC. Impact of spinal anaesthesia and obesity on maternal respiratory function during elective Caesarean section. Anaesthesia 2004;59:743–9.

97. Harrop-Griffiths AW, Ravalia A, Browne DA, Robinson PN. Regional anaesthesia and cough effectiveness. A study in patients undergoing caesarean section. Anaesthesia 1991;46:11–13.

98. Yun E, Topulos GP, Body SC, Datta S, Bader AM. Pulmonary function changes during epidural anesthesia for cesarean delivery. Anesth Analg 1996;82:750–3.

99. Bardoczky GI, Engelman E, d'Hollander A. Continuous spirometry: an aid to monitoring ventilation during operation. Br J Anaesth 1993;71:747–51.

Juniper EF, Daniel EE, Roberts RS, Kline PA, Hargreave FE, Newhouse MT. Improvement in airway responsiveness and asthma severity during pregnancy. A prospective study. Am Rev Respir Dis 1989;140(4):924–31.

Sims CD, Chamberlain GV, de Swiet M. Lung function tests in bronchial asthma during and after pregnancy. Br J Obstet Gynaecol 1976;83(6):434–7.

Lao TT, Huengsburg M. Labour and delivery in mothers with asthma. Eur J Obstet Gynecol Reprod Biol 1990;35(2–3):183–90.

Useful resources

American Lung Association – www.lungusa.org

1800-LUNG-USA, Freedom from Smoking – www.ffsonline.org

March of Dimes – www.marchofdimes.com

National Partnership for Smoke-free Families

American Legacy Foundation

www.smokefree.gov

1800quitnow.cancer.gov

Toll Free Quit Line: 800-QUITNOW

www.helppregnantsmokersquit.org

American Academy of Allergy, Asthma, and Immunology – www.aaaai.org

American Thoracic Society – www.thoracic.org

American Association for Respiratory Care – www.aarc.org/links/links.asp

American College of Chest Physicians – www.chestnet.org/about/links/index.php

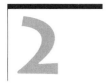

Hematologic disease in pregnancy

Claire McLintock[1], John T. Repke[2] with Brenda Bucklin[3]

[1]National Women's Health, Auckland City Hospital, Auckland, New Zealand
[2]Penn State Milton S. Hershey Medical Center, MSHMC Maternal Fetal Medicine, Hershey, PA, USA
[3]Department of Anesthesiology, University of Colorado Health Sciences Center, Denver, CO, USA

Anemia

Physiologic anemia is well recognized during pregnancy, resulting from an expansion of maternal plasma volume that occurs to a greater degree than the pregnancy-induced expansion of red cell mass. Maternal anemia can also be present or develop during pregnancy because of deficiencies of essential hematinics such as iron, vitamin B12 and folate. Such pathologic anemia can adversely affect fetal growth and development and also increases the risk of maternal morbidity and mortality mainly at delivery if postpartum hemorrhage occurs. Severe anemia is common in women from resource-poor countries with an estimated 75% of women having anemia. However, even in industrialized countries, anemia mainly due to iron deficiency is common, especially in less advantaged groups. The increased hematinic requirements during normal pregnancy can further compound deficiency states and anemia in women. Correction of anemia in the antenatal period may improve maternal and fetal outcomes. The WHO definition of anemia in pregnancy is a hemoglobin of less than 110 g/L (11 g/dL) but many laboratories will define their own pregnancy normal ranges that may be as low as 100 g/L (10 g/dL).

Iron and iron deficiency

Iron is an essential component of hemoglobin and deficiency of iron will ultimately lead to anemia. In the absence of bleeding, only a small amount of iron is lost daily, mainly through shedding of intestinal mucosal cells so that iron deficiency is uncommon in men who have a diet with high iron bio-availability. In women menstrual blood loss places a continual demand on iron stores so that iron deficiency is much more common

if dietary iron intake is insufficient to offset losses due to menstruation, especially in women with menorrhagia. Studies suggest that one in 10 women of reproductive age in developed countries is iron deficient, with iron deficiency anemia (IDA) present in 2–5% [1]. Adolescent women have a higher prevalence of iron deficiency and IDA likely to reflect iron requirements for growth during this period coupled with less reliable dietary intake of iron.

Iron requirements in pregnancy

The additional iron requirements for pregnancy are estimated to be around 1000 mg, with 45% of the total required for expansion of the maternal red blood cell mass, about one-third for fetal and placental growth and the remainder made up of obligatory basal intestinal losses and maternal blood loss at delivery. The increased demand is not uniform throughout pregnancy, with the greatest fetal demand for iron occurring in the last trimester of pregnancy. Iron requirements during the first trimester of pregnancy are estimated to be 0.8 mg/day of elemental iron, 4–6 mg/day from the second trimester onwards increasing to as high as 8–10 mg/day in the last 6 weeks of pregnancy. The term elemental iron refers to the amount of absorbable iron in any supplement and varies with formulation of iron used (see below). The predominant transfer of iron to the fetus occurs in the third trimester. There is active placental transport of iron via specific placental iron receptors ensuring continued supply of iron for fetal development [2].

For women who eat a diet with high iron bio-availability, pre-pregnancy iron stores of around 300 mg are thought to be sufficient to prevent iron deficiency developing during pregnancy. Iron stores are dependent on factors such as dietary intake, degree of menstrual blood loss, number of previous pregnancies and lactation. Iron deficiency and IDA are more common in adolescents and women with a higher parity. Median iron stores in women from industrialized countries vary between 150 mg and 300 mg but an alarming 20% of

de Swiet's Medical Disorders in Obstetric Practice, 5th edition. Edited by R. O. Powrie, M. F. Greene, W. Camann. © 2010 Blackwell Publishing.

women enter pregnancy with no iron stores. In less developed countries with low bio-availability iron diets and other factors that contribute to anemia, a very high proportion of women can be expected to enter pregnancy with low or no iron stores.

Iron deficiency and iron deficiency anemia: prevention and treatment

Dietary intervention

Iron deficiency itself leads to increased absorption of dietary iron and there is also increased absorption during pregnancy. Even with these physiologic changes, women are unable to maintain a positive iron balance during pregnancy and it is not surprising that at least 40% of women will be iron deficient by the third trimester. A diet with high iron bio-availability provides an estimated 3–4 mg of iron each day and absorption can increase to 5 mg/day in the third trimester. The most bio-available food source of iron is heme iron that is derived from hemoglobin-containing animal foods. Around 20–30% of heme iron in food can be absorbed compared to absorption of 2–10% of nonheme dietary iron, i.e. from plant foods. Consumption of food containing heme iron will augment the absorption of iron from nonheme sources. Certain foods inhibit absorption of dietary nonheme iron but with the exception of calcium, foods do not affect absorption of heme iron (Table 2.1). Simple dietary advice can help optimize women's dietary iron intake and reduce their requirements for iron supplementation. However, given the considerable demands for iron in the second half of pregnancy, one can appreciate how depletion of iron stores occurs during pregnancy and understand why many women will require dietary iron supplements. Women who enter pregnancy with iron deficiency and those with a diet with low bio-availability are at much greater risk of developing iron deficiency and anemia.

Table 2.1 Food factors that modify absorption of dietary iron

Inhibitors of absorption of dietary nonheme iron	Example of food source	Enhancers of absorption of dietary nonheme iron	Example of food source
Tannins	Tea	Vitamin C	Citrus fruit, strawberries, kiwifruit, capsicum, tomatoes, broccoli
Oxalates	Spinach	Meat proteins	
Phytates	Cereals, legumes, nuts		
Polyphenols	Tea, coffee, red wine		
Calcium*	Dairy foods		

*Also inhibits absorption of heme iron.

Dietary iron supplements: targeted or universal?

Studies have consistently shown that anemia and iron deficiency anemia are risk factors for preterm delivery and for small-for-gestational age infants [3]. The adverse impact of anemia is mainly restricted to anemia present in early pregnancy. It is interesting that correction of iron deficiency anemia with iron supplementation has not lead to reductions in these adverse fetal outcomes; however, the majority of clinical trials were carried out in women who were not anemic early in pregnancy thereby excluding those women who were likely to have shown most benefit from intervention [4]. Similarly, routine iron supplementation in pregnant women who are not iron deficient has not been shown to impact on fetal outcome although it does improve maternal iron stores and hemoglobin levels [5]. Given the absence of evidence of benefit of routine iron supplementation in pregnancy and the potential for adverse effects such as increasing oxidative stress, iron supplementation should be directed to those women who have iron deficiency or IDA.

Despite lack of evidence of improved pregnancy outcome, the US Centers for Disease Control and Prevention (CDC) recommend 30 mg/day elemental iron supplements (e.g. 150 mg of ferrous sulfate) for all pregnant women, with higher doses in women who are iron deficient or have IDA. Although treatment of iron deficiency and iron deficiency anemia does not impact on fetal outcome, correction of maternal anemia and iron deficiency contributes to improved maternal well-being and mortality outcomes. Women who are anemic should be treated to restore the hemoglobin to normal levels in preparation for delivery. Hemorrhage complicating delivery is likely to pose more of a problem for a woman who has pre-existing anemia. In addition, correction of anemia will improve maternal well-being. Iron deficiency even in the absence of anemia can cause maternal symptoms such as fatigue and restless legs and supplementary iron can alleviate these symptoms. Iron deficiency may also have detrimental effects on the immune system and reduce healing.

Commonly available iron supplements are usually the ferrous form of iron coupled with inorganic salts – ferrous fumarate, ferrous sulfate and ferrous gluconate, containing 33%, 20% and 11% elemental iron, respectively; 300 mg of each of these formulations therefore contain approximately 100 mg, 60 mg and 33 mg of elemental iron respectively. Ferrous sulfate is the most readily absorbed form but causes more gastric irritation than the other forms. A typical dose for treatment of IDA would be ferrous sulfate 325 mg PO two to three times a day taken, if possible, on an empty stomach. There is little capacity for the gastrointestinal system to absorb doses significantly above this level. Vitamin C supplementation or consuming the iron supplementation with red meat will increase absorption of supplemental iron. Simultaneous intake of calcium supplementation will decrease iron absorption. Side effects of iron supplements include nausea, vomiting, constipation, and dark stools and are dose related. Hemoglobin levels rise within 2–3 weeks of starting iron therapy and one of the most common causes of lack of response is noncompliance, mainly because of side effects. In such cases it may be helpful to prescribe a formulation that has a lower concentration of elemental iron to reduce side effects and improve compliance.

Of note, high hemoglobin later in pregnancy is also associated with adverse pregnancy outcome, which is likely to reflect the plasma volume contraction that occurs in placental insufficiency syndromes such as pre-eclampsia [6].

Diagnosis of iron deficiency and iron deficiency anemia

While the functional compartments of iron are contained in hemoglobin and myoglobin, ferritin is the predominant storage compartment for excess iron. Transferrin is the transport molecule that shuttles iron between the storage and functional compartments. Serum ferritin generally provides the most easily assessable measure of total body iron stores. However, ferritin is an acute-phase protein that will increase in the presence of acute or chronic inflammation or infection so will be unreliable in these clinical circumstances. A reduction in serum ferritin is usually the earliest indication of iron deficiency. Low iron stores will reduce the amount (saturation) of iron bound to transferrin, the iron transport protein, so that its capacity to bind iron is increased. A low transferrin saturation or increased total iron-binding capacity is often present in iron deficiency but on their own are unhelpful in diagnosis of iron deficiency because of rapid fluctuations in levels. A newer, more accurate laboratory measure of iron deficiency is the soluble form of the cellular transferrin receptor that binds and internalizes transferrin, thus facilitating intracellular transportation of iron. The solubilized serum transferrin receptor is a truncated form of the receptor that increases in concentration when iron deficiency develops, but only once the storage compartment of iron is exhausted and depletion of the functional iron compartment begins. Measurement of serum transferrin receptor is particularly useful in diagnosing iron deficiency in anemia of chronic disease where the ferritin level increases as an acute-phase response. Not all laboratories provide routine analysis of the serum transferrin receptor.

In pregnancy, the serum ferritin is the most useful measure of iron deficiency. Transferrin levels increase during pregnancy, making measurement of the total iron-binding capacity unhelpful in the diagnosis of iron deficiency.

Continued iron deficiency leads to depletion of the functional compartment of iron that initially leads to production of microcytic, hypochromic red cells and ultimately development of anemia, i.e. low hemoglobin and hematocrit (Figure 2.1).

Assessment of iron status in pregnancy

Assessment of iron status and identification of women at risk of developing iron deficiency in pregnancy are an essential

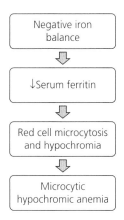

Figure 2.1 Stages in development of iron deficiency anemia.

part of antenatal care. Booking bloods traditionally include complete blood count (CBC) that can identify anemia and microcytic (cells with a low mean cellular volume or MCV), hypochromic red blood cells in women who already have a significant negative iron balance. These women require urgent treatment to restore iron stores and reverse anemia and should receive relatively high-dose inorganic iron supplementation. Intravenous iron supplementation with iron polymaltose should be reserved for those women who are unable to absorb iron due to gastrointestinal disease or surgical resection. In addition, parenteral iron may be considered for the unusual case where a woman with severe iron deficiency anemia is seen for the first time late in pregnancy and is unlikely to have sufficient time for oral iron replacement to be effective. Parenteral iron is available as iron dextran, iron sucrose, ferric gluconate complex and iron polymaltose. Severe adverse drug reactions including death from anaphylaxis are reported with iron dextran but appear to be far less common with the other forms of parenteral iron. Iron can also be given by intramuscular injection; however, not only is absorption variable but this method of administration leaves permanent stains on the skin. Blood transfusion should be reserved for women with severe symptomatic anemia or other medical conditions such as cardiac disease that will be compounded by maternal anemia.

Measurement of serum ferritin with booking bloods is not a universal recommendation but does provide the opportunity to identify women with marginal iron stores who are likely to become iron deficient earlier in pregnancy. Iron deficiency is diagnosed with a serum ferritin of <12–15 μg/L (12–15 ng/mL or 27–33 pmol/L) in the absence of inflammation.

Vitamin B12: cobalamin

Vitamin B12 belongs to the cobalamin family of compounds which together with folate are a vital part of the so-called one-carbon metabolism cycle that provides methyl groups required for synthesis of DNA, formation of myelin and neurotransmitters such as dopamine. Strictly speaking, vitamin B12 refers only to cyanocobalamin, a form of cobalamin that exists only *in vitro*. For clarity, the term cobalamin will be used in this text to refer to all members of this vitamin group including vitamin B12.

Cobalamin (Cbl) in humans is derived entirely from the diet, from vegetable sources via cobalamin-producing bacteria on leguminous plants and from animal sources through the cobalamin present in muscle and tissues. The major dietary source of Cbl is animal protein with fish, animal muscle, milk products and egg yolk providing about 1–10 μg cobalamin/100 g wet weight of food. Cobalamin is very effectively stored with total body stores of 2–5mg in adults. It takes about 3–4 years to deplete cobalamin stores if dietary intake is interrupted but the deficiency state takes longer to manifest due to enterohepatic circulation of cobalamin.

Cobalamin in food undergoes peptic digestion at acid pH in the stomach and is released when it initially binds to R-protein (haptocorrin) prior to its passage to the duodenum. There, pancreatic proteases degrade the R-proteins, allowing transfer of Cbl to intrinsic factor (IF) produced by gastric parietal cells. Cbl bound to IF then continues down the small intestine to be bound by specific IF receptors on the terminal ileum to deliver to plasma. Cbl in plasma is wholly bound to transport proteins, transcobalamins, with 10–30% bound to transcobalamin II and most of the remainder to transcobalamin I. Lysosomal transfer of Cbl to the intracellular compartment provides Cbl that is modified and acts as a co-enzyme for the intracellular enzymes methylmalonyl-CoA mutase and methionine synthetase required for one-carbon metabolism [7].

Cobalamin deficiency

Cobalamin deficiency can occur due to inadequate dietary intake, defective absorption or, rarely, defective plasma transportation. Given the availability of cobalamin in food sources of animal origin, it is clear that dietary deficiency will mainly be a problem for individuals who adhere to a strict vegan diet, i.e. one that contains no animal products. However, low levels of B12 are reported in lacto-vegetarians (diet includes dairy products) and also ovo-lacto-vegetarians (diet includes dairy products and eggs) [8]. The most common cause of defective absorption is likely to be gastric achlorhydria that results in the loss of the acidic gastric milieu essential for initial release of Cbl from food sources and reduced transfer of Cbl to binding proteins in the stomach. Achlorhydria can be the result of drug treatment with gastric acid pump inhibitors such as omeprazole but also occurs with aging. Pernicious anemia is an autoimmune disorder in which the autoantibodies are formed to the gastric parietal cells that produce intrinsic factor, thus preventing transportation and transfer of Cbl to the terminal ileum for cellular uptake. Other causes of cobalamin deficiency include gastric or intestinal surgery, blind loop syndrome.

Cobalamin requirements and cobalamin deficiency in pregnancy

A mixed Western diet provides about 5–7 μg/day of Cbl, well above the recommended daily intake of 2 μg/day for adults that increases to 2.2–2.6 μg/day during pregnancy and lactation. Given the minimal fetal Cbl requirements of 60–100 μg during pregnancy and a relative abundance of dietary cobalamin and maternal stores of around 3000 μg, it seems unlikely that cellular Cbl deficiency will develop in pregnant women who eat a mixed diet so that supplementation of dietary vitamin B12 is unlikely to be necessary. However, a lower dietary cobalamin intake in women who eat ovo-lacto, lacto-vegetarian or vegan diets will result in lower cobalamin stores and dietary intake may not meet the recommended daily requirement [9].

These factors and therefore the potential for cellular deficiency of cobalamin and its resultant effect on DNA synthesis are important when interpreting serum vitamin B12 results during pregnancy. A number of studies have reported a reduction in serum B12 levels during pregnancy but whether this represents a true cellular deficiency of B12 is not clear. The low levels may represent no more than the dilutional effect of plasma volume expansion on serum B12 levels. In contrast to the assessment of iron stores, there is no ferritin equivalent to confirm that there is insufficient cobalamin available for essential cellular functions. However, increases in other intermediates in the one-carbon pathway that require cobalamin and folate have been shown to support a diagnosis of deficiency of one of these vitamins. Typically, cobalamin deficiency will lead to increased levels of methylmalonic acid (MMA) and homocysteine whereas folate deficiency will lead to increases in homocysteine levels. However, the pregnancy-related reduction in homocysteine levels makes interpretation of laboratory measurements of these metabolites difficult during pregnancy. The hematologic effects of Cbl deficiency initially include development of red cell macrocytosis (an elevation in mean cell volume (MCV)) and eventually megaloblastic anemia with characteristic blood film features (Box 2.1). It is important to note that blood film features cannot distinguish between the megaloblastic anemias caused by cobalamin or folate deficiency. Neurologic sequelae include sensory disturbances and confusion.

Box 2.1 Hematologic features of B12 and folate deficiency

- Oval macrocytes
- Hypersegmented neutrophils
- Howell-Jolly bodies
- Thrombocytopenia
- Red cell fragments and tear drop red cells

In clinical practice, screening measurement of serum B12 levels should be restricted to women with significant gastric resections or a low dietary intake of cobalamin, i.e. women on ovo-lacto, lacto-vegetarian or vegan diets. Otherwise testing should be limited to patients with unexplained elevations in MCV on a complete blood count. If reduced serum B12 levels are detected in vegetarian women, they should be offered oral B12 supplements. As their low levels are due to a low dietary intake and not malabsorption, parenteral cobalamin is not essential. However, some women may prefer a single intramuscular injection of 1000 μg of hydroxycobalamin that may be sufficient for the entire pregnancy. Patients with B12 deficiency due to pernicioius anemia or gastrectomy may be treated with 1000 μg every day for 1 week, followed by 1000 μg every week for 4 weeks and then 1000 μg every month thereafter.

Breastfeeding

An adequate dietary intake of cobalamin is essential during breastfeeding to ensure sufficient quantities of cobalamin for the developing infant. Megaloblastic anemia, neurologic abnormalities and developmental delay have been described in breastfed infants of strictly vegetarian mothers and dietary supplementation is essential [10]. Malabsorption of cobalamin can also occur in patients after gastric bypass surgery and these women may require parenteral supplementation of B12 to prevent B12 deficiency in their breastfed infants [11].

Folate

Folate is the generic term for the vitamin that is an essential co-enzyme in the one-carbon metabolism cycle that provides methyl groups required for DNA synthesis and cell division. Synthetic folic acid, used in vitamin preparations and for food fortification, is a monoglutamic acid and is the most active form of the vitamin. It is also the most readily absorbed and has 100% absorption and bio-availability when taken on an empty stomach that is reduced to about 85% when taken with food. Food sources of folate provide the polyglutamate form of the vitamin that is much less readily absorbed, with ≤50% bio-availability. Food sources of folate include green leafy vegetables, mushrooms, yeast and fruit, with high levels present in animal protein such as liver and kidney. Ingested folate is absorbed via specific transport mechanisms in the small intestine and in addition to dietary folate, normal serum folate levels are maintained by the enterohepatic circulation. Cellular transport of folate is mediated by specific folate receptors. Folate is stored in the liver with total body stores of only 8–20 mg, which is small relative to recommended daily requirements, i.e. 100 μg/day (nonpregnant). Serum folate levels fall within a few days of interruption of dietary folate intake even though folate stores are not exhausted. Folate is incorporated into red blood cells early in their production and given their ≈120 day lifespan, red blood cell folate levels will give an indication of folate intake for the 2–3 months prior to blood sampling and red cell folate levels are thought to more accurately reflect total body folate stores than serum levels.

Folate requirements and supplementation during pregnancy

Daily folate requirements increase during pregnancy to 600 μg/day and 300 μg/day during lactation, the additional folate being required for nucleotide synthesis, cell division and increased red cell production. Given the relative small size of folate stores, ongoing severe reduction in dietary folate intake or increased utilization of folate will manifest within a few months [7].

The efficacy of preconceptual folic acid supplementation for primary and secondary prevention of neural tube defects (NTD) is well established. Daily supplements of 0.4 mg folic acid are recommended for low-risk women and 5 mg daily for women at higher risk. Despite this, a significant reduction in the incidence of NTD was not reported until mandatory folate fortification of foods was introduced in 1998. Closure of the neural tube occurs early in gestation, at around 21–28 days post conception, perhaps only 1–2 weeks after an expected missed period. For the many women for whom pregnancy is an unplanned event, this important opportunity for preconceptual folate supplementation would be missed [12].

In addition to folic acid supplementation for prevention of NTD, women with a low dietary intake of folate may require ongoing supplementation to prevent development of anemia. As with Cbl deficiency, the initial hematologic manifestation of folate deficiency is usually development of macrocytosis and if left untreated, megaloblastic anemia ensues.

Folate deficiency: laboratory investigation

Investigation of folate deficiency includes CBC, measurement of serum and occasionally red cell folate levels. The serum folate level is less expensive than the red cell folate level and reflects recent dietary intake and in an otherwise well person, deficiency is unlikely if serum folate levels are normal. Low serum folate levels are commonly found in hospitalized patients and confirmation of low serum levels by measurement of the more expensive red cell folate is recommended before making a diagnosis of deficiency but otherwise the serum folate alone can be used for diagnosis [13]. Of note, serum folate levels may be increased with cobalamin deficiency as a result of the block in the one-carbon metabolism pathway. Development of macrocytic red cells induced by deficiencies of folate and/or cobalamin may not occur in the presence of co-existing iron deficiency or the presence of a thalassemia or hemoglobinopathy. Careful examination of the peripheral blood smear may reveal other abnormalities suggestive of a deficiency such as hypersegmented neutrophils.

Confirmation of folate deficiency and differentiating it from cobalamin deficiency can be problematic as none of the commonly used laboratory tests is 100% sensitive and specific for diagnosis of a cellular deficiency of either vitamin. Measurement of other intermediates in the one-carbon cycle such as MMA and homocyteine (Hcy) have been suggested to be more specific and sensitive methods of determining a deficiency state and of differentiating between cobalamin and folate deficiency. Blocks in the one-carbon cycle due to deficiency of cobalamin will lead to increased levels of both MMA and Hcy whereas folate deficiency will only increase levels of Hcy. A reduction in Hcy levels in pregnancy due to increased glomerular filtration rates and lack of a defined normal range for pregnancy may limit the utility of these laboratory analytes in pregnancy, apart from the expense and limited availability of the tests themselves [14].

It is worth mentioning here that although macrocytosis may be caused by either or both folate and B12 deficiency, other causes include alcoholism, hypothyroidism, liver disease, hyperlipidemia and some medications (including phenytoin, azathioprine and zidovudine). The macrocytosis that occurs in some individuals who take anticonvulsant drugs is mediated by undefined mechanisms that are not due to folate or B12 deficiency and therefore does not respond to vitamin supplementation.

Summary

Anemia is the most prevalent hematologic abnormality in pregnancy, one that most commonly is caused by factors associated with poverty and social deprivation. It is associated with significant fetal and maternal morbidity and mortality, it can be easily diagnosed and responds quickly to intervention and treatment that is both inexpensive and readily available. Efforts to improve maternal and infant mortality could be addressed by diagnosis and treatment of anemia that on a global scale will have most impact in resource-poor countries but that could also lead to significant improvements in pregnancy outcome and maternal well-being for less advantaged women in more industrialized countries.

The hemoglobinopathies and thalassemias

Hemoglobinopathies and thalassemias are structural and quantitative abnormalities of hemoglobin. Together, they are the most common single-gene disorders affecting humans, found in almost 5% of the world's population. Originally described

in people from the Mediterranean and South East Asia, it was later recognized that hemoglobinopathies were common in people from Africa, the Indian subcontinent and the Pacific, with marked differences in prevalence existing within regions. The original geographical distribution of hemoglobin variants is thought to be due to the protective effect that the heterozygous state confers against malaria, the mosquito-borne disease that is a major cause of mortality and morbidity in these regions. Demographic changes have resulted in major increases in the number of individuals with hemoglobinopathies and thalassemia in North America and Northern Europe [15] Such changes require that, globally, clinicians involved in obstetric care develop an understanding of the potential health consequences of these disorders for mother and child.

Structure of hemoglobin

Hemoglobin is the iron-containing compound in red blood cells that is responsible for oxygen transfer in vertebrates and mammals, including humans. The hemoglobin molecule is a tetramer composed of two different pairs of globular protein subunits, i.e. globins, each of which is covalently attached to a nonprotein heme moiety that carries iron and is responsible for binding oxygen. In adult life the predominant hemoglobin type is Hb A, made up of two α and two β chains ($\alpha_2\beta_2$), accounting for around 95–97% of adult hemoglobin, with 1.5–3.5% Hb A_2 ($\alpha_2\gamma_2$) and HbF ($\alpha_2\delta_2$) making up the remainder. Different globin chains are expressed in embryonic and fetal development so that in embryogenesis the hemoglobins are Hb Gower 1 ($\zeta_2\varepsilon_2$), Hb Gower 2 ($\alpha_2\varepsilon_2$) and Hb Portland 1 ($\zeta_2\delta_2$). By 8–9 weeks gestation, the embryonic ζ – and ε-globin chains are no longer detectable and Hb F ($\alpha_2\delta_2$) is the predominant hemoglobin during fetal development. Synthesis of the β-globin chain begins from around 7 weeks gestation with Hb A accounting for around 10% of total hemoglobin at birth, reaching normal adult levels by 6 months to 1 year of age. Chromosome 16 is the site of the α-globin gene cluster composed of two α-globin genes and a single ζ-globin gene with the non-α chains, β, ε, and γ encoded by single genes on chromosome 11. Normal individuals therefore express four α-globin genes and two β-like genes. Deletions or mutations of the α- or β-globin genes will lead to α- or β-thalassemia, respectively, with most hemoglobinopathies occurring as a result of mutations affecting the β-globin gene cluster [16].

Thalassemias and hemoglobinopathies can be categorized in a number of ways. Firstly, according to the severity of clinical manifestations, i.e. the phenotypic expression, ranging from the most severe (thalassemia major) to that of moderate severity (thalassemia intermedia) to a mild or clinically silent phenotype (thalassemia minor). Thalassemias can be also grouped by whether the mutation affects the α- or β-globin chain with the specific mutations or deletions described.

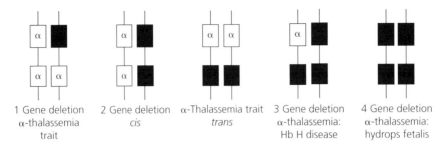

Figure 2.2 Genotypes of α-thalassemia.

Disorders of α-globin synthesis

α-Thalassemia results from reduced production of α-globin chains due mainly to deletions of one or more of the four α- globin genes (Figure 2.2). The length of the deletion determines whether one or both α-globin genes are missing from the same chromosome. The South East Asian (SEA), Philippino (FIL), Thai (THAI) Mediterranean (MED) and $-(\alpha)^{20.5}$ genotypes cause loss of both α-chains from a single chromosome, leading to *cis* 2-gene deletion α-thalassemia known as α^0-thalassemia (*cis* refers to the fact that the two mutations are both on the same chromosome). These mutations are particularly common in South East Asia, the Mediterranean and the Middle East. Single α-globin gene deletions are also prevalent in these geographical areas but also in the Pacific region and include $-\alpha^{4.2}$ and $-\alpha^{3.7}$ and lead to one-gene deletion denoted by α^+- thalassemia. Nondeletional α-thalassemia also occurs, the most common defect being Hb Constant Spring where the mutation leads to formation of unstable extended α-globin chains. Carrier rates of α-thalassemia show marked geographical variation, with rates of up to 25% reported in Thailand, around 3% in China, with the α^+-thalassemia described in 10–15% of people of Pacific origin [17].

Hydrops fetalis, the most severe form of α-thalassemia, results from deletion of all four α-globin genes. Although the literature reports a small number of survivors with this condition [18], it is usually lethal *in utero* as α-globin chains are required for formation of fetal hemoglobin from very early in fetal life. Absence of α-globin results in the formation of Hb Barts made by tetramers of the γ-globin chain (γ_4), the fetal equivalent of the β-globin chain. Hb Barts has a very high oxygen affinity and does not release oxygen to fetal tissues, leading to severe hypoxia and ultimately fetal hydrops. Hydrops fetalis most commonly results from inheritance of α^0-thalassemia from each parent (Figure 2.3). The geographical distribution of these genotypes means that hydrops fetalis is therefore particularly common in South East Asia where it poses a major health problem.

Hb H disease is due to loss of three α-globin genes ($--/-\alpha$) (see Figure 2.3). Deficiency of α-globin chains with excess of β-globin chains leads to formation of Hb H, a tetramer of β-globin (β_4) which is relatively unstable and forms intracellular precipitates that ultimately shorten red

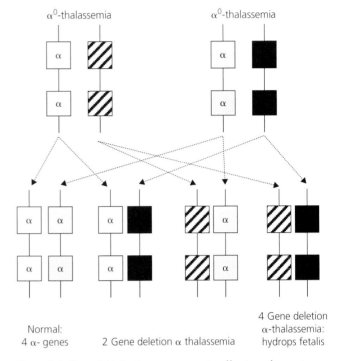

Figure 2.3 Potential inheritance patterns in offspring of parents with α^0-thalassemia traits demonstrating a one in four chance of development of hydrops fetalis due to absence of four α-chains.

cell survival. Hb H disease generally exhibits a mild clinical phenotype with mild anemia that is not usually transfusion dependent although in some patients anemia is more severe, requiring transfusion.

Two-gene deletion α-thalassemia or α-thalassemia trait can be due to deletions of α-globin genes from the same chromosome ($--/\alpha\alpha$) or to single gene deletions from both chromosomes ($-\alpha/-\alpha$). α-Thalassemia trait is phenotypically mild with microcytic, hypochromic red cell indices and occasionally mild anemia. It is not possible to distinguish between the two types of two-gene deletion α-thalassemia using basic hematologic indices and special molecular studies are required.

Single gene deletion α-thalassemia or α^+-thalassemia ($-\alpha/\alpha\alpha$) is clinically silent and may present only with mild red cell microcytosis and hypochromia. It is the predominant form of α-thalassemia trait in people of Pacific origin but is in Africa, the Mediterranean and South East Asia.

Disorders of β-globin synthesis

Disordered synthesis of the β-globin chain usually results from point mutations of the β-globin gene, of which over 200 different mutations have been described. β-Thalassemia is caused by mutations that lead to reduced (β^+) or absent (β^0) production of structurally normal β-globin chains. In contrast, the hemoglobinopathies result from mutations that produce usually normal amounts of structurally abnormal or variant hemoglobins.

β-Thalassemia

β-Thalassemia trait, prevalent in the Mediterranean, North Africa, the Middle East, the Indian subcontinent and South East Asia, is due to inheritance of one of nearly 200 single β-globin gene mutations, usually a point mutation or single amino acid change that leads to reduced production of a normal β-globin chain. It exhibits a clinically mild phenotype but with microcytic, hypochromic red cells seen in the peripheral blood smear. Inheritance of two abnormal β-globin genes leads to thalassemia major or thalassemia intermedia, depending on the combination of β-globin gene mutations inherited. One of the most severe clinical phenotypes occurs in individuals homozygous for β^0 mutations resulting in complete absence of β-globin chain production. This presents in the first year of life with severe anemia, hepatosplenomegaly, bone deformities and growth delay. Individuals who are compound heterozygotes for β^0 and β^+ mutations show variable clinical manifestations ranging from those with severe transfusion-dependent anemia to those who require only periodic transfusions. More recently, it has been recognized that β-thalassemia major or intermedia is associated with an increased risk of venous thromboembolism, especially in individuals who have had a splenectomy. The anemia in β-thalassemia is due to ineffective erythropoiesis and hemolysis, both of which are the result of an excess of α-chains. There is considerable variation in the prevalence of β-thalassemia among different countries, ranging from 2–3% in the Middle East to 17% in Cyprus. Also marked variations are described within individual countries; for example, in Greece the prevalence ranges from 6% to 19% and in Italy from 7% to 19%. Clinically significant interactions of β-thalassemia trait with other hemoglobin variants, such as Hb S and Hb E, are described under the individual hemoglobinopathies.

Hemoglobinopathies

Of the greater than 200 different β-globin gene mutations, only a very small number, i.e. Hb E, Hb C, Hb S, and Hb

Lepore, cause clinically significant abnormalities. This occurs most commonly in the compound heterozygous state with other β-chain abnormalities but importantly sickle cell disease develops in individuals homozygous for Hb S. These mutations show quite marked geographical variability: Hb E is particularly prevalent in South East Asia, with carrier rates of 20–60%, and Hb S and Hb C are common in Africa with carrier rates of 12% and 3%, respectively. In the heterozygous or carrier state these hemoglobinopathies do not cause clinical abnormalities but a high carrier frequency in certain populations leads to perpetuation of severe thalassemia syndromes in the children of asymptomatic carriers. Carriers are frequently undiagnosed when embarking on pregnancy, do not receive pre-pregnancy or antenatal counseling or may choose not to have antenatal testing for social or cultural reasons.

Hb E

Hb E is caused by a single point mutation at position 26 on the β-chain (β^E) where glutamine is replaced by lysine, resulting in reduced synthesis of the β-globin chain. Individuals who are heterozygous or even homozygous for HbE are completely asymptomatic and its clinical relevance stems from the consequences that occur when this very common hemoglobin variant combines with β-thalassemia trait. Compound heterozygotes for HbE and β-thalassemia have a wide range of clinical manifestations from mild anemia to the most severe form of thalassemia major. Such marked phenotypic variability is not well understood and, in particular, does not seem to be related to the specific mutation responsible for the β-thalassemia trait. So even among individuals with the same β-chain mutation in combination with Hb E, there are major differences in the clinical severity of the thalassemia that results.

Hb C

Hb C is caused by a single point mutation at position 6 on the β-chain where glutamine is replaced by lysine, resulting in a variant Hb (β^c) that is less soluble than Hb A and also has a lower oxygen affinity. Thought to have originated in West Africa, the heterozygous state has an overall prevalence of around 3% that reaches as high as 40% in Burkina Faso and 50% in Ivory Coast. Individuals heterozygous for Hb C are clinically well and homozygotes exhibit mild, chronic hemolytic anemia. Combinations of Hb C with β-thalassemia or other variant hemoglobins, especially Hb S, lead to clinically significant disorders. Compound heterozygotes for Hb C and β^0-thalassemia have moderately severe anemia with splenomegaly whereas those with Hb C and mild β^+-thalassemia have mild to moderate hemolytic anemia. The clinical implications for individuals who are compound heterozygotes for Hb C and Hb S are discussed later.

Hb Lepore

Hb Lepore is a hemoglobin variant that results from creation of a fusion δβ-globin gene, due to abnormal cross-over during meiosis. There is inefficient synthesis of the δβ-chain of Hb Lepore that leads to a thalassemia phenotype. Individuals heterozygous for Hb Lepore are asymptomatic with microcytic, hypochromic red blood cell indices similar to those found in β-thalassemia trait. The homozygous state varies between transfusion-dependent thalassemia major and thalassemia intermedia. Compound heterozygotes for Hb Lepore and β-thalassemia manifest as thalassemia major.

Hb S

Hb S or sickle cell trait results from replacement of glutamine by valine on position 6 of the β-globin chain (β^S). It is particularly common in sub-Saharan Africa but also occurs in the Indian subcontinent, the Middle East and the Mediterranean. The carrier frequency in African Americans is 8%. The deleterious effects of Hb S result from polymerization of Hb S that occurs when the Hb molecule is deoxygenated, leading to reduced deformability of the red cell and increased adhesion to endothelial cells. This results in reduced red cell survival due to hemolysis and also vaso-occlusive events, especially in the low oxygen environment of the capillary circulation. The polymerization of Hb S is particularly slowed by the presence of Hb F but also to a lesser degree by Hb A_2 and Hb A [19].

Sickle cell disease

Red cell sickling does not occur in individuals who have sickle cell trait except in conditions of extremely low oxygen tension, such as travel by air, especially in unpressurized cabins, vigorous exercise or high fever. Patients homozygous for Hb S ($\alpha_2\beta^S_2$) have sickle cell disease (SCD) although, as seen later, SCD also occurs in patients who are compound heterozygotes for Hb S and other β-chain abnormalities such as β-thalassemia trait. The major clinical manifestations of SCD are due to vaso-occlusive events that either present acutely as a sickle cell or vaso-occlusive crisis or as the result of chronic vascular occlusion. Most individuals have chronic hemolysis with a hemoglobin in the order of 6–9 g/dL but symptomatic anemia is uncommon as patients compensate well for their degree of anemia, especially as Hb S has a relatively low oxygen affinity. The skeletal and growth abnormalities seen with β-thalassemia major do not develop and overall patients go through normal puberty. The most significant clinical problems are the result of acute and sometimes life-threatening vaso-occlusive sickling crises that can affect bones, lungs, the brain, spleen, liver and in men can cause recurrent priapism. Crises can be provoked by cold, dehydration and infection but are self-limiting, usually lasting a few days. About 20% of patients with SCD suffer from recurrent severe events and 50% have about one crisis per year. Vaso-occlusion of the bone marrow leads to severe bone pain usually requiring narcotic analgesia. Lung crises or acute chest syndrome, a common cause of mortality, presents with hypoxia, dyspnea and pulmonary infiltrates on X-ray due to sequestration of sickled cells in the pulmonary circulation. Brain syndrome with stroke or hemorrhage is described in 11% of patients by the age of 20 years and in 24% by the age of 45 years. Manifestations of chronic vascular occlusion include aseptic necrosis of the femoral or humeral head, pulmonary hypertension, leg ulcers, proliferative retinopathy and progressive renal failure. Sepsis is an important cause of morbidity and mortality for individuals with SCD at all ages, in particular due to *Strep. pneumoniae*, *Salmonella* and *Klebsiella*, and pneumococcal vaccination is recommended.

The pathophysiology of vaso-occlusion in SCD is more complex than simple mechanical obstruction by rigid, sickled red cells. Sickled red cells are also more likely to adhere to vascular endothelium due to their innate properties and also to increased expression of inflammatory markers and adhesion molecules on leukocytes and the endothelial surface. Ischemia-reperfusion injury is thought to be a major contributor to the proinflammatory state in SCD [20].

Hb F inhibits polymer formation of the β^S-globin chains so that individuals with increased levels of Hb F have a less severe clinical phenotype of SCD. The level of Hb F has been shown to be a prognostic factor for complications of SCD. Certain ethnic subgroups, for example people from India and Saudi Arabia, record higher levels of Hb F and a very mild clinical phenotype. As mentioned previously, SCD also occurs when Hb S is co-inherited with other abnormalities of the β-chain. Compound heterozygotes of β-thalassemia and Hb S show a very variable clinical phenotype ranging from mild disease in patients of African origin with Hb S-β^+thalassemia to more severe forms of when combined with β^0-thalassemia and even β^+-thalassemia from other ethnic groups. In general, it is not possible to predict the clinical course of SCD in compound heterozygotes of β-thalassemia and Hb S on the basis of the β-thalassemia genotype, thus making genetic counseling particularly problematic. Individuals who inherit both Hb S and Hb C have milder, chronic hemolytic anemia and although they experience fewer sickle cell crises, they are more prone to vaso-occlusive osteonecrosis and also retinal disease.

Treatment of SCD

Increased levels of Hb F are associated with a less severe clinical phenotype and studies have shown that treatment with the cytotoxic agent hydroxyurea increases expression of Hb F, leading to a reduction in frequency of sickling crises, acute chest syndrome and overall mortality [21]. Treatment of an acute crisis involves maternal oxygen supplementation, rapid relief of pain (usually requiring opioid analgesics) and maintenance of good oral fluid intake with intravenous fluids if required. Blood transfusion is not routinely required in an uncomplicated sickling crisis but in severe chest crises, cerebrovascular events or multiorgan failure, exchange transfusion is indicated [22].

Interaction of α-thalassemia with β-chain abnormalities

The clinical consequences of the thalassemias result from an imbalance of α-chains relative to β-chains. Given the geographical distribution of these mutations, co-inheritance of both α-thalassemia traits and β-thalassemia major or minor is therefore not surprising. When this occurs, a less severe clinical phenotype is present as there is an overall reduction in α-chains relative to β-chains which protects against the effects of excess globin chains. When α-thalassemia is inherited with β-chain hemoglobin variants, lower amounts of the abnormal Hb are formed overall as the α-chains preferentially bind to normal β-chains.

Diagnosis of thalassemias and hemoglobinopathies

The diagnosis of thalassemias and hemoglobinopathies requires a combination of laboratory tests. In the absence of iron deficiency, the finding of microcytic, hypochromic red cell indices on an automated CBC are strongly suggestive of the diagnosis of a hemoglobin disorder. Mean cell volume (MCV) describes red cell size (normal range ≈80–100 fL) with microcytosis referring to small red cells. An MCV <78 fL is suggestive of a thalassemia or hemoglobinopathy although the MCV does increase with storage of blood samples and can lead to falsely high results. The mean

corpuscular hemoglobin (MCH) is a more stable analytic variable so provides more reliable results. Testing for hemoglobinopathies is recommended if the MCH is less than 27 pg [23]. The peripheral blood smear should be examined for abnormal red cell morphology, such as target cells (red blood cells characterized by a densely stained center surrounded by a pale unstained ring that is encircled by a dark irregular band), stippled cells (small basophilic inclusions distributed throughout the cytoplasm), sickle cells (the characteristic sickle-shaped cell), nucleated red cells and red cell inclusions (round dense bodies of variable size, usually single and staining similarly to a nucleus, also known as Howell Jolly bodies). The Hb H inclusions of α-thalassemia (globular bodies scattered throughout the red cell cytoplasm) can be generated *in vitro* by using an oxidative dye such as new methylene blue and the peripheral blood smear reviewed to determine their presence and the number of red cells affected. Hemoglobin electrophoresis is routinely used to detect the presence and quantity of normal and abnormal hemoglobins although high-performance liquid chromatography (HPLC) is a useful tool for this purpose. And serendipitous discovery of variant hemoglobins is becoming more frequent as HPLC is also used to quantify glycosylated Hb (Hb A1c) in people with diabetes. Specific laboratory tests are used to detect sickle cell trait and disease. A diagnostic pathway for investigation of hemoglobinopathies and thalassemias is given in Figure 2.4 with a summary of helpful laboratory findings with specific disorders listed in Table 2.2.

Pregnancy and the thalassemias and hemoglobinopathies

The relevance of the thalassemias and hemoglobinopathies in obstetrics relates to the potential impact on fertility and pregnancy complications in women who have these disorders,

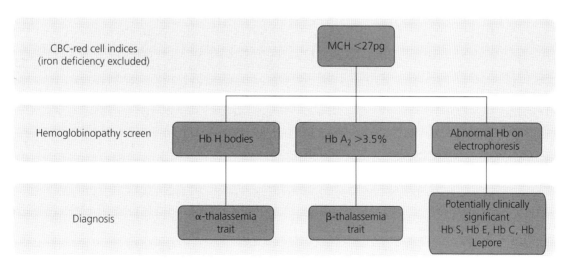

Figure 2.4 Diagnostic pathway for thalassemias and hemoglobinopathies. CBC, complete blood count; MCH, mean corpuscular hemoglobin.

Table 2.2 Hematologic, blood film and hemoglobinopathy findings for certain thalassemias and hemoglobinopathies

	Complete blood count	Blood film	Hemoglobinopathy screen
α-Thalassemia trait	Normal Hb or mild anemia ↓MCV, ↓MCH	Microcytosis, hypochromia	Small numbers of Hb H bodies
Hb H disease	Moderately severe anemia Hb 7–10 g/dL, MCV 50–65 fL, MCH 15–20 pg	Variable red cell shape and size with red cell fragments, teardrop red cells, hypochromia, microcytosis Nucleated red cells unusual	Moderate numbers of Hb H bodies Hb H 8–10% Hb A$_2$ 1–2% Hb F 1–3%
β-Thalassemia trait	Mild anemia ↓MCV, ↓MCH	Microcytosis and hypochromia Stippled red cells	Hb A2 >3.5%
β-Thalassemia major	Hb 3–7 g/dL, MCV 50–60 fL, MCH 12–18 pg	Variable red cell shape and size with red cell fragments, teardrop red cells, hypochromia, microcytosis, stippled cells, nucleated red cells	β^{0}β^0 – Hb F, Hb A$_2$ β^{0}β$^+$ or β$^+$β$^+$ – Hb F, Hb A$_2$ variable Hb A
Hb E – heterozygous	Normal Hb, ↓MCV	Microcytosis, stippled cells, target cells	Hb E ≤30%
Hb E – homozygous	Normal Hb or very mild anemia ↓MCV, ↓MCH	Microcytosis, target cells	Hb E + Hb A$_2$ 85–99%[§] Hb F 1–15%
Hb C – heterozygous	Normal Hb, ↓MCV	Microcytosis, target cells	Hb A >50% Hb C <50%
Hb C – homozygous	Mild anemia, ↓↓ MCV	Microcytosis, target cells ++, occasional Hb crystals	Hb C 97% Hb F ≤3%
Hb S – heterozygous (sickle cell trait)	Normal Hb and MCV, MCH[§]	Normal	Hb S 40% Hb A 60%
Hb S – homozygous (sickle cell disease)	Hb 6–9 g/dL MCV 70–100 fL	Sickle cells, target cells, Howell-Jolly bodies, polychromasia	Hb S 90–95% Hb A$_2$ 2–4% *Hb F 5–10%

*Variable can be up to 25% depending on haplotype of β^S gene.
[§]Hb E and Hb A$_2$ co-migrate so it is not possible to easily determine the respective amounts of each Hb.
MCH, mean corpuscular hemoglobin; MCV, mean cell volume.

especially those who have clinical manifestations. Of equal importance, given the prevalence of these hemoglobin mutations, is the risk of abnormal genes being passed from parents to children resulting in the perpetuation of clinical disease in the next generation. Pre-pregnancy counseling and antenatal diagnosis are key aspects of management in these conditions.

Impact of the thalassemias and hemoglobinopathies on fertility and pregnancy outcome

Thalassemia major

In the developed world, the major clinical complications of transfusion-dependent β-thalassemia result from iron overload due to the disease itself and also secondary to blood transfusions. Chelation therapy (the use of binding agents to remove heavy metals from the body) plays a vital role in minimizing iron overload but if inadequate, leads to iron deposition and ultimately dysfunction of the liver, heart and endocrine organs. Even with tertiary care, the majority of adult patients with transfusion-dependent β-thalassemia

have hypogonadotropic hypogonadism that may not always respond to gonadotropins. Other important endocrine disorders relating to pregnancy include diabetes and hypothyroidism as well as liver disease or transfusion-transmitted viral infections such as HIV and hepatitis C.

Tuck described the outcome of 29 pregnancies in 22 women with transfusion-dependent thalassemia major [24]. He suggests that assessment of cardiac function is the most important pre-pregnancy investigation as the presence of cardiac impairment is a poor prognostic factor that is associated with a significant risk of premature death. Both of the maternal deaths in their patient population were due to cardiac failure and they would discourage pregnancy in women with cardiac impairment. Other important pre-pregnancy care includes optimization of diabetic control, thyroid replacement and, importantly, determination of the hemoglobinopathy status of the male partner. Calcium and vitamin D supplements should be given during pregnancy in view of the high incidence of reduced bone mineral density in these patients. Tuck did not report an increased incidence of fetal growth restriction or preterm delivery as has been reported by other centers but put this down to maintaining the maternal hemoglobin above 10 g/dL during pregnancy. He emphasizes the importance of thorough pre-pregnancy assessment to determine maternal risks during pregnancy and whether pregnancy is even advisable, as well as close antenatal monitoring for development of maternal complications.

Sickle cell disease

A large cohort study from birth through young adulthood [25] reported a significantly reduced livebirth rate of 57% (48/94 pregnancies) in 52 women with sickle cell disease compared to a livebirth rate of 89% (128/157) in 68 control women. The difference in outcome was due primarily to an increase in spontaneous miscarriage in women with SCD: 36% (30/94 pregnancies) compared to 10.4% (15/157 pregnancies) in controls. Six stillbirths were reported in the women with SCD compared to only one in the control group. There were no differences in development of pregnancy-induced hypertension, pre-eclampsia or antepartum or postpartum hemorrhage between groups. Other studies have reported high rates of pre-eclampsia in the order of 15–20% in multiparous women with sickle cell disease with histopathologic evidence of placental fibrosis, infarction and thrombosis in the majority of cases. An increased incidence of sickle cell crises is described, particularly in the last trimester of pregnancy and the postpartum period. Women with SCD are advised to ensure they remain well hydrated during pregnancy. The increased risk of infection in SCD should be remembered, especially as it can trigger an acute sickling crisis. Additional folate supplementation (1 mg daily) is required because of chronic hemolysis in SCD. The use of hydroxyurea in pregnancy to increase the levels of hemoglobin F is not justifiable in pregnancy due to the potential teratogenic effects of this agent.

Crises should be managed as in nonpregnant patients but clinicians should be aware that episodes are often more prolonged than those outside pregnancy. Acute crises are managed with aggressive pain control, hydration, oxygen supplementation, continued folate and a careful search for and treatment of any underlying infection. Severe crises may warrant transfusion therapy with the goal being to achieve at least 50% normal hemoglobin, i.e. Hb A.

The role of prophylactic blood transfusions in pregnant women with SCD has been controversial [26]. A randomized trial demonstrated no improvement in maternal and fetal outcome when comparing prophylactic blood transfusions to emergency transfusion for sickle cell crises. Women who received prophylactic red cell transfusions experienced fewer painful crises during pregnancy but women were exposed to four times as many units of blood [27]. In the absence of an improvement in maternal or fetal outcome, prophylactic red cell transfusion during pregnancy is not recommended.

The peridelivery period is associated with a particularly high risk of provoking a sickling crisis. Management of labor includes maintaining adequate hydration and oxygenation and providing good pain relief. Mode of delivery should be determined by obstetric indications.

Hb H disease and thalassemia traits

Worsening anemia is not usually a problem in women with Hb H disease or thalassemia traits but occasionally evidence of hemolysis with anemia is reported in women with thalassemia traits, especially β-thalassemia trait. This may be due to the effect of increased oxidative stress in pregnancy causing destruction of red cells made more fragile by the inclusion bodies formed by excess α-globin chains. Women with these conditions are not themselves at an increased risk of adverse pregnancy outcome.

There is no increased risk of pregnancy complications for women who are carrying an infant that will develop thalassemia major due to abnormalities of the β-globin genes. Infants develop normally in utero as the predominant fetal hemoglobin is Hb F ($\alpha_2\gamma_2$) and the abnormal β-chains are not produced in significant numbers until around 6 months of age which is when these disorders begin to manifest. In contrast, infants who inherit α-thalassemia trait from each parent in cis form, where the two α-genes are deleted from the same chromosome, will have fetal hydrops. In this condition, the predominant hemoglobin in fetal life is Hb Barts which is formed by γ_4 tetramers and has a very high oxygen affinity (and therefore does not deliver oxygen to fetal tissue). In very early gestation the embryonic hemoglobins Hb Gower 1 ($\zeta_2\varepsilon_2$) and Hb Portland 1 ($\zeta_2\delta_2$) are present and can deliver oxygen to the fetal tissues. The condition is generally thought to be incompatible with survival, with most pregnancies ending in stillbirth or premature delivery of an infant who survives for only a very short time. However, there are a few cases reports of infants who have survived beyond delivery and a very small number of transfusion-dependent long-term survivors [28]. Fetal anomalies are frequently described and include hypospadias, ambiguous genitalia and limb defects. Women carrying an affected infant are at increased risk of developing complications such as pre-eclampsia, placental abruption, polyhydramnios and premature labor.

Table 2.3 Hemoglobin types

Hemoglobin	Symbol	Normal levels present	
		Adult Hb	Newborn Hb
Hb A	$\alpha_2\beta_2$	95–97%	10%
Hb A$_2$	$\alpha_2\delta_2$	1.5–3.5%	
Hb F	$\alpha_2\gamma_2$	<2%	90%
Hb Gower 1*	$\zeta_2\varepsilon_2$	–	–
Hb Gower 2*	$\alpha_2\varepsilon_2$	–	–
Hb Portland*	$\zeta_2\delta_2$	–	–

*Embryonic Hb present until 8–9 weeks gestation.

Prenatal diagnosis

The high prevalence of hemoglobinopathies and thalassemias worldwide has major implications for the global health burden. This is felt most strongly in the developing world but demographic changes mean that the number of births of children affected by major thalassemia is also increasing in developed countries. Worldwide, Hb E β-thalassemia is the most important cause of thalassemia major due to the high gene frequencies of Hb E, reaching 60% in some areas of Thailand, Laos and Cambodia, with the prevalence of β-thalassemia trait ranging from 3% to 6%. Effective strategies for antenatal screening and prenatal diagnosis to help reduce the numbers of affected children have been established in areas of particularly high prevalence, such as Cyprus. Increased migration from South East Asia prompted development of a newborn screening program in California for Hb H disease, testing heel-prick samples for Hb Barts. The authors reported a prevalence of Hb H disease in 1 in 15,000 newborns and recommended that screening programs be implemented in areas with significant South East Asian populations [29].

A key component to prevention is increasing awareness of these disorders and ensuring that simple baseline investigations such as CBC are carried out in all women, especially those from ethnic groups with a high prevalence of the disorders. Women with red cell indices suggestive of an abnormality should have confirmatory testing to determine the clinical significance of a hemoglobin variant (see Figure 2.4). Partners should also be tested to identify couples at risk of having a child with a clinically significant thalassemia syndrome. In regions where there is a high prevalence of both α- and βthalassemia, molecular studies may be required to exclude co-inheritance of the disorders [30]. Careful discussion of the potential outcomes and recommendations for prenatal diagnosis is required. For some, religious, spiritual or personal beliefs may preclude consideration of termination of pregnancy even if the fetus was found to be severely affected but it is important to ensure that all prospective parents are informed of the risks.

Standard prenatal diagnostic techniques include amniocentesis and chorionic villus sampling (CVS) that can detect disorders where the genetic abnormality has been identified, such as the deletions that cause α-thalassemia or mutations leading to β-thalassemia, β^S or β^E. However, these diagnostic methods generally imply the parents' willingness to make a decision regarding termination of pregnancy if a major abnormality is detected. Techniques for detection of fetal DNA in maternal blood early in pregnancy are increasingly being explored but termination of pregnancy, albeit at an earlier gestation, is still the only option if the fetus is found to be affected. Preimplantation genetic diagnosis (PGD) uses *in vitro* fertilization (IVF) technology to produce embryos that are then tested for the specific genetic abnormality. Unaffected embryos are then implanted into the uterus. However, the relative inefficiency of IVF and its associated costs, especially when PGD is carried out in tandem, limits the ability of widespread adoption of this technique [31–33]. Antenatal fetal ultrasound looking for cardiomegaly is used in some centers for antenatal detection of hydrops fetalis [34].

Thrombocytopenia and other platelet disorders in pregnancy

Thrombocytopenia in pregnancy

Thrombocytopenia in pregnancy is defined as a platelet count less than 150×10^9/L. Such a diagnosis in a pregnant woman can often lead to considerable clinician anxiety that in turn may be passed onto the patient. The concerns are driven by the perception of an increased risk of bleeding for mother and baby, in particular the threat of fetal or neonatal intracranial hemorrhage due to thrombocytopenia in the infant. Indeed, medical literature from the 1980s warned of this risk and recommended variously that all women with thrombocytopenia in pregnancy be delivered by cesarean section to reduce the risk of intracranial hemorrhage or that the mode of delivery be decided by using invasive methods such as percutaneous umbilical blood sampling (PUBS) or fetal scalp vein sampling to determine which infants had thrombocytopenia [35]. By the 1990s, a shift in recommendations for management of women with thrombocytopenia in pregnancy was occurring. The risk of fetal intracranial hemorrhage in infants born to these women was downgraded as was the incidence of severe thrombocytopenia in infants [36]. Decisions regarding the mode of delivery in women with ITP, in particular delivery by cesarean section, were recommended to be guided by obstetric indications alone because of the growing recognition that the majority of profoundly thrombocytopenic infants were born to mothers with normal platelet counts and that delivery by cesarean section did not necessarily prevent bleeding complications in thrombocytopenic infants. Such a paradigm shift is likely in part to have been due to an increasing use of automated full blood count analyzers in clinical care so that all pregnant women and their newborns had routine full blood count analysis, thus providing more

---

Box 2.2 Practice point: thalassemia and CBC

Co-inheritance of β-thalassemia and α-thalassemia traits leads to normalization of the red cell indices. In high-risk ethnic groups a laboratory report of an increased Hb A_2 with near normal MCV and MCH should prompt a careful search for Hb H bodies. If none are found, molecular genetic testing for α-thalassemia may be required to exclude co-existence of α^0-thalassemia and β-thalassemia.

complete data regarding the prevalence of thrombocytopenia in these patients and its clinical impact. Prior to this only symptomatic women or infants would have been tested, thus potentially exaggerating the clinical impact of thrombocytopenia in this setting.

The aim of this section is to clarify when thrombocytopenia in pregnancy is clinically important, to provide guidance regarding diagnosis and management of thrombocytopenia in pregnancy, and information to advise women about potential risks to themselves and their babies. It is important to be aware that the majority of women with thrombocytopenia in pregnancy require no additional special care, but even those who do should be reassured that risks to themselves and their baby are low.

Prevalence of thrombocytopenia during pregnancy

During pregnancy, hemodilution caused by the relative increase in plasma volume coupled with increased platelet turnover leads to development of so-called gestational or incidental thrombocytopenia that accounts for three-quarters of cases of thrombocytopenia detected during pregnancy. The largest cross-sectional study to report the prevalence of maternal thrombocytopenia in pregnancy recorded platelet counts taken on admission to the labor ward in 15,471 women who delivered consecutively over a 7-year period in a tertiary care obstetric center [37]. Mild thrombocytopenia, i.e. platelet count of $<150 \times 10^9/L$ was recorded in 6.6% (n=1027) of women, with 1.2% (n=181) having moderate thrombocytopenia, i.e. platelets of $<100 \times 10^9/L$. A smaller study of 4382 Finnish women [38] reported similar prevalence of mild thrombocytopenia in 317 women (7.3%) and moderate thrombocytopenia in 25 women (0.6%).

Diagnostic approach to thrombocytopenia in pregnancy

Detection of a low platelet count in pregnancy should initiate a clear diagnostic pathway to elucidate the cause of the thrombocytopenia to allow a management plan to be developed (Table 2.4). The first step is confirmation that the low platelet count is real and not spurious due to a clotted specimen or anticoagulant-mediated platelet clumping. Review of the peripheral blood smear is essential to exclude fibrin clots, EDTA-mediated platelet clumping (ethylenediamine tetra-acetic acid (EDTA) is an anticoagulant often used in blood specimen collection vials) and also allow review of morphology of platelet and other blood cells. If platelet clumping or platelet satellitism due to the EDTA is suspected, a repeat CBC can be taken in a citrated anticoagulant specimen tube. If there are concerns that the specimen is clotted, a repeat sample should be taken. Certain rare inherited platelet disorders have specific morphologic features such as the Gray platelet syndrome characterized by the presence of large agranular platelets or the May – Hegglin anomaly where inclusion bodies are seen in the granulocytic cells.

Women should be questioned to see if they have a history suggestive of a bleeding disorder, i.e. symptoms such as menorrhagia (especially if severe enough to cause anemia), bleeding following surgical procedures or tooth extraction. Bleeding disorders associated with low platelet counts include the Bernard – Soulier syndrome and type 2B von Willebrand's disease.

Confirmation of previously undiagnosed thrombocytopenia warrants further investigation (see Table 2.5). An attempt should be made to review prior maternal platelet counts. A previously detected and unexplained low platelet count either before pregnancy or very early in pregnancy

Table 2.4 Investigation pathway for thrombocytopenia detected in pregnancy

Low platelet count in pregnancy $<150 \times 10^9/L$	
Confirm low result and review blood smear	? Specimen clotted ?Platelet aggregation or satellitism: EDTA anticoagulant-mediated effect
Large platelets on blood smear	ITP Bernard–Soulier syndrome (inherited) May–Hegglin anomaly – abnormal inclusion bodies in granulocytic cells (inherited)
Previous platelet results available Maternal bleeding history	Known diagnosis ITP or inherited platelet disorder Known or previously undiagnosed disorder i.e. Bernard–Soulier syndrome, type 2B von Willebrand's disease
Exclude hypertensive complication of pregnancy i.e pre-eclampsia, HELLP Autoimmune disorder	Usually present only after 20th week Check blood pressure, urine for protein, AST, uric acid, creatinine ?Clinical symptoms Tests for ANA, lupus anticoagulant and anticardiolipin antibodies
Other	Obtain HIV serology, review medication and alcohol history, examine for evidence of liver disease or splenomegaly

ANA, antinuclear antibody; AST, aspartate aminotransferase; EDTA, ethylenediamine tetra-acetic acid; HELLP, *h*emolysis, *e*levated *l*iver enzymes, *l*ow *p*latelet count; ITP, immune-mediated thrombocytopenia.

Table 2.5 Comparison between gestational thrombocytopenia and ITP

Gestational thrombocytopenia	ITP
Platelet count usually 100–149 $\times$ 10^9/L; rarely <80 $\times$ 10^9/L	Platelet count often <80 $\times$ 10^9/L
Due to increased platelet turnover and hemodilution	Induced by platelet-specific IgG antibodies
No treatment of maternal thrombocytopenia required	Treatment of maternal thrombocytopenia may be required (see Figures 2.5, 2.6)
Does not cause neonatal thrombocytopenia	Neonatal thrombocytopenia may develop. Platelets <150 $\times$ 10^9/L in 28% infants, <50 $\times$ 10^9/L in 11% infants

is suggestive of immune-mediated thrombocytopenia (ITP). A diagnosis of ITP may have been established prior to pregnancy or a woman may be known to have an autoimmune condition that is associated with thrombocytopenia, such as systemic lupus erythematosus (SLE) or the antiphospholipid antibody syndrome. In the second half of pregnancy, pre-eclampsia and HELLP (hemolysis, elevated liver enzymes, low platelets) should be excluded by assessing maternal blood pressure, testing for proteinuria and measuring aspartate aminotransferase (AST), alanine aminotransferase (ALT), creatinine and urate. While a number of women will enter pregnancy with a known diagnosis of a platelet disorder, pregnancy will often provide the first opportunity for diagnosis of these important clinical problems.

Gestational thrombocytopenia versus ITP

Differentiation of gestational thrombocytopenia from ITP can be problematic as there is no diagnostic test for ITP (Table 2.5). The degree of thrombocytopenia may be helpful in diagnosis as in gestational thrombocytopenia the platelet count is usually in the range of 100–150$\times$$10^9$/L and a platelet count of <80 $\times$ 10^9/L is unlikely to be due to gestational thrombocytopenia. A platelet count of <80 $\times$ 10^9/L is strongly suggestive of ITP but a platelet count >80 $\times$ 10^9/L does not exclude a diagnosis of ITP. The original promise of platelet-associated antibodies and serum platelet antibodies as diagnostic tests for ITP has not been realized. They are neither sensitive nor specific for ITP and are not a recommended part of investigations. The infants of all women with low platelets in pregnancy should have a platelet count measured on a cord blood.

Relevance of thrombocytopenia in pregnancy in a general obstetric population

In two population studies [38,39] thrombocytopenia was diagnosed as "gestational" in 77.3% of women, as a result of ITP in 3.5% of women and occurring in association with pre-eclampsia or HELLP in 18.5%. Both studies determined the prevalence of neonatal thrombocytopenia by measuring platelet counts from cord blood samples. Sainio and co-workers

[38] reported platelet counts of <150 $\times$ 10^9/L in 2% (n = 89) of 3944 infants where cord blood samples were taken; 0.7% (n = 33) of infants had platelet counts of <100 $\times$ 10^9/L and 0.24% (n = 17) had platelet counts of <50 $\times$ 10^9/L. Maternal thrombocytopenia did not predict the development of thrombocytopenia in the infants, with low platelets detected in 2.1% of infants (6 of 292) born to women with thrombocytopenia and 2% of infants (73 of 3653) born to women without thrombocytopenia.

Burrows & Kelton [39] used a platelet level of <50 $\times$ 10^9/L to identify significant neonatal thrombocytopenia and reported this degree of thrombocytopenia in 19 out of 15,932 infants (0.12%). An analysis of the relationship between neonatal and maternal thrombocytopenia reported that only three of 19 infants with cord blood platelets <50 $\times$ 10^9/L were born to mothers with platelet counts of <100 $\times$ 10^9/L. It is important to remember that in a general obstetric population, where gestational thrombocytopenia accounts for the majority of women with low platelets in pregnancy, 99% of women with a platelet count of <150 $\times$ 10^9/L at delivery will have an infant with platelets of >50 $\times$ 10^9/L and even for women with platelet counts of <100 $\times$ 10^9/L, 98.3% will have an infant with platelets of >50 $\times$ 10^9/L. Thus, detection of maternal thrombocytopenia defined as platelet count of <150 $\times$ 10^9/L does not help identify which infants will have severe thrombocytopenia. Invasive antenatal testing such as PUBS and fetal scalp vein sampling to determine the degree of thrombocytopenia in the infants of women with thrombocytopenia in pregnancy is not therefore recommended. Whether it is possible to identify a subgroup where antenatal testing is recommended is discussed below.

Specific causes of thrombocytopenia: immune-mediated thrombocytopenia

Immune-mediated thrombocytopenia is a common disorder in adults, with an incidence of around 50–60 new cases per million population per year, and women of childbearing age account for the majority of cases. It is not uncommon therefore for a woman to enter pregnancy with a known diagnosis of ITP or to develop *de novo* ITP during pregnancy itself.

Unlike in children, in whom the disorder invariably presents and resolves rapidly following a viral disorder, ITP in adults is commonly a chronic disorder that often presents with no preceding viral illness. Presenting symptoms include bruising, epistaxis, gum bleeding or a petechial rash, although more significant hemorrhage can occur; however, increasingly, asymptomatic patients are diagnosed when routine blood tests reveal a low platelet count. Spontaneous bleeding is unusual with platelet counts $>20 \times 10^9/L$.

Immune-mediated thrombocytopenia is an autoimmune disorder caused by development of IgG autoantibodies that are directed against a number of platelet glycoproteins. Antibody-bound platelets are rapidly cleared from the maternal circulation once they bind to specific antibody receptors on macrophages, mainly found in the spleen but also in the liver. The bone marrow usually responds by increasing megakaryocyte platelet production but in affected patients, even increased production is insufficient to maintain platelet counts within the normal range.

Diagnosis

The diagnostic approach to ITP in a pregnant woman does not differ from that of a nonpregnant patient. A diagnosis of ITP is reached after exclusion of other potential causes of thrombocytopenia using clinical history and examination, analysis of the CBC and peripheral blood smear. Additional laboratory tests include investigation of possible autoimmune disorders, and exclusion of HIV is important. In patients under the age of 60 years, bone marrow biopsy is not routinely recommended unless there are atypical features [40]. The initial promise of diagnostic tests for ITP looking for either platelet-associated antibodies or serum platelet antibodies has not been realized. Tests to detect platelet-associated IgG antibodies, although sensitive, lack the specificity to be diagnostically helpful. Platelet-bound IgG is frequently present in thrombocytopenia that is not thought to have an immune origin and the tests are unable to distinguish between pathologic and nonpathologic antibodies. False-negative results with platelet-associated antibodies are reported in 34–50% of patients and false-positive results in 8–22%. Serum platelet antibodies are even less helpful. Tests that look for antibodies directed at platelet glycoproteins, i.e. monoclonal antibody immobilization of platelet antibodies (MAIPA), are more specific, with a false-positive rate of only 7–22% but are insufficiently sensitive (49–66%) to exclude a diagnosis of ITP if the test is negative [41]. Platelet antibody testing is therefore not recommended in the diagnosis of ITP.

Treatment

First-line treatment of adult ITP is with tapered doses of corticosteroids (prednisone 1 mg/kg daily), effective in around 80% of patients. Splenectomy is reserved for those patients who either do not respond or who do not maintain a response

---

Box 2.3 Practice point: management of severe or refractory thrombocytopenia in pregnancy

Don't panic – remember that maternal bleeding risk is low even with platelet count $<20 \times 10^9/L$.

A maintenance dose of corticosteroids of around 10 mg daily often improves mucocutaneous bleeding, i.e. development of fresh or "wet" purpura and mucous membrane bleeding, even if it causes no increase in the platelet count.

Box 2.4 Practice point: management of severe hemorrhage in ITP

Transfuse platelets: 2 adult doses (typically "12 units" in the US) – platelets will last only a short time in maternal circulation but should be sufficient to help with hemostasis.

IVIG (1 mg/kg daily for 2 days) provides more rapid increase in maternal platelet count than corticosteroids.

---

to prednisone. Intravenous immunoglobulin (IVIG) can also be used, but in adults its response is usually short-lived, lasting around 2–4 weeks. A number of other therapeutic agents including anti-D, vincristine, dexamethasone and danazol, have been used to treat adult ITP, with varying success rates [42].

Effect of pregnancy on ITP

Immune-mediated thrombocytopenia accounts for 3–4% of the cases of thrombocytopenia detected in pregnancy. There are no data to suggest that pregnancy *per se* alters the natural course of ITP by increasing antibody production. However, given the increase in platelet turnover that occurs in pregnancy, it seems plausible that the bone marrow may struggle to compensate for this increased turnover and that this may lead to a lower platelet count than outside pregnancy.

Effect of ITP on pregnancy

Major clinical concerns when managing ITP in pregnancy include the following.

Risk of thrombocytopenia in the infant
- How commonly does it occur?
- Can we predict which infants will develop clinically important thrombocytopenia?
- Is antenatal assessment of fetal platelet count required?
- What is the risk of clinically severe bleeding *in utero* and/or during delivery and is this modified by mode of delivery?

Risk of maternal bleeding as a result of thrombocytopenia

• What platelet level is safe during pregnancy to prevent spontaneous bleeding?

• Should a diagnosis of ITP influence mode of delivery?

• What platelet level is safe for delivery either vaginally or via cesarean section?

• At what platelet level can regional anesthesia safely be used?

Complications of thrombocytopenia in the infant

The autoantibodies responsible for ITP can passively diffuse across the placenta. Being directed against platelet glycoproteins that are common to maternal and fetal platelets, these IgG antibodies can therefore induce thrombocytopenia in the fetus. Our review of 10 studies [35,43–51] of 600 pregnancies in 469 women with known ITP reported neonatal thrombocytopenia, i.e. platelets $<150 \times 10^9$/L, in a mean of 28% of infants (range 12.9–56.3%) with severe thrombocytopenia, i.e. platelets $<50 \times 10^9$/L occurring in 11% (range 4.9–20.5%) (Table 2.6). Intracranial hemorrhage (ICH), the most feared complication of neonatal thrombocytopenia, was reported in seven infants, accounting for 1.2% of births, although in at least two of the infants there were other significant risk factors for ICH.

Many investigators have attempted to determine methods that can predict which infants of women with ITP will develop severe thrombocytopenia. It is well recognized that the maternal platelet count at delivery is not predictive of neonatal platelet count. This is not surprising as women with marked thrombocytopenia will usually have been treated during pregnancy and especially close to delivery to increase the platelet count. While the degree of thrombocytopenia at delivery is not helpful, a study by Valat and co-workers [49] showed that women with more severe thrombocytopenia, identified as those with a platelet nadir of $<50 \times 10^9$/L during pregnancy, were more likely to have an infant with severe thrombocytopenia at birth, i.e. platelets $<50 \times 10^9$/l. The risk of neonatal thrombocytopenia was further increased if the women had severe thrombocytopenia and had a prior splenectomy, which again is a marker of more significant maternal disease. Severe neonatal thrombocytopenia was not reported in any of the women with ITP whose platelet count during pregnancy had remained above 50×10^9/L and who had not had a prior splenectomy. Of note, women who have had a splenectomy for ITP may still have circulating antiplatelet antibodies that can cross the placenta. It is important to ensure that a cord blood is done in the infants of these women.

The study by Samuels and co-workers [47] provoked a move to using the presence of circulating antiplatelet antibodies to recommend delivery by cesarean section because of their ability to predict which women with ITP were at risk of having infants with severe thrombocytopenia. Circulating antiplatelet antibodies were positive in 70 of 88 women with a diagnosis of ITP prior to pregnancy and 46 of 74 women with ITP diagnosed in the index pregnancy. Neonatal thrombocytopenia was reported in a total of 38 infants, 35 to women with previously diagnosed ITP and only three with newly diagnosed ITP. Circulating antiplatelet antibodies were present in all 35 women with previously diagnosed ITP who had infants with thrombocytopenia and no woman in this group without circulating antiplatelet antibodies had an infant with thrombocytopenia. In the group of women with ITP diagnosed in the index pregnancy, two of the three infants with thrombocytopenia were born to women with circulating antiplatelet antibodies. This lead the authors to conclude that detection of circulating antiplatelet antibodies could identify women with ITP who were at risk of having an infant with thrombocytopenia and who would potentially benefit from treatment, PUBS or operative delivery. Improved understanding

Table 2.6 Summary of neonatal thrombocytopenia in studies of maternal ITP in pregnancy

Study author	Pregnancies (women) n	Infants, n	Neonatal thrombocytopenia, n (%)			Neonatal ICH, n
			Platelets <150	Platelets 50–100	Platelets <50	
Kaplan[35]	33 (33)	33	11 (33.3)	-	4 (21.1)	0
Samuels[47]	88 (88)	88		17 (19.3)	18 (20.5)	2
Burrows[44]	60 (50)	61	9 (14.8)	3 (4.9)	3 (4.9)	0
Yamada[51]	52 (52)	54		8 (14.8)	4 (7.4)	0
Sharon[48]	72 (46)	72	-	18 (25)	11 (15.3)	1
Al-Mofada[43]	26 (26)	32	18 (56.3)	14 (43.8)	4 (12.5)	0
Payne[46]	55 (41)	55	14 (25.5)	-	4 (7.3)	1
Moutet[45]	37 (36)	37	4 (12.9)	1 (3.2)	3 (9.7)	1
Valat[49]	64 (57)	64	16 (25)	4 (6.3)	8 (12.5)	0
Webert[50]	119 (92)	109	31 (28.4)		11 (10.1)	2
Mean incidence neonatal thrombocytopenia			28.0%	16.8%	11.2%	7 (1.2%)

ICH, intracranial hemorrhage.

about poor specificity of antiplatelet antibody tests [52] and the recognition that delivery by cesarean section does not influence the risk of intracranial hemorrhage in infants with thrombocytopenia from any cause have led to a reduction in the influence of this study on clinical practice.

Currently, testing of maternal platelet antibodies is not recommended in the diagnostic work-up of thrombocytopenia in pregnancy nor does it play a role in predicting which women with ITP are at risk of having an infant with severe thrombocytopenia. The most useful factor in predicting the severity of neonatal thrombocytopenia is a history of severe thrombocytopenia in a previous sibling. Christiaens and co-workers [53] reported a strong correlation between the cord blood platelet count and the platelet count nadir in consecutive siblings of women with ITP.

Percutaneous umbilical blood sampling and fetal scalp vein sampling are no longer recommended as measures to determine the presence and degree of neonatal thrombocytopenia in infants of women with ITP. This is because of the relatively low probability of severe thrombocytopenia but, more importantly, the very low risk of clinically significant bleeding in the infant and the risks to the infant of the procedures themselves. Moreover, detection of severe thrombocytopenia should not influence the mode of delivery as there is no evidence that the risk of intracranial hemorrhage in infants with severe thrombocytopenia is reduced by avoiding vaginal delivery by carrying out elective cesarean section.

Maternal issues

The risk of spontaneous bleeding in patients with ITP, including pregnant women, is low. In a retrospective chart review of 92 women with ITP in pregnancy from a single center [50], the majority of women had no symptoms of hemostatic impairment during pregnancy. Mild symptoms such as easy bruising and purpura were reported in 12.9% of pregnancies (n = 15); epistaxis, bleeding after trauma or mucous membrane bleeding was reported in 18.1% of pregnancies (n = 21) with severe bleeding reported in four women (two had hematuria, one had hematoma formation and one had gastrointestinal bleeding). The authors reported that no woman required hospitalization as a result of bleeding.

In asymptomatic, nonpregnant patients, a platelet count $<20 \times 10^9$/L is the threshold below which hospitalization and treatment are recommended. In pregnancy, this threshold has somewhat arbitrarily been raised to a platelet count $<30 \times 10^9$/L in the antenatal period. The reason for this higher target platelet level is not evidence based but is presumably driven by the potential risk of massive bleeding should hemorrhage from the placental bed occur. After 34 weeks gestation, in women in whom vaginal delivery is anticipated, a platelet count $>50 \times 10^9$/L is recommended in preparation for delivery. This platelet level should also be sufficient for adequate hemostasis in the event of an emergency cesarean

section but most anesthetists are reluctant to use regional anesthesia unless the platelet count is $>80–100 \times 10^9$/L so that if elective cesarean section is planned the target platelet count is usually $80–100 \times 10^9$/L. What constitutes a safe platelet level for pregnancy and delivery has not been determined. The study by Webert and co-workers is reassuring in that although 17 women had platelet counts of $<50 \times 10^9$/L at the time of delivery, bleeding complications were uncommon and not related to the degree of thrombocytopenia [50].

Treatment

Both clinicians and patients are likely to be more reassured if target platelet counts can be achieved. A scheme for treatment of ITP is outlined in Figure 2.5, and Figure 2.6 summarizes aspects of individual therapies. First-line treatment is usually with corticosteroids at a dose of 1 mg/kg daily, usually given at this high dose for 7–10 days and then gradually tapered to keep the platelet count above the desired threshold. Prednisone is metabolized by the placenta so has minimal fetal effects but corticosteroid treatment in pregnancy increases the risk of gestational diabetes, hypertension, maternal infection and preterm delivery and so the lowest possible dose should be aimed for, preferably <10 mg daily. The majority of patients will respond to corticosteroids but some women require relatively high doses to maintain a platelet count above the desired level. Azathioprine is a steroid-sparing agent that can be used in pregnancy in conjunction with corticosteroids in women with refractory ITP. Outside pregnancy, splenectomy is the next treatment of choice for patients who either do not respond to corticosteroids or who require very high doses to maintain platelet counts. In pregnancy, laparoscopic splenectomy has been safely carried out, mainly in the second trimester.

Intravenous immunoglobulin (IVIG) provides effective but temporary improvements in the platelet count in a number of patients who do not respond to corticosteroids. Its mechanism of action is thought to be to swamp the IgG Fc receptors of macrophages, principally in the spleen. The recommended dose is 1 g/kg (pre-pregnancy maternal weight) given daily for 2 days and is effective in about 80% of patients. However, the duration of effect is variable, usually lasting about 2–4 weeks, and IVIG is expensive and time-consuming to administer. It does produce a more rapid increase in the platelet count and should be given in preference to corticosteroids for women with moderate or severe bleeding symptoms or who have a platelet count $<10 \times 10^9$/L. Repeated doses of IVIG can be given but after multiple doses the IVIG effect may become attenuated, perhaps because a consistently high level of immunoglobulin upregulates its natural clearance mechanism from the maternal circulation. In practice, if this occurs, a break from treatment for a few weeks often allows the IVIG to be effective once more. Despite early claims to the contrary, neither prednisone nor IVIG has any effect on the fetal platelet count.

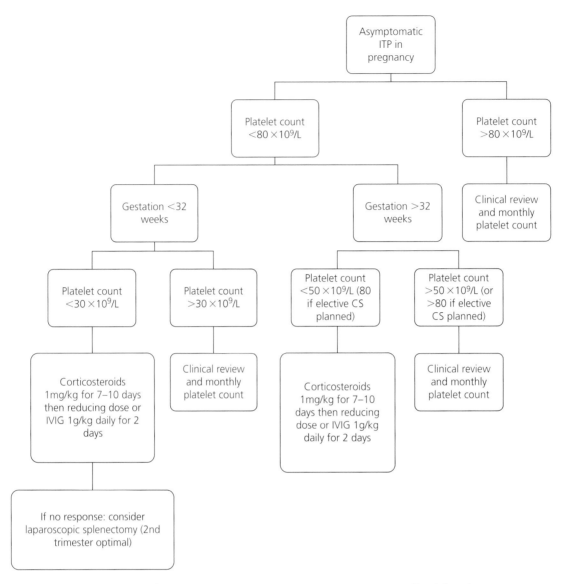

Figure 2.5 Management of ITP in pregnancy. CS, cesarean section; ITP, immune-mediated thrombocytopenia; IVIG, intravenous immunoglobulin.

High-dose methylprednisone, 1 g given intravenously, is a potential agent in women who do not respond to these measures. Dexamethasone, 40 mg daily for 4 days, has been used with good effect as first-line treatment of ITP outside pregnancy but crosses the placenta and will have fetal effects. Other agents such as vincristine and danazol are best avoided in pregnancy.

Immune-mediated thrombocytopenia is an autoimmune disorder mediated by antibodies produced by B lymphocytes. Rituxumab is a monoclonal antibody therapy developed for treatment of lymphomas of B cell origin that specifically targets B cells and, in the nonpregnant population, its use is increasingly being explored in treatment of resistant autoimmune conditions including ITP [54]. Although it is reportedly effective in resistant ITP, it should be used with caution in pregnancy as it crosses the placenta and has been shown to cause temporary suppression of B lymphocytes and the long-term effect of this on development of the infant's immune system is not clear.

Delivery

Mode of delivery should be determined by obstetric indications. Most women with ITP in pregnancy will have babies with normal platelet counts but even where the platelet count is low, delivery by cesarean section has not been shown to reduce the risk of intracranial hemorrhage. Given the potential risk of bleeding if an infant is thrombocytopenic, it is generally recommended that vacuum-assisted delivery is avoided although

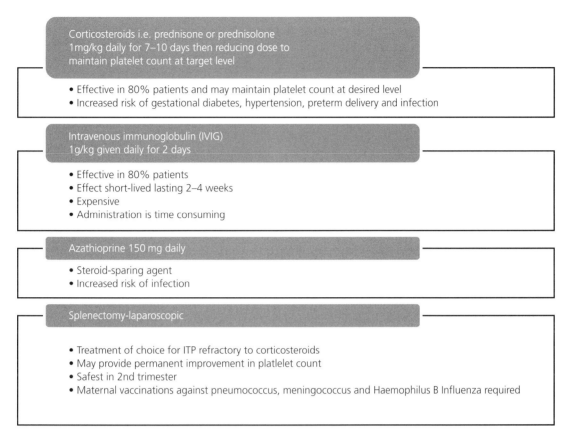

Corticosteroids i.e. prednisone or prednisolone
1mg/kg daily for 7–10 days then reducing dose to
maintain platelet count at target level

- Effective in 80% patients and may maintain platelet count at desired level
- Increased risk of gestational diabetes, hypertension, preterm delivery and infection

Intravenous immunoglobulin (IVIG)
1g/kg given daily for 2 days

- Effective in 80% patients
- Effect short-lived lasting 2–4 weeks
- Expensive
- Administration is time consuming

Azathioprine 150 mg daily

- Steroid-sparing agent
- Increased risk of infection

Splenectomy-laparoscopic

- Treatment of choice for ITP refractory to corticosteroids
- May provide permanent improvement in platlelet count
- Safest in 2nd trimester
- Maternal vaccinations against pneumococcus, meningococcus and Haemophilus B Influenza required

Figure 2.6 Therapeutic agents recommended for management of ITP in pregnancy.

this recommendation is not supported by strong clinical data. In women with known ITP, monthly platelet counts are recommended but the frequency of testing should be increased if the degree of thrombocytopenia worsens (see Figure 2.5). Women who maintain a platelet count $>50 \times 10^9/$ L will not require treatment to increase their platelet count unless there is anticipation of the need for regional anesthesia, such as a planned delivery by cesarean section. Some centers will treat platelet counts of $<80 \times 10^9/$L for patients desiring an epidural for pain control with a vaginal delivery. Women who have maintained a platelet count between 30 and $50 \times 10^9/$L in the antenatal period should be offered a trial of corticosteroids at around 30–32 weeks gestation to allow time for a trial of IVIG should steroids prove ineffective.

Anesthetic management

While platelets are an integral component of coagulation, they are just one indicator of a patient's coagulation status. During spinal or epidural placement, venepuncture occurs in up to 20% of patients [55,56]. In the presence of thrombocytopenia or other coagulopathy, trauma within the epidural or spinal space can result in neuraxial hematoma formation. Although reports of spinal/epidural hematoma are rare, this complication can result in permanent neurologic injury [57,58].

Anesthesiologists have attempted to answer the longstanding question, "What is the lowest acceptable platelet count for spinal or epidural anesthesia without risking epidural hematoma?" The actual platelet count safe for neuraxial needle placement is unknown. Although an arbitrary platelet count of $100 \times 10^9/$L is often suggested prior to spinal or epidural needle placement, there are no outcome data suggesting that lower counts are associated with increased complications. To definitely determine whether it is safe to place a neuraxial anesthetic in patients with platelet counts less than 80 or $100 \times 10^9/$L, large prospective studies would be required. The American Society of Anesthesiologists practice guidelines on obstetric anesthesia state that a specific platelet count predictive of neuraxial anesthetic complications has not been determined [59]. The anesthesiologist's decision to order or require a platelet count should be individualized and based on a patient's history, physical examination, and clinical signs. A routine platelet count is unnecessary in the healthy parturient [59].

The widespread belief that the risk of epidural hematoma formation is increased with platelet counts of less than $100 \times 10^9/$L is based on a study correlating platelet counts and bleeding times [60]. However, bleeding time has been abandoned in many institutions because of its failure to predict surgical bleeding. Reviews of the literature demonstrate that there are no existing data to support the bleeding time's ability to predict adequacy of hemostasis [61]. If there is obvious evidence of clinical bleeding, e.g. petechiae, ecchymoses, other coagulation tests may be indicated to exclude disseminated intravascular coagulation. If the platelet count is greater than 100×10^9/L and there is no evidence of clinical bleeding, it is unlikely that the prothrombin time (PT) or activated partial thromboplastin time (APPT) will be prolonged. In a study of pre-eclamptic patients without evidence of hemorrhage or abruption but with platelet counts less than 100×10^9/L, there were no other abnormal coagulation tests, i.e. PT, partial thromboplastin time (PTT), fibrinogen. However, many centers would recommend obtaining these tests when possible prior to caesarean delivery in any pre-eclamptic patient with thrombocytopenia [62].

Several studies have tried to assess the risk of epidural hematoma when the platelet count was between 50 and 100×10^9/L. In two retrospective reports, there were no complications when the platelet count was less than 100×10^9/L [63,64]. Similarly, in a study of 24 patients with thrombocytopenia and regional anesthesia, there were no complications when the platelet count was less than 100×10^9/L [65]. Beilin *et al.* reported a case series of 30 patients with platelet counts 69–98×10^9/L over a 3-year period who had received epidural anesthesia without complications [66]. However, a more difficult situation is the patient who has significant decreases in platelet count over a short time-period, e.g. 150×10^9/L to 100×10^9/L. In fact, neuraxial anesthesia may be contraindicated in some patients when there is evidence of a dynamic consumptive process. Administration of regional anesthesia in these patients is dependent on clinical judgment. The very low likelihood of epidural hematoma must be weighed against the benefits of regional anesthesia.

Besides the platelet count, other tests of coagulation (e.g. thromboelastography (TEG) and the platelet function analyzer (PFA-100)) have also been used to assess platelet function and coagulation in patients with thrombocytopenia. Despite their simplicity, further studies are needed to determine their ability to predict risk of epidural hematoma formation in patients with thrombocytopenia. The choice of anesthetic technique in pregnant women with thrombocytopenia depends on the planned method of delivery, coagulation status, history of recent or current bleeding, associated co-morbidities and the entire clinical picture.

Management of infants in neonatal period

All infants born to women with ITP should have a cord blood taken to check the platelet count. Infants who are destined to develop thrombocytopenia usually manifest low platelet counts at time of delivery. The platelet count nadir usually occurs about 4–7 days post delivery with platelet counts increasing after about 10–14 days. Most pediatricians and neonatologists would treat asymptomatic infants with platelet counts $<20 \times 10^9$/L but parents and clinicians should be

---

Box 2.5 Helpful hint: ITP or NAIT?

A frequent source of confusion for clinicians seems to be the clinical implications to the fetus of maternal ITP and that of neonatal alloimmune thrombocytopenia (NAIT). NAIT is the platelet equivalent of Rh disease and is caused by development of a maternal alloantibody that reacts with the fetal platelets leading to, often profound, thrombocytopenia that is associated with a high risk of fetal intracranial hemorrhage. Of note, there is even a move away from elective cesarean section in pregnancies severely affected by NAIT given our current understanding of the limited impact of mode of delivery on development of fetal intracranial hemorrhage. The maternal platelet count in NAIT is usually normal unless there is co-existent gestational thrombocytopenia or ITP.

---

reassured of the relatively low bleeding risk and spontaneous resolution of the thrombocytopenia. IVIG is usually first-line treatment for symptomatic thrombocytopenic infants but platelet transfusions can also be given. For severely affected infants, either those with profound thrombocytopenia or those with clinically severe bleeding, the parents should be tested to exclude the rare possibility of co-existent neonatal alloimmune thrombocytopenia (NAIT).

Other platelet disorders

May–Hegglin anomaly

The May–Hegglin anomaly is an autosomal dominant disorder marked by thrombocytopenia where the peripheral blood smear shows morphologically normal large platelets but characteristic inclusion bodies in white blood cells. There is no abnormality of platelet function and the variable bleeding tendency reported is thought to relate to the degree of thrombocytopenia. The risk of bleeding during pregnancy, at delivery and post partum is low. Mode of delivery should be determined by obstetric indications. Neither corticosteroids nor IVIG will affect the maternal platelet count and should not be given. Prophylactic platelet transfusion should not be required but platelets should be on standby in case of bleeding [67]. As it is an autosomal dominant disorder, 50% of infants will be affected and have a low platelet count but again the platelets will be functionally normal and platelet transfusions should only be given for clinically significant bleeding.

Bernard–Soulier syndrome

The Bernard–Soulier syndrome is a rare autosomal recessive disorder characterized by thrombocytopenia and clinically significant bleeding symptoms that are usually out of keeping with the degree of thrombocytopenia [68]. The peripheral blood smear shows morphologically normal large platelets and the platelets are functionally abnormal with defects in the platelet glycoprotein, GPIb-V-IXa, responsible for platelet adhesion to collagen in vessel walls, an essential first step in primary hemostasis. The diagnosis can be made by demonstrating absence of platelet agglutination to ristocetin (an antibiotic that normally causes platelet agglutination *in vitro*). Patients with Bernard–Soulier syndrome usually develop symptoms early in life and in women severe menorrhagia from the time of menarche is common. The risk of bleeding during pregnancy in affected women is low but there is an increased risk of postpartum hemorrhage [69,70]. Again, the mode of delivery should be determined by obstetric indications and prophylactic platelet transfusions are not recommended but platelets should be available in case of bleeding. Regional anesthesia is generally not provided to these patients. Active management of the third stage of labor with prompt administration of oxytocic agents immediately following delivery of the baby is essential to reduce the risk of postpartum hemorrhage. It is unlikely that the infant will be affected as this is a rare autosomal recessive disorder but the risk should be borne in mind in a consanguineous relationship.

Glanzmann's thrombasthenia

Glanzmann's thrombasthenia (GT) is a rare autosomal recessive disorder characterized by severe bleeding due to quantitative or qualitative abnormalities in the platelet membrane glycoprotein complex IIb-IIIa (GPIIb-IIIa). Type 1 GT describes a complete absence of GPIIb-IIIa while in type 2 the glycoproteins are present at 10–20% normal levels. Patients usually present early in life with mucocutaneous bleeding, epistaxis and gingival hemorrhages, with women experiencing severe menorrhagia usually present from menarche [71]. Confirmation of the disorder requires demonstration of a long bleeding time; absent platelet aggregation to the agonists adenosine diphosphate (ADP), adrenaline, thrombin and collagen; defective clot retraction; and flow cytometry studies demonstrating an absence or reduction in platelet glycoproteins using specific monoclonal antibodies [72]. Platelet number and morphology are normal. The bleeding risk cannot be predicted by clinical history or laboratory tests so care is mainly supportive to enable sufficient hemostasis in the event of bleeding. For more minor bleeds antifibrinolytic agents such as tranexamic acid can be given. Platelet transfusions were, for a long time, the only option for treatment of severe bleeds but carry the risk of formation of alloantibodies to platelet glycoproteins that leads to refractoriness to platelet transfusions. More recently, recombinant FVIIa has been successfully used in patients with severe bleeding or who are refractory to platelet transfusions. The optimal dose of rFVIIa for this indication has not been determined but generally doses of 90 μg/kg are recommended but lower doses have been used successfully, including in pregnancy [73].

Glanzmann's thrombasthenia and pregnancy

Pregnancy itself has no direct effect on platelet function in women with GT. While the risk of bleeding during pregnancy does not appear to be increased, there is a significant risk of major hemorrhage immediately following delivery and in the postpartum period. As in nonpregnant patients, treatment options include human leukocyte antigen (HLA)-matched platelet transfusions with or without recombinant FVIIa and antifibrinolytic agents. It should be recognized that even with these measures, the risk of bleeding remains high. As Glanzmann's is an autosomal recessive disorder, the infant will only be affected if the father is heterozygous for a GPIIb-IIIa mutation.

Bleeding disorders

Pregnancy, and in particular childbirth, pose an enormous hemostatic challenge to any woman. When faced with a pregnant woman with a known bleeding disorder, most obstetricians are justifiably concerned. How will the bleeding disorder affect this woman during pregnancy, at delivery and in the postpartum period? What are the risks to the fetus or infant in the neonatal period? What specific management is required? Should any procedures be avoided?

During pregnancy and in preparation for childbirth, the body responds by inducing a hypercoagulable state. This effect on the hemostatic system means that for the majority of women with bleeding disorders, pregnancy and childbirth are not associated with a significant bleeding risk and with prior knowledge of the disorder, clinicians can be vigilant at times when hemorrhagic risk is present. Some disorders will not be corrected by the hypercoagulable state induced by pregnancy and require specific measures to prevent maternal and fetal bleeding complications, especially at the time of delivery.

This section will discuss how inherited and acquired bleeding disorders are affected by pregnancy, which of the disorders are clinically important in pregnancy, and the management of women with bleeding disorders during pregnancy and at delivery. Potential risks to the fetus and infant will also be addressed.

Antenatal assessment for possible bleeding disorders

In a significant number of cases, a definitive diagnosis of a bleeding disorder will not have been made prior to pregnancy. A woman's personal bleeding history and any family history should be recorded at the first antenatal visit. Symptoms such as frequent easy bruising, especially without injury, bleeding following dental work or surgery, gingival bleeding and menorrhagia, especially when it leads to iron deficiency, are reported more frequently in women with a defect in hemostasis. Other symptoms such as epistaxis, hematuria or rectal bleeding may not be as discriminatory. Laboratory studies of coagulation including a CBC, APTT, prothrombin ratio (PR) and possibly a bleeding time or PFA-100 (see below) are indicated in women who report symptoms suggestive of a bleeding disorder. Further testing will be guided by the results of these tests and will often include specific investigations for von Willebrand's diease (discussed below) [74].

Von Willebrand's disease

Von Willebrand's disease (VWD) is the most common inherited bleeding disorder, affecting about 1% of the population, and marked by either a quantitative or qualitative deficiency in von Willebrand factor (VWF). VWF plays a key role in primary hemostasis by facilitating platelet adherence to damaged subendothelium, platelet–platelet interaction and binding of platelets to fibrinogen. A second role of VWF is to act as a carrier protein for clotting factor VIII (FVIII), protecting FVIII from proteolysis and thus prolonging its half-life in the circulation.

Von Willebrand factor is synthesized by endothelial cells and also in the bone marrow by platelet precursors, i.e. megakaryocytes. Pro-VWF first forms dimers that are then assembled into variably sized high molecular weight multimers that are secreted or stored in Weibel–Palade bodies (an organelle) of endothelial cells and in platelet α-granules. The highest molecular weight multimers play the most important role in adherence of VWF to the subendothelial cells, platelets and fibrinogen.

Quantitative or qualitative deficiencies in VWF can be caused by mutations or deletions in the VWF gene on chromosome 12. In addition, it has more recently been accepted that abnormalities in the cellular processing of VWF or increased degradation of VWF can also lead to a clinical phenotype of VWD. The updated classification of VWD [75] concentrates on laboratory tests that identify the VWF protein phenotype and subdivides VWD (Table 2.7).

- *Type 1 VWD*: a partial quantitative deficiency of VWF with functional activity of VWF proportional to the level of VWF antigen. Accounts for ~70–80% of VWD.
- *Type 2 VWD*: a qualitative deficiency of VWF further subclassified into 2A, 2B, 2M and 2N, reflecting specific functional abnormalities.
- *Type 3 VWD*: characterized by almost complete absence of VWF.

In VWD, the deficiency or defect in VWF impacts upon primary hemostasis, causing problems with mucocutaneous bleeding, such as frequent spontaneous bruising or epistaxis. Menorrhagia is a frequent symptom in women and postsurgical bleeding or bleeding following dental extraction is common. Spontaneous muscle bleeds or hemarthroses that can be seen in patients with hemophilia are rare. There is variable clinical expression of VWD even within the same family kindred.

In an individual with a bleeding history suggestive of a problem with primary hemostasis, especially if supported by a positive family history, laboratory tests to confirm a possible diagnosis of VWD are required (Table 2.8). A prolonged skin bleeding time is the classic laboratory test for a defect in primary hemostasis. In many centers this been superseded by an automated measurement of platelet function using a platelet function analyzer such as the PFA-100 because the bleeding time is neither sensitive nor specific. The PFA-100 is a combined measure of platelet aggregation and adhesion. It is an *in vitro* test that measures the time taken for blood, drawn through a fine capillary, to block a membrane coated with ADP, collagen and epinephrine. The result is measured in seconds and is reported as the closure time. PFA-100 has nearly a 100% sensitivity for VWD, in comparison to bleeding time which can be normal in 25–50% of patients with VWD.

More specific laboratory tests are reviewed in Table 2.9. VWD patients will typically demonstrate either a low level of the VWF antigen (VWF:Ag) or a low level of VWF activity, i.e. ristocetin co-factor assay (RiCoF) or collagen-binding assay (CBA), in conjunction with reduced levels of FVIII.

Table 2.7 Von Willebrand's disease subtypes

VWD subtype			Inheritance pattern
Type 1	Quantitative reduction in VWF		Autosomal dominant
Type 2	Functional abnormality of VWF		Autosomal dominant
	2A	Selective reduction high molecular weight multimers → reduced VWF-dependent platelet adhesion	
	2B	Increased affinity for platelet glycoprotein Ib	
	2M	Reduced VWF-dependent platelet adhesion with normal levels of high molecular weight multimers	
	2N	Reduced binding affinity for FVIII	
Type 3	Almost complete absence of VWF		Autosomal recessive

VWF, von Willebrand factor.

Table 2.8 Screening tests for detection of hemostatic defects

Category or test	Specific tests	Comments
Clinical history	Ask patient about whether they have or have had any of the following:	
	1. a blood relative with a history of a bleeding disorder	
	2. prolonged bleeding from a trivial injury that lasted longer than 15 minutes or recurred spontaneously over the next 7 days	
	3. heavy, prolonged or recurrent bleeding after a surgical procedure	
	4. bruising with minimal or no trauma, particularly that caused a lump under the skin	
	5. spontaneous nosebleeds that lasted longer than 10 minutes or required medical attention to stop	
	6. heavy prolonged bleeding after dental extractions that required medical attention	
	7. gastrointestinal bleeding not associated with any specific gastrointestinal lesion	
	8. anemia requiring treatment or transfusion	
	9. heavy periods, particularly that involved passing clots greater than 2.5 cm in length or the need to change tampons or pads on an hourly basis or that caused anemia	
Basic hematologic tests	CBC APTT PR	
Assessment of primary hemostasis (platelet function)	Skin bleeding time	Lacks both sensitivity and specificity. Results may vary considerably with technique
	PFA-100	Measures both platelet aggregationand adhesion and is highly sensitive for VWD
Standard tests for VWD	Factor VIII antigen (FVIII)	Measures the amount of FVIII in the serum. In the context of VWD, this assay measures the ability of VWF to bind and maintain circulating FVIII
	VWF antigen (VWF:Ag)	Measures the amount of VWF protein in the serum
	VWF ristocetin co-factor activity (VWF:RCoA or RiCoF)	Measures the ability of VWF to interact with normal platelets
Other available tests for VWD	Collagen-binding assay (VWF:CB or CBA)	This test has a less well-established role in the initial diagnosis of VWD than the three tests listed above. It assesses the ability of VWF to bind to collagen. In some cases of VWD VWF:RCo will be normal and this test abnormal. The test may be helpful in distinguishing VWD type 1 from the subtypes of type 2
	Low-dose ristocetin platelet aggregation study	The ability of very low doses of ristocetin to cause platelet aggregation suggests type 2B VWD
	VWF:Ag/VWF:CBA ratio	Used to help distinguish between type 1 VWD and the subtypes of type 2 VWD

Ag, antigen; APTT, activated partial thromboplastin time; CB/CBA, collagen binding assay; CBC, complete blood count; PR, prothrombin ratio; RCoA/ RiCoF, ristocetin co-factor assay; VWD, von Willebrand's disease; VWF, von Willebrand factor.

A significant reduction in FVIII level will lead to a prolonged APTT (Table 2.9).

The diagnosis may not always be straightforward due to variations in VWF antigen levels. VWF antigen and activity levels are dependent on blood group with individuals who are blood group O having the lowest levels of VWF antigen and activity, followed by higher levels in groups A, B and the highest VWF levels in individuals with blood group AB. Some laboratories report blood group-dependent VWF normal ranges. Increases in VWF level can also be induced by stress, such as that of illness. Importantly, pregnancy-induced increases in VWF and FVIII make it difficult to diagnose type 1 VWD in pregnancy.

Table 2.9 Summary of laboratory results for diagnosis of VWD

	Test Von Willebrand's disease subtype					
	1	2A	2B	2M	2N	3
Platelet count	N	N	N or ↓	N	N	N
Bleeding time	N or ↑	N or ↑	N or ↑	N or ↑	N or ↑	N or ↑
PFA-100 closure time	↑	↑	↑	↑	N	↑
APTT	N or ↑	N or ↑	N or ↑	N or ↑	N or ↑	N or ↑
FVIII Ag	N or ↓	N or ↓	N or ↓	N	↓	↓↓
VWF Ag*	↓	N or ↓	↓	N or ↓	N or ↓	↓↓
RiCoF (RCoA) activity	↓	↓	↓	N or ↓	↓ or N	↓↓
Collagen-binding assay (CBA or VWF:CB)	↓ or N	↓↓	↓	N or ↓	N or ↓	↓↓
VWF Ag/CBA ratio	<2	>2	>2	<2	Variable	Not used
Low-dose RIPA	Absent	Absent	Present	Absent	Absent	Absent

VWF Ag, VWF antigenic level; VWF:RCoA or RiCoF, ristocetin co-factor activity, measure of functional activity of VWF; low-dose RIPA, ability of low doses of ristocetin to cause platelet aggregation.

Other disorders of primary hemostasis, such as platelet granule release defects, should be considered in the presence of clinical symptoms and an abnormal skin bleeding time or PFA-100 result and normal VWF tests if stress- or pregnancy-induced increases can be excluded.

Effect of pregnancy on VWD

Type 1 VWD

FVIII and VWF increase progressively throughout pregnancy so levels are within the normal range in most women with type 1 VWD. As a result, type 1 VWD does not cause bleeding complications in the majority of women. Levels of VWF and FVIII begin to rise from the 10th week of gestation and are maximal by 34 weeks gestation. The risk of intrapartum bleeding is thought to be low if VWF ristocetin co-factor activity levels are greater than 50 IU/dL and treatment to increase factor levels is not required. Levels return to those present pre-pregnancy in the first few days following delivery [76] and women with VWD have an increased risk of postpartum hemorrhage, especially delayed postpartum hemorrhage.

Type 2 VWD

Pregnancy-induced increases in VWF in women with type 2 VWD will lead to increased levels of the functionally abnormal VWF, so correction of the clinical phenotype may not occur. The increased levels of FVIII may help to ameliorate the bleeding risk but postpartum bleeding is more common in women with these subtypes of VWD than in type 1 VWD. Women with type 2B VWD may develop progressive and severe thrombocytopenia during pregnancy as pregnancy-induced increases in the abnormal VWF with its increased platelet affinity will accelerate platelet clearance [77].

Type 3 VWD

A clinically significant increase in VWF and FVIII levels is not reported in women with type 3 VWD.

Effect of VWD on pregnancy

The rate of spontaneous miscarriage in women with VWD is not thought to be higher than in women without the disorder. However, the incidence of bleeding following miscarriage and also termination of pregnancy in the first trimester is higher in women with VWD [78] as the pregnancy-induced increases in VWF and FVIII are unlikely to have occurred to any significant degree. The mode of delivery for women with VWD should be dictated by obstetric indications.

Management of VWD in pregnancy

The majority of women with VWD have an uncomplicated pregnancy and with close liaison between the obstetrician, hematologist and anesthesiologist, potential problems can be anticipated and prevented (Table 2.10). An approach to management of women with VWD is outlined in Figure 2.7. The risk of bleeding is thought to be low if VWF ristocetin co factor assay is >50 IU/dL. Below this level, treatment may be required to either prevent or treat bleeding problems such as early pregnancy bleeding or prior to invasive procedures, including CVS or amniocentesis. Measurement of VWF and FVIII levels at booking and then at 34 weeks gestation should be adequate for the majority of women if pregnancy is uncomplicated. If at 34 weeks levels of VWF or FVIII are less than 50 IU/dL, treatment to increase VWF and FVIII should be considered for delivery.

In the postpartum period, women with VWD should be watched for evidence of abnormal bleeding. The usual obstetric interventions should occur to prevent postpartum haemorrhage. Some centers would recommend measuring VWF ristocetin co-factor assay daily in the first 3–5 postpartum days and that the patient be treated if levels fall below 50 IU/dL. Since it may take up to 3 weeks for VWF levels to return

Table 2.10 Checklist for obstetric management of women with von Willebrand's disease (VWD)

1. Review VWF test results from prior to pregnancy and confirm VWD subtype
2. Obtain accurate bleeding history and prior response to DDAVP
3. VWF laboratory tests at booking
4. Arrange anesthesiology consult
5. Hematology consult especially if VWD other than type 1
6. Repeat VWF laboratory tests at 34 weeks gestation
   Treatment at delivery required if FVIII or VWF levels < 50 IU/dl
7. Ensure group and hold specimen for blood transfusion if required at delivery
8. Active management of 3rd stage of labor
9. Clinical vigilance for 1° or 2° postpartum hemorrhage. Consider monitoring of FVIII and VWF: Ag levels for first three days postpartum if patient required DDAVP or factor replacement for delivery

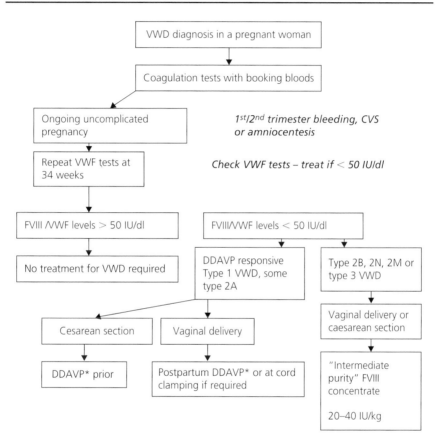

Figure 2.7 Management of pregnancy in women with VWD. *Repeat doses of DDAVP at 24-hour intervals may be required to ensure VWF levels are maintained following delivery. The majority of women require only two or three repeat doses. With repeat doses the DDAVP effect may be blunted and monitoring of factor levels may be helpful. CVS, chorionic villus sampling; DDAVP, 1-desmopressin-8-D-arginine vasopressin; VWD, von willebrand's disease; VWF, von willebrand factor.

to their pre-pregnancy levels, these patients should be told to watch for and report early any excessive bleeding or vaginal bruising in the weeks following delivery so that treatment can occur promptly.

1-Desmopressin-8-D-arginine vasopressin (DDAVP), a synthetic vasopressin agonist that promotes release of preformed VWF from storage bodies in endothelial cells, is effective in the majority of patients with type 1 VWD. It is used to increase VWF and FVIII levels in patients with type 1 VWD

and some patients with type 2 VWD. It can be administered intravenously or subcutaneously at a dose of 0.3 μg/kg or intranasally using 1–2 sprays of a 1.5 mg/mL preparation [79]. Peak levels of VWF and FVIII are reached within 30–60 minutes of intravenous administration and 60–120 minutes if given subcutaneously. Repeated doses of DDAVP given at 24-hour intervals are usually effective although the response may be blunted due to depletion of VWF stores. It is specific for V2 vasopressin receptors so does not cause uterine contraction or vasoconstriction that are mediated by V1 vasopressin receptors on smooth muscle. Side effects include mild tachycardia, facial flushing and headache that can be quite troublesome for some women. Antidiuretic effects of DDAVP (hyponatremia and volume overload) rarely cause maternal problems if fluid intake is restricted. In clinical practice fetal hyponatremia has not been reported [80].

1-Desmopressin-8-D-arginine vasopressin is ineffective in women with type 3 VWD and should be used with caution in women with type 2B VWD as it can cause profound thrombocytopenia by increasing release of the abnormal VWF and accelerating platelet clumping and destruction. It can be effective in women with type 2A VWD but shows variable efficacy in type 2N or 2M VWD.

Alternatives to DDAVP that allow direct replacement of VWF are cryoprecipitate and plasma-derived FVIII ("intermediate purity FVIII"). Cryoprecipitate carries a risk of blood-borne pathogens and its use in settings where alternatives exist is to be discouraged. Plasma-derived FVIII, so-called "intermediate purity FVIII," is marketed in the US in two different preparations: Humate-P and Alphanate SD/HT. These agents are both lyophilized concentrates of plasma-derived FVIII, VWF and other plasma proteins. The preparation of these products inactivates most viruses. They should be used as an alternative to DDAVP in women with type 3 and type 2B VWD, as well as known DDAVP nonresponders with type 1, 2A, 2N or 2M VWD. Doses are given intravenously and if repeated dosing is given, some experts would recommend monitoring FVIII and VWF levels to avoid overtreatment as the use of these agents has been associated with venous thromboembolism. More highly purified FVIII concentrates contain very little VWF and recombinant FVIII contains none and therefore these are not recommended for treatment of women with VWD.

Regional analgesia and anesthesia

Anesthesiologists will certainly encounter parturients with VWD since it is the most commonly inherited bleeding disorder. Although there are several case reports describing the safe administration of neuraxial analgesia for labor and delivery in patients with VWD [77,81–83], there are no clear guidelines for laboratory monitoring or indications for neuraxial or general anesthesia. The greatest anesthetic risk for parturients with VWD is spinal epidural hematoma, with the potential for permanent neurologic injury. In obstetric patients overall, the reported risk of such complications is around 1 in 200,000, with most cases occurring in patients with coagulopathy [58,84].

In patients with VWD, FVIII activity and FVIII ristocetin co-factor activity should be within the normal range before spinal or epidural needle placement [88]. The decision to administer a neuraxial technique should be individualized and made after phenotype identification, treatment planning, and careful evaluation. Central to this decision is whether the risk of general anesthesia outweighs the risk of neuraxial hematoma. Clinical judgment represents the most important means of assessing the risk for spinal epidural hematoma in an individual patient [89].

As mentioned previously, type 1 VWD patients are likely to demonstrate a good response to DDAVP. In these patients, DDAVP should be administered prior to neuraxial anesthesia to maintain VWF ristocetin co-factor assay levels >50 IU/dL. In cases where FVIII and VWF levels are inadequate or there is concern about risk of spinal epidural hematoma, patient-controlled analgesia (PCA) fentanyl is an alternative labor analgesic [85]. In cases where spinal or epidural anesthesia is contraindicated for cesarean delivery, general anesthesia will be required.

More challenges may be encountered in providing neuraxial analgesia/anesthesia in parturients with the other VWD subtypes. Although type 2A VWD patients may respond to DDAVP, type 2B VWD patients may respond with thrombocytopenia due to increased levels of abnormal VWF. Because patients with type 3 VWD have near absent levels of plasma, there will be no response to DDAVP. In cases unresponsive to DDAVP, Humate P or Alphanate SD/HT can be administered to increase levels of FVIII [86]. Administration of Humate P has been previously described for patients with VWD who were receiving neuraxial labor analgesia [81,87]. No complications were reported in either case. The use of neuraxial anesthesia in such patients should likely be limited to patients for whom documentation of normalization of VWF:Ag and FVIII levels can be demonstrated. General anesthesia is recommended in cases where neuraxial anesthesia is contraindicated [89].

Effects on the fetus

Von Willebrand's disease is usually inherited in an autosomal dominant pattern so that infants born to women with VWD have a 50% chance of having the disorder. Bleeding complications are rare during delivery of affected infants. Healthy neonates show elevated levels of VWF antigen [90], perhaps leading to a relative increase in VWF in infants affected by type 1 VWD. Increased numbers of very large VWF multimers are also reported in normal infants and may explain the moderate to severe thrombocytopenia that may be found in infants affected by type 2B VWD.

Elective delivery by cesarean section is not required, except for specific obstetric indications. Fetal scalp monitoring is not contraindicated in infants who may be affected by type 1 VWD but should not be used in cases where infants may be affected by type 2B or type 3 VWD. Instrumental delivery with low forceps is permissible and although neonatal bleeding is rare, delivery by Ventouse (vacuum) extraction or midcavity or rotational forceps delivery is not recommended. Prenatal testing, if available, is advocated only for severe cases.

Hemophilia

Hemophilia A and B are X-linked recessive bleeding disorders caused by mutations in the genes for factors VIII and IX, respectively, that result in reduced levels of blood clotting factors. As X-linked disorders, they predominantly manifest clinically in males, with the majority of affected females being carriers of the disorder. In most cases, the normal X chromosome in carrier women produces sufficient FVIII or IX so that overall clotting factor levels are at least 50 IU/dL (i.e. 50%). Extreme lyonization or inactivation of the normal X chromosome occurs in some women, resulting in low clotting factor levels. These women have symptoms similar to affected males with mild to moderate and rarely even severe hemophilia. Daughters of men with hemophilia A or B are obligate carriers of the disorder but sons are not affected. Female carriers of hemophilia A or B have a 50% chance of passing the abnormal X chromosome to their children, leading to hemophilia in their sons and carrier status in their daughters. The availability of plasma-derived and recombinant clotting factor concentrates has lead to improvements in quality of life and life expectancy in affected males, with an increase in the numbers of children and in particular carrier females born to men with hemophilia.

Increasingly obstetricians are faced with managing pregnancy in women who are carriers of severe hemophilia and whose male children may be affected. This has implications for issues related to prenatal testing, management of pregnancy and delivery. Of note, as many as 30% of cases of hemophilia are due to new mutations so that often neither maternal problems nor fetal complications can be anticipated.

Hemophilia A

Expected course through pregnancy

Pregnancy complications are not increased in the majority of women who are carriers of hemophilia A. FVIII levels steadily increase as gestation advances, usually reaching normal levels by the third trimester with maximal levels reached at around 34 weeks gestation. Hemophilia is an X-linked disorder so there is a 50% chance that male infants born to carrier women will have hemophilia. Some parents will choose to have prenatal testing to determine if their child is affected. Fetal sex can be determined by ultrasound and in the case of a male fetus, further testing with CVS or amniocentesis can be helpful if the causative mutation has been identified. Positive identification of an affected male infant by these techniques leaves parents with the difficult decision of whether to terminate the pregnancy. Measurement of maternal FVIII levels should be carried out prior to invasive procedures and if levels are >50 IU/dL (i.e. 50%), no treatment is necessary but DDAVP or FVIII concentrate, plasma derived or recombinant, should be given for levels lower than this. Fresh-frozen plasma also contains significant amounts of FVIII but because of a small risk of transmission of blood-borne pathogens, its use should be limited to settings where the more expensive purified plasma or recombinant products are not available. A recent advance in prenatal testing is the availability of preimplantation genetic diagnosis (PGD), a technique where following *in vitro* fertilization, embryos are tested for the genetic mutation and only female embryos or unaffected males are transferred to the uterus for implantation [91].

Management at delivery

From a maternal perspective, delivery is usually uncomplicated with no increased bleeding risk if the management plan outlined above is followed. The risk of bleeding complications at delivery is not increased in women who have FVIII levels greater than 50 IU/dL (i.e. 50%) and these women require no additional treatment but should have active management of the third stage of labor with prompt administration of oxytocic agents immediately following delivery of the baby and close observation for delayed postpartum hemorrhage as FVIII levels fall in the postpartum period. If FVIII levels are <50 IU/dL (i.e. 50%) at around 34 weeks gestation, treatment to increase factor levels is recommended (Table 2.11). DDAVP may often be sufficient to increase FVIII levels to the normal range. As with treatment for VWD, a dose of 0.3 µg/kg is given intravenously or subcutaneously. There are concerns that DDAVP use during pregnancy may cause maternal or fetal hyponatremia and stimulate uterine contraction. Maternal hyponatremia can be avoided by restricting fluid intake and as previously mentioned, DDAVP is selective for V2 vasopressin receptors and does not activate the vasopressin V1 receptors that have an oxytocic effect or cause vasoconstriction. If DDAVP is given at the time of cord clamping, fetal hyponatremia will not be an issue but even if its use is required at an earlier stage, it is reassuring that hyponatremia was not described in the infants of women who have received DDAVP for diabetes insipidus during pregnancy [92].

Hemophilia B

Expected course during pregnancy

Factor IX, unlike FVIII, does not increase during pregnancy so that symptomatic carriers with low levels of FIX are more likely to develop bleeding problems during pregnancy and at delivery. Spontaneous bleeding is uncommon but treatment is recommended prior to any invasive procedures, such as CVS and amniocentesis, and at delivery for women with factor levels of <50 IU/dL (i.e. 50%) (see Table 2.12). FIX levels should be measured at booking. DDAVP has no effect on FIX levels and clotting factor concentrates, either highly purified plasma-derived FIX concentrate or recombinant FIX, should be used. The aim with factor replacement is to attain a factor level of around 50 IU/dL (i.e. 50%) so the dosage required will depend on the mother's baseline FIX level, but 20–40 IU/

Table 2.11 Labor and delivery checklist for female hemophilia A or B carrier

1. Measure clotting factor level at 34 weeks gestation

  FVIII or FIX levels > 50 IU/dL (i.e. >50%)
  √ Treatment to increase clotting factor level not required

- **Hemophilia A carrier**
  FVIII < 50 IU/dL (i.e. <50%)
  √ DDAVP (0.3 µg/kg intravenously or subcutaneously) or recombinant or plasma- derived FVIII concentrate (10–20 IU/kg) required for delivery

- **Hemophilia B carrier**
  FIX < 50 IU/dL (i.e. <50%)
  √ Recombinant or plasma-derived FIX concentrate (20–40 IU /kg) required for delivery

2. All women
  √ Active management 3rd stage
  √ Close observation for postpartum hemorrhage

DDAVP, 1-desmopressin-8-D-arginine vasopressin.

Table 2.12 Labor and delivery checklist: fetal issues

Fetal sex determined by prenatal testing
✓ Female infant – follow routine obstetric delivery plan
✓ Male infant- unaffected - follow routine obstetric delivery plan
✓ Male infant- affected *OR* fetal sex not determined antenatally
- Decision re vaginal delivery or caesarean section to be made for obstetric indications
- Assisted delivery with outlet forceps is possible
- Ventouse or vacuum delivery contraindicated
- Cord blood (citrate tube) for APTT and FVIII or FIX levels
- No intramuscular injections until hemophilia status known
- Clotting factor concentrates only if clinical bleeding

APTT, activated partial thromboplastin time.

kg generally is sufficient. Individual responses to recombinant FIX are variable and should be determined before delivery.

Hemophilia A and B: regional analgesia and anaesthesia

Successful neuraxial anesthesia without complications has been reported in nonpregnant patients with either hemophilia A or B [93]. In these cases there were adequate levels of FVIII or FIX prior to needle placement. Neuraxial anesthesia is possible in patients with hemophilia A or B if coagulation is normal and factor levels are >50 IU/dL (i.e. 50%). However, if there is concern about risk of spinal epidural hematoma, PCA fentanyl is an alternative labor analgesic [85]. If cesarean delivery becomes necessary in cases where spinal or epidural anesthesia is contraindicated, general anesthesia will be required.

Termination of pregnancy

If termination of pregnancy is required for medical or social reasons, FVIII or FIX levels, as appropriate, should be determined. Treatment may be required prior to the procedure if levels are <50 IU/dL (i.e. 50%) to reduce the risk of bleeding.

Hemophilia A and B: fetal concerns during delivery

As outlined in Table 2.12, prenatal identification that the infant is female is reassuring, as is prior knowledge that a male infant is unaffected. However, for technical reasons or as a result of parental choice, the fetal sex may not have been determined antenatally or the hemophilia status of a male infant may not have been established. In these situations there is no choice but to assume that the infant is affected and plan delivery accordingly. If parents do not wish to know the fetal sex, it may be helpful if the obstetrician can be made aware as this information can modify decisions taken during delivery.

Intracranial hemorrhage, potentially the most devastating fetal complication, is reported in 1–4% of severely affected male infants and occurs more commonly with traumatic delivery. The risk is not modified by elective cesarean delivery and mode of delivery should be determined by obstetric indications. Outlet forceps delivery is unlikely to cause significant trauma and would be preferable to cesarean delivery if the head is deep in the pelvis. Midcavity and rotational forceps delivery should not be done. Ventouse delivery (vacuum extraction) is contraindicated as it carries a substantial risk of cephalohematoma that can be severe. Placement of fetal scalp electrodes does not appear to cause major bleeding problems but routine use should be discouraged.

Following delivery, a cord blood sample should be taken in a citrated tube to measure the APTT and FVIII or FIX levels, as appropriate, thus avoiding the need for later venepuncture. Intramuscular vitamin K injections should be withheld until the hemophilia status of a male infant is known and repeated doses of oral vitamin K should be given to affected infants. Prophylactic treatment with clotting factor concentrates is only required if there are concerns of bleeding symptoms in the infant. Early exposure to clotting factor concentrates may be a risk factor for inhibitor development, especially in infants with severe hemophilia or if there is a family history of inhibitors.

Factor XI deficiency

Factor XI (FXI) deficiency is a rare bleeding disorder that has an autosomal recessive pattern of inheritance. It is described in all races but has a particularly high frequency in Ashkenazi Jews with a heterozygote frequency of 9% [94]. Heterozygotes have FXI levels of 20–70 IU/dL (i.e. 20–70%) with levels in homozygotes of less than 20 IU/dL (i.e. <20%) . Severe deficiency is described with FXI levels <15 IU/dL. Spontaneous bleeding is uncommon and bleeding typically occurs following trauma or surgery, in particular in areas with high fibrinolytic activity, such as the oral cavity, genitourinary tract and nasal cavity. Menorrhagia is a frequent complication in women with FXI deficiency and is reported in up to 59% of women [95]. FXI levels are not predictive of bleeding risk and this may reflect *in vivo* properties of FXI that are not measured by *in vitro* APTT clotting assays. Although FXI levels are not predictive of the bleeding risk, patients self-segregate into "bleeder" and "nonbleeder" groups, which is helpful for management.

Expected course during pregnancy

Factor XI levels do not significantly increase during pregnancy [78]. Miscarriage and antenatal bleeding rates are not increased but excessive bleeding following miscarriage has been reported and correction of FXI levels may be required prior to invasive antenatal procedures such as amniocentesis or chorionic villus sampling. Primary and secondary postpartum hemorrhage rates of 16% and 24% respectively have been reported in women with FXI deficiency in the absence of prophylaxis to increase factor levels [78]. In a study of 105 pregnancies in 33 women with FXI deficiency [96], women were subgrouped into known "bleeders" and "nonbleeders." The majority of women (71%) had uncomplicated pregnancies and deliveries and the overall rate of postpartum hemorrhage (PPH) was 13% (n=9) with only one PPH occurring in a "nonbleeder."

Management at delivery

Women who have severe FXI deficiency (FXI <15 IU/dL, i.e. <20% of normal range) who have a history of abnormal bleeding are usually given blood product support with either fresh-frozen plasma (FFP) or FXI concentrate for delivery, especially if operative delivery is planned. However, there is no clear consensus regarding the FXI level that allows for adequate surgical hemostasis but some centers recommend a level of >50 IU/dL (i.e. >50% of normal range) during labor, continuing for 3–4 days after vaginal delivery and 7 days following cesarean delivery [95]. FXI has a long half-life of 60– 80 hours so that plasma may only be required every 2–3 days. FXI concentrate was developed to avoid exposure of patients to FFP with its potential complications such as volume overload and transfusion-transmitted diseases but reports of thromboembolic events following use of the concentrate have tempered more widespread use.

Regional analgesia/anaesthesia

Factor XI deficiency is a rare inherited bleeding disorder and not frequently encountered by anesthesiologists. The risk/benefit ratio for neuraxial anesthesia is influenced by the fact that the bleeding tendency in these patients is unpredictable since factor levels are not always predictive of bleeding risk. Neuraxial anesthesia may be administered if normalized coagulation status is confirmed [97].

Fetal concerns during delivery

Given the autosomal recessive form of inheritance, an infant born to a woman with FXI will inherit only a single abnormal gene from its mother and would only be affected if the father also carried an abnormal gene. An infant with a single abnormal gene would not be at increased risk of bleeding. In populations with a high frequency of FXI deficiency, such as Ashkenazi Jews, antenatal screening may be clinically useful [98].

Factor VII deficiency

Factor VII plays a pivotal role in the initiation stage of coagulation *in vivo*. It forms a complex with exposed tissue factor leading to activation of FIX and FX and generation of thrombin that in turn cleaves fibrinogen to allow formation of a fibrin clot. FVII deficiency is an autosomal recessive disorder and is the most common of the rare bleeding disorders with a prevalence of 1 in 500,000. Most patients have a quantitative deficiency with low levels of FVII but a small number of patients have functional abnormalities. Patients with FVII deficiency demonstrate marked variability in bleeding symptoms. Factor VII levels do not correlate with the severity of symptoms although bleeding usually occurs with factor levels <10 IU/dL (i.e. <10% of normal range) but individuals with higher levels may also be symptomatic. The most frequent bleeding symptoms are menorrhagia, epistaxis and easy bruising but severe bleeding such as intracranial hemorrhage, gastrointestinal bleeding and rarely hemarthrosis may occur. Postoperative bleeding particularly following dental extraction is common. FVII deficiency should be considered in patients with bleeding symptoms who have a normal APTT and prolonged prothrombin ratio that is corrected by mixing patient's plasma with normal plasma and the diagnosis is confirmed by factor-specific assays.

Pregnancy and FVII deficiency

Factor VII levels normally increase up to fourfold during pregnancy but this rise may not occur in women with severe deficiency of FVII. Kulkarni and co-workers reviewed pregnancy outcome in 14 pregnancies in seven women with FVII deficiency [99]. Three women with a known diagnosis of mild-to-moderate deficiency prior to pregnancy demonstrated an increase in FVII from a mean baseline of 33 IU/dL to a mean of 73 IU /dL at term (i.e. from 33% to 73% of normal range). All three women were given recombinant FVII (rFVII) and a postpartum hemorrhage of 1400 mL was reported in one woman following her second cesarean delivery. The remaining four women had entered pregnancy with an unknown diagnosis of FVII deficiency and therefore did not receive treatment with rFVIIa at delivery. Of 10 pregnancies, eight progressed to term and no bleeding complications were reported in five spontaneous vaginal deliveries and three cesarean deliveries. The remaining two pregnancies ended in the first trimester and were complicated by significant hemorrhage. One woman had a surgical termination of pregnancy complicated by hemorrhage requiring multiple blood transfusions. The other (who had had two previously uncomplicated term pregnancies) had a miscarriage complicated by excessive blood loss requiring surgical evacuation [99].

Treatment options in FVII deficiency include FFP, prothrombin complex concentrate, FVII concentrates and recombinant FVII. Recombinant FVII is the treatment of choice and has been approved for this indication in many countries. Replacement therapy is thought to be indicated for delivery in women with severe deficiency but there is no agreed dosing schedule. For surgical procedures in nonpregnant patients, a dose of 15–30 μg/kg repeated every 4–6 hours until hemostasis is achieved is recommended [100]. This should be sufficient for vaginal delivery and probably delivery by cesarean section but definitive data are not available. No clear guidelines exist for replacement therapy in women with mild-to-moderate FVII deficiency and perhaps clinicians should be guided by increases in FVII levels during pregnancy and whether there is a prior maternal history of bleeding following previous surgical or dental challenges.

FXIII deficiency

Factor XIII is a transglutaminase enzyme that is involved in the last steps of the coagulation cascade covalently cross-linking α- and γ-fibrin chains, thus stabilizing the fibrin clot and protecting it from fibrinolytic degradation. Other substrates for FXIII include the adhesive proteins fibronectin and vitronectin, involved in wound healing and also contractile or cytoskeletal proteins. Factor XIII is mainly present in plasma, platelets and monocytes/macrophages with small amounts expressed in the liver. In plasma, it circulates as a complex of the two enzymatically active A subunits (FXIIIA) coupled with the two B carrier subunits (FXIIIB). In the placenta, high concentrations of FXIIIA are expressed in tissue macrophages.

Factor XIII deficiency is an autosomal recessive disorder with a population prevalence of around one in 2 million. Deficiency is most commonly due to mutations that affect

FXIIIA subunit production but a minority of patients have defects in hepatic production of the FXIIIB carrier subunit, resulting in increased destruction of the A subunit and reduced FXIII activity. The archetypal clinical presentation of FXIII deficiency is delayed umbilical cord healing. Intracranial hemorrhage is a frequent complication occurring in 25–60% of patients and is significantly more common than in individuals with other severe bleeding disorders such as hemophilia and type 3 VWD. Delayed wound healing is common and is usually the cause of postsurgical bleeding.

Pregnancy and FXIII deficiency

A high rate of spontaneous abortion is reported in women with FXIII deficiency with the exception of women with deficiency due to defects in the FXIIIB carrier subunit. This suggests that the enzymatically active subunit FXIIIA is critical for placental development and maintenance of pregnancy. In the absence of FXIII replacement therapy, miscarriage usually occurs after the sixth week of gestation, indicating that FXIIIA is not required for fertilization or very early placental development [101].

Factor XIII plasma levels of 2–5% are thought to be sufficient for hemostasis and prevention of spontaneous bleeding. If bleeding occurs or is anticipated, higher levels will be required, i.e. 10% for minor bleeding, 20–30% for ovarian bleeding, 50% for minor surgery and 100% for critical bleeding such as intracranial hemorrhage or major surgery.

Although cryoprecipitate or FFP can be used to treat FXIII deficiency in settings where alternatives are not available, the use of FXIII concentrate is highly preferable. Fibrogammin P® is a plasma-derived, heat-treated purified FXIII concentrate that, outside pregnancy, is given every 4–6 weeks at a dose of 10 IU/kg to maintain FXIII levels in the target range. The long dosing interval is possible because of the long half-life of 5–11 days in nonpregnant individuals. The optimal dose and frequency of dosing during pregnancy have not been established but recent review articles recommend maintaining FXIII above 10% during pregnancy with levels of 20–30% at the time of delivery. In normal individuals FXIII levels fall with advancing gestation, reaching around 70% of normal by term and pregnancy appears to shorten the half-life of FXIII, necessitating more frequent dosing. Some authors recommend one vial (250 IU) every 7 days, increasing to two vials (500 IU) after 23 weeks gestation with a 1000 IU bolus during active labor [102].

References

1. Scholl TO. Iron status during pregnancy: setting the stage for mother and infant. Am J Clin Nutr 2005;81:1218S–22S.
2. Beard JL. Effectiveness and strategies of iron supplementation during pregnancy. Am J Clin Nutr 2000;71:1288S–94S.
3. Allen LH. Anemia and iron deficiency: effects on pregnancy outcome. Am J Clin Nutr 2000;71:1280S–4S.

4. Scholl TO, Reilly T. Anemia, iron and pregnancy outcome. J Nutr 2000;130:443S–7S.

5. Pena-Rosas JP, Viteri FE. Effects of routine oral iron supplementation with or without folic acid for women during pregnancy. Cochrane Database of Systematic Reviews, 2006;3:CD004736.

6. Steer PJ. Maternal hemoglobin concentration and birth weight. Am J Clin Nutr 2000;71:1285S–7S.

7. Hoffman R, Benz EJ, Shattil SJ, Furie B, Cohen HJ, Silberstein LE. Hematology: basic principles and practice. Churchill Livingstone, Edinburgh, 1995.

8. Hokin BD, Butler T. Cyanocobalamin (vitamin B–12) status in seventh-day adventist ministers in Australia. Am J Clin Nutr 1999;70:576S–8S.

9. Koebnick C, Hoffmann I, Dagnelie PC, Heins UA, Wickramasinghe SN, Ratnayaka ID, et al. Long-term ovo-lacto vegetarian diet impairs vitamin B-12 status in pregnant women. J Nutr 2004; 134(12):3319–26.

10. Kuhne T, Bubl R, Baumgartner R. Maternal vegan diet causing a serious infantile neurological disroder due to vitamin B12 deficiency. Eur J Pediatr 1991;150:205–8.

11. Wardinsky TD, Montes RG, Friederich RL, Broadhurst RB, Sinnhuber V, Bartholomew D. Vitamin B12 deficiency associated with low breast-milk vitamin B12 concentration in an infant following maternal gastric bypass surgery. Arch Pediatr Adol Med 1995;149:1281–4.

12. Pitkin RM. Folate and neural tube defects. Am J Clin Nutr 2007;85:285S–8S.

13. Galloway MJ, Rushworth L. Red cell or serum folate? Results from the National Pathology Alliance benchmarking review. J Clin Pathol 2003;56:924–6.

14. Zittoun J, Zittoun R. Modern clinical testing strategies in cobalamin and folate deficiency. Semin Hematol 1999;36:35–46.

15. Vichinsky EP. Changing patterns of thalassemia worldwide. Ann NY Acad Sci 2005;1054:18–24.

16. Weatherall DJ, Clegg JB. The thalassemia syndromes, 4th edn. Blackwell Science, Oxford, 2001.

17. Angastiniotis M, Modell B. Global epidemiology of hemoglobin disorders. Ann NY Acad Sci 1998;850:251–69.

18. Lucke T, Pfister S, Durken M. Neurodevelopmental outcome and haematological course of a long-time survivor with homozygous alpha-thalassaemia: case report and review of the literature. Acta Paediatr 2005;94:1330–3.

19. Frenette PS, Atweh GF. Sickle cell disease: old discoveries, new concepts, and future promises. J Clin Invest 2007;117:850–8.

20. Madigan C, Malik P. Pathophysiology and therapy for haemoglobinopathies. Part I: sickle cell disease. Exp Rev Mol Med 2006;8:1–23.

21. Davies SC, Gilmore A. The role of hydroxyurea in the management of sickle cell disease. Blood Rev 2003;17:99–109.

22. Rees D, Olujohungbe AD, Parker NE, Stephens AD, Telfer P, Wright J. Guidelines for the management of the acute painful crisis in sickle cell disease. Br J Haematol 2003;120:744–52.

23. Leung TN, Lau TK, Chung TK. Thalassaemia screening in pregnancy. Curr Opin Obstet Gynecol 2005;17:129–34.

24. Tuck SM. Fertility and pregnancy in thalassemia major. Ann NY Acad Sci 2005;1054:300–7.

25. Serjeant GR, Loy LL, Crowther M, Hambleton IR, Thame M. Outcome of pregnancy in homozygous sickle cell disease. Obstet Gynecol 2004;103:1278–85.

26. Koshy M. Sickle cell disease and pregnancy. Blood Rev 1995;9:157–64.

27. Koshy M, Burd L, Wallace D, Moawad A, Baron J. Prophylactic red-cell transfusions in pregnant patients with sickle cell disease: a randomized cooperative study. N Engl J Med 1988;319:1447–52.

28. Lorey F, Charoenkwan P, Witkowska HE, Lafferty J, Patterson M, Eng B, et al. Hb H hydrops foetalis syndrome: a case report and review of literature. Br J Haematol 2001;115:72–8.

29. Lorey F, Cunningham G, Vichinsky EP, Lubin BH, Witkowska HE, Matsunaga A, et al. Universal newborn screening for Hb H disease in California. Genet Test 2001;5:93–100.

30. Li D, Liao C, Li J, Xie X, Huang Y, Zhong H. Detection of alpha-thalassemia in beta-thalassemia carriers and prevention of Hb Bart's hydrops fetalis through prenatal screening. Haematologica 2006;91:649–51.

31. Chan V, Ng EHY, Yam I, Yeung WSB, Ho PC, Chan TK. Experience in preimplantation genetic diagnosis for exclusion of homozygous α^0 thalassemia. Prenat Diagn 2006;26:1029–36.

32. Qureshi N, Foote D, Walters MC, Singer ST, Quirolo K, Vichinsky EP. Outcomes of preimplantation genetic diagnosis therapy in treatment of beta-thalassemia: a retrospective analysis. Ann NY Acad Sci 2005;1054:500–3.

33. Kuliev A, Rechitsky S, Verlinsky O, Ivakhnenko V, Evsikov S, Wolf G, et al. Preimplantation diagnosis of thalassemias. J Assist Reprod Genet 1998;15:219–25.

34. Phupong V. An increase of the cardiothoracic ratio leads to a diagnosis of Bart's hydrops. J Med Assoc Thai 2006;89:509–12.

35. Kaplan C, Daffos F, Forestier F, Tertian G, Catherine N, Pons JC, et al. Fetal platelet counts in thrombocytopenic pregnancy. Lancet 1990;336:979–82.

36. Burrows RF, Kelton JG. Incidentally detected thrombocytopenia in healthy mothers and their infants. N Engl J Med 1988;319(3):142–5.

37. Burrows RF, Kelton JG. Pregnancy in patients with idiopathic thrombocytopenic purpura: assessing the risks for the infant at delivery. Obstet Gynecol Surv 1993;48:781–8.

38. Sainio S, Kekomaki R, Riikonen S, Teramo K. Maternal thrombocytopenia at term: a population-based study. Acta Obstet Gynecol Scand 2000;79:744–9.

39. Burrows RF, Kelton JG. Fetal thrombocytopenia and its relation to maternal thrombocytopenia. N Engl J Med 1993;329:1463–6.

40. George JN, Woolf SH, Raskob GE, Wasser JS, Aledort LM, Ballem PJ, et al. Idiopathic thrombocytopenic purpura: a practice guideline developed by explicit methods for the American Society of Hematology. Blood 1996;88:3–40.

41. Brighton TA, Evans S, Castaldi PA, Chesterman CN, Chong BH. Prospective evaluation of the clinical usefulness of an antigen-specific assay (MAIPA) in idiopathic thrombocytopenic purpura and other immune thrombocytopenias. Blood 1996;88:194–201.

42. Cines DB, Dusak B, Tomaski A, Mennuti M, Schreiber AD. Immune thrombocytopenic purpura and pregnancy. N Engl J Med 1982;306:826–31.

43. Al-Mofada SM, Osman ME, Kides E, Al-Momen AK, Al-Herbish AS, Al-Mobaireek K. Risk of thrombocytopenia in the infants of mothers with idiopathic thrombocytopenia. Am J Perinat 1994;11:423–6.

44. Burrows RF, Kelton JG. Low fetal risks in pregnancies associated with idiopathic thrombocytopenic purpura. Am J Obstet Gynecol 1990;163:1147–50.

45. Moutet A, Fromont P, Farcet JP, Rotten D, Bettaieb A, Duedari N, et al. Pregnancy in women with immune thrombocytopenic purpura. Arch Intern Med 1990;150:2141–5.

46. Payne SD, Resnik R, Moore TR, Hedriana HL, Kelly TF. Maternal characteristics and risk of severe neonatal thrombocytopenia and intracranial hemorrhage in pregnancies

complicated by autoimmune thrombocytopenia. Am J Obstet Gynecol 1997;177:149–55.

47. Samuels P, Bussel JB, Braitman LE, Tomaski A, Druzin ML, Mennuti MT, *et al.* Estimation of the risk of thrombocytopenia in the offspring of pregnant women with presumed immune thrombocytopenic purpura. N Engl J Med 1990;323:229–35.

48. Sharon R, Tatarsky I. Low fetal morbidity in pregnancy associated with acute and chronic idiopathic thrombocytopenic purpura. Am J Hematol 1994;46:87–90.

49. Valat AS, Caulier MT, Devos P, Rugeri L, Wibaut B, Vaast P, *et al.* Relationships between severe neonatal thrombocytopenia and maternal characteristics in pregnancies associated with autoimmune thrombocytopenia. Br J Haematol 1998;103:397–401.

50. Webert KE, Mittal R, Sigouin C, Heddle NM, Kelton JG. A retrospective 11–year analysis of obstetric patients with idiopathic thrombocytopenic purpura. Blood 2003;102:4306–11.

51. Yamada H, Kato EH, Kishida T, Negishi H, Makinoda S, Fujimoto S. Risk factors for neonatal thrombocytopenia in pregnancy complicated by idiopathic thrombocytopenic purpura. Ann Hematol 1998;76:211–14.

52. British Committee for Standards in Haematology General Haematology Task Force. Guidelines for the investigation and management of idiopathic thrombocytopenic purpura in adults, children and in pregnancy. Br J Haematol 2003;120:574–96.

53. Christiaens GC, Nieuwenhuis HK, Bussel JB. Comparison of platelet counts in first and second newborns of mothers with immune thrombocytopenic purpura. Obstet Gynecol 1997;90:546–52.

54. Arnold DM, Dentali F, Crowther MA, Meyer RM, Cook RJ, Sigouin C, *et al.* Systematic review: efficacy and safety of rituximab for adults with idiopathic thrombocytopenic purpura. Ann Intern Med 2007;146:25–33.

55. McNeill MJ, Thorburn J. Cannulation of the epidural space. A comparison of 18– and 16-gauge needles. Anaesthesia 1988; 43:154–5.

56. Verniquet AJ. Vessel puncture with epidural catheters. Experience in obstetric patients. Anaesthesia 1980;35:660–2.

57. Lee LA, Posner KL, Domino KB, Caplan RA, Cheney FW. Injuries associated with regional anesthesia in the 1980s and 1990s: a closed claims analysis. Anesthesiology 2004;101:143–52.

58. Moen V, Dahlgren N, Irestedt L. Severe neurological complications after central neuraxial blockades in Sweden 1990–1999. Anesthesiology 2004;101:950–9.

59. American Society of Anesthesiologists Task Force on Obstetric Anesthesia. Practice guidelines for obstetric anesthesia: an updated report by the American Society of Anesthesiologists Task Force on Obstetric Anesthesia. Anesthesiology 2007;106:843–63.

60. Ramanathan J, Sibai BM, Vu T, Chauhan D. Correlation between bleeding times and platelet counts in women with preeclampsia undergoing cesarean section. Anesthesiology 1989;71:188–91.

61. Rodgers RP, Levin J. A critical reappraisal of the bleeding time. Semin Thromb Hemostas 1990;16:1–20.

62. Prieto JA, Mastrobattista JM, Blanco JD. Coagulation studies in patients with marked thrombocytopenia due to severe preeclampsia. Am J Perinatol 1995;12:220–2.

63. McCrae KR, Samuels P, Schreiber AD. Pregnancy-associated thrombocytopenia: pathogenesis and management. Blood 1992;80:2697–714.

64. Rolbin SH, Abbott D, Musclow E, Papsin F, Lie LM, Freedman J. Epidural anesthesia in pregnant patients with low platelet counts. Obstet Gynecol 1988;71:918–20.

65. Rasmus KT, Rottman RL, Kotelko DM, Wright WC, Stone JJ, Rosenblatt RM. Unrecognized thrombocytopenia and regional anesthesia in parturients: a retrospective review. Obstet Gynecol 1989;73:943–6.

66. Beilin Y, Zahn J, Comerford M. Safe epidural analgesia in thirty parturients with platelet counts between 69,000 and 98,000 mm(-3). Anesth Analg 1997;85:385–8.

67. Urato AC, Repke JT. May–Hegglin anomaly: a case of vaginal delivery when both mother and fetus are affected. Am J Obstet Gynecol 1998;179:260–1.

68. Lopez JA, Andrews RK, Afshar-Kharghan V, Berndt MC. Bernard – Soulier syndrome. Blood 1998;91:4397–418.

69. Khalil A, Seoud M, Tannous R, Usta I, Shamseddine A. Bernard – Soulier syndrome in pregnancy: case report and review of the literature. Clin Lab Haematol 1998;20:125–8.

70. Peng TC, Kickler TS, Bell WR, Haller E. Obstetric complications in a patient with Bernard–Soulier syndrome. Am J Obstet Gynecol 1991;165:425–6.

71. George JN, Caen JP, Nurden AT. Glanzmann's thrombasthenia: the spectrum of clinical disease. Blood 1990;75:1383–95.

72. Bellucci S, Caen J. Molecular basis of Glanzmann's thrombasthenia and current strategies in treatment. Blood Rev 2002;16:193–202.

73. Kale A, Bayhan G, Yalinkaya A, Yayla M. The use of recombinant factor VIIa in a primigravida with Glanzmann's thrombasthenia during delivery. J Perinat Med 2004;32:456–8.

74. Kouides PA, Phatak PD, Burkart P, Braggins C, Cox C, Bernstein Z, *et al.* Gynaecological and obstetrical morbidity in women with type I von Willebrand disease: results of a patient survey. Haemophilia 2000;6:643–8.

75. Sadler JE, Budde U, Eikenboom JCJ, Favaloro EJ, Hill FGH, Holmberg L, *et al.* Update on the pathophysiology and classification of von Willebrand disease: a report of the Subcommittee on von Willebrand Factor. J Thromb Haemost 2006;4:2103–14.

76. Sanchez-Luceros A, Meschengieser SS, Marchese C, Votta R, Casais P, Woods AI, *et al.* Factor VIII and von Willebrand factor changes during normal pregnancy and puerperium. Blood Coag Fibrinol 2003;14:647–51.

77. Hepner DL, Tsen LC. Severe thrombocytopenia, type 2B von Willebrand disease and pregnancy. Anesthesiology 2004;101: 1465–7.

78. Kadir RA, Lee CA, Sabin CA, Pollard D, Economides DL. Pregnancy in women with von Willebrand's disease or factor XI deficiency. Br J Obstet Gynaecol 1998;105:314–21.

79. Mannucci PM. Treatment of von Willebrand's disease. J Intern Med 1997;740:129–32.

80. Sanchez-Luceros A, Meschengieser SS, Turdo K, Arizo A, Woods AI, Casais P, *et al.* Evaluation of the clinical safety of desmopressin during pregnancy in women with a low plasmatic von Willebrand factor level and bleeding history. Thromb Res 2007;120:387–90.

81. Jones BP, Bell EA, Maroof M. Epidural labor analgesia in a parturient with von Willebrand's disease type IIA and severe preeclampsia. Anesthesiology 1999;90:1219–20.

82. Milaskiewicz RM, Holdcroft A, Letsky E. Epidural anaesthesia and von Willebrand's disease. Anaesthesia 1990;45:462–4.

83. Stedeford JC, Pittman JA. Von Willebrand's disease and neuroaxial anaesthesia. Anaesthesia 2000;55:1228–9.

84. Ruppen W, Derry S, McQuay H, Moore RA. Incidence of epidural hematoma, infection, and neurological injury in obstetric pateints with epidural analgesia/anaesthesia. Anesthesiology 2006;105:394–9.

85. Campbell DC. Parenteral opioids for labor analgesia. Clin Obstet Gynecol 2003;46:616–22.

86. Rodeghiero F, Castaman G. Treatment of von Willebrand disease. Semin Hematol 2005;42:29–35.

87. Cohen S, Zada Y. Neuroaxial block for von Willebrand's disease. Anaesthesia 2001;56:397.

88. Roque H, Funai E, Lockwood CJ. von Willebrand disease and pregnancy. J Matern Fetal Med 2000;9:257–66.

89. Sharma SK LR. Hematologic and coagulation disorders. In: Chestnut DH (ed) Obstetric anesthesia: principles and practice, 3rd edn. Elsevier Mosby, Philadelphia, 2004.

90. Andrew M, Paes B, Milner R, Johnston M, Mitchell L, Tollefsen DM, et al. Development of the human coagulation system in the full-term infant. Blood 1987;70:165–72.

91. Lavery S. Preimplantation genetic diagnosis: new reproductive options for carriers of haemophilia. Haemophilia 2004;10:126–32.

92. Ray JG. DDAVP use during pregnancy: an analysis of its safety for mother and child. Obstet Gynecol Surv 1998;53:450–5.

93. Hack G, Hofmann P, Brackmann HH, Stoeckel H, Pichotka H. Regional anaesthesia in haemophiliacs. Anasth Intensivther Notfallmed 1980;15:45–51.

94. O'Connell NM. Factor XI deficiency. Semin Hematol 2004;41:76–81.

95. Kadir RA. Women and inherited bleeding disorders: pregnancy and delivery. Semin Hematol 1999;36:28–35.

96. Myers B, Pavord S, Kean L, Hill M, Dolan G. Pregnancy outcome in Factor XI deficiency: incidence of miscarriage, antenatal and postnatal haemorrhage in 33 women with Factor XI deficiency. Br J Obstet Gynecol 2007;114:643–6.

97. Singh AJ, Harnet MJ, Connors MJ, Camman WR. Factor XI deficiency and obstetrical anesthesia. Anesth Analg 2009;108:1882–5.

98. Kadir RA, Kingman CEC, Chi C, O'Connell NM, Riddell A, Lee CA, et al. Screening for factor XI deficiency amongst pregnant women of Ashkenazi Jewish origin. Haemophilia 2006;12:625–8.

99. Kulkarni AA, Lee CA, Kadir RA. Pregnancy in women with congenital factor VII deficiency. Haemophilia 2006;12:413–16.

100. Mariani G, Dolce A, Marchetti G, Bernardi F. Clinical picture and management of congenital factor VII deficiency. Haemophilia 2004;10:180–3.

101. Ichinose A, Asahina T, Kobayashi T. Congenital blood coagulation factor XIII deficiency and perinatal management. Curr Drug Targ 2005;6:541–9.

102. Asahina T, Kobayashi T, Takeuchi K, Kanayama N. Congenital blood coagulation factor XIII deficiency and successful deliveries: a review of the literature. Obstet Gynecol Surv 2007;62:255–60.

Thromboembolic disease in pregnancy

Catherine Nelson-Piercy[1] *and Ian Greer*[2]

[1]Guy's & St Thomas' Foundation Trust and Queen Charlotte's & Chelsea Hospital, London, UK
[2]Faculty of Health and Life Sciences, University of Liverpool, Liverpool, UK

Introduction

Pulmonary thromboembolism (PTE) remains a major cause of direct maternal mortality. The UK Confidential Enquiries into Maternal Deaths have highlighted failures in providing appropriate prophylaxis for women at risk, in obtaining objective diagnoses, and employing adequate treatment [1]. Thus the management of these patients is important for the obstetrician, medical consultant and anesthesiologist. Venous thromboembolism (VTE) is up to 10 times more common in pregnant women (defined to include the puerperium and 6–8 weeks post partum) than in nonpregnant women of the same age and complicates about 1/1000 pregnancies [2–4]. Around 85% of these gestational VTE are deep venous thrombosis (DVT) rather than PTE [4–6], as compared to 70% DVT in nonpregnant patients with VTE [7].

The majority of these DVT occur antenatally (65.5%), with distribution across the three trimesters of pregnancy [8,9]. Indeed, almost half of antenatal VTE occurs before 15 weeks gestation [5], emphasizing the need for risk assessment pre-pregnancy and prophylaxis in early pregnancy. However, the rate of VTE is greatest in the puerperium, being almost fourfold that during pregnancy [4–6,8]. Interestingly, almost 90% of pregnancy-associated DVT occur on the left side in contrast to the non-pregnant situation, where only 55% of DVT occur on the left. This may reflect some compression of the left common iliac vein by the right iliac artery. Over 70% of gestational DVT are ileofemoral in their location, which contrasts with around a 9% rate of ileofemoral DVT in the nonpregnant, in whom calf vein DVT predominate [10]. This is important as ileofemoral DVT are more likely to embolize than calf vein thromboses. In the most recent report of the UK Confidential Enquiries into Maternal Deaths, the mortality rate for PTE, the leading cause of direct maternal death, was 1.6 per 100,000 maternities [1]. In the United States,

the CDC Pregnancy Mortality Surveillance System (PMSS) has reported rates of fatal VTE during pregnancy of 1.8 and 2.3 per 100,000 livebirths for the periods of 1987–1990 and 1991–1999 respectively [11,12] and PTE was the most frequent cause of maternal death.

Previous VTE is associated with an increased risk of future VTE. The risk of a recurrence of an idiopathic deep venous thrombosis in the general medical population is 10% per year for the first 2 years and 3% per year thereafter. There is also a risk of deep venous insufficiency known as "post-thrombotic syndrome" [13]. This is characterized by chronic persistent leg swelling, pain, a feeling of heaviness, dependent cyanosis, telangiectasia, chronic pigmentation, eczema, associated varicose veins and in some cases lipodermatosclerosis and chronic ulceration. Symptoms are worsened by standing or walking and improve with rest and recumbency. The syndrome is more common where there is a recurrent DVT, with obesity, and where there has been inadequate anticoagulation. Up to 80% of women with VTE develop post-thrombotic syndrome and over 60% will develop objectively confirmed deep venous insufficiency following a treated DVT [14]. The risk of developing venous insufficiency after DVT is greater than with PTE (odds ratio 10.9, 95% confidence interval (CI) 4.2–28.0) for DVT (compared to 3.8 (95% CI 1.2–12.3)) after PTE [14]. This may be due to the thrombus clearing from the leg veins in those with PTE, leading to less extensive venous damage. Berqvist *et al.* reported that up to 21% of women with a treated DVT in pregnancy required a compression bandage and 6% had venous ulcers at a median follow-up of 10 years [15]. Historical data show rates for venous ulceration following untreated DVT to be 19–28% on follow-up periods ranging from 6 to 31 years [15].

Investigation for venous thromboembolism in pregnancy

Clinical diagnosis of VTE is unreliable, especially in pregnancy. Presenting features (reviewed in Table 3.1) such as dyspnea, cough, chest pain, leg swelling and presyncope/syncope are

de Swiet's Medical Disorders in Obstetric Practice, 5th edition.
Edited by R. O. Powrie, M. F. Greene, W. Camann. © 2010 Blackwell Publishing.

Table 3.1 Presenting features of pulmonary embolism in nonpregnant patients

Symptom/sign	Frequency
Shortness of breath	73%
Tachypnea	70%
Pleuritic type chest pain	66%
Crackles on chest auscultation	51%
Cough	37%
Tachycardia	30%
Hemoptysis	13%
Cardiovascular collapse	8%

Reproduced with permission from Stein *et al.* [90].

common in pregnancy. Many young patients with pulmonary embolism may not manifest the typical features of tachypnea, tachycardia, hypotension or hypoxia. Thus any woman with signs and symptoms suggestive of VTE without obvious explanation should have an objective diagnostic investigation performed. Where the likelihood is considered high or there is any delay in such investigation, treatment with low molecular weight heparin (LMWH) should be given until the diagnosis is excluded, unless LMWH treatment is strongly contraindicated.

Compression duplex ultrasound is the primary diagnostic test for DVT [16]. If the diagnosis is confirmed, therapeutic LMWH should be continued. In the event that the ultrasound venogram is negative and there is a reasonable alternative explanation for the patient's symptoms, the investigations may be complete. However, if a high level of clinical suspicion exists, the ultrasound should be repeated in 1 week or an alternative diagnostic test (such as magnetic resonance imagining (MRI) venography, computed tomography (CT) of the iliac veins, pulsed Doppler studies or even conventional venography) employed [16]. If the clinicial suspicion is high enough in some circumstances it may be advisable to continue anticoagulation until this second investigation is completed. If on repeat testing there is no evidence of DVT, treatment can be discontinued [17].

Where PTE is suspected, anticoagulant treatment should be continued until PTE is objectively excluded unless bleeding is considered to be a likely alternative diagnosis. A chest X-ray (CXR) and a duplex ultrasound examination should be conducted. The CXR may identify other pulmonary disease such as pneumonia or pneumothorax [18]. CXR is normal in over half of pregnant patients with objectively proven PTE, but abnormalities suggestive of pulmonary embolism such as atelectasis, pleural effusion, focal opacities, and regional oligemia may be seen [19]. The radiation dose to the fetus from a CXR performed at any stage of pregnancy is negligible [20]. If the CXR does not provide a definitive diagnosis (and it usually will not), bilateral lower limb duplex ultrasound or definitive testing for pulmonary embolism with a CT pulmonary angiogram (CTPA) or ventilation perfusion scan (V/Q) should be carried out. Doppler ultrasound of the legs for the investigation of PTE has not been validated in pregnancy, but several

studies in nonpregnant patients with suspected PTE have shown its value [21–23]. The diagnosis of DVT will indirectly confirm a likely PTE. Anticoagulant treatment is the same for both conditions and further investigation may not be necessary, so reducing the number of diagnostic tests and radiation exposure (see below). If the leg compression ultrasounds have not confirmed the presence of thromboembolic disease, or a compression ultrasound is not readily available, then a CT angiogram or ventilation perfusion scan should be obtained.

Currently the decision about whether to use a CTPA or V/Q scan as the primary investigation for PTE will often be determined by local availability and practice patterns. Both are acceptable options with their own advantages and disadvantages. Their relative merits are reviewed in Table 3.2 and discussed below.

Computed tomography pulmonary angiogram is increasingly recommended as the first-line investigation for nonmassive PTE in nonpregnant patients. CTPA has several advantages over V/Q scan, including better sensitivity and specificity, and a lower radiation dose to the fetus. In addition, it can identify alternative diagnoses which may present similarly to PTE such as pulmonary edema, pneumonia or aortic dissection. However, CTPA may not identify small peripheral PTE although modern multidetector-row spiral CT systems now offer increasingly accurate detection of central and peripheral emboli. Despite these potential advantages of CTPA, many authorities continue to recommend V/Q scanning as the first-line investigation in pregnancy because of the low prevalence of chronic chest disease in young women and its high negative predictive value and also its substantially lower radiation dose to pregnant breast tissue.

The average fetal radiation dose with CTPA is less than 10% of that with V/Q scanning during all trimesters of pregnancy [24–26] with estimates that the risk of this translating into a fatal cancer to the age of 15 years in the child is <1/1,000,000 after *in utero* exposure to CTPA and 1/280,000 following a perfusion lung scan. Thus in the context of a possible PTE which may have fatal consequences, the risk to the fetus from such investigations should not prevent these investigations being conducted.

The main disadvantage of CTPA is the significant radiation dose (of the order of 20 mGy) to the maternal breasts, which is associated with an increased lifetime risk of developing breast cancer. This is particularly relevant, as around 90–95% of such investigations will have a negative result in pregnancy. The delivery of 10 mGy of radiation to a woman's breast is estimated to increase her lifetime risk of developing breast cancer, possibly by as much as 13.6% [27], but more recently it has been suggested that this is an overestimate [28] and breast shields may be used with CTPA to limit this exposure further. Nevertheless, breast tissue may be especially sensitive to radiation exposure during pregnancy. Thus, many still consider V/Q scans to be the investigation of first choice for young women with a normal CXR, especially if there is a family history of breast cancer or the patient has had a previous chest CT scan [24].

Table 3.2 Relative merits of V/Q scan and computed tomography pulmonary angiogram (CTPA) in the investigation of pulmonary thromboembolism (PTE)

Parameter	V/Q scan	CTPA
Radiation exposure	Minimal radiation to fetus (0.064–0.08 rads). Ventilation scan may be withheld in patients with a normal perfusion scan, further decreasing radiation exposure. Minimal radiation (1.4 mSv) to maternal breast	Minimal radiation to fetus (0.003–0.0131 rads [91]). Significant radiation to maternal breast (2.2–6.0 mSv) that increases risk of breast cancer by 13%. Risk can be decreased by the use of breast shields
Ability to offer alternative diagnosis	No	Yes, CTPA diagnoses can identify pulmonary edema, pneumonia and some cases of aortic dissection
Ability to offer definitive diagnosis	High probability scan fairly definitive for presence of pulmonary embolism. Low and intermediate probability scan may or may not represent pulmonary embolism with interpretation varying with underlying likelihood of PTE. Normal scan has excellent negative predictive value for PTE [16]. Pregnant patients more likely than general population to have definitive studies. V/Q scan unlikely to be normal in the setting of an abnormal chest X-ray	CTPA likely has better sensitivity and specificity for moderate to large PTE if study is of high quality. Patient movement or variations in timing of intravenous contrast or type of scanner may lead to difficult to interpret studies, especially for smaller peripheral PTE. "Multidetector" CT more likely to identify small PTE than a single-detector CT
Need for patient cooperation	Requires considerable time to perform and patient cooperation with positioning and breathing	Relatively brief study that only requires that patient be able to hold breath briefly and lie still on table
Invasiveness	Requires intravenous injection and (if perfusion scan abnormal) inhalation of radionuclide	Requires intravenous injection of contrast
Ease of access	Varies by institution- handling of radionuclide requires special technician who may not be in hospital after hours.	Varies by institution
Ease of interpretation	Interpretation fairly standardized	Interobserver variation in interpretation is considerable. Reading best done by experienced personnel [92]

Reproduced with permission from Bourjeily *et al*. [93].

What is our practice? We support using whichever test is readily available at the hospital where the patient is receiving care. When both studies are readily available, we obtain a V/Q scan if the CXR is normal because of the lower dose of radiation to the breast and its strong negative predictive value. If the CXR is abnormal (making a normal V/Q scan highly unlikely), if the patient is unstable or if the patient is in labor, our preference is to obtain a CTPA.

While pulmonary angiography remains the gold standard for diagnosing pulmonary embolism, the test is increasingly less commonly done as confidence in CTPA increases. This is partly because pulmonary angiography is a much more invasive test and partly because, although the radiation dose is still well below the acceptable limits in pregnancy, it does involve the highest radiation exposure to mother and fetus of all the available testing modalities.

D-dimer is a degradation product of cross-linked fibrin that is elevated in up to 75% of hospitalized medical patients due to a wide variety of conditions. The role outside pregnancy of the two most commonly available D-dimer assays is reviewed in Table 3.3. D-dimer, however, is of very limited value in pregnancy. It is increased by the physiologic changes in the coagulation system in pregnancy and so levels become "abnormal" by term and in the postnatal period in most pregnant women, with all of 23 women tested in the third trimester in one study exhibiting elevated D-dimer levels [29]. Furthermore, D-dimer levels can increase if there is a concomitant problem such as threatened

Table 3.3 D-dimer testing in nonpregnant patients

D-dimer test	Characteristics
Semi-quantitative latex agglutination assay	Rapid but far less accurate than the ELISA test. Can be used to rule out PTE in nonpregnant patients with a low probability of PTE only
Quantitative ELISA	More time intensive but increased sensitivity and specificity. Can be used to rule out PTE in nonpregnant patients except for those with a high probability of PTE.

ELISA, enzyme-linked immunosorbent assay; PTE, pulmonary thromboembolism. Reproduced with permission from Righini *et al*. [94].

miscarriage or pre-eclampsia [30]. Thus a "positive" D-dimer test in pregnancy is not necessarily consistent with VTE and objective testing remains necessary. A low level of D-dimer in pregnancy is compatible, as in the nonpregnant patient, with no VTE being present. Even then, the D-dimer test is not completely reliable; in the nonpregnant patient with a high pretest probability and a highly sensitive D-dimer assay, 4% of DVT will not be identified by the ELISA D-dimer test, increasing to 17% with a moderately sensitive latex agglutination D-dimer assay. Although some have advocated a role for a negative D-dimer test in the investigation of VTE in pregnancy [31], we believe that D-dimer is of no value [32] in this population. In the presence of clinical suspicion of such an important diagnosis, it does not avoid

Table 3.4 Inherited and acquired tendencies to thrombosis and how to test for them in pregnancy

Thrombophilia	Test	Effect of pregnancy on assay	Meaningful in the setting of acute thrombotic event?	Meaningful in the setting of heparin therapy?
Protein C deficiency	Functional protein C assay	None	No	Yes
Protein S deficiency	Free protein S antigenic assay	Decreases levels	No	Yes
Antithrombin (AT) deficiency (aka AT III deficiency)	AT-heparin co-factor assay	None	No	No
Factor V Leiden mutation (90% of R-APC)	PCR for factor V Leiden mutation	None	Yes	Yes
Functional resistance to activated protein C (R-APC)	Factor V deficient assay for R-APC	None[a]	Yes	No
Prothrombin gene mutation G20210A	PCR for prothrombin gene mutation G20201A	None	Yes	Yes
Antiphospholipid antibodies	Anticardiolipin and anti-B2 glycoprotein I antibody ELISA (IgM and IgG)	None	Yes	Yes
Lupus like inhibitor	Phospholipid-dependent clotting assay (APTT, kaolin clotting time (KCT), dilute Russel viper venom time (DRVVT), and dilute prothrombin time)	None	Yes	No
Factor VIII level	Plasma factor VIII coagulant activity (VIII:C)	Increased	No	Yes

[a]Other assays for R-APC will show increased resistance to APC (i.e. a decreased ratio) in pregnancy, however. APPT, activated partial thromboplastin time; ELISA enzyme-linked immunosorbent assay; PCR, polymerase chain reaction.

objective diagnostic testing in pregnancy where the patient will usually have an increased pretest probability for VTE in view of the pregnancy-associated risk factors.

When considering starting anticoagulation, a baseline complete blood count (hemoglobin and platelet count), prothrombin time (international normalized ratio – INR) and activated partial thromboplastin time (APTT) should be obtained. As anticoagulant therapy can be influenced by renal and hepatic function, a creatinine and aspartate aminotransferase (AST) should also be obtained. Performing a thrombophilia screen prior to therapy is a controversial area and therefore is not routinely recommended. The most commonly ordered thrombophilia tests are reviewed in Table 3.4 along with the effects of acute VTE and heparinization on the results. Whether obtaining a thrombophilia screen acutely is warranted in all patients with PTE is controversial because the results of a thrombophilia screen will not influence immediate management of acute VTE. However, it can provide information that can influence the duration and intensity of anticoagulation, such as when antithrombin deficiency or antiphospholipid syndrome is identified.

It is important to be aware of the effects of pregnancy and thrombus on the results of a thrombophilia screen. For example, protein S levels fall in normal pregnancy, making it difficult to make a diagnosis of protein S deficiency during pregnancy. Acquired activated protein C resistance is found with the APC sensitivity ratio (a functional assay sometimes used to identify the probability of factor V Leiden gene

polymorphism) test in around 40% of pregnancies, linked to the physiologic changes of pregnancy on the coagulation system. Antithrombin may be reduced when extensive thrombus is present. In nephrotic syndrome and pre-eclampsia (conditions associated with an increased risk of thrombosis), antithrombin levels are reduced and in liver disease protein C and S will be reduced. It is important, therefore, that thrombophilia screens are interpreted by clinicians with specific expertise in the area.

Acute treatment of venous thromboembolism

The treatment of VTE in pregnancy is heparin, either in the form of unfractionated heparin (UFH) or LMWH. Potential complications of heparin therapy are reviewed in Table 3.5. The most dangerous of these complications is heparin-induced thrombocytopenia (HIT) and is reviewed in Table 3.6. Meta-analyses of randomized controlled trials (RCT) indicate that LMWH are more effective, are associated with a lower risk of hemorrhagic complications and are associated with lower mortality than UFH in the initial treatment of DVT in nonpregnant patients, and also that LMWH is of equivalent efficacy to UFH in the initial treatment of PTE [33,34]. A large systematic review has concluded that LMWH is a safe alternative to UFH as an anticoagulant during pregnancy [35]. This review found a risk of recurrent VTE of 1.15% when treatment doses of LMWH were

Table 3.5 Complications of heparin therapy and their likelihood in unfractionated heparin (UFH) versus low molecular weight heparin (LMWH)

Risk	Comments	Relative frequency with UFH versus LMWH
Bleeding	Can occur in up to 5.5% of medical patients on heparin	LMWH less likely to be associated with major hemorrhage [95]
Heparin-induced thrombocytopenia (HIT)	Well-recognized complication usually occurring 5–10 days after initiating therapy	HIT is rare in pregnant patients on LMWH
Skin necrosis	Rare. Typically occurs in fat-rich areas. Begins with erythema followed by bruising, and then necrosis.	Not known
Osteoporosis	Reported in patients on heparin for more than 6 months. Can cause pathologic fractures (in one report in 2.2% of recipients) [96]. Generally felt to be reversible after stopping medication	LMWH causes less osteoclast activation and appears to be much less likely to cause osteoporosis [97]
Heparin contamination	Contamination of UFH with oversulfated chondroitin sulfate led to many deaths in 2007. Assays are now used by manufacturers which screen for this contaminant	Contamination has also occurred with some LMWH products

Table 3.6 Heparin-induced thrombocytopenia (HIT)

Type of HIT	Characteristics
Type 1	Usually occurs in the first 2 days of heparin therapy Nonimmune mechanism likely related to platelet activation by heparin Drop in platelet counts is usually small and resolves when heparin is stopped Not clinically significant except as part of the differential diagnosis of type 2 HIT
Type 2	Usually occurs in the first 5–10 days of heparin therapy Occurs in 0.2–5% of nonpregnant patients on heparin for more than 4 days and is more common in surgical than medical patients Immune-mediated disorder characterized by formation of antibodies againt the heparin-platelet factor 4 complex (platelet factor 4 complex is a heparin-neutralizing protein released from platelet granules when platelets are activated) that leads to widespread platelet activation, aggregation, destruction and often subsequent venous or less commonly arterial thrombosis (HITT) Platelet counts typically drop no more than 60,000/uL and almost never <20,000/uL Diagnosis is largely a clinical one but supported by the 14C-serotonin release assay (which has a 95% sensitivity and specificity), heparin-induced platelet aggregation studies and/or solid phase immunoassays Treatment involves immediate withdrawal of heparin and use of alternative anticoagulants (reviewed in Table 3.7)

Reproduced with permission from Hassell [98].

used to manage VTE in pregnancy. This compares favorably with recurrence rates of 5–8% reported in trials carried out in nonpregnant patients treated with LMWH or UFH followed by coumarin therapy who are followed up for 3–6 months [36,37] and confirms that LMWH are effective in the treatment of acute VTE in pregnancy. Further, there is evidence that LMWH do not cross the placenta and appear to pose no direct risk to the fetus [38]. LMWH are not associated with an increased risk of severe bleeding peripartum and the risk of HIT is substantially lower compared with UFH [35]. Indeed, in women who have not been exposed to UFH and who are treated with LMWH, some experts believe it may not be necessary to monitor the platelet count (although a baseline platelet count before starting is still advisable) [38,39]. Compared with UFH, LMWH also has a much reduced risk of heparin-induced osteoporosis [35,40].

In nonpregnant patients, the recommended therapeutic dose of LMWH varies according to the manufacturer (enoxaparin 1.5 mg/kg once daily, dalteparin 10,000–18,000 units once daily depending on body weight, tinzaparin 175 units/kg once daily). In view of recognized alterations in the pharmacokinetics of daltaparin and enoxaparin during pregnancy, a twice-daily dosage regimen (enoxaparin 1 mg/kg twice daily, dalteparin 100 units/kg twice daily) is usually recommended for these LMWH in the treatment of VTE in pregnancy [17,38]. There are insufficient data to determine if a once-daily dose is adequate and once-daily dosing therefore remains controversial [41]. Preliminary biochemical data from a relatively small number of patients suggest that once-daily administration of tinzaparin (175 units/kg) may be appropriate in terms of anti-Xa acivity in the treatment of VTE in pregnancy [42].

If the diagnosis of VTE is confirmed, treatment with LMWH should be continued. The APTT is not meaningfully changed in patients on LMWH and cannot be used to guide therapy as is done with UFH therapy. Monitoring anti-FXa levels, although still done as an alternative to APTT for patients on LMWH by some groups, is no longer recommended [17] due to the satisfactory results obtained with weight-based dosing and also because anti-Xa monitoring does not predict either recurrent thrombosis or bleeding risk well, at least in part because of variability in the assay [41]. There may be a case for monitoring levels at extremes of body weight (<50 kg and ≥90 kg), and women with other complicating factors including renal disease and recurrent VTE. As noted above, routine platelet count monitoring for evidence of HIT is likely not required in obstetric patients who have received only LMWH. However, if the obstetric patient is receiving LMWH after first receiving UFH, or if she has received UFH in the past, making HIT more likely, the platelet count should be monitored every 2 days from day 4 to day 14, or until LMWH is stopped, whichever occurs first [39,43]. Since UFH is used for a wide variety of medical purposes in which the patient may not always be aware that she has received it, it is the practice of the editors, but not the authors, to monitor platelets in all patients in whom therapeutic LMWH has been initiated.

Intravenous UFH was the traditional method of heparin administration in acute VTE and remains the preferred treatment in massive PTE because of its rapid effect and extensive experience of its use in this situation. In contrast to LMWH, UFH must be monitored and the therapeutic target for the APTT ratio is usually 1.5–2.5 times the average laboratory control value. It should be administered by a weight-based standardized protocol, beginning with a loading bolus of 80 units/kg/h followed by a maintenance infusion of 18 units/kg/h. The first APTT should be checked 4–6 hours after the loading dose, 6 hours after any dose change and then at least daily when in the therapeutic range. However, APTT monitoring of UFH is technically problematic, particularly in late pregnancy when an apparent heparin resistance occurs due to increased nonspecific plasma binding and increased factor VIII and fibrinogen which influence the APTT [17,38]. Therefore, if UFH dose adjustments during the third trimester are based upon a nonpregnant APTT therapeutic range, systematic overdosing of pregnant women could result, possibly increasing the risk of bleeding and osteoporosis. The use of anti-factor Xa heparin assays (target range 0.35–0.67 U/mL, equivalent to heparin level of 0.2–0.4 U/mL by protamine titration) to monitor UFH results in less dose escalation than monitoring with APTT [44]. A variety of nomograms exist for dose adjustment of UFH; however, given that APTT reagents and coagulometers vary markedly in their sensitivity to UFH, institution-specific nomograms should probably be utilized. When patients are converted from intravenous to subcutaneous UFH, a typical approach is to calculate the total 24-hour UFH dose, divide it by two (or three) and administer the dose obtained from this calculation every 12 (or 8 hours). Subsequent adjustments can be based on either the APTT 6 hours after injection or the anti-factor Xa level 2–4 hours after injection. HIT is a real possibility with UFH and platelet count in these patients must be monitored at baseline and every 2–3 days for the first 14 days. Thereafter, we monitor them monthly but HIT becomes very unlikely after the initial 2 weeks. The features of HIT and alternative anticoagulants to use if HIT develops are reviewed in Tables 3.6 and 3.7 respectively.

Table 3.7 Newer anticoagulants and their use in pregnancy

Agent	Route of administration	Monitoring	Clearance	Half-life	Additional comments
Heparinoids					
Danaparoid	IV bolus followed by Q12 H SC injections	Anti-Xa levels	Renal	25 +/− 100 hours	Probably the preferred newer anticoagulation in pregnancy due to preliminary but encouraging published reports. Not available in the US. May have a 5–10% risk of cross-reactivity with HIT antibodies. Expensive
Direct thrombin inhibitors					
Lepirudin	IV infusion	PTT	Renal	60 minute	Recombinant hirudin. Approved for treatment of HIT by the US Food and Drug Administration. Unlike UFH and LMWH, this agent binds both free and clot-bound thrombin. Does not cause HIT and works in patients with AT deficiency
Bivalirudin	IV infusion	ACT, APTT or PT	Renal	25 minutes	Approved only for use for unstable angina patients undergoing coronary angioplasty. Human pregnancy data extremely limited
Argatroban	IV infusion	PTT	Hepatic (no renal adjustment needed)	28 minutes	Human pregnancy data limited but given its low molecular weight, it probably readily crosses the placenta
Anti-Xa inhibitors					
Fondaparinux	Subcutaneous injections once daily	Anti-Xa level	Renal	17–21 hours	Placental transfer appears to be minimal, suggesting this may be the best newer anticoagulant for pregnant patients with HIT when there is no access to danaparoid

APTT, activated partial thromboplastin time; HIT, heparin-induced thrombocytopenia; IV intravenous; LMWH, low molecular weight heparin; PT, prothrombin time; PTT, partial thromboplastin time; UFH, unfractionated heparin. Reproduced with permission from Gibson PS, Powrie RO. Anticoagulants and pregnancy: when are they safe? Cleve Clin J Med 2009;76(2):113–27.

In massive life-threatening PTE with hemodynamic compromise, there is a case for considering thrombolytic therapy as anticoagulant therapy will not reduce the obstruction of the pulmonary circulation. RCT using thrombolytic agents for PTE in nonpregnant patients have established that thrombolysis is more effective than heparin in reducing clot burden and rapidly improving hemodynamics but have not shown any impact on long-term survival [45]. A systematic review of thrombolytic therapy in pregnancy reported on 172 women: 164 treated with streptokinase, three with urokinase and five with rt-PA. There were five nonfatal maternal bleeding complications (2.9%) and three fetal deaths (1.7%) [46]. Overall, data suggest that the maternal bleeding complication rate is in the range of 1–6%, which is consistent with that in nonpregnant patients receiving thrombolytic therapy. It is not known whether these agents cross the placenta but their high molecular weight makes this unlikely. Most bleeding events occur around catheter and puncture sites and, in pregnant women, there have been no reports of intracranial bleeding. If thrombolytic therapy has been given, an infusion of UFH is then started but the loading dose should be omitted.

Pain and swelling in the affected leg are debilitating symptoms of DVT. In patients with proximal DVT, pain and swelling improve faster in mobile patients wearing compression hosiery than in those resting in bed without any compression. Studies in nonpregnant persons have shown that early mobilization, with compression therapy, does not increase the likelihood of developing PTE. Thus there is no requirement for bed rest in a stable patient on anticoagulant treatment with acute DVT [47,48]. Where DVT threatens leg viability through venous gangrene, the leg should be elevated, anticoagulation given and consideration given to surgical embolectomy or thrombolytic therapy.

Maintenance treatment of venous thromboembolism

Antepartum

From the discussion above, it is clear that LMWH has significant advantages over APTT-monitored UFH in the maintenance treatment of VTE in pregnancy. Thus women with antenatal VTE should be managed with subcutaneous LMWH for the remainder of the pregnancy [17,35,38,49]. If LMWH therapy requires monitoring (e.g. extremes of body weight or renal impairment) the aim is for a peak anti-Xa level (measured 2–4 hours after the injection) between 0.4 and 1.2 IU/mL. Once stable, the woman can be managed as an outpatient until delivery. It is not yet established whether the dose of LMWH can be reduced to an intermediate dose or once-daily dose after an initial period of several weeks of therapeutic anticoagulation. However, such regimens have been successfully used in patients with contraindications to

warfarin and in patients with underlying malignancy [50]. Outside pregnancy, the duration of anticoagulation reflects the balance between the risk of thrombosis recurrence and the risk of serious bleeding on oral anticoagulants. In pregnancy, oral anticoagulants are not used.

As LMWH is not associated with a significant bleeding risk and there are significant ongoing risk factors for VTE recurrence including pregnancy-related changes in the coagulation system, reduced venous flow velocity, and presence of a thrombophilia in at least 50% of pregnant patients with PTE, LMWH should be given throughout pregnancy. In addition, the location of the thrombus is important with regard to recurrence risk. In contrast to the nonpregnant where the vast majority of DVT are popliteofemoral, the majority of DVT in pregnancy are ileofemoral with a greater risk of both embolization and recurrence. Thus, the balance of risks for recurrence versus bleeding on oral anticoagulants in nonpregnant patients is not directly applicable to pregnancy, emphasizing the need for a longer duration of treatment.

While some experts will decrease the dose of anticoagulation close to term to decrease the risk of bleeding, this is not our practice or recommendation. Therapeutic anticoagulant therapy should be continued for the duration of the pregnancy and for at least 6 weeks postnatally and until at least 3 months of treatment has been given in total because of the presence of ongoing risk factors and the safety of LWMH. Note that prolonged UFH use during pregnancy may result in osteoporosis and fractures [38,51]. Allergic skin reactions to heparin can occur and may require the heparin preparation to be changed; the platelet count should also be checked as this may herald HIT.

Peripartum

Management of full therapeutic anticoagulation at the time of delivery is complicated because of the wide number of variables that need to be considered. Factors contributing to planning for delivery in a woman on therapeutic anticoagulation include: mode of delivery, the degree to which regional anesthesia is desired by the patient, the individual patient's risk of thrombosis during the period off anticoagulation, the risk of the individual patient for postpartum bleeding and the possibility of obstetric complications that precipitate the need to alter even the most carefully considered plans. While there is very little evidence and little in the way of guidelines to help with decisions on how to manage anticoagulation in the puerperium, Table 3.8 reviews some possible options for patients on therapeutic anticoagulation.

A particularly challenging situation arises when a patient has an acute thromboembolism in the weeks or days prior to an anticipated (or unanticipated) delivery. Again, while there is very little evidence to guide decisions about how to manage this situation in pregnancy, there is some experience and there are guidelines with respect to the management of nonpregnant patients with recent VTE who require emergency surgery.

Table 3.8 Management options for therapeutic anticoagulation and delivery

Mode of full anticoagulation	Comments	Specific intrapartum and postpartum strategies for this option
Full anticoagulation with UFH	Regional anesthesia must be delayed until PTT is normalized Consider intermittent compression stockings during cesarean delivery	Choose one of the following options: 1. For most patients, hold subcutaneous therapeutic UFH with onset of labor/12–24 hours before induction/cesarean. Check APTT prior to delivery and insertion of epidural. PTT will take ~12 hours to normalize. Can use protamine to reverse UFH if necessary 2. For patients at lower risk of recurrent VTE: and remote from acute event, consider reducing dose of subcutaneous UFH at 36–38 weeks to prophylactic range (10,000 units SC q12h) and manage delivery as described below for patients on prophylactic UFH in Table 3.11 If patient is on IV UFH, can stop intravenous therapeutic UFH with well-established labor or 4–6 h prior to planned cesarean. Check APTT prior to delivery/insertion of epidural. PTT will take ~2 hours to normalize. Can use protamine to reverse UFH Postpartum: Resume therapeutic anticoagulation postpartum in one of the following timeframes. 1. If thrombosis risk is deemed low to moderate: resume anticoagulation when hemostasis well established and ideally at least 12 hours after epidural has been removed 2. If thrombosis risk is high to highest, resume anticoagulation as soon as possible postpartum but no sooner than 2 hours after removal of the regional anesthesia catheter Resume therapeutic anticoagulation postpartum employing one of the following strategies. 1. UFH 80 mg/kg IV UFH bolus followed by 18 mg/kg/h. Check PTT in 6 hours and adjust per protocol 2. UFH 12–18 mg/kg/h with NO UFH boluses. Check PTT at 6-hour intervals and adjust infusion rate up or down without boluses until therapeutic PTT achieved 3. Begin LMWH in therapeutic doses (usually enoxaparin 1 mg/kg every 12 hours) To transition patient from heparin to warfarin, begin 5 mg of warfarin on the third day postpartum (or later if risk of bleeding is deemed to be particularly high) and titrate dose to achieve an INR of 2–3. Overlap warfarin with UFH/LMWH until INR is in this range for 2 days.
Full anticoagulation with LMWH	Regional anesthesia cannot be administered until 24 hours after last dose of LMWH LMWH monitored with heparin level (anti-Xa level) not PTT	Follow one of the following strategies. 1. Continue LMWH until patient is in labor. Patient may not be a candidate for regional anesthesia if less than 24 hours have elapsed since time of last injection. PTT not helpful in assessing anticoagulant activity of LMWH and heparin level (anti-Xa level) cannot be used to guide timing of epidural 2. Switch patient from LMWH to UFH at 36 weeks and follow one of the protocols described above for UFH 3. Stop LMWH for 24 hours and then induce delivery/perform cesarean delivery 4. Reduce therapeutic dose of subcutaneous LMWH at 36–38 weeks to a prophylactic dose of LMWH. Follow one of the options for LMWH prophylaxis listed in Table 3.11 5. Switch patient from therapeutic LMWH to prophylactic UFH at 36–38 weeks. Check platelet count every 2–3 days and day of delivery because of risk of HIT. Manage prophylactic UFH with one of the options listed in Table 3.11

(Continued on p. 90)

Table 3.8 (Continued)

Mode of full anticoagulation	Comments	Specific intrapartum and postpartum strategies for this option
	LMWH only partially reversible with protamine

LMWH SC injections can last for 12 hours

Consider intermittent compression stockings during cesarean delivery | Postpartum:
Resume therapeutic anticoagulation postpartum in one of the following timeframes.
1. If thrombosis risk is low to moderate: resume anticoagulation when hemostasis well established and ideally at least 12 hours after epidural has been removed
2. If thrombosis risk is high to highest, resume anticoagulation as soon as possible postpartum but no sooner than 2 hours after removal of regional anesthesia catheter

Resume therapeutic anticoagulation postpartum employing one of the following strategies.
1. UFH 80 mg/kg IV UFH bolus followed by 18 mg/kg/h. Check PTT in 6 hours and adjust per protocol
2. UFH 18 mg/kg/h with NO UFH boluses. Check PTT in 6 hours and adjust up or down without boluses, checking PTT at 6-hour intervals
3. Begin LMWH in therapeutic doses (usually enoxaparin 1.5 mg/kg every 24 hours)
To transition patient from heparin to warfarin, employ the following strategy.
1. Begin 5 mg of warfarin third day postpartum (or later if bleeding risk deemed to be high) and titrate dose to achieve an INR of 2–3. Overlap with UFH/LMWH until INR therapeutic for 2 days |
| Patient on full anticoagulation because of new VTE in 4 weeks prior to anticipated delivery | Risk of pulmonary embolism off anticoagulation is highest in weeks following formation of new thrombosis | Patient who has had a new DVT/PE diagnosed in 0–2 weeks prior to an anticipated delivery should be considered for either (1) continuing anticoagulation during delivery or stopping it for the briefest possible period, or (2) the placement of a temporary IVC filter. The patient can then otherwise be managed as above but with the added security of a filter to protect the patient from major pulmonary embolism during the hours that the patient is off heparin for delivery |

APTT, activated partial thromboplastin time; DVT/PE, deep venous thrombosis/pulmonary embolism; INR, international normalized ratio; IV, intravenous; IVC, inferior vena cava; LMWH, low molecular weight heparin; PTT, partial thromboplastin time; SC, subcutaneous; UFH, unfractionated heparin; VTE, venous thromboembolism.

In general, the practice for these patients is to not interrupt heparin therapy at all, to interrupt it for as brief a period as possible or to consider placement of a temporary or permanent inferior vena caval (IVC) filter if it has been less than 2 weeks since treatment for the thrombosis was begun. The justification for this recommendation is that "fresh" clot (before it has had time to organize and begun to resolve) is deemed more friable and therefore more likely to embolize. Unprotected periods without anticoagulation in the first few weeks are therefore more likely to lead to clot propagation and embolization than is the case after months of treatment [52]. For this reason, it is the practice of the editors to consider placement of a temporary (also known as retrievable) IVC filter in women who are delivering or are expected to deliver having had less than 2 weeks of anticoagulation for acute VTE. The authors, however, favor continuing LMWH peripartum in these patients and not subjecting the patient to the risk of IVC filter.

Complications of IVC filters in the nonpregnant population include a fatality rate of 0.12–0.3% with insertion [53,54]. This fatality rate occurred in a population with many more co-morbid conditions than will be typically seen in the pregnant population. All types of filters also carry the risk of migration of the filter, bleeding at the site of insertion and acute thrombosis at the site of insertion. Permanent filters also carry a higher risk of subsequent DVT [55], a risk of erosion through the IVC wall and obstruction of the IVC if thrombosis accumulates distal to the filter. Temporary filters do not carry these risks if removed but they are not always retrievable. The published experience with their use in pregnancy has been largely favorable [56,57].

In rare circumstances, patients on full anticoagulation with UFH or LMWH may need urgent delivery within hours of receiving a full anticoagulant dose of heparin or may experience significant bleeding in the postpartum weeks and the obstetrician may want to attempt to reverse the heparin. While UFH is fully reversible with protamine, LMWH is only partially reversible with this agent. A protocol for heparin reversal with protamine is reviewed in Box 3.1.

Postpartum

Coumarins, unlike the heparins, cross the placenta readily and are associated with a characteristic embryopathy in the first trimester, central nervous system abnormalities which occur during any trimester, fetal hemorrhage and neonatal hemorrhage following the trauma of delivery [38,51]. Thus, they are not usually used for the management of VTE in pregnancy. However, following delivery, women should be offered a choice of heparin or warfarin for postnatal therapy after discussion about the need for regular blood tests for monitoring of warfarin, particularly during the first 10 days of treatment. Note that neither heparin (UFH or LMWH) nor warfarin is contraindicated in breastfeeding as there is no evidence of a significant amount of any of these agents in breast milk and the heparins are not orally active in any event. If the woman

---

Box 3.1 Protamine reversal of heparin

- UFH completely reversible with protamine
- LMWH only partially reversible with protamine
- Effects can be measured immediately
- Excessive dosing may increase bleeding
- 1% risk of anaphylaxis if prior exposure (including exposure to protamine in NPH (neutral protamine hagedorn) intermediate duration of action insulin)
- 1:1000 epinephrine should be available

Dosing and administration

1 mg of protamine sulfate
Per 100 units heparin
Per 1 mg of enoxaparin
Per 100 IU of dalteparin or tinzaparin

- Must be given SLOWLY IV (not >20 mg/min and never >50 mg over 10 min)
- Rarely need more than 25–50 mg as total treatment
- In patients on SC heparin, protamine may warrant a divided dose repeated over time due to the ongoing absorption of the subcutaneous heparin

---

chooses to continue with LMWH postnatally, then the recommended doses for the nonpregnant patient can confidently be employed (enoxaparin 1.5 mg/kg once daily, dalteparin 10,000–18,000 units once daily depending on body weight, tinzaparin 175 units/kg once daily). If the woman chooses to commence warfarin postpartum, it is our practice to delay the concomitant use of warfarin and heparin until at least the third postnatal day (and longer for women at higher risk of bleeding because of delivery complications) because of the risk of postpartum hemorrhage (PPH). Daily testing of the INR is recommended during the transfer from LMWH to warfarin to avoid overanticoagulation. The INR should be checked on day 2 of warfarin treatment and subsequent warfarin doses titrated to maintain the INR between 2.0 and 3.0. Heparin treatment should be continued until the INR is >2.0 on two successive days. Arrangements should be made for completion of the thrombophilia testing after anticoagulants are stopped.

Periodically, postpartum patients on warfarin may experience abnormal bleeding unresponsive to the usual obstetric interventions and warrant reversal of warfarin. A protocol for warfarin reversal with vitamin K is reviewed in Table 3.9.

Graduated elastic compression stockings should be worn on the affected leg for 2 years after the acute event to reduce the risk of post-thrombotic syndrome. A RCT in nonpregnant patients has shown that such therapy can reduce the incidence of mild to moderate post-thrombotic syndrome from 47% to 20%, and severe post thrombotic syndrome from 23% to 11% over this period [48].

Table 3.9 Warfarin reversal

Timeframe	Options
Gradual	By stopping the warfarin, most patients will have a near normal INR within 4 days
Over 24 hours	Three options: 1. 0.5–1 mg of IV vitamin K1. Reversal of INR to <1.4 in 57% by 27 hours. 2% risk of reaction [99]. Median elapsed time when reintroducing warfarin to obtain an INR >2.0 is 4.1 days 2. fresh-frozen plasma 2–3 units 3. vitamin K 1–2.5 mg PO. SC unnecessary if able to take PO but since pills typically come as 5 mg, may want to give 1 mg of IV preparation orally
In emergency	Two options: 1. 10 mg of vitamin K over 20–60 minutes, and/or 2. fresh-frozen plasma 2–3 units or prothrombin complex concentrate or recombinant factor VIIa

Prevention of venous thromboembolism in pregnancy

Pregnancy increases the risk of VTE 10-fold [2–4] but some women are at further increased risk in the antenatal or postnatal period because of one or more well-documented risk factors [6,58,59]. These risk factors are listed in Box 3.2. Several advances in antenatal, intrapartum and postnatal care over the last 50 years have reduced the risk of venous thrombosis in association with pregnancy, particularly early mobilization and adequate hydration following delivery, and abandoning the practice of using estrogen therapy to suppress lactation. However, other sociologic and demographic changes, as well as advances in assisted reproductive techniques, have led to increasing age, obesity, co-morbidities and increasing cesarean delivery rates in the pregnant population, all of which significantly increase the risk of venous thrombosis.

Effective preventive therapy is available in the form of LMWH. A systematic review of the efficacy and safety of LMWH to prevent VTE in pregnancy has shown that in 30 studies of 1348 patients where prophylactic doses of LMWH were used for prevention of VTE in pregnancy, only 0.84% of pregnancies were complicated by VTE [35]. However, LMWH is expensive and inconvenient and may be associated with mild side effects such as bruising and allergic skin reactions. Therefore, rather than offering LMWH to every pregnant or recently delivered woman, consideration of the risk versus the benefit for each individual is appropriate.

In order to determine which women should receive thromboprophylaxis in pregnancy and the puerperium, an individual assessment of thrombotic risk should be undertaken ideally before pregnancy, or at least in early pregnancy, during each antenatal admission and prior to and after delivery. Women at high risk of VTE (including those with previous confirmed VTE) should be offered pre-pregnancy counseling with a prospective

management plan. This is particularly important in view of the increased thrombotic risks associated with complications in the first trimester (see Table 3.10) and the fact that women may not meet their primary or secondary care provider until the end of the first trimester, after the stage at which thromboprophylaxis should have ideally begun. Since intercurrent illness (especially if associated with dehydration), enforced immobility, pre-eclampsia and other factors can superimpose extra thromboembolic risk upon the woman as pregnancy progresses, repeated risk assessment is vital; a young slim woman with no previous history of venous thrombosis at low risk early in gestation may become high risk if she develops hyperemesis gravidarum or pre-eclampsia with nephrotic range proteinuria or has a prolonged admission following an antepartum hemorrhage complicated by a urinary tract infection. Similarly, although thromboprophylaxis may not be warranted antenatally, the risk of VTE increases dramatically post partum [4–6,8] and a much lower threshold for LMWH use is therefore appropriate at that time.

The following guidance for thromboprophylaxis is taken from several well-established international peer-reviewed guidelines [38,43,60–62] but is necessarily only guidance and the principle of assessing individual risk is paramount.

Women with previous confirmed VTE and/or thrombophilia

Women who have a history of previous VTE should have a careful history documented and where objective documentation of previous VTE is not available, the previous diagnosis of VTE can be assumed in cases where the woman gives a good history and received prolonged (6–12 weeks) therapeutic anticoagulation.

Women with previous VTE have an increased risk of recurrence in pregnancy [63]. A retrospective comparison of VTE in 109 women during pregnancy and the nonpregnant period revealed recurrence rates of 10.9% during and 3.7% outside pregnancy, giving a relative risk during pregnancy of 3.5 (95% CI 1.6–7.8) [63]. So, one strategy would be to offer antenatal thromboprophylaxis to all women with a previous documented episode of VTE. However, in a small Canadian study investigating the safety of withholding antepartum heparin in women with a single previous episode of VTE, there were no recurrent episodes of VTE in 44 women (0%, 95% CI 0–8%) with no known thrombophilia and in whom the previous VTE was associated with a temporary risk factor (such as surgery, a fracture or the oral contraceptive pill)[64]. The risk of recurrence in pregnancy was increased to 5.9% (95% CI 1.2–16.2%) in women with thrombophilia and/or previous idiopathic VTE [51,64]. Another large retrospective cohort study evaluated the risk of recurrent pregnancy-associated thrombosis in 159 women with previous VTE [65]. Eight recurrent events occurred during 197 pregnancies without thrombosis

Box 3.2 Risk factors for VTE associated with pregnancy

Pre-existing	Previous VTE	
	Thrombophilia	Heritable
		Antithrombin deficiency
		Protein C deficiency
		Protein S deficiency
		Factor V Leiden
		Prothrombin gene variant (G20210A)
		Acquired (antiphospholipid syndrome)
		Lupus anticoagulant
		Anticardiolipin antibodies
	Age over 35 years	
	Obesity (BMI >30 kg/m^2) either pre-pregnancy or in early pregnancy	
	Parity greater than 2	
	Gross varicose veins	
	Paraplegia	
	Sickle cell disease	
	Inflammatory disorders	e.g. inflammatory bowel disease
New onset/transient	Some medical disorders	e.g. nephrotic syndrome, cancer, certain cardiac diseases
These risk factors are potentially reversible and may develop at later stages in gestation than the initial risk assessment or may resolve and therefore what is important is an ongoing individual risk assessment	Surgical procedure in pregnancy or puerperium	e.g. evacuation of retained products of conception (ERPC), postpartum sterilization
	Hyperemesis	
	Dehydration	
	Ovarian hyperstimulation syndrome	
	Infection	e.g. urinary tract infection
	Immobility (>4 days bed rest)	
	Pre-eclampsia	
	Excessive blood loss	
	Long distance travel	

Adapted from RCOG Green Top Guideline [60].

prophylaxis. The probability of VTE during pregnancy without thrombosis prophylaxis was 6.2% (95% CI 1.6–10.9%). The risk was constant over the whole period of pregnancy. But four of these eight women with VTE during pregnancy were heterozygous for factor V Leiden (FVL). No VTE occurred during 87 pregnancies with thrombosis prophylaxis.

Therefore, since the presence of thrombophilia influences the risk of recurrent events in pregnancy, any woman with objective documentation of previous VTE should undergo screening for both heritable and acquired thrombophilia,

ideally before pregnancy. As stated above, thrombophilia screens performed in pregnancy should be interpreted by those with expertise in this area as the results may be influenced by the pregnancy.

Women with thrombophilia have an increased risk of VTE in pregnancy [64,71,72]. This risk varies depending on the specific thrombophilia [71]. A case–control study compared the presence of thrombophilia in 119 women with and 233 without VTE in pregnancy. The relative risk for VTE was 7 for FVL, 9.5 for prothrombin G20210A (PT), 10 for

Table 3.10 Doses of LMWH for thromboprophylaxis in pregnancy and the puerperium

Anticoagulant		Enoxaparin	Dalteparin	UFH
Standard dose	50–90 kg Most patients requiring thromboprophylaxis fit into this category (see Table 3.5)	40 mg daily or 30 mg twice daily (with some experts increasing this to 40 mg twice daily at 28 weeks gestation)	5000 units daily	5000 units twice daily throughout (some experts increasing this to 7500 units twice daily at 14 weeks and to 10000 units twice daily at 28 weeks)
Low dose	<50 kg	20 mg daily	2500 units daily	5000 units twice daily throughout
Intermediate dose	>90 kg Asymptomatic antithrombin deficiency Previous VTE on long-term warfarin (some would place this scenario in the "high-dose" category below)	40 mg twice daily throughout the pregnancy Or some experts advise 60 mg once daily if 90–130 kg 80 mg once daily if 130–180 kg (promoted as an option in the UK RCOG 2009 Green Top Guidelines)	5000 units twice daily	UFH subcutaneously every 12 hours in doses adjusted to target an anti-Xa level of 0.1 to 0.3 units/mL
High dose	VTE in this pregnancy Symptomatic antithrombin deficiency Patient has indication for lifelong full anticoagulation	1 mg/kg twice daily in pregnancy 1.5 mg/kg once daily post partum	90 u/kg twice daily	UFH SC every 12 hours in doses adjusted to target a mid-interval (12 hours after injection) APTT and/or a peak (2–4 hours after injection) anti-Xa level in the therapeutic range

antithrombin deficiency and 107 for the combination of FVL and PT [71]. The risk is also influenced by whether the woman or her family are symptomatic, i.e. whether she has suffered a previous VTE or not [1,73,74]. Current evidence supports, and existing guidelines recommend, that women with previous VTE and an identifiable thrombophilia should receive antenatal thromboprophylaxis with LMWH [38,60,61,64,74].

Since a positive family history of VTE, particularly in a first-degree relative, is suggestive of heritable thrombophilia, even if none is detectable, it is our practice to manage such women in the same manner as those with known thrombophilia.

The latest American College of Chest Physicians (ACCP) and Royal College of Obstetricians and Gynaecologists (RCOG) guidelines also recommend prophylaxis be given to women whose previous VTE was estrogen (i.e. pregnancy or pill) related even if there is no identifiable thrombophilia. This is because recent studies have suggested that these women are at increased risk of recurrence during pregnancy [65–68].

Sometimes women will present in pregnancy with a known thrombophilia, usually detected because of screening following identification of heritable thrombophilia in a family member. The risk of VTE associated with thrombophilic defects varies considerably, as discussed above [72,74]. Antithrombin deficiency is associated with a very high risk (30%) [75] of VTE in pregnancy and retrospective data support a higher risk of VTE for antithrombin deficiency than other thrombophilias [76]. Asymptomatic women with antithrombin, protein C or protein S deficiencies have an eightfold increased risk of VTE

associated with pregnancy, but most events occur post partum [77]. Women heterozygous for the FVL mutation or the PT gene variant are at considerably lower risk [71]. Prospective data examining the incidence of VTE in pregnant women with thrombophilia and no prior VTE are lacking, but there are now several cohorts showing that the risk of VTE is low in women from asymptomatic kindred with minor thrombophilias, e.g. heterozygotes for FVL and PT mutations [78–80]. Patients should be stratified according to the level of risk associated with their thrombophilia. Since the risk of VTE is lower in asymptomatic women, antenatal thromboprophylaxis is not usually necessary except in those with combined defects (i.e. more than one defect), those homozygous for defects or those with antithrombin deficiency [71,73,81,82]. However, VTE is a multifactorial disease – the greater the number of risk factors, the greater the likelihood of an event and since asymptomatic thrombophilia is a risk factor, if combined with other risk factors such as increasing age, obesity or immobility, there may be a justification for the use of antenatal thromboprophylaxis in individual circumstances.

A summary of recommendations for thromboprophylaxis in women with previous VTE and/or thrombophilia is given in Box 3.3.

Women without previous VTE or thrombophilia

Most women who develop VTE in pregnancy have not had prior VTE and are not known to have thrombophilia.

Box 3.3 Summary of protocol for thromboprophylaxis in women with previous VTE and/or thrombophilia

Very high risk	Previous VTE on long-term warfarin (usually for life-threatening thrombosis or recurrent VTE)	Antenatal therapeutic LMWH and at least 6 weeks postnatal warfarin. These women require specialist management by experts in hemostasis and pregnancy
High risk	Previous unprovoked VTE or estrogen-associated VTE	Antenatal and 6 weeks postnatal prophylactic LMWH
	Previous VTE + thrombophilia	
	Previous VTE + family history of VTE	
	Asymptomatic thrombophilia (combined defects, homozygous FVL, antithrombin deficiency)	
Moderate risk	Single previous provoked (by a transient risk factor that is no longer present) VTE without thrombophilia, family history or other risk factors	Six weeks postnatal prophylactic LMWH and close antenatal surveillance for other risk factors
	Asymptomatic thrombophilia (except antithrombin deficiency, combined defects, homozygous FVL)	One week postnatal prophylactic LMWH

Adapted from RCOG Greentop Guideline [60].

Therefore a strategy is needed to assess which women without a prior history require thromboprophylaxis. One approach is to look at the number of risk factors listed in Table 3.10 and the British RCOG guidelines [60] suggest that the presence of three or more risk factors (excluding previous VTE and thrombophilia) is an indication for the use of prophylactic LMWH antenatally. The problem with this approach is that a woman may have only one risk factor but this in itself is associated with a high risk of VTE (for example, morbid obesity or nephrotic syndrome with heavy proteinuria, hypoalbuminemia, associated reduced levels of antithrombin (AT) and edema). Similarly, in certain circumstances, only two risk factors may be sufficient justification for the use of LMWH (for example, an obese woman admitted to hospital). Whatever decision is made prior to pregnancy and in early gestation, it is imperative that the risk assessment is repeated with each contact with healthcare professionals, since the development of pregnancy complications, such as pre-eclampsia or urinary tract infection, and the woman's own circumstances (e.g. long-distance travel) further increase the thromboembolic risk.

When to start thromboprophylaxis

It is commonly erroneously thought that the risk of VTE increases with gestation. Data from recent confidential enquiries in the UK of fatal PTE [1], data from the UK obstetric surveillance system [83] of all antenatal pulmonary emboli in the UK, data from retrospective analysis of VTE recurrence risks [65] and data from meta-analysis of period of risk of VTE in pregnancy [8] show that prevalence of VTE is equally distributed throughout the three trimesters. A Norwegian study has alternatively suggested a bimodal distribution for antenatal VTE with peaks in the first and third trimesters [69]. In another study from the US of 268,525 deliveries [5], there were 165 (0.06%) episodes of venous thromboembolism (one per 1627 births). Three-quarters of DVT (94 of 127, 74.8%) occurred during the antepartum period. Furthermore, among cases of antepartum DVT, half were detected before 15 weeks gestation (47 of 95, 49.5%), and only 28 cases occurred after 20 weeks (P < 0.001) [5]. The risk of fatal PTE is highest in the first trimester [8]. This is likely at least in part to be related to the occurrence early in gestation of other associated conditions that confer an increased thromboembolic risk. These include hyperemesis gravidarum that may lead to profound dehydration, ovarian hyperstimulation that is particularly associated with internal jugular vein [84] and superior vena caval thrombosis, miscarriage and early pregnancy surgery.

Therefore if a decision is made to initiate thromboprophylaxis antenatally, this should begin as early in pregnancy as practical [60]. For women with recurrent previous VTE on long-term warfarin, the change to LMWH should be made as soon as possible after a pregnancy has been recognized and not later than 6 weeks gestation. Women at high risk of VTE in pregnancy such as those with previous VTE should be offered pre-pregnancy counseling and a prospective management plan for thromboprophylaxis in pregnancy [60].

In the retrospective study of VTE recurrence [65], the majority of events occurred after delivery, reflecting the very high risk during the postpartum period. In that study, 15 VTEs occurred: two (2.4%) following 83 pregnancy terminations, one (1.9%) following 53 miscarriages, three (30%) following 10 stillbirths and nine (6.5%) following 138 livebirths. The Norwegian study mentioned above [69] also demonstrated a much higher risk in the postpartum period, particularly in the first 2 weeks but lasting until 6 weeks post partum [69]. For women with previous VTE or thrombophilia, in whom LMWH is not required antenatally, postpartum thromboprophylaxis is essential [79] and this should begin as soon as is practical following delivery and be continued for 6 weeks postpartum or one week in the case of asymptomatic low risk thrombophilia.

What agent to use for thromboprophylaxis and in what dose

The benefits of LMWH over UFH for thromboprophylaxis in pregnancy in terms of convenience, safety and efficacy are now well established [35,39,40,85–87]. LMWHs are, however, more expensive and although used extensively in Europe and Canada, in the US some units still use UFH. There are few circumstances where oral anticoagulants are indicated and these mostly relate to particularly high-risk mechanical heart valves.

Some practitioners will use low-dose aspirin as thromboprophylaxis in pregnancy in situations that do not warrant use of LMWH, but although there are data to support this strategy outside pregnancy [88], there are few data relating to pregnancy and current guidelines do not recommend the use of aspirin for thromboprophylaxis in pregnancy. Graduated compression stockings (GCS) may be used antenatally and postnatally. There are no trials to support such practice in pregnancy but the British Society for Haematology guidelines [82] give a grade C recommendation (evidence level IV) that all women with previous VTE or a thrombophilia should be encouraged to wear GCS throughout their pregnancy and for 6–12 weeks after delivery. The use of properly applied GCS of appropriate strength is recommended in pregnancy and the puerperium for:
- those who are hospitalized and have a contraindication to LMWH
- those who are hospitalized post- cesarean section (combined with LMWH) and considered to be at particularly high risk of VTE (e.g. previous VTE, more than three risk factors)
- outpatients with prior VTE (usually combined with LMWH)
- women traveling by air in medium to long haul flights of more than 4 hours duration [70].

Appropriate doses for thromboprophylaxis are given in Table 3.10. Mostly a standard fixed dose is used, except at the extremes of weight or in the presence of severe renal impairment. Higher prophylactic doses may be indicated for women with antithrombin deficiency (where antithrombin concentrates may also be used) and for those with combined defects (for example, homozygous FVL or compound heterozygote, e.g. FVL plus PT gene mutation) and those who are on long-term warfarin outside pregnancy. Full anticoagulant doses are rarely indicated for thromboprophylaxis but may be used for symptomatic AT deficiency.

Monitoring of LMWH in patients on prophylactic doses

As stated for full therapeutic doses of LMWH, extensive experience of LMWH use for prophylaxis in pregnancy indicates that monitoring of anti-Xa levels is not required, provided the woman has normal renal function and that the dose is adjusted for the extremes of weight. In antithrombin deficiency anti-Xa monitoring is critical, higher doses of LMWH may be necessary and the patient should be monitored by a clinician with expertise in hemostasis.

The risk of HIT is extremely low with LMWH [35,39] and substantially lower with LMWH use compared with UFH. In the 2777 pregnancies treated with LMWH and reviewed by Greer & Nelson Piercy [35], no cases of HIT associated with thrombosis were reported. Therefore, as discussed above, monitoring of platelet counts after verifying that the initial baseline is normal is not warranted unless there has been prior exposure to UFH [39].

Thromboprophyaxis during and after delivery

There are profound hemostatic changes after delivery and the prothrombotic physiologic adaptations to pregnancy are maximal in the immediate puerperium. Consequently, this is the time of greatest risk of VTE. Although most VTE occurs antenatally [5], the risk per day is greatest in the weeks immediately after delivery [8]. Furthermore, the risk of VTE is up to 20-fold higher following delivery by cesarean delivery. In one study the incidence of postpartum PTE was 0.052% post cesarean delivery and 0.0017% (P < 0.001) [5] after vaginal delivery. The mean time of postpartum VTE post cesarean delivery was later than post vaginal delivery (6.3 vs 2.3 days, P = 0.004) [5].

For patients who have been on prophylactic anticoagulation throughout the pregnancy and enter the peripartum period, there is little evidence to guide the management. Given the increased risk in the postpartum period, however, it does appear that prolonged withdrawal of thromboembolic prophylaxis is ill advised. Again, there are many factors to consider when deciding how to approach the management of peripartum thromboprophylaxis, including risk of recurrent thrombosis, risk of bleeding, patient preference for regional anesthesia, mode of delivery and unanticipated obstetric complications that may alter delivery plans. Perhaps most difficult of these considerations are the limitations associated with LMWH use and regional anesthesia, discussed in Chapter 4.

Preventing VTE in patients who did not require antepartum thromboprophylaxis

Despite VTE being a leading cause of maternal mortality in the developed world, the absolute rate of VTE is low and universal thromboprophylaxis with heparin is not warranted. All guidelines [38,43,60,61] agree that early mobilization and avoidance of dehydration are important measures that should be adopted universally to reduce the postpartum risk of VTE. Guidelines also agree about the use of UFH or LMWH or warfarin for 6 weeks after delivery in women with previous VTE and those with high risk thrombophilia (see above). Warfarin, UFH or LMWH may be used safely in the breastfeeding mother. However, there is no consensus about which women without a prior history of VTE or thrombophilia should receive UFH or LMWH post partum. One study screening women who underwent cesarean delivery for VTE found an incidence of 0.5% (95% CI 0.1–2.8%), not enough to support universal use of LMWH/UFH in patients undergoing cesarean delivery [71]. The 2008 recommendations by the ACCP [43] and the updated 2009 Green Top Guideline from the RCOG both use the principle of risk assessment for thromboprophylaxis. For cesarean delivery, the presence of one of the risk factors (other than previous VTE or thrombophilia) listed in Table 3.10 justifies the use of LMWH prophylaxis for 7 days. The UK guidelines [60] also advocate the use of prophylactic doses of heparin for 7 days following a vaginal delivery in women with two or more persisting risk factors (again, listed in Table 3.10). The recommendation to continue prophylaxis for 7 days will typically extend beyond hospitalization and will necessitate women being taught how to self-administer LMWH prior to discharge in the UK.

The first thromboprophylactic dose of LMWH should be given as soon as possible after delivery provided there is no postpartum hemorrhage and regional analgesia has not been used (or 2 hours after removal of the epidural/spinal catheter in patients who did receive regional anesthesia – see Chapter 4). Despite the recommendations given in the preceding paragraph, the optimal duration of thromboprophylaxis post partum is not known. This is because it is difficult to determine when the increased VTE risk is reduced enough to discontinue thromboprophylaxis. Preliminary data using thromboelastography (TEG) suggest that by the end of postpartum week 3, blood coagulation has returned to nonpregnant levels, but most of this resolution has occurred by the end of week 1 [89]. Also, time to resolution of hypercoagulability to a nonpregnant state was unaffected by mode of delivery. This provided the rationale for the updated recommendation to continue LMWH for 7 days after both vaginal and cesarean delivery in women with additional risk factors, rather than 3–5 days. More research is needed in this area since TEG is only a very limited evaluation of only one of the three elements of Virchow's triad.

Just as circumstances and risk factors can change antenatally, so too may they in the postpartum period. Therefore puerperal women undergoing surgery for any reason or those who develop severe infection or who choose to travel long distance are at increased risk of VTE even though they may have been discharged from hospital following normal vaginal delivery several weeks before. Consideration should be given to reintroducing LMWH in these circumstances.

Anesthetic issues related to venous thromboembolism and anticoagulation

Anesthetic issues related to thromboembolism and anticoagulation are discussed at the end of Chapter 4.

Table 3.11 Options for managing prophylactic UFH/LMWH in the peripartum period

Antepartum VTE prophylaxis mode	General comments	Specific intrapartum and postpartum strategies for this option
UFH prophylactic doses	Prophylactic UFH can be administered concomitantly with epidural anesthesia if PTT is normal. All patients should be on intermittent compression stockings during cesarean delivery	Hold UFH with onset of labor or on morning of planned cesarean/induction and check platelet count and PTT prior to delivery/epidural
LMWH prophylactic doses	LMWH must be held for 10–12 hours prior to insertion of an epidural catheter and must not be administered postpartum until 2 hours after removal of the epidural All patients should be on intermittent compression stockings during cesarean delivery.	Choose one of the following strategies. 1. Continue prophylactic LMWH until patient in labor and then stop. Patient can only receive regional anesthesia if 12 hours have elapsed since last dose, regardless of anti-Xa level 2. Switch patients from prophylactic LMWH to prophylactic UFH at 36 weeks. Check platelets on day every 2 days for 14 days after initiating UFH (and on day of delivery) because of risk of HIT on UFH. Peripartum management strategies as per option 1 above 3. Hold LMWH for 12–24 hours and then induce delivery 4. Stop LMWH 12–24 hours prior to scheduled cesarean

References

1. Lewis G (ed). The confidential enquiry into maternal and child health (CEMACH). Saving mothers' lives: reviewing maternal deaths to make motherhood safer 2003–2005. The Seventh Report on Confidential Enquiries into Maternal Deaths in the UK. Department of Health, London, 2007.
2. Macklon NS, Greer IA. Venous thromboembolic disease in obstetrics and gynaecology: the Scottish experience. Scott Med J 1996;41:83–86.
3. Lindqvist P, Dahlback B, Marsal K. Thrombotic risk during pregnancy: a population study. Obstet Gynecol 1999;94: 595–9.
4. Andersen BS, Steffensen FH, Sorensen HT, Nielsen GL, Olsen J. The cumulative incidence of venous thromboembolism during pregnancy and puerperium – an 11 year Danish population-based study of 63,300 pregnancies. Acta Obstet Gynecol Scand 1998;77:170–3.
5. Gherman RB, Goodwin TM, Leung T, et al. Incidence, clinical characteristics, and timing of objectively diagnosed venous thromboembolism during pregnancy. Obstet Gynecol 1999;94:730–4.
6. McColl MD, Ramsay JE, Tait RC, et al. Risk factors for pregnancy associated venous thromboembolism. Thromb Haemost 1997;78:1183–8.
7. White RH. The epidemiology of venous thromboembolism. Circulation 2003;107:14–18.
8. Ray JG, Chan WS. Deep vein thrombosis during pregnancy and the puerperium: a meta-analysis of the period of risk and the leg of presentation. Obstet Gynecol Surv 1999;54:265–71.
9. Blanco-Molina A, Trujillo-Santos J, Criado J, et al. Venous thromboembolism during pregnancy or postpartum: findings from the RIETE Registry. Thromb Haemost 2007;97:186–90.
10. Greer IA, Thomson AJ. Management of venous thromboembolism in pregnancy. Best Pract Res Clin Obstet Gynaecol 2001;15:583–603.
11. Berg CJ, Atrash HK, Koonin LM, Tucker M. Pregnancy-related mortality in the United States, 1987–1990. Obstet Gynecol 1996;88:161–7.
12. Chang J, Elam-Evans LD, Berg CJ, et al. Pregnancy-related mortality surveillance – United States, 1991–1999. MMWR Surveill Summ 2003;52:1–8.
13. Bounameaux H, Perrier A. Duration of anticoagulation therapy for venous thromboembolism. Hematol Am Soc Hematol Educ Program 2008;2008:252–8.
14. McColl M, Ellison J, Greer IA, et al. Prevalence of the post-thrombotic syndrome in young women with previous venous thromboembolism. Br J Haematol 2000;108:272–4.
15. Bergqvist D, Bergqvist A, Lindhagen A, et al. Long-term outcome of patients with venous thromboembolism during pregnancy. In: Greer IA, Turpie AGG, Forbes CD (eds) Haemostasis and thrombosis in obstetrics and gynaecology. Chapman and Hall, London, 1992: 349–59.
16. Scarsbrook AF, Evans AL, Owen AR, Gleeson FV. Diagnosis of suspected venous thromboembolic disease in pregnancy. Clin Radiol 2006;61:1–12.
17. Thomson AJ, Greer IA. Acute management of venous thromboembolism in pregnancy. Royal College of Obstetricians and Gynaecologists, London, 2007.
18. Ferrari E, Baudout M, Cerboni P, et al. Clinical epidemiology of venous thromboembolic disease: results of a French multicentre registry. Eur Heart J 1997;18:685–91.
19. Fidler JL, Patz Jr EF, Ravin CE. Cardiopulmonary complications of pregnancy: radiographic findings. Am J Roentgenol 1993:161:937–42.
20. Damilakis J, Perisinakis K, Prassopoulos P, Dimovasili E, Varveris H, Gourtsoyiannis N. Conceptus radiation dose and risk from chest screen-film radiography. Eur Radiol 2003;13(2):406–12.
21. Wells PS, Ginsberg JS, Anderson DR, et al. Utility of ultrasound imaging of the lower extremities in the diagnostic approach in patients with suspected pulmonary embolism. J Intern Med 2001;250:262–4.
22. MacGillavry MR, Sanson BJ, Buller HR, et al. Compression ultrasonography of the leg veins in patients with clinically suspected pulmonary embolism: is a more extensive assessment of compressibility useful? Thromb Haemostas 2000;84:973–6.
23. Turkstra F, Kuijer PM, van Beek EJ, et al. Diagnostic utility of ultrasonography of leg veins in patients suspected of having pulmonary embolism. Ann Intern Med 1997;126:775–81.
24. Cook JV, Kyrion J. Radiation from CT and perfusion scanning in pregnancy. BMJ 2005;331:350.
25. Nijkeuter M, Geleijns J, de Roos A, Meinders AE, Huisman MV. Diagnosing pulmonary embolism in pregnancy: rationalizing fetal radiation exposure in radiological procedures. J Thromb Haemost 2004;2(10):1857.
26. Winer-Muram HT, Boone JM, Brown HL, Jennings SG, Mabie WC, Lombardo GT. Pulmonary embolism in pregnant patients: fetal radiation dose with helical CT. Radiology 2002;224(2):487–9.
27. Remy-Jardin M, Remy J. Spiral CT angiography of the pulmonary circulation. Radiology 1999;212(3):615–36.
28. Allen C, Demetriades T. Radiation risk overestimated. Radiology 2006;240(2):613–14.
29. Francalanci I, Comeglio P, Alessandrello Liotta A, et al. D-dimer plasma levels during normal pregnancy measured by specific ELISA. Int J Clin Lab Res 1997;27(1):65–7.
30. Kline JA, Williams GW, Hernandez-Nino J. D-dimer concentrations in normal pregnancy: new diagnostic thresholds are needed. Clin Chem 2005;51(5):825–9.
31. Chan WS, Chunilal S, Lee A, Crowther M, Rodger M, Ginsberg JS. A red blood cell agglutination D-dimer test to exclude deep venous thrombosis in pregnancy. Ann Intern Med 2007;147(3):165–70.
32. Damodaram M, Kaladindi M, Luckit J, Yoong W. D-dimers as a screening test for venous thromboembolism in pregnancy: is it of any use? J Obstet Gynaecol 2009;29(2):101–3.
33. Gould MK, Dembitzer AD, Doyle RL, et al. Low molecular weight heparins compared with unfractionated heparin for treatment of acute deep venous thrombosis. A meta-analysis of randomized, controlled trials. Ann Intern Med 1999;130: 800–9.
34. Quinlan DJ, McQuillan A, Eikelboom JW. Low-molecular-weight heparin compared with intravenous unfractionated heparin for treatment of pulmonary embolism: a meta-analysis of randomized, controlled trials. Ann Intern Med 2004;140:175–83.
35. Greer IA, Nelson-Piercy C. Low-molecular-weight heparins for thromboprophylaxis and treatment of venous thromboembolism in pregnancy: a systematic review of safety and efficacy. Blood 2005;106:401–7.
36. Yusen RD, Gage BF. Outpatient treatment of acute thromboembolic disease. Clin Chest Med 2003;24:46–61.
37. Hirsh, J. Warkentin TE, Shaughnessy SG, et al. Heparin and low–molecular weight heparin: mechanism of action, pharmacokinetics, dosing, monitoring, efficacy, and safety. Chest. 2001;119(suppl 1):64S–94S.
38. Bates SM, Greer IA, Hirsh J, Ginsberg JS. Use of antithrombotic agents during pregnancy: the Seventh ACCP Conference on Antithrombotic and thrombolytic therapy. Chest 2004;163:627S–644S.

39. Warkentin TE, Greinacher A. Heparin-induced thrombocytopenia: recognition, treatment, and prevention: the Seventh ACCP Conference on Antithrombotic and Thrombolytic Therapy. Chest 2004;126(3 suppl):311S–337.

40. Pettila V, Leinonen P, Markkola A, Hiilesmaa V, Kaaja R. Postpartum bone mineral density in women treated for thromboprophylaxis with unfractionated heparin or LMW heparin. Thromb Haemost 2002;87(2):182–6.

41. Greer I, Hunt BJ. Low molecular weight heparin in pregnancy: current issues. Br J Haematol 2005;128:593–601.

42. Smith MP, Norris LA, Steer PJ, Savidge GF, Bonnar J. Tinzaparin sodium for thrombosis treatment and prevention during pregnancy. Am J Obstet Gynecol 2004;190:495–501.

43. Bates SM, Greer IA, Pabinger I, Sofaer S, Hirsh J, American College of Chest Physicians. Venous thromboembolism, thrombophilia, antithrombotic therapy, and pregnancy: American College of Chest Physicians Evidence-Based Clinical Practice Guidelines (8th edition). Chest 2008;133(6 suppl):844S–886S.

44. Levine MN, Hirsh J, Gent M, et al. A randomized trial comparing activated thromboplastin time with heparin assay in patients with acute venous thromboembolism requiring large daily doses of heparin. Arch Intern Med 1994;154:49–56.

45. Wan S, Quinlan DJ, Agnelli G, Eikelboom JW. Thrombolysis compared with heparin for the initial treatment of pulmonary embolism: a meta–analysis of the randomized controlled trials. Circulation 2004;110:744–9.

46. Ahearn GS, Hadjiliadis MD, Govert JA, Tapson VF. Massive pulmonary embolism during pregnancy successfully treated with recombinant tissue plasminogen activator. Arch Intern Med 2002;162:1221–7.

47. Blättler W, Partsch H. Leg compression and ambulation is better than bed rest for the treatment of acute deep vein thrombosis. Int Angiol 2003;22:393–400.

48. Brandjes DP, Buller HR, Heijboer H, et al. Randomised trial of effect of compression stockings in patients with symptomatic proximal-vein thrombosis. Lancet 1997;349:759–62.

49. Rodie VA, Thomson AJ, Stewart FM, et al. Low molecular weight heparin for the treatment of venous thromboembolism in pregnancy– case series. Br J Obstet Gynaecol 2002;109:1020–4.

50. Lee AY, Levine MN, Baker RI, et al., Randomized Comparison of Low-Molecular-Weight Heparin versus Oral Anticoagulant Therapy for the Prevention of Recurrent Venous Thromboembolism in Patients with Cancer (CLOT) Investigators. Low-molecular-weight heparin versus a coumarin for the prevention of recurrent venous thromboembolism in patients with cancer. N Engl J Med 2003;349:146–53.

51. Greer IA.Thrombosis in pregnancy: maternal and fetal issues. Lancet 1999;353:1258–65.

52. Kearon C, Hirsh J. Management of anticoagulation before and after elective surgery. N Engl J Med 1997;336:1506–11.

53. Becker DM, Philbrick JT, Selby JB. Inferior vena cava filters. Indications, safety, effectivemess. Arch Intern Med 1992;152(10):1985–94.

54. Athanasoulis CA, Kaufman JA, Halpern EF, Waltman AC, Geller SC, Fan CM. Inferior vena caval filters: review of a 26-year single-center clinical experience. Radiology 2000;216(1):54–66.

55. Decousus H, Leizorovicz A, Pretn F, et al. A clinical trial of vena caval filters in the prevention of pulmonary embolism in patients with proximal deep-vein thrombosis. Prevention du Risque d'Embolie Pulmonaire par Interruption Cave Study Group. N Engl J Med 1998;338(7):409–15.

56. Kawamata K, Chiba Y, Tanaka R, Higashi M, Nishigami K. Experience of temporary inferior vena caval filters inserted in the perinatal period to prevent pulmonary embolism in pregnant women with deep vein thrombosis. J Vasc Surg 2005;41(4):652–6.

57. Jamjute P, Reed N, Hinwood D. Use of inferior vena cava filters in thromboembolic disease during labor: case report with a literature review. J Matern Fetal Neonatal Med 2006;19(11):741–4.

58. Jacobsen AF, Skjeldestad FE, Sandset PM. Ante- and postnatal risk factors of venous thrombosis: a hospital-based case-control study. J Thromb Haemost 2008;6(6):905–12.

59. Simpson EL, Lawrenson RA, Nightingale AL, Farmer RDT. Venous thromboembolism in pregnancy and the puerperium: incidence and additional risk factors from a London perinatal database. Br J Obstet Gynaecol 2001;108:56–60.

60. RCOG. Reducing the risk of thrombosis and embolism during pregnancy and the puerperium. Green Top Guideline No 37. Royal College of obstetricians and Gynaecologists, London, 2009.

61. Scottish Intercollegiate Guidelines Network. Pregnancy and the puerperium. Scottish Intercollegiate Guidelines Network, Edinburgh, 2002.

62. Bates SM, Greer IA, Pabinger I, Sofaer S, Hirsh J. Venous thromboembolism, thrombophilia, antithrombotic therapy, and pregnancy: American College of Chest Physicians Evidence-Based Clinical Practice Guidelines (8th Edition). Chest 2008;133 (6 suppl):844S–886S.

63. Pabinger I, Grafenhofer H, Kyrle PA, et al. Temporary increase in the risk for recurrence during pregnancy in women with a history of venous thromboembolism. Blood 2002;100: 1060–2.

64. Brill-Edwards P, Ginsberg JS, for the Recurrence Of Clot In This Pregnancy (ROCIT) Study Group. Safety of withholding antepartum heparin in women with a previous episode of venous thromboembolism. N Engl J Med 2000;343:1439–44.

65. Pabinger I, Grafenhofer H, Kaider A, et al. Risk of pregnancy-associated recurrent venous thromboembolism in women with a history of venous thrombosis. J Thromb Haemost 2005;3:949–54.

66. Duhl AJ, Paidas MJ, Ural SH, et al. Antithrombotic therapy and pregnancy: consensus report and recommendations for prevention and treatment of venous thromboembolism and adverse pregnancy outcomes. Am J Obstet Gynecol 2007;197(5):457–21.

67. De Stefano V, Martinelli I, Rossi E, et al. The risk of recurrent venous thromboembolism in pregnancy and puerperium without antithrombotic prophylaxis. Br J Haematol 2006;135(3):386–91.

68. White RH, Chan WS, Zhou H, Ginsberg JS. Recurrent venous thromboembolism after pregnancy-associated versus unprovoked thromboembolism. Thromb Haemost 2008;100(2):246–52.

69. Jacobsen AF, Skjeldestad FE, Sandet PM. Incidence and risk patters of venous thromboemolism in pregnancy and puerperium – a register-based case-control study. Am J Ostet Gynecol 2008;198:223e.1–223e.7.

70. Royal College of Obstetricians and Gynaecologists. Air travel and pregnancy. Scientific Advisory Committee Opinion Paper 1. Royal College of Obstetricians and Gynaecologists, London, 2008.

71. Sia WW, Powrie RO, Cooper AB, et al. Incidence of deep vein thrombosis in women undergoing cesarean delivery. Thromb Res 2009;123(3):550–5.

72. Gerhardt A, Scharf RE, Beckman MW, et al. Prothrombin and factor V mutations in women with thrombosis during pregnancy and the puerperium. N Engl J Med 2000;342:374–80.

73. Greer IA. The challenge of thrombophilia in maternal–fetal medicine. N Engl J Med 2000;342:424–5.

74. McColl MD, Ellison J, Reid F, et al. Prothrombin 20210GA, MTHFR C677T mutations in women with venous thromboembolism associated with pregnancy. Br J Obstet Gynaecol 2000;107:565–9.

75. McColl MD, Walker ID, Greer IA. The role of inherited thrombophilia in venous thromboembolism associated with pregnancy. Br J Obstet Gynaecol 1999;75:387–8.

76. McLintock, North RA, Dekker G. Inherited thrombophilias: associated venous thromboembolism and obstetric complications. Curr Prob Obstet Gynecol Fertil 2001;24:109–52.

77. Conard J, Horellou MH, van Dreden P, Le Compte T, Samama M. Thrombosis in pregnancy and congenital deficiencies in AT III, protein C or protein S: study of 78 women. Thromb Haemost 1990;63:319–20.

78. Friederich PW, Sanson BJ, Simioni P, et al. Frequency of pregnancy–related venous thromboembolism in anticoagulant factor–deficient women: implications for prophylaxis. Arch Intern Med 1996;125:955–60.

79. Lim W, Eikelboom JW, Ginsberg J. Inherited thrombophilia and pregnancy associated thromboembolism. BMJ 2007;443:1318–21.

80. Dizon-Towson D, Miller C, Sibai B, et al. The relationship of the factor V Leiden mutation and pregnancy outcomes for mother and fetus. Obstet Gynecol 2005;106:517–24.

81. Simioni P, Tormene D, Prandoni P, Girolami A. Pregnancy related recurrent events in thrombophilic women with previous venous thromboembolism. Thromb Haemost 2001;86:929.

82. Walker ID, Greaves M, Preston FE. British Society for Haematology Guideline. Investigation and management of heritable thrombophilia. Br J Haematol 2001;114:512–28.

83. Knight M, UKOSS. Antenatal pulmonary embolism: risk factors, management and outcomes. Br J Obstet Gynecol 2008;115(4):453–61.

84. Arya R, Shehata HA, Patel RK, et al. Internal jugular vein thrombosis following assisted conception therapy. Br J Haematol 2001;115:153–6.

85. Sanson BJ, Lensing AWA, Prins MH, et al. Safety of low-molecular-weight heparin in pregnancy: a systematic review. Thromb Haemost 1999;81:668–72.

86. Ensom MHH, Stephenson MD. Low molecular weight heparins in pregnancy. Pharmacotherapy 1999;19:1013–25.

87. Lepercq J, Conard J, Borel-Derlon A, et al. Venous thromboembolism during pregnancy: a retrospective study of enoxaparin safety in 624 pregnancies. Br J Obstet Gynaecol 2001;108(11):1134–40.

88. Pulmonary Embolism Prevention (PEP) Trial Collaborative Group. Prevention of pulmonary embolism and deep venous thrombosis with low dose aspirin: Pulmonary Embolism Prevention (PEP) trial. Lancet 2000;355:1295–302.

89. Maybury H, Waugh JJ, Gornall AS, Pavord S,. There is a return to non–pregnant coagulation parameters after four not six weeks postpartum following spontaneous vaginal delivery. Obstet Med 2008;1:92–4.

90. Stein PD , Terrin ML, Hales CA, et al Clinical, laboratory, roentgenographic and electrocardiographic findings in patients with acute pulmonary embolism and no pre-existing cardiac or pulmonary disase. Chest 1991;100(3):598–603.

91. Marik PE, Plante LA. Venous thromboembolic disease and pregnancy. N Engl J Med 2008;359:2025–33.

92. Pahde JK, Litmanovich D, Pedrosa I, Romero J, Bankier AA, Boiselle PM. Quality initiatives: imaging patients with suspected pulmonary embolism: what the radiologist needs to know. Radiographics 2009;29(3):639–54.

93. Bourjeily G, Rosene–Montella K. Venous thromboembolism in pregnancy. In: Pulmonary Problems in Pregnancy. Humana Press, New York, 2009.

94. Righini M, Perrier A, de Moerloose P, Bounameaux H. D-dimer for venous thromboembolism diagnosis: 20 years later. J Thromb Haemost 2008; 6(7):1059–71.

95. van Dongen CJ, van den Belt AG, Prins MH, Lensing AW. Fixed dose subcutaneous low molecular weight heparins versus adjusted dose unfractionated heparin for venous thromboembolism. Cochrane Database of Systematic Reviews, 2004;4: CD001100.

96. Dahlman TC. Osteoporotic fractures and the recurrence of thromboembolism during pregnancy and the puerperium in 184 women undergoing thromboprophylaxis with heparin. Am J Obstet Gynecol 1993;168(4):1265–70.

97. Le Templier G, Rodger MA. Heparin–induced osteoporosis and pregnancy. Curr Opin Pulm Med 2008;14(5):403–7.

98. Hassell K. Heparin-induced thrombocytopenia: diagnosis and management. Thromb Res 2008;123(suppl 1):S16–21.

99. Shields RC, McBane RD, Kuiper JD, Li H, Heit JA. Efficacy and safety of intravenous phytonadione (vitamin K1) in patients on long-term oral anticoagulant therapy. Mayo Clin Proc 2001;76(3):260–6.

Thrombophilias and pregnancy

Marc A. Rodger[1], Michael Paidas[2] with Lawrence Tsen[3] and Joanne Douglas[4]

[1]Division of Hematology, The Ottawa Hospital, University of Ottawa; Clinical Epidemiology Program, Ottawa Health Research Institute, Ottawa, Ontario, Canada
[2]Department of Obstetrics, Gynecology, and Reproductive Sciences, Yale Women and Children's Center for Blood Disorders, Yale-New Haven Hospital, New Haven, CT, USA
[3]Department of Anesthesiology, Center for Reproductive Medicine, Perioperative and Pain Medicine, Brigham and Women's Hospital, Boston, MA, USA
[4]Department of Anesthesia, British Columbia Women's Hospital, Vancouver, BC, Canada

Physiologic changes of the hemostatic system in pregnancy

Understanding disease in pregnancy requires knowledge of the normal physiologic changes occurring in pregnancy (Table 4.1). The hemostatic system is a physiologic system designed to limit bleeding at sites of vascular injury. Hemostasis, involving vasoconstriction, platelet plug formation through platelet aggregation, fibrin clot formation through coagulation activation, and fibrinolysis or clot dissolution, is normally limited to sites of vascular injury. Each of these processes is classically thought to occur in sequence (in phases) but a more modern understanding is that these steps occur in varying sequence and at varying rates in different vascular beds in a time, flow and interdependent manner. The hemostatic system undergoes many physiologic changes in an effort to prepare the parturient for the hemostatic challenge of delivery. These changes have likely evolved due to the tremendous selective pressure from maternal mortality caused by hemorrhage at childbirth throughout evolution. As recently as the 17th century, more than 10% of parturients died at childbirth from hemorrhage.

Hypercoagulability of pregnancy

Pregnancy is associated with increased levels of procoagulant factors and decreases in anticoagulant factors, resulting in increased thrombin generation [2,3]. This increased thrombin generation coupled with a decrease in fibrinolysis results in hypercoagulability that prepares expectant mothers for the hemostatic challenge of delivery. Progressively throughout gestation, some procoagulant factors including factor VIII, factor V and fibrinogen increase while the anticoagulant mechanisms are reduced, including increasing resistance to activated protein C and reduced protein S levels. Antithrombin and protein C levels are not reduced in pregnancy [2]. The gradual increase in thrombin activation throughout gestation is evidenced by increases in coagulation activation markers including thrombin antithrombin complex (TAT) levels and F1.2 (a byproduct of thrombin acting on fibrinogen) [4]. Von Willebrand factor (vWF) is involved in two components of the hemostatic mechanism: coagulation, in which vWF acts as a plasma carrier protein for FVIII, and platelet plug formation where vWF permits adhesion of platelets to the subendothelial matrix proteins. Von Willebrand factor levels also increase throughout pregnancy. Fibrinolytic activity (mediated by plasmin) is reduced in pregnancy most likely due to increased levels of plasminogen activator inhibitor (PAI) type 1 and type 2 (produced mainly by the placenta). Thrombin activatable fibrinolysis inhibitor (TAFI) has been demonstrated to be a key component of the reduced fibrinolysis seen with increasing gestation [5]. D-dimers are byproducts of fibrinolysis created by the action of plasmin on cross-linked fibrin. These increasing D-dimer levels may not appear consistent with the previously mentioned decreased fibrinolysis observed in pregnancy but are likely due to the increased thrombin generation as gestation progresses resulting in greater fibrin formation (i.e. increased substrate for fibrinolysis).

All the above changes in the hemostatic system normalize to the nonpregnant state by 6–8 weeks post partum.

de Swiet's Medical Disorders in Obstetric Practice, 5th edition.
Edited by R. O. Powrie, M. F. Greene, W. Camann. © 2010 Blackwell Publishing.

Table 4.1 Hemostatic changes in pregnancy. Adapted from Bremme [1]

Variables (mean ± SD)	1st Trimester	2nd Trimester	3rd Trimester	Nonpregnant normal range
Platelets (×10⁹/L)	275 ± 64	256 ± 49	244 ± 52	125–400
Fibrinogen (g/L)	3.7 ± 0.6	4.4 ± 1.2	5.4 ± 0.8	2.1–4.2
PTT	↔	↔	↔	24–36s
INR	↔	↔	↔	0.9–1.2
Antithrombin (U/mL)	1.02 ± 0.10	1.07 ± 0.14	1.07 ± 0.11	0.85–1.25
Protein C (U/ mL)	0.92 ± 0.13	1.06 ± 0.17	.94 ± 0.2	0.68–1.25
Protein S, total (U/ mL)	0.83 ± 0.11	0.73 ± 0.11	0.77 ± 0.10	0.70–1.70
Protein S, free (U/ mL)	0.26 ± 0.07	0.17 ± 0.04	0.14 ± 0.04	0.20–0.50
Soluble fibrin (nmol/L)	9.2 ± 8.6	11.8 ± 7.7	13.4 ± 5.2	<15
Thrombin-antithrombin (μg/L)	3.1 ± 1.4	5.9 ± 2.6	7.1 ± 2.4	<2.7
D-dimers (μg/L)	91 ± 24	128 ± 49	198 ± 59	<250
Plasminogen activator inhibitor 1 (AU/ mL)	7.4 ± 4.9	14.9 ± 5.2	37.8 ± 19.4	<15
Plasminogen activator inhibitor 2 (μg/L)	31 ± 14	84 ± 16	160 ± 31	<5
Cardiolipin antibodies positive	2/25	2/25	3/23	0
Von Willebrand factor antigen (vWF)	↑	↑	↑	Subjects with blood group O: 0.40–1.75 U/mL Subjects with blood group A, B or AB: 0.70–2.10 U/mL

Introduction to thrombophilia

Thrombophilias are acquired or inherited predispositions to developing venous thrombosis (deep vein thrombosis or pulmonary embolism). These prevalent conditions may have given women a selective evolutionary advantage over non-thrombophilic women by allowing them to cope better with the hemostatic challenge of delivery. For example, it has been demonstrated that women with factor V Leiden (see below) have a reduced risk of intrapartum bleeding compared to normal women [6]. However, in the present day, with modern obstetric practice, this advantage is likely less important than in the past. The downside is that thrombophilias predispose women to venous thrombosis in pregnancy and, as reviewed below, may increase their risk of developing the placenta-mediated pregnancy complications (intrauterine growth restriction (IUGR), pregnancy loss, pre-eclampsia and placental abruption).

Thrombophilias can be acquired or inherited. The known acquired (or partly acquired) thrombophilias include hyperhomocysteinemia, elevated levels of factor VIII and the antiphospholipid antibodies. The known inherited thrombophilias are factor V Leiden (FVL), prothrombin gene variant (PGV), protein C, protein S and antithrombin deficiencies. These inherited thrombophilias are inherited in an autosomal dominant fashion. FVL and PGV are each the result of a single specific mutation, unlike the protein deficiencies which can be caused by multiple different mutations.

Epidemiology

Thrombophilias are common, with a combined general population prevalence of the known thrombophilias over 15%

(Table 4.2) [7–15]. Given that they are so common, the obstetric care provider will frequently encounter pregnant patients with thrombophilia. The prevalence of thrombophilias varies greatly in populations of different ethnicity [16]. The most common thrombophilias in Caucasian populations are FVL and PGV. However, in one study, while the carrier frequency of FVL was 5.27% in 2468 Caucasian Americans, the prevalence was much lower in other ethnic populations (2.21% in 407 Hispanic Americans, 1.25% in 80 Native Americans, 1.23% in 650 African Americans, and 0.45% in 442 Asian Americans) [16].

Diagnosis and pathophysiology

Our knowledge about thrombophilia has grown enormously in the past decade; however, because thrombophilia testing is expensive, it is recommended that screening be directed at specific populations where the yield of thrombophilia testing will be higher than for an unselected population (Box 4.1). All women with a previous venous thromboembolism (VTE) who are contemplating pregnancy should be tested for thrombophilia as this will permit better risk stratification. Screening should also be considered in women with a positive family history for thrombophilia or thrombosis (i.e. two or more first-degree relatives affected by thrombosis) where the prevalence of thrombophilia is likely to be increased. A history of placenta-mediated pregnancy complications may be as important as family history when the likelihood of an inherited or acquired thrombophilia is being considered.

The recommended panel of thrombophilia screening tests is presented in Box 4.2. In asymptomatic women with a positive family history for thrombophilia, testing can be limited to the specific thrombophilia identified in the first-degree relative.

Table 4.2 Prevalence of inherited and acquired thrombophilias

Thrombophilia	Among persons with idiopathic VTE	Normal population	References
Antithrombin	3%	0.2%	[7,8]
Protein C	2%	0.3–0.4%	[7,8]
Protein S	2%	0.7%	[7,8]
Factor V Leiden	20–40%	3–9%	[7,8]
Prothrombin defect	6–8%	2–6%	[9,11]
Factor VIII >150%	15–25%	5–11%	[7,13]
Antiphospholipid antibodies	10–15%	2%	[7,14]
Hyperhomocysteinemia (levels >95th percentile of the general population)	10%	3–10%	[7,15]

Box 4.1 Indications for diagnostic evaluation for thrombophilia

Non-obstetric

- Family history of thrombophilia
- Family history with two or more first-degree relatives with thromboembolism
- History of venous thromboembolism

Obstetric

- Early-onset severe pre-eclampsia <34 wks
- Recurrent early pregnancy loss (2 or more losses less than 10 weeks)
- Unexplained fetal demise >10 wks
- Intrauterine growth restriction <10th percentile adjusted for gender and gestational age
- Placental abruption leading to delivery

Box 4.2 Thrombophilias to be screened for in patients with an indication for thrombophilia testing (see also Table 3.4)

- Factor V Leiden (FVL)
- PCR for prothrombin gene mutation G20210A (PGV)
- Protein S deficiency (PS)
- Protein C deficiency (PC)
- Antithrombin deficiency (AT)
- Antiphospholipid antibodies
  - Anticardiolipin antibodies (ACLA), anti-beta-2 glycoprotein I antibodies and lupus antico-agulant (LA)
- Hyperhomocysteinemia (HCY)

A careful history and physical exam should be performed on all pregnant women suspected of having a thrombophilia. Any history suggestive of thrombophilia should be elicited, including a personal history of venous thrombosis, recurrent thrombosis or thrombosis at an unusual site. A personal history of arterial thrombosis and previous pregnancy complications are also pertinent. The presence of a family history of venous thrombosis or thrombophilia should be determined. Patients with a personal and family history of thrombosis often have more than one thrombophilic state and therefore should be tested for all thrombophilias.

Diagnostic tests for thrombophilia and the effects of pregnancy on these tests are discussed in detail below. The definitive diagnosis of thrombophilia can only be made by laboratory testing in a laboratory that is skilled at handling such requests. When a reliable laboratory is not available, the managing physician should refer patients to a thrombosis specialist. A specialist should also be consulted when the thrombophilia test results are confusing, ambiguous or equivocal.

Activated protein C resistance and factor V Leiden

Activated protein C (APC) is an important element in the coagulation cascade, in which it functions to suppress activated coagulation. APC, with its co-factors protein S and factor V, forms a complex that dampens coagulation through proteolytic action on factor Va and factor VIIIa [17–19]. APC resistance (APCR) results in less dampening of activated coagulation, leading to an increased propensity for abnormal thrombosis. APCR in 90% of cases is due to a mutation referred to as factor V Leiden (FVL) after the city in The Netherlands where it was initially described. FVL is a a single missense mutation in the factor V gene that renders the gene resistant to cleavage and inactivation by APC.

Factor V Leiden should be diagnosed in a laboratory with the appropriate expertise. The following approach should be considered.

- Measure the resistance to activated protein C (PCR) in plasma diluted with FV-deficient plasma as an initial screening test. FV-deficient APCR assays for FVL are highly sensitive and specific [20] and are unmodified by pregnancy [2], oral anticoagulants [21] or factor VIII levels [21]. FV-deficient APCR assays are less expensive to perform than DNA-based PCR assays but may not be readily available in all labs. Other assays may show increased resistance to AP C during pregnancy that will not be present in the nonpregnant state and therefore should not be used.

- Confirm the diagnosis (or if the FV-deficient assay is not available, begin your investigations during pregnancy) with DNA testing using direct PCR testing to determine hetero- or homozygous state and exclude false positives. False positives secondary to antiphospholipid antibodies can occur so all positive APCR tests should be confirmed with DNA testing.

Prothrombin gene variant

Prothrombin, the precursor to thrombin, is encoded by a gene on the long arm of chromosome 11. In 1996, a mutation in the prothrombin gene, called G20210A or PGV, was identified which results in a single base substitution from guanine to adenosine on the 3' untranslated end at nucleotide 20210 [11]. PGV results in increased prothrombin levels and a predisposition to venous thromboembolic disease [22].

Prothrombin gene variant should be diagnosed in a laboratory with the appropriate expertise and should be tested with DNA-based PCR testing.

Protein C, protein S and antithrombin deficiencies

These anticoagulant proteins all suppress activated coagulation and deficiency results in increased risk of venous thrombosis, with lifetime VTE risk in the 50–60% range. These deficiencies, like FVL and PGV, have autosomal-dominant inheritance, with variable penetrance (i.e. they are tendencies to develop VTE, not certainties). However, unlike the unique mutations that lead to FVL and PGV, hundreds of rare insertions, deletions and point mutations account for these protein deficiencies. Patients with antithrombin deficiency seem to have the highest risk for thrombosis (~65% lifetime risk).

Protein C should be tested in an accredited lab with the appropriate expertise. The following approach should be considered and pitfalls avoided.
• Recognize that at least two abnormally low results (and no normal results) are required to make the diagnosis of protein C deficiency.
• Perform a functional assay (preferably an amidolytic assay) as a screening test. Antigenic assays help distinguish between quantitative and qualitative deficiencies, but the vast majority of patients have both low activity and low antigen levels. Distinguishing between quantitative and qualitative deficiencies is of little clinical value and a functional assay is the appropriate test to begin with.
• Avoid testing patients on oral anticoagulants as protein C levels decrease with oral anticoagulants [23]. Protein C levels can also decrease with acute thrombosis [24], liver disease [25], vitamin K deficiency and sepsis [25]. Protein C levels are not influenced by pregnancy [2]. False positives secondary to APCR and elevated FVIII levels can be minimized by using amidolytic assays with snake venom as the activator [26].

Protein S should be tested in an accredited lab with the appropriate expertise. The following approach should be considered and pitfalls avoided.
• At least two abnormally low results (and no normal results) are required to make the diagnosis of protein S deficiency.
• Perform antigenic assays for free protein S when screening for protein S deficiency. Recognize that the antigenic assay should be a free protein S assay. Free protein S levels are more sensitive and specific than total protein S levels in patients with genotypically confirmed protein S deficiency [27,28].
• Functional assays are not specific or sensitive for protein S deficiency and should not be used to diagnose protein S deficiency [29].
• Avoid testing patients on oral anticoagulants [23], oral contraceptives, hormone replacement therapy or during pregnancy [2] or acute thrombotic events [24], which can all lead to decreased protein S levels. Protein S levels are also decreased by liver disease, vitamin K deficiency, disseminated intravascular coagulation (DIC) and nephrotic syndrome [25,30]. Functional protein S assays can be falsely low in patients with APCR [31].

Antithrombin deficiency should be diagnosed in a lab with the appropriate expertise. The following approach should be considered and pitfalls avoided.
• Recognize that at least two abnormally low results (and no normal results) are required to make the diagnosis.
• Perform a heparin co-factor activity-based functional assay. These assays can detect all cases of clinically relevant antithrombin (AT) deficiency [32]. Patients with AT deficiency may have low activity and low antigen levels or low activity and normal antigen levels. Hence, functional testing is adequate to detect all relevant AT deficiency.
• Avoid testing patients on oral anticoagulants or heparin therapy; false-positive results are common with heparin therapy [33]. False-negative results can result from vitamin K antagonist therapy [34]. False-positive results (low levels) can also be seen with pre-eclampsia, liver disease, DIC, nephrotic syndrome and acute thrombosis [25].
• Acquired antithrombin deficiency may occur with nephrotic syndrome or pre-eclampsia.

Antiphospholipid antibodies

Antiphospholipid antibodies predispose to venous and arterial thrombosis and recurrent miscarriage. The exact mechanism by which antiphospholipid antibodies (lupus anticoagulants, anti-beta-2 glycoprotein I antibodies and anticardiolipin antibodies (ACLA)) predispose to thrombosis or miscarriage is unknown.

Antiphospholipid antibody testing is complex and confusing in the best of hands. The lab diagnosis of antiphospholipid antibody syndrome is complicated by the lack of specific tests, the heterogeneity of the antibodies and problems with test standardization. While the following approach and pitfalls must be considered, if results are ambiguous a thrombosis expert should be consulted.
• Perform anticardiolipin and anti-beta-2 glycoprotein I antibody testing (IgG and IgM) by enzyme-linked immunosorbent assay (ELISA). Test for lupus anticoagulant (LA) activity with a phospholipid-dependent clotting assay (activated partial thromboplastin time (aPTT), kaolin clotting time (KCT), dilute Russell's viper venom time (DRVVT),

dilute prothrombin time). LA is diagnosed if the following criteria are met: one or more phospholipid-dependent test(s) is prolonged; the above prolongation is not corrected when patient and healthy control plasma are mixed (i.e. do not correct with a mixing study); the prolongation for patient plasma is corrected by adding phospholipid in the test system (platelet phospholipid neutralization) [35]. Testing for other antiphospholipid antibodies is not usually necessary as they are far less likely to be of clinical significance.

• Recognize that a "positive" result requires at least one abnormal result but that persistently positive results, higher titers (for ACLA) or greater prolongation of phospholipid-dependent tests (for LA) are more specific [36]. Positive anticardiolipin results can be transient and may be related to acute infection or other illness. Mild elevations of ACLA antibodies are nonspecific and do not necessarily indicate a hypercoagulable state. Positive results should be confirmed over time to ensure that they are not transient [37].

Hyperhomocysteinemia

Hyperhomocysteinemia is a common cause of hypercoagulability and a risk factor for VTE and arterial thrombosis. Homocysteine levels are usually maintained within a narrow range of concentrations via a complex series of enzymes and co-factors. These include folic acid, vitamin B12 and vitamin B6. It has long been known that the severe form of hyperhomocysteinemia, an inborn error of metabolism, causes both arterial and venous thrombosis. However, more recently it was discovered that mild acquired hyperhomocysteinemia, at times resulting from folic acid, vitamin B6 or vitamin B12 deficiency, renal failure or certain drugs, was also associated with an increased risk for thrombosis [15].

The common C677T mutation (and the less common a1A298C mutation) for methylenetetra-hydrofolate reductase (MTHFR) is associated with hyperhomocysteinemia; however, its correlation with VTE remains controversial. Meta-analyses have failed to find a strong association between VTE and homozygosity for MTHFR C677T [38]. Similarly, this mutation has not been clearly implicated in placenta-mediated pregnancy complications (see Table 4.2). Homocysteine levels decrease in pregnancy, probably related to increased circulating volume, decreased albumin levels and the use of prenatal vitamins containing folic acid [39].

The following diagnostic approach and pitfalls should be considered.

• Perform fasting homocysteine levels as they are simpler than and as reliable as postmethionine loading tests [40]. The risk of VTE and cardiovascular disease begins to increase as fasting plasma homocysteine levels exceed 10 μmol/L. Do not test for the MTHFR gene mutation (MTHFR) as the association appears to be with homocysteine and not MTHFR.

• Plasma homocysteine levels increase with age, renal impairment and low dietary B6, B12 and folate intake [40].

If hyperhomocysteinemia is diagnosed, exclude B12 and folate deficiency by testing these levels as other important underlying diseases need to be excluded (e.g. celiac disease, pernicious anemia).

Elevated factor VIII

Elevated FVIII levels have been identified as a risk factor for a first VTE and a predictor of recurrent VTE in those that have had VTE. However, the appropriate upper cut-off level for defining a FVIII thrombophilia is debated and inter-reagent and intermachine variability is very high, currently limiting the clinical utility of elevated FVIII levels and confidence in establishing or excluding this thrombophilia [41]. Also, it is well recognized (see above) that FVIII levels increase in pregnancy, further hampering the ability to make an accurate diagnosis of pathologically elevated FVIII levels. Furthermore, elevated FVIII levels and association with placenta-mediated pregnancy complications have received little attention in the literature thus far and we do not recommend this testing during pregnancy at the time of writing.

Clinical presentations

Thrombophilia as a predisposing factor for VTE in pregnancy

Pregnancy and thrombophilia act as synergistic risks and increase the risk of thrombosis during pregnancy. Case–control evidence indicates that women with thrombophilia have a 3–15-fold higher risk of VTE during pregnancy [22,42,43]. Although asymptomatic thrombophilic women (i.e. no prior VTE) are at greater relative risk of developing VTE, what is known about absolute risks of antepartum VTE is reassuring, with absolute risks of VTE in pregnant thrombophilic women being low with the common thrombophilias (e.g. ~1% with FVL) [44,45]. These absolute risks are poorly defined with the less common and more potent thrombophilias (e.g. AT deficiency) because large prospective cohort studies have not been conducted.

In women with previous VTE (proximal deep vein thrombosis (DVT) or pulmonary embolism (PE)) who are no longer on anticoagulants, the absolute risks are more of a concern. In a study of 125 untreated women with a single previous VTE, 1/10 (10%, 95% confidence interval (CI) 0.3–44%) women with a prior unprovoked VTE and thrombophilia and 2/21(10%, 95% CI 1–30%) women with a prior VTE and an identifiable thrombophilia had antepartum recurrences [46]. These women had a risk of postpartum recurrence of 2.4% (3/125) (95% CI 0.5–7.0%) despite all study participants being recommended postpartum prophylaxis, demonstrating the even higher risk during this brief period when delivery and immobilization are added to the synergistic risks of thrombophilia and the hypercoagulability of pregnancy. In women with combined thrombophilic defects, homozygosity for genetic thrombophilias or type 1 antithrombin deficiency (abnormal functional and antigenic levels of antithrombin), absolute risks have been reported to be as high as 10–35% [47].

Thrombophilia as a predisposing factor for placenta-mediated pregnancy complications

Venous thromboembolism is the most common cause of maternal mortality in developed countries but placenta-mediated pregnancy complications are also significant causes of maternal and fetal mortality and morbidity. These complications include IUGR, pre-eclampsia, and pregnancy loss (embryonic and fetal loss and placental abruption) [48–50]. The placenta-mediated pregnancy complications, like thrombophilias, are common, occurring in over 1/6 pregnancies, and are important conditions with a large impact on maternal and fetal health. Pre-eclampsia is a frequent cause of fetal and neonatal morbidity and mortality [51]. IUGR is associated with increased risk for fetal demise and may result in long-term effects in children, including developmental delay and poor school performance. Those afflicted by IUGR are also significantly less likely to attain higher academic and professional achievement as adults [52]. Pregnancy loss is a devastating event for pregnant women and their families.

A successful pregnancy demands the development of adequate placental circulation. The placenta-mediated pregnancy complications are thought to be due to inadequate placenta circulation (in part due to thrombosis) [53–56] and/or abnormal placentation (which is likely influenced by coagulation activation and fibrinolysis at the maternal/fetal interface) [57,58]. While all placenta-related complications are likely multifactorial, and most happen in the absence of a thrombophilia, it is biologically plausible that thrombophilia may increase the risk of both placental insufficiency due to placental micro- and/or macrovascular thrombosis and abnormal placentation due to alterations in coagulation and fibrinolysis at the maternal/fetal interface.

Factor V Leiden and PGV are the best studied thrombophilias to date (due to their high prevalence and the ability to simply and reliably test for them in large populations with PCR assays). As FVL and PGV are the least potent of the thrombophilias, it should follow that if they cause the placenta-mediated pregnancy complications then the more potent thrombophilias may also cause these complications. Similarly, if it is demonstrated that anticoagulants reduce the risk of placenta-mediated pregnancy complications in FVL or PGV pregnancies then it is likely that they will be beneficial in women with more potent thrombophilias.

Thrombophilia and placenta-mediated pregnancy complications: a causality assessment

To begin a causality assessment, statistical association in case–control or cohort studies is required. While statistical association may be a matter of fact, causation is a matter of opinion. Statistical association is but one criterion that is used to establish causation. As in criminal courts, a case for causal association is developed and opinion rendered by expert interpreters but ultimately clinicians must be judge and jury and determine for themselves whether causation has been proven. As detailed below, we submit that the case for thrombophilias causing placenta-mediated complications is at best weak and does not yet meet the criteria to establish causality.

The definitions of causation [59] and criteria for causality assessment are hotly debated in epidemiologic literature but Hill's criteria [60] are widely used and have withstood the test of time. Hill's criteria include strength of association, consistency of association, temporal relationship, specificity, biologic plausibility, biologic gradient, coherence, analogy, and experimentation.

• *Strength of association*: this criterion states that if factor X causes disease Y then variation of factor X will influence the probability of disease Y [61]. Furthermore, if X and Y are strongly linked then the case for causation is improved. The statistical association between factor X and disease Y can be studied in observational studies (case–control and cohort studies). In case–control studies, the prevalence of factor X is measured in those who did and did not develop disease Y. In cohort studies, those with and without factor X are followed over time to see who develops disease Y. Meta-analyses of observational studies suggest that women with thrombophilia are at increased risk of pre-eclampsia (see Table 4.2) [62,63], IUGR [63,64], abruptio placentae [65], miscarriage, and stillbirth [63,66]. However, on close inspection of these meta-analyses where the confidence intervals are narrow (i.e. where there are a larger number of events available for study), the point estimates of the odds ratios (effect sizes) are small (1.5–4 range), suggesting that the association is weak. To put these absolute odds ratios in context, odds ratios in the 1000 range are seen in single-gene diseases like hemochromatosis [67]. The prospective cohort studies conducted to date have suggested no association and have been large enough to exclude relative risks >4 (see below).

• *Consistency of association*: this criterion states that if an observed effect of factor X on disease Y is consistently shown in studies of different designs and in different populations then causation is more likely [61]. While the meta-analyses and systematic reviews of case–control studies have overall suggested an association, many individual studies have not (see Table 4.2). To be adequately powered (>80%) to detect an odds ratio of 2 or greater with a risk factor that has a prevalence of less than 5%, a sample size of greater than 1000 is required in a 1:1 case–control study. With but one exception [68], all the case–control studies published to date have been smaller than 1000 patients. It follows that the inconsistency seen in the case–control studies published to date may be due to small actual effect sizes combined with insufficient power (i.e. type II error). If we turn our attention to other study designs, as introduced above, none of the published prospective cohort studies examining the association between thrombophilia and the placenta-mediated pregnancy complications have demonstrated a statistical association. However, if an increase in relative risk truly exists, and the increase is of the order of twofold, then the individual prospective cohort studies have been underpowered.

• *Temporal relationship*: this criterion is considered by definition necessary and states that exposure to risk factor X should precede disease Y. Clearly, this criterion is met for the inherited thrombophilias, but for elevated FVIII, hyperhomocysteinemia and the antiphospholipid antibodies, this criterion has not been necessarily met in investigations conducted to date.

• *Specificity*: this controversial criterion is met if factor X is the sole cause of disease Y and if disease Y is only caused by factor X. When one examines the etiologic literature for each of the placenta-mediated pregnancy complications, it is clear that for each of these there are multiple recognized risk factors and that thrombophilia is almost certainly not the sole cause. Conversely, thrombophilias by definition cause other diseases (VTE).

• *Biologic plausibility*: this criterion requires that factor X causing disease Y should make biologic sense. It is biologically plausible that if thrombophilias predispose to the development of thrombosis in the slow flow circulation of the legs, they will also predispose to development of thrombosis in the slower flow circulation of many parts of the placenta. In the intervillous space of the placenta, the flow is slower than in the lower extremity veins. Placental thrombosis is a common hallmark of the placental pathology for each of the placenta-mediated pregnancy complications [53–56]. Thrombotic lesions of the placenta have various pathologic features and can arise either from the maternal supply line or in the fetal vasculature. Lesions that are maternal in origin include villous infarction, perivillous fibrin deposition, intervillous thrombosis and maternal floor infarction. Fetal side lesions or fetal thrombo-occlusive lesions include chorionic plate and fetal stem vessel thrombosis and hyalinized avascular villi. Fibrinoid necrosis, villous infarcts, and avascular terminal villi were demonstrated in one study to be independent predictors of restricted fetal growth in placentas of preterm intrauterine growth-restricted babies [53]. Pregnancies with placental thrombotic lesions are more likely to have complications than those pregnancies without placental abnormalities [69]. In one study, a very high incidence of vascular lesions in severe early-onset pre-eclampsia was found compared with preterm placentas without severe pre-eclampsia [70]. Several studies have been conducted to date exploring whether thrombophilic women with pregnancy complications are more likely to have placental thrombotic lesions compared to women without thrombophilia. Some suggest that thrombophilias cause placental thrombosis and others do not. However, these studies were retrospective, limited by small sample sizes and selection bias, and not controlled for known confounders

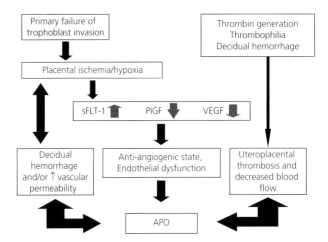

Figure 4.1 Proposed pathophysiology of adverse pregnancy outcome (APO). A primary failure of trophoblast invasion occurs (still of unknown etiology), which results in placental ischemia and hypoxia. Increases in soluble fms-like tyrosine kinase-1 (sFLT-1) with decreases in placental growth factor (PlGF) and vascular endothelial growth factor (VEGF) follow, creating an antiangiogenic state with endothelial dysfunction. In a parallel pathway, maternal factors result in thrombin generation and thrombophilia, and decidual hemorrhage. Ultimately, uteroplacental thrombosis and diminished uteroplacental blood flow result. Both primary trophoblast insults and maternal tendencies toward thrombosis lead to the syndrome of adverse pregnancy outcome.

(e.g. maternal age and smoking). Hence, no definitive answer to the question of whether thrombophilic women have more placental thrombosis than nonthrombophilic women has been provided by the literature to date.

• *Biologic gradient*: this criterion states that increasing dose exposure to factor X (longer duration and/or intensity) should result in a higher risk of disease Y or a worse manifestation of disease Y. Some evidence suggests that having multiple thrombophilias results in a higher risk of placenta-mediated pregnancy complications or worse manifestations. However, due to the relative rarity of combined or homozygous thrombophilias (<1% in the general population), very large case–control (n > 4000) or cohort studies (n > 10,000 if prevalence of placenta-mediated pregnancy complications in unexposed population is 15%) are required to even detect an association, let alone compare odds ratios or relative risk with odds ratios or relative risks in those with heterozygous thrombophilias.

• *Coherence*: for this criterion, risk factor X causing disease Y should be congruent with generally known facts of the biology of disease Y. As a contributor in the causal chain, thrombophilia makes sense and is coherent with current theories for causation of placenta-mediated pregnancy complications. Thrombophilias as a sole cause may make sense but would require that we discount multiple other theories. The "web of causation" concept, whereby causal pathways are complex and interconnected [59], is a more inclusive and likely more accurate view of the pathophysiology of the placenta-mediated pregnancy complications.

Table 4.3 Association between thrombophilias and placenta-mediated pregnancy complications

	Severe pre-eclampsia OR (95% CI)	IUGR* OR (95% CI)	Abruptio placentae OR (95% CI)	Recurrent miscarriage* OR (95% CI)	Late fetal loss* OR (95% CI)
Factor V Leiden	2.24 (1.28–3.94)	2.7 (1.3–5.5)	6.7 (2.0–21.6)	2.0 (1.5–2.7)	3.26 (1.82–5.83)
Prothrombin G20210A	1.98 (0.94–4.17)	2.5 (1.3–5.0)	28.9 (3.5–236.7)	2.0 (1.0–4.0)	2.3 (1.09–4.87)
Protein C deficiency	21.5 (not severe) (1.1–414.4)	–	–	1.57 (0.23–10.54)	1.41 (0.96–2.07)
Protein S deficiency	12.7 (not severe) (4–39.7)	10.2 (1.1–91)	–	14.72 (0.99–218.01)	7.39 (1.28–42.83)
Antithrombin deficiency	7.1 (not severe) (0.4–117.4)	–	4.1 (0.3–49.9)	–	–
ACA IgG antibodies	4.0 (not severe) (0.4–44.5)	33.9 (1.6–735.8)	20.8 (2.5–175.8)	–	5.6 (2.6–11.7)
Lupus anticoagulant	0.1 (not severe) (0–6.8)	–	–	–	3.2 (1.2–9.0)
Hyperhomocysteinemia	2.2 (not severe) (0.9–5.2)	–	3.5 (1.5–8.1)	–	–
MTHFR C677T (homozygosity)	1.38 (0.93–2.06)	5.0 (1.8–13.8)	2.2 (0.4–11.6)	0.98 (0.55–1.72)	1.4 (0.9–2.1)

*When pooled data were available from more than one meta-analysis, data from the most recent were included.
ACA, anticardiolipin antibodies; CI, confidence interval; IUGR, intrauterine growth restriction; MTHFR, methylenetetrahydrofolate reductase; OR, odds ratio.

• *Analogy*: this criterion is met if there exist risk factors similar to factor X that cause diseases similar to disease Y. Other thrombotic tendencies have been implicated as potential causal agents for the placenta-mediated pregnancy complications, including the myeloproliferative disorders and paroxysmal nocturnal hemoglobinuria.

• *Experimentation*: Hill's strongest criterion for causation requires that removing or reducing risk factor X reduces disease Y. Often this is the most difficult criterion to study. With the hereditary thrombophilias, it is obviously not possible to randomize women to exposure and no exposure. However, we can examine the effect of anticoagulants on the risk of development of the placenta-mediated pregnancy complications in thrombophilic women as a surrogate for removing or reducing the thrombophilias. That is, if anticoagulants can negate the increase in thrombotic tendency in thrombophilic women and reduce their risk of development of placenta-mediated pregnancy complications then the case for causation will be strengthened. As outlined in the management sections, the literature on anticoagulant treatment for thrombophilic pregnancies is too immature (i.e. insufficient controlled trials) to claim that this criterion has been met.

In summary, causation is not proven. Thrombophilias are potentially a weak contributor to the placenta-mediated pregnancy complications. To firmly establish that thrombophilias are a contributor requires:

• more large prospective cohort studies demonstrating a consistent association (even if the association is weak) and biologic gradient (higher risk with multiple thrombophilias)

• further experimentation to establish a clear biologic rationale for implicating thrombophilias in the causal web for each of the placenta-mediated pregnancy complications

• well-conducted controlled trials comparing anticoagulants to no intervention, demonstrating a clear reduction in risk of placenta-mediated pregnancy complications in thrombophilic pregnancies.

Management of thrombophilic pregnancies

The specific content of management discussions is based on the thrombophilia(s) identified and is influenced by a personal history of VTE and/or pregnancy complications. From the venous disease literature we know that not all thrombophilias are of equal potency. For instance, women with antithrombin deficiency have a lifetime risk of developing VTE of 65% compared to 35% with FVL. Homozygosity for antithrombin deficiency is incompatible with life, whereas homozygosity for FVL is compatible with life and is only associated with a 60% lifetime VTE risk. The potency of the thrombophilia needs to color the recommendations considered below.

Preconception counseling

Preconception counseling for women with thrombophilia should include a discussion about the uncertainty surrounding the association between thrombophilia and pregnancy complications and the certainty of increased risk, albeit low in absolute risk, of VTE. Thrombophilic women should be reassured that thrombophilias are only *possibly* weakly associated with pregnancy complications. The level of risk is not high enough to dissuade thrombophilic women from getting pregnant. Patients should be encouraged, however, to address any concomitant modifiable risk factors for thromboembolic disease such as physical inactivity, obesity or smoking.

Genetic counseling

Referral of women with a genetic thrombophilia for preconception genetic counseling is uncommon. In theory, a genetic counselor can inform couples about how thrombophilia is inherited and give estimates of the likelihood of thrombophilia in their children [71]. In practice, pregnancies are very rarely terminated or prevented due to maternal (or paternal) thrombophilia because penetrance is variable and affected offspring may never develop thrombosis. Furthermore, there is no prenatal benefit to determining if a fetus has inherited a thrombophilia and this knowledge would not influence the management of the pregnancy or care of the neonate. The exception to the latter may be homozygosity for defects associated with protein C or protein S deficiency. While homozygosity is extremely uncommon, if the pregnancy progresses to term, neonates present at birth with massive VTE or purpura fulminans. Homozygous antithrombin deficiency is not compatible with life. Hence, in couples where one partner has one of these anticoagulant deficiencies, the other partner should be tested to exclude the same anticoagulant deficiency.

Antenatal care of thrombophilic women

Nonpharmacologic management

It is appropriate to review the symptoms of DVT and PE with all thrombophilic women so that diagnosis and treatment can be initiated promptly if these symptoms arise. DVT symptoms that should prompt medical attention include leg swelling, calf, thigh, groin or buttock pain (especially unilateral) that does not improve within an hour lying down with the leg up. PE symptoms that should prompt medical attention include chest pain (especially pleuritic) and/or shortness of breath that lasts longer than 15 minutes.

Women with thrombophilia and prior pregnancy complications should be considered for referral to an obstetrician or clinic with special expertise in high-risk pregnancy for monitoring throughout pregnancy, including ultrasound examinations to assess fetal growth and placental function. It is our practice to initiate monthly fetal growth ultrasound examinations after 24 weeks and to increase the frequency of these examinations to include assessments of fetal well-being for patients for whom there is any concern of impaired fetal growth.

Antepartum thromboprophylaxis

The potential benefits of heparin or low molecular weight heparin (LMWH) thromboprophylaxis for pregnant thrombophilic women must be weighed against the costs and potential risks of prophylactic LMWH administration. Prolonged LMWH use throughout pregnancy is expensive, inconvenient and may cause serious (albeit rare) complications, including heparin-induced thrombocytopenia (HIT), osteoporotic fractures and bleeding (reviewed below and in Tables 3.5 and 3.6). Therefore, before using LMWH to prevent pregnancy complications in thrombophilic women, it is crucial to determine whether LMWH is safe and effective in these women and for what indications. As detailed below, efficacy data are lacking for most indications, leaving clinicians with significant therapeutic uncertainty.

Maternal considerations for thromboprophylaxis

Low molecular weight heparin has become the gold standard for thromboprophylaxis in pregnancy. This is primarily due to ease of administration (longer half-life and greater bio-availability allow once-daily injections) and favorable safety profile. Although complications of LMWH for pregnant women are uncommon, they can be serious and life-threatening. None of the individual studies examining LMWH use in pregnancy has been adequately powered to provide accurate estimates of the incidence of HIT, bleeding and osteoporosis after prolonged LMWH therapy in pregnancy. A recent systematic review by Greer, including 64 reports documenting 2777 pregnancies, concluded that LMWH is safe during pregnancy [72]. In this review, there were no deaths and serious side effects were rare.

Heparin-induced thrombocytopenia is a clinical syndrome resulting from development of platelet-activating anti-PF4/heparin complex antibodies. The diagnosis is made by documenting HIT antibody formation in addition to arterial or venous thromboembolism or unexplained thrombocytopenia or skin lesions at heparin injection sites or acute systemic reactions after administration of an IV heparin bolus [73]. Careful review of the literature reveals two cases of HIT in pregnancy with LMWH use [74,75]. In the Greer review, allergic skin reactions to LMWH were reported in 50 women (1.8%) [72], some of which may be associated with HIT antibodies [76]. Long-term LMWH can result in osteoporosis and osteoporotic fractures (reported in one patient (0.04%) in Greer's review). Significant bleeding was more common (1.98% overall; 55 events), with 12 (22%) cases of significant antenatal bleeding, 26 (47%) cases of postpartum hemorrhage, and 17 (31%) wound hematomas. Therapy with heparin near the time of delivery has been shown to reduce the likelihood of obtaining epidural anesthesia [77], after reports of epidural hematomas and hemiplegia in nonobstetric patients on LMWH undergoing epidural anesthesia [78,79]. Furthermore, the American Society of Regional Anesthesia currently recommends withholding regional anesthesia in patients who have had prophylactic-dose LMWH injections in the 10–12 hours prior to the procedure (and 24 hours for patients who have received therapeutic doses of LMWH) [80]. Thus, use of LMWH in pregnant women at term potentially severely limits their analgesic options at the time of delivery.

Fetal/neonatal considerations for thromboprophylaxis

Low molecular weight heparins do not cross the placental barrier, thereby making them safe for the fetus when administered during pregnancy. A small study that specifically examined the teratogenic potential of LMWH found no difference in the incidence of congenital malformations between women receiving LMWH and those receiving low-dose aspirin [84]. Greer's systematic review had limited data on fetal outcomes; of 2215 pregnancies treated with LMWH, 94.7% were reported to have successful outcomes, defined as livebirth [72]. LMWH is only minimally secreted in the breast milk [85]. Furthermore, LMWH, including dalteparin, are not significantly orally bio-available; hence, any LMWH in the breast milk would not be absorbed in the infant's GI tract. The ACCP consensus guidelines on antithrombotic therapy conclude that LMWH is safe to use in the nursing mother [86].

Asymptomatic thrombophilic pregnancies (no prior VTE or placenta-mediated pregnancy complications)

In thrombophilic women without prior thrombosis, no antepartum prophylaxis is recommended given low absolute antepartum VTE risks (<1%), with few exceptions. These exceptions include women with combined thrombophilic defects, homozygosity for genetic thrombophilias or type 1 antithrombin deficiency, where absolute risks of VTE have been reported to be as high as 10–35% [47] and warrant closer follow-up, and the case for antepartum thromboprophylaxis is strong (see Table 3.11). Given that we have not clearly demonstrated that thrombophilias cause placenta-mediated pregnancy complications, it is definitely premature to recommend antepartum anticoagulant prophylaxis in asymptomatic thrombophilic pregnant women to prevent placenta-mediated pregnancy complications. It is, however, recommended that women with known thrombophilias receive thromboprophylaxis for 4–6 weeks post partum with either once-daily preventive-dose LMWH or warfarin.

Thrombophilic women with prior placenta-mediated pregnancy complications

Antiphospholipid antibody syndrome/recurrent pregnancy loss

Two randomized trials have shown a significant increase in livebirth rates using the combination of heparin and aspirin in women with previous fetal loss (three or more) who have antiphospholipid antibody syndrome (APLA) [87,88]. Specific shortcomings of these studies include small samples in both studies and quasi-randomized allocation was used for one study [88]. A more recent randomized trial examining the combination of aspirin and LMWH did not demonstrate this benefit in women with recurrent pregnancy loss and APLA [89]. This trial, however, had a high cross-over rate (25% did not receive allocated treatment), limiting power to demonstrate a difference. A Cochrane review suggested that further study of heparin is warranted to prevent recurrent miscarriage in women with antiphospholipid antibodies [90]. We currently recommend aspirin (81 mg per day after conceiving), given the relatively benign nature of this intervention, and discuss the limitations of the literature supporting the addition of heparin/LMWH to aspirin. After discussing the uncertain benefit, the risks and inconveniences of heparin/LMWH use, some centers support patients in choosing these therapeutic options. We note, however, that in recent consensus recommendations, thromboprophylaxis for women with previous pregnancy losses and APLA with low-dose aspirin in combination with heparin (Grade 1B) [86] is advised, a recommendation that is followed by many centers.

Thrombophilia and pregnancy loss

Very few completed trials have examined thromboprophylaxis in women with pregnancy loss and the other thrombophilias. A recent randomized study suggests benefit of LMWH prophylaxis in women with a single previous unexplained late fetal loss (>8 weeks) and selected thrombophilias (FVL, prothrombin G20210A or protein S deficiency) [91]. This trial requires validation [92]. A 2003 Cochrane review, while not recent, still appropriately summarizes the present state of the literature when it concludes: "The evidence on the efficacy and safety of thromboprophylaxis with aspirin and heparin in women with a history of at least two spontaneous miscarriages or one later intrauterine fetal death without apparent causes other than inherited thrombophilias is too limited to recommend the use of anticoagulants in this setting. Large, randomized, placebo-controlled trials are urgently needed" [93].

Even if we assume that thrombophilias are weakly causal, there currently exist insufficient RCT data to recommend anticoagulant antepartum prophylaxis to prevent placenta-mediated pregnancy complications. This is the position taken by the American College of Chest Physicians in 2008, although recommendations from some experts have supported the use of LMWH in patients with thrombophilia and recurrent pregnancy loss while still acknowledging the lack of adequate evidence to support this practice [94].

Thrombophilia and other placenta-mediated pregnancy complications (pre-eclampsia, IUGR, abruption)

A 2005 Cochrane review similarly concluded that there are insufficient trials to determine the effects of heparin on other pregnancy outcomes in thrombophilic women [95] despite small nonrandomized studies that suggest LMWH is of benefit in preventing pregnancy complications [96]. Many experts advocate administering LMWH to thrombophilic women in pregnancy despite the lack of substantive evidence to support this practice. Considering the absence of randomized controlled trials demonstrating benefit, thromboprophylaxis must be considered experimental in this population and treatment decisions should be made by individual clinicians and patients bearing this in mind. The 2008 ACCP recommendations do not support the use of UFH/LMWH to prevent any of these obstetric complications [94].

Thrombophilic women with prior VTE

In general, thromboprophylaxis is recommended during pregnancy if a thrombophilic woman has had a prior VTE, due to the high rate of recurrence in this group The role of antepartum and postpartum thromboprophylaxis for women with a history of VTE with and without an identifiable thrombophilia is discussed in Chapter 3.

Labor and delivery

In those patients for whom thromboprophylaxis is recommended, one must consider the absolute risks of thrombophilia-associated complications after 37 weeks and counterbalance these with the risks of continuing anticoagulants to term. The risks of continuing anticoagulants to term include major hemorrhage at the time of delivery of approximately 1% [72] and limiting epidural analgesic use because of the very real, albeit very rare complication of epidural hematoma with LMWH use in the period prior to needle placement [80]. These downsides can lead to planned delivery via induction or C-section. Both induction and C-section are associated with a higher risk of complications compared to spontaneous vaginal birth. Management of both therapeutic and prophylactic-dose anticoagulation is discussed in detail in Chapter 3 and in Tables 3.8 and 3.11.

Postpartum considerations

Postpartum VTE risk

More than a third of pregnancy-related VTE occur during the postpartum period, highlighting the increased daily risk of thrombosis in the brief 6-week postpartum period compared to the 40-week antepartum period [97]. The daily risk of VTE is fourfold higher in the postpartum period compared to the antepartum period. These risks are amplified in women with thrombophilia and it is generally accepted that thromboprophylaxis is appropriate at this time. The duration of postpartum prophylaxis is controversial and should probably

be continued throughout the entire postpartum period (6–8 weeks) until coagulation factors return to pre-pregnant levels. Either LMWH or vitamin K antagonists (warfarin) can be used post partum although most women prefer LMWH injections in order to avoid going to the lab for INR monitoring for vitamin K antagonists with a newborn at home. While both drugs enter the breast milk, they do not influence the baby's coagulation system.

Contraceptive recommendations

Contraceptive pills containing estrogen increase the relative risk of VTE in patients with thrombophilias [98–102]. Of the thrombophilias, FVL has been the most studied and this has allowed relative risks to be accurately estimated. The increased risk of VTE with estrogen-containing oral contraceptive pill (OCP) use is approximately fourfold; with the addition of FVL this increases to 20–30-fold. However, the absolute increases in risk are small. Women of childbearing age have a yearly incidence of VTE of 10–20/100,000 patient-years (i.e. 0.01–0.02% per year); with estrogen-containing OCP use and FVL, this increases at most 30-fold to 0.6% per year. While this increase in risk should not be ignored, it is not considered high enough by most women with FVL to avoid using estrogen-containing OCP when these risks are counterbalanced with the risk and burdens of an unwanted pregnancy.

We do encourage patients who are heterozygotes for FVL to consider use of progesterone-only OCP or progesterone-containing intrauterine device as alternatives to estrogen-containing OCP. However, we do not refuse estrogen-containing OCP use in women with asymptomatic heterozygous FVL but to those to whom it is prescribed, we emphasize their increased risk of VTE, review the symptoms of VTE with them and instruct them to seek medical attention should they arise. Similar advice is suggested for women who are heterozygotes for the prothrombin gene mutation where concomitant estrogen-containing OCP use increases by 16-fold the risk of VTE compared to noncarriers and non-OCP users. In a study of first-degree relatives with AT, PC or PS deficiency who were OCP users, the absolute risk of VTE was estimated at 4.3% per year (95% CI 1.4–9.7%) [103]. These absolute risks are more concerning and in these patients we advise against oral contraceptives.

Clinicians should discuss these absolute risks with thrombophilic women to allow them to make an enlightened and informed choice about OCP use. The lowest possible estrogen dose should be recommended as low-dose estrogen pills are associated with a lower risk of VTE. Patients with prior VTE and thrombophilia should be strongly discouraged from using estrogen-containing OCP as they will have absolute risks estimated to be 8.5% per year [104]. See also Chapter 33.

Anesthetic concerns related to thrombophilias and thromboembolic disease in pregnancy

Thrombophilias have special relevance to the provision of analgesia and anesthesia during pregnancy [105]. As anticoagulant agents are utilized to prevent or treat these conditions in thrombophilic women, algorithms for the discontinuation or reversal of these agents must be considered, particularly if epidural or spinal anesthetic techniques are to be used for analgesia during labor or anesthesia for operative deliveries.

Anticoagulation, reversal, and timing of neuraxial technique

Regional anesthesia is desirable in obstetric patients because it provides pain relief in labor and also can obviate the need for (and thus the risks of) general anesthesia (see Chapter 29). However, anticoagulation therapy, particularly with LMWH, can increase the risks of complications from regional anesthesia to a degree that may prohibit regional anesthesia. Therefore, when regional anesthesia is desired for delivery and anticoagulation is not deemed essential for the patient's safety, stopping anticoagulation at 37 weeks gestation should be considered. If regional anesthesia is desired for delivery but cessation of anticoagulants is deemed inappropriate, many centers, particularly in North America, transition their patients from LMWH to unfractionated heparin (UFH) approximately 2–4 weeks prior to a scheduled induction or delivery [106]. Patients on UFH may be more likely to be candidates for regional anesthesia for several reasons. First, when given in a prophylactic low dose of 5000 U every 12 hours subcutaneously, UFH seldom leads to significant changes in coagulation parameters. Second, UFH is more rapidly and predictably reversed with time, or more actively, with protamine. Third, UFH's anticoagulant effect as measured by the aPTT is more rapidly ascertainable in most laboratories than is the anti-factor Xa level used to assess the effects of LMWH. Despite these advantages of UFH, its use does require the monitoring of platelet counts for evidence of HIT and the measuring of the aPTT for patients on doses higher than 5000 U SC every 12 hours. In Europe, where insistence

upon epidural anesthesia may be less common than in the US, this approach of switching from UFH to LMWH is not usually employed because of the hazards (HIT) and difficulties (the need for monitoring of aPTT) of using UFH. The authors also use UFH infrequently and either continue LMWH at reduced doses or favor strong consideration of whether continued anticoagulation is necessary in the weeks leading up to delivery.

While not specific to the parturient population, a consensus statement from the American Society of Regional Anesthesia and Pain Medicine (ASRA) recommends that patients on LMWH prophylaxis or treatment doses wait at least 10–12 hours or 24 hours, respectively, from the last dose before attempting neuraxial anesthesia [107]. The measurement and reversal of anti-Xa levels below a certain threshold value (e.g. <0.2 IU/mL) has not been recommended, as such a level has yet to be correlated with the absence of spinal or epidural bleeding and the ability to provide the testing is not uniformly available. LMWH can be reinstituted 2 hours after needle placement or catheter removal. With UFH used in prophylactic doses of 5000 U SC/12 h, regional anesthesia can proceed once a normal platelet count is verified. With UFH used at higher prophylactic doses (up to 10,000 units SC/12 h) it is our practice to wait 4–6 hours after injection and verify a normal aPTT but the ASRA does not provide guidance on this matter. When unfractionated heparin is given intravenously for therapeutic effect, 4–6 hours should elapse after cessation of the intravenous dosing and a normal aPTT and platelet count verified prior to neuraxial technique placement. Full-dose therapeutic anticoagulation with UFH administered subcutaneously likely requires a delay of 12–24 hours and verification of a normal aPTT and platelet count prior to regional anesthesia. The ASRA recommendations are summarized in Table 4.4.

Neuraxial hematomas

The bony vertebrae traditionally protect the spinal cord from trauma but on rare occasions, space-occupying lesions (e.g. abscesses and hematomas) within the vertebral canal may result in spinal cord or cauda equina compression and/or ischemia. The patient on anticoagulants is at increased risk for this outcome and consequently, the perceived risks and

Table 4.4 Heparin and regional anesthesia: American Society of Regional Anesthesia (ASRA) recommendations

Mode of anticoagulation	ASRA recommendations as to whether regional anesthesia may be given
UFH prophylactic	Normal PTT and platelet count should be verified but otherwise regional anesthesia can proceed without limitations on timing
UFH therapeutic	Normal PTT and platelet count needed before proceeding with regional anesthesia. Ideally 6 hours should have elapsed since cessation of IV UFH or 12 hours since administration of therapeutic dose SC UFH
LMWH prophylactic	Patient should be off LMWH for 10–12 hours before regional anesthesia is provided. Do not restart LMWH until 2 hours after withdrawal of regional anesthesia catheter. Anti-Xa levels not relevant to whether regional anesthesia can be given
LMWH therapeutic	Patient should be off LMWH for 24 hours before regional anesthesia is provided. Do not restart LMWH until 2 hours after withdrawal of regional anesthesia catheter. Anti-Xa levels not relevant to whether regional anesthesia can be given

IV, intravenous; LMWH, low molecular weight heparin; PTT, partial thromboplastin time; SC, subcutaneous; UFH, unfractionated heparin.

benefits of their baseline disorder, the anticoagulated state, and available anesthetic options must be evaluated.

Although the exact incidence of hematomas associated with neuraxial blockade is unknown, it has been estimated to be less than 1 in 150,000 and less than 1 in 220,000 epidural and spinal anesthetic techniques, respectively [108,109]. The risk appears higher with the epidural technique, likely owing to the larger needle and the presence of a catheter-based technique; 46 of 61 reported cases of spinal hematoma from 1906 to 1994 were associated with epidural, versus spinal, anesthesia [108,109]. In addition, the hematoma occurred immediately following the removal of the catheter in 15 of the 32 patients with an epidural catheter-based technique. Additional risk factors appear to have included hemostatic abnormalities and difficult or bloody needle or epidural catheter insertions [108,109].

The recovery of adequate hemostasis following the cessation of anticoagulation agents is not always straightforward. The regeneration of functional clotting factors occurs at different rates, and thus the recovery and onset phases of anticoagulation may yield similar coagulation testing results but different hemostatic states [107]. In addition, the concurrent use of more than one antihemostatic agent, even aspirin, makes the integrity of the hemostatic system less predictable. Of interest, although clinical reports have observed excessive blood loss in the perioperative period in individuals taking aspirin, the associated risk for developing an epidural hematoma with neuraxial techniques appears very low. In two trials with 1422 and 891 pregnant women, respectively, taking low-dose aspirin therapy, no adverse effects related to the epidural technique occurred [110.111]. Overall, the hemostatic status should be optimized at the time of neuraxial technique initiation and catheter removal, and sensory and motor function and neurologic testing should be frequently and routinely evaluated.

Early signs of spinal cord compression include progressive motor or sensory blockade and complaints of back pain or pressure. The onset of bowel or bladder incontinence or urinary retention, radicular pain or increasing anesthetic blockade or neurologic deficits warrants a consultation with a neurologist and/or neurosurgeon. Space-occupying lesions are best confirmed by urgent magnetic resonance imaging (MRI) scanning as they are initially undetectable on plain radiographs and computed tomography (CT) scans do not reliably distinguish hematoma from adjacent bone. Surgical decompression is usually indicated and neurologic outcome is improved if decompression occurs within 6–12 hours of onset of symptoms [107].

Acute pulmonary embolism in pregnancy: an anesthesiologist's perspective

When a pregnant woman suffers a massive pulmonary embolus, the anesthesiologist may need to assist with resuscitation. Pulmonary thromboembolism has a greater impact on the pregnant compared to the nonpregnant woman due to the physiologic changes of pregnancy. Increased oxygen consumption and decreased functional residual capacity mean that there is less oxygen reserve during pregnancy, enhancing the risk to mother and fetus.

The general principles of resuscitation are similar to those in nonpregnant patients with the exception that one has to be aware of the presence of the fetus and if the woman is beyond 20 weeks gestation, aortocaval compression may impact on the success of resuscitation, so left lateral tilt to ensure uterine displacement is essential. If the woman fails to respond to resuscitation, it may be necessary to deliver the fetus in order to enhance venous return through relieving aortocaval compression.

Although pulmonary embolectomy during pregnancy has the highest maternal mortality rate of all procedures performed during pregnancy, it sometimes is required in a life-threatening situation. The anesthesiologist may be required to provide anesthesia for thrombectomy or embolectomy during pregnancy [112–117]. Anesthesia is similar to that in any other pregnant woman undergoing nonobstetric surgery, with the exception that central neuraxial (spinal, epidural) anesthesia will be contraindicated due to the need for therapeutic anticoagulation. Additionally, there will be a high risk of hemorrhage and appropriate blood products should be available. Pillny *et al.* described 97 cases of successful thrombectomy during pregnancy, of which there were 11 cases of thrombectomy coincident with cesarean delivery [113]. The authors note that pulmonary artery catheters were used routinely in all cases, but there is no information regarding anesthetic management.

When pulmonary embolism unexpectedly occurs during cesarean delivery, a major problem is whether the profound cardiovascular changes are due to a thrombus, amniotic fluid or air. Resuscitation is similar but with amniotic fluid embolism one has to be prepared for DIC, in addition to right and left heart dysfunction. In most cases reported in the literature of pulmonary embolism occurring during cesarean delivery, the diagnosis had been made preoperatively [112–115]. In some of these cases embolectomy was performed after delivery of the baby and the decision to remove the embolus was based on a deterioration in the woman's condition. Recombinant tissue plasminogen activator (rt-PA) has been used successfully for life-threatening pulmonary embolism during and following cesarean delivery [116,117].

Conclusion

Thrombophilias are major causes of pregnancy-related VTE and possibly a weak cause of placenta-mediated pregnancy complications. Laboratory evaluation is indicated in pregnant women with previous VTE and possibly in women with placenta-mediated pregnancy complications (pregnancy loss, IUGR, pre-eclampsia and placental abruption) to define the potential etiology of prior complications, allow tailoring of pre-pregnancy counseling, and guide general counseling for nonpregnancy issues in thrombophilics and to discuss the potential benefits and risks of thromboprophylaxis.

References

1. Bremme KA. Haemostatic changes in pregnancy. Best Pract Res Clin Haematol 2003;16(2):153–68.

2. Clark P, Brennand J, Conkie JA, McCall F, Greer IA, Walker ID. Activated protein C sensitivity, protein C, protein S and coagulation in normal pregnancy. Thromb Haemost 1998;79(6):1166–70.

3. Comeglio P, Fedi S, Liotta AA, Cellai AP, Chiarantini E, Prisco D, et al. Blood clotting activation during normal pregnancy. Thromb Res 1996;84(3):199–202.

4. Eichinger S, Weltermann A, Phillipp K, Hafner E, Kaider A, Kittl E-M, et al. Prospective evaluation of hemostatic system activation and thrombin potential in healthy pregnant women with and without factor V leiden. Thromb Haemost 1999;82:1232–6.

5. Mousa HA, Downey C, Alfirevic Z, Toh CH. Thrombin activatable fibrinolysis inhibitor and its fibrinolytic effect in normal pregnancy. Thromb Haemost 2004;92(5):1025–31.

6. Lindqvist PG, Svensson PJ, Dahlback B, Marsal K. Factor V Q^{506} mutation (Activated Protein C Resistance) associated with reduced intrapartum blood loss – a possible evolutionary selection mechanism. Thromb Haemost 1998;79:69–73.

7. van der Meer FJ, Koster T, Vandenbroucke JP, Briet E, Rosendaal FR. The Leiden Thrombophilia Study (LETS). Thromb Haemost 1997;78:631–5.

8. Rodeghiero F, Tosetto A. The epidemiology of inherited thrombophilia: the VITA Project. Vicenza Thrombophilia and Atherosclerosis Project. Thromb Haemost 1997;78(1):636–40.

9. Souto JC, Coll I, Llobet D, del Rio E, Oliver A, Mateo J, et al. The prothrombin 20210A allele is the most prevalent genetic risk factor for venous thromboembolism in the Spanish population. Thromb Haemost 1998;80:366–9.

10. Brown K, Luddington R, Williamson D, Baker P, Baglin T. Risk of venous thromboembolism associated with a G to A transition at position 20210 in the 3'-untranslated region of the prothrombin gene. Br J Haematol 1997;98:907–9.

11. Poort SW, Rosendaal FR, Reitsma PH, Bertina RM. A common genetic variation in the 3'-untranslated region of the prothrombin gene is associated with elevated plasma prothrombin levels and an increase in venous thrombosis. Blood 1996;88:3698–703.

12. Koster T, Blann AD, Briet E, Vandenbroucke JP, Rosendaal FR. Role of clotting factor VIII in effect of von Willebrand factor on occurrence of DVT. Lancet 1995;345:152–5.

13. Kraaijenhagen RA, Anker PS, Koopman MMW, Reitsma PH, Prins MH, van den Ende A, et al. High plasma concentration of Factor VIIIc is a major risk factor for venous thromboembolism. Thromb Haemost 2000;83(1):5–9.

14. Halbmayer WM, Haushofer A, Schon R, Mannhalter C, Strohmer E, Baumgarten K, et al. The prevalence of moderate and severe FXII (Hageman factor) deficiency among the normal population: evaluation of the incidence of FXII deficiency among 300 healthy blood donors. Thromb Haemost 1994;71:68–72.

15. den Heijer M, Koster T, Blom HJ, Bos GM, Briet E, Reitsma PH, et al. Hyperhomocysteinemia as a risk factor for deep-vein thrombosis. N Engl J Med 1996;334(12):759–62.

16. Ridker PM, Miletich JP, Hennekens CH, Buring JE. Ethnic distribution of factor V Leiden in 4047 men and women. Implications for venous thromboembolism screening. JAMA 1997;277:1305–7.

17. Bertina RM, Koeleman BP, Koster T, Rosendaal FR, Dirven RJ, de Ronde H, et al. Mutation in blood coagulation factor V associated with resistance to activated protein C. Nature 1994;369(6475):64–7.

18. Dahlback B. Factor V gene mutation causing inherited resistance to activated protein C as a basis for venous thromboembolism. J Intern Med 1995;237:221–7.

19. Svensson PJ, Dahlback B. Resistance to activated protein C as a basis for venous thrombosis. N Engl J Med 1994;330:517–22.

20. Strobl FJ, Hoffman S, Huber S, Williams EC, Voelkerding KV. Activated protein C resistance assay performance: improvement by sample dilution with factor V-deficient plasma. Arch Pathol Lab Med 1998;122(5):430–3.

21. Chitolie A, Lawrie AS, Mackie IJ, Harrison P, Machin SJ. The impact of oral anticoagulant therapy, factor VIII level and quality of factor V-deficient plasma on three commercial methods for activated protein C resistance. Blood Coagul Fibrinolysis 2001;12(3):179–86.

22. Gerhardt A, Scharf RE, Beckmann MW, Struve S, Bender HG, Pillny M, et al. Prothrombin and factor V mutations in women with a history of thrombosis during pregnancy and the puerperium. N Engl J Med 2000;342(6):374–80.

23. Harrison L, Johnston M, Massicotte MP, Crowther MA, Moffat K, Hirsh J. Comparison of 5-mg and 10-mg loading doses in initiation of warfarin therapy. Ann Intern Med 1997;126:133–6.

24. Reiter W, Ehrensberger H, Steinbruckner B, Keller F. Parameters of haemostasis during acute venous thrombosis. Thromb Haemost 1995;74:596–601.

25. Humphries JE. Thrombophilia and complex acquired deficiencies of antithrombin, protein C, and protein S. Semin Hematol 1995;32(4 suppl 2):8–16.

26. Ireland H, Bayston T, Thompson E, Adami A, Goncalves C, Lane DA, et al. Apparent heterozygous type II protein C deficiency caused by the factor V 506 Arg to Gln mutation. Thromb Haemost 1995;73(4):731–2.

27. Simmonds RE, Ireland H, Lane DA, Zoller B, de Frutos PG, Dahlback B. Clarification of the risk for venous thrombosis associated with hereditary protein S deficiency by investigation of a large kindred with a characterized gene defect. Ann Intern Med 1998;128:8–14.

28. Makris M, Leach M, Beauchamp NJ, Daly ME, Cooper PC, Hampton KK, et al. Genetic analysis, phenotypic diagnosis, and risk of venous thrombosis, in families with inherited deficiencies of protein S. Blood 2000;95:1935–41.

29. Rodger MA, Carrier M, Gervais M, Rock G. Normal functional protein S activity does not exclude protein S deficiency. Pathophysiol Haemost Thromb 2003;33(4):202–5.

30. Kanfer A. Coagulation factors in nephrotic syndrome. Am J Nephrol 1990;10(suppl 1):63–8.

31. Faioni EM, Franchi F, Asti D, Sacchi E, Bernardi F, Mannucci PM. Resistance to activated protein C in nine thrombophilic families: interference in a protein S functional assay. Thromb Haemost 1993;70:1067–71.

32. Friberger P, Egberg N, Holmer E, Hellgren M, Blomback M. Antithrombin assay – the use of human or bovine thrombin and the observation of a "second" heparin cofactor. Thromb Res 1982;25(5):433–6.

33. Marciniak E, Gockerman JP. Heparin-induced decrease in circulating antithrombin-III. Lancet 1977;2(8038):581–4.

34. Marciniak E, Farley CH, DeSimone PA. Familial thrombosis due to antithrombin 3 deficiency. Blood 1974;43(2):219–31.

35. Brandt JT, Barna LK, Triplett DA. Laboratory identification of lupus anticoagulants: results of the Second International Workshop for Identification of Lupus Anticoagulants. Thromb Haemost 1995;74(6):1597–603.

36. Escalante A, Brey RL, Mitchell BD Jr, Dreiner U. Accuracy of anticardiolipin antibodies in identifying a history of thrombosis among patients with systemic lupus erythematosus. Am J Med 1995;98(6):559–65.

37. Josephson C, Nuss R, Jacobson L, Hacker MR, Murphy J, Weinberg A, et al. The varicella-autoantibody syndrome. Pediatr Res 2001;50(3):345–52.

38. Ray JG, Shmorgun D, Chan WS. Common C677T polymorphism of the methylenetetrahydrofolate reductase gene and the risk of venous thromboembolism: meta-analysis of 31 studies. Pathophysiol Haemost Thromb 2002;32:51–8.

39. Walker MC, Smith GN, Perkins SL, Keely EJ, Garner PR. Changes in homocysteine levels during normal pregnancy. Am J Obstet Gynecol 1999;180:660–4.

40. Cattaneo M. Hyperhomocysteinemia, atherosclerosis and thrombosis. Thromb Haemost 1999;81(2):165–76.

41. Wells PS, Langlois NJ, Webster MA, Jaffey J, Anderson JL. Elevated factor VIII is a risk factor for idiopathic venous thromboembolism in Canada – is it necessary to define a new upper reference range for factor VIII? Thromb Haemost 2005;93:842–6.

42. Martinelli I, de Stefano V, Taioli E, Paciaroni K, Rossi E, Mannucci PM. Inherited thrombophilia and first venous thromboembolism during pregnancy and puerperium. Thromb Haemost 2002;87:791–5.

43. Friederich PW, Sanson BJ, Simioni P, Zanardi S, Huisman MV, Kindt I, et al. Frequency of pregnancy-related venous thromboembolism in anticoagulant factor-deficient women: implications for prophylaxis. Ann Intern Med 1996;125:955–60.

44. Lindqvist PG, Svensson PJ, Marsaal K, Grennert L, Luterkort M, Dahlback B. Activated protein C resistance (FV:Q506) and pregnancy. Thromb Haemost 1999;81(4):532–7.

45. Dizon-Townson D, Miller C, Sibai B, Spong CY, Thom E, Wendel G Jr, et al. The relationship of the factor V Leiden mutation and pregnancy outcomes for mother and fetus. Obstet Gynecol 2005;106(3):517–24.

46. Brill-Edwards P, Ginsberg JS, Gent M, Hirsh J, Burrows RF, Kearon C, et al. Safety of withholding heparin in pregnant women with a history of venous thromboembolism. Recurrence of Clot in This Pregnancy Study Group. N Engl J Med 2000;343:1439–44.

47. McColl MD, Ramsay JE, Tait RC, Walker ID, McCall F, Conkie JA, et al. Risk factors for pregnancy associated venous thromboembolism. Thromb Haemost 1997;78(4):1183–8.

48. Department of Health, Scottish Department of Health, Drife J, Lewis G (eds). Why mothers die. Report on Confidential Enquiries into Maternal Deaths in the United Kingdom 1994–1996. Stationary Office, London, 1998.

49. Berg CJ, Atrash HK, Koonin LM, Tucker M. Pregnancy-related mortality in the United States, 1987–1990. Obstet Gynecol 1996;88:161–7.

50. Rusen ID, Liston R, Wen SW, Bartholomew S. Special Report on Maternal Mortality and Severe Morbidity in Canada. Enhanced surveillance: the path to prevention. Minister of Public Works and Government Services, Ottawa, Canada.

51. Helewa ME, Burrows RF, Smith J, Williams K, Brain P, Rabkin SW. Report of the Canadian Hypertension Society Consensus Conference: 1. Definitions, evaluation and classification of hypertensive disorders in pregnancy. CMAJ 1997;157:715–25.

52. Strauss RS. Adult functional outcome of those born small for gestational age: twenty-six-year follow-up of the 1970 British Birth Cohort. JAMA 2000;283:625–32.

53. Salafia CM, Minior VK, Pezzullo JC, Popek EJ, Rosenkrantz TS, Vintzileos AM. Intrauterine growth restriction in infants of less than thirty-two weeks' gestation: associated placental pathologic features. Am J Obstet Gynecol 1995;173(4):1049–57.

54. Salafia CM, Pezzullo JC, Lopez-Zeno JA, Simmens S, Minior VK, Vintzileos AM. Placental pathologic features of preterm preeclampsia. Am J Obstet Gynecol 1995;173(4):1097–105.

55. Roberts JM, Redman CW. Pre-eclampsia: more than pregnancy-induced hypertension. Lancet 1993;341(8858):1447–51.

56. Khong TY, de Wolf F, Robertson WB, Brosens I. Inadequate maternal vascular response to placentation in pregnancies complicated by pre-eclampsia and by small-for-gestational age infants. Br J Obstet Gynaecol 1986;93(10):1049–59.

57. Isermann B, Sood R, Pawlinski R, Zogg M, Kalloway S, Degen JL, et al. The thrombomodulin-protein C system is essential for the maintenance of pregnancy. Nat Med 2003;9(3):331–7.

58. Li W, Zheng X, Gu JM, Ferrell GL, Brady M, Esmon NL, et al. Extraembryonic expression of EPCR is essential for embryonic viability. Blood 2005;106(8):2716–22.

59. Parascandola M, Weed DL. Causation in epidemiology. J Epidemiol Commun Health 2001;55(12):905–12.

60. Hill AB. The environment and disease: association or causation? Proc R Soc Med 1965;58:295–300.

61. Thygesen LC, Andersen GS, Andersen H. A philosophical analysis of the Hill criteria. J Epidemiol Commun Health 2005;59(6):512–16.

62. Lin J, August P. Genetic thrombophilias and preeclampsia: a meta-analysis. Obstet Gynecol 2005;105(1):182–92.

63. Wu O, Robertson L, Twaddle S, Lowe GD, Clark P, Greaves M, et al. Screening for thrombophilia in high-risk situations: systematic review and cost-effectiveness analysis. The Thrombosis: Risk and Economic Assessment of Thrombophilia Screening (TREATS) study. Health Technol Assess 2006;10:1–110.

64. Howley HE, Walker M, Rodger MA. A systematic review of the association between factor V Leiden or prothrombin gene variant and intrauterine growth restriction. Am J Obstet Gynecol 2005;192:694–708.

65. Alfirevic Z, Roberts D, Martlew V. How strong is the association between maternal thrombophilia and adverse pregnancy outcome? A systematic review. Eur J Obstet Gynecol Reprod Biol 2002;101(1):6–14.

66. Rey E, Kahn SR, David M, Shrier I. Thrombophilic disorders and fetal loss: a meta-analysis. Lancet 2003;361(9361):901–8.

67. Burke W, Thomson E, Khoury MJ, McDonnell SM, Press N, Adams PC, et al. Hereditary hemochromatosis. Gene discovery and its implications for population-based screening. JAMA 1998;280:172–8.

68. Infante-Rivard C, Rivard GE, Yotov WV, Genin E, Guiguet M, Weinberg C, et al. Absence of association of thrombophilia polymorphisms with intrauterine growth restriction. N Engl J Med 2002;347(1):19–25.

69. Ogueh O, Chen MF, Spurll G, Benjamin A. Outcome of pregnancy in women with hereditary thrombophilia. Int J Gynaecol Obstet 2001;74(3):247–53.

70. Ghidini A, Salafia CM, Pezzullo JC. Placental vascular lesions and likelihood of diagnosis of preeclampsia. Obstet Gynecol 1997;90(4 Pt 1):542–5.

71. Reich LM, Bower M, Key NS. Role of the geneticist in testing and counseling for inherited thrombophilia. Genet Med 2003;5:133–43.

72. Greer IA, Nelson-Piercy C. Low-molecular-weight heparins for thromboprophylaxis and treatment of venous thromboembolism in pregnancy: a systematic review of safety and efficacy. Blood 2005;106:401–7.

73. Warkentin TE, Greinacher A. Heparin-induced thrombocytopenia: recognition, treatment, and prevention: the Seventh ACCP Conference on Antithrombotic and Thrombolytic Therapy. Chest 2004;126(3 suppl):311S-337S.

74. Lepercq J, Conard J, Borel-Derlon A, Darmon JY, Boudignat O, Francoual C, et al. Venous thromboembolism during pregnancy: a retrospective study of enoxaparin safety in 624 pregnancies. Br J Obstet Gynaecol 2001;108:1134–40.

75. Huhle G, Geberth M, Hoffmann U, Heene DL, Harenberg J. Management of heparin-associated thrombocytopenia in pregnancy with subcutaneous r-hirudin. Gynecol Obstet Invest 2000;49(1):67–9.

76. Payne SM, Kovacs MJ. Cutaneous dalteparin reactions associated with antibodies of heparin-induced thrombocytopenia. Ann Pharmacother 2003;37(5):655–8.

77. Howell R, Fidler J, Letsky E, de Swiet M. The risks of antenatal subcutaneous heparin prophylaxis: a controlled trial. Br J Obstet Gynaecol 1983;90(12):1124–8.

78. Wysowski DK, Talarico L, Bacsanyi J, Botstein P. Spinal and epidural hematoma and low-molecular-weight heparin. N Engl J Med 1998;338(24):1774–5.

79. Herbstreit F, Kienbaum P, Merguet P, Peters J. Conservative treatment of paraplegia after removal of an epidural catheter during low-molecular-weight heparin treatment. Anesthesiology 2002;97(3):733–4.

80. ASRA Second Consensus Conference on Neuraxial Anesthesia and Anticoagulation. Regional Anesthesia in the Anticoagulated Patient: Anesthetic Management of the Patient Receiving Low Molecular Weight Heparin (LMWH). American Society of Regional Anesthesia and Pain Medicine, 28th April 2002.

81. Schambeck CM, Eberl E, Geisen U, Grossmann R, Keller F. The impact of dalteparin (Fragmin) on thrombin generation in pregnant women with venous thromboembolism: significance of the factor V Leiden mutation. Thromb Haemost 2001;85: 782–6.

82. Bombeli T, Raddatz MP, Fehr J. Evaluation of an optimal dose of low-molecular-weight heparin for thromboprophylaxis in pregnant women at risk of thrombosis using coagulation activation markers. Haemostasis 2001;31:90–8.

83. Hunt BJ, Doughty HA, Majumdar G, Copplestone A, Kerslake S, Buchanan N, et al. Thromboprophylaxis with low molecular weight heparin (Fragmin) in high risk pregnancies. Thromb Haemost 1997;77:39–43.

84. Bar J, Cohen-Sacher B, Hod M, Blickstein D, Lahav J, Merlob P. Low-molecular-weight heparin for thrombophilia in pregnant women. Int J Gynaecol Obstet 2000;69:209–13.

85. Richter C, Sitzmann J, Lang P, Weitzel H, Huch A, Huch R. Excretion of low molecular weight heparin in human milk. Br J Clin Pharmacol 2001;52:708–10.

86. Bates SM, Greer IA, Pabinger I, Soafer S, Hirsh J. Venous thromboembolism, thrombophilia, antithrombotic therapy and pregnancy. ACCP Evidence-Based Clinical Practice Guidelines, 8th edn. Chest 2008;133(6 suppl):844S-886S.

87. Rai R, Cohen H, Dave M, Regan L. Randomised controlled trial of aspirin and aspirin plus heparin in pregnant women with recurrent miscarriage associated with phospholipid antibodies (or anti-phospholipid antibodies). BMJ 1997;314:253–7.

88. Kutteh WH. Anti-phospholipid antibody-associated recurrent pregnancy loss: treatment with heparin and low-dose aspirin is superior to low-dose aspirin alone. Am J Obstet Gynecol 1996;174(5):1584–9.

89. Farquharson RG, Quenby S, Greaves M. Anti-phospholipid syndrome in pregnancy: a randomized, controlled trial of treatment. Obstet Gynecol 2002;100:408–13.

90. Empson M, Lassere M, Craig J, Scott J. Prevention of recurrent miscarriage for women with anti-phospholipid antibody or lupus anticoagulant. Cochrane Database of Systematic Reviews, 2005;2:CD002859.

91. Gris J-C, Mercier E, Quéré I, Lavigne-Lissalde G, Cochery-Nouvellon E, Hoffet M, et al. Low-molecular-weight heparin versus low-dose aspirin in women with one fetal loss and a constitutional thrombophilic disorder. Blood 2004;103:3695–9.

92. Rodger MA, Gris J-C, Quere I, Dauzat M, Mares P. Important publication missing key information. Blood 2004;104(10): 3413–14.

93. Di Nisio M, Peters L, Middeldorp S. Anticoagulants for the treatment of recurrent pregnancy loss in women without anti-phospholipid syndrome. Cochrane Database of Systematic Reviews, 2005;2:CD004734.

94. Duhl AJ, Paidas MJ, Ural SH, et al, Pregnancy and Thrombosis Working Group. Antithrombotic therapy and pregnancy: consensus report and recommendations for prevention and treatment of venous thromboembolism and adverse pregnancy outcomes. Am J Obstet Gynecol 2007;197(5):457.

95. Walker MC, Ferguson SE, Allen VM. Heparin for pregnant women with acquired or inherited thrombophilias. Cochrane Database of Systematic Reviews, 2003;2:CD003580.

96. Paidas M, Ku DH, Triche E, Lockwood C, Arkel Y. Does heparin therapy improve pregnancy outcome in patients with thrombophilias? J Thromb Haemost 2004;2(7):1194–5.

97. Ray JG, Chan WS. Deep vein thrombosis during pregnancy and the puerperium: a meta-analysis of the period of risk and the leg of presentation. Obstet Gynecol Surv 1999;54: 265–71.

98. Vandenbroucke JP, Koster T, Briet E, Reitsma PH, Bertina RM, Rosendaal FR. Increased risk of venous thrombosis in oral-contraceptive users who are carriers of factor V Leiden mutation. Lancet 1994;344(8935):1453–7.

99. Martinelli I, Taioli E, Bucciarelli P, Akhavan S, Mannucci PM. Interaction between the G20210A mutation of the prothrombin gene and oral contraceptive use in deep vein thrombosis. Arterioscler Thromb Vasc Biol 1999;19(3):700–3.

100. Pabinger I, Schneider B. Thrombotic risk of women with hereditary antithrombin III-, protein C- and protein S-deficiency taking oral contraceptive medication. The GTH Study Group on Natural Inhibitors. Thromb Haemost 1994;71:548–52.

101. Rintelen C, Pabinger I, Knobl P, Lechner K, Mannhalter C. Probability of recurrence of thrombosis in patients with and without factor V Leiden. Thromb Haemost 1996;75:229–32.

102. Rosendaal FR, Helmerhorst FM, Vandenbroucke JP. Oral contraceptives, hormone replacement therapy and thrombosis. Thromb Haemost 2001;86(1):112–23.

103. Simioni P, Sanson BJ, Prandoni P, Tormene D, Friederich PW, Girolami B, et al. Incidence of venous thromboembolism in families with inherited thrombophilia. Thromb Haemost 1999;81(2):198–202.

104. Hoibraaten E, Qvigstad E, Arnesen H, Larsen S, Wickstrom E, Sandset PM. Increased risk of recurrent venous thromboembolism during hormone replacement therapy – results of the randomized, double-blind, placebo-controlled Estrogen in Venous Thromboembolism Trial (EVTET). Thromb Haemost 2000;84(6):961–7.

105. Cook TM, Counsell D, Wildsmith JAW. Major complications of central neuraxial block: report on the third national audit project of the Royal College of Anaesthestists. Br J Anaesth 2009;102:179–90.

106. Harnett MJ, Walsh ME, McElrath TF, Tsen LC. The use of central neuraxial techniques in parturients with Factor V Leiden muation. Anesth Analg 2005;101(6):1821–3.

107. Horlocker TT, Wedel DJ, Rowlingson JC, et al. Regional anesthesia in the patient receiving antithrombotic or thrombolytic therapy. American Society of Regional Anesthesia and Pain Medicine Evidence-Based Guidelines, 3rd edn. Reg Anesth Pain Med 2010;35:64–101.

108. Vandermuelen EP, van Aken H, Vermylen J. Anticoagulants and spinal-epidural anesthesia. Anesth Analg 1994;79:1165–77.

109. Tryba M. Epidural regional anesthesia and low molecular weight heparin: Pro (German). Anasth Intensivmed Notfallmed Schemerzther 1993;28:179–81.

110. CLASP Collaborative Group. A randomized trial of low-dose aspirin for the prevention and treatement of pre-eclampsia amoung 9364 pregnant women. Lancet 1994;343:619–29.

111. Sibai BM Caritis SN, Thom E, et al. and the National Institue of Child Health and Human Development Maternal-Fetal Network. Low-dose aspirin in nulliparous women: safety of continuous epidural block and correlation between bleeding time and maternal-neonatal bleeding complications. Am J Obstet Gynecol 1994;172:1553–7.

112. Woodward DK, Birks RJS, Granger KA. Massive pulmonary embolism in late pregnancy. Can J Anaesth 1998;45:888–92.

113. Pillny M, Sandmann W, Luther B, et al. Deep venous thrombosis during pregnancy and after delivery: indications for and results of thrombectomy. J Vasc Surg 2003;37:528–32.

114. Funakoshi Y, Kato M, Kuratani T, Shigemura N, Kaneko M. Successful treatment of massive pulmonary embolism in the 38th week of pregnancy. Ann Thorac Surg 2004;77:694–5.

115. Splinter WM, Dwane PD, Wigle RD, McGrath MJ. Anaesthetic management of emergency caesarean section followed by pulmonary embolectomy. Can J Anaesth 1989;36:689–92.

116. Nishimura K, Kawaguchi M, Shimokawa M, Kitaguchi K, Furuya H. Treatment of pulmonary embolism during cesarean section with recombinant tissue plasminogen activator. Anesthesiology 1998;89:1027–8.

117. Aya AGM, Saissi G, Eledjam J-J. In situ pulmonary thrombolysis using recombinant tissue plasminogen activator after cesarean delivery. Anesthesiology 1999;91:578–9.

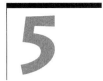

Heart disease in pregnancy

*Cynthia Maxwell[1], Athena Poppas[2], Mathew Sermer[3]
with Elizabeth McGrady[4]*

[1]Obstetrics and Maternal Fetal Medicine, Mount Sinai Hospital, Toronto, Ontario, Canada
[2]Division of Cardiology, Department of Medicine, Warren Alpert Medical School of Brown University and Echocardiography Laboratory, Rhode Island Hospital, Providence, RI, USA
[3]Department of Obstetrics and Gynecology, University of Toronto, and Obstetrics and Maternal Fetal Medicine, Mount Sinai Hospital, Toronto, Ontario, Canada
[4]Department of Anesthesia, Princess Royal Maternity Unit, Glasgow Royal Infirmary, Glasgow, Scotland, UK

Introduction

Heart disease affecting women in reproductive age continues to be a challenge to providers of pregnancy care. To the obstetrician, heart disease provides a special challenge, as it is a leading cause of maternal mortality internationally. In the most recent Confidential Enquiry into Maternal and Child Health (CEMACH) report from the United Kingdom in 2007, cardiovascular disease was the most common cause of indirect maternal mortality, with a maternal mortality rate (MMR) of 2.27 per 100,000 livebirths [1]. Furthermore, this report confirmed a continued rise in mortality related to cardiac disease in pregnancy since the 1980s. The leading causes of cardiac death were found to be myocardial infarction related to ischemic heart disease, followed by dissection of the thoracic aorta. In Canada, the Maternal Health Study Group of the Canadian Perinatal Surveillance System generated the Special Report on Maternal Mortality and Severe Morbidity in 2004, following the principles of the CEMACH reporting system [2]. This group concluded that while the overall MMR was low (6.1 per 100,000 livebirths), cardiovascular disease was the leading cause of indirect maternal deaths, accounting for 60% of indirect deaths, and associated with an MMR of 1.1 per 100,000 livebirth. Again, coronary artery disease was the most common cause of cardiac death. Thus, care of the pregnant patient with cardiovascular disease requires special attention to diagnosis, treatment and multidisciplinary management by the obstetric and medical teams.

Physiologic changes of pregnancy

A multitude of physiologic adaptations of the cardiovascular system to pregnancy influence the impact of heart disease in the pregnant woman. The most notable changes are the increases in intravascular volume and cardiac output. Early estimates obtained via invasive cardiac testing suggest that cardiac output increases from 3.5 to 6.0 L/min at rest, a rise of close to 40% [3]. These changes begin as early as the first trimester of pregnancy. Several noninvasive studies suggest that cardiac output may decrease in the latter portion of the third trimester [4–7]. The changes in cardiac output are related to increases in maternal heart rate as well as stroke volume [8]. As blood pressure typically decreases during early pregnancy, the rise in cardiac output is accompanied by a dramatic fall in peripheral vascular resistance. Interestingly, the fall in peripheral vascular resistance contributes minimally to the overall rise in cardiac output [9,10]. Various mediators, including estrogens, prostaglandins, and nitric oxide, likely contribute to these changes [11–13]. During labor and delivery, uterine contractions result in an additional increase of cardiac output and blood pressure, the increase in cardiac output approaching 20% [14,15]. Following delivery, relief of vena caval compression and autotransfusion from the emptied and contracted uterus cause additional rises in cardiac output. Most hemodynamic alterations resolve rapidly post partum and are near normal by 6 weeks though structural cardiac changes may not return completely to normal until 6 months.

Counseling patients

The key to safe pregnancy care in the context of cardiac disease is prenatal assessment. The initial approach to obstetric patients should include an appropriate obstetric and cardiac history, as

de Swiet's Medical Disorders in Obstetric Practice, 5th edition.
Edited by R. O. Powrie, M. F. Greene, W. Camann. © 2010 Blackwell Publishing.

well as physical examination. Appendix 5.1, at the end of this chapter, provides a review of the basics of the cardiac examination. Laboratory investigations will include hemoglobin and platelet count. Specific cardiac testing will generally include electrocardiography and echocardiography. Where appropriate, oxygen saturation, Holter monitoring, exercise stress testing, chest X-ray, CT scanning, and cardiac catheterization can and should be performed. Should this assessment reveal that the cardiac condition can be optimized by medical or surgical means, then these measures should be performed, ideally prior to conception. It has been demonstrated that corrective surgery, or even palliative surgery, when appropriate, improves both maternal and fetal outcome [16,17].

Although most diagnostic radiation is associated with minimal exposure and hence risk to the developing fetus, it is preferable to perform such examinations prior to conception and, for reasons more cultural than scientific, to avoid the first trimester. However, most cardiac diagnostic tests can be safely carried out in pregnancy when indicated (see Chapter 32). No increase in the congenital abnormality rate has been documented with radiation exposure of less than 10 rads (0.1 Gy) [18,19]. A chest X-ray delivers less than 0.005 rads (0.00005 Gy) to the pelvis, while cardiac catheterization delivers about 1–2 rads (0.01–0.02 Gy) to the pelvis. Thus these tests should not be withheld during pregnancy if the benefit is deemed to outweigh the potential risk [20]. Echocardiography has proven to be a very useful and safe diagnostic test, regardless of pregnancy state, and it should be used liberally when indicated. Magnetic resonance imaging has not been linked to unfavorable fetal effects, and recent reports suggest minimal fetal risks associated with gadolinium exposure, commonly utilized to enhance diagnostic capability [21].

Following review and discussion of the assessment with the patient and her family, the risks to mother and fetus require careful consideration. Occasionally, the risks are so great that pregnancy may be discouraged. In such cases, other options such as gestational carriers can be discussed. However, in the majority of cases, the likelihood of unfavorable outcome is relatively low. Thus patients and their families can be cautioned yet reassured. Box 5.1 summarizes the high-, intermediate- and low-risk conditions [22].

In the prediction of adverse maternal and fetal outcome, it is helpful to focus on maternal functional status (Box 5.2) in addition to:
- the type of cardiac abnormality
- whether the patient has undergone corrective surgery or procedure to correct the underlying condition
- whether other risk factors are present
- assessment of maternal prognosis and expected survival, and the maternal ability to engage in childrearing
- the heredity of the cardiac lesion in the offspring, if applicable.

Maternal and fetal outcome can be linked to functional status. Maternal mortality may be as high as 7% when class III and IV patients are combined. In contrast, classes I and II combined yield a mortality of 0.5%. Similarly, fetal mortality may be as a high as 30% in class III and IV patients, in contrast to 2% for classes I and II [17]. In situations where maternal mortality risks are considerable, appropriate counseling and social support for the pregnant woman and her family are critical, including frank discussions about who will be involved in the care of the child should maternal demise occur. The context of the birth must also be taken into consideration, for example,

---

Box 5.1 Risk classification of conditions in patients with congenital heart disease

High-risk conditions	• NYHA functional classes III and IV • Significant pulmonary hypertension (defined as >75% of systemic) • Marfan's syndrome with significant aortic root or aortic valve involvement • Severe or symptomatic aortic stenosis
Intermediate-risk conditions	• Uncorrected defects with cyanosis • Large left-to-right shunt • Uncorrected coarctation • Mitral stenosis • Aortic stenosis • Prosthetic valves
Low-risk conditions	• Repaired congenital heart disease without residual cardiac dysfunction • Small to moderate left-to-right shunts • Mitral valve prolapse • Bicuspid aortic valve with normal aorta • Pulmonic stenosis • Aortic or mitral regurgitation with good ventricular function

I	Patients with cardiac disease but without limitations of physical activity. Ordinary physical activity does not cause undue fatigue, palpitation, dyspnea or anginal pain
II	Patients with cardiac disease resulting in slight limitation of physical activity. They are comfortable at rest. Ordinary physical activity results in fatigue, palpitation, dyspnea or anginal pain
III	Patients with cardiac disease resulting in marked limitation of physical activity. They are comfortable at rest. Less than ordinary physical activity causes fatigue, palpitation, dyspnea or anginal pain
IV	Patients with cardiac disease resulting in inability to carry on any physical activity without discomfort. Symptoms may be present even at rest. If any physical activity is undertaken, discomfort is increased

if the child is born prematurely or in the setting of perimortem cesarean delivery.

Prenatal diagnosis and genetic counseling are important components of pre-pregnancy and early pregnancy management. The incidence of congenital heart disease in the offspring of women with congenital heart disease is increased. Autosomal dominant conditions such as Marfan's syndrome carry a 50% recurrence rate. The association between maternal and fetal congenital and inherited heart disease is discussed below in the section on fetal considerations.

Management: general principles

Maternal considerations

In cases where continuing the pregnancy poses significant risk to the pregnant woman with cardiac disease, termination of pregnancy should be discussed. If the woman opts to continue, as is the case in most situations when the risks are deemed acceptable, a management plan is formulated and discussed. Antepartum surveillance seeks to prevent, identify and treat maternal complications including congestive heart failure, arrhythmias, and thromboembolism.

Certain complications, such as congestive heart failure, may be avoidable despite the potential for the physiologic changes of pregnancy to overwhelm the compromised heart's ability to adapt. In such cases, reduction in physical activity, such as work and exercise cessation, may be indicated. It may also be advisable for the pregnant patient to seek methods of stress reduction, avoid excessive atmospheric heat and humidity, and decrease consumption of salt and large meals. In order to avoid unnecessary Valsalva maneuver, constipation should be avoided by increasing dietary fiber intake and the use of stool softeners. Patients belonging to class III–IV as well as those with significant pulmonary hypertension often require inpatient admission during the mid-second trimester for the duration of the pregnancy. Patients should be counseled to watch for signs and symptoms of arrhythmias (particularly palpitations, presyncope or syncope), as tachyarrhythmias commonly occur in pregnant women with congenital heart disease, and may lead to congestive heart failure. Common third-trimester pregnancy complications can pose significant risks to the gravida with heart disease, including conditions such as gestational hypertension, infection, and anemia. Assessment of hemoglobin and urine cultures in each trimester are reasonable approaches to surveillance for these conditions.

Healthy pregnant women often experience fatigue, chest discomfort, dyspnea, palpitations and even syncope. However, in the setting of cardiac disease, these symptoms may represent signs of decompensation. Careful evaluation in normal pregnancies may reveal any of the following: peripheral edema, prominent neck vein pulsations, a diffuse apical impulse, a systolic pulsation along the left sternal border, a split first heart sound, a third heart sound, a systolic murmur that is less than 3/6 in intensity, an accentuated second heart sound, a venous hum, and mammary arterial murmurs [24]. However, identification of severe or progressive dyspnea, orthopnea particularly with paroxysmal nocturnal dyspnea, hemoptysis, syncope with exertion, chest pain related to effort or emotion, development of cyanosis, persistent neck vein distension, systolic murmur grade 3/6 or more in intensity, any diastolic murmur, cardiomegaly, sustained arrhythmia, a fixed split second sound, and left parasternal lift or loud P2 suggestive of pulmonary hypertension should initiate further investigation as to the likely indicated underlying cardiac abnormalities [25].

Fetal considerations

Given the recurrence risk associated with maternal congenital heart disease, fetal assessment includes diagnosis and management of cardiac lesions, as well as detection of pregnancy complications such as intrauterine growth restriction and preterm birth. Infants of mothers with congenital heart disease are more likely to be growth restricted [26], be premature [26,27] and have congenital cardiac anomalies [28,29]. In the general population, the incidence of congenital heart disease (CHD) is 0.7–0.8%, but the incidence has been reported to be as high as 3.4–14.2% for patients with congenital heart conditions, depending on the particular cardiac lesion [17, 30–32]. In a recent literature review of 48 studies including 2491 pregnancies, the recurrence rate for CHD was lowest in patients with corrected transposition of the great arteries (0.6%) and highest in those with atrioventricular septal defects (8%) [33]. In one comprehensive study from the 1960s, the reported recurrence rate was 17.9–23% for women with uncorrected lesions, but this report was likely confounded by genetic syndromes [17].

Fetal cardiac anomalies are best assessed through echocardiography at 18–20 weeks gestation. Smoking cessation, correction of maternal anemia and rest may be employed to minimize the risks of intrauterine growth restriction and preterm birth [34–38]. Aggressive measures to reduce maternal activity, such as hospital admission, as well as continuous oxygen therapy, may lessen risks of fetal growth restriction and preterm birth in cases of cyanotic maternal heart disease or pulmonary hypertension. For the same reason, in-hospital management should be considered for patients who belong to New York Heart Association (NYHA) functional class III or IV. Fetal well-being, growth, and Amniotic Fluid Index can be assessed with serial fetal ultrasound and biophysical testing beginning as early as 24–26 weeks gestation. The frequency of testing depends on the patient's presenting symptoms and underlying cardiac condition. Early preterm labor can be detected with fundal palpation for uterine contractions, pelvic exam to assess cervical dilation, and, in certain cases, cervical length measurement using vaginal ultrasound. Administration of antenatal corticosteroids for fetal lung maturity should be considered when preterm birth prior to 32–24 weeks is anticipated.

The interval between prenatal visits may need to be as frequent as every 2 weeks until 32 weeks, and weekly to delivery to ensure adequate surveillance of maternal and fetal status.

Depending on the maternal cardiac status and fetal well-being, this surveillance may need to be increased or decreased accordingly.

Multidisciplinary approach

Managing pregnant patients with complex cardiac disease mandates participation from a multidisciplinary medical team. When potential exists for maternal compromise, the management is best delivered in a tertiary-level perinatal center with availability of obstetricians, cardiologists, pediatricians, anesthesiologists, and obstetric nursing. Early in the pregnancy, a patient care meeting is arranged to chart a course of management for the antepartum, peripartum and postpartum phases of care. Anticipation and contingency planning for obstetric, cardiac or pediatric emergencies are articulated in advance. Given the infrequent nature of these cases and that some or much of the care will be occurring on units that do not routinely care for cardiac patients, it is important that the plan be as specific and detailed as possible. Should the patient be on a cardiac monitor? What training should the nurse have who is caring for the patient? What medications might be needed for potential complications and how are these medications administered? These are all examples of the specific questions the care plan should address. A checklist of items to consider and/or carry out when caring for pregnant women with cardiac disease is given in Box 5.3. Such directives are placed in writing in the patient's medical record and are communicated to medical and nursing staff in the maternity units

---

Box 5.3 Cardiac patient care considerations checklist

Antepartum care considerations

Is additional testing needed to assess risk or guide therapy peripartum?
- Baseline EKG done in third trimester
- Echocardiogram at any time in the past for lowest risk lesions, in this pregnancy for moderate-risk lesions and in the third trimester for high- and highest risk lesions
- Stress testing (exercise echo or dobutamine echo in past year for patients with known or suspected ischemic heart disease or more recently if they are symptomatic)
- EP testing for life-threatening arrhythmia investigation (often deferred until post partum but can be done in pregnancy if warranted)
- Has fetus of mother with congenital heart disease had fetal survey by ultrasound to indentify congenital malformations?

Has the patient's cardiac status been optimized?
- Is medical therapy optimized and have appropriate dose adjustments been made for pharmacokinetics of pregnancy?
- Are there interventions that would be done if the woman was not pregnant that should be done while she is pregnant to optimize patient's status for delivery, e.g. diagnostic or therapeutic cardiac catheterization (angioplasty, stent), valvuloplasty, valve replacement., diagnostic or therapeutic EP studies, AICD or pacemaker placement or adjustment?

(Continued on p. 122)

Box 5.3 (Continued)

Multidisciplinary team meeting needed and arranged (generally should have occurred by 34 weeks). Team should include:
- Nursing (LDR and postpartum care RN +/− ICU/CCU nursing)
- Maternal fetal medicine
- Anesthesia (ideally obstetric anesthesia, also consider cardiac anesthesia for high- and highest risk cases)
- Cardiology
- ICU/CCU doctor
- Neonatology
- Written delivery plan should be generated and distributed and made available to all relevant parties including nursing (should include **who to call and how to do so** when the patient comes in)
- Case-specific nursing education should occur in advance of delivery

Intrapartum care considerations

Determine mode and timing of delivery (decision based on obstetric, medical and logistical issues to ensure the availability of the necessary caregivers):
- Planned induction at what gestation/cervical status
- Planned cesarean delivery at what gestation
- Spontaneous delivery

Determine delivery location (decision based on local facilities and expertise. In general, care prior to delivery is best provided in LDR and afterwards in medical setting):
- Standard LDR
- Specialized LDR
- Obstetric ICU
- MICU
- CCU

Delivery personnel who should be notified of admission (make sure needed parties available on day of any planned delivery)

Medical attendants:
- Obstetrician
- Cardiologist
- Anesthesia (ideally obstetric anesthesia, also consider cardiac anesthesia for high- and highest risk cases)
- Intensivist

Nursing (consider need for team approach of ICU/CCU/recovery room/ER nurse with LDR nurse. Define necessary nurse-to-patient ratio):
- LDR nurse
- LDR nurse with Advanced Cardiac Life Support (ACLS) recovery room training
- LDR nurse with ACLS and special critical care training
- Critical care nurse (ICU/CCU/recovery room/ER) nurse

Required response time of ACLS trained personnel if nursing team caring for patient is not ACLS certified/experienced?

Education:
- Verify written care plan is available to all team members
- Is a "recap" in-service for care team advisable on day of delivery?

Monitoring:

Cardiac monitor options (choose one)
- Not necessary
- To be in room but does not need to be on if patient asymptomatic
- To be on patient at all times but not continuously observed
- To be on patient at all times and should be continually observed by ACLS trained individual

- To be on patient at all times and should be observed at all times by critical care nurse/MD/physician assistant or nurse practitioner

Many cardiac patients aside from the highest risk patients or those with a history of life-threatening hemodynamically unstable arrhythmias will not need continuous nursing by ACLS trained personnel. Nursing should, however, have ready access to ACLS trained individuals if patient has any change in status or there is any bradycardia or tachycardia warranting expert interpretation

Pulse oximeter (choose one)
- Not necessary
- Readily available but use only with symptoms
- In room and check hourly
- In room and on continuously

Pulse oximeter may provide evidence of CHF but should always be interpreted in view of strength of pulse signal

Fetal monitoring

Obtain explicit plan from obstetric team including who will read the fetal monitoring strips and the plan of action should they be concerning

Defibrillator (choose one)
- On the unit with ready access to defibrillator pads
- Defibrillator and defibrillator pads in the room
- Defibrillator pads on patient but machine not hooked up
- Patient to be monitored using defibrillator with defibrillator pads

IV access (choose one)
- No IV necessary
- Single peripheral IV lines needed
- Two peripheral IV lines needed
- Central line
- Central line with CVP
- Central line with pulmonary artery catheter

All patients need strict ins and outs measured throughout hospitalization. We will want to keep most cardiac patients in a neutral fluid balance during hospitalization (+800–1000 mL/day to account for insensible loss)

Fluid to be run: _____
Rate: _____

Make sure to add in all fluids given with medications and for regional anesthesia

Arterial line (choose one)
- No arterial line needed
- Arterial line warranted

Arterial line advisable when hemodynamics make moment-to-moment monitoring of blood pressure useful, e.g. aortic stenosis

Medications:
- Need for SBE prophylaxis to be determined by care team but may not be necessary for most patients. If decision is made to give, the standard regimens are as follows:
  - Standard dosing: ampicillin 2 g IV plus gentamicin 1.5 mg/kg within 30 minutes of delivery; ampicillin 1 g IV 6 hours after delivery
  - Pen allergy: vancomycin 1 g IV over 1–2 hours plus gentamicin 1.5 mg/kg IV within 30 minutes of delivery
- Consider any special issues related to interactions with commonly used obstetric medications
- Consider all possibly necessary cardiac medications not routinely used on obstetric units.
- Plan RN/MD education regarding these medications
- Develop written instructions with respect to preparation and administration of this medication
- Consider need for medication to be at bedside
- Notify pharmacy in advance of request (esp. if free-standing obstetrics hospital)

(*Continued on p. 124*)

Box 5.3 (Continued)

Anesthetic concerns:
- Consider special issues related to anesthesia

Anesthesia department to determine preferred modality of anesthesia timing and precautions in technique

- Are there special issues with respect to cautery for cesarean delivery?

Implanted defibrillators may need to be turned off prior to surgery because of interference from cautery

Thromboprophylaxis (choose one)
- Intermittent compression stockings
- Heparin 5000 units SQ q12 h
- Heparin 5000 units SQ q8 h
- Enoxaparin 40 units SQ daily
- Enoxaparin 30 units SQ q12 h
- Full anticoagulation necessary in peripartum period (please see peripartum anticoagulation protocol)

Options 1 and 2 compatible with epidural anesthesia. Options 3–6 should only be done after the epidural catheter is removed. Consider option 1 or 2 antepartum and option 2, 3, 4 or 5 for most patients while in hospital

Postpartum care considerations

How long post partum will patient require special observation? (choose one)
- Usual period of postpartum observation
- 6 hours
- 12 hours
- 24 hours
- 48 hours
- 72 hours
- 96 hours

Low-risk patients probably only warrant the usual period of observation given to all patients. Moderate-risk patients warrant 6 hours. High-risk patients warrant between 6 and 48 hours and highest risk 72–96 hours.

Location of special postpartum observation (choose one)
- Room on regular postpartum floor
- Room on high-risk antenatal floor
- Standard LDR/postoperative CS area
- Specialized LDR/postoperative CS area
- Obstetric ICU
- MICU
- CCU
- Other_____

Option 1, 2 or 3 for low-risk, 2, 3 or 4 for moderate-risk, 4, 5, 6 or 7 for high and highest risk patients

Monitoring:
Cardiac monitor options (choose one)
- Not necessary
- To be in room but does not need to be on if patient asymptomatic
- To be on patient at all times but not continuously observed
- To be on patient at all times and should be continually observed by ACLS trained individual
- To be on patient at all times and should be observed at all times by critical care nurse/MD/PA/RNP

Option 1 or 2 for low-risk, 2 or 3 for moderate-risk, 3 for high-risk and 3, 4 or 5 for highest risk patients

Postpartum monitoring/interventions recommended and for how long (choose one and recommend a duration)
- Peripheral IV
- Central line
- CVP

- Arterial line
- Pulmonary artery catheter

All patients need strict ins and outs measured throughout hospitalization. We will want to keep most cardiac patients in a neutral fluid balance during hospitalization (+800–1000mL/day to account for insensible loss)

Fluid to be run: _____

Rate: _____

Make sure to add in all fluids given with medications and for regional anesthesia

Pulse oximeter in room and checked how often
- Not necessary
- In room but use only with symptoms
- In room and check hourly
- In room and on continuously

Availability of ACLS trained physician/PA/RNP
- Special availability not necessary
- Special availability necessary with what maximum response time

Postpartum care team: identify the care team and indicate who will be the initial contact should medical problems arise. Make sure the person's name and contact numbers are clearly documented in the chart

Medical attendants:
- Obstetrician
- Cardiologist
- Anesthesia (ideally obstetric anesthesia, also consider cardiac anesthesia for high and highest risk cases)
- General internist
- ICU team
- CCU team
- Medical ICU versus LDR with cardiac nursing (consider need for team approach and necessary nurse-to-patient ratio)
- LDR nurse
- LDR nurse with ACLS training
- LDR nurse with ACLS and special critical care training
- Critical care (ICU/CCU/recovery room/ER) nurse

Required response time of ACLS trained personnel if nursing/MD attendant not present (choose one)
- 1 minute
- 5 minutes

Defibrillator (choose one)
- On the unit
- In the room
- Pads on patient
- Patient to be monitored with defibrillator with defibrillator pads on
- Special issues related to interactions with commonly used obstetric medications

Thromboprophylaxis

Start: _____

Duration: _____
- Intermittent compression stockings
- Heparin 5000 units SQ q12 h
- Heparin 5000 units 5000 Units SQ q8 h
- Enoxaparin 40 units SQ daily
- Enoxaparin 30 units SQ q12 h
- Full anticoagulation will be needed postpartum

Possibly necessary cardiac medications not routinely used on obstetric units
- Need for RN/MD education regarding these medications
- Need for written instructions with respect to preparation and administration of this medication

(*Continued on p. 126*)

Box 5.3 (Continued)

- Need for medication to be at bedside
- Pharmacy notified in advance of request (esp. if free-standing obstetrics hospital)

Discharge planning care considerations

Will there be any adjustments to medication necessary post partum (e.g. resumption/replacing of medications stopped/started because of pregnancy OR dosing adjustments necessary in postpartum period because of increases made during pregnancy)?

Who will follow the patient after discharge and when will they need to be seen (letter or phone call should be sent/made to receiving MD)

- Cardiology
- Primary care doctor
- Obstetrics
- Obstetric medicine (where available)

---

as well as cardiology and intensive care units, so that everyone is familiar with the contingency planning. As nursing staff are most often the healthcare providers who first identify such emergency situations, it is imperative they be informed and incorporated into the multidisciplinary planning process.

Peripartum management

Labor and delivery management usually follows the standard obstetric indications for induction and mode of delivery. Rarely is a cesarean delivery indicated solely due to maternal cardiac disease. However, elective induction is often advocated to ensure that the necessary staff are readily available for management of peripartum complications. Furthermore, advanced delivery planning allows for the necessary adjuncts to care, such as insertion of monitoring lines and epidural anesthesia, both of which can be introduced in a controlled environment.

If the patient is receiving full therapeutic doses of anticoagulation, delivery may need to be timed such that anticoagulation can be stopped shortly prior to delivery. Unfractionated intravenous heparin (UFH) is usually stopped 4–6 hours prior to induction of labor, cesarean delivery and/or regional anesthesia to allow normalization of partial thrombin time (PTT). If the patient has received full-dose low molecular weight heparin (LMWH), the recommended waiting period extends to 24 hours [39]. This allows safe insertion of regional anesthesia and decreases potential for peripartum hemorrhage. If an anticoagulated patient goes into spontaneous labor, protamine can be given intravenously to reverse heparinization. Protamine can completely reverse UFH and partially reverse LMWH. Anticoagulation can usually be restarted 6–12 hours after the delivery depending on the patient's condition and the amount of bleeding (see Chapters 3, 4 and 46).

The American Heart Association and the American College of Cardiology now recommend that infective endocarditis (IE) prophylaxis be given only for patients undergoing dental or respiratory procedures who have a cardiac lesion deemed to be at very high risk for IE. They no longer recommend IE prophylaxis for patients with congenital or valvular heart disease undergoing genitourinary procedures, including vaginal or cesarean deliveries [40]. IE prevention in obstetric patients with cardiac lesions should be restricted to antibiotic prophylaxis for dental and respiratory procedures and the prompt and consistent use of antibiotics to prevent and treat noncardiac infections just as would be done in obstetric patients without cardiac disease. This recommendation is based on both the lack of evidence of benefit of IE prophylaxis in uncomplicated vaginal and cesarean deliveries and the real but small possibility that IE prophyaxis will cause harm. However, many obstetric physicians and centers have been reluctant to adopt this recommendation. The widespread use of antibiotics in the delivery suite both to treat group B streptococcal colonization and prevent wound infections in cesarean deliveries makes many clinicians skeptical about the risks of IE prophylaxis and even in the absence of good evidence of their benefit, the practice continues.

Although present recommendations do not support its use, if the decision is made to give IE prophylaxis, it is increasingly clear that it should be reserved for those patients with cardiac lesions that are at a particularly high risk of IE. This does not include the majority of the cardiac lesions discussed in this chapter and is limited to patients with the following conditions:
- a prior history of IE
- unrepaired or incompletely repaired cyanotic congenital heart disease (including those with palliative shunts and conduits)
- completely repaired congenital heart defects with prosthetic material or devices during the first 6 months after insertion
- any residual defect near the site of a prosthetic patch or device
- cardiac transplant patients who have valvular regurgitation through structurally abnormal valves.

Patients with known arrhythmias or who are at risk for rate or rhythm disturbances are monitored with telemetry, or a bedside monitor and nurse when telemetry facilities are not available. The treatment for arrhythmias is similar to that in the nonpregnant state. Persons caring for such patients should be educated on the preparation and use of cardiac medications that may be required and ready access to these medications ensured.

For pregnant patients with intracardiac shunts, it is critical to avoid decreases in left-sided filling pressures. Reversal of left to right flow or exacerbation of existing right to left flow may lead to pulmonary thrombosis and/or cardiopulmonary collapse. Oxygen desaturation can be monitored with continuous pulse oximetry. Maternal expulsive efforts are minimized in the second stage of labor to avoid the Valsalva maneuver. Peripartum hemorrhage should be identified and managed promptly. In cases where mothers have previously experienced peripartum hemorrhage, are receiving anticoagulation or have Eisenmenger's syndrome, cross-matching for blood products before labor and delivery admission is advisable. To prevent paradoxic air emboli in cyanotic patients with intracardiac shunts, an air filter is placed in all intravenous lines.

Congestive heart failure is another peripartum complication requiring immediate identification and treatment. When the laboring woman is in the supine position, uterine contractions increase the maternal cardiac output by 24% [41], due to the repeated autotransfusion of blood from the contracting uterus into the intravascular space, as well as catecholamine release and attendant increase in the arterial blood pressure [42,43]. Thus, laboring in the left lateral position is most appropriate, as the increase in cardiac output is closer to 10%, and there is a lesser increase in arterial blood pressure [41,44]. If ventricular function is known to be compromised on echocardiographic assessment, or if the patient has known class II–IV functional status, labor should take place with carefully titrated epidural anesthesia. The anesthesia will lessen the catecholamine release, attenuating the rise in arterial blood pressure. Uterine contractions, under epidural coverage, should be allowed to facilitate the descent of the presenting part in the early phase of the second stage of labor. This process often takes several hours and the second stage of labor may in fact be prolonged. Maternal expulsive efforts are then minimized in the latter portion of the second stage with the aid of assisted vaginal delivery, with either forceps or a vacuum device.

As there is further autotransfusion of blood from the contracting uterus and the vena caval compression is simultaneously relieved, the period immediately following delivery is when the largest increase in cardiac output may be anticipated [45]. These changes will occur irrespective of mode of delivery, so cesarean delivery is normally reserved for the usual obstetric indications rather than maternal cardiac status.

Complications such as pulmonary edema and congestive heart failure (CHF) are treated in the standard fashion. Features of CHF include tachypnea, tachycardia, elevations in jugular venous pulse, rales on lung examination, peripheral edema, hypoxia and chest X-ray changes which may include an enlarged heart, increased vascular markings in the upper lung fields, pleural effusion and bilateral fluffy interstitial infiltrates. Acute treatment includes oxygen, an intravenous diuretic such as furosemide with aggressive dosing to maintain a 1–2 liter/day negative fluid balance, and careful documentation of all fluid intake and output. Delivery is generally not expedited until the maternal hemodynamic status is stabilized, unless fetal compromise is detected. In some cases, precipitous delivery by cesarean section may actual destabilize the maternal status, by exacerbating cardiac output and thus cardiac work. If aggressive pharmacologic measures to treat pulmonary edema are not rapidly successful, noninvasive ventilation such as biphasic positive airway pressure (BiPAP) or intubation and mechanical ventilation are appropriate. In emergency situations where pulmonary edema occurs at cesarean delivery, following the delivery of the neonate, the obstetrician may perform manual compression of the vena cava to decrease the preload as a temporizing measure [22].

Invasive hemodynamic monitoring (through the use of pulmonary artery or Swan–Ganz catheters) is rarely needed for the intrapartum care of most cardiac patients. Increasing data have brought into question the use of these monitors for the management of nonpregnant surgical and intensive care patients (even in very experienced hands) and many experts (including the editors) believe the risk/benefit ratio is not favorable to their use in the obstetric setting. However, other experts would recommend the use of invasive monitoring for patients with conditions such as pulmonary hypertension, severe aortic or mitral stenosis, patients with uncorrected cyanotic lesions, patients with NYHA functional class III–IV status, and high-grade ventricular dysfunction. Therefore final decisions on the use of these devices in the peripartum period should be made on the basis of both the patient's clinical condition and the quality and availability of local expertise and support.

Peri- or postmortem cesarean delivery should be discussed in advance with patients and the multidisciplinary team in circumstances of severe or complex congenital heart disease or other lesions associated with a high maternal mortality rate.

Contraceptive counseling

In cases where women of reproductive age have significant cardiac lesions or for those who develop life-threatening cardiac complications during pregnancy, it is critical that counseling regarding effective contraception occurs. Furthermore, as most pregnancies in the general population are unplanned, women with congenital or acquired heart disease require special attention. Options for contraception include barrier methods, hormonal contraception, and sterilization. The choice of method depends on the maternal cardiac status, associated risk factors and consideration of the consequences of unplanned pregnancies in life-threatening situations [46]. The reader is directed to Chapter 33 and Trussell [47] for further reading on contraceptive efficacy.

As most barrier methods are associated with a high failure rate (up to 26%), they cannot be recommended alone as ideal contraception. However, when used in conjunction with other methods, they may confer greater confidence in conception control. The standard combined oral contraceptive tablets are highly effective, with typical failure rates less than 1%. Vaginal rings and combined injectable forms of combined estrogen/progestin preparations are available in some areas, but have less established use in the setting of women with heart disease. All contraceptives containing estrogen carry risks of arterial and venous thrombosis and are generally to be avoided in women with significant valvular heart disease associated with the risk of valvular or mural thrombosis or in patients with cyanotic heart disease with the potential for paradoxic embolism. Although women taking coumadin for prothrombotic heart conditions have a relative contraindication to estrogen-containing contraceptives, the efficacy of these agents may justify their use when a patient is reliably protected by anticoagulation but desiring a reversible mode of contraception.

Progestin-only preparations are not contraindicated in cardiac disease as they carry minimal thrombotic risk [48,49]. The failure rates associated with progestin-only preparations are slightly higher than for combined oral contraceptives and are associated with higher vaginal breakthrough bleeding rates. However, with careful use and barrier method back-up, they may provide an ideal solution for women with complex heart disease. The long-acting injectable form, depot medroxyprogesterone, provides a high degree of protection, but may be a source of bleeding and/or hematoma formation at the site of injection in women who are anticoagulated.

Intrauterine devices (IUD), such as the copper device or progestin-containing intrauterine system (IUS), have very low failure rates, approaching the rates seen with sterilization procedures. Placement of these devices may theoretically predispose to bacterial endocarditis, but a similar situation applies here as to the role of IE prophylaxis as was previously discussed for vaginal and cesarean deliveries. The editors and the World Health Organization support their use in women with cardiac disease. At the time of insertion, clinicians should be aware that a vagal response may occur, and the resulting decrease in left-sided pressures may be undesirable in patients with intracardiac shunts. Arrhythmias at the time of IUD insertion have been reported as well [50]. Thus, in patients with shunts and those at higher risk of developing bacterial endocarditis (Eisenmenger's syndrome, uncorrected tetralogy of Fallot, patent ductus arteriosus, coarctation of the aorta, and significant mitral and aortic valve disease), IUD should be inserted with caution or placed carefully (due to the risk of uterine perforation) in the immediate postpartum period [51].

For patients who have completed their families or where the medical condition cannot be repaired and is perceived to be associated with high maternal and fetal morbidity and mortality (severe pulmonary hypertension, left ventricular dysfunction, NYHA class III and IV), vasectomy or tubal ligation should be offered. As tubal ligations are typically performed via a laparoscopic approach, the effect of intraperitoneal carbon dioxide insufflation and general anesthesia on cardiac output, as well as the possibility of air embolism, must be considered in patients with cyanotic lesions or pulmonary hypertension. Laparoscopic procedures usually require general anesthesia, as insufflation of the abdomen and pressure on the diaphragm is poorly tolerated by awake patients under neuraxial anesthesia. It may be a safer approach to consider a mini-laparotomy as the preferred approach, under slowly titrated neuraxial anesthesia.

Specific lesions

With continued advances in the early diagnosis and definitive treatment of CHD, women with a variety of heart defects now live longer, into their childbearing years. Furthermore, as women delay childbearing, there are more women with acquired heart disease who choose to become pregnant. Although the cardiac effects and outcome of pregnancy in these women and their offspring have improved, the risk of pregnancy remains significant. The care and management of patients with heart disease require a clear understanding of how each type of defect responds to the known physiologic alterations of pregnancy. Both maternal and neonatal morbidity and mortality can be predicted using a risk index derived from a prospective study of 562 women with a broad range of congenital and acquired heart disease. Complications of pulmonary edema, arrhythmias, stroke and cardiac death were increased in women with prior cardiac events, poor functional class, left ventricular dysfunction and left heart obstruction [52].

The normal hemodynamic adaptations to pregnancy are well defined, with a marked increase in blood volume, vascular compliance, heart rate and cardiac output. The impact of these physiologic changes on the pathologic cardiovascular system can be anticipated. Therefore, it is helpful to group the different acquired and congenital heart defects by pathophysiologic characteristics into categories that have similar treatments, outcomes, and labor and delivery options. The three categories are lesions that produce volume overload, lesions that produce pressure overload, and lesions that produce cyanosis. Other cardiac conditions which have their own unique issues are cardiomyopathy, coronary artery disease and Marfan's syndrome.

The congenital volume overload lesions are due to left-to-right shunts and include atrial septal defects (ASD), ventricular septal defects (VSD), and patent ductus arteriosus. Uncorrected lesions are generally well tolerated in pregnancy. However, in rare cases, chronic volume overload of the right heart from the shunted blood leads to increased right-sided heart pressures and pulmonary hypertension. If right heart and pulmonary pressures begin to approach the pressures of the left side of the heart, right-to-left shunting of blood can occur, resulting in systemic desaturation (cyanosis). This is Eisenmenger's syndrome physiology with a very different and elevated risk and is discussed separately below [33,52]. Acquired volume overload lesions are due to valvular insufficiency.

Stenotic lesions produce pressure load on the preceding chamber. They include aortic stenosis, mitral stenosis, coarctation of the aorta, and pulmonary valve stenosis. They are generally moderately well tolerated in pregnancy unless the obstruction is severe. The obstructive lesion idiopathic hypertrophic subaortic stenosis (IHSS, a type of hypertrophic cardiomyopathy or HCM) may actually experience some lessening of obstruction in pregnancy due to the fact that increased blood volume in this particular lesion leads to lessening of outflow tract obstruction.

Cyanotic heart disease results from right-to-left shunts because shunt flow is increased. These patients are usually corrected or palliated at a young age, and uncorrected patients rarely survive to adulthood and childbearing years. These diseases include tetralogy of Fallot, more severe degrees of Ebstein's anomaly, tricuspid atresia, transposition of the great vessels (TGV), truncus arteriosus, and univentricles. Maternal and fetal morbidity and mortality correlate with the degree of cyanosis as expressed by the maternal hematocrit and arterial PO_2. Patients with severe pulmonary hypertension or Eisenmenger's syndrome have a maternal mortality rate approaching 50% [53].

Volume overload lesions

Atrial septal defects

The most common congenital lesions in adults are atrial septal defects and they may be first diagnosed during pregnancy. There are three types of ASD classified by their location and embryology; the most common, accounting for approximately 80%, is the secundum type. The secundum ASD (located in the central portion of the atrial septum) is associated with myxomatous mitral valve disease and prolapse in 20–30% of cases. The more unusual types are primum, or endocardial cushion, defects (located in the lower portion of the atrial septum), which are most commonly associated with Down's syndrome, and sinus venosus defects (located in the upper portion of the atrial septum) in which the right upper pulmonary vein is usually emptying into the superior vena cava and right atrium. The uncorrected left-to-right shunt produces a volume load on the right side with enlargement of the right atrium and ventricle.

The flow across an ASD is not very turbulent and runs down a low gradient and hence does not directly cause an audible murmur; however, increased flow across the pulmonary valve may cause a 2/6 systolic ejection flow murmur. Classically, an ASD causes a wide fixed split second heart sound with the patient in the sitting/standing position. Signs of right ventricular hypertrophy and pulmonary

hypertension can be present in advanced and severe cases. ASD are typically asymptomatic but may be associated with atrial arrhythmias, stroke from paradoxic emboli, migraine and right heart failure. The diagnosis can usually be made on transthoracic echocardiography but may require transesophageal echocardiography to detect some smaller shunts and sinus venosus defects.

The expected 50% increase in blood volume during pregnancy causes further volume loading, although usually without a concomitant increase in pulmonary artery pressures. Most patients with an isolated ASD tolerate pregnancy well; good left ventricular ejection fraction and NYHA functional status are predictive of uncomplicated and successful outcomes [52,54]. With larger defects and shunts, there is risk for congestive heart failure, atrial arrhythmias, peripheral venous thrombosis or embolism, cerebral vascular accidents, and shunt reversal with cyanosis from sudden systemic hypotension [52, 54–56]. Congestive heart failure can be treated medically with digoxin and diuretics. Atrial arrhythmias can worsen or precipitate heart failure and should be treated with beta-blockers and digoxin. Due to the relative hypercoagulable state of pregnancy, empiric use of low-dose aspirin after the first trimester is advocated to reduce the risk of venous thrombosis and hence paradoxic emboli. Systemic hypotension, which can occur during parturition and epidural anesthesia, should be anticipated and rapidly corrected with pressors and volume to prevent possible shunt reversal and oxygen desaturation. Preconception closure of the defect is recommended for women with symptoms, arrhythmias or significant right-to-left shunts where the ratio of pulmonary to systemic blood flow (the Qp to Qs ratio, which is normally 1:1) is >1.5:1. For moderate-sized, secundum ASD, surgical patch or transcatheter devices have been shown to have equivalent short- and long-term success [57,58].

Ventricular septal defects

Ventricular septal defects (VSD) are common at birth (0.3–3 per 1000 livebirths) but many close spontaneously in childhood [59]. The size and location of the defect affect the clinical course. The most common type of defect occurs in the membranous septum or left ventricular outflow tract; they may be associated with aortic insufficiency due to prolapse of the adjacent aortic cusp.

The flow across a VSD produces a loud (typically 4–6/6) systolic ejection murmur and hence most VSD in the developed world are identified and repaired in infancy or childhood. Those that are left unrepaired in adulthood are small, without significant volume of shunting; these are often asymptomatic unless the patient develops IE or the effects of chronic volume overload and secondary pulmonary hypertension begin to manifest as exercise intolerance, dyspnea or congestive heart failure. Clinical sequelae and symptoms are most likely to happen if the VSD is large in size and therefore exerts a hemodynamic effect. Infective endocarditis, however, can occur with any size of VSD. Similarly to ASD, VSD should be repaired if symptomatic, large (a Qp:QS ratio of >1.5:1) or associated with an elevation in pulmonary artery pressure.

Isolated VSD are usually well tolerated in pregnancy unless the size is large and degree of shunting places a large volume burden on the system; peripartum risks are determined by parameters which reflect the degree of shunting: left ventricular size and function, pulmonary artery pressures, and the patient's functional class [52,60,61]. In hemodynamically significant shunts, complications include congestive heart failure, atrial arrhythmias, worsening pulmonary artery hypertension, and shunt reversal with cyanosis due to systemic hypotension. In a study from Connecticut, USA, in the 1970s, there were no maternal deaths reported in 98 pregnancies resulting in 78 liveborn infants in 50 women with VSD [17]. In women with corrected lesions, no increased risks are associated with gestation.

Patent ductus arteriosus

Patent ductus arteriosus is the persistence after birth of the direct connection between the pulmonary and arterial circulation that is an essential part of the normal fetal circulation. Isolated, persistent patent ductus arteriosus may be found in approximately 1:2000 newborns, but rarely in adults. The residual embryonic shunt is from the descending aorta at the isthmus to the proximal left pulmonary artery. Similar to above, the risks of pregnancy are related to shunt size and degree of pulmonary hypertension. Clinical symptoms and complications are also similar to those associated with VSD. Physical examination classically reveals a grade 4–6/6 continuous (diastolic and systolic), "machinery" (i.e rumbling) murmur that is best heard at the upper left sternal border or infraclavicular area. In asymptomatic women with normal pulmonary artery pressures and small shunts, maternal and fetal outcomes are not altered. As with other left-to-right shunts, there is still a theoretical risk of shunt reversal and cyanosis from sudden, systemic hypotension. Patients with large shunts have enlargement of the pulmonary artery and left-sided chambers and can develop high-output heart failure. In corrected or uncorrected patent ductus arteriosus, pulmonary hypertension significantly increases maternal and fetal morbidity and mortality rates [56].

Mitral and aortic regurgitation (insufficiency)

Valvular regurgitation may be due to rheumatic disease, prolapse or endocarditis. It can also occur in relation to ischemic heart disease and dilated cardiomyopathies. Trivial or physiologic regurgitation of the mitral valve is present in up to 70% of normal patients on echocardiography; it is not audible and is of no clinical signficance. Complications occur from valvular regurgitation as a result of chronic volume overload and related atrial or ventricular strain and can include arrhythmias (especially atrial fibrillation in the setting of mitral regurgitation), pulmonary hypertension (particularly from chronic severe mitral insufficiency or congestive heart failure. Mitral regurgitation typically causes a blowing or high-pitched holosystolic murmur (2–4/6) heard best at the apex of the heart and radiating to the left axilla. S1 may be diminished and S2 may have a fixed split as can be seen with both a VSD and an ASD (see Appendix 5.1 at the end of this chapter). Surgical valve repair or replacement is typically done if the patient is symptomatic, has left ventricular enlargement or dysfunction or pulmonary hypertension.

Aortic regurgitation typically causes a blowing diastolic (1–4/4) murmur heard best at the right upper sternal border at end expiration with the patient leaning forward. Severe, chronic insufficiency is most classically characterized by the many manifestations of high cardiac output with bounding pulses and a widened pulse pressure (a large difference between systolic and diastolic blood pressure).

If found in isolation, these lesions are usually well tolerated in pregnancy. Due to the favorable effects of decreased systemic vascular resistance and consequent afterload reduction in pregnancy, even severe regurgitation does not exhaust the cardiac reserve. On the other hand, those patients with chamber enlargement or ventricular dysfunction have higher rates of peripartum heart failure and this should be anticipated. For symptomatic patients, treatment includes digoxin and diuretics. For aortic insufficiency, afterload reduction, preferably with dihydropyridine calcium channel blockers (e.g. nifedipine), is preferred, as angiotensin-converting enzyme (ACE) inhibitors are contraindicated due to known teratogenic effects [62,63]. Mitral or aortic valve repair or replacement is rarely indicated during pregnancy. Cardiopulmonary bypass surgery done with high flow rates, normothermia, and fetal heart rate monitoring may decrease the reported 3–6% maternal mortality rate but a 20–29% fetal and neonatal mortality rate may be unavoidable [64,65]. Vaginal delivery is safe and is preferred. In the symptomatic patient, the expected increase in volume and cardiac output during labor and delivery can be attenuated by epidural anesthetics, limiting volume resuscitation and the judicious use of diuretics. In patients with functional class I–II, regurgitant lesions are not associated with adverse fetal outcome.

Mitral regurgitation due to mitral valve prolapse is due to congenital, developmental or degenerative processes. It is common in adults; the reported incidence is 3–6% [63,66]. The characteristic exam findings of a mid-systolic click and late systolic murmur as well as symptoms are reduced in pregnancy due to the favorable effects of normal hemodynamic changes [67]. Regardless of severity, isolated mitral valve prolapse is well tolerated in pregnancy and has no adverse maternal or fetal effects, though a possible increase in supraventricular arrhythmias has been noted in some centers [67,68].

Pressure overload lesions

Congenital aortic stenosis

The most common congenital heart disease found in adulthood is bicuspid aortic valve, occurring in 1–2% of the population [69]. Rarer causes of obstruction of left ventricular outflow include unicuspid aortic valves and supra- and subvalvular membranes. Importantly, bicuspid aortic valves are associated with coarctation and an aortopathy, predisposing these patients to aneurysm and dissection [69]. These patients typically have a harsh systolic murmur(2–5/6) at the right upper sternal border which is transmitted to both carotid arteries. Severe aortic stenosis is associated with a softened and single S2 and a slow rate of rise of the carotid pulse. Patients with severe aortic stenosis can remain asymptomatic for years. The development of symptoms portends an ominous prognosis; classic signs and symptoms include dyspnea on exertion, paroxysmal nocturnal dyspnea (congestive heart failure), exertional presyncope or syncope and angina. These patients should undergo aortic valve replacement.

Isolated mild-to-moderate valvular aortic stenosis is well tolerated in pregnancy, but severe aortic stenosis (aortic valve area (AVA) <1.0 cm^2 – the normal aortic valve area is 3–4 cm^2) is associated with increased maternal and fetal morbidity and mortality rates. Studies from the 1970s reported mortality rates of 17% for mothers and 32% for fetuses [70]. The Connecticut study spanning the 1970s reported 59 pregnancies with 46 liveborn infants in 27 women with no maternal deaths but with an increased rate of cardiovascular complications in women with worse functional class [17]. A study from 1993 evaluated 25 pregnancies in 13 patients of whom seven had AVA 0.7–0.9 cm^2 and four had repaired coarctations. It found no maternal deaths, but 31% of patients had functional deterioration; one patient required percutaneous balloon valvuloplasty and another required pregnancy termination and five pregnancy terminations were performed early. Among the 20 liveborn infants, no perinatal deaths or illnesses were seen [71]. The most recent series of 49 pregnancies in 39 women found a 10% incidence of heart failure or arrhythmias in the patients with severe stenosis. One patient with AVA 0.5 cm^2 required valvuloplasty but there was no morbidity in the group with mild-to-moderate disease [72].

Thus, women with severe valvular aortic stenosis should undergo percutaneous or surgical repair or replacement before conception, if possible, or mid-gestation if symptomatic and resistant to medical therapy (NYHA class III–IV) and for those in whom early termination is not an option. In symptomatic patients with severe aortic stenosis, late second-trimester terminations may, however, carry many of the risks associated with a term delivery – an increased risk with less benefit because the hemodynamic alterations are near maximum and late terminations can be associated with increased blood loss and resultant, sudden hypotension. Due to fixed outflow tract obstruction, these patients may not meet the increased demand and myocardial ischemia and hemodynamic collapse may ensue. Physical exertion, particularly recreational exercise, should be limited. In the symptomatic patient, labor and delivery may require management with invasive hemodynamic monitoring [73].

Coarctation of the aorta

Coarctation of the aorta is an abnormal ridge of smooth muscle, fibrous and elastic tissue typically in the descending thoracic aorta that produces a discrete narrowing, usually just distal to the left subclavian artery at the ligament arteriosum (Figure 5.1). There is hypertension above the narrowing and hypoperfusion and sometimes dilation below. Commonly associated anomalies include bicuspid aortic valve (85%) and cerebral aneurysms [69]. A systolic or occasionally continuous murmur can be heard in the infraclavicular or scapular area. Most patients present in infancy due to the murmur or, if the gradient is severe, with symptoms of acute CHF, and undergo repair. Some patients will only present later in life with hypertension and a delay between brachial and femoral pulses and a large drop in blood pressure between the upper and lower limbs (lower limb blood pressures are obtained by inflating a large cuff above the knee and auscultating in the popliteal fossa). True claudication is rare due to collateral circulation.

The risks of pregnancy in women with aortic coarctation include worsening hypertension, new-onset heart failure and, rarely but ominously, aortic dissection and rupture [17,33,52]. Ideally, moderate-to-severe aortic coarctation should be repaired, with balloon angioplasty or stenting, or replacement prior to pregnancy (although correction will not always result in resolution of the hypertension). In a review of 50 patients with corrected and uncorrected coarctation over a

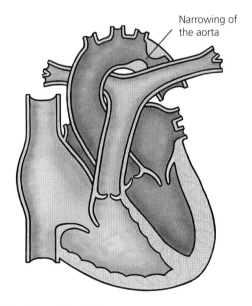

Figure 5.1 Coarctation of the aorta.

20-year period at the Mayo Clinic, the incidence of systemic hypertension was 30% and was associated with significant, residual gradients of over 20 mmHg (normally there should be no gradient between the ascending and descending aorta). Furthermore, the authors reported one maternal death from a dissection of the ascending aorta in the third trimester [74]. In patients with aortic or cerebral aneurysms or associated cardiac anomalies, maternal morbidity and mortality are increased. In one large study of women with corrected and uncorrected coarctation, no maternal deaths occurred, although nine of 74 pregnant women developed hypertension. The prospective study by Siu *et al.* included women with 43 repaired and eight unrepaired coarctations, of which two developed heart failure [52]. Data from the Dutch national registry included 54 women with a history of aortic coarctation repair and 126 pregnancies; there were 98 livebirths (78%) and 22 spontaneous and six elective abortions. Maternal complications (a total of 21%) included hypertension in 21 pregnancies and preeclampsia in five pregnancies [75]. There is a theoretical risk for decreased placental perfusion causing increased fetal morbidity and mortality, fetal loss, intrauterine growth restriction and congenital heart disease being more common. Data from both the Mayo Clinic and the Dutch registry noted a 4% incidence of congenital heart defects in the children [74,75]. Serial fetal monitoring that includes placental Doppler velocimetry may be warranted.

Maternal management includes limitation of physical activity and maintenance of systolic blood pressure close to 140 mmHg; beta-blockers are the agent of choice. Blood pressure control may be important to decrease the risk of aortic dissection or rupture. However, the blood pressures in the upper limbs (particularly the right arm) will be higher by as much as the measured gradient (say 20 mmHg) and hence will not be reflective of the uterine artery pressures. Periodically measuring blood pressure in the lower limbs may help prevent excessive lowering of blood pressure distal to the coarctation. Successful surgical repair and percutaneous stenting have been reported during gestation but should be reserved for patients with uncontrolled hypertension or heart failure. Vaginal delivery, with an assisted second stage to reduce Valsalva, is preferred; increased hypertension and myocardial oxygen demand can be reduced by the use of beta-blockers and adequate pain control, particularly with the use of epidural anesthetics.

Pulmonary valve stenosis

Pulmonary valve stenosis is the most common type of isolated right ventricular outflow tract obstruction. It is almost always congenital in origin. It is associated with a systolic ejection murmur at the left upper sternal border and often a fixed split S2. Severe stenosis is usually associated with right-sided heart failure and is typically repaired with surgical or balloon valvotomy in childhood. Ideally, patients with isolated, congenital pulmonary valve stenosis should have

percutaneous balloon valvuloplasty before conception. These patients are often left with some degree of insufficiency, but if it is mild to moderate in degree, it is well tolerated in pregnancy [52,76].

Patients with unrepaired mild-to-moderate pulmonary stenosis (gradients less than 40 mmHg; normally there should be no gradient across any valve) are usually asymptomatic and tolerate the hemodynamic burden of pregnancy with a low incidence of complications [33,76,77]. In a study of 46 pregnancies resulting in 36 livebirths in 24 women with pulmonary stenosis, no maternal deaths occurred, although there was one report of congestive heart failure [17,77]. The prospective study by Siu *et al.* included women with pulmonary stenosis, of whom 23 had been repaired and 35 were unrepaired; only one woman had deterioration in functional class during pregnancy and there were no cardiac events [52]. In patients with more severe obstruction and worsening clinical function, percutaneous balloon valvuloplasty can be done during pregnancy with appropriate abdominal shielding.

Rheumatic mitral stenosis

Most mitral stenosis is caused by rheumatic fever. Rheumatic fever results in leaflet thickening, commissural fusion, and retraction of the chordae tendineae and, in those native to a developed country, usually does not present until after age 30. On the other hand, the disease is more rapidly progressive in the developing world and one should have a higher index of suspicion in new immigrants in their 20s. Mitral stenosis restricts left ventricular inflow, with resultant elevation of the left atrial and pulmonary venous pressures. The diagnosis is made on echocardiography and classified as follows: mild mitral stenosis is valve area 1.5–2.0 cm^2 (normal is 4–6), moderate mitral stenosis is 1–1.5 cm^2 and severe mitral stenosis is <1.0 cm^2. Cardiac examination may reveal a loud S1 (S1 is as loud or louder than S2 when listening over the aortic or pulmonary area), an opening snap (a sound heard shortly after S2, similar in timing to the S3 but much more distinct) and a diastolic rumbling murmur (heard best with the bell of the stethoscope at the point of maximal impulse). Later, signs of right ventricular strain and pulmonary hypertension may become apparent (see Appendix 5.1 at the end of this chapter).

Patients with mild stenosis are asymptomatic. Those with moderate stenosis are asymptomatic at rest. Symptoms can include limited exercise tolerance, dyspnea on exertion or, when supine, hemoptysis, and pedal edema. Unless the mitral stenosis is severe, most patients are asymptomatic. Medical treatment can include diuretics, beta-blockers, digoxin and anticoagulation. Its most common complications are atrial fibrillation (with the possibility of systemic thromboembolization), CHF and pulmonary hypertension. Patients usually undergo percutaneous mitral valve balloon valvotomy or surgery when symptomatic or the stenosis is severe.

The predictable changes of pregnancy with both increased volume and heart rate adversely affect cardiovascular hemodyanmics in rheumatic mitral stenosis, and clinical deterioration during gestation should be expected. Patients with mild-to-moderate or occult mitral stenosis may first become symptomatic during pregnancy and, thus, may first be diagnosed during pregnancy. The risks of mitral stenosis to the mother include atrial arrhythmias, thromboembolic events, and pulmonary edema and are greatest in the third trimester and the puerperium; the incidence of complications is related to the severity of mitral stenosis and the patient's functional class [62,77,78]. In a study of 46 pregnancies in 44 women, heart failure requiring hospitalization occurred in 61% of those with moderate stenosis (mitral valve area (MVA)1.0–1.5 cm^2) and 78% of those with severe stenosis (<1.0 cm^2). Furthermore, clinical deterioration was noted in 82% of NYHA class I and 61% of class II patients [77]. A broader study of 80 pregnancies in 74 women found a lower incidence of overall complications of 38% and 67% in those with moderate and severe stenosis respectively [78]. Treatment should include continued antibiotic prophylaxis for streptococcal pharyngitis. which is usually continued until age 20 or 25 and given as either 1.2 million units of benzathine penicillin G every 3–4 weeks or Pen V 500 mg PO two to three times a day. Restriction of physical activity and treatment with beta-blockade will reduce heart rate (allowing more time for blood to pass through the stenotic valve) and thereby symptoms in moderate-to-severe mitral stenosis. In one study of 25 pregnant patients with symptomatic mitral stenosis (mean MVA 1.1cm^2), 92% noted significant improvement with beta-blockade [79].

Patients should be followed closely with repeat echocardiography to assess pulmonary artery pressures; mitral valve gradients may be falsely elevated due to increased cardiac output and pressure half time and planimetered valve area (specific echocardiographic methods for estimating valvular area) are more reliable. Atrial fibrillation will cause rapid clinical deterioration due to tachycardia and the loss of the atrial "kick" that assists in movement of blood across the stenotic valve. Atrial fibrillation also increases the risk of systemic thromboembolism. It should be treated aggressively with digoxin and beta-blockade to slow the ventricular response and full anticoagulation with a heparin. DC cardioversion may be carried out in pregnancy for new-onset atrial fibrillation but recurrence is common. Anticoagulation is important in preventing thromboembolic stroke but can be safely held in the peripartum period for a few days. The fetal risks include intrauterine growth restriction in patients with more than moderate stenosis and regular ultrasound examinations to assess fetal growth are recommended [77].

In patients with NYHA class III–IV status who do not respond to medical therapy, percutaneous balloon valvuloplasty with pelvic shielding is safe and has fewer fetal complications than surgery [80,81]. A study from Brazil compared 21 consecutive women who had percutaneous valvuloplasty from 1990 to 1995 with a historic control group of 25 consecutive women with open commissurotomy from the preceding 5 years. The hemodynamic success was equivalent but there was one neonatal death in the first group and six fetal and two neonatal deaths among the historic controls. Of note, only one-third of the patients in either group had been treated with beta-blockers, which might have improved their clinical status [81]. In hospitals without expertise in this procedure, surgical commissurotomy carries a maternal mortality rate of approximately 1–2% and a fetal mortality rate of 10% [82,83].

Finally, if significant mitral insufficiency precludes commissurotomy, mitral valve replacement can be performed, recognizing the risks of cardiopulmonary bypass [82]. A review of published reports from 1984 to 1996 found 161 cases of cardiac surgery performed during pregnancy, of which 137 required cardiopulmonary bypass. For the patients with valvular indications for surgery, the maternal morbidity and mortality were 19% and 9% respectively [65].

In all patients with mitral stenosis, very careful attention to fluid administration is essential to avoid congestive heart failure and Swan–Ganz catheterization for hemodynamic monitoring should be considered when managing labor and delivery in patients with severe mitral stenosis. Rheumatic mitral stenosis frequently occurs in association with some degree of mitral insufficiency and this can make interpretation of the Swan–Ganz catheter waveforms challenging and requires physicians and nurses with considerable expertise and experience. Carefully titrated epidural anesthesia and instrumental delivery should be considered in all patients with mitral stenosis to control catecholamine release and decrease expulsive efforts of the mother in the second stage of labor [62,84]. There is a high risk of pulmonary edema in these patients in the postpartum period and some centers routinely administer intravenous furosemide shortly after delivery in an attempt to circumvent this possibility.

Cyanotic congenital disease heart

Ebstein's anomaly

In this uncommon congenital heart lesion, a malformed tricuspid valve is apically displaced to a variable extent with resultant tricuspid regurgitation, atrial dilation, and limited right ventricular function (Figure 5.2). Severe cases present in infancy, but many cases will first present in teenagers or adults. Complications include CHF, arrhythmias, and paradoxic embolism. Associated abnormalities are frequent and include ASD (50%) and the Wolff–Parkinson–White (WPW) syndrome (30%) [57]. Most patients can be treated medically but more severe forms may develop right heart failure and require surgical correction.

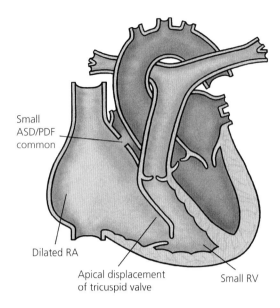

Figure 5.2 Ebstein's anomaly.

Preconception repair is preferable, particularly for patients with an interatrial communication; this nearly eliminates the maternal and fetal risks, though the risk of congenital heart disease in the offspring remains high at 6% [57,85,86]. The maternal risks of pregnancy are low and correspond with the degree of tricuspid regurgitation, right ventricular function, and presence of cyanosis [85,86]. The significant increase in circulating volume during gestation will predictably cause worsening of tricuspid regurgitation and right ventricular function; if an interatrial shunt is present, right-sided heart failure can result in increased right-to-left shunting and cyanosis. Also, atrial arrhythmias may occur; in the presence of an accessory path of Wolf-Parkinson White (WPW) syndrome, atrioventricular conduction can become exceedingly rapid with resultant hemodynamic collapse. Approximately 70% of women with Ebstein's anomaly have an interatrial shunt, and therefore these women are also at risk for paradoxic emboli (venous thromboembolism that passes through an ASD into the left atrium and thereby the systemic-arterial circulation to cause stroke or peripheral embolism). In a recent review of 111 pregnancies that resulted in 85 livebirths in 44 women, no maternal deaths or cardiovascular complications were seen. Conversely, increased rates of fetal loss, prematurity, and, in cyanotic patients, lower neonatal birth weight were seen [33,85].

Tetralogy of Fallot

The most common cyanotic congenital heart defect found in children, adults, and pregnant women is tetralogy of Fallot. It occurs in 3.9 per 10,000 births and accounts for up to 10% of congenital heart disease. The four diagnostic abnormalities are a VSD, deviation of the aorta to the right

so that it over-rides the VSD, infundibular pulmonic stenosis causing right-sided outflow obstruction, and secondary right ventricular hypertrophy (Figure 5.3). Repair usually involves relief of the right ventricular outflow obstruction (ideally with some preservation of the pulmonary valve) and closure of the VSD. Patients with repaired tetralogy of Fallot have good survival rates, with 90% survival at 30 years and an annual death rate of 0.94% per year after age 25. Usual causes of death in these patients are heart failure or sudden cardiac death presumably from arrhythmia [87].

Preconception repair is preferred to reduce morbidity and mortality; corrected patients should have a preconception functional assessment to further define risk. Patients with corrected lesions, good residual right ventricular function and good functional status usually tolerate the increased hemodynamic stress of pregnancy. Prophylaxis with aspirin to reduce the risk of thrombosis and paradoxic emboli may be indicated for those with residual shunts. In a recent retrospective study of 50 pregnancies that did not end in abortions in 26 women, the maternal complication rate was 12% (of pregnancies) and 19% (of patients); cardiac complications included symptomatic right-sided heart failure in two cases and arrhythmias (three ventricular and three supraventricular). All patients were NYHA class I prior to pregnancy. The two patients with heart failure were noted to have severe pulmonary insufficiency which would further increase the volume load on the right ventricle [88]. On the other hand, uncorrected or palliated lesions can be expected to have clinical deterioration during pregnancy, resulting in increased maternal and fetal complications [89]. In these patients, maternal risks include increased right-to-left shunting via a residual VSD

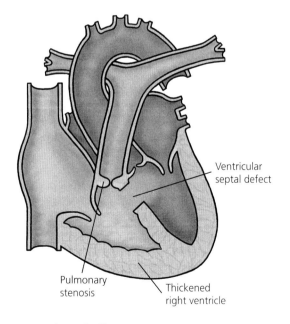

Figure 5.3 Tetralogy of Fallot.

due to the normal fall in systemic vascular resistance and, thus, worsening cyanosis during gestation and delivery; biventricular heart failure; arrhythmias; and cerebral vascular accidents from paradoxic emboli. Fetal risk is correlated with maternal hypoxia and includes a very high rate of prematurity, low birthweight, and spontaneous abortion [89–91]. In a 1994 review of 46 pregnancies in 21 uncorrected cyanotic patients seen over the preceding 20 years, 38% of patients had cardiovascular complications and there were only 15 livebirths, 60% of which were premature [89]. Pregnancy is to be discouraged in severe cyanosis, which is defined by a preconception maternal hematocrit greater than 60% and by an arterial saturation less than 80–85%.

Complex cyanotic congenital heart disease

Survival after repair of complex, cyanotic congenital heart disease has been extended into the reproductive years and pregnancy is now possible, albeit rare. The maternal morbidity and fetal mortality remain high. There have been a number of small series reported in the literature from which we can infer risk to the mother and fetus. In patients with single ventricles, a Fontan repair (Figures 5.4 and 5.5) allows the right atrium to empty directly into the pulmonary arteries without passing through the ventricle and thereby allows the single ventricle to have the sole task of generating systemic blood flow. It is generally viewed as a palliative procedure but increasing numbers of children who have undergone this procedure are reaching adulthood and pregnancy. Expected sequelae both in and out of pregnancy include venous congestion, arrhythmia and systemic ventricular dysfunction.

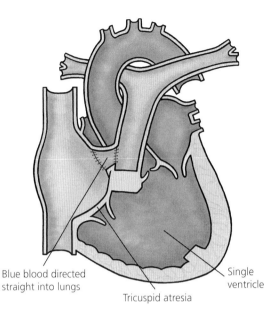

Blue blood directed straight into lungs

Tricuspid atresia

Single ventricle

Figure 5.5 Fontan procedure.

In a review which mailed questionnaires to patients who had univentricles corrected by the Fontan procedure, 33 pregnancies resulted in 15 livebirths (45%) in 14 women. The only reported maternal complication was one episode of supraventricular tachycardia (SVT); spontaneous abortions (13) and elective terminations (5) were common [92]. Similarly, in an older review of 26 pregnancies in 10 women with cyanosis from univentricles or tricuspid atresia, there were eight livebirths (31%), two cardiovascular complications (25%) and no maternal deaths [89].

There are conflicting findings in patients with complete transposition of the great vessels (the aorta arises from the right ventricle and the pulmonary artery arises from the left ventricle – see Figure 5.6). Prior to 1982 most patients with this anomaly were corrected by the Mustard procedure (atrial repair which redirects pulmonary venous return to the right ventricle and systemic venous return to the left ventricle) but since that time increasing numbers of patients have undergone the arterial switch procedure (Jatene). Most of the published data to date involve patients who have undergone the Mustard procedure (Figure 5.7). In a report of 15 pregnancies in nine asymptomatic women, no cardiovascular complications were seen [93]. However, in smaller series of similar patients, the morphologic right ventricle, functioning as the systemic ventricle, deteriorated and/or preterm delivery ensued [94,95]. Conversely, patients with congenitally corrected transposition of the great vessels (circulation is physiologic but the morphologic right ventricle supports systemic output) tend to do well. In a series of 60 pregnancies in 22 women, two patients (11%) developed congestive heart failure [96]. In summary, in surgically corrected patients complications that should be anticipated include functional deterioration and CHF due to limited cardiac reserve, tachyarrhythmias, and paradoxic emboli.

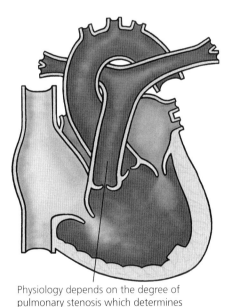

Physiology depends on the degree of pulmonary stenosis which determines the amount of pulmonary blood flow

Figure 5.4 Single ventricle.

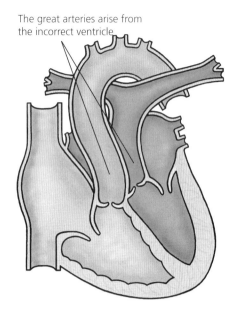

Figure 5.6 Transposition of the great vessels.

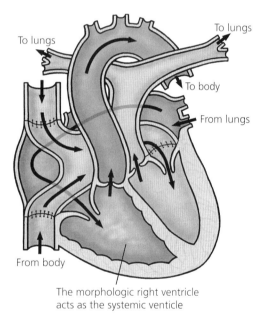

Figure 5.7 Mustard/Senning procedure to repair transposition of the great vessels.

The fetal prognosis remains poor, with mortality close to 50% and prematurity and intrauterine growth restriction ranging from 30% to 50% [33].

Eisenmenger's syndrome and pulmonary hypertension

Severe pulmonary vascular obstructive disease and hypertension resulting from septal communication between the systemic and pulmonary circulations is termed Eisenmenger's syndrome. Eventually the normally "lower pressure" right ventricle and

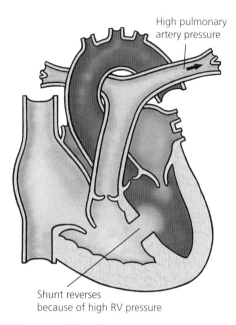

Figure 5.8 Eisenmenger's syndrome.

pulmonary circulation begin to see pressures that approach the pressures on the normally "higher pressure" left heart. Eisenmenger's syndrome refers to the endstage of this process when equalization of pressures in the right and left heart causes the previous shunting to reverse so that unoxygenated blood that was intended for the pulmonary circulation enters the systemic circulation (Figure 5.8). The degree of pulmonary hypertension determines the amount of right-to-left shunting and, thus, cyanosis. The prognosis for patients with Eisenmenger's syndrome is poor, with a very limited exercise capacity and very few surviving into the fifth decade of life.

The hemodynamic and hemostatic changes of pregnancy and parturition are poorly tolerated in Eisenmenger's syndrome and contribute to the high incidence of death. The maternal mortality rate may be as high as 39–52%; thus, pregnancy is contraindicated [53]. In one report following a series of 13 pregnancies in 12 women with Eisenmenger's syndrome (where mean pulmonary artery pressure was 113/62 mmHg) who declined termination, there were three (25%) maternal deaths. Seven patients who reached the end of the second trimester were hospitalized, treated with heparin and oxygen, but all were delivered by cesarean section due to worsening maternal and/or fetal function [53]. In a questionnaire-based study spanning 1991–1995, 15 pregnancies in patients with Eisenmenger's syndrome resulted in a maternal mortality of 40% [90]. Pregnancy termination carries a relatively lower risk, especially if carried out early in gestation, and should be recommended. Sterilization should also be recommended and can be done laparoscopically. In patients who decline termination, empiric management should include strict limitation of physical activity, oxygen for dyspnea, and heparin prophylaxis throughout pregnancy and for 4–6 weeks after delivery. Many of these patients may need to be managed in hospital on bedrest for a considerable portion of the pregnancy. In addition to the maternal risks of these pregnancies, the risks to the fetus are substantial. The fetal mortality rate is 40%, and prematurity and intrauterine growth restriction predominate in survivors [97,98]. Serial ultrasound examinations for fetal growth should be considered.

Labor, delivery and the early peripartum period carry the highest risk. Central hemodyanamic monitoring with Swan–Ganz catheterization has not been shown to improve outcome and carries significant risks and we generally discourage it [90,97]. Vaginal delivery is preferred, as cesarean delivery does not confer additional maternal benefit; however, many patients require cesarean delivery due to deterioration in fetal status [90,97]. Many of the maternal mortalities associated with Eisenmenger's syndrome occur in the hours and days following delivery and hence these patients are commonly treated with full-dose anticoagulation post partum and carefully monitored in the hospital. The efficacy of these interventions has not been established and the risk of maternal mortality remains high regardless of treatment.

Other cardiovascular disease

Coronary artery disease

Atherosclerotic coronary artery disease is rare in premenopausal women, but with increases in smoking, obesity, diabetes and delayed childbearing, ischemic heart disease is now being seen in pregnancy more frequently. Pregnancy increases the risk of myocardial infarction 3–4-fold [99]. Acute myocardial infarction was reported to occur with a frequency of 10/100,000 deliveries and a Medline search of case reports suggests a very high maternal mortality rate (19–35%) [100,101]. More recent and rigorous database searches found a lower frequency and mortality. In a review of hospital records linked to birth and death certificates in California from 1991 to 2000, the incidence was 1/35,700 deliveries which likely represents a less biased estimate. Furthermore, of the 151 women with acute myocardial infarctions, the mortality rate was substantially lower at 7.3%. Interestingly, the deaths occurred in those presenting before or at delivery [102]. Similarly, in a recent national query of pregnancy-related discharge codes from 2000 to 2002, the incidence of myocardial infarction was 6.2/100,000 (95% confidence interval (CI) 3–9.4) deliveries and the case fatality rate was 5%. By regression analysis, significant risk factors included hypertension, thrombophilia, diabetes, smoking and age greater than 30 years [99].

Approximately half of reported cases of myocardial infarction are due to atherosclerotic disease in older women with established cardiovascular risk factors, but other cases have been ascribed to a host of rare causes including: oral contraceptives, ergotamine derivatives, cocaine, amphetamines, collagen vascular disease, Kawasaki's disease, spontaneous arterial dissection, vasospasm, thromboembolism, and hypercoagulable states [100,101,103]. When available, coronary angiography was normal in 29–47% of patients. Most cases, especially those caused by coronary artery dissection, occur in the third trimester or puerperium.

Importantly, medical therapy is the same as that in the non-pregnant patient and includes oxygen, aspirin, beta-blockers, heparin, and nitrates. Thrombolytic agents, particularly streptokinase and tissue plasminogen activator, have been used in pregnancy for massive pulmonary embolism and prosthetic valve thrombosis with no maternal mortality, but significant morbidity from hemorrhage was seen when these agents were used in the peripartum period [104]. Because of the increased incidence of arterial dissections in this population, cardiac catheterization, if available, would be preferable over thrombolysis. There are case reports of successful outcome with angioplasty or stent placement during gestation and the postpartum period [105–107]. In the recent national survey mentioned above, cardiac catheterization was performed in 45% of cases and stenting, angioplasty or bypass surgery in 37% [99]. In a pregnant patient presenting with an acute myocardial infarction, urgent angiography should be performed to define the cause of the infarction and the best treatment options.

For women who have had a prior myocardial infarction and wish to become pregnant, preconception evaluation is imperative. There are close to 30 case reports of successful pregnancies in women after myocardial infarction. Careful preconception evaluation of ventricular function and ischemic burden can help guide recommendations and management. Patients with reduced left ventricular systolic function should be discouraged from conceiving as they will have increased risks similar to those with dilated cardiomyopathies, as outlined in the following section. In general, physical activity should be limited and use of cardiovascular medications should generally be continued. Beta-blockers and low-dose aspirin (<100 mg/day) significantly affect outcome in these patients and have a good safety record in pregnancy. ACE inhibitors and angiotensin receptor blockers are contraindicated in pregnancy. The HMG-CoA reductase inhibitors are generally avoided in pregnancy but their use may be justifiable, after the first trimester, in cases where the cardiologist feels they are likely to cause significant improvements in outcome over the duration of the pregnancy. When left ventricular function is preserved and the patient is vigilantly monitored for cardiovascular complications, maternal and fetal prognosis appears favorable [108,109]. Cardiac stress testing should be performed before conception but if needed can and should be carried out in pregnancy. Although most available modalities for cardiac stress testing are justifiable, exercise echocardiography (or dobutamine echocardiography in those patients who cannot exercise) has the advantage of not requiring any exposure to radiation. When considering the possibility of acute myocardial infarction in peripartum patients, it is important to recognize that the cardiac isoenzyme CPK-MB can show mild elevations after vaginal and cesarean deliveries in healthy patients and therefore troponin is the preferred assay in this setting.

Cardiomyopathy

Dilated cardiomyopathy (DCM) with left ventricular systolic dysfunction and CHF is rare in women of childbearing age. Etiologies include hypertension, toxins (such as alcohol or prior cardiotoxic chemotherapeutic agents), viral myocarditis, and familial/genetic cases; half of cases are deemed idiopathic. Maternal and fetal risks are related to severity of ventricular dysfunction and degree of functional limitation as assessed by the NYHA classification. One should expect worsening left ventricular dilation, dysfunction and symptoms due to the metabolic and volume stress of pregnancy and the puerperium. Other risks include those for thromboembolism, ventricular arrhythmias, sudden death, and shortened life expectancy. The prospective, multicenter trial of Siu et al. included 23 patients with dilated cardiomyopathy and noted 12 cardiac events (52%) including seven cases of CHF, five cases of arrhythmia, one stroke and one death. In all 523 cardiac patients, the multivariate predictors of complications included NYHA >II (odds ratio 6) and ventricular dysfunction (ejection fraction (EF) <40%) (odds ratio 11) [52].

Though etiology of cardiomyopathy in general has been clearly shown to affect long-term prognosis, there are conflicting data concerning pregnancy risks, likely due to the small numbers prohibiting powerful subgroup analysis. In a retrospective, university-based study in the US comparing idiopathic and peripartum cardiomyopathy patients, there were three deaths and four transplants among the 23 women with peripartum cardiomyopathy (PPCM), whereas only one of the eight DCM patients had an event (transplant). The high event rate of 30% in the PPCM group may be due to selection bias at tertiary referral centers [110]. Conversely, in a study from Brazil comparing 26 women with PPCM (42% with persistent left ventricular (LV) dysfunction) to eight women with DCM, a higher adverse event rate was reported, including two deaths, in the DCM group [111].

Treatment is similar to that in the nonpregnant patient, with one important exception: ACE inhibitors can cause fetal oligohydramnios and anuria and should be discontinued before conception or when pregnancy is diagnosed. Beta-blockers should be continued, dietary salt intake should be restricted to less than 2 g/d, and physical exertion should be limited. If clinical deterioration or congestive heart failure ensues, digoxin and diuretics should be added. Heparin anticoagulation should be instituted if bedrest is required and left ventricular ejection fraction is significantly decreased (<35%). Management during labor and delivery and the first 48 hours post partum should include good pain control, careful attention to fluid balance and consideration of continuous cardiac monitoring. Some experts would consider the use of invasive hemodynamic monitoring (Swan–Ganz catheters) for patients who are NYHA class III–IV.

Hypertrophic cardiomyopathy (of which idiopathic hypertrophic subaortic stenosis is the most well-known subtype) is a primary myocardial disorder caused by mutations in a number of different genes coding for contractile proteins. It can occur sporadically or in an autosomal-dominant pattern of inheritance. Patients have normal left ventricular systolic function but abnormal diastolic function from marked myocardial hypertrophy and in addition may have outflow tract obstruction. The thickened, noncompliant ventricle causes dyspnea, angina, syncope, arrhythmias, and sudden cardiac death [112]. Women with HCM usually tolerate the hemodynamic stress of pregnancy well; the favorable effects of increased preload (which helps to "keep open" the outflow obstruction) offset the negative effects of tachycardia and vasodilation. Maternal morbidity includes new or worsening congestive heart failure and, more rarely, chest pain, syncope, ventricular tachycardia (VT), SVT, and sudden cardiac death. In a report of 199 livebirths in 100 women from Italy with familial HCM, there was sudden death in two patients, both of whom were at deemed high risk. The report also included morbidity data on 40 women and noted that 5% of asymptomatic and 42% of the 12 symptomatic patients progressed to NYHA class III–IV during gestation (overall event rate 15%) [113]. A lower incidence of events was reported from a tertiary referral center in England. In 271 pregnancies in 127 consecutive women with HCM, there was no maternal mortality, though the authors did note that in all of England during an earlier time span 5 years earlier, 2/446 maternal deaths were ascribed to HCM. In a British study of 127 patients referred for evaluation of HCM, pregnancy was associated with worsening functional status in 10% and postpartum heart failure in 2% [114].

Treatment should include continuation of cardioselective beta-blockers and verapamil, and avoidance of drugs that increase heart rate, such as tocolytics, sympathomimetic agents, and digoxin. In patients with heart failure, diuretics can be added judiciously [112]. Labor and delivery should be managed with electrocardiographic monitoring, use of the left lateral decubitus position, avoidance of the Valsalva maneuver, and assisted vaginal delivery. Epidural anesthetics can be used with caution, utilizing small incremental doses and favoring narcotics over local anesthetics [114]. The primary fetal risks appear to be those of inheriting the disorder.

Peripartum cardiomyopathy

Peripartum cardiomyopathy (PPCM) is defined by the National Heart, Lung, Blood Institute (NHLBI) as the new onset of systolic dysfunction occurring in the absence of other plausible causes any time between the final month of pregnancy up to 5 months post partum. It occurs in between 1 in 3000 and 1 in 15000 pregnancies and the incidence may be increasing [110,111]. It is more common in women who have twins, pre-eclampsia/eclampsia and older multiparous women. Patients who are black are more likely than whites to develop PPCM or have complications. In the current era of heart failure medications, the mortality rate in the US is 3–9% which is much lower than previously reported and includes transplant rates of 4–10% [115–117]. Also, 41–62% of patients with PPCM show significant improvement in left ventricular function by 6 months [118]. In most studies the degree of left ventricular dilation and dysfunction, either initially or at 2–6 months, was predictive of those who would recover function.

Pathologic evaluation of patients who die from PPCM reveals four-chamber enlargement with normal coronary arteries and valves. Light microscopy reveals myocardial hypertrophy and fibrosis with scattered mononuclear infiltrates. Patients may present with ventricular failure, arrhythmias and/or pulmonary/systemic emboli. Clinical symptoms of PPCM are those of congestive heart failure: shortness of breath, paroxysmal nocturnal dyspnea, orthopnea, fatigue and edema. Clinical signs may include rales, elevated jugular venous pressue (JVP), and lower extremity edema. Treatment includes bedrest, sodium restriction, aggressive diuresis, beta-blockade and afterload reduction (calcium channel blocker and hydralazine while pregnant and ACE inhibitors post partum). It is not clear if early delivery changes the course of this illness but many practitioners will deliver women with PPCM once fetal lung maturity can be assured or if the mother's status is deteriorating despite good medical therapy. ACE inhibitor therapy should begin promptly in the postpartum period. If the patient's cardiac ejection fraction is less than 35%, consideration should be given to anticoagulation with LMWH while pregnant and warfarin post partum.

In those patients who have persistent left ventricular dysfunction, maternal risk associated with another pregnancy is high. One retrospective survey sent to US cardiologists reported 16 patients with PPCM and low EF (mean 36%) who underwent a second pregnancy: 25% underwent therapeutic abortions, 44% developed heart failure and 19% died [119]. Other complications to be expected include arrhythmias. In those patients who have recovered ventricular function, there may be subclinical dysfunction which is unmasked by a subsequent pregnancy. In the same survey, there were 28 patients with PPCM and recovered LV function; of these, 21% developed CHF and there was no mortality [120].

Cardiac transplantation

The number of women deciding to become pregnant after cardiac transplantation has increased as more recipients are surviving longer and with an improved quality of life. Recent statistics suggest that once past the first 6 months after transplantation, the yearly mortality rate of all heart transplant recipients is 3.4%, with an average survival of 11 years. The prognosis is even better for young patients with no concurrent medical illness. Death, when it does occur, is usually due to allograft rejection, allograft vasculopathy or immunosuppressive agent-related infections or malignancy [121]. Cardiac transplantation confers increased risk for hypertension in the mother (44%) and for prematurity in the fetus (40–50%), but in patients with preserved ventricular function, pregnancy seems to be well tolerated.

The most robust data on outcomes, rejection, and medications come from the larger population of solid-organ transplant recipients. In an Italian retrospective survey of pregnancies in kidney, liver and heart transplant patients, 17/67 women (25%) developed complications and more than half of these were hypertension. The risks to the fetus were greater; the incidence of miscarriages was 29% and 41% of liveborn infants were premature. Though 59% of the patients were on triple-drug immunosuppression (azathioprine, corticosteroids and cyclosporins) there were no fetal anomalies [122]. In a smaller population of 32 heart recipients surveyed from US transplant centers, maternal complications were more common and included hypertension (44%), pre-eclampsia (22%), rejection (22%), infections (13%) and worsening renal function (13%); there were no peripartum deaths but three late deaths. Neonatal complications were similar to the larger, Italian data and included prematurity (41%) and low birthweight (17%) [123]. Cardiac function and the possibility of rejection should be assessed before conception and some advocate waiting for 2 years after transplant to ensure stability of the graft and immunosuppressive regimen. Pregnancy does not appear to have an adverse effect with respect to cardiac function or episodes of rejection [123,124]. Immunosuppression regimens must be closely monitored, and medications adjusted to achieve the lowest possible therapeutic dose, although they do not appear to be associated with an increased incidence of congenital anomalies [122,124]. Labor and delivery should be planned, and vaginal delivery should be attempted. Invasive hemodynamic monitoring is only indicated for patients with significant left ventricular dysfunction.

Marfan's syndrome

Marfan's syndrome is one of the most common inherited disorders of connective tissue and is caused by mutations in the fibrillin gene on chromosome 15. It is present in 1 in 3000–5000 individuals. In over 70% of cases, it follows an autosomal-dominant pattern of inheritance with a high degree of penetrance [125]. It manifests with classic ocular (lens displacement, myopia, retinal detachments) musculoskeletal (large arm span, pectus excavatum or carinatum, hypermobile joints and long thin fingers) and cardiac abnormalities. The cardiovascular manifestations of the disease include dilation of the aorta, aortic regurgitation, mitral valve prolapse, and regurgitation. Pregnancy in women with the Marfan syndrome carries risk for worsening aortic dilation, aortic valve regurgitation, congestive heart failure, and, more ominously, acute aortic dissection and death. Older reports suggest high peripartum morbidity and mortality when patients have an aortic root diameter greater than 4.0–4.5 cm or significant, concomitant cardiovascular abnormalities, such as aortic regurgitation, left ventricular dilation and dysfunction, hypertension or coarctation [126,127].

Robust data on risk are available from three studies of women with Marfan's syndrome which included 45 pregnancies in 21 patients, 91 pregnancies in 36 patients, and 78 pregnancies in 44 patients. In these 101 patients, there was a consistent incidence of acute aortic dissection of 10–11% during gestation [128–131]. Preconception aortic replacement or pregnancy termination should be strongly considered for patients with ascending aortic diameters greater than or equal to 4.5 cm [63,127,131]. On the other hand, women without aortic dilation or cardiovascular complications appear to tolerate pregnancy well [126,130]. These patients require serial echocardiography to monitor for aortic root dilation and if noted during gestation, elective surgical repair is indicated to reduce the risk of rupture [63]. The primary risk to the fetus is a 50% chance of inheriting the syndrome.

Management during pregnancy includes limitation of physical activity and use of beta-blockers (usually metoprolol or labetalol in pregnancy at doses that keep heart rate <110 minute with submaximal exertion) to reduce shear stress along the aortic vessel wall. Vigilance for evidence of aortic dissection is important in patients with Marfan's syndrome and particularly in those with larger aortic diameters. Aortic dissection classically presents as an intermittent tearing chest pain that radiates to the back. It may be associated with a disparity between the blood pressures in the right and left arms (<20 mmHg) and/or the new onset of the murmur or aortic insufficiency (a diastolic murmur heard best by having the patient lean forward and exhale). Dissections of the aortic root may result in rupture into the pericardial sac, causing tamponade or occlusion of the coronary ostia, resulting in myocardial infarction. Diagnosis may be suggested by widening of the aorta or mediastinum on chest X-ray but is most consistently identified by transesophageal echocardiography or CT scan of the chest. Patients with Marfan's syndrome presenting with symptoms possibly attributable to an aortic dissection warrant emergency imaging even if the presentation is not typical for aortic dissection.

In low-risk women, vaginal delivery with adequate pain control and assisted second stage of labor is appropriate. In high-risk patients with aortic diameters greater than 4.0 cm or cardiovascular complications, cesarean delivery may be preferable to vaginal birth [126] although the evidence for this recommendation remains scant.

Ehlers–Danlos type IV

Ehlers–Danlos syndrome (EDS) is a heterogeneous group of inherited connective tissue disorders caused by defects in collagen and characterized by joint hypermobility, skin hyperelasticity, tissue fragility, easy bruising and poor wound healing. It occurs in approximately 1 in 40,000 Americans. There are presently 11 types of Ehlers–Danlos syndrome and any of them may be associated with pelvic instability or pain in pregnancy, and postpartum problems with hemorrhage and wound healing. Type IV or vascular EDS is the most dangerous type of EDS and may result in death related to arterial, intestinal and uterine fragility or rupture. The heredity pattern is autosomal dominant. Overall life expectancy is estimated to be 40–50 years, and most deaths are secondary to arterial rupture. Maternal mortality rate is approximately 12%, with the greatest risk of complications occurring during labor, delivery and early postpartum periods. Although uterine rupture has been cited as the most common cause of maternal mortality related to EDS type IV, these patients are also at risk for cardiac-related events and death. The largest series from The Netherlands reported 128 pregnancies in 46 women, 11% of whom had EDS type IV [132]. There was one maternal death related to bowel rupture. Another report describes a woman at 30 weeks gestation with EDS type IV who presented in preterm labor and died due to a coronary artery dissection and myocardial infarction [133]. There is another case report of a woman 1 week post partum presenting with pulmonary edema, severe mitral regurgitation, and rupture of a papillary muscle. She was successfully treated with valvuloplasty [134].

Intrauterine growth restriction and intrauterine fetal demise have been reported [135,136]. The safest mode of delivery is generally agreed to be cesarean, as the force of uterine contractions may lead to uterine rupture, and could theoretically increase the chance of vascular rupture. As these patients are at risk of bleeding from puncture sites, regional anesthesia is usually avoided, and general anesthesia is preferred. Although there are no specific preventive treatments available, pregnant women with EDS type IV are usually cautioned to rest and avoid exertion. In cases of hemorrhage, 1-desamino-8d-arginine vasopressin (DDAVP) has been used to control bleeding. Due to the risks of labor, elective admission to the hospital in the third trimester has been suggested by some. Serial echocardiography to monitor cardiac function and aortic dilation may be helpful. Continuous cardiac monitoring is suggested during labor, delivery and the initial postpartum period. Invasive cardiac monitoring is to be avoided given the risks of vascular rupture and hemorrhage.

Mechanical and bioprosthetic heart valves

Women of reproductive age are more likely to receive mechanical heart valves as compared to tissue valves, given their greater longevity. Bioprosthetic valves have the advantage of not requiring long-term anticoagulation, but are subject to more rapid deterioration, perhaps accelerated by pregnancy [137–140]. Certain types of mechanical heart valves carry a greater risk of thrombosis and subsequent valve failure, such as the caged ball and single tilting disk varieties [141]. Therefore, they require lifelong anticoagulation with coumadin. As pregnancy creates a prothrombotic state, there is substantial risk to the pregnant woman with a mechanical heart valve, and thus the need for vigilance in her anticoagulation regimen. Coumadin unfortunately has an associated embryopathy when used in the first trimester of pregnancy, and may have additional fetal effects such as hemorrhage, optic atrophy and growth restriction when exposure occurs later in pregnancy [142–145]. Thus obstetricians and cardiologists have debated whether unfractionated (UFH) or low molecular weight heparin (LMWH) might be better alternatives, given lack of transplacental transport and fetal safety. At the time of this writing, expert opinion supports the use of any of these options although opinions vary as to which option would be preferable in a given clinical setting. This topic is covered in some detail in Chapter 46.

Arrhythmias

The physiologic and anatomic changes of pregnancy shift the heart such that the normal electrocardiogram (EKG) is altered. There may be a shift in the QRS complex in the frontal plane, along with inverted T waves as well as small Q waves in lead III [146]. Nonspecific changes in the ST segments and T waves are commonly seen [147,148]. As palpitations are a common complaint during pregnancy, assessment for arrhythmia may be important in the diagnosis of new-onset conditions. In fact, there is an increased incidence of arrhythmias in pregnancy with and without identifiable conditions [149].

The most common arrhythmia in pregnancy is supraventricular tachycardia (SVT). In a study of 207 women with symptomatic paroxysmal SVT, one group found that the rate of new-onset SVT during pregnancy was 4%, while the rate of exacerbation was 22% [150]. Similarly, another group reported on 38 pregnant women with SVT and noted an exacerbation rate of 29% [151]. In a more recent prospective series of 31 pregnant women, a higher rate of exacerbation was noted (44%), thought in part to be due to the higher proportion of patients with underlying structural heart disease [152]. Standard approaches to treatment of SVT during pregnancy include vagal maneuvers such as carotid massage, adenosine, beta-blockers, calcium channel blockers, and antiarrhythmic agents where appropriate.

Pregnant women with WPW syndrome (a congenital condition associated with an accessory conduction pathway between the atrium and the ventricles that is characterized by a short PR interval on EKG) have been reported to have a higher incidence of paroxysmal SVT during pregnancy [153].

Ventricular tachycardia (VT) rarely occurs in pregnancy. When present, it is usually related to cardiac conditions such as hypertrophic or peripartum cardiomyopathy, myocardial ischemia or underlying arrhythmia (such as long QT syndrome). Standard treatment for unstable VT is emergency cardioversion. Cases of idiopathic left-sided VT can occur in pregnancy, and can usually be treated with beta-blockade or other antiarrhythmic medication [154,155].

Several series show that long QT syndrome (a congenital cardiac conduction abnormality typically associated with a prolonged QT interval on EKG and placing the patient at increased risk of the life-threatening ventricular arrhythmia torsades de pointe) is well tolerated during pregnancy. One series examining pregnancies in 111 pregnant women and another following 115 pregnancies showed no serious cardiac events during pregnancy [156,157]. Beta-blockers are the mainstay of treatment for these patients as they appear to decrease the patient's propensity for arrhythmia and these agents should be continued during pregnancy.

Atrial flutter and fibrillation are most likely to occur in pregnant women with underlying structural heart disease [73]. Investigation of any significant arrhythmia should include an echocardiogram. If structural heart disease is not present, evaluation should include screening for hypertension, thyroid disease, alcohol or drug misuse and consideration of ischemic heart disease. A more recent series reported 23 pregnancies in 18 women with either atrial fibrillation or flutter. All except one patient had underlying structural heart disease. Arrhythmias occurred during 52% of the pregnancies [152]. Treatment usually consists of correction of any underlying endocrinopathy or calcium channel blockers, beta-blockers, digoxin and chemical or electrical cardioversion as needed [158,159].

Anesthetic concerns for pregnant women with cardiac disease

Key points in anesthetic care of parturients with cardiac disease

- An obstetric anesthesiologist should review the mother in the prenatal period as part of the multidisciplinary team.
- Regional analgesia and anesthesia are suitable for all but the most severe disease and provide good pain control that may decrease cardiac work and thereby improve outcome.
- Manipulate timing of anticoagulant drugs to allow a "window" for siting a regional block and minimize concerns about spinal hematoma.
- Slow, cautious, incremental onset of regional block is essential.
- The aim is to minimize hemodynamic changes.
- The obstetric anesthesiologist must use techniques they are familiar with.

Maternal death from cardiac disease is becoming more common [160] and parturient women with cardiac disease do present the obstetric anesthesiologist with a number of problems, requiring meticulous care to minimize morbidity

Table 5.1 Differences between regional analgesia and anesthesia

Block characteristics	Regional analgesia	Regional anesthesia
Sensory lock	Low-dose local anesthetic/opioid	Strong local anesthetic – dense block
Height	T10 upper limit	T4 upper limit
Sympathetic block	+	+++
Motor block	+/−	+++
Hemodynamic changes	+	+++

[161]. There is no rigorous evidence (i.e. meta-analysis or randomized controlled trials) available to guide anesthetic management of parturients with cardiac disease, so the following observations are based on case reports, observational studies and expert opinion.

Cesarean section (CS) rates are higher in women with cardiac disease, but there is a growing trend towards vaginal deliveries, which have a lower risk of many complications, particularly hemorrhage and infection. For both vaginal and cesarean deliveries, regional analgesia or anesthesia can be used; the term "regional" includes epidural, spinal, combined spinal-epidural (CSE) or in some centers intrathecal catheters [162]. Regional *analgesia* refers to a low-density block with limited spread, used for pain relief in labor, and regional *anesthesia* to a dense block to the fourth thoracic dermatome, with dense motor block, suitable for surgery (Table 5.1).

Prenatal assessment

All parturients with cardiac disease should receive regular cardiology and obstetric review but the obstetric anesthesiologist must also be part of the multidisciplinary team [163,164]. The obstetric anesthesiologist's assessment should include preparation for a number of different potential scenarios as plans often need to be changed in obstetrics. Some mothers scheduled for induction of labor or CS may go into labor before the planned delivery date, and contingency plans must be made to ensure safe emergency delivery at any time and by any route.

Anesthesiology assessment – things to consider

- Severity of illness – is NYHA status worsening during pregnancy?
- Anticoagulation therapy – can this be withheld to allow for regional analgesia/anesthesia?
- Plan for elective vaginal delivery +/− emergency CS.
- Plan for elective CS.
- Plan for unscheduled labor.
- Plan for emergency "stat" CS.
- Antibiotic prophylaxis – consult local protocol.

Although regional blocks have been used successfully there are contraindications to their use which are specific to cardiac disease:

- full anticoagulation

- maternal refusal or extreme anxiety
- severe stenotic valves with low, fixed output (this may be a relative contraindication).

Regional analgesia in labor

Regional analgesia in labor (CSE or epidural) can provide good pain relief while attenuating the labor-induced catecholamine rise. Epidural analgesia with low-dose local anesthesia combined with an opioid provides excellent pain relief with little cardiovascular instability. Although there will be some associated sympathetic block, this can be minimized with care. The reduction in preload may be beneficial after delivery, as it will increase venous capacitance and limit the adverse effect of the autotransfusion of blood associated with uterine contraction (Box 5.4).

Mothers who have severe disease may be suitable for regional analgesia, but extreme caution should be used. If an arterial line is inserted it is important to ensure that staff in the delivery suite are competent and familiar with their use.

Important points to consider with epidural analgesia in labor include the following.
- Bupivacaine or equivalent ≤0.1% with fentanyl 2–4 μg/mL.
- Minimize aortocaval compression by having the mother's right side tilted upwards on a wedge or placing the mother in the left lateral decubitus position.

Box 5.4 Pros and cons of regional analgesia in labor in the mother with a prosthetic valve

Advantages	Disadvantages
• Excellent pain relief	• Vasodilation from sympathetic block may decrease venous return and adversely affect patients with pressure overload lesions
• Attenuates maternal catecholamine rise	• Timing of anticoagulation important – to allow "window" for epidural block
• Vasodilation will increase venous capacity – may be beneficial during uterine contractions and after delivery	
• "Low dose" can minimize sympathetic block	

- Inject local anesthesia in a slow, incremental fashion.
- Use caution if using a test dose (e.g. 3 mL 2% lidocaine) which may cause some sympathetic block.
- Consider invasive monitoring of blood pressure in severe cases but care is required if delivery suite staff are unfamiliar with arterial lines.

Anesthesia for cesarean section

There is no evidence available to support either regional or general anesthesia as being the safer option for women with cardiac disease who require CS. Each case must be assessed individually.

Traditionally women with cardiac disease received general anesthesia (GA) because of concerns that the sympathetic block associated with regional anesthesia could be catastrophic in women with cardiac disease. However, this view has been repeatedly challenged, mainly by a plethora of case reports describing women with severe cardiac compromise receiving regional anesthesia safely for labor and delivery. As in all areas of medicine, practice is constantly changing and in many centers only those women with the most severe disease, or who are fully anticoagulated, will receive general anesthesia. There is a very important proviso, though: neuraxial block must be induced in a slow, incremental, cautious way as the sudden induction of a T4 block, with its associated sympathectomy, could indeed be catastrophic. The most important thing is that the anesthesiologist uses a technique they are familiar with, rather than one they use rarely, and that they are extremely cautious. An emergency "stat" cesarean section is the most risky situation though concerns for fetal well-being should not compromise the mother's care.

Regional anesthesia for CS

There is a growing trend towards the slow, careful induction of regional block, with a variety of techniques. "Single shot" spinal (SSS) anesthesia is contraindicated in anyone with symptomatic cardiac disease. The sudden onset of sympathetic block to T4, causing a dramatic fall in systemic vascular resistance, together with inferior vena caval compression, which is only partly obtunded by lateral tilt, may lead to irretrievable cardiovascular collapse. Safer options are available and should be used for any women with cardiac disease – either CSE or epidural alone – in all but the most severely compromised mothers with cardiac disease.

The advantages of regional anesthesia for CS are as follows.
- Avoid the catecholamine rise associated with endotracheal intubation and extubation.
- Good postoperative analgesia if a neuraxial opioid is used.
- Neonate less likely to require ventilatory support.
- Mother awake for delivery, and partner able to be present.
- Avoids GA risks – see later.

The cornerstone of regional block in women with cardiac disease is an extremely cautious introduction of sensory block. As the block has to be more extensive than that required for analgesia in labor, i.e. T4, and has to be more profound, there is an inevitable almost complete sympathectomy which will cause a significant drop in venous return and therefore cardiac preload. However, in skilled hands, with very slow induction of block and appropriate use of vasopressors to maintain vascular tone, regional block had been used successfully in a number of women with severe cardiovascular compromise.

It is important to allocate extra time to these cases – rushing this type of procedure is likely to be detrimental.

Most case reports describe the use of an arterial line for blood pressure monitoring, allowing for beat-to-beat pressure monitoring. The use of central venous pressure monitoring or a pulmonary artery catheter is more controversial, and may be unnecessary. Some mothers may find it difficult to lie supine or in the Trendelenburg position for line placement. There is always the option of placing a central line from the antecubital fossa, if measurement of CVP is considered essential.

Intravenous fluids should be given cautiously – there is little evidence that a fluid load prevents hypotension, and fluid overload is a risk to most of these patients.

While epidural block has been used, there is a growing trend to use CSE. CSE has a faster onset and is more reliable than an epidural alone, but can be administered in an incremental fashion, avoiding the precipitate onset of a SSS. The initial intrathecal injection can be low volume – usually 0.5–1.0 mL hyperbaric bupivacaine, and the block extended slowly with the epidural catheter. The sympathetic block also develops slowly, allowing vasopressors to be used to limit falls in blood pressure (Table 5.2).

There is increasing evidence that phenylephrine is a safer vasoconstrictor than ephedrine; it is a pure α-agonist and in equipotent doses as ephedrine it maintains maternal blood pressure but is associated with a superior fetal acid–base status, and avoids maternal tachycardia [161].

Key points in regional anesthesia for cesarean section
- Modifications in technique are needed to ensure maintenance of cardiovascular stability.
- Consider arterial line for beat-to-beat blood pressure monitoring.

Table 5.2 Block characteristics of SSS, epidural and CSE for CS

Block characteristics	Single-shot spinal (SSS)	Epidural anesthesia	Combined spinal-epidural
Onset time	Fast: 5–10 min	Slow: 30–50 min	Titrate as required
Reliability	Very good	Around 10% failure rate	Very good – if familiar with technique
Hypotension	+ + +	+	Slower onset, less hypotension than SSS

- Cautious intravenous fluid loading.
- Slow incremental induction of anesthesia.
- Avoid aortocaval compression by positioning mother with a 15° lateral tilt.
- Minimize sympathetic block.
- Administer appropriate vasoconstrictors (phenylephrine being preferred).
- Maintain preload and afterload.

General anesthesia for CS

The traditional rapid-sequence induction used for CS, which ensures early endotracheal intubation and limits the risks of aspiration of gastric contents, is associated with a hypertensive response to intubation and extubation, so should be modified in cardiac parturients to limit cardiovascular changes. It may be appropriate to involve a cardiac anesthesiologist who is more familiar with techniques which minimize cardiovascular changes at induction of anesthesia. Antacid prophylaxis is of course essential. Women receiving GA may benefit from intraoperative transesophageal echocardiography (TEE). A "cardiac" anaesthetic, which aims to limit hemodynamic changes, may involve high doses of opioid. Both mother and neonate may require ventilatory support postoperatively.

The disadvantages of GA for CS are as follows.
- Risk of aspiration of gastric contents.
- One in 300 risk of failed intubation.
- Hypertension and tachycardia on intubation.
- Reduction in venous return with mechanical ventilation.
- Negative inotropic effect of inhalational anesthetic agents.
- Neonatal sedation.

Key points for GA for cesarean delivery of patients with cardiac disease
- Arterial line usually helpful.
- Antacid prophylaxis essential for all.
- Position mother with a 15° lateral tilt.
- Use GA technique that will minimize cardiovascular changes.
- Consult cardiac anesthesiologist about optimum technique.
- If high-dose opioid technique used, inform neonatologist.
- Mother may require postoperative ventilation.
- Transesophageal echocardiography may help guide management.

Management of third stage

All drugs which promote uterine contractility have hemodynamic effects. Bolus administration of oxytocin is associated with a fall in systemic vascular resistance, hypotension and maternal tachycardia [158]. A syntocinon infusion should be administered cautiously. Ergometrine causes coronary vasospasm and raises systemic vascular resistance so will increase afterload.

Antibiotics

Infective endocarditis prophylaxis is needed far less commonly in the most recent recommendations from the American Heart Association and this issue has been discussed previously in this chapter.

Monitoring

Most women with prosthetic heart valves will have reasonable cardiac reserve, but it is limited. As a minimum, they require EKG and pulse oximetry. Further monitoring will depend on the severity of disease. An arterial line allows for beat-to-beat monitoring of blood pressure and therefore can detect cardiovascular changes early. If these are used in the delivery suite for laboring women, extreme care should be taken; obstetric nurses, obstetricians and midwives may be unfamiliar with them, and there is always the potential for inadvertent intra-arterial injections and potentially catastrophic disconnections. Early involvement and education of the nursing team are essential.

Central venous pressure monitoring probably is not needed in NYHA I or II parturients. The more compromised mother may not tolerate lying head down for line insertion; if a cardiac anesthesiologist is in attendance they may be the best person to insert a central line expeditiously. TEE may be considered in mothers receiving GA.

Areas requiring meticulous attention include:
- care of intravenous lines – remember potential for endocarditis
- potential for paradoxic air emboli – women with complex disease may have persistent right-to-left shunts; ensure no air in injections/infusions.

Women with severe disease

As a practical matter, women with severe disease can be broadly categorized into two groups: those who tolerate volume reduction poorly and those who tolerate excessive volume poorly. A patient with a relatively fixed obstruction (e.g. aortic stenosis) following a high pressure chamber (left ventricle) needs substantial preload to distend the ventricle to make use of Starling's curve to generate enough force to pump her cardiac output past the obstruction. In this situation, a fall in volume or preload (as can happen with bleeding or some regional anesthesia techniques) will compromise her ability to maintain her cardiac output. If she is taking a beta-blocker with negative chronotropic and inotropic effects, this may further compromise her output. A woman with a variable degree of obstruction in her left ventricular outflow tract, as is seen with idiopathic hypertrophic subaortic stenosis, depends upon adequate preload to distend her ventricle to minimize the degree of outflow obstruction. Finally, volume loss and a fall in pressure on the left side of the heart may increase shunting and cyanosis in women with intracardiac shunts and right-sided pressures equal to or greater than left-sided pressures. In all of these examples, a fall in preload or systemic blood pressure, as might occur with compression of the inferior vena cava, placement of a spinal anesthetic or postpartum hemorrhage, will exacerbate the pathophysiology of their lesions. Thus loss of preload must be avoided by avoiding caval compression, ensuring adequate volume loading prior to induction of conduction anesthesia, gradual induction of the anesthetic block and replacing hemorrhage.

The alternative problem would be encountered in a woman with a relatively fixed obstruction (e.g. mitral stenosis) following a low pressure chamber (left atrium) which forces a relatively small percentage of her cardiac output across her valve with each atrial contraction but needs more time in the cardiac cycle for the blood to cross the valve passively. With severe disease and left atrial enlargement, the atrium functions less well because it must generate greater tension in its wall to develop the same amount of pressure as a smaller atrium (an example of Laplace's law). With more severe disease, left atrial enlargement and/or atrial fibrillation, the left atrial contraction ("kick") is lost entirely, further compromising the patient's ability to move volume past the stenotic valve. This physiology tolerates excessive volume (preload) very poorly because there is no good way to force the extra volume across the stenotic valve. For these women, it is critical to avoid volume overload by parsimonious fluid administration during labor (including use of concentrated medication solutions whenever possible) and attending promptly to the fluid shifts that occur immediately post partum with diuretic therapy as needed [158].

It is uncommon to see pregnant women at term with severe cardiac lesions in need of urgent surgical intervention. Many such patients will now undergo intervention during gestation. However, in rare cases, cesarean delivery and cardiac surgery may be undertaken sequentially and will require the combined involvement of an obstetric and cardiac anesthesiologist. In these cases general anesthesia will normally be used.

Acknowledgment

The figures in this chapter are copyrighted materials adapted from the Yorkshire and Humber Adult Congenital Heart Disease Network website http://www.yorksandhumberhearts. nhs.uk/templates/Page.aspx?id=415

References

1. Lewis G (ed) The Confidential Enquiry into Maternal and Child Health (CEMACH). Saving mothers' lives: reviewing maternal deaths to make motherhood safer – 2003–2005. CEMACH, London, 2007: 117–30.
2. Health Canada. Special report on maternal mortality and severe morbidity in Canada – enhanced surveillance: the path to prevention. Minister of Public Works and Government Services Canada, Ottawa, 2004.
3. Bader RA, Bader ME, Rose DF, Braunwald E. Haemodynamics at rest and during exercise in normal pregnancy as studied by cardiac catheterization. J Clin Invest 1955;34:1524–36.
4. Davies P, Francis RI, Docker MF, Watt JM, Crawford JS. Analysis of impedance cardiography longitudinally applied in pregnancy. Br J Obstet Gynaecol 1986;93:717–20.
5. Ueland K, McAnulty JH, Ueland FR, Metcalfe J. Special considerations in the use of cardiovascular drugs. Clin Obstet Gynecol 1981;24:809–23.
6. Morton MJ, Paul MS, Campos GR, Hart MV, Metcalfe J. Exercise dynamics in late gestation: effects of physical training. Am J Obstet Gynecol 1985;152:91–7.
7. James CF, Banner T, Caton D. Cardiac output in women undergoing cesarean section with epidural or general anesthesia. Am J Obstet Gynecol 1989;160(5 Pt 1):1178-84.
8. Clapp JF III. Maternal heart rate in pregnancy. Am J Obstet Gynecol 1985;152:659–60.
9. Phippard AF, Horvath JS, Glynn EM, Garner MG, Fletcher PJ, Duggin GG, Tiller DJ. Circulatory adaptation to pregnancy – serial studies of haemodyamics, blood volume, renin and aldosterone in the baboon (Papio–hamadryas). J Hypertens 1986;4:773–9.
10. Schrier RW. A unifying hypothesis of body fluid volume regulation. J R Coll Phys Lond 1992;26:295–306.
11. Sanders SP, Levy RJ, Freed MD, Norwood WI, Castaneda AR. Use of Hancock porcine xenografts in children and adolescents. Am J Cardiol 1980;46:429–38.
12. De Swiet M. The cardiovascular system. In: Hytten F, Chamberlain GVP (eds) Clinical physiology in obstetrics. Blackwell Scientific, Oxford, 1980.
13. De Swiet M. The physiology of normal pregnancy. In: Rubin PC (ed) Hypertension in pregnancy, Volume 12. Handbook of hypertension. Elsevier, Amsterdam, 1998.
14. Elkayam U, Gleicher N. Hemodynamic and cardiac function during normal pregnancy and the puerperium. In: Cardiac problems in pregnancy: diagnosis and management of maternal and fetal disease, 3rd edn. Wiley-Liss, New York, 1998:139.
15. Hunter S, Robson SC. Adaptation of the maternal heart in pregnancy. Br Heart J 1992;68:540–3.
16. Cooley DA, Chapman DW. Mitral commissurotomy during pregnancy. JAMA 1952;150:1113.
17. Whittemore R, Hobbins JC, Engle MA. Pregnancy and its outcome in women with and without surgical treatment of congenital heart disease. Am J Cardiol 1982;50:641.
18. Barron WM. The pregnant surgical patient: medical evaluation and management. Ann Intern Med 1984;101:683.
19. Mossman KL, Hill LT. Radiation risks in pregnancy. Obstet Gynecol 1982;60:237.
20. Metcalfe J, McAnulty JH, Ueland K. Heart disease and pregnancy: physiology and management, 2nd edn. Little, Brown, Boston, 1986:116.
21. De Santis M, Straface G, Cavaliere A, Carducci B, Caruso A. Gadolinium periconceptional exposure: pregnancy and neonatal outcome. Acta Obstet Gynecol Scand 2007;86(1):99–101.
22. Elkayam U, Gleicher N. Hemodynamic and cardiac function during normal pregnancy and the puerperium. In: Cardiac problems in pregnancy: diagnosis and management of maternal and fetal disease, 3rd edn. Wiley-Liss, New York, 1998:3.
23. Braunwald E. Heart failure. In: Zipes D, Liddy P, Bonow R, Braunwald E (eds) Braunwald's heart disease: a textbook of cardiovascular medicine, 7th edn. Elsevier-Saunders, New York, 2005:603.
24. Metcalfe J, McAnulty JH, Ueland K. Heart disease and pregnancy: physiology and management, 2nd edn. Little, Brown, Boston, 1986:56.

25. Metcalfe J, McAnulty JH, Ueland K. Heart disease and pregnancy: physiology and management, 2nd edn. Little, Brown, Boston, 1986:61.

26. Niswander KR, Berendes H, Deutschberger J, et al. Fetal morbidity following potentially anoxigenic obstetric conditions: V. Organic heart disease. Am J Obstet Gynecol 1967;98:871.

27. Ueland K, Novy MJ, Metcalfe J. Hemodynamic responses of patients with heart disease to pregnancy and exercise. Am J Obstet Gynecol 1972;113:47.

28. Morris CD, Menashe VD. Recurrence of congenital heart disease in offspring of parents with surgical correction. Clin Res 1985;33:68A.

29. Rose V, Gold RJM, Lindsay G, Allen MA. Possible increase in the incidence of congenital heart defects among the offspring of affected parents. J Am Coll Cardiol 1985;6:376.

30. Dennis NR, Warren J. Risks to the offspring of patients with some common congenital heart defects. J Med Genet 1981;18:8–16.

31. Driscoll DJ, Michels VV, Gersony WM, et al. Occurrence risk for congenital heart defects in relatives of patients with aortic stenosis, pulmonary stenosis, or ventricular septal defect. Circulation 1993;87:I114–20.

32. Kaemmerer H, Bauer U, Stein JI, et al. Pregnancy in congenital cardiac disease: an increasing challenge for cardiologists and obstetricians—a prospective multicenter study. Zeitschr Kardiol 2003;92:16–23.

33. Drenthen W, Pieper PG, Roos-Hesselink JW, et al. Outcome of pregnancy in women with congenital heart disease. J Am Coll Cardiol 2007;49:2303–11.

34. Abboud TK, Raya J, Noueihed R, Daniel J. Smoking during pregnancy: a review of effects on growth and development of offspring. Hum Biol 1980;52:593.

35. Eckhardt MJ, Harford TC, Kaelber CT, et al. Health hazards associated with alcohol consumption. JAMA 1981;246:648.

36. Elliot J. Maternal smoking and the fetus: one fear buried but others arise. JAMA 1979;241:867.

37. Naeye RL, Peters EC. Working during pregnancy: effects on the fetus. Pediatrics 1982;69:724.

38. Nieburg P, Marks JS, McLaren NM, Remington PL. The fetal tobacco syndrome. JAMA 1985;253:2998.

39. Horlocker TT, Wedel DJ, Benzon H, et al. Regional anesthesia in the anticoagulated patient: defining the risks (the Second ASRA Consensus Conference on Neuraxial Anesthesia and Anticoagulation). Reg Anesth Pain Med 2003;28(3):172–97.

40. Nishimura RA, Carabello BA, Faxon DP, et al., American College of Cardiology/American Heart Association Task Force. ACC/AHA 2008 guideline update on valvular heart disease: focused update on infective endocarditis: a report of the American College of Cardiology/American Heart Association Task Force on Practice Guidelines: endorsed by the Society of Cardiovascular Anesthesiologists, Society for Cardiovascular Angiography and Interventions, and Society of Thoracic Surgeons. Circulation 2008;118(8):887–96.

41. Ueland K, Hansen JM. Maternal cardiovascular dynamics. II. Posture and uterine contractions. Am J Obstet Gynecol 1969;103:1.

42. Cunningham I. Cardiovascular physiology of labor and delivery. J Obstet Gynecol Br Comm 1966;73:500.

43. Winner W, Romney SL. Cardiovascular responses to labor and delivery. Am J Obstet Gynecol 1966;95:1104.

44. Knuttgen HG, Emerson K Jr. Physiological response to pregnancy at rest and during exercise. J Appl Physiol 1974;36:549.

45. Ueland K, Hansen JM. Maternal cardiovascular dynamics. III. Labor and delivery under local and caudal analgesia. Am J Obstet Gynecol 1969;103:8.

46. Thorne S, MacGregor A, Nelson-Piercy C. Risks of contraception and pregnancy in heart disease. Heart 2006;92:1520–5.

47. Trussell J. Contraceptive efficacy. In: Hatcher R, Trussell J, Stewart F, et al. (eds) Contraceptive technology, 18th edn. Ardent Media, New York, 2004.

48. Vasilakis C, Jick H, del Mar Melero-Montes M. Risk of idiopathic venous thromboembolism in users of progestogens alone. Lancet 1999;354:1610–11.

49. World Health Organization. Cardiovascular disease and use of oral and injectable progestogen-only contraceptives and combined injectable contraceptives. Results of an international, multicenter, case-control study. World Health Organization Collaborative Study of Cardiovascular Disease and Steroid Hormone Contraception. Contraception 1998;57:315–24.

50. Acker D, Boehm FH, Askew DE, Rothman H. Electrocardiogram changes with intrauterine contraceptive device insertion. Am J Obstet Gynecol 1973;115:458.

51. Metcalfe J, McAnulty JH, Ueland K. Heart disease and pregnancy: physiology and management, 2nd edn. Little, Brown, Boston, 1986:116.

52. Siu SC, Sermer M, Colman JM, et al. Prospective multicenter study of pregnancy outcomes in women with heart disease. Circulation 2001;104:515–21.

53. Gleicher N, Midwall J, Hochberger D, Jaffin H. Eisenmenger's syndrome and pregnancy. Obstet Gynecol Surv 1979;34:721–41.

54. Zuber M, Gautschi N, Oechslin E, Widmer V, Kiowski W, Jenni R. Outcome of pregnancy in women with congenital shunt lesions. Heart 1999;81(3):271–5.

55. Whittemore R. Congenital heart disease: its impact on pregnancy. Hosp Pract (Off Ed) 1983;18:65–74.

56. Pitkin RM, Perloff JK, Koos BJ. Pregnancy and congenital heart disease. Ann Intern Med 1990;112:445–54.

57. Driscoll D, Allen HD, Atkins DL, et al. Guidelines for evaluation and management of common congenital cardiac problems in infants, children, and adolescents. A statement for healthcare professionals from the Committee on Congenital Cardiac Defects of the Council on Cardiovascular Disease in the Young, American Heart Association. Circulation 1994;90(4):2180–8.

58. Du ZD, Hijazi ZM, Kleinman CS, Silverman NH, Larntz K. Comparison between transcatheter and surgical closure of secundum atrial septal defect in children and adults: results of a multicenter nonrandomized trial. J Am Coll Cardiol 2002;39(11):1836–44.

59. Perloff JK. Ventricular septal defects. In: The clinical recognition of congenital heart disease. WB Saunders, Philadelphia, 1994.

60. Pitkin RM, Perloff JK, Koos BJ. Pregnancy and congenital heart disease. Ann Intern Med 1990;112:445–54.

61. Whittemore R, Hobbins JC, Engle MA. Pregnancy and its outcome in women with and without surgical treatment of congenital heart disease. Am J Cardiol 1982;50:641–51.

62. Elkayam U, Bitar F. Valvular heart disease and pregnancy. J Am Coll Cardiol 2005;46:223–30.

63. Carabello BA, Chatterjee K, de Leon AC, et al. ACC/AHA 2006 guidelines for the management of patients with valvular heart disease. J Am Coll Cardiol 2006;48:1–148.

64. Sullivan HJ. Valvular heart surgery during pregnancy. Surg Clin North Am 1995;75:59–75.

65. Weiss BM, son Segesser LK, Eli A, et al. Outcome of cardiovascular surgery and pregnancy: a systematic review of the period 1984–1996. Am J Obset Gynecol 1998;179:1643–53.

66. Devereux RB, Kramer R, Kligfield P. Mitral valve prolapse: causes, clinical manifestations and management. Ann Intern Med 1989;111:305–17.

67. Cowles T, Gunik B. Mitral valve prolapse in pregnancy. Semin Perinatol 1990;14:34–41.

68. Chia YT, Yeoh SC, Viegas OA, Lim M, Ratnam SS. Maternal congenital heart disease and pregnancy outcome. J Obstetric Gynaecol Res 1996;22:185–91.

69. Fedak PWM, Verma S, David TE, Leask RL, Weisel RD, Butany J. Clinical and pathophysiological implications of a bicuspid aortic valve. Circulation 2002;106:900–4.

70. Arias F, Pineda J. Aortic stenosis and pregnancy. J Reprod Med 1978;4:229–32.

71. Lao TT, Sermer M, MaGee L, Farine D, Colman JM. Congenital aortic stenosis. Am J Obstet Gynecol 1993;169:540–5.

72. Silversides CK, Colman JM, Sermer M, Farine D, Siu SC. Early and intermediate–term outcomes of pregnancy with congenital aortic stenosis. Am J Cardiol 2003;91(11):1386–9.

73. Oakley C, Child A, Jung B. Expert consensus document on management of cardiovascular disease during pregnancy. Eur Heart J 2003;24:761–81.

74. Beauchesne LM, Connolly HM, Ammash NM, Warnes CA. Coarctation of the aorta: outcome of pregnancy. J Am Coll Cardiol 2001;38(6):1728–33.

75. Vriend JW, Drenthen W, Pieper PG, et al. Outcome in pregnancy in patients after repair of aortic coarctation. Eur Heart J 2005;26(20):2173–8.

76. Drenthen W, Pieper PG, Roos-Hesselink JW, et al. Non-cardiac complications during pregnancy in women with isolated congenital pulmonary valve stenosis. Heart 2006;92:1838–43.

77. Hameed A, Karaalp IS, Tummala PP, et al. The effect of valvular heart disease on maternal and fetal outcome of pregnancy. J Am Coll Cardiol 2001;37:893–9

78. Silversides CK, Colman JM, Sermer M, et al. Cardiac risk in pregnant women with rheumatic mitral stenosis. Am J Cardiol 2003;91:1382–5.

79. Al Kasab SM, Sabag T, al Zaibag M, et al. Beta-adrenergic receptor blockade in the management of pregnant women with mitral stenosis. Am J Obstet Gynecol 1990;163:37–40.

80. Esteves CA, Ramos AL, Braga SL. Effectiveness of percutaneous balloon mitral valvotomy during pregnancy. Am J Cardiol 1991;68:930–4.

81. De Souza JAM, Martinez EE, Ambrose JA, et al. Percutaneous balloon mitral valvuloplasty in comparison with open mitral valve commissurotomy for mitral stenosis during pregnancy. J Am Coll Cardiol 2001;37:900–3.

82. Sullivan HJ. Valvular heart surgery during pregnancy. Surg Clin North Am 1995;75:59–75.

83. Vosloo S, Reichard B. The feasibility of closed mitral valvotomy in pregnancy. J Thorac Cardiovasc Surg 1987;93:675–9.

84. Oakley C, Child A, Jung B. Expert consensus document on management of cardiovascular disease during pregnancy. Eur Heart J 2003;24:761–81.

85. Connolly HM, Warnes CA. Ebstein's anomaly: outcome of pregnancy. J Am Coll Cardiol 1994;23:1194–8.

86. Donnelly JE, Brown JM, Radford DJ. Pregnancy outcome and Ebstein's anomaly. Br Heart J 1991;66:368.

87. Nollert G, Fischlein T, Bouterwek S, Böhmer C, Klinner W, Reichart B. Long-term survival in patients with repair of tetralogy of Fallot: 36–year follow-up of 490 survivors of the first year after surgical repair. J Am Coll Cardiol 1997;30(5):1374–83.

88. Meijer JM, Pieper PG, Drenthen W, et al. Pregnancy, fertility and recurrence risk in corrected tetralogy of Fallot. Heart 2005;91:801–5.

89. Presbitero P, Somerville J, Stone S, Aruta E, Spiegelhalter D, Rabajoli F. Pregnancy in cyanotic congenital heart disease: outcome of mother and fetus. Circulation 1994;89:2673–6.

90. Whittemore R. Congenital heart disease: its impact on pregnancy. Hosp Pract (Off Ed) 1983;18:65–74.

91. Patton DE, Lee W, Cotton DB, et al. Cyanotic maternal heart disease in pregnancy. Obstet Gynecol Surv 1990;45:594–600.

92. Canobbio MM, Mair DD, van der Velde M, Koos BJ. Pregnancy outcomes after the Fontan repair. J Am Coll Cardiol 1996;28:763–7.

93. Clarkson PM, Wilson NJ, Neutze JM, North RA, Calder AL, Barratt-Boyes BG. Outcome of pregnancy after the Mustard operation for transposition of the great arteries with intact ventricular septum. J Am Coll Cardiol 1994;24:190–3.

94. Lynch-Salamon DI, Maze SS, Combs CA. Pregnancy after Mustard repair for transposition of the great arteries. Obstet Gynecol 1993;82:676–9.

95. Lao TT, Sermer M, Colman JM. Pregnancy following surgical correction for transposition of the great arteries. Obstet Gynecol 1994;83:665–8.

96. Connolly HM, Gorgan M, Warnes CA. Pregnancy among women with congenitally corrected transposition of the great arteries. J Am Coll Cardiol 1999;33:1693–5.

97. Avila WS, Grinberg M, Snitcowsky R, et al. Maternal and fetal outcome in pregnant women with Eisenmenger's syndrome. Eur Heart J 1995;16:460–4.

98. Yentis SM, Steer PJ, Plaat F. Eisenmenger's syndrome in pregnancy; maternal and fetal mortality in the 1990s. Br J Obstet Gynaecol 1998;105:921–2.

99. James AH, Jamison MG, Biswas MS, et al. Acute myocardial infarction in pregnancy: a United States population-based study. Circulation 2006;113:1564–71.

100. Badin E, Enciso R. Acute myocardial infarction during pregnancy and puerperium: a review. Angiology 1996;47:739–56.

101. Hankins GD, Wendel GDJ, Leveno KF. Myocardial infarction during pregnancy. A review. Obstet Gynecol 1985;65:139–46.

102. Ladner HE, Danielsen B, Gilbert WM. Acute myocardial infarction in pregnancy and the puerperium: a population-based study. Obstet Gynecol 2005;105:480–4.

103. Donnelly S, McKenna P, McGing P, Sugrue D. Myocardial infarction during pregnancy. Br J Obstet Gynaecol 1993;100:781–2.

104. Turrentine MA, Braems G, Ramirez MM. Use of thrombolytics for the treatment of thromboembolic disease during pregnancy. Obstet Gynecol Surv 1995;50:534–41.

105. Cowan NC, de Belder MA, Rothman MT. Coronary angioplasty in pregnancy. Br Heart J 1988;59:588–92.

106. Giudici MC, Artis AK, Webel RR, Alpert MA. Postpartum myocardial infarction treated with balloon coronary angioplasty. Am Heart J 1989;118:614–16.

107. Saxena R, Nolan TE, von Dohlen T, Houghton JL. Postpartum myocardial infarction treated by balloon coronary angioplasty. Obstet Gynecol 1992;79:810–12.

108. Frenkel Y, Barkai G, Reisin L, Rath S, Mashiach S, Battler A. Pregnancy after myocardial infarction: are we playing it safe? Obstet Gynecol 1991;77:822–5.

109. Vinatier D, Virelizier S, Depret-Mosser S, et al. Pregnancy after myocardial infarction. Eur J Obstet Gynecol Reprod Biol 1994;56:89–93.

110. Bernstein PS, Magriples U. Cardiomyopathy in pregnancy: a retrospective study. Am J Perinatol 2001;18:163–8.

111. Avila WS, de Carvalho ME, Tschaen CK, et al. Pregnancy and peripartum cardiomyopathy. A comparative and prospective study. Arq Bras Cardiol 2002;79:484–93.

112. Wigle ED, Rakowski H, Kimball BP, William WG. Hypertrophic cardiomyopathy: clinical spectrum and treatment. Circulation 1995;92:1680–92.

113. Autore C, Conte MR, Piccininno M, *et al*. Risk associated with pregnancy in hypertrophic cardiomyopathy. J Am Coll Cardiol 2002;40:1864–9.

114. Thaman R, Varnava A, Hamid MS, *et al*. Pregnancy related complications in women with hypertrophic cardiomyopathy. Heart 2003;89:752–6.

115. Amos AM, Jaber WA, Russell SD. Improved outcomes in peripartum cardiomyopathy with contemporary. Am Heart J 2006;152(3):509–13.

116. Elkayam U, Akhter MW, Singh H, Khan S, Bitar F, Hameed A, Shotan A. Pregnancy-associated cardiomyopathy: clinical characteristics and a comparison between early and late presentation. Circulation 2005;111(16):2050–55.

117. Brar SS, Khan SS, Sandhu GK, Jorgensen MB, Parikh N, Hsu JW, Shen AY. Incidence, mortality, and racial differences in peripartum cardiomyopathy. Am J Cardiol 2007;100(2):302–4.

118. Amos AM, Jaber WA, Russell SD. Improved outcomes in peripartum cardiomyopathy with contemporary. Am Heart J 2006;152(3):509–13.

119. Elkayam U, Tummala PP, Rao K, *et al*. Maternal and fetal outcomes of subsequent pregnancies in women with peripartum cardiomyopathy. N Engl J Med 2001;344(21):1567–71.

120. Sliwa K, Fett J, Elkayam U. Peripartum cardiomyopathy. Lancet 2006;368(9536):687.

121. Taylor DO, Edwards LB, Boucek MM, *et al*. Registry of the International Society for Heart and Lung Transplantation: twenty-fourth official adult heart transplant report – 2007. J Heart Lung Transplant 2007;26(8):769–81.

122. Miniero R, Tardivo I, Curtoni ES, *et al*. Outcome of pregnancy after organ transplantation: a retrospective survey in Italy. Transplant Int 2005;17:724–9.

123. Wagoner L, Taylor D, Olson S, *et al*. Immunosuppressive therapy, management and outcomes of heart transplant recipients during pregnancy. J Heart Lung Transplant 1993;12:993–1001.

124. Branch KR, Wagoner LE, McGrory CH, *et al*. Risk of subsequent pregnancies on mother and newborn in female heart transplant recipients. J Heart Lung Transplant 1998;17:698–702.

125. Dietz HC, Cutting GR, Pyerutzm RE, *et al*. Marfan syndrome caused by a recurrent de novo missense mutation in the fibrillin gene. Nature 1991;352:337–9.

126. Elkayam U, Ostzega A, Shotan A, Mehra A. Cardiovascular problems in pregnant women with the Marfan syndrome. Ann Intern Med 1995;123:117–22.

127. Pyertiz RE. Maternal and fetal complications of pregnancy in the Marfan syndrome. Am J Med 1981;71:784–90.

128. Lipscomb KJ, Smith JC, Clarke B, *et al*. Outcome of pregnancy in women with Marfan's syndrome. Br J Obstet Gynaecol 1997;104:201–6.

129. Lind J, Wallenburg HC. The Marfan syndrome and pregnancy: a retrospective study in a Dutch population. Eur J Obstet Gynecol Reprod Biol 2001;98:28–35.

130. Rossiter JP, Repke JT, Morales AJ, Murphy EA, Pyertiz RA. A prospective longitudinal evaluation of pregnancy in the Marfan syndrome. Am J Obstet Gynecol 1995;173:1599–606.

131. Oakley C, Child A, Jung B. Expert consensus document on management of cardiovascular disease during pregnancy. Eur Heart J 2003;34:761–81.

132. Lind J, Wallenburg HC. Pregnancy and the Ehlers–Danlos syndrome: a retrospective study in a Dutch population. Acta Obstet Gynecol Scand 2002;81:293–300.

133. Athanassiou AM, Turrentine MA. Myocardial infarction and coronary artery dissection during pregnancy associated with type IV Ehlers–Danlos syndrome. Am J Perinatol 1996;13(3):181–3.

134. Seve P, Dubreuil O, Farhat F, *et al*. Acute mitral regurgitation caused by papillary muscle rupture in the immediate postpartum period revealing Ehlers–Danlos syndrome type IV. J Thorac Cardiovasc Surg 2005;129:680–1.

135. Kundu AK, Chattopadhyay P, Kundu S, Choudhury S. Pregnancy in Ehlers–Danlos syndrome. J Assoc Physicians India 2006;54:938.

136. De Paepe A, Thaler B, van Gijsegem M, van Hoecke D, Matton M. Obstetrical problems in patients with Ehlers–Danlos syndrome type IV: a case report. Eur J Obstet Gynecol Reprod Biol 1989;33:189–93.

137. Born D, Martinez EE, Almeida PAM, Santos DV, Carvalho ACC, Moron AF. Pregnancy in patients with prosthetic heart valves: the effect of anticoagulation on mother, fetus and neonate. Am Heart J 1992;124:413–17.

138. Sbarouni E, Oakley CM. Outcome of pregnancy in women with valve prostheses. Br Heart J 1994;71:196–201.

139. Hanania G, Thomas D, Michel PL, *et al*. Grossesses chez les porteuses de prostheses valvulaires: etude cooperative retrospective francaise (155 cas). [Pregnancy in patients with heart valve prosthesis. A French retrospective cooperative study (155 cases)] Arch Mal Coeur Vaiss 1994;87:429–37.

140. Lee CN, Wu CC, Lin PY, Hsieh FJ, Chen HY. Pregnancy following cardiac prosthetic valve replacement. Obstet Gynecol 1994;83:353–6.

141. Goldsmith I, Turpie AGG, Lip GYH. ABC of antithrombotic therapy. Valvuar heart disease and prosthetic heart valves. BMJ 2002;325(7374):1228–31.

142. Ginsberg JS, Hirsh J, Turner DC, Levine MN, Burrows R. Risks to the fetus of anticoagulant therapy during pregnancy. Thromb Haemost 1989;61:197–203.

143. Hall JAG, Paul RM, Wilson KM. Maternal and fetal sequelae of anticoagulation during pregnancy. Am J Med 1980;68:122–40.

144. Chan WS, Anand S, Ginsberg JS. Anticoagulation of pregnant women with mechanical heart valves: a systematic review of the literature. Arch Intern Med 2000;160:191–6.

145. Robin F, Lecuru F, Desfeux P, Boucaya B, Taurelle R. Anticoagualation therapy in pregnancy. Eur J Obstet Gynecol Reprod Biol 1999;83:171–7.

146. Nihoyannopoulos P. Cardiovascular examination in pregnancy and the approach to diagnosis of cardiac disorder. In: Oakley C (ed) Heart disease in pregnancy. BMJ Books, London, 1997: 52–62.

147. Boyle DM, Lloyd-Jones RL. The electrocardiographic ST segment in pregnancy. J Obstet Gynaecol Br Comm 1966;73(6):986–7.

148. Oram S, Holt M. Innocent depression of the S-T segment and flattening of the T-wave during pregnancy. J Obstet Gynaecol Br Empire 1961:68:765–70.

149. Shotan A, Ostrzega E, Mehra A, Johnson JV, Elkayam U. Incidence of arrhythmias in normal pregnancy and relation to palpitations, dizziness, and syncope. Am J Cardiol 1997;79:1061–4.

150. Lee SH, Chen SA, Wu TJ, *et al*. Effects of pregnancy on first onset and symptoms of paroxysmal supraventricular tachycardia. Am J Cardiol 1995;76:675–8.

151. Tawam M, Levine J, Mendelson M, Goldberger J, Dyer A, Kadish A. Effect of pregnancy on paroxysmal supraventricular tachycardia. Am J Cardiol 1993;72:838–40.

152. Silversides CK, Harris L, Haberer K, *et al*. Recurrence rates of arrhythmias during pregnancy in women with previous tachyarrhythmia and impact on fetal and neonatal outcomes. Am J Cardiol 2006;97:1206–12.

153. Widerhorn J, Widerhorn AL, Rahimtoola SH, Elkayam U. WPW syndrome during pregnancy: increased incidence of supraventricular arrhythmias. Am Heart J 1992;123(3):796–8.

154. Page RL, Shenasa H, Evans J, Sorrentino RA, Wharton JM, Prystowsky EN. Radiofrequency catheter ablation of idiopathic recurrent ventricular tachycardia with a right bundle branch block, left axis pattern. Pace Clin Electrophysiol 1993;16:327–36.

155. Brodsky M, Doria R, Allen B, Sato D, Thomas G, Sada M. New-onset ventricular tachycardia during pregnancy. Am Heart J 1992;123(4 Pt 1):933–41.

156. Rashba EJ, Zareba W, Moss AJ, et al. Influence of pregnancy on the risk for cardiac events in patients with hereditary long QT syndrome. LQTS Investigators. Circulation 1998;97(5):451–6.

157. Heradien MJ, Goosen A, Crotti L, et al. Does pregnancy increase cardiac risk for LQT1 patients with the KCNQ1-A341V mutation? J Am Coll Cardiol 1996;48(7):1410–15.

158. Kron J, Conti JB. Arrhythmias in the pregnant patient: current concepts in evaluation and management. J Interv Card Electrophysiol 2007;19:95–107.

159. Trappe HJ. Acute therapy of maternal and fetal arrhythmias during pregnancy. J Intens Care Med 2006;21:305–15.

160. Malhotra S, Yentis SM. Report on Confidential Enquiries into Maternal Deaths: management strategies based on trends in maternal cardiac deaths over 30 years. Int J Obstet Anesth 2006;15:223–6.

161. Reimold SC, Rutherford JD. Valvular heart disease in pregnancy. N Engl J Med 2003;349:52–9.

162. Dob DP, Yentis SM. Practical management of the parturient with congenital heart disease. Int J Obstet Anesth 2006;15:137–44.

163. Ray P, Murphy GJ, Shutt LE. Recognition and management of maternal cardiac disease in pregnancy. Br J Anaesth 2004;93:428–39.

164. Saravanan S, Kocarev M, Wilson RC, Watkins E, Columb MO, Lyons G. Equivalent dose of ephedrine and phenylephrine in the prevention of post–spinal hypotension in Caesarean section. Br J Anaesth 2006;96:95–9.

Appendix 5.1 Cardiac examination: a helpful review

This appendix reviews some of the cardiac examination techniques most relevant to the care of the pregnant woman. It is essential to emphasize, however, that perhaps the most important part of the examination in these patients is measurement of the *pulse rate* and *respiratory rate* on every antenatal visit. Changes in cardiac status will usually be hallmarked by some degree of tachypnea or tachycardia and these measurements, particularly the direct counting of a patient's respiratory rate, are often neglected in ambulatory antenatal care.

Inspection

Jugular venous pulse

Jugular venous pulse (JVP) examination is a critical aspect of assessing cardiac status. Elevations of JVP suggest right ventricular overload. The internal jugular vein begins between the sternal and clavicular heads of the sternocleidomastoid muscle and runs in a straight line up to the front of the ear. It can be difficult to see because the vein itself is a deep structure and it is the vein's pulsations through the overlying structures that are being visualized, rather than the actual vein itself.

Right JVP is assessed as follows.
• Raise the head of the bed/examining table to 30–45°.
• Turn the patient's head slightly to the left.
• Look for the flickering pulsations of the internal jugular vein being transmitted through overlying tissue. If you are not sure whether what you are seeing is internal jugular or carotid pulsation, the internal jugular pulsations should have the following distinctive characteristics.
   • The JVP is NOT palpable.
   • The JVP is flickering (like a candle flame) rather than bounding in quality.
   • The JVP can be readily eliminated by light pressure just above the sternal end of the clavicle.

• The JVP will change in height with the patient's positioning, dropping as the patient becomes more upright and rising as the patient lies down more.
• The JVP will descend with inspiration.
• The JVP will rise transiently with pressure on the right upper quadrant. If the rise is sustained, hepatojugular reflux is present, another sign of right-sided volume overload.
• The JVP is measured as a horizontal line starting at the angle of Louis of the sternum (the point where the upper portion of the sternum meets, at an angle, with the manubrium) (see Figures A5.1 and A5.2). Normally the JVP is 1–3 cm in height. It is often more prominent in pregnant women but it is not typically higher. The JVP may be reported as the central venous pressure (CVP) by adding 5 cm to the measurement of the JVP to incorporate the distance from the angle of Louis to the right atrium.

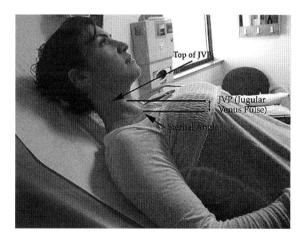

Figure A5.1 Locating the JVP.

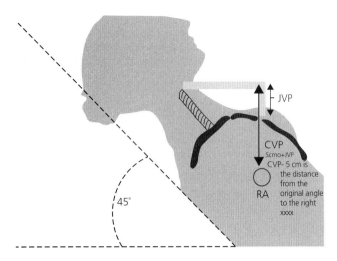

Figure A5.2 Measuring the JVP.

Palpation

The *right ventricle heave/parasternal lift* is assessed by placing your fingertips or the heel of your hand along the the left sternal border in the third, fourth and fifth intercostal spaces with the patient supine. If an impulse or "lift" is palpable, this is evidence of right ventricular overload as can be seen with an ASD, VSD, pulmonary hypertension or pulmonary stenosis. If you are not sure if the impulse is really there, the impulse can often be confirmed by placing one end of a pen or tongue depressor along the left sternal border and watching the other end for pulsatile movement.

A *palpable pulmonary heart sound* ("palpable P2") is detected by placing your fingertips in the pulmonic area (second left intercostal space) and feeling for a pulsation. A palpable pulmonic heart sound (P2) suggests dilation or increased flow in the pulmonary artery. This pulsation can also be confirmed with a pen or tongue blade using the same technique as described above for the right ventricular heave.

The left ventricle is assessed by examining the *apical beat* or point of maximal impulse (PMI). The apical beat is assessed by having the patient lie in the supine position and palpating below and to the left of the patient's breast. The normal apical beat has the following characteristics.
• *Location*: the fifth intercostal space in the mid-clavicular line. Left ventricular hypertrophy is suggested if the apical beat is shifted to the left.
• *Size*: usually about the size of a US 1 cent piece in diameter and occupies only one interspace. Left ventricular hypertrophy or dilation is suggested if the apical beat is larger than this.
• *Character/duration*: usually feels brisk and tapping and lasts less than two-thirds of the time between S1 and S2. A sustained apical beat, where the impulse seems to last longer, suggests either LVH or left ventricular dilation/dysfunction.

Auscultation

Heart sounds

The four areas for listening to the four heart valves are shown in Figure A5.3 and described as follows.
• *Aortic*: second intercostal space, right sternal border
• *Pulmonary*: second intercostal space, left sternal border
• *Tricuspid*: fourth intercostal space, left sternal border
• *Mitral*: fifth intercostal space just lateral to the mid-clavicular line

Auscultation of the heart involves listening to the heart sounds and for murmurs. The auscultatory findings for the normal cardiac cycle are depicted in Figure A5.4.
• S1 is the sound made by the closure of the mitral and tricuspid valve.
• S2 is the sound made by the closure of the aortic and pulmonary valve.
  • The sounds from the closure of the aortic and pulmonary valves are typically simultaneous during expiration but become separate and distinct (the A2 and the P2) during inspiration. This is known as "physiologic splitting of the second heart sound" (see Figure A5.5).

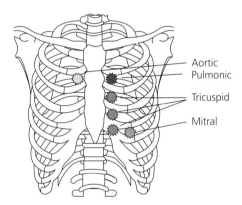

Figure A5.3 Areas for auscultation of valves on precordium.

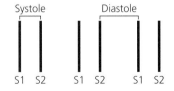

Figure A5.4 Normal cardiac cycle.

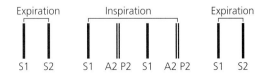

Figure A5.5 Physiologic splitting of S2.

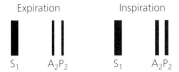

Figure A5.6 Fixed splitting of S2.

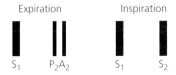

Figure A5.7 Reversed splitting of S2.

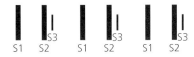

Figure A5.8 S3.

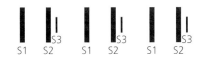

Figure A5.9 S4.

- If the aortic and pulmonary component of S2 are separate and distinct both in inspiration and expiration ("*fixed split S2*"), this suggests right-sided volume overload typically from an ASD (see Figure A5.6).
- If the aortic and pulmonary components of S2 are separate and distinct in expiration but not in inspiration (*paradoxic splitting*), this suggests left bundle branch block or aortic outflow obstruction from aortic stenosis or hypertrophic cardiomyopathy (see Figure A5.7).
- S3 is a sound made by the sudden filling of the ventricle when the mitral valve first opens (like wind catching a sail) and is most commonly heard when the left ventricle is overloaded due to failure. It is best heard with the bell of the stethoscope over the apex of the heart. The S3 when present closely follows the S2. In the US, students are taught to think of the S3 following the S2 in a rhythm similar to the final syllable of the word Kentucky where "Ken" is the S1 and "tuck" is the S2 (see Figure A5.8).
- S4 is a sound made by the filling of the ventricle by the atrial contraction. It is most commonly heard when a patient has a stiff ventricle from left ventricular hypertrophy. It is best heard with the bell of the stethoscope over the apex of the heart. It immediately precedes the closure of the mitral valve and therefore S1. In the US, students are taught to think of the S4 preceeding the S1 in a rhythm similar to the first syllable of the word Tennessee where "es" is the S1 and "see" is the S2. (see Figure A5.9).
- A "gallop rhythm" is when both S3 and S4 are audible.

Benign Flow Murmurs

Mitral or pulmonary regurgitation

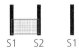

Mitral valve prolapse with regurgitation

Aortic regurgitation

Mitrial or tricuspid stenosis

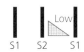

Mitral stenosis with opening snap and diastolic rumble

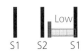

Figure A5.10 Benign and pathologic cardiac murmurs.

Murmurs

Murmurs are graded from I to VI.
- Grade I is only audible with very careful listening
- Grade II is readily audible
- Grade III is louder than grade II but not palpable
- Grade IV is palpable when the fingertips are placed over the place where the sound is heard
- Grade V is audible even when the edge of the stethoscope touches the chest wall
- Grade VI is audible to the naked ear

Distinguishing benign flow murmurs from pathologic murmurs

The normal flow murmur of pregnancy is from flow across the pulmonic valve. It has the following characteristics.
- It is usually grade I–II and never >III/VI.
- It is heard best at the left upper sternal border and does not radiate beyond this area.

• It is soft and blowing in quality.

• It occurs immediately following the S1, quickly gets louder and then rapidly dissipates ("crescendo, decrescendo") and disappears well before S2 is heard ("early systolic").

Any murmur heard in pregnancy that does not clearly fit this description should lead to the consideration of an EKG and echocardiogram when feasible. Murmurs that are louder than grade III, heard in multiple areas or that occur in diastole are most likely to represent underlying pathology. Figure A5.10 illustrates the typical auscultation findings of benign flow murmurs and some of the valvular lesions reviewed in this chapter.

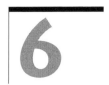

Hypertension in pregnancy

Christopher W.G. Redman[1], Sig-Linda Jacobson[2]
with Robin Russell[3]

[1]Nuffield Department of Obstetrics and Gynaecology, University of Oxford, Oxford, UK
[2]Department of Obstetrics and Gynecology, Oregon Health and Science University,
 Division of Maternal-Fetal Medicine, Portland, OR, USA
[3]Nuffield Department of Anaesthetics, John Radcliffe Hospital, Oxford, UK

Cardiovascular changes in pregnancy

Cardiovascular adaptations to pregnancy (Box 6.1) begin early, persist to an extent post partum, and appear to be enhanced by a subsequent pregnancy [1]. Cardiac output may decline during the third trimester [2]. This is partly because, in the supine position, the venous return to the heart is obstructed by the gravid uterus. This reduces cardiac output acutely by 20% or more [3], which may produce the supine hypotensive syndrome.

Arterial pressure falls during pregnancy (Figure 6.1), beginning in the first trimester, when the cardiac output is rising, and reaching a nadir in mid-pregnancy [4]. During the third trimester both systolic and diastolic readings slowly rise to about the pre-pregnant levels [4]. The reduced peripheral resistance of normal pregnancy appears to depend largely on increases in endothelial production of vasodilating factors.

In nongravid women, blood pressures depend on age, sex, body build and other factors including the circumstances under which the measurement is taken and the time of day.

Pregnant women are affected by many of these factors but with a narrower range of blood pressures than in the general population.

Measurement of blood pressure

The indirect method of measuring blood pressure gives an estimate of the true intra-arterial pressure. The auscultatory technique with a trained observer and mercury sphygmomanometer

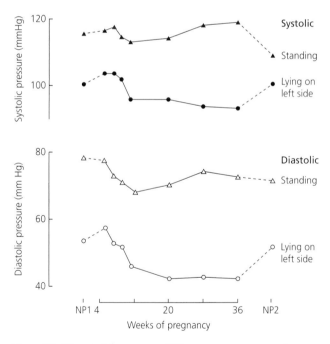

Figure 6.1 The arterial pressures of 10 women were measured using a London School of Hygiene sphygmomanometer to reduce observer bias. Readings were taken in the right arm and phase IV of the Korotkoff sounds defined the diastolic pressures. Pressures taken before conception (NP1), during pregnancy, and 6 weeks after delivery (NP2) are shown, both standing and supine on the left side ({black dot}, {white dot}) (C.W.G. Redman, unpublished observations).

> **Box 6.1** Cardiovascular changes in pregnancy
>
> - Increased cardiac output
> - Increased plasma volume
> - Increase heart rate
> - Increased stroke volume
> - Reduced arterial pressure (mainly in second trimester)
> - Reduced peripheral resistance

---

de Swiet's Medical Disorders in Obstetric Practice, 5th edition.
Edited by R. O. Powrie, M. F. Greene, W. Camann. © 2010 Blackwell Publishing.

- *Intra-arterial catheter with pressure transducer*: accurate, no observer error, but not applicable in general clinical practice.
- *Mercury sphygmomanometry in upper arm*: the gold standard of indirect measurement of blood pressure, although the use of mercury is being phased out.
- *Aneroid sphygmomanometry*: inaccurate and requires frequent calibration (often not done at many centers).
- *Hybrid manometry*: indirect measurement via arm cuff with electronic transducer; uncommon but better than aneroid manometry.
- *Oscillometric automatic devices*: variable accuracy; no observer bias; each marketed device type needs validation for use in pregnancy.

Box 6.3 Technique of indirect blood pressure measurement

- The observer must be fully trained.
- Ideally, the patient should have rested for 10 minutes before measurement. Phase 1 (onset) and phase 5 (disappearance) of Korotkoff sounds should be used to record systolic and diastolic pressures respectively.
- The arm cuff should be level with the heart.
- The cuff size should be appropriate for arm size with a length that is 1.5 times the circumference of the upper arm or a bladder at least 80% of the arm. (Many cuffs are marked to show whether the size is appropriate.) Too small a cuff will overestimate blood pressure and too large a cuff will underestimate it. Practitioners caring for pregnant women should have ready access to small, medium and large cuffs.
- The patient's position should be standardized as follows:
  Outpatients: the woman should be seated
  Inpatients: the woman may be either sitting or lying in the left lateral recumbent position; in either position, the arm cuff must be level with the heart. If it is above the heart the reading will be falsely low.
- The cuff pressure should be deflated slowly.
- Observer bias, especially digit preference, is a problem.
- Single readings can have large sampling errors.
- Clinic readings may be atypically high – white coat hypertension (see text).
- Readings in the third trimester, taken with the patient prone, may be atypically low because of the supine hypotension syndrome (see text).

remains the gold standard for clinical blood pressure measurement. The requirements for other instrumentation and standardized techniques are reviewed in Boxes 6.2 and 6.3. Figure 6.2 shows the preferred and the more commonly used techniques for blood pressure measurement.

The time of day is an important determinant of blood pressure (Figure 6.3). As in nongravid individuals, the major change occurs in sleep. During waking hours, the patient's blood pressure fluctuates minute by minute. Hence blood pressure measurements have large sampling errors that are distinct from the possible technical errors of measurement and can be reduced by averaging many readings. Ambulatory monitors can now be used for this purpose. A number of devices have been validated for use, and tested, in pregnancy and reference ranges have been published [5]. In general medical practice, ambulatory monitoring is the best way of diagnosing hypertension which predicts long-term cardiovascular risk and is useful for diagnosing white coat hypertension. However, it is expensive and cannot be recommended for routine use to screen pregnant women [6].

Arterial pressure is distributed continuously in the general population. The dividing line between normotension and hypertension is an artificial concept, used for pregnant and nonpregnant individuals alike. An arbitrary threshold is imposed which divides the population quantitatively but not qualitatively – an important but frequently forgotten distinction. A high blood pressure may be unusual but not necessarily abnormal. This threshold is conventionally taken as ≥ 140 mmHg systolic or ≥ 90 mmHg diastolic.

The average blood pressure of more than 6000 women booking before 20 weeks for delivery in Oxford was 120/70. Two and three standard deviations above this mean were 144/87 and 156/95, respectively. The actual distribution of the readings is shown in Table 6.1. Later in pregnancy the blood pressure rises. A maximum antenatal reading (excluding those taken in labor) of 140/90 or more was found in 21.6% of all women and of 170/110 or more in 1.2%. By convention, the threshold for "diagnosing" hypertension in pregnancy is 140/90 mmHg. In the first half of pregnancy this identifies a small group (<2.0%) of hypertensive individuals. In the second half, a much greater proportion (21.6%) exceeds this limit at least once. So although 140/90 is an appropriate limit in the second half of pregnancy, it would be better to use a cut-off of 170/110 (maximum antenatal

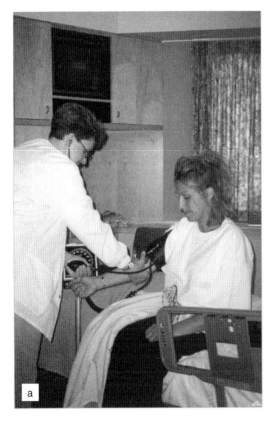
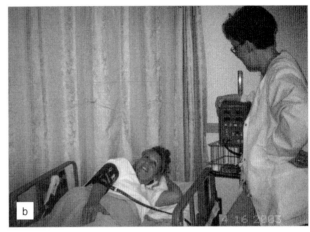

Figure 6.2 (A) Blood pressure in pregnancy should be measured in the sitting position with the cuff at the level of the heart. The cuff should be appropriate for the arm circumference: with the increasing prevalence of obesity, this aspect of proper measurement is important. Ideally a mercury manometer should be used. If an aneroid sphygmomanometer is used it should be calibrated regularly against mercury. If an automated oscillometric technique is used, it should be a machine that has been validated for use in pregnancy. (B) The common practice of measuring blood pressure in the uppermost arm of women lyin`g on their left sides is not recommended. The arm is elevated above the level of the heart, which leads to an underestimate of the true blood pressure.

reading) to identify the extreme end of the distribution in populations that resemble the Oxford population. However, more usually, 160/110 or higher is considered to be "severe" hypertension [7].

Hypertension in pregnancy: introduction

Hypertension in pregnancy occurs in three contexts: chronic hypertension, pre-eclampsia-eclampsia and gestational hypertension. Chronic hypertension and pre-eclampsia are not mutually exclusive so that the two occur together as superimposed pre-eclampsia (Box 6.4). The incidence of all hypertensive disorders in pregnancy is about 6% [8]. The term hypertensive disease of pregnancy (HDP) is sometimes used to include all hypertension recorded during pregnancy regardless of its chronicity. This is imprecise and unhelpful since medical forms of hypertension are not diseases of pregnancy but of the affected woman regardless of pregnancy. Pregnancy-induced hypertension (PIH) is a term commonly used outside North America and means the same as gestational hypertension. Whether or not hypertension is truly gestational (or "pregnancy induced")

cannot, in fact, be known until nonpregnancy blood pressures have been defined in the remote puerperium.

Pre-eclampsia

Hypertension and blood pressure measurement would be of limited importance to obstetricians were it not for the syndrome of pre-eclampsia, which has also been called pre-eclamptic toxemia (PET) or gestosis. It is common, becomes detectable in the second half of pregnancy (although its origins may lie in the first half) and has been defined in terms of the development of new hypertension and proteinuria, which resolve after delivery. It is dangerous to both mother and baby, and of unknown cause. It is a difficult and elusive condition even for experienced clinicians. Toxemia is an obsolete expression, previously used to describe any hypertension or proteinuria in pregnancy, whether pregnancy induced or not. Pre-eclampsia is so called because it precedes eclampsia, which is characterised by grand mal convulsions, associated with signs of pre-eclampsia. In ensuing sections we shall see that the terminology is inexact. Eclampsia is not the only

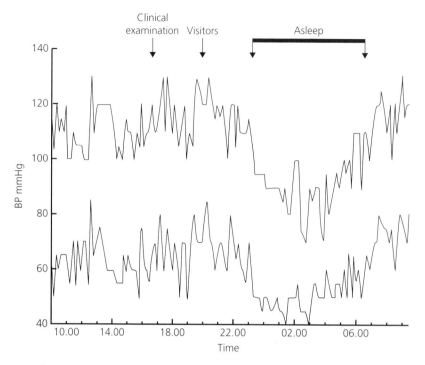

Figure 6.3 The circadian pattern of the arterial pressure of a pregnant woman at rest in bed during the third trimester is shown. The major change in the levels is the normal fall which occurs during sleep (C.W.G. Redman, unpublished observations).

Table 6.1 Blood pressures of 6790 women in pregnancy (cumulative frequency distribution)

At booking before 20 weeks		Maximum during antenatal period
(mmHg)	(%)	(%)
170/110	(0.0)	1.2
160/100	(0.1)	3.7
150/95	(0.4)	8.7
140/90	(2.0)	21.5
130/85	(5.0)	38.7
120/80	(21.0)	76.7

crisis of the condition, may occur without prodromal signs of pre-eclampsia, and is by no means the inevitable endstage of pre-eclampsia. Pre-eclampsia affects 2–5% of the pregnant population.

Etiology and pathogenesis of pre-eclampsia

Pre-eclampsia is a placental disease that evolves in two stages

Although the etiology of pre-eclampsia is not understood, the presence of a placenta is necessary and sufficient to cause the disorder [9,10]. A fetus is not required because pre-eclampsia can occur with hydatidiform mole. A uterus is probably not required because pre-eclampsia may develop with abdominal pregnancy. Central to management is delivery, which removes the causative organ, namely the placenta.

The disorder evolves in two stages [9] (Figure 6.4). The placental problem appears to be an inadequate maternal (uteroplacental) circulation leading to placental hypoxia, oxidative stress and infarction [11]. The uteroplacental

> **Box 6.4 Classification of hypertension in pregnancy**
>
> - *Hypertension*: a blood pressure >140 mmHg systolic or >90 mmHg diastolic.
> - *Chronic hypertension*: hypertension that is present before pregnancy or is diagnosed before the 20th week of gestation. The hypertension may be primary or secondary to medical conditions such as pheochromocytoma.
> - *Gestational hypertension (also called pregnancy-induced hypertension)*: new-onset hypertension after mid-pregnancy without proteinuria. This is a nonspecific term that includes women with incipient pre-eclampsia as well as those who do not develop pre-eclampsia.
> - *Pre-eclampsia-eclampsia*: a pregnancy-specific syndrome that usually occurs after 20 weeks gestation and is characterized by new-onset hypertension and proteinuria, which regresses remotely after delivery.
> - *Pre-eclampsia superimposed on chronic hypertension* may be more severe than simple pre-eclampsia.

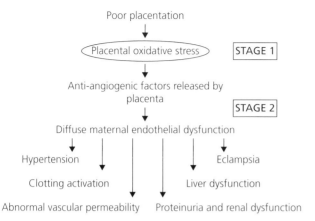

Figure 6.4 Pre-eclampsia evolves in two stages: poor placentation and then an excessive systemic inflammatory response of which maternal endothelial dysfunction in stage 2 explains the diversity of the pre-eclampsia syndrome.

circulation is unique because it lacks arterioles, capillaries or venules. Instead, about 40–50 spiral arteries deliver the 500 mL/min of blood required at the end of term pregnancy, directly into the intervillous space. In pre-eclampsia, two lesions may affect the spiral arteries. The first, called deficient placentation, comprises a relative lack of the structural remodeling and dilation that develop between weeks 8 and 18 [12] so that in normal pregnancy the arteries can transmit the expanded uteroplacental blood flow of the second half of gestation. At this time there is no clinical disease. The problem is not specific to pre-eclampsia; it is also found in some cases of intrauterine growth restriction (IUGR) without a maternal syndrome.

The second lesion in the spiral arteries is "acute atherosis" – aggregates of fibrin, platelets and lipid-loaded macrophages (foam cells), which partially or completely block the arteries [12]. The time course of development is unknown, but it is likely that acute atherosis is a late pathologic feature. The cause is not known. The lesions are not the consequence of hypertensive injury. Acute atherosis and the associated thromboses are the cause of placental infarctions, which are more common in pre-eclampsia. The two spiral artery pathologies also can explain the reduced uteroplacental blood flow of pre-eclampsia. All these changes are consistent with an underlying placental ischemia to which the maternal signs of pre-eclampsia are secondary.

Impairment of the uteroplacental circulation affects the placental functions that sustain the fetus. Pre-eclampsia is conventionally considered to be a maternal disorder in which the fetus is an incidental participant. A more complete perception is that the placental problem causes both maternal and fetal syndromes [9]. The balance of the two syndromes varies: in some cases there is a major fetal problem and the maternal features are relatively trivial; in others the converse picture may be seen.

There are numerous animal models of pre-eclampsia, but differences in placentation between species limit their value.

The clinical features of pre-eclampsia are secondary to systemic endothelial dysfunction

The second stage of pre-eclampsia, the maternal syndrome, is surprisingly variable in the time of onset, speed of progression and the extent to which it involves different systems. It can cause hypertension, renal impairment and proteinuria, convulsions, hepatic dysfunction and necrosis, jaundice, abdominal pain, disseminated intravascular coagulation (DIC) or normotensive proteinuria (among others – see Box 6.5). Until relatively recently it was impossible to explain this astounding variability by a single underlying pathologic process; certainly hypertension could not account for all these features. But the concept that the maternal endothelium is the target organ for the pre-eclampsia process has resolved this difficulty [13]. In short, the maternal syndrome can be explained if it is seen

---

Box 6.5 Complications of pre-eclampsia

Central nervous system

- Eclamptic convulsions
- Cerebral hemorrhage
- Cerebral edema
- Cortical blindness
- Retinal edema
- Retinal detachment

Renal system

- Renal cortical necrosis
- Renal tubular necrosis

Respiratory system

- Laryngeal edema
- Pulmonary edema

Liver

- Jaundice
- Hepatic infarction
- HELLP syndrome (see text)
- Hepatic rupture

Coagulation system

- DIC
- Microangiopathic hemolysis
- HELLP syndrome

Placenta

- Placental infarction
- Retroplacental bleeding and abruptio placentae

not as a hypertensive problem, but as the sum of the consequences of systemic maternal endothelial dysfunction.

Endothelial dysfunction appears to be caused by increased circulating levels of antiendothelial factors produced in excess by the oxidatively stressed placenta, namely the soluble vascular endothelial growth factor receptor 1 (also called sFlt-1) [14] and soluble endoglin [15]. There is also reduced availability of the angiogenic factor placental growth factor. Together, these factors synergize in their effects on the endothelium. These factors provide links between the pre-eclampsia placenta and the maternal disorder. A direct example of endothelial pathology of pre-eclampsia is the renal lesion of glomerular endotheliosis ([16] and see below).

In pre-eclampsia, endothelial dysfunction is one aspect of a maternal systemic inflammatory response

Systemic inflammation comprises multiple changes in the inflammatory network of the circulatory compartment. Apart from endothelial dysfunction, there is activation of circulating leukocytes (especially granulocytes and monocytes) and of the clotting and complement systems. All such changes have been demonstrated in pre-eclampsia [17]. Hence, it has been concluded that the endothelial dysfunction is one aspect of a more generalized process [17].

Pre-eclampsia and normal pregnancy are part of the same continuum

A maternal systemic inflammatory response is also detected in normal third-trimester pregnancy when it is not intrinsically different from that in pre-eclampsia except that it is milder. It has been suggested that pre-eclampsia develops when the systemic inflammatory process causes one or other maternal system to decompensate [17]. In other words, the disorder is not a separate condition but the extreme end of a range of maternal systemic inflammatory responses engendered by pregnancy. The problem is not the pre-eclampsia but pregnancy itself. This explains why, in clinical practice, it is often extraordinarily difficult to decide whether an atypical presentation is, or is not, pre-eclampsia.

Pre-eclampsia is heterogeneous and cannot be distinguished completely from normal pregnancy

This concept suggests that pre-eclampsia is the outcome of two opposing factors: a proinflammatory stimulus released by the placenta and a mother's ability to respond and accommodate to the stimulus. Excessive inflammatory stimuli from the placenta could vary with either its physical size or a change in the intensity of (unknown) proinflammatory signals from the placenta. The larger the placenta, the larger the inflammatory burden – as, for example, with multiple pregnancy, a well-known predisposition to pre-eclampsia.

In addition, advancing gestational age, which increases the physical bulk of the placenta, is itself a major risk factor for pre-eclampsia. Near term, normal pregnancy is characterized by many changes that are so well known that they are taken for granted, for example a rising diastolic pressure [4], which blur the distinction between normality and pre-eclampsia. In other words, during the last few weeks of normal pregnancy, more and more women appear to be driven towards the margin that distinguishes normal pregnancy from pre-eclamptic pregnancy.

Factors other than placental size must also be involved. With regard to the intensity of the proinflammatory stimulus of pregnancy, there are situations when, even from a small placenta, the inflammatory stimulus is excessive. It is suggested that, in this case, placental hypoxia, secondary to uteroplacental arterial insufficiency, amplifies release of inflammatory stimuli into the maternal circulation. These concepts imply that there cannot be a single cause of pre-eclampsia [17,18]. Different factors, particularly genetic factors that alter maternal inflammatory responses, will contribute. If the mother is genetically susceptible to inflammatory stimuli her constitution becomes the main determinant of the disorder (maternal pre-eclampsia). The other end of the spectrum is when the placenta is the main determinant (placental pre-eclampsia).

Heterogeneity of cause will lead to heterogeneity of clinical presentation. This is a main characteristic of the disorder that will be constantly emphasized in the ensuing sections. Furthermore, these considerations also lead to the conclusion that there can be no single preventive measure. Different prophylactic strategies will need to be targeted to the needs of different women.

The second stage of pre-eclampsia

Cardiovascular changes

The hypertension of pre-eclampsia is usually an early feature, not associated with a single hemodynamic pattern. Some investigators find increased cardiac output, others the converse. It is, however, agreed that peripheral resistance is increased once the condition is clinically apparent. The blood pressure is typically unstable at rest. Circadian variation is altered with, first, a loss of the normal fall in blood pressure at night and then, in the worst cases, a reversed pattern with the highest readings during sleep [19].

Pre-eclamptic hypertension is a form of secondary hypertension, arising from pathology in the placenta. Antihypertensive treatment is therefore not a cure; the definitive treatment is to remove the causative organ, the placenta, which means delivery. The hypertension is important because it is an accessible and early diagnostic sign of pre-eclampsia. In addition, if it is extreme, it may predispose to cerebral hemorrhage.

Complications of the hypertension

A sudden increase of blood pressure above a critical threshold causes acute arterial damage and loss of vascular autoregulation. The central nervous system appears to be particularly sensitive to hypertensive pathology, including cerebral hemorrhage, which antihypertensive treatment helps to prevent.

Pre-eclampsia may cause blood pressures which are well above the threshold (i.e. a mean arterial pressure of about 140 mmHg) at which organ damage would be expected. Cerebral hemorrhage remains a prominent cause of maternal death from pre-eclampsia and eclampsia in England and Wales [20], with a similar pathology to other hypertensive states. For this reason, adequate blood pressure control remains a priority. There is evidence that systolic rather than diastolic hypertension may be more important and the editors, but not the senior author, believe, but do not have published evidence, that the degree to which the blood pressure has increased acutely may also play a role independent of the absolute number.

Renal involvement (Box 6.6)

Glomerular filtration rate and renal plasma flow increase by 40–65% and 50–85%, respectively, during normal pregnancy [21]. Plasma creatinine and urea fall such that a plasma creatinine of more than 100 μmol/l (1.1 mg/dL) is always abnormal. Proteinuria is used as a defining sign of pre-eclampsia. Once present, it indicates a poorer prognosis for both mother and baby than when it is absent. It may be heavy (greater than 5.0 g/day). Overall, pre-eclampsia is the most common cause of nephrotic syndrome in pregnancy [22].

Proteinuria is one of several signs of involvement of the kidney in pre-eclampsia. Glomerular endotheliosis is a non-inflammatory lesion that underlies this proteinuria [16]. However, renal biopsy is only indicated where the presentation strongly suggests an underlying glomerular pathology that could benefit from treatment. Otherwise, the investigation is reserved for those who continue to have significant proteinuric renal impairment at a remote time after delivery or very occasionally in early pregnancy where the specific

diagnosis of renal disease will alter management in the short term (see Chapter 7).

Renal function is also impaired. Often the changes are biphasic, involving first tubular dysfunction and later glomerular dysfunction. A common early feature of pre-eclampsia is a reduced uric acid clearance, reflecting altered tubular function and causing a reciprocal rise in plasma urate. Later, at about the time that proteinuria develops, glomerular filtration becomes impaired. At this point the plasma creatinine rises and clearance falls. A rising plasma urate may be an early sign of pre-eclampsia but it is not always demonstrated, reflecting the heterogeneity of the disease (see above). Another relatively early but inconsistent change in renal function is hypocalciuria [23], which is not a feature of pregnant women with other forms of hypertension. The endstage of renal involvement is acute renal failure, with tubular or partial cortical or total cortical necrosis. In relation to management, it is important to note that reduced renal function is rarely due to hypovolemia, but results from structural changes in the renal glomeruli [24].

Plasma volume, colloid osmotic pressure and edema

Maternal plasma volume increases during the second and third trimesters of normal pregnancy but is reduced in pre-eclampsia relative to normal pregnancy [25]. The vascular system in pre-eclampsia becomes "leaky", with maldistribution of fluid: too much in the interstitial spaces (edema) and too little in the vascular compartment (hypovolemia). Hypoalbuminemia is also characteristic of the disorder, which causes a lower colloid osmotic pressure that may contribute to the problem.

Most women with proteinuric pre-eclampsia have edema. However, pre-eclampsia without edema – "dry pre-eclampsia" – has long been recognized as a particularly dangerous variant. Edema is difficult to quantify objectively. The best way is to chart weight gain. Those with excessive gain have an increased risk of pre-eclampsia [26]. Complications of the fluid retention include ascites, which is more common than generally recognized, affecting 13 of 99 women seen personally with severe pre-eclampsia. Pulmonary edema is a rare but life-threatening complication presenting before or after delivery [27]. Laryngeal edema may cause respiratory obstruction as well as difficulties at intubation if a general anesthetic is required.

Box 6.6 Renal system and pre-eclampsia

- Proteinuria
- Glomerular endotheliosis
- Reduced uric acid clearance
- Hypocalciuria
- Moderately reduced renal plasma flow
- Moderately reduced glomerular filtration
- Renal tubular necrosis
- Renal cortical necrosis

Coagulation system (Box 6.7)

During normal pregnancy, the clotting system is activated such that pregnancy becomes a "hypercoagulable" state (see Chapters 3 and 4). This would be expected as part of the systemic inflammatory response that is intrinsic to late normal pregnancy (see above). The blood response to clotting stimuli is brisker and the natural "turnover" of the system is enhanced. Standard clinical tests do not detect these changes

Box 6.7 Coagulation in pre-eclampsia compared to normal pregnancy*

Platelet activation

- Reduced platelet count
- Higher circulating beta thromboglobulin, platelet factor 4
- Younger, larger platelets
- Increased activation marker (CD63)

Plasma markers of activation of coagulation cascade

- Increased soluble fibrin
- Increased thrombin-antithrombin complexes
- Increased fibrinopeptide A (marker of thrombin activation)
- Increased circulating tissue factor (produced by activated endothelium)

Changes in fibrinolytic system

- Increased plasminogen activator type 1 antigen
- Increased d-dimer
- Reduced alpha-2 antiplasmin

Changes in clotting inhibitors

- Decreased antithrombin
- Decreased protein S

*None of these changes is diagnostic of pre-eclampsia. Absence of any one change does not exclude the diagnosis.

readily. In parallel, circulating platelets are also progressively activated.

Consistent with the continuum between normal pregnancy and pre-eclampsia, the activation of the clotting system is exaggerated in pre-eclampsia and may, in severe cases, decompensate as DIC. Activation causes changes in several tests of coagulation that are accessible in clinical laboratories, especially reductions of the platelet count. In the earlier stages, this is a chronic, fully compensated process which cannot be labeled as pathologic DIC, which is a late but inconstant feature of preictal pre-eclampsia and eclampsia. DIC is a condition in which intravascular activation of the clotting cascade leads to pathologic formation of fibrin within the circulation, with consumption and depletion of clotting factors. Complications can come both from bleeding and *in situ* microthrombi in the kidneys, brain, lungs and peripheral circulation. Microangiopathic hemolysis is a complication of DIC, associated with hemoglobinemia and a sudden fall in the hemoglobin concentration (see discussion of HELLP syndrome in the next section).

Liver dysfunction and the HELLP syndrome
(see also Chapter 9)

Liver dysfunction is a feature of pre-eclampsia detected by elevations of circulating hepatic enzymes [28]. Epigastric pain and vomiting are the typical symptoms but are not always present. About two-thirds of women dying from eclampsia have specific lesions in the liver, which are periportal "lake" hemorrhages and various grades of ischemic damage, including complete infarction. Most of this pathology has been defined post mortem, although it has been confirmed in biopsy studies.

Liver damage is particularly associated with DIC in pre-eclampsia. If this occurs together with hemolysis, the acronym HELLP syndrome has been used to label the concurrence of Hemolysis, Elevated Liver enzymes and Low Platelet counts [29]. It is a dangerous complication that is often not associated with marked hypertension [28,29]. The severity of the presentation may be graded by the intensity of the laboratory changes. Hemolysis is detected by the presence of fragmented red cells (schistocytes) on a blood film, by the disappearance of haptoglobin (which binds and clears free hemoglobin from the circulation) or, less precisely, by acute increases of plasma lactate dehydrogenase (LDH), which is a nonspecific marker of cell necrosis.

Maternal mortality is of the order of 1% [28] and is commonly associated with cerebral hemorrhage. Recovery from the primary problem may take a week or longer if there is renal failure and be complicated by rebound hypercoagulability, which can cause fatal thrombosis. In rare cases, typically of multiparae rather than primiparae, there may be bleeding under the liver capsule. Subsequently this may rupture to cause massive hemoperitoneum, shock and (possibly) maternal death [30]. There may well be an overlap between the liver involvement in pre-eclampsia and acute fatty liver of pregnancy [31] as described in Chapter 9, which may depend on impaired fatty acid metabolism.

Eclampsia

Eclampsia is a form of hypertensive encephalopathy, an acute or subacute syndrome of diffuse cerebral dysfunction not ascribable to uremia or hypertension but commonly associated with both. Hypertensive encephalopathy is part of a wider syndrome – reversible posterior leukoencephalopathy (also known as PRES – posterior reversible encephalopathic syndrome) [32]. The latter describes the commonly seen changes on magnetic resonance imaging of the brain which may occur not only with hypertensive encephalopathy in nonpregnant individuals but in eclampsia, lupus or in those who require immunosuppressive treatment. The term is a misnomer, because the lesions may not be fully reversible nor confined to the posterior cortex or the white matter.

The symptoms include headaches, nausea, vomiting and cortical blindness. Convulsions commonly but not invariably occur. Blood pressure may be relatively low or normal [32]. This is not, therefore, a form of malignant hypertension which is characterized by gross papilledema and retinopathy, secondary to extreme hypertension, and are lesions which are rare in eclampsia.

The pathophysiology is thought to be vasogenic edema secondary to loss of autoregulation combined with endothelial dysfunction [33]. Autopsies on patients with hypertensive encephalopathy have demonstrated arteriolar fibrinoid necrosis with microinfarcts and failed to show brain edema; however, brain biopsy has shown edematous white matter with no evidence of vessel wall damage or infarction [34].

The role of hypertension in the genesis of pre-eclampsia associated encephalopathy is uncertain, since it may not be present in all cases. Protective vasospasm of cerebral vessels is sustained by myogenic tone and lost with pressure-forced dilation. Pregnant animals seem more susceptible to this type of damage and even in pre-eclampsia without convulsions, there is increased cerebral arterial flow [35]. Hypertension will certainly extend the problem even if it is not the primary cause.

Fetal and neonatal issues

Fetal and neonatal issues are discussed later in the chapter in a section entitled "The fetus in hypertensive pregnancies."

Maternal mortality in pre-eclampsia

Pre-eclampsia and hypertensive diseases of pregnancy remain a prominent cause of maternal death worldwide. In relation to other causes, they are most important in Latin America and the Caribbean [36]. In undeveloped countries the main problems are access to medical services, the organization and range of available facilities, and the training of medical and paramedical staff [37]. In the UK pre-eclampsia is now a more important antecedent than eclampsia, in contrast to previous years. Cerebral hemorrhage continues to be the predominant cause of death in the UK [20]. In the USA higher mortality among black women is attributable not to a greater incidence of eclampsia but to higher case fatality rates [38].

Maternal risk factors (Box 6.8)

Risk factors may be specific to the mother or her pregnancy. Some, such as primigravidity or a past history of pre-eclampsia, are well known. The subject is systematically reviewed by Duckett & Harrington [39].

The predisposition to pre-eclampsia is, in part, inherited so that a positive family history is a risk factor. However, there is poor concordance between identical twin sisters so that maternal genes are not a dominant factor. Obese women are particularly susceptible but not to the variant of the HELLP

Box 6.8 Risk factors for pre-eclampsia

Maternal factors

- Primigravidity
- Primipaternity*
- Short period of cohabitation[†]
- Increasing maternal age
- Previous pre-eclampsia
- Obesity (syndrome X, polycystic ovarian syndrome)
- Medical disorders
  - Diabetes
  - Chronic hypertension
  - Chronic renal disease
  - Antiphospholipid antibody syndromes
  - Thrombophilia
  - Migraines
  - Asthma
- Family history of pre-eclampsia
- Stressful job

Placental/fetal factors

- Advancing gestational age
- Poor placentation‡
- Multiple pregnancy
- Hydatidiform mole
- Triploidy
- Trisomy 13
- Trisomy 16 mosaic
- Placental hydrops

---

*There may be partner specificity so it is not simply the first pregnancy that is an important risk factor but the first by the current partner.
[†]Stable cohabitation with a single partner seems to reduce the risk of pre-eclampsia in the first pregnancy by that partner.
‡See text for explanation of terminology.

---

syndrome. Obesity is associated with a constellation of other medical problems including type 2 diabetes and hypertension (syndrome X or metabolic syndrome). The separate parts of this constellation have all been associated with an increased tendency to pre-eclampsia [40]. The importance of renal disease increases with the degree of renal dysfunction and hypertension. The association with antiphospholipid antibodies is strong although the condition itself is rare. Antiphospholipid antibodies are an acquired cause of thrombophilia, which is a constitutional tendency to thromboembolism, some of which are genetically determined, for example possession of the Factor V Leiden gene or antithrombin (previously known as antithrombin III) deficiency. Thrombophilia is associated with more pregnancy complications and perinatal losses, including pre-eclampsia [41,42].

Chronically hypertensive women are 3–7 times more likely to develop higher blood pressure combined with proteinuria or "superimposed pre-eclampsia" than are normotensive women. If hypertension is combined with renal disease, then the risk is particularly high. Since the first report [43], it has been repeatedly shown that cigarette smoking, for unknown reasons, is associated with a reduced incidence of pre-eclampsia, albeit with an increased perinatal mortality from other causes.

It is now known that nonpregnant individuals suffering obesity, syndrome X, type 2 diabetes or hypertension show evidence of endothelial dysfunction or systemic inflammation [44]. Thus, it is possible that these conditions all predispose to pre-eclampsia because they cause high susceptibility to processes that are important in pre-eclampsia.

There are a number of reports suggesting that stress at work may increase the risk of pre-eclampsia. This tends to become an issue after an episode of pre-eclampsia when women wish to review whether their lifestyle contributed to their problem.

Because pre-eclampsia is primarily a placental disease (see above), it is not surprising that placental/fetal factors may increase risk. Some are associated with larger than average placentas. One example is advancing gestational age, which is such a basic feature of the disease that it is rarely considered in this context. The other associations are listed in Box 6.8. If it is considered that poor placentation is a separate condition that may or may not be associated with pre-eclampsia, then it must be also considered to be a powerful predisposing factor [17].

It is not know whether all these risk factors can be formally combined to give clinically useful predictions of the onset of pre-eclampsia.

How can pre-eclampsia be defined? (Box 6.9)

The only consistent feature of pre-eclampsia is its inconsistency. There are many possible features, but no set pattern in the way that they occur. Definitions therefore are limited in their usefulness. For the clinician, they should point to situations that are dangerous, regardless of the fine detail found in various formal definitions. As already stated, pre-eclampsia is primarily a placental disorder. Hence, although it is defined by hypertension, it is not primarily a hypertensive disease. The raised blood pressure and other maternal signs by which it is recognized are secondary to intrauterine problems. Because the placenta is affected, the fetus may suffer its own morbidity or mortality. The mother suffers diffuse circulatory dysfunction secondary to endothelial involvement. Hence pre-eclampsia affects many maternal systems (see above) causing different presentations which are not included in the simple epidemiologic definition of pre-eclampsia. These problems have been recognized by proposing two definitions – a narrow one for research purposes and a broader one for clinical purposes.

Box 6.9 Research and clinical definitions of pre-eclampsia

Strict research definition of pre-eclampsia (International Society for the Study of Hypertension in Pregnancy [7,45])
- New hypertension after 24 weeks: diastolic pressure ≥90 mmHg on two or more consecutive occasions >4 hours apart or >110 mmHg once AND
- New proteinuria after 24 weeks: 24-hour urine collection ≥300 mg protein or two mid-stream samples of urine collected more than 4 hours apart with >+ on stick test

Both features must be present.

Broad clinical definition of pre-eclampsia (adapted from Australasian Society for the Study of Hypertension in Pregnancy [46]

Hypertension arising after 20 weeks gestation and the new onset of one or more of:
- Proteinuria
- Renal insufficiency
- Hepatocellular dysfunction and/or severe epigastric/right upper quadrant pain
- Neurologic problems – convulsions (eclampsia); severe headaches; persistent scotomata
- Hematologic disturbances – thrombocytopenia; DIC; hemolysis
- Fetal growth restriction

The hypertension of pre-eclampsia will have returned to normal within 3 months post partum in both definitions.

In clinical practice, pre-eclampsia is better sought using the broader definition (Box 6.9).

The research definition is based on the presence of hypertension (see above) and new-onset proteinuria after 24 weeks gestation [7,45]. The idea that new hypertension is a mandatory part of the syndrome is historical, not logical. It is the focus of interest because this is what clinicians measure at the bedside. A syndrome requires at least two specific features before it can be recognized. Thus, new-onset hypertension (PIH) on its own (a common clinical presentation) is not pre-eclampsia; at least one more sign (by convention, pregnancy-induced proteinuria) is required. Some clinicians and investigators fail to appreciate this fact and use PIH and pre-eclampsia interchangeably, which confuses further an already confused subject. The clinical definition (Box 6.9) emphasizes the broader features of the disorder. It is to guide inexperienced clinicians and alert them to dangerous situations. With this approach, the term "nonproteinuric pre-eclampsia" in this chapter means new-onset or worsening hypertension in the second half of pregnancy combined with other features of pre-eclampsia, but without proteinuria.

Definitions are chosen for convenience, by consensus [46]. They describe outward appearances and embody no special truth about the underlying disease or diseases. When a syndrome such as pre-eclampsia is "defined," rules are set that bring consistency to what is being discussed. The rules may be sensible or not, but their validity cannot be tested because there is no standard to which to refer. All definitions of pre-eclampsia have these limitations. Real progress is impossible until the mechanisms of the disease or diseases that contribute to the syndrome are fully understood.

Incidence of pre-eclampsia and eclampsia

The incidence of pre-eclampsia depends on how it is defined, how assiduously the signs are sought and how accurately the diagnoses are recorded on large databases. Some reports are of hospital-based incidences which may be biased by selective referral or incomplete ascertainment. The size of the problem can be estimated, but it is always approximate. A population with a higher proportion of primigravidae will have more pre-eclampsia. The current epidemic of obesity [47] would be expected to have the same effect. The incidence of pre-eclampsia is affected to an unknown extent by interventions to end a pregnancy, particularly at term for gestational hypertension (PIH) to prevent possible progression to pre-eclampsia. Just as the classification of hypertension has many observational problems, so does that of proteinuria, which is the second, defining feature of the syndrome. Urine testing is more often omitted than blood pressure measurements, particularly during labor or the early puerperium when significant pre-eclampsia may occur for the first time.

In Aberdeen the incidence in primigravidae has fluctuated between 3.0% and 7.7% since 1950. In the same study the incidence in multiparae was 0.8–2.6% [48]. The incidence was 5.3% in Norway in 1991–2003 [49] and 2.3% in the USA in 1979–86 [50]. Hence, the incidence of proteinuric pre-eclampsia is of the order of one in 20–40 maternities.

Eclampsia complicates one in 2000 pregnancies in the UK [51] and one in 1000 in the USA [8]. In about 10% of cases it is unheralded, without prodromal signs or symptoms [51]. In 10% of cases the only warning sign is proteinuria and in another 20% there is hypertension only [51]. Hence, extreme hypertension is not a necessary (or indeed sufficient) predisposing factor. This said, eclampsia occurs 7–8 times more commonly in the contexts of proteinuric than of nonproteinuric pre-eclampsia [52] and the average blood pressures of women with eclampsia are higher than those with severe pre-eclampsia.

In the UK (and probably other Western countries), the majority of cases occur during labor or after delivery. Such presentations are mostly at term and occur in hospital.

Preterm eclampsia is more likely to be antepartum [51]. Eclampsia has been observed as early as 16 weeks of pregnancy [53]. Most postpartum fits occur within 24 hours of delivery but about one-fifth are defined as late post partum and occur more than 48 hours after delivery [54].

Screening for and prediction of pre-eclampsia

If the continuum theory of pre-eclampsia described above is accepted, then it is to be expected that there can be no reliable predictive test and indeed, this is the case to date, although numerous variables have been investigated. In brief, the maternal syndrome is too heterogeneous in its origins to be anticipated by a single test. Measurement of blood pressure and urine testing for proteinuria are the basic screening modes because they are relatively cheap, noninvasive and give an immediate result. Ways of improving their precision have been sought. Thus, 24-hour blood pressure monitoring (see above) eliminates many of the sampling errors of single measurements and provides a better estimate of the true blood pressure and may detect the changes of pre-eclampsia earlier. However, it is neither cheap nor simple to use and not all investigators agree that the information obtained is useful [6].

The different ways of assessing proteinuria have been summarized elsewhere [55] and are discussed in Chapter 7. A measurement of 24-hour protein excretion remains the gold standard but is too cumbersome and expensive for routine screening.

Dipsticks are the quickest and easiest but are not accurate for quantification because of natural variations in the degree of urinary dilution. This problem can be largely corrected by measuring urinary protein/creatinine ratios which can be obtained quickly from most laboratories from a small, randomly collected urine sample. Dipsticks for protein/creatinine ratio are also available that give convenient point-of-care estimates but may not be designed and calibrated to identify the mild level of proteinuria that is of concern in early pre-eclampsia. Any measurement based on single samples of urine will be affected to an unknown extent by variations in the rate of protein excretion. For the time being, standard dipsticks must remain the standard screening tool but positive results should be followed up by laboratory confirmation.

There are many possible circulating markers for pre-eclampsia reflecting endothelial dysfunction, activation of the clotting or inflammatory systems, renal or liver dysfunction. Their diversity reflects the huge range of systemic pathophysiology in pre-eclampsia. However, for prediction they have limited usefulness [56]. It is more logical to get as close to the primary pathology, the placenta, as possible. This can be done in two ways. The first is by ultrasound Doppler assessment for the presence of high-resistance blood flow patterns in the uterine arteries in mid-pregnancy which is gaining increasing acceptance as a moderately reliable technique [57]. A second way is to measure products of the placenta, secreted into maternal blood, that reflect the placental ischemia. These include factors that sustain or impair endothelial viability, including placental growth factor, soluble fms-like tyrosine kinase-1 (sFlt-1) and endoglin [14,58]. Further refinements of these techniques involve combining the Doppler measures and blood tests [57,59] or extending the screening from the second trimester to the end of the first trimester [60]. These techniques are under development and promise well for the future.

Diagnosis of pre-eclampsia

None of the signs of pre-eclampsia is specific; even convulsions in pregnancy are, in modern practice, more likely to have causes other than eclampsia. Diagnosis depends on finding a coincidence of several pre-eclamptic features. The final proof is their regression after delivery.

There are two ways to make the diagnosis. For research purposes, the rules have to be followed which require the presence of new hypertension in pregnancy and pregnancy-induced proteinuria. In practice, clinicians must seek features that indicate possible danger and be aware of atypical presentations [61]. This requires a broader view of a wider range of combinations of the possible features of the syndrome, as already discussed (Box 6.9). As with all syndromes, the more of the features that are clustered together, the more certain is the diagnosis. But, and this is not always appreciated, the absence of any one feature does not exclude the diagnosis. For example, eclampsia can occur without proteinuria. Even hypertension seems not to be essential. To diagnose pre-eclampsia superimposed on long-term hypertension or renal disease, there are, as stated already, no clear rules. In these circumstances, the diagnosis has to be made intuitively by judging the exacerbation of the long-term hypertension or proteinuria, in association with the appearance of other associated signs. In practice, hypertension and proteinuria have to be the signs of interest for screening in routine antenatal clinics.

Pre-eclampsia is usually initially symptomless and becomes symptomatic late in its course. Its detection depends on signs or investigations. One symptom is crucially important, because it is often misinterpreted. The epigastric pain, which reflects hepatic involvement and is the typical presentation of the HELLP syndrome, may easily be confused with heartburn, which is very common in pregnancy. However, it is not burning in quality, does not spread upwards towards the throat, is associated with hepatic tenderness, may radiate through to the back, and is not relieved by antacid. It is often very severe – described by sufferers as the worst pain that they have ever experienced. Affected women are not uncommonly referred to general surgeons as suffering from an acute abdomen, for example, acute cholecystitis.

New-onset hypertension in pregnancy on its own is not pre-eclampsia, although the term is commonly, but wrongly, used to mean mild or early pre-eclampsia. It is true that isolated hypertension may be the first indication of the onset of pre-eclampsia, but until other signs appear this remains unconfirmed. Often spontaneous or induced delivery prevents further developments so that a final certain diagnosis cannot be made.

Making the diagnosis

In most situations new or worsening hypertension and new proteinuria have to be present. One or more of the ancillary features listed (Box 6.10) may also suggest the diagnosis. Their absence never excludes the diagnosis; their presence is consistent with it. Different definitions have been proposed for what constitutes hypertension. The details are less important than the principle of an increment from a recording taken in the first half of pregnancy; this establishes the existence of new

---

Box 6.10 Clinical features of pre-eclampsia

Maternal syndrome

Pregnancy-induced hypertension*
Excessive weight gain (>1.0 kg/week)
Generalized edema

Evidence for hemoconcentration:
- Increased hematocrit
- Disturbances of renal function:
- Hyperuricaemia
- Proteinuria#
- Raised plasma creatinine, reduced creatinine clearance
- Hypocalciuria

Increased circulating markers of endothelial dysfunction:
- von Willebrand factor
- Cellular fibronectin

Laboratory evidence of excessive activation of the clotting system:
- Reduced plasma concentration of antithrombin III
- Thrombocytopenia
- Increased circulating fibrin d-dimer
- Increased circulating concentrations of liver enzymes

Fetal syndrome

Intrauterine growth restriction
Evidence for intrauterine hypoxemia

---

*Mandatory.
Usually mandatory unless several other ancillary features strongly suggest diagnosis.

or worsening hypertension in pregnancy. Between weeks 20 and 30 the blood pressure is normally steady so that even a small consistent rise is clinically important. Between week 30 and term, the diastolic will rise by about 10 mmHg on average [4] (Figure 6.5). A sustained rise of at least 25 mmHg to a threshold of 90 mmHg or more correlates broadly with the occurrence of proteinuria and the occurrence of pre-eclampsia [62]. However, these are guidelines; there is no clinical situation in which rigid interpretation of the blood pressure is helpful. Although the concept of new or worsening hypertension in pregnancy depends on measured increases in blood pressure, previously used definitions of increments have not proved helpful [63]. The systolic pressure should be given equal emphasis with the diastolic.

Before 20 weeks, hypertension usually reflects a problem that preceded pregnancy. After 20 weeks, it may represent a continuation of chronic hypertension or a new event. Given the technical and sampling errors of blood pressure measurement, small increases of pre-eclamptic origin are difficult to detect. It may be possible to improve diagnostic accuracy by rigid standardization of the methods of measurement or by ambulatory monitoring (see above) but no practical way of achieving this is currently available.

A normal blood pressure in the first half of pregnancy does not necessarily mean long-term normotension because the fall in blood pressure induced in early pregnancy may be exaggerated in some women. Many with relatively severe hypertension may have normal blood pressures by 12 weeks, without treatment. In other words, some women enjoy the benefits of pregnancy-induced normotension just as others suffer the disadvantages of new or worsening hypertension in pregnancy. Pregnancy-induced normotension tends to be lost in the third trimester. If the pre-pregnancy blood pressures are unknown then this development may be misinterpreted as pre-eclampsia or gestational hypertension. In an extreme case, a woman had pre-pregnancy readings of 224–280/140–180 mmHg; during pregnancy the pressure fell, without treatment, which was not available at that time, to normal levels of 110–130/60–80 mmHg7 [64]. During the third trimester extreme hypertension developed as the woman's normal cardiovascular status reappeared. This case report demonstrates clearly how chronic hypertension can masquerade as pre-eclampsia or gestational hypertension – a common problem in clinical practice, although its exact extent has never been assessed.

Proteinuria and evidence of a reduced glomerular filtration rate usually become evident after the onset of hypertension although the converse sequence may happen. It is agreed that the progression from new-onset hypertension to pre-eclampsia denotes a worsening perinatal outcome [65]. A diagnostic criterion for pre-eclampsia is proteinuria in excess of 0.3 g/24 h. In terms of stick testing, 0.5 g/24 h corresponds to at least "+" in every specimen of urine that is tested. When this point is reached, the disease can be said to have entered its proteinuric phase. Measurements of glomerular function are usually within the normal range for nonpregnant individuals. In general, abnormal concentrations of plasma creatinine and blood urea nitrogen (BUN) are above 100 μmol/L (1.1. mg/dL) and 6.0 mmol/L (17 mg/dL), respectively. These parameters are measured to monitor the progression of the disorder, not to screen for its occurrence, nor to predict its outcome except in respect of anticipating early renal failure. An increased plasma uric acid may indicate incipient pre-eclampsia in the context of new or worsening blood pressures. However, it is inconsistently present which accounts for the conclusions that it has poor predictive power [66]. It can precede proteinuria and is a simple investigation, which can suggest the later development of pre-eclampsia in the presence of new or worsening hypertension [67]. Plasma uric acid depends on both renal glomerular and tubular function

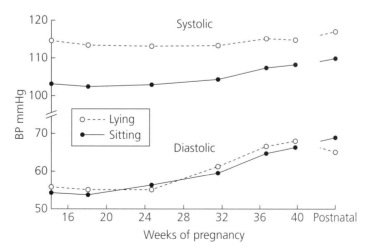

Figure 6.5 Serial arterial pressures in 226 primigravidae taken both lying and sitting. Reproduced with permission from MacGillivray *et al.* [4].

[68] and reflects a different aspect of renal involvement from plasma creatinine or urea.

The pathologic edema of pre-eclampsia is easily confused with the physiologic edema found in 80% of normal pregnant women and is therefore not now considered to be a mandatory feature for diagnosing pre-eclampsia. Development of edema is associated with a higher rate of weight gain; hence the reports associating excessive weight gain with the development of pre-eclampsia. Routine weighing during antenatal care is now not practiced in the UK but remains routine in the US. But it is cheap and noninvasive and, as already indicated, excessive gain is associated with pre-eclampsia. In general, if weight gain is consistently more than 1 kg per week then incipient pre-eclampsia can be suspected.

Pre-eclampsia is associated with an exaggeration of the activation of the clotting system intrinsic to normal pregnancy. In this context, platelet counts are useful because they are routinely available, not because they give the most insight into the condition. Although a declining platelet count may be an early feature of pre-eclampsia, it has limited diagnostic value because of the large variability between individuals in normal pregnancy. Prospective serial counts in selected high-risk patients are more useful when the patient's own baseline is established early in pregnancy.

Thrombocytopenia ($<100 \times 10^9$/L) tends to be a late development and can occur suddenly with the acute onset of HELLP syndrome. The same is true for raised liver enzymes. In regard to the latter, it should be noted that plasma alkaline phosphatase is often elevated in late pregnancy because of the contribution from the placental isoenzyme so that its measurement is not a useful guide to hepatic function. Therefore the appropriate simple tests are plasma aspartate aminotransferase (AST) or alanaine aminotransferase (ALT).

Epigastric pain is an important symptom of the HELLP syndrome. It may be so severe and sudden in onset that it is misinterpreted as a surgical emergency. Less severe pain is often mistreated as heartburn. Signs of pre-eclampsia may not be evident at first presentation [28]. Other symptoms include headache, vomiting and malaise. It may very rarely occur as early as 17 weeks but 30% of cases present after delivery, sometimes very suddenly. Eclampsia, pulmonary edema and acute renal failure are associated complications. Platelet counts and ALT or AST should be checked urgently in the context of epigastric pain. Lactate dehydrogenase (LDH) is a ubiquitous intracellular enzyme released on cell death. It therefore increases in the circulation with any form of tissue necrosis. In the HELLP syndrome, this is useful when an acute increase indicates red cell necrosis (hemolysis). Reduced haptoglobin is a more specific test for hemolysis but is usually not available in an emergency situation. A blood film shows fragmented red cells (schistocytes) which are diagnostic of hemolysis. Serum bilirubin may be abnormal, secondary to hepatic metabolism of hemoglobin released during acute hemolysis. Gamma-glutamyl transferase (GGT) is increased only late in the evolution of the condition.

Partial variants of the syndrome occur when only two features are present (ELLP, HEL, LP and EL). They are, in general, less severe [61,69].

Management of pre-eclamptic hypertension and associated problems

Pre-eclampsia is probably the most common cause of secondary hypertension in clinical practice; delivery always reverses the problem because it removes the causative organ – the placenta. The principles of management are screening of the symptomless patient, diagnosis and well-timed delivery. Interposed between diagnosis and delivery is the need for hospital admission to monitor a condition that may change rapidly and unpredictably. It is essential for the correct timing and management of pre-emptive delivery. The problem is to decide at what stage the pre-eclamptic patient should be admitted. In general, symptomatic pre-eclampsia (symptoms, hypertension and proteinuria) justifies an emergency admission. Symptomless but definite proteinuric pre-eclampsia is best managed as an inpatient because of the sudden, unpredictable and dangerous crises that can occur. New hypertension without proteinuria, in which developing pre-eclampsia is suspected (for example, due to hyperuricemia), is usually best managed in a day assessment unit where frequent detailed checks are routine. Mild hypertension with no other complicating factor can be managed conservatively in routine clinics.

Antihypertensive drugs

Antihypertensive treatment will prevent only those problems directly caused by maternal hypertension. Pre-eclamptic hypertension is a secondary or peripheral feature of a placental problem but extreme pre-eclamptic hypertension causes direct arterial injury that predisposes to cerebral hemorrhages and is therefore dangerous. The threshold at which this will typically occur has been said to be at a mean arterial pressure of 140 mmHg (180–190/120–130) but the majority of cases in one recent series happened at much lower blood pressures and the degree to which the blood pressure has changed from its baseline may be as important as the absolute number. Definitive treatment is delivery, but antihypertensive agents are used to protect the mother before, during and afterwards [70]. Our aim is to keep all blood pressure readings below 160/110; hence treatment is started if blood pressures repeatedly reach or exceed this value. Others have different thresholds; the exact levels are less important than understanding the principles that determine the need for treatment.

Acute control of severe hypertension

The arterial spasm of pre-eclampsia responds best to the drugs that directly relax vascular smooth muscle. A smooth and sustained reduction is to be preferred to sudden short-term changes. A number of vasodilating agents given parenterally have been used, including hydralazine, labetalol, and nitroglycerine or sodium nitroprusside. In addition, oral calcium channel-blocking agents are increasingly administered for this purpose.

Hydralazine has previously been the preferred antihypertensive agent for the treatment of acute severe pre-eclampsia. It is usually given intravenously by continuous infusion or intermittent boluses, or by intramuscular or subcutaneous injections. After intravenous administration there is a substantial delay in the onset of action of 20–30 minutes. Hydralazine directly relaxes vascular smooth muscle. A common side effect is severe headache. It also causes prolonged release of noradrenaline (norepinephrine), which correlates closely with the tachycardia that usually develops, and could also explain the anxiety, restlessness and hyper-reflexia which are common side effects. These symptoms and signs, together with headaches, may affect 50% of women and simulate the features of impending eclampsia. Then the symptoms of the disease cannot be disentangled from those caused by the treatment.

It is relevant that hydralazine stimulates the release of norepiephrine which vasoconstricts the uteroplacental circulation. Thus, although it increases cardiac output, hydralazine fails to improve indices of uteroplacental perfusion in pre-eclamptic women and thus is not an ideal drug. A meta-analysis leads to the conclusion that it should not be the drug of first choice for acute hypertension in pregnancy [71] and gives inferior blood pressure control when compared to oral calcium channel blockers [72]. It is easier to use if the sympathetic nervous system is already inhibited by methyldopa or adrenergic blocking agents. A continuous infusion is not a rational way to achieve control of the blood pressure for more than 4–6 hours except in intensive care situations. Monitoring of the fetus is essential but in our experience fetal distress is rare, and more related to the severity of the pre-eclampsia than to the administration of the hydralazine.

Labetalol is a combined alpha- and beta-adrenergic blocking agent, which can be given intravenously or orally. After parenteral administration it lowers the blood pressure smoothly but rapidly, without the tachycardia characteristic of treatment with hydralazine. Although the data are not extensive, what is known does not suggest that it causes fetal harm. The typical oral dose begins with 100–200 mg orally, twice a day, and can be gradually titrated up to 800 mg orally three times a day. A typical intravenous regimen starts with a 20 mg IV bolus over 2 minutes that can be doubled every 10 minutes to a maximum single dose of 80 mg and/or a total dose of 300 mg. Another less aggressive regimen is an IV infusion starting with 20 mg/h, which is doubled every 30 min until control has been gained or a maximum of 120 mg/h is reached. (Labetalol infusions are typically run at 0.5–2 mg/min. Labetalol comes in vials of 100 mg/20 mL in the US and the infusion can be mixed by putting five vials (100 mL) of labetalol into 150 mL of IV fluid to get a solution of 2 mg/mL. An infusion of 15 mL/h will then be 0.5 mg/min and 60 mL/h will be 2 mg/min). As alpha-adrenergic stimulation is thought to constrict the uteroplacental circulation, labetalol (alpha-blockade) would be expected to enhance flow; in fact, no effect, good or bad, has been observed. There are reports of symptomatic neonatal beta-adrenergic blockade after *in utero* exposure. Single case reports may be misleading and there are no adequate trials of its parenteral use in pregnancy to show how it might affect perinatal outcome. Other vasodilators include sodium nitroprusside and nitroglycerine, given intravenously to severely hypertensive pregnant women. Neither is to be recommended except in extreme circumstances and in specialist intensive care.

The calcium channel-blocking agent nifedipine is an effective vasodilator that acts rapidly when given orally. Nifedipine capsules, which act within 10–15 min, cause dangerously abrupt blood pressure reductions in nonpregnant individuals and are no longer used. Slow-release tablets begin to act within about 60 minutes and have a more prolonged effect sustained by administration 3–4 times a day. Nifedipine appears to be at least as safe as hydralazine and, with respect to blood pressure control, superior [73]. Tachycardia occurs but is less of a problem than with hydralazine. In theory, there could be a problem if given with parenteral magnesium sulfate. In practice, this seems not to be the case [73]. The advantage of nifedipine over hydralazine is its ease of administration. It can also cause severe headaches like hydralazine. An antitocolytic effect on uterine muscle [74] might predispose to postpartum hemorrhage, although this complication has not been reported.

The acute management of severe hypertension is discussed in additional detail in Chapter 39.

Conservative management of severe pre-eclampsia (blood pressure ≥170/110)

There have to be compelling reasons to leave women with proteinuric pre-eclampsia undelivered after 36 weeks gestation. Even after 34 weeks it becomes increasingly difficult to justify conservative management. The same arguments can be transposed to women with evolving pre-eclampsia at 38–40 weeks even in the absence of proteinuria.

Proteinuric pre-eclampsia, without symptoms, that presents at 26–34 weeks of pregnancy presents challenges. Although delivery is desirable, it may not be essential. If it can be deferred for 2 weeks or longer, significant maturation of the fetus may be achieved to reduce the problems of immaturity after birth. Conservative management of proteinuric pre-eclampsia demands an experienced team offering close monitoring and specialized care. It is not easy, and sometimes impossible in understaffed, busy units with heavy routine commitments. It is thus desirable that such patients are moved at an early stage to specialized regional centers. It is also necessary that such centers have adequately skilled staff and appropriate resources.

Conservative management needs to be used with discretion and in the knowledge that it will achieve little or no gain for some women. It should be carried out only for patients for whom it is believed there is a reasonable chance of prolonging gestation long enough to improve neonatal morbidity and mortality. To defer delivery safely, it is essential to know how all maternal systems are affected by the disorder. The fetus must be reviewed frequently also. Delivery is necessary if the maternal blood pressure cannot be controlled, if the platelet count is $<50 \times 10^9$/L, if the plasma creatinine has risen from normal levels to ≥ 120 μmol/L (1.3–1.4 mg/dL), if there is evidence of liver damage or if the woman has symptoms that are clearly caused by her condition. In some cases, increasing fetal problems may make extrauterine life safer. Any of these developments can happen unpredictably and suddenly, and will be missed unless the monitoring and care are maintained at a high level.

Two trials comparing conservative management with immediate delivery have suggested the potential advantages of a cautious expectant approach [75,76], as has our own experience at Oxford. While the authors are comfortable with the above described approach, the editors remain skeptical about the role of expectant management of severe pre-eclampsia as they feel the published experience remains both small and devoid of long-term follow-up data.

Longer term control of severe pre-eclamptic hypertension

Good blood pressure control is mandatory for conservative management of pre-eclampsia. It can reduce the dangers of severe hypertension but not the other problems of pre-eclampsia (abnormalities of renal, coagulation and placental function). Thus treatment only suppresses one dangerous manifestation of this disorder. Parenteral therapy is inappropriate for ongoing conservative management and oral agents need to be used. Labetalol 200 mg PO twice a day is one such typical initial regimen. The issues of drug use become those of the management of chronic hypertension in pregnancy (see below). The special requirements are for a fast onset of action and rapid responses changes in dose (titration). Methyldopa is the drug with the most extensive pregnancy safety data [77] but needs to be used with an initial loading dose (500–750 mg) and at 1.0–3.0 g per day, a dose that some women may find intolerable due to the side effect of somnolence. Labetalol is an alternative faster-acting agent and nifedipine is useful as a second-line supplementary agent. The evidence for choices of drugs is not detailed. Which of the pregnancy-compatible agents (Table 6.2) is preferred probably matters less than the clinician's familiarity with its use.

Table 6.2 Antihypertensive drugs in pregnancy

Stage of pregnancy	Relatively contraindicated[1]	Absolutely contraindicated	Drugs that may be used
First trimester[2]	–	ACE inhibitors A-II receptor antagonists	Methyldopa Labetalol and beta-blockers Calcium channel blockers
Second trimester	Beta-blockers Diuretics	ACE inhibitors A-II antagonists	Methyldopa Nifedipine Labetalol
Third trimester	Beta-blockers Diuretics	ACE inhibitors A-II receptor antagonists	Methyldopa Nifedipine Labetalol Doxazosin Prazosin
Puerperium	Methyldopa[3]	None known	Beta-blockers Labetalol Nifedipine ACE inhibitors A-II receptor antagonists Diuretics

[1] Can be used but avoid unless necessary.
[2] Avoid all drugs in the first trimester unless necessary.
[3] Side effect profile and efficacy make this agent less desirable for long-term use.

Escape from blood pressure control

So long as pregnancy continues, pre-eclampsia is relentlessly progressive, so that escape from blood pressure control can be expected. In general, the maternal and fetal conditions deteriorate together and it is not difficult to see when the limits of conservative management have been reached and delivery is indicated. Oral vasodilators, especially nifedipine (up to 120 mg in total per day, in slow-release tablet form), may be usefully added to either methyldopa or labetalol to prevent loss of blood pressure control. Antihypertensive treatment would be expected to help prevent cerebral hemorrhages but not eclampsia (see above).

Fluid balance and oliguria

Pre-eclampsia is associated with a contracted but full intravascular space. It has been claimed that plasma volume expansion is beneficial to correct poor renal and placental function. The evidence in favor is not supported by recent evidence [78]. The possibility that it could cause circulatory overload and pulmonary edema makes the treatment potentially dangerous [79]. It cannot therefore be considered to be a part of routine management.

The renal problem that causes oliguria and anuria in pre-eclampsia arises from structural disease in the glomeruli and not hemodynamic factors [24]; hence it cannot be resolved by fluid administration. Hypovolemia secondary to blood loss associated with bleeding at delivery clearly must be excluded, and for this a central venous line can be very helpful. But once the cardiac return is assured by adequate venous filling, fluid replacement must be used with caution. In particular, the intensive care unit convention that urine output must be seen to be at least 30 mL/h is inapplicable. With an adequate central venous pressure, additional fluid loading is unlikely to be of benefit. If plasma creatinine is less than 100 mmol/L (1.1 mg/dL) and there are no signs of HELLP, there is no problem even if urine output drops to the range 10–20 mL/h, providing there is no evidence for blood loss. Such reduced urinary output is transient and self-correcting. However, in the presence of a rising plasma creatinine (>100 mmol/L) with hemolysis, poor urine output is highly likely to be secondary to structural deficits in the kidneys, which are not corrected by infusion of fluids. Indeed, all that can happen is that the infusions will overflow into the lungs. Genuine anuria, even for as short a time as 1 hour, is always abnormal and may herald total renal failure.

Prevention and treatment of eclampsia

The patient is symptomless for most of the course of pre-eclampsia – a critical feature where diagnosis and management are concerned. Terminally symptoms may include headaches, visual disturbances, nausea, vomiting, epigastric pain and neurologic irritability (clonus and shaking). At this point convulsions may occur.

Eclampsia is rare so that, in the first world, few obstetricians except in big tertiary centers have extensive experience of its management. About 40% of cases are either completely unheralded or only partially heralded. More cases occur in labor or after delivery than antepartum, for which reason alone the first eclamptic convulsion occurs after admission to hospital in the majority of women. The aim of management is to protect the maternal airway, control convulsions, control extreme hypertension and expedite delivery.

If a patient needs anticonvulsant medication she also needs urgent delivery. Most eclamptic convulsions stop spontaneously and therefore no acute medical treatment is necessary. If the seizure persists, a benzodiazepine may be administered. Intravenous lorazepam is preferred to diazepam, because of its shorter half-life. An aliquot of 4 mg can be given by cautious slow intravenous injection with attention to avoiding oversedation and respiratory depression. Benzodiazepines are, however, inappropriate to prevent recurrent convulsions, for which purpose magnesium sulfate is indicated. It is more effective than either parenteral phenytoin or long-term diazepam [80]. Magnesium sulfate can be given intravenously or by intramuscular injection, although with both regimens an initial loading dose (usually 4 g) is given. The advantage of the former is more precise control of dosage. The disadvantage is the risk of overdose. This is highest if there is renal impairment when a continuous infusion causes rapid accumulation of magnesium and toxic side effects, including muscular weakness, respiratory paralysis, heart failure and death. Hence blood levels of magnesium should be monitored when there is any suspicion of renal impairment Therapeutic levels are 2–3.5 mmol/L (4–7 mEq/L or 4.9–8.5 mg/dL).

Whether magnesium levels need to be followed routinely in patients with good renal function remains unclear. A simple clinical test to screen for magnesium toxicity is to check the deep tendon reflexes. If they are suppressed, no more magnesium should be given pending more accurate knowledge of what the plasma concentrations are. The antidote for magnesium sulfate is calcium gluconate (1 g calcium gluconate IV; 10 mL ampoule of 10% calcium gluconate administered over 10 min).

Continuous monitoring of urine output from an indwelling catheter is essential, as is knowing the plasma creatinine. Oliguria (<10 mL/h) or anuria is a reason to stop giving magnesium, as is a high plasma creatinine (>150 mmol/L or 1.7 mg/dL). Extreme caution should be exercised if the urine output is 10–20 mL/h or the plasma creatinine is 100–150 mmol/L (1.1–1.7 mg/dL) when the rate of infusion should be slowed, if not stopped. To minimize the risk of accidental infusion of overdoses, 10 g of magnesium sulfate in a 50 mL solution of 0.9% (1 g in 5 mL) saline should be given by an infusion pump. In the USA the preferred rate of administration is 2 g/h whereas in the UK it is 1 g/h.

Intramuscular magnesium sulfate is easier to manage but achieves a less precise dosage regimen. Because it is easy to give overdoses, which are potentially lethal, magnesium sulfate should not be used indiscriminately. Magnesium sulfate has long been used in the USA for prophylaxis in pre-eclamptic women who have not had a convulsion. A large trial (MAGPIE [81]) justifies this practice. In fact, the problem is not its efficacy but who to treat. In the MAGPIE trial, the number needed to treat to prevent one case of eclampsia varied according to the economic status of the participating country. In developed countries (defined by low perinatal mortality rates), it was nearly 400 but lower in less developed countries. Symptoms of impending eclampsia (severe headaches, blurred vision or epigastric pain) defined a higher risk group of which 36 women needed to be treated to prevent one case of eclampsia. HELLP syndrome is a very high-risk group in which nearly one in 25 women has eclampsia [28]. These groups clearly justify routine prophylaxis. About 40% of cases are either partially or totally unheralded and it is difficult to envisage how these might be prevented. Moreover, the use of magnesium sulfate does not guarantee prevention [81]. There are many side effects, which are listed in Table 6.3. The mechanism of action of magnesium sulfate is not known.

Other measures for the treatment of pre-eclampsia and its complications

There is no evidence to justify the routine use of diuretics to prevent or treat pre-eclampsia [91]. They can be safely used, however, for treating the rare complication of pulmonary edema. In general, the only remedy for DIC is to correct the underlying problem. In pre-eclampsia this means delivery. The poor hemostasis of women recovering from severe DIC post partum can cause intractable hemorrhage. Transfusions of platelets and fresh-frozen plasma may be needed in addition to the replacement of whole blood as supportive treatment.

Prevention of pre-eclampsia

No totally effective measure for the primary prevention of pre-eclampsia has been found. If the concepts of pathogenesis are correct (see above), it is unlikely that any single measure will ever be identified that is effective for all susceptible women. But specific measures of reducing the susceptibilities among subgroups of women may be developed. Measures which may be effective or are probably or definitely ineffective are summarized in Table 6.4. Antiplatelet agents, in particular low doses of aspirin, confer a small but statistically significant benefit with a relative risk of developing pre-eclampsia in women who took aspirin during pregnancy (versus those who did not) of 0.90 (95% confidence interval

Table 6.4 Primary prevention of pre-eclampsia

Probably or definitely ineffective	May be effective for at least some women
Weight restriction	Low-dose aspirin and other antiplatelet agents
Salt restriction	Calcium supplements
Antioxidant vitamins (vitamins C and E)	
Diuretics	
Antihypertensive agents	
Fish oil supplements	

(CI) 0.84–0.97) or of having a serious adverse pregnancy outcome of 0.90 (0.85–0.96) but no reduction in the risk of perinatal death [92]. Calcium supplements appear to confer benefit but this may be confined to areas where calcium intake is low [93]. Antihypertensive agents do not prevent pre-eclampsia but significantly reduce the risk of severe hypertension [92].

Secondary prevention – the importance of antenatal care

There is no evidence that, once it becomes overt, pre-eclampsia can be reversed except by delivery. Pre-eclampsia cannot be predicted accurately (see above). Hence, by far the most important part of secondary prevention is regular antenatal care to screen for asymptomatic incipient or early pre-eclampsia and therefore to allow timely delivery before the disease becomes dangerous. This simple concept has not been formally tested but it works and provides a safety net for all pregnant women who have access to antenatal care. Screening assessments have to be repeatedly updated during the second half of pregnancy because pre-eclampsia can evolve quickly, rarely in 1 week or, at times, within 2 weeks. The key is the regularity of repeated checks, the backbone of antenatal care. The longer the interval between one check and the next, the greater the risk of a serious episode of pre-eclampsia developing undetected. The critical issue is therefore the duration of the screening interval. One longer than 4 weeks is always too long except for the lowest risk group, which comprises normal multiparae with singleton pregnancies, and no past history of hypertension in pregnancy.

Longer screening intervals at gestations between 20 and 28 weeks are a feature of most patterns of antenatal care. But early-onset pre-eclampsia and eclampsia at this time are the most dangerous, both for the mother and in terms of perinatal outcome. The disease is characterized by more intrauterine growth restriction, a substantially higher perinatal mortality and more maternal complications [51].

One needs to view with caution claims that it is possible to reduce antenatal care, which in practice involves minimizing the number of visits between 20 and 36 weeks, at this time of

Table 6.3 Side effects of magnesium sulfate given for preventing or treating eclampsia

Side effect	Reference
Flushing	81
Nausea and/or vomiting	81
Muscle weakness	81
Respiratory depression or other problems	81
Thirst	81
Hypotension, palpitations or tachycardia	81
Dizziness	81
Drowsiness or confusion	81
Itching or tingling	81
Overdose and maternal death	82
Overdose and cardiac arrest	83
Diminished pulmonary function	84
Paralysis in women with neuromuscular disorders	85
Recurrent convulsions	80
Increased rates of prolonged labor, cesarean delivery, postpartum bleeding	86
Prolonged bleeding time	87
Maternal hypocalcemia and tetany	88
Neonatal hypotonia and lower APGAR scores	89
Reduced fetal heart rate variation	90

greatest risk. In four studies no, or inadequate, care has been statistically associated with the risks of eclampsia [94–97]. This highlights the role of good antenatal care as the primary effective measure in secondary prevention.

Of the other measures, there is no evidence that blood pressure control attenuates the progression of early pre-eclampsia or that it prevents superimposition of pre-eclampsia in chronically hypertensive women, who otherwise are more susceptible to the disorder [98]. The only clear advantage of antihypertensive treatment is where the hypertension is so severe that delivery is essential to preserve maternal safety. At early gestational ages, antihypertensive treatment can allow prolongation of pregnancy in this context. The benefit is not from prevention but palliation. The extent of the presumed benefit has not been measured because severe hypertension is a reason for exclusion from randomized trials of treatment. Hence, in all contexts antihypertensive treatment helps to protect the mother from the consequences of her problem, but not from the problem itself. Undoubtedly, treatment can lower the blood pressure in early pre-eclampsia; by so doing, it can modify the medical interventions that are triggered when hypertension of a particular severity is encountered. If the interventions are, in reality, unnecessary then all that the treatment achieves is to protect the patient from her doctors.

Postpartum hypertension

The arterial pressure progressively rises during the first 5 days after normal delivery [99]. This trend may be exaggerated in hypertensive women, so that the highest readings of all may be recorded during this period. Concurrently, the signs and symptoms of severe pre-eclampsia may or may not appear for the first time, with the onset of epigastric pain or eclampsia.

Postpartum hypertension needs to be managed, as is antepartum hypertension, with treatment titrated to prevent severe hypertension. What is ideally needed is a rapid-onset agent that allows rapid titration in the rapidly changing circumstances of the immediate puerperium. It is better not to use methyldopa because of the tiredness and depression that it can cause. Of the beta-blocking agents, oxprenolol (not available in the US), labetalol and short-acting nifedipine (10–20 mg orally three times a day) have the advantage of a quick onset of action but postural hypotension can be a problem, particularly with labetalol. The patient can usually be discharged 5–6 days after delivery, generally once blood pressure has been consistently <160/100 for 24 hours. Within 2–3 weeks of discharge antihypertensive treatment can usually be reduced or stopped, a decision that can be delegated to the general practitioner. Whereas angiotensin-converting enzyme (ACE) inhibitors are contraindicated during pregnancy, they can be used in the puerperium. There is no clear evidence that treatment interferes with breastfeeding. What is known is summarized in Table 6.5.

Table 6.5 Antihypertensive drugs and breastfeeding

Drug	Secretion in breast milk	Position of American Academy of Pediatrics on use of agent with breastfeeding
Methyldopa	Minimal secretion; too small to be harmful	Approved
Labetalol	Secreted in breast milk in small amounts	Approved
Atenolol, acebutolol, nadolol, metoprolol	Secreted in breast milk. Atenolol and nadolol are found in higher concetrations in breast milk than other beta-blockers so they may not be first-line agents within this class	Approved
Nifedipine	Secreted in breast milk	Approved
Diltiazem	Secreted in breast milk in higher concentrations than many other agents	Approved
Hydrochlorothiazide	Secreted in breast milk to a small degree. No evidence that it impairs milk production	Approved
ACE inhibitors	Secreted in breast milk but in small amounts that are unlikely to be harmful	Enalapril and captopril approved but no comment on other ACE inhibitors or the angiotensin receptor blockers

ACE, angiotensin-converting enzymes.

Remote postpartum assessment and recurrent pre-eclampsia

Women who have suffered pre-eclampsia and its complications always ask for information about the likelihood of recurrence. The outlook is better than they think but not as good as they would like. In general, if all grades of pre-eclampsia are considered, the recurrence rate is 7.5% [100]. The risk increases with the severity of the disease [101] and the earlier its onset [102]. Recurrent eclampsia is rare. The HELLP syndrome recurs in about 3% of women, the rate being unaffected by whether the woman has underlying CHT or not [101].

It is necessary to determine what, if any, long-term medical problems underlie an episode of severe pre-eclampsia. These include CHT, chronic renal disease, the antiphospholipid antibody syndrome and possibly thrombophilia. This is important not only to determine the risk of recurrence (higher if there are such underlying medical problems) but to discuss contraception options and to give advice about lifestyle and medical surveillance in relation to long-term medical health.

Oral contraceptives containing estrogen sometimes cause hypertension, which can be severe or, very rarely, malignant.

For this reason, poorly controlled hypertension is a relative contraindication to their use. The advice given to postpartum women should therefore be guided by whether or not hypertension persists as a chronic problem. Women with thrombophilia including antiphospholipid antibodies should avoid estrogen-containing oral contraceptives, although progestogen-only preparations are deemed to be safe. For the rest, if a pre-eclamptic woman's blood pressure returns to normal, there seems little reason to deny her the benefits of oral contraceptives provided adequate and continuing medical supervision is available. Likewise, an episode of HELLP syndrome is unlikely to be a contraindication to use of estrogen-containing oral contraceptives. Chronic hypertension, when well controlled, is not a contraindication to estrogen-containing oral contraceptives.

Severe pre-eclampsia and eclampsia can cause irreversible maternal damage, particularly acute renal cortical necrosis or cerebral hemorrhage. In the absence of these complications, there is no clear information of the impact of a pre-eclamptic episode on long-term maternal health. In terms of later life, women with pre-eclampsia as a group have a higher than normal incidence of arterial disease [103]. In this regard, pregnancy is an ideal screening test for long-term health. Given the fact that many of the conditions that predispose to pre-eclampsia are those that predispose to later arterial disease, it is difficult to disentangle the relative contributions of an episode of pre-eclampsia itself from these underlying risk factors with regard to the long-term maternal risks.

There may be considerable residual distress and anxiety for both a mother and her partner after she has endured a severe episode of pre-eclampsia. Events such as emergency cesarean deliveries, perinatal death or severe perinatal complications such as prematurity or neonatal intensive care, even at term, markedly increase the likelihood of puerperal post-traumatic stress reactions, which have been documented in relation to pre-eclampsia [104]. It is essential to recognize the problem, to offer appropriate counseling or to help the sufferers gain professional counseling.

Other causes of hypertension in pregnancy

This group comprises women with essential and renal hypertension, and hypertension caused by miscellaneous but rare conditions.

Chronic (essential) hypertension

Women with essential hypertension tend to be older, hence more likely to be parous, heavier and to have a family history of hypertension. Chronic hypertension (CHT) is detected either by an antecedent medical history or by a raised blood pressure (140/90 mmHg or more) in the first half of pregnancy.

As stated earlier, the physiologic decline in the blood pressure in early pregnancy is exaggerated in women with CHT so that they may become normotensive. Conversely, in later pregnancy the normal rise in blood pressure is exaggerated. Thus, a woman with CHT may be normotensive when she starts antenatal care early in the second trimester, but then develop hypertension in the third trimester; she thus presents as gestational hypertension or evolving pre-eclampsia. Not uncommonly, the presentation is of mild hypertension alone in the second half of pregnancy without antecedent readings. Then it is not possible to distinguish CHT from incipient pre-eclampsia with certainty.

The specific problem of CHT in pregnancy is that it is one of the major predisposing factors to pre-eclampsia. Among women with a blood pressure of 140/90 mmHg or more in the first half of pregnancy, the likelihood of developing pre-eclampsia is about five times more than in normotensive individuals [42]. The signs of pre-eclampsia in chronically hypertensive women are the same as in other women except that the blood pressure levels start from a higher baseline; in addition, there may be progressive hyperuricemia or abnormal activation of the clotting system and, more definitively, proteinuria.

Chronically hypertensive women who do not get pre-eclampsia can usually expect an uncomplicated perinatal outcome. It is generally believed that CHT predisposes to abruption [105]. It is a relatively rare complication (about 1%). There is some evidence for a modestly increased incidence of fetal growth restriction associated with CHT.

Treatment

If antihypertensive treatment has been started before conception, the patient may seek advice about the possible effects of her medication on the growth and development of her fetus. Only ACE inhibitors and angiotensin receptor blockers are thought to be teratogenic [106,107] and are definitely fetotoxic in the second and third trimesters[108], as discussed below. It is appropriate that women with no more than moderate hypertension should stop treatment before conception, so that only those whose hypertension is an immediate health hazard continue on medication throughout the first trimester. By the 12th week the normal fall in blood pressure may enable all treatment to be temporarily reduced or stopped, to be restarted as the blood pressure rises again during the third trimester.

If CHT is diagnosed for the first time in pregnancy, it is necessary to treat those in whom it presents an immediate (as opposed to a long-term) hazard. The approach to hypertension remote from term is reviewed in Chapter 42 and should include some basic investigations to look for evidence of secondary causes of hypertension such as a complete blood count, creatinine, calcium, thyroid-stimulating hormone, urinalysis and serum potassium. The precise levels for treatment have not been agreed upon; we take a cut-off point of peak readings at or above 160/110 mmHg while the US national recommendations and common practice favor a cut-off point of 160/100 mmHg. The problem of less severe CHT (i.e. 140–160/90–110 mmHg) needs to be considered. In general medical practice, the purpose of treating this degree of hypertension is to prevent long-term complications, which are not relevant for the brief period of gestation. For this reason, the only indication for antihypertensive treatment in these women would be if it could prevent the superimposition of pre-eclampsia, which is the major short-term problem. There is no evidence that this is the case [98].

The choice of drugs is dictated by fetal considerations. Methyldopa is preferred because its fetal effects have been defined much more clearly than those of any other drug. There are follow-up data showing no short- or long-term problems up to 7 years of age from exposure *in utero* [109]. Its antihypertensive action and side effects are the same as in nonpregnant individuals and no serious adverse fetal effects have yet been documented. Its use not only relieves the patient of the problems of parenteral therapy but if, at a later time, hydralazine or another vasodilator, such as nifedipine, is needed, its action is potentiated. An adequate therapeutic response can be achieved within 12 hours of starting oral treatment with a loading dose of 500 mg. Usually this is not necessary and the initial regimen can be 250 mg 2–3 times a day. This can be increased to 1–2 g/day (500–1000 mg PO bid). Only rarely should a further increase, to 3 g/day (1000 mg PO tid), be needed. A satisfactory drop in the blood pressure tends to provoke transient oliguria, which may cause anxiety about renal failure – a complication discounted by measuring the plasma creatinine. The treatment regimen may need to anticipate nocturnal hypertension [19] by a variable schedule with the largest doses at night.

The beta-adrenergic antagonists (beta-blockers) have the advantage of causing fewer subjective sideeffects but their safety in pregnancy has not been so exhaustively investigated. A preparation such as atenolol has a slow onset of action and a flat dose–response curve, which make the day-to-day titration of blood pressure control almost impossible. The use of other drugs such as labetalol and the conventional beta-blockers has been fully discussed above and is endorsed at many centers. There has been a tendency for beta-blockers, particularly atenolol, to be associated with smaller fetuses [110–113]. This does not preclude their short-term use in the third trimester for the treatment of pre-eclampsia or gestational hypertension. Among the calcium channel blockers, nifedipine has the broadest experience in pregnancy and is used at many centers as a first- or second-line agent for treatment of chronic hypertension in pregnancy. If diuretics are essential for good blood pressure control, they can be continued throughout pregnancy but their use carries certain disadvantages if pre-eclampsia should supervene, as already discussed. ACE inhibitors are, as already stated, contraindicated.

Long-term use of antihypertensive agents of all sorts has been associated with modest fetal growth restriction [114]. This may be because lowering the arterial pressure reduces placental perfusion or because other effects of the drugs, all of which must be assumed to cross the placenta, have a separate effect on the growth rates of exposed fetuses. This is an excellent justification for the conservative criteria for using these agents, described in this chapter. They should be limited to the treatment of women with severe, rather than mild or moderate, hypertension.

The selection of antihypertensive drugs for use in pregnancy is summarized in Table 6.2.

Secondary hypertension

Women with secondary hypertension in pregnancy are rare but important to detect. All patients with hypertension should have some formal consideration of secondary causes of hypertension and this is reviewed in Chapter 42. Standard recommended testing and evaluation of patients with hypertension as well as the features of the known secondary causes of hypertension are found in the tables and boxes in that chapter.

Pheochromocytoma is a dangerous complication of pregnancy [115] and is discussed in detail in Chapter 13. Maternal mortality is higher if it is not diagnosed before the peripartum period. Its presentation is variable but includes extreme hypertension, severe pre-eclampsia, cardiomyopathy with heart failure, cardiovascular collapse or diabetes mellitus. Diagnosis depends primarily on the appropriate level of clinical suspicion and investigations as are used in nonpregnant individuals, including biochemical measures of catecholamine secretion and examination of the adrenals by ultrasound, magnetic resonance imaging or computed tomography. Conditions with an added risk of the condition include multiple endocrine neoplasia types 2a and 2b, neurofibromatosis type 1, tuberous sclerosis and von Hippel–Lindau syndrome. Ten percent of pheochromocytomas are extramedullary and these are the ones that are more likely to be or become malignant. It has been reported that if the condition is identified and treated before delivery, the maternal mortality is reduced, especially if alpha-adrenergic blockade has been used. Treatment with alpha-adrenergic blockade (phenoxybenzamine) with or without addition of beta-adrenergic blockade is compatible with normal fetal survival. Given adequate medical treatment, tumor resection (preferably laparoscopically) can be successfully accomplished early in pregnancy, at delivery or at a later elective date. Women with severe pre-eclampsia and extremely unstable hypertension, tachycardia without obvious cause or very early-onset pre-eclampsia should at least be screened for pheochromocytoma.

Coarctation of the aorta (see Chapter 5 for more details) may present for the first time in pregnancy or after earlier surgical correction. In the latter case, the advisability of a pregnancy depends more on related factors such as associated cardiac malformation than on the presence of the coarctation. A previous successful resection is not a contraindication to undertaking pregnancy but consideration of the possible long-term complications following a previous repair should be undertaken. They include recurrent hypertension, recoarctation, repair site aneurysms, and aortic root problems, which are best reassessed before pregnancy. Surgical resection during pregnancy is not advisable, but has been reported.

Cushing's syndrome is rare in pregnancy especially because it is associated with amenorrhea. It usually presents in pregnant women with hypertension, often associated with diabetes and other clinical features [116] (see Chapter 13 for more details). Diagnosis should take account of the increased urinary free cortisol of normal pregnancy associated with some blunting of its diurnal variation. Suppression of cortisol production by dexamethasone is the appropriate diagnostic test although normally this is less complete than in nonpregnant subjects. There is a relatively high incidence of primary adrenal tumors, including carcinoma in rare instances. For these reasons, surgical exploration and removal should be considered once the diagnosis is made.

Conn's syndrome or hyperaldosteronism is also rare in pregnancy [117] and is also discussed in detail in Chapter 13. It has usually been diagnosed on the basis of hypokalemia combined with hypertension. The diagnosis should be considered in any hypertensive women with persistent, otherwise unexplained hypokalemia. During pregnancy, both plasma concentrations and urinary excretion of aldosterone are increased which makes diagnosis difficult. Remission of the disorder may occur during pregnancy, possibly caused by progesterone, which antagonizes the renal action of aldosterone but then presents as postpartum hypertension. Successful pregnancies with and without medical treatment have been reported.

Renovascular hypertension in pregnancy may be due to stenosis, thrombosis or embolism and is one of the most common secondary causes of hypertension in women of reproductive age. The diagnosis needs to be considered for atypical severe hypertension. Renal bruits (audible when listening to the abdomen or flanks) may be present but lack both sensitivity and specificity. Renal ultrasound may reveal one or two small kidneys. Diagnosis can be made with duplex Doppler ultrasound (in very experienced hands), renal angiography, magnetic resonance angiography or spiral CT with CT angiography. Percutaneous renal artery angioplasty has been safely completed during pregnancy.

Hypercalcemia, thyroid disease, sleep apnea, cocaine or alcohol use and any underlying renal disease may also cause secondary hypertension and are discussed in the relevant chapters. A simple screening approach to this considerable list of possible underlying causes of hypertension is provided in Chapter 42.

The fetus in hypertensive pregnancies

When compared to normotensive pregnancies, the fetus and newborn are at increased risk of adverse outcomes when gestation is complicated by hypertension, whether pre-existing CHT, gestational hypertension (GH), pre-eclampsia or pre-eclampsia superimposed on chronic hypertension.

It is now thought that decreased blood flow to the uteroplacental bed, secondary to abnormal placentation, is central to the pathophysiology of pre-eclampsia (see above). In some cases the lack of oxygen and nutrients causes intrauterine fetal growth restriction that, in severe cases, can result in intrauterine fetal death. With enhanced fetal surveillance, the baby can often be delivered prior to severe compromise or death, but may then have to cope with the consequences of prematurity – respiratory distress syndrome, bronchopulmonary dysplasia, intraventricular hemorrhage, necrotizing enterocolitis, hearing or visual deficits, cerebral palsy and neurodevelopmental delay. Fetal mortality and morbidity are highest when hypertension is severe and levels of proteinuria high.

Risks to the fetus

Intrauterine fetal growth restriction

Overall, fetal growth restriction is thought to occur in about 30% of women with pre-eclampsia [118]. Ray [119] studied 1948 (9%) of 21,723 singleton gestations which were complicated by hypertension. The incidence of small for gestational age (SGA) newborns, defined as a birthweight below the 10th centile for age, was 9.6% in women with GH, 12.2% in CHT, 25.9% in pre-eclampsia alone and 24.4% when pre-eclampsia was superimposed on CHT. Lydakis [120] reported incidences of 19.7%, 29.6%, 21% and 17.6% respectively. In another report of 598 pregnancies [121], SGA was present in 6.5% in mild GH, 4.8% in mild pre-eclampsia and 11.4% in severe pre-eclampsia. In isolated CHT the odds ratio for fetal growth restriction ranges from 2.0 to 4.4 [122–124]. McCowan [125] and Sibai [126] found higher rates of IUGR in pregnancies complicated by pre-eclampsia superimposed on CHT than in isolated CHT. When compared to women with gestational hypertension alone, women with CHT have less risk of delivering a small baby [127].

Pre-eclampsia and gestational hypertension that occur earlier in pregnancy are more likely to be associated with IUGR and SGA than when these conditions occur close to term. Clausson et al. found that SGA babies were seen in 40.5% of women with pre-eclampsia prior to 32 weeks, 17.4% at 33–36 weeks and 2.3% at >37 weeks [128].

Gestational age is the factor most highly correlated with outcome in preterm infants. At one time it was thought that growth-restricted preterm babies fared better in the neonatal intensive care unit than normally grown infants of the same gestational age. Now that gestational age can be assessed more accurately, it is known that growth-restricted newborns actually have more problems than gestationally age-matched, normally grown infants [129]. Short-term problems include hypoglycemia, hypothermia and necrotizing enterocolitis. In addition, being born small is now known to be associated with an increased risk of hypertension and glucose intolerance later in life [130].

Preterm birth

The major cause of perinatal morbidity and mortality, prematurity, is primarily from spontaneous preterm labor or preterm, premature rupture of membranes. However, up to 30% of preterm births are iatrogenic, indicated deliveries [131] and hypertension is involved in up to 40% of them [132].

Several authors have reported that in the setting of CHT, the odds ratio of delivering at <37 weeks was 1.8–2.4 [122–124]. Buchbinder [121] found that the incidence of preterm birth in pregnancies complicated by hypertension was 6.2% in women with mild GH, 25.8% with mild pre-eclampsia and 66.7% in severe pre-eclampsia. The odds ratio for delivery <37 weeks was 3.8 (95% CI 3.3–4.5) and 3.0 (95% CI 2.2–4.2) for delivery <32 weeks in women with pre-eclampsia compared to normotensive women. The incidence of preterm birth <32 weeks was 4.4% in presence of GH, 5.1% with mild CHT, 28.5% with severe pre-eclampsia and 30.5% where pre-eclampsia was superimposed on CHT. McCowan [125] and Sibai [126] also found higher rates of preterm birth in women with pre-eclampsia superimposed on CHT than women with isolated pre-eclampsia.

Abruption

Abruption is involved in 0.5% of all births >35 weeks gestation, 5.8% of all births <35 weeks but 11.9% of indicated preterm births <35 weeks gestation [134]. Buchbinder [121] found abruption occurred in 1.3% of women with mild GH, 3.2% in mild pre-eclampsia and 6.7% in severe pre-eclampsia. In the setting of CHT, 0.7–3.0% suffer abruption [123,125–127] but when superimposed pre-eclampsia is present, rates increase to 3–12% [125–127].

Perinatal death

Perinatal mortality increases as the maximum diastolic pressure rises above 90 mmHg even when controlled for various confounders and in the absence of proteinuria or CHT. Ray [119] found that perinatal morbidity or mortality occurs in 25.4% of women with GH, 25.5% with isolated CHT, 59.7% in pre-eclampsia and 57.6% when pre-eclampsia was superimposed on CHT. Perinatal mortality was 28.1/1000 in 211 women

with mild CHT, but most deaths occurred in the setting of superimposed pre-eclampsia, while in women without superimposed pre-eclampsia there was only one perinatal death [134].

In summary, the rates of perinatal morbidity and mortality are increased whenever pregnancy is complicated by hypertension, but are the highest when pre-eclampsia develops in a woman with chronic hypertension. Risks are also high in women with pre-eclampsia who were previously normotensive.

Effects on the fetus from the treatment of hypertension in pregnancy

Treating mild to moderate chronic hypertension has not been shown to improve perinatal outcomes [135]. In fact, treatment may have the adverse effect of decreasing birthweight. In a recent meta-analysis, von Dadelzson et al. [136] have shown that there is a direct relationship between the decrease in maternal blood pressure and birthweight. Moreover, there is an apparent inverse association of adverse outcomes with maternal blood pressure in the absence of hypertensive disease. One study found an increase in the rate of stillbirth when the highest maternal diastolic BP was <70 [138] and another reported a higher risk of preterm birth if blood pressure was controlled to near normal levels than if women were allowed to remain mildly hypertensive [127].

Surveillance of the fetus during hypertensive pregnancy

There is a consensus that fetuses of pregnancies complicated by hypertension should be followed carefully to detect signs of growth restriction or fetal compromise, although recommendations vary widely on which tests, how often and when.

The Royal College of Obstetricians and Gynaecologists [138] recommends that for mild gestational hypertension, "… a clinical appraisal of fetal size and well-being (i.e. abdominal palpation, fundal height measurement and inquiry into fetal movements)" should be done. The document further states that "… scan assessment of fetal growth and liquor volume and assessment by cardiotocography (or other means, e.g. Doppler ultrasound as favoured locally) of fetal well-being" is appropriate "when BP elevations are >25 mmHg increase of diastolic BP over baseline values or sustained >100."

The American College of Obstetricians and Gynecologists (ACOG) states that adverse outcomes in women with chronic hypertension are mostly due to superimposed pre-eclampsia and/or fetal growth restriction and therefore "antepartum fetal assessment should be directed at early detection of superimposed pre-eclampsia and fetal growth restriction. If these are not present then extensive antepartum testing is less essential." The ACOG [139] recommends an ultrasound at 18–20 weeks and monthly assessment of growth thereafter, usually by ultrasound. If there is evidence of fetal growth restriction, then other methods of antepartum fetal assessment should be employed including nonstress tests, contraction stress tests and/or biophysical profile (BPP). If pre-eclampsia cannot be excluded then the most prudent approach is to follow the recommendations for pre-eclampsia, but "If the infant is normally grown and pre-eclampsia can be excluded, however, there is no indication for these studies."

When pre-eclampsia is diagnosed, whether in the setting of CHT or not, an ultrasound should be performed to assess fetal growth and amniotic fluid volume [139]. If these are normal then a repeat scan should be done every 2–3 weeks. In addition, a cardiotocogram (nonstress test), ultrasound of fetal activity and amniotic fluid volume, i.e. BPP and/or fetal movement counts are often used.

Umbilical artery Doppler ultrasound is also used to assess fetal well-being. The frequency of formal testing varies with the clinical condition and gestational age, but is usually once or twice weekly. In the setting of no abnormality of fetal growth or fluid volume and normal fetal heart rate monitoring, then tests need be repeated only weekly.

In the presence of GH (hypertension, with no proteinuria, normal laboratory values and no symptoms), the ACOG [139] suggests an ultrasound for growth and fluid volume at the time of diagnosis. If normal, then a repeat ultrasound for growth and/or fluid need only be done if there is a change in maternal condition. If the clinical condition of a woman with any diagnosis of hypertension deteriorates or the estimated fetal weight is <10th percentile for gestational age or the amniotic fluid index is less than 5 cm, then testing should be twice weekly at a minimum.

Delivery

Although continuing the pregnancy to gain further growth and maturation of the fetus is desirable, there are situations where delivery cannot be postponed. These include absence of fetal growth over a 1–2-week interval, cardiotocogram with decreased to absent variability, an abnormal BPP and absent or reverse diastolic flow on Doppler assessment of the umbilical artery. The decision to deliver is greatly influenced by gestational age. At early gestational ages the risks of prematurity may outweigh the risks of remaining *in utero* while later in gestation, when the risks of prematurity are less, the decision to delivery may be made more promptly.

Anesthesia concerns for women with pre-eclampsia

Recent editions of the Confidential Enquiries into Maternal and Child Health (CEMACH) have highlighted the need for a multidisciplinary approach to the management of high-risk pregnancy [20]. Hypertensive disease remains one of the leading causes of maternal mortality and consequently effective communication and team working are vital. Early referral and assessment by a senior obstetric anesthesiologist are recommended, allowing adequate time to discuss labor analgesia and where necessary anesthesia for cesarean section. When requesting anesthetic assessment, it is helpful to signify the severity of the condition and current treatment, and the time frame for labor and delivery as these determine anesthetic management. If vaginal delivery is planned, a discussion with the patient of the various methods of analgesia and their suitability is helpful. For cesarean section, assessment to determine the most appropriate technique is required. To help in the decision-making process, up-to-date blood tests should be available to check for thrombocytopenia, clotting status and renal function. Where there is significant impairment of coagulation, not uncommon in severe hypertensive disease, regional blocks are contraindicated for fear of producing an epidural hematoma and neurologic damage.

Labor analgesia

Regional analgesia is recommended in labor for women with hypertensive disease. It provides superior pain relief when compared to systemic or inhalational analgesia [140] and prevents further surges in blood pressure associated with autonomic activity. Epidural analgesia promotes uteroplacental blood flow [141] and results in improved umbilical blood gases [142]. Furthermore, epidural analgesia in labor can be easily extended to provide regional anesthesia for instrumental delivery or cesarean section.

For women with severe hypertension, a recent platelet count should be performed to assess the suitability of regional analgesia. Ideally this should be performed on admission to the labor ward and repeated every 6 hours. Both the absolute number and rate of decline may guide the anesthetist as to safety of the procedure. If the total platelet count is below 80×10^9/L or the number has dropped by more than 50×10^9/L in the previous 12 hours, many anesthesiologists are not prepared to perform a regional block. Faced with such results, the risks and benefits should be assessed on an individual basis by senior clinicians [143]. It is important for obstetricians to recognize that the risk of epidural hematoma exists with both insertion and subsequent removal of the catheter. It is therefore important that anesthesiologists consider the trend in platelet count as the number at removal is important as the number at the time of insertion. Other assessments of coagulation such as bleeding times, thromboelastography and platelet function analyzers have failed to gain widespread popularity. A further assessment of coagulation is also necessary before removing an epidural catheter for the reason mentioned above.

Early placement of an epidural catheter and the administration of low-dose local anesthetic and opioid mixture is not associated with an increase in obstetric intervention [141]. Intravenous fluid preloading, which carries the risk of pulmonary edema especially in the pre-eclamptic patient, is not required to prevent maternal hypotension when low-dose regimens are used. Once established, analgesia may be maintained with intermittent boluses, continuous infusion or patient-controlled epidural analgesia (PCEA). The use of a continuous infusion may reduce the incidence of hypotension although at the expense of greater total drug administration.

Cesarean section anesthesia

The decision on whether to use regional or general anesthesia is based on both the clinical features of the underlying disease and the urgency for surgery. Regional block is preferred as it is considered to be associated with reduced maternal mortality. General anesthesia is usually used only when regional techniques are contraindicated, have failed or there is inadequate time to perform a block. In the presence of pulmonary edema, general anesthesia may also be preferred.

Epidural anesthesia has traditionally been the preferred technique, with small incremental dosing considered to provide greater control of maternal blood pressure whilst maintaining placental blood flow. With early placement of an epidural catheter in labor, analgesia may be readily extended if cesarean section is required. There have been concerns that the rapid onset of spinal anesthesia might cause profound maternal hypotension as a result of the sympathectomy in the presence of a reduced intravascular volume. However, recent studies have found this not to be so, and that hypotension is less frequent with spinal anesthesia in the hypertensive patient [144,145] and that neonatal outcome is not impaired [146]. It should be noted that in these studies, the mixed alpha- and beta-agonist ephedrine was used to treat maternal hypotension and pure alpha-agonists such as phenylephrine and metaraminol, which produce less umbilical arterial acidosis in studies in healthy pregnancy [147], are now more widely used. The effects of pure alpha-agonists in hypertensive disease are currently under evaluation.

General anesthesia has additional risks in the hypertensive patient. Transient but severe hypertension may occur during laryngoscopy and intubation. A number of intravenous agents have been tried to attenuate this response including labetalol, short-acting opioids such as alfenantil and remifentanil, magnesium, lidocaine and nitrates. The choice of agent is usually dictated by local policy. Difficulty with tracheal intubation is more common in pregnancy and airway management may be more challenging in the hypertensive patient as a result of airway edema. Upper airway narrowing is increased in pre-eclampsia [148] and the anesthesiologist must be prepared with appropriate equipment for difficult intubation. Magnesium therapy interferes with pre- and postsynaptic neuromuscular transmission and so doses of nondepolarizing muscle relaxant should be reduced and their effect monitored

with a peripheral nerve stimulator. The combined tocolytic effects of magnesium and volatile anesthetic agents increase the risk of uterine atony for which an oxytocic infusion is usually necessary.

Intravenous fluids must be given with great caution in the peri- and postoperative period regardless of which anesthetic technique is employed. Preloading the circulation with large volumes, a common practice in healthy parturients, should be avoided to minimize the risk of precipitating pulmonary edema, especially when renal function is compromised. Invasive hemodynamic monitoring may be warranted in severe hypertension but its place is controversial. Noninvasive blood pressure techniques have a tendency to overestimate blood pressure when it is low and underestimate when high. Invasive arterial pressure is therefore helpful in refractory hypertension and during induction of anesthesia. It provides real-time representation of maternal hemodynamics and enables repeated samples to be taken for blood gas analysis. As with noninvasive techniques, mean arterial pressure is the most accurate measurement. Central venous pressure (CVP) may help guide management in the oliguric patient, although excessive fluid administration, in an effort to increase CVP, may precipitate pulmonary edema. This results from low oncotic pressure secondary to loss of plasma proteins and the presence of endothelial damage which facilitates passage of fluid into the lung interstitium. In the presence of impaired coagulation, peripherally inserted central venous access may be safer as inadvertent arterial puncture is avoided. The role of pulmonary artery catheters in pre-eclampsia is more controversial as their use does not appear to influence maternal and neonatal outcome.

All patients receiving either general or regional anesthesia must receive appropriate postoperative care, which may range from admission to an ICU to routine recovery room care. For the latter, location may vary depending on local facilities but should conform to national standards. Measurements of pulse, blood pressure, respiratory rate, temperature and oxygen saturation should be documented in addition to an assessment of analgesia. Supplemental oxygen is given as required and intravenous fluids and analgesics should be prescribed. Assessment of risk for thromboembolic disease and uterine atony should be made and heparin and oxytocin used as indicated.

The provision of postoperative pain relief is more challenging in the hypertensive patient. Effective analgesia facilitates blood pressure control and allows early ambulation, thereby decreasing the risk of thromboembolism. Pain is initially controlled with either spinal opioids, if a regional technique has been used, or alternatively with intravenous opioids, usually with a patient-controlled analgesia device. Supplemental acetaminophen reduces opioid requirements but nonsteriodal anti-inflammatory drugs should not be given if there is evidence of renal impairment. Not infrequently, deterioration in clotting mechanisms follows delivery and if an epidural catheter has been sited for labor or delivery, it should not be removed until coagulation has returned to normal.

Conclusions

- Hypertension is a sign, not a disorder.
- Hypertension in pregnancy arises from the pregnancy-specific disorder of pre-eclampsia or a long-term maternal attribute, most commonly CHT, or a new medical cause of secondary hypertension.
- New-onset or worsening hypertension in pregnancy is not pre-eclampsia. It may signify a prodromal phase that evolves into pre-eclampsia or underlying long-term hypertension revealed by the pregnancy.
- Pre-eclampsia arises from a systemic inflammatory response that causes endothelial dysfunction. The response is common to all pregnancies, and pre-eclampsia is simply the extreme end of the spectrum.
- With pre-eclampsia, the main differential diagnosis is from CHT which in its pure form does not share the renal, coagulation, hepatic and placental abnormalities of pre-eclampsia.
- The principal perinatal risks of CHT in pregnancy result from superimposed pre-eclampsia.
- Extreme hypertension in pregnancy ($\geq 160/110$ mmHg) is as dangerous as it is in any other medical situation and demands urgent treatment.
- There is no case for antihypertensive treatment for mild to moderate hypertension (140–155/90–105 mmHg). There is evidence that long-term antihypertensive treatment in pregnancy causes a degree of fetal growth restriction.
- Methyldopa is the most thoroughly tested antihypertensive agent in pregnancy. Beta-blocking agents are safe for short-term use but cause significant fetal growth restriction if administered over longer periods (from the second trimester onwards).
- Nifedipine and labetalol appear to be safe.
- Diuretics should primarily be reserved for the treatment of heart failure complicating pre-eclampsia.
- ACE inhibitors and angiotensin receptor blockers are contraindicated for use in pregnancy because of teratogenesis and adverse effects on fetal renal function.

References

1. Clapp JF, Capeless E. Cardiovascular function before, during, and after the first and subsequent pregnancies. Am J Cardiol 1997;80:1469–73.
2. van Oppen AC, Stigter RH, Bruinse HW. Cardiac output in normal pregnancy: a critical review. Obstet Gynecol 1996;87:310–18.
3. Lanni SM, Tillinghast J, Silver HM. Hemodynamic changes and baroreflex gain in the supine hypotensive syndrome. Am J Obstet Gynecol 2002;187:1636–41.
4. MacGillivray I, Rose GA, Rowe B. Blood pressure survey in pregnancy. Clin Sci 1969;37:395–407.
5. Brown MA, Robinson A, Bowyer L, et al. Ambulatory blood pressure monitoring in pregnancy: what is normal? Am J Obstet Gynecol 1998;178:836–42.
6. Higgins JR, Walshe JJ, Halligan A O'Brien E, Conroy R, Darling MR. Can 24-hour ambulatory blood pressure measurement predict the development of hypertension in primigravidae? Br J Obstet Gynaecol 1997;104:356–62.
7. Davey DA, MacGillivray I. The classification and definition of the hypertensive disorders of pregnancy. Am J Obstet Gynecol 1988;158: 892–8.
8. Zhang J, Meikle S, Trumble A. Severe maternal morbidity associated with hypertensive disorders in pregnancy in the United States. Hypertens Pregnancy 2003;22:203–12.
9. Redman CW. Current topic: pre-eclampsia and the placenta. Placenta 1991;12:301–8.
10. Redman CW, Sargent IL. Latest advances in understanding pre-eclampsia. Science 2005;308:1592–4.
11. Lain KY, Roberts JM. Contemporary concepts of the pathogenesis and management of pre-eclampsia. JAMA 2002;287:3183–6.
12. Pijnenborg R, Vercruysse L, Hanssens M. The uterine spiral arteries in human pregnancy: facts and controversies. Placenta 2006;27:939–58.
13. Roberts JM, Taylor RN, Musci TJ, Rodgers GM, Hubel CA, McLaughlin MK. Pre-eclampsia: an endothelial cell disorder. Am J Obstet Gynecol 1989;161:1200–4.
14. Widmer M, Villar J, Benigni A, Conde-Agudelo A, Karumanchi SA, Lindheimer M. Mapping the theories of pre-eclampsia and the role of angiogenic factors: a systematic review. Obstet Gynecol 2007;109:168–80.
15. Venkatesha S, Toporsian M, Lam C, et al. Soluble endoglin contributes to the pathogenesis of pre-eclampsia. Nat Med 2006;12:642–9.
16. Gaber LW, Spargo BH, Lindheimer MD. Renal pathology in pre-eclampsia. Baillière's Clin Obstet Gynaecol 1994;8:443–68.
17. Redman CW, Sacks GP, Sargent IL. Pre-eclampsia: an excessive maternal inflammatory response to pregnancy. Am J Obstet Gynecol 1999;180:499–506.
18. Ness RB, Roberts JM. Heterogeneous causes constituting the single syndrome of pre-eclampsia: a hypothesis and its implications. Am J Obstet Gynecol 1996;175:1365–70.
19. Redman CW, Beilin LJ, Bonnar J. Variability of blood pressure in normal and abnormal pregnancy . In: Lindheimer MD, Katz AI, Zuspan FP (eds) Hypertension in pregnancy. John Wiley, New York, 1976: 53–60.
20. CEMACH. Why mothers die 2000–2002. RCOG Press, London, 2004.
21. Jeyabalan A, Conrad KP. Renal function during normal pregnancy and pre-eclampsia. Front Biosci 2007;12:2425–37.
22. Fisher KA, Ahuja S, Luger A, Spargo B, Lindheimer M. Nephrotic proteinuria with pre-eclampsia. Am J Obstet Gynecol 1977;129: 643–6.
23. Taufield PA, Ales KL, Resnick LM, Druzin ML, Gertner JM, Laragh JH. Hypocalciuria in pre-eclampsia. N Engl J Med 1987;316:715–18.
24. Lafayette RA, Druzin M, Sibley R, et al. Nature of glomerular dysfunction in pre-eclampsia. Kidney Int 1998;54:1240–9.
25. Gallery ED, Saunders DM, Hunyor SN, Gyory AZ. Randomised comparison of methyldopa and oxprenolol for treatment of hypertension in pregnancy. BMJ 1979;1:1591–4.
26. Cedergren M. Effects of gestational weight gain and Body Mass Index on obstetric outcome in Sweden. Int J Gynaecol Obstet 2006;93:269–74.
27. Tuffnell DJ, Jankowicz D, Lindow SW, et al. Yorkshire Obstetric Critical Care Group. Outcomes of severe pre-eclampsia/eclampsia in Yorkshire 1999/2003. Br J Obstet Gynaecol 2005; 112:875–80.
28. Sibai BM, Ramadan MK, Usta I, et al. Maternal morbidity and mortality in 442 pregnancies with hemolysis, elevated liver enzymes, and low platelets HELLP syndrome. Am J Obstet Gynecol 1993;169:1000–6.

29. Weinstein L. Syndrome of hemolysis, elevated liver enzymes, low platelet count: a severe consequence of hypertension on pregnancy. Am J Obstet Gynecol 1982;142:159–67.

30. Araujo AC, Leao MD, Nobrega MH, et al. Characteristics and treatment of hepatic rupture caused by HELLP syndrome. Am J Obstet Gynecol 2006;195:129–33.

31. Dani R, Mendes GS, Medeiros JD, Peret FJ, Nunes A. Study of the liver changes occurring in pre-eclampsia and their possible pathogenetic connection with acute fatty liver of pregnancy. Am J Gastroenterol 1996;91:292–4.

32. Hinchey J, Chaves C. Appignani B, et al. A reversible posterior leukoencephalopathy syndrome. N Engl J Med 1996;334:494–500.

33. Lamy C, Oppenheim C, Meder JF, Mas JL. Neuroimaging in posterior reversible encephalopathy syndrome. J Neuroimaging 2004;14:89–96.

34. Oehm E, Hetzel A, Els T, et al. Cerebral hemodynamics and autoregulation in reversible posterior leukoencephalopathy syndrome caused by pre-/eclampsia. Cerebrovasc Dis 2006;22:204–8.

35. Zeeman GG, Hatab MR, Twickler DM. Increased cerebral blood flow in pre-eclampsia with magnetic resonance imaging. Am J Obstet Gynecol 2004;191:1425–9.

36. Khan KS, Wojdyla D, Say L, Gulmezoglu AM, van Look PF. WHO analysis of causes of maternal death: a systematic review. Lancet 2006;367:1066–74.

37. Moodley J. Maternal deaths associated with hypertensive disorders of pregnancy: a population-based study. Hypertens Pregnancy 2004;23:247–56.

38. Tucker MJ, Berg CJ, Callaghan WM, Hsia J. The black-white disparity in pregnancy-related mortality from 5 conditions: differences in prevalence and case-fatality rates. Am J Public Health 2007;97:247–51.

39. Duckitt K, Harrington D. Risk factors for pre-eclampsia at antenatal booking: systematic review of controlled studies. BMJ 2005;330:565.

40. Kaaja R, Laivuori H, Laakso M, Tikkanen MJ, Ylikorkala O. Evidence of a state of increased insulin resistance in pre-eclampsia. Metabolism 1999;48:892–6.

41. Robertson L, Wu O, Langhorne P, et al. The Thrombosis: Risk and Economic Assessment of Thrombophilia Screening (TREATS) Study. Thrombophilia in pregnancy: a systematic review. Br J Haematol 2006;132:171–96.

42. Butler NR, Bonham DG. Perinatal mortality. E and S Livingstone, Edinburgh, 1963

43. Zabriskie JR. Effect of cigarette smoking during pregnancy. Study of 2000 cases. Obstet Gynecol 1963;21:405–11.

44. Barden A. Pre-eclampsia: contribution of maternal constitutional factors and the consequences for cardiovascular health. Clin Exp Pharmacol Physiol 2006;33:826–30.

45. American College of Obstetrics and Gynecology. Hypertension in pregnancy. Technical Bulletin Number 21. American College of Obstetrics and Gynecology, Washington, DC, 1996.

46. Australasian Society for the Study of Hypertension Consensus Statement. Management of hypertension in pregnancy: executive summary. Australasian Society for the Study of Hypertension in Pregnancy. Med J Aust 1993;158: 700–2.

47. Hill JO. Understanding and addressing the epidemic of obesity: an energy balance perspective. Endocr Rev 2006;27:750–61.

48. Campbell DM, MacGillivray I. Pre-eclampsia in twin pregnancies: incidence and outcome. Hypertens Pregnancy 1999;18:197–207.

49. Basso O, Rasmussen S, Weinberg CR, Wilcox AJ, Irgens LM, Skjaerven R. Trends in fetal and infant survival following pre-eclampsia. JAMA 2006;296:1357–62.

50. Saftlas AF, Olson DR, Franks AL, Atrash HK, Pokras R. Epidemiology of pre-eclampsia and eclampsia in the United States, 1979–1986. Am J Obstet Gynecol 1990;163:460–5.

51. Douglas KA, Redman CWG. Eclampsia in the United Kingdom. BMJ 1994;309:1395–400.

52. Nelson TR. A clinical study of pre-eclampsia. J Obstet Gynaecol Br Emp 1955;62:48–57.

53. Lindheimer MD, Spargo BH, Katz AI. Eclampsia during the 16th week of gestation. J Am Med Assoc 1974;230:1006–8.

54. Hirshfeld-Cytron J, Lam C, Karumanchi SA, Lindheimer M. Late postpartum eclampsia: examples and review. Obstet Gynecol Surv 2006;61:471–80.

55. Villar J, Say L, Shennan A, et al. Methodological and technical issues related to the diagnosis, screening, prevention, and treatment of pre-eclampsia and eclampsia. Int J Gynaecol Obstet 2004;85(suppl 1): S28–S41.

56. Lyell DJ, Lambert-Messerlian GM, Giudice LC. Prenatal screening, epidemiology, diagnosis, and management of pre-eclampsia. Clin Lab Med 2003;23:413–42.

57. Papageorghiou AT, Roberts N. Uterine artery Doppler screening for adverse pregnancy outcome. Curr Opin Obstet Gynecol 2005;17:584–90.

58. Levine RJ, Lam C, Qian C, et al. CPEP Study Group. Soluble endoglin and other circulating antiangiogenic factors in pre-eclampsia. N Engl J Med 2006;355:992–1005.

59. Stepan H, Unversucht A, Wessel N, Faber R. Predictive value of maternal angiogenic factors in second trimester pregnancies with abnormal uterine perfusion. Hypertension 2007;49:818–24.

60. Staboulidou I, Soergel P, Schippert C, Hertel H, Hillemanns P, Scharf A. The significance of uterine notching in Doppler sonography in early pregnancy as a predictor for pathologic outcome of the pregnancy. Arch Gynecol Obstet 2007;276(1):21–8.

61. Stella CL, Sibai BM. Pre-eclampsia: diagnosis and management of the atypical presentation. J Matern Fetal Neonatal Med 2006;19:381–6.

62. Redman CWG, Jefferies M. Revised definition of pre-eclampsia. Lancet 1988;1:809–12.

63. Levine RJ, Ewell MG, Hauth JC, et al. Should the definition of pre-eclampsia include a rise in diastolic blood pressure of >/=15 mm Hg to a level <90 mm Hg in association with proteinuria? Am J Obstet Gynecol 2000;183:787–92.

64. Chesley LC, Annitto JE. Pregnancy in the patient with hypertensive disease. Am J Obstet Gynecol 1947;53:372–81.

65. North RA, Taylor RS, Schellenberg JC. Evaluation of a definition of pre-eclampsia. Br Obstet Gynaecol 1999;106:767–73.

66. Cnossen JS, de Ruyter-Hanhijarvi H, van der Post JA, Mol BW, Khan KS, ter Riet G. Accuracy of serum uric acid determination in predicting pre-eclampsia: a systematic review. Acta Obstet Gynecol Scand 2006;85:519–25.

67. Roberts JM, Bodnar LM, Lain KY, et al. Uric acid is as important as proteinuria in identifying fetal risk in women with gestational hypertension. Hypertension 2005;46:1263–9.

68. Broughton Pipkin F. Uric acid, endothelial dysfunction and pre-eclampsia. J Hypertens 2004;22:237–9.

69. Audibert F, Friedman SA, Frangieh AY, Sibai BM. Clinical utility of strict diagnostic criteria for the HELLP (hemolysis, elevated liver enzymes, and low platelets) syndrome. Am J Obstet Gynecol 1996;175:460–4.

70. Martin JN Jr, Thigpen BD, Moore RC, Rose CH, Cushman J, May W. Stroke and severe pre-eclampsia and eclampsia: a paradigm shift focusing on systolic blood pressure. Obstet Gynecol 2005;105(2):246–54.

71. Magee LA, Cham C, Waterman EJ, Ohlsson A, von Dadelszen P. Hydralazine for treatment of severe hypertension in pregnancy: meta-analysis. BMJ 2003;327:955–60.

72. Duley L, Henderson-Smart DJ, Meher S. Drugs for treatment of very high blood pressure during pregnancy. Cochrane Database of Systematic Review, 2006;3:CD001449.

73. Magee LA, Miremadi S, Li J, *et al*. Therapy with both magnesium sulfate and nifedipine does not increase the risk of serious magnesium-related maternal side effects in women with pre-eclampsia. Am J Obstet Gynecol 2005;193:153–63.

74. van Geijn HP, Lenglet JE, Bolte AC. Nifedipine trials: effectiveness and safety aspects. Br J Obstet Gynaecol 2005;112(suppl 1):79–83.

75. Odendaal HJ, Pattinson RC, Bam R, Grove D, Kotze TJ. Aggressive or expectant management for patients with severe pre-eclampsia between 28 and 34 weeks' gestation: a randomized controlled trial. Obstet Gynecol 1990;76:1070–5.

76. Sibai BM, Mercer BM, Schiff E, Friedman SA. Aggressive versus expectant management of severe pre-eclampsia at 28–32 weeks' gestation: a randomized controlled trial. Am J Obstet Gynecol 1994;171:818–22.

77. Podymow T, August P. Hypertension in pregnancy. Adv Chronic Kidney Dis 2007;14:178–90.

78. Ganzevoort W, Rep A, Bonsel GJ, *et al*. A randomised controlled trial comparing two temporising management strategies, one with and one without plasma volume expansion, for severe and early onset pre-eclampsia. Br J Obstet Gynaecol 2005;112:1358–68.

79. Sibai B, Dekker G, Kupferminc M. Pre-eclampsia. Lancet 2005;365:785–99.

80. Collaborative Eclampsia Trial. Which anticonvulsant for women with eclampsia? Evidence from the Collaborative Eclampsia Trial. Lancet 1995;345:1455–63.

81. Altman D, Carroli G, Duley L, *et al*. Do women with pre-eclampsia, and their babies, benefit from magnesium sulphate? The Magpie Trial: a randomised placebo-controlled trial. Lancet 2002;359:1877–90.

82. Pritchard JA, Cunningham F, Pritchard SA. The Parkland Memorial Hospital protocol for treatment of eclampsia: evaluation of 245 cases. Am J Obstet Gynecol 1984;148:951–63.

83. Swartjes JM, Schutte MF, Bleker OP. Management of eclampsia: cardiopulmonary arrest resulting from magnesium sulfate overdose. Eur J Obstet Gynecol Reprod Biol 1992;47:73–5.

84. Herpolsheimer A, Brady K, Yancey MK, Pandian M, Duff P. Pulmonary function of preeclamptic women receiving intravenous magnesium sulfate seizure prophylaxis. Obstet Gynecol 1991;78:241–4.

85. Bruner JP, Yeast JD. Pregnancy associated with Friedreich ataxia. Obstet Gynecol 1990;76:976–7.

86. Witlin AG, Sibai BM. Magnesium sulfate therapy in pre-eclampsia and eclampsia. Obstet Gynecol 1998;92:883–9.

87. Fuentes A, Rojas A, Porter KB, Saviello G, O'Brien WF. The effect of magnesium sulfate on bleeding time in pregnancy. Am J Obstet Gynecol 1995;173:1246–9.

88. Cruikshank DP, Chan GM, Doerrfeld D. Alterations in vitamin D and calcium metabolism with magnesium sulfate treatment of pre-eclampsia. Am J Obstet Gynecol 1993;168:1170–6.

89. Riaz M, Porat R, Brodsky NL, Hurt H. The effects of maternal magnesium sulfate treatment on newborns: a prospective controlled study. J Perinatol 1998;18:449–54.

90. Hiett AK, Devoe LD, Brown HL, Watson J. Effect of magnesium on fetal heart rate variability using computer analysis. Am J Perinatol 1995;12:259–61.

91. Churchill D, Beevers G, Meher S, Rhodes C. Diuretics for preventing pre-eclampsia. Cochrane Database of Systematic Reviews, 2007;1:CD004451.

92. Askie LM, Duley L, Henderson-Smart DJ, Stewart LA, PARIS Collaborative Group. Antiplatelet agents for prevention of pre-eclampsia: a meta-analysis of individual patient data. Lancet 2007;369(9575):1791–8.

93. Hofmeyr GJ, Atallah AN, Duley L. Calcium supplementation during pregnancy for preventing hypertensive disorders and related problems. Cochrane Database of Systematic Reviews, 2006; 3: CD001059.

94. Abi Said D, Annegers JF, Combs Cantrell D, Frankowski RF, Willmore LJ. Case-control study of the risk factors for eclampsia. Am J Obstet Gynecol 1995;142:437–41.

95. Ansari MZ, Mueller BA, Krohn MA. Epidemiology of eclampsia. Eur J Epidemiol 1995;11:447–51.

96. Conde Agudelo A, Kafury GA. Case-control study of risk factors for complicated eclampsia. Obstet Gynecol 1997;90:172–5.

97. Witlin AG, Saade GR, Mattar F, Sibai BM. Risk factors for abruptio placentae and eclampsia: analysis of 445 consecutively managed women with severe pre-eclampsia and eclampsia. Am J Obstet Gynecol 1999;180:1322–9.

98. Abalos E, Duley L, Steyn D, Henderson-Smart D. Antihypertensive drug therapy for mild to moderate hypertension during pregnancy. Cochrane Database of Systematic Reviews, 2007;1:CD002252.

99. Walters BNJ, Thompson ME, Lee A, de Swiet M. Blood pressure in the puerperium. Clin Sci 1986;71:589–94.

100. Campbell DM, MacGillivray I, Carr Hill R. Pre-eclampsia in second pregnancy. Br J Obstet Gynaecol 1985;82:131–40.

101. Sibai BM, El Nazer A, Gonzalez Ruiz A. Severe pre-eclampsia-eclampsia in young primigravid women: subsequent pregnancy outcome and remote prognosis. Am J Obstet Gynecol 1986;155:1011–16.

102. Sibai BM, Ramadan MK, Chari RS, Friedman SA. Pregnancies complicated by HELLP syndrome (hemolysis, elevated liver enzymes, and low platelets): subsequent pregnancy outcome and long-term prognosis. Am J Obstet Gynecol 1995;172:125–9.

103. Sattar N, Greer IA. Pregnancy complications and maternal cardiovascular risk: opportunities for intervention and screening? BMJ 2002;325:157–60.

104. van Pampus MG, Wolf H, Weijmar Schultz WC, Neeleman J, Aarnoudse JG. Post-traumatic stress disorder following pre-eclampsia and HELLP syndrome. J Psychosom Obstet Gynaecol 2004;25:183–7.

105. Oyelese Y, Ananth CV. Placental abruption. Obstet Gynecol 2006;108:1005–16.

106. Cooper WO, Hernandez-Diaz S, Arbogast PG, *et al*. Major congenital malformations after first-trimester exposure to ACE inhibitors. N Engl J Med 2006;354:2443–51.

107. Pryde PG, Sedman AB, Nugent CE, Barr M Jr. Angiotensin-converting enzyme inhibitor fetopathy. J Am Soc Nephrol 1993;3:1575–82.

108. Cooper W, Hernandez-Diaz S, Arogast PG, *et al*. Major congenital malformations after first-trimester exposure to ACE inhibitors. N Engl J Med 2006;354:2443–51.

109. Cockburn J, Moar VA, Ounsted M, Redman CWG. Final report of study on hypertension during pregnancy: the effects of specific treatment on the growth and development of the children. Lancet 1982;1:647–9.

110. Magee LA, Duley L. Oral beta-blockers for mild to moderate hypertension during pregnancy. Cochrane Database of Systematic Reviews, 2003;3:CD002863.

111. Lip YH, Beevers SRN, Churchill D, Shaffer LM, Beevers DG. Effect of atenolol on birth weight. Am J Cardiol 1997;79:1436–8.

112. Butters L, Kennedy S, Rubin PC. Atenolol in essential hypertension during pregnancy. BMJ 1990;301:587–9.

113. Montan S, Ingermarsson I, Marsal K, Sjoberg NO. Randomised controlled trial of atenolol and pinodol in human pregnancy: effects on fetal haemodynamics. BMJ 1992;304:946–9.

114. von Dadelszen P, Ornstein MP, Bull SB, Logan AG, Koren G, Magee LA. Fall in mean arterial pressure and fetal growth restriction in pregnancy hypertension: a meta-analysis. Lancet 2000;355:87–92.

115. Ahlawat SK, Jain S, Kumari S, Varma S, Sharma BK. Pheochromocytoma associated with pregnancy: case report and review of the literature. Obstet Gynecol Surv 1999; 54:728–37.

116. Polli N, Giraldi FP, Cavagnini F. Cushing's disease and pregnancy. Pituitary 2004;7:237–41.

117. Okawa T, Asano K, Hashimoto T, Fujimori K, Yanagida K, Sato A. Diagnosis and management of primary aldosteronism in pregnancy: case report and review of the literature. Am J Perinatol 2002;19:31–6.

118. Eskenazi B, Fenster L, Sidney S, Elkin EP. Fetal growth retardation in infants of multiparous and nulliparous women with pre-eclampsia. Am J Obstet Gynecol 1993;169:1112–18.

119. Ray JG, Burrows RF, Burrows EA, Mermeulen M J. MOS HIP: McMaster outcome study of hypertension in pregnancy. Early Hum Dev 2001;64:129–43.

120. Lydakis C, Beevers M, Beevers DG, Lip G. The prevalence of pre-eclampsia and obstetric outcome in pregnancies of normotensive and hypertensive women attending a hospital specialist clinic. Int J Clin Pract 2001;55:361–7.

121. Buchbinder A, Sibai GH, Caritis S, MacPherson C, Hauth J, Lindheimer MD, et al. Adverse perinatal outcomes are significantly higher in severe gestational hypertension than in mild pre-eclampsia. Am J Obstet Gynecol 2002;186:66–71.

122. Samadi AR, Mayberry RM, Zaide AA, Pleasant JC, McGhee N, Rice RJ. Maternal hypertension and associated pregnancy complications among African-American and other women in the United States. Obstet Gynecol 1996;87:557–63.

123. Rey E, Couturier A. The prognosis of pregnancy in women with chronic hypertension. Am J Obstet Gynecol 1994;171:410–16.

124. Sibai BM, Caritis SN, Hauth JC, MacPherson C, van Dorsten JP, et al. Preterm delivery in women with pregestational diabetes mellitus or chronic hypertension relative to women with uncomplicated pregnancies. Am J Obstet Gynecol 2000;183:1520–4.

125. McCowan LME, Buist RG, North RA, Gamble G. Perinatal morbidity in chronic hypertension. Br J Obstet Gynaecol 1996;103:123–9.

126. Sibai BM, Lindheimer M, Hauth J, et al. Risk factors for pre-eclampsia, abruption placentae, and adverse neonatal outcomes among women with chronic hypertension. N Engl J Med 1998;339:667–71.

127. Magee LA, von Dadelszen P, Bohun CM, et al. Serious perinatal complications of non-proteinuric hypertension: an international, multicentre, retrospective cohort study. J Obstet Gynaecol Can 2003;25:372–82.

128. Clausson B, Cnattingius S, Axelsson O. Preterm and term births of small for gestational age infants: a population-based study of risk factors among nulliparous women. Br J Obstet Gynaecol 1998; 105:1011–17.

129. Chari RS, Friedman SA, Schiff E, Frangieh AY, Sibai B. Is fetal neurologic and physical development accelerated in pre-eclampsia? Am J Obstet Gynecol 1996;174:829–32.

130. Barker DJP, Eriksson JG, Forsen T, Osmond C. Fetal origins of adult disease: strength of effects and biological basis. Int J Epidemiol 2002;31:1235–9.

131. Savitz DA, Blackmore CA, Thorp JM. Epidemiologic characteristics of preterm delivery: etiologic heterogeneity. Am J Obstet Gynecol 1991;164:467–71.

132. Steer PJ. The epidemiology of preterm labour – why have advances not equated to reduced incidence? Br J Obstet Gynaecol 2006;113(suppl):1–3.

133. Ananth CV, Vintzileos AM. Maternal-fetal conditions necessitating a medical intervention resulting in preterm birth. Am J Obstet Gynecol 2006;195:1557–63.

134. Sibai BM, Abdella TN, Anderson GD. Pregnancy outcome in 211 patients with mild chronic hypertension. Am J Obstet Gynecol 1983;61:571–6.

135. Duley L, Henderson-Smart DJ, Meher S. Drugs for treatment of very high blood pressure during pregnancy. Cochrane Database of Systematic Reviews, 2006;3:CD001449.

136. von Dadelszen P, Magee LA. Fall in mean arterial pressure and fetal growth restriction in pregnancy hypertension: an updated metaregression analysis. J Obstet Gynaecol Can 2004;24:941–5.

137. Steer P, Little MP, Kold-Jensen T, Chapple J, Elliott P. Maternal blood pressure in pregnancy, birth weight, and perinatal mortality in first births: prospective study. BMJ 2004;329:1312–17.

138. Royal College of Obstetricians and Gynaecologists; Scottish Obstetric Guidelines and Audit Project. The management of mild, on-proteinuric hypertension in pregnancy. SPCERH Publication Number 2. Royal College of Obstetricians and Gynaecologists, London, 1997.

139. American College of Obstetricians and Gynecologists. Practice Bulletin Number 29. Chronic Hypertension in Pregnancy. American College of Obstetricians and Gynecologists, Washington, DC, 2001.

140. Halpern SH, Leighton BL, Ohlsson A, Barrett JFR, Rice A. Effect of epidural vs parenteral opioid analgesia on the progress of labor. JAMA 1998;280:2105–10.

141. Jouppila P, Jouppila R, Hollmen A, et al. Lumbar epidural analgesia to improve intervillous blood flow during labor in severe pre-eclampsia. Obstet Gynecol 1982;59:158–61.

142. Reynolds F, Sharma SK, Seed PT. Analgesia in labour and fetal acid-base balance: a meta-analysis comparing epidural with systemic opioid analgesia Br J Obstet Gynaecol 2002;109:1344–53.

143. Wong CA, Scavone BM, Peaceman AM, et al. The risk of cesarean delivery with neuraxial analgesia given early versus late in labor. N Engl J Med 2005;352:655–65.

144. Aya AGM, Mangin R, Vialles N, et al. Patients with severe pre-eclampsia experience less hypotension during spinal anesthesia for elective cesarean delivery than healthy parturients: a prospective cohort comparison. Anesth Analg 2003;97:867–72.

145. Santos AC, Birnbach DJ. Spinal anesthesia for cesarean delivery in severely preeclamptic women: don't throw out the baby with bathwater! Anesth Analg 2005;101:859–61.

146. Visalyaputra S, Rodanant O, Somboonviboon W, et al. Spinal versus epidural anesthesia for cesarean delivery in severe pre-eclampsia: a prospective randomized multicenter study. Anesth Analg 2005;101:862–8.

147. Reynolds F, Seed PT. Anaesthesia for Caesarean section and neonatal acid-base status: a meta-analysis. Anaesthesia 2005;60:636–53.

148. Iczi B, Riha RL, Martin SE, et al. The upper airway in pregnancy and pre-eclampsia. Am J Respir Crit Care Med 2003;167:137–40.

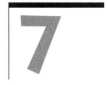

Renal disease in pregnancy

Mark A. Brown[1], *George J. Mangos*[1], *Michael Peek*[2]
with Felicity Plaat[3]

[1]Department of Renal Medicine, St George Hospital and University of New South Wales, Sydney, Australia
[2]Department of Obstetrics and Gynaecology, University of Sydney and Nepean Hospital, Sydney, Australia
[3]Department of Anaesthesia, Queen Charlotte's and Hammersmith Hospitals, London, UK

Introduction

Many women with renal disease wish to have a baby. In the past renal disease was often considered a contraindication to pregnancy, but times have changed and many women with significant renal problems now embark on a pregnancy.

This chapter provides clinicians with practical advice in relation to management and counseling of such women. We begin with a description of renal physiology and anatomic changes in normal pregnancy and relate these to clinical interpretation issues. We then focus on how to counsel the woman with known renal disease in advance of a pregnancy about likely pregnancy outcomes and how she will be managed during the pregnancy. The following sections deal with those renal problems which arise *de novo* during pregnancy and then the less common but important areas of managing women on dialysis or with a renal transplant before and throughout their pregnancy. The final section provides suggested models of care, emphasizing the team-based approach to management, integral to any successful "high-risk" pregnancy.

Changes in renal physiology in normal pregnancy

Management of renal disorders in pregnancy begins with an understanding of what changes usually occur in kidney function and structure in normal pregnancy.

Pregnancy causes a major change in systemic hemodynamics, detectable as early as 8 weeks gestation, characterized by reduced systemic vascular resistance and increased cardiac output with resting tachycardia [1]. These changes result in a small reduction in arterial blood pressure, typically reaching a nadir in the mid-trimester of about 10 mmHg systolic, rising towards pre-pregnancy levels at term.

de Swiet's Medical Disorders in Obstetric Practice, 5th edition.
Edited by R. O. Powrie, M. F. Greene, W. Camann. © 2010 Blackwell Publishing.

Renal tract anatomy

The kidneys enlarge during normal pregnancy, increasing in length (by up to 1.5 cm) and volume towards term, due to tissue hypertrophy and greater water content. More important from a clinical perspective is the increase in size of the renal pelvices and ureters, occurring in the first trimester and generally detectable by the second. Hydroureter is often observed by ultrasound, more often on the right than on the left. A number of factors are thought to be important in this change. Progesterone, a smooth muscle relaxant, reduces ureteric tone and peristalsis. The asymmetric dilation of the ureters suggests that extrinsic compression by the enlarging uterus at the pelvic brim, hypertrophy of surrounding connective tissue (Waldeyer's sheath) and kinking due to ligaments or compression by iliac blood vessels all may contribute to this change.

The clinical relevance is that these changes promote urinary stasis and therefore increase the risk of bacterial growth; this also means that any 24-hour urine collection may be incomplete. A second relevance is to the management of pregnant women who present with symptoms that suggest renal colic but no stone is detectable by ultrasound or by radiographic imaging. In these women, it is imperative to exclude urinary tract infection and to avoid the temptation to insert a nephrostomy tube, despite the hydroureter. Firstly, acute renal failure as a consequence of ureteric obstruction in pregnancy is uncommon; secondly, ureteric dilation is part of normal pregnancy and it is not usually possible to distinguish between this and pathologic dilation. Observation of ureteral "jets" (echogenic streams on ultrasound arising from ureteral orifices and entering the bladder) can suggest that there is no significant upstream ureteric obstruction but they must be done in the patient with a full bladder and are even then not always readily visible [2,3]. The only compelling indications for percutaneous nephrostomy or stenting of hydronephrosis associated with calculi in pregnancy are advancing renal failure for no other reason and pyelonephritis failing to respond to antibiotics. Even very large hydroureter resolves quickly after delivery in normal pregnancy [4].

Progesterone also relaxes the bladder wall. However, the gravid uterus displaces the bladder anteriorly and may result in reduced total capacity. Consequently, symptoms of urinary frequency, a feeling of pressure on the bladder and stress incontinence, dysuria and nocturia are commonly reported. In the absence of urine infection, further investigation of these symptoms during pregnancy is not indicated.

Glomerular filtration rate

Renal plasma flow (RPF) and glomerular filtration rate (GFR) increase early in pregnancy, and by the end of the first trimester RPF increases by as much as 80% and glomerular filtration rate by 50% above baseline levels [5]. Increased RPF is thought to be due to reduced renal vascular resistance, possibly mediated by relaxin. This persists through the mid-trimester, with some reports indicating that GFR falls by 20% towards term, but not necessarily returning to baseline until after delivery [6]. The increment in GFR is mostly due to hemodynamic changes with a small change in ultrafiltration coefficient [7]. The fall in plasma oncotic pressure accompanying the fall in serum albumin may also contribute slightly to this increase in GFR. Generally the hemodynamic changes of pregnancy have resolved by 3 months post partum.

Sodium and water balance

Sodium and water retention occur during pregnancy, partly due to stimulation of the renin-aldosterone system, resulting in increased total body water and plasma volume [8]. A relative hyponatremia occurs, with a fall in sodium of about 5 mmol/L, thought to be due to a "reset osmostat" mechanism (i.e. a lower threshold for release of vasopressin, also known as antidiuretic hormone). This is a normal pregnancy-related physiologic adaptation, which correlates with the rise in release of circulating placental human chorionic gonadotropin but the exact mechanism remains unknown [9]. The normal pregnant woman develops thirst at a lower plasma osmolality and retains water, leading to a new equilibrium around a lower plasma sodium concentration.

Tubular function during pregnancy

Serum potassium usually remains in the low normal range, a balance between increased excretion due to both increased urine flow rate and aldosterone, offset by the antimineralocorticoid effect of progesterone [10]. Serum bicarbonate falls slightly as a consequence of a mild respiratory alkalosis induced by progesterone-mediated hyperventilation which then stimulates bicarbonaturia. There is an accompanying metabolic acidosis, probably of fetal origin. The anion gap is slightly reduced in normal pregnancy despite the reduction in serum bicarbonate [11]. Plasma urea falls in association with plasma volume expansion, as does serum albumin, but the fractional excretion of albumin is unchanged, suggesting intact tubular catabolism [12].

Glucose excretion increases during pregnancy, as a consequence of both increased filtered load and altered tubular handling, the latter related somehow to volume expansion.

Urate excretion rises during pregnancy, due to increased filtration, incompletely offset by increased reabsorption, leading to a fall in serum urate of about 25%. Ethnic differences affect serum urate concentration, with higher levels in Pacific Islanders, and higher serum urate levels are also observed in multiple pregnancies, probably due to increased production by placental tissue.

The net result of these changes in normal pregnancy is a slight reduction in serum albumin, hematocrit and hemoglobin, a low normal serum potassium value and reduced plasma sodium and bicarbonate concentration. Plasma pH rises to 7.42–7.44 and arterial PCO_2 falls from about 39 to 30 mmHg. Urinary acidification remains normal during pregnancy but there is no indication to test this in usual clinical practice.

Clinical significance of blood tests (Table 7.1)

The clinical consequences of the above changes are important. First, the definition of renal impairment is modified. The majority of pregnant patients will have creatinines under 76 μmol per litre (1.0 mg/dL) and a serum creatinine above 90 umol/L (1.2 mg/dL) is generally reflective of impaired GFR during pregnancy. A rising urea or creatinine concentration, even within the "normal" range used outside pregnancy, should alert the clinician to the possibility of pre-renal problems such as "effective" or true intravascular volume contraction. Plasma sodium and bicarbonate are typically slightly reduced, potassium should remain low normal, and albumin and urate should be lower than in the nonpregnant state. Increases in plasma sodium to those of nonpregnant women

Table 7.1 Biochemical changes during normal pregnancy* (see also Chapter 34)

Parameter	Pregnant	Nonpregnant
Plasma urea	3.2–4.4 mmol/L	4–11 mmol/L
	9–12 mg/dL	11.2–31 mg/dL
Plasma creatinine	<90 μmol/L	<120 μmol/L
	<1.0 mg/dL	<1.3 mg/dL
Urinary protein excretion (mg/day)	<300	<150
Plasma Na	130–140 mmol/L	135–145 mmol/L
	130–140 mEq/L	135–145 mEq/L
Plasma HCO3	18–20 mmol/L	22–28 mmol/L
	18–20 mEq/L	22–28 mEq/L
Plasma albumin	25–35 g/L	35–45 g/L
	2.5–3.5 g/dL	3.5–4.5 g/dL

*These ranges are approximate and listed in both SI and conventional units.

should raise the possibility of (reversible) pregnancy-specific diabetes insipidus (due to excess vasopressinase breaking down vasopressin) [13]. Increments in serum urea, particularly when accompanied by rising hemoglobin or hematocrit, may represent intravascular contraction, typically seen in pre-eclampsia.

Protein excretion

Protein excretion increases in normal pregnancy, predominantly due to an increase in the porosity of the glomerular basement membrane, though the mechanisms leading to this are unknown [7,14]. In association with increased glomerular filtration rate, protein excretion increases such that normal protein excretion during pregnancy is about 200 mg/day, with the upper limit defined as 300 mg per day [15]. Measurement of threshold protein excretion during pregnancy is reliably and rapidly achieved using a mid-stream specimen of urine, a protein/creatinine ratio >30 mg/mmol correlating with >300 mg/day proteinuria [16].

Urine testing in pregnancy

The dipstick urine test is a reasonable screening tool for proteinuria but should not be used alone for this purpose. A dipstick test of "negative" or "trace" protein in most (but not all) studies has a high negative predictive value to exclude proteinuria, whereas "2+" (1 g/L) protein or above strongly correlates with >300 mg/day proteinuria. However, in view of the unreliability of the dipstick, any woman with "1+" (0.3 g/L) protein or above should have formal quantification of protein excretion either with a spot protein/creatinine ratio or 24-hour urinary protein collection. It is important to emphasize that a urinary protein/creatinine ratio above 30 mg/mmol is a good test for detecting proteinuria above the threshold excretion of 300 mg/day but is unproven as being accurate enough to reflect increasing protein excretion as pregnancy progresses, discussed below.

The appearance of glucose in the urine may be normal and is not diagnostic of diabetes mellitus; a formal oral glucose challenge test should be arranged if diabetes is suspected.

Dipstick hematuria during pregnancy is common. Provided the urine sediment is not active, i.e. there are no casts, and the serum creatinine is normal, this is not associated with adverse maternal or fetal outcomes during pregnancy and can be investigated if persistent post partum [17]. Many such cases will resolve after pregnancy. However, the appearance of proteinuria on dipstick or hematuria on microscopic examination of the urine requires further evaluation, and exclusion of urinary tract infection is imperative. Pregnancy may be the first time a woman's urine is examined, offering the opportunity to diagnose previously undetected renal parenchymal disorders, which may have consequences not only for the pregnancy but for later life.

Chronic kidney disease outside pregnancy

Epidemiology

Chronic kidney disease (CKD) is present in 13.1% of the US population and is increasing in incidence. Although there are many known associations, diabetes, hypertension and cardiovascular disease appear to be the most significant risk factors. Table 7.2 reviews a common classification system for severity of CKD and the estimated prevalence in the US population. Although the minority of these cases occur in women of reproductive age, 1–7% of women of reproductive age on dialysis will become pregnant at some point in their care.

Etiology

The leading causes of chronic renal failure in the US are diabetic nephropathy, hypertensive or ischemic nephrosclerosis and various primary and secondary glomerulopathies. Table 7.3 delineates the distinctions between nephrotic and nephritic

Table 7.2 Staging of chronic kidney disease using the National Health and Nutrition Examination Survey (NHANES)

Stage	GFR in mL/min/1.73 m²	Estimated prevalence in the US
Stage 1	GFR is >90 and persistent microalbuminuria	1.8%
Stage 2	GFR is 60–89 and persistent microalbuminuria	3.2%
Stage 3	GFR is 30–59	7.7%
Stage 4	GFR is 15–29	0.35%
Stage 5	GFR is 0–14 (also known as endstage kidney disease (ESKD))	2.4%

GFR, glomerular filtration rate.

Table 7.3 Features of nephrotic and nephritic renal disease

Syndrome	Features	Typical causes seen in women of reproductive age
Nephrotic syndrome	Urine sediment: inactive Heavy proteinuria (>3.5 g/24 h) Edema, hyperlipidemia, hypoalbuminemia (<30g/L) Biopsy generally does not show prominent inflammation	Minimal change disease Focal glomerulosclerosis Mesangial IgA proliferative GN SLE
Nephritic syndrome	Urine sediment: active (i.e. red cells, white cells, granular and red cell casts seen on urine microscopy) Renal insufficiency with variable proteinuria Biopsy does show prominent inflammation	SLE Crescentic GN Postinfectious GN Vasculitis

GN, glomerulonephritis; SLE, systemic lupus erythematosus.

Table 7.4 Causes of chronic kidney disease (CKD)

General category	Some specific etiologies that may be seen in women of reproductive age
Primary glomerulopathies	Focal glomerulosclerosis Crescentic glomerulonephritis IgA nephropathy Membranoproliferative glomerulonephritis Fibrillary glomerulonephritis Membranous nephropathy
Glomerulopathies associated with systemic disease	Diabetes mellitus Hemolytic uremic syndrome Postinfectious glomerulonephritis SLE Wegener's granulomatosis
Hypertension	Ischemic (hypertensive) nephrosclerosis
Chronic tubulointerstitial nephropathies	Broad range of causes including: – reflux nephropathy, – medications (e.g. cisplatin, cyclosporine, tacrolimus and lithium) more often a cause of acute kidney injury rather than CKD – genetic (e.g. polycystic kidney disease) – metabolic disturbances (e.g. hypokalemia, hypercalcemia, hyperuricemia)
Obstructive uropathies (rare)	Ureteral obstruction (congenital, calculi) Vesicoureteral reflux
Renovascular disease	Renal artery stenosis caused by fibromuscular dysplasia in this age group – rarely causes ESKD
Hereditary nephropathies	Polycystic kidney disease Alport's syndrome Familial hyperuricemic nephropathy

ESKD, endstage kidney disease; SLE, systemic lupus erythematosus; TB, tuberculosis.

glomerular renal disease (although there is considerable overlap between these two syndromes) and lists the most common causes of each inx women of reproductive age. Other possible causes of CKD in women of reproductive age are reviewed in Table 7.4, and Table 7.5 reviews the clinical features of four of the most common causes of CKD in patients of reproductive age. Renal biopsy may be necessary to make a definitive diagnosis and is usually warranted for cases of unexplained or rapidly progressive renal failure, in adults with nephrotic syndrome, acute nephritic syndromes or isolated glomerular hematuria with significant proteinuria.

Management of CKD outside pregnancy

Management of patients with CKD involves treating or removing any underlying cause (e.g. obstruction, recurrent urinary infections, HIV, SLE, chronic infection) and preventing or slowing progression. The treatment of specific etiologies of CKD varies considerably and is not suitable for a summary, but the general management of established CKD is more uniform and is summarized in Table 7.6 both for the nonpregnant patient and with any modifications for pregnancy. The rate of progression of CKD is highly variable even for specific etiologies but each of the interventions listed in the table is viewed to have some role in preventing progression to endstage renal disease.

In addition to the complications listed in Table 7.6, patients with endstage kidney disease (ESKD) may also suffer from uremic bleeding due to platelet dysfunction, uremic pericarditis, uremic neuropathy, thyroid dysfunction and malnutrition. In general, these complications are avoided with current

Table 7.5 Clinical features of four of the more common causes of renal disease in women of reproductive age

Disease	Clinical features
IgA nephropathy	IgA nephropathy is the most common primary GN in the developed world. It presents typically in the second of third decade of life Presentation is typically with hematuria following a viral upper respiratory tract infection or on the basis of a routine screening urinalysis. Diagnosis is made on immunoflourescence staining of renal biopsy which reveals prominent clumps of IgA deposits in the mesangium
	Most patients have slowly progressing disease, although those with proteinuria tend to have worse prognosis. 25–50% of patients with IgA nephropathy have renal insufficiency or ESKD 20 years into the diagnosis
	Most patients are managed with risk factor modifications listed in Table 7.6
SLE-related nephropathy	SLE is associated with 6 distinct types of glomerular disease, each with its own prognosis and management. These types are: I. minimal mesangial, II. mesangial proliferative, III. focal, IV. diffuse, V. membranous, VI. advanced sclerosing lupus nephritis. This has been further classified according to chronicity and whether changes are global or segmental
	Class I and II have a good prognosis and do not require treatment. Classes III–IV require steroid and other immunosuppression therapy such as mycophenolate or cyclophosphamide. Class V may sometimes need this therapy if the nephrotic syndrome is severe or progressive. Class VI has a high risk of ESKD and does not respond to immunosuppressive treatment as the sclerosis changes are not reversible
Reflux nephropathy	Renal damage that occurs from childhood vesicoureteral reflux with or without associated recurrent urinary tract infections leading to interstitial scarring and presenting as asymptomatic renal insufficiency and scarred small kidney(s) in an adult who may or may not have been known to have recurrent UTI in childhood. Urine sediment is often not active but proteinuria is apparent as CKD progresses and there is typically hypertension
Focal segmental glomerulosclerosis	The most common cause of nephrotic syndrome in adults and the most common primary glomerular disease to cause ESKD in the US
	It presents typically as nephrotic syndrome or at least heavy proteinuria and will generally lead to ESKD if not treated
	Treatment is often with prednisone, with cyclosporine an option for steroid-resistant cases

CKD, chronic kidney disease; ESKD, endstage kidney disease; GN, glomerulonephritis; IgA, immunoglobulin A; SLE, systemic lupus erythenatosus; UTI, uterine infection.

Table 7.6 Management of CKD in nonpregnant patients

Intervention	Method	Modification of intervention for pregnancy
Interventions to prevent progression of CKD		
Maintain good blood pressure	Antihypertensive therapy to bring BP <130/80 or lower (an ACE inhibitor or ARB is preferred in diabetic patients)	Stop ACE inhibitors and ARB prior to conception or early in pregnancy Not clear what goal BP should be in pregnancy but consider target of 130/80 and avoid hypotension Methyldopa, labetalol or oxprenolol probably preferred agents in pregnancy
Quit smoking		No change
Nutrition	Keep at least 0.8–1.0 g/kg per day to avoid protein malnutrition and ensure adequate calorie and nutrient intake	Liberalize dietary protein to at least 1–1.2 g/kg/day of preconception weight
Treat hyperlipidemia	Typically achieved with both diet and a statin to bring the LDL to <70–100 mg/dL or 1.8–2.6 mmol/L. This guideline is the subject of ongoing clinical trials and not yet of proven benefit	Stop statins and other lipid-lowering drugs after first missed period or positive pregnancy test Correct hyperglycemia (which can cause hypertriglyceridemia) with insulin in a patient with diabetes
Correct metabolic acidosis	Typically done by administering sodium bicarbonate in a daily dose of 0.5–1 mEq/kg/day to maintain a serum bicarbonate of >22 mEq/L	Serum bicarbonate normally drops in pregnancy to 18–20 mEq/L and should not be corrected above this level
Interventions to prevent complications of CKD		
Potential complications	*Preventive measure/treatment*	*Pregnancy adjustments*
Volume overload	Salt and fluid restriction Loop diuretics	Use diuretics with caution to ensure no decrease in intravascular volume that could impair placental perfusion. Avoid diuretics in the setting of preeclampsia where intravascular volume is likely to be decreased
Hyperkalemia	Dietary potassium restriction If necessary, low-dose daily administration of a potassium-binding resin (e.g. kayexalate)	No change
Hyperphosphatemia	Dietary restriction of phosphate to <800 mg/day Administration with each meal of a phosphate binder such as calcium phosphate	No change
Renal osteodystrophy (a bone disease related to alterations in phosphate and vitamin D metabolism in CKD)	Dietary restriction of phosphate to <800 mg/day and phosphate binders as above Administration of the vitamin D metabolite calcitriol	No change
Anemia	Managed when necessary with administration of erythropoietin	No change

ACE, angiotensin-converting enzyme; ARB, angiotensin receptor blocker; LDL, low-density lipoprotein.

treatment by early dietary intervention and commencement of dialysis before such a late stage of CKD. Patients with ESKD and these complications are managed with hemodialysis, peritoneal dialysis or renal transplant. The usual indications for beginning dialysis in nonpregnant patients with CKD are listed in Box 7.1.

Management of pre-existing renal disease in pregnancy

Management of the pregnant woman with chronic renal disease ideally begins prior to pregnancy with time for appropriate counseling regarding the potential risks and likely outcomes not only of the pregnancy but for the woman post partum. Attitudes have changed over the past 20–30 years, with chronic renal disease no longer seen as an automatic contraindication to pregnancy [18]. However, the data we

use to counsel women today are still those derived from a few key studies published 10–20 years ago [19–26], summarized clearly in two key reviews [5,27]. A recent review searched the literature from January 1990 through December 2005 and found 23 publications relevant to this topic [28]. None were randomized clinical trials or meta-analyses and the comment was made that most outcome studies lacked an appropriate control group. Nevertheless, these authors agreed with previous reviewers that the two key issues in pre-pregnancy counseling are assessment of:
• the degree of renal insufficiency at the time of conception
• control of hypertension pre-pregnancy and throughout pregnancy.
Imbasciati *et al.* [29] recently reviewed 49 women with GFR less than 60 mL/min before conception, (i.e. at least stage 3 chronic kidney disease), whose pregnancy proceeded beyond 20 weeks. They noted that as a group, GFR was lower after

Box 7.1 Indications for renal replacement therapy in nonpregnant patients with endstage renal disease

Life-threatening clinical indications

- Fluid overload unresponsive to diuretics
- Hypertension refractory to medication
- Uremic pericarditis or pleuritis
- Uremic encephalopathy or neuropathy
- Clinically significant bleeding due to uremia
- Metabolic disturbances refractory to medical treatment (hyperkalemia, acidosis, hyperphosphatemia, hyper/hypocalcemia)
- Malnutrition or weight loss

Laboratory parameters

- GFR <15 mL/min/1.73 m^2 (National Kidney Foundation
- Dialysis Outcomes Quality Initiative) or <8–10 mL/min/1.73 m^2 (European Best Practice Guidelines)

GFR, glomerular filtration rate.

pregnancy than before conception but the fall in GFR was predicted by the combined presence of a preconception GFR below 40 mL/min and proteinuria greater than 1 g per day, not by GFR alone.

In broad terms, women with mild renal impairment and controlled hypertension will have a successful pregnancy outcome while those with moderate to severe renal insufficiency, particularly when accompanied by hypertension, have a lower chance of having a live baby, will certainly have more maternal complications during the pregnancy and have an accelerated rate towards dialysis or transplantation following the pregnancy. Some believe that only pre-existing hypertension predicts the pregnancy outcome [30] but the study quoted as evidence for this opinion was conducted largely in women with mild renal impairment. Counseling needs to occur around the following issues:

- chances of fertility in relation to the degree of renal impairment
- progress of renal disease during the pregnancy
- likelihood of prematurity or fetal growth restriction
- likelihood of livebirth
- control of hypertension and development of superimposed pre-eclampsia
- progression to endstage renal failure after delivery.

There are no true estimates of the likelihood of fertility in women with moderate to severe renal impairment; in general, these women have a reduced fertility rate though even women on dialysis may become pregnant and should be advised to use contraception unless truly planning a pregnancy. Contraceptive

options for women with renal insufficiency include barrier methods, progesterone-only pills, injections and implants and tubal ligation. The use of the combined oral contraceptive pill is reasonable in women with renal disease who do not have nephrotic range proteinuria, have well-controlled hypertension and no history of thrombosis.

The likelihood of progression of renal disease during the pregnancy depends only partly on the intrinsic nature of the renal disorder but significantly on the baseline GFR (Boxes 7.2 and 7.3), control of hypertension and the development of superimposed pre-eclampsia. The natural history of most chronic renal disorders during pregnancy is that progressive deterioration during a 40-week interval is unlikely, the main

Box 7.2 Maternal renal outcomes according to pre-pregnancy serum creatinine

Creatinine <130 μmol/L (<1.5 mg/dL)

- Permanent loss of GFR in <10% women
- Major determinant of ESRF progression is hypertension

Creatinine 130–220 μmol/L (1.5–2.5 mg/dL)

- Expect initial pregnancy increase in GFR then decline
- Permanent loss of GFR in 30% (increased to 50% if uncontrolled hypertension)
- 10% ESRF soon after pregnancy

Creatinine >220 μmol/L (>2.5 mg/dL)

- Progression to ESRF highly likely during or soon after pregnancy

ESRF, endstage renal failure; GFR, glomerular filtration rate.

Box 7.3 Fetal outcomes according to maternal serum creatinine before pregnancy

Creatinine <130 mmol/L (<1.5 mg/dL)

- Livebirths in >90%

Creatinine 130–220 mmol/L (1.5–2.5 mg/dL)

- Livebirths in about 85% unless uncontrolled hypertension (MAP >105 mmHg) at conception
- Sixty percent prematurity, mainly iatrogenic (pre-eclampsia/fetal growth restriction)

Creatinine >220 mmol/L (>2.5 mg/dL)

- fetal loss high – estimates uncertain

MAP, mean arterial pressure.

exception being SLE which by its nature can flare, leading to accelerated renal disease during the pregnancy. About 50% of women with moderate renal insufficiency have a significant rise in serum creatinine in the third trimester and if this occurs, almost one in four progresses to endstage renal disease within 6 months after delivery.

Prematurity, fetal growth restriction and stillbirth are not major concerns for women with mild renal impairment unless superimposed pre-eclampsia develops. On the other hand, fetal survival ranges from 65% to 85%, fetal growth restriction 35–45% and prematurity 30–85% in the group with moderate to severe renal impairment [28]. Uncontrolled hypertension at conception is a poor prognostic feature in terms of fetal outcome.

Based upon these estimates of outcomes for mother and baby, the key principles of antenatal care in women with pre-existing chronic renal disease are:
• management of hypertension
• interpretation and management of changes in GFR
• measurement, interpretation and management of proteinuria, including nephrotic syndrome
• consideration of the primary underlying renal disease and its peculiar problems
• identification and management of urinary tract infection
• clinical assessment and maintenance of volume homeostasis
• consideration of appropriate "renal" and antihypertensive medications throughout pregnancy
• identification of superimposed pre-eclampsia
• assessment of fetal well-being.
Each of these items is discussed below.

Hypertension

Most women with chronic renal disease will not exhibit the usual early fall in blood pressure and many will undergo an increase in blood pressure as the pregnancy progresses. Pregnancy is accompanied by significant volume expansion which under normal circumstances does not induce hypertension. However, in the context of chronic renal impairment outside pregnancy, there is often an inability to excrete a sodium load, with accompanying hypertension, and it is likely that this mechanism is partly involved in the development of hypertension in these women during pregnancy. Regardless of the cause, persistence of hypertension is an adverse factor in pregnancy outcome [31] and it is therefore imperative that considerable attention is paid to the blood pressure of women with chronic renal disease during their antenatal care.

Measurement of blood pressure has been traditionally done by mercury sphygmomanometry but this is slowly being replaced by a range of automated blood pressure recorders. It is probable that most of the automated blood pressure recorders used in routine clinical practice have not been validated for use in pregnancy. Where possible, blood pressure should still be recorded using mercury sphygmomanometry,

recording the phase 5 sound (the pressure at which the sounds disappear) as the true diastolic pressure [32]. Hypertension is generally defined as a blood pressure above 140/90 mmHg and in pregnancy treatment is generally reserved for blood pressures above this level. However, it is important to remember that the target blood pressure for most women with chronic renal impairment is below 130/80 mmHg and a period of 40 weeks or so of blood pressures above this level may lead to progressive renal impairment after the pregnancy.

Most women with chronic renal impairment, particularly those with proteinuria above 1 g per day, will be receiving angiotensin-converting enzyme (ACE) inhibitors or angiotensin 2 receptor antagonists before pregnancy. These must be discontinued, preferably before pregnancy and certainly once pregnancy is diagnosed, due to increased risks of fetal growth restriction, oligohydramnios, neonatal renal failure and probably cardiac and neurologic development abnormalities [33,34]. Suitable antihypertensives include methyldopa, labetalol, nifedipine, hydralazine and the beta-blockers oxprenolol (where available), pindolol and (from the editors' perspective but not the authors') metoprolol. Failure to use antihypertensives in pregnancy can be associated with poorer pregnancy outcomes, at least in women with renal transplants [35]. Target blood pressures in this population should probably be in the order of 110–140/80–90 mmHg, though there is no solid research to support this recommendation.

It is important to appreciate that blood pressure will often rise significantly soon after delivery; therefore blood pressure measurement should be just as diligent in the early postpartum period as during pregnancy.

Glomerular filtration rate

Glomerular filtration rate should rise by about 50% during normal pregnancy, typically apparent by the end of the first trimester. Under experimental conditions, ensuring both adequate hydration and urine output, GFR is measured as either creatinine clearance or inulin clearance. From a practical point of view, clinicians rely upon serum creatinine as the main measurement of GFR during pregnancy, discussed above. Measurement of creatinine clearance requires 24-hour urine collection, which is cumbersome and even when conducted diligently may be inaccurate due to ureteric dilation which results in pooling of urine and an incomplete collection, as outlined above. Cystatin C has been used to measure GFR during pregnancy [36] as has beta-2 microglobulin. However, there are problems with both measurements and serum creatinine remains the standard of assessing GFR during pregnancy.

Several equations have been developed to estimate GFR without collecting a 24-hour urine. The MDRD (modification of diet in renal disease study equation) formula for estimating GFR is now used widely outside pregnancy [37] but has not been validated for use in pregnant women. Similarly, the Cockcroft–Gault [38] formula has not been validated for use in pregnancy; this formula depends on bodyweight as a reflection of muscle mass and bodyweight changes considerably during pregnancy, not so much due to changes in body muscle mass but largely due to volume expansion, maternal fat and the fetus.

For practical purposes, serum creatinine should still be used to assess GFR in pregnancy despite the fact that it will not identify patients with mild decreases in GFR. Although the majority of pregnant women will have creatinines under 76 μmol/L (1.0 mg/dL), a value above 90 μmol/L (1.2 mg/dL) is definitely abnormal for pregnancy, reflecting impaired GFR, as above.

Proteinuria and nephrotic syndrome

In the nonpregnant woman daily protein excretion is generally less than 150 mg per day, composed of up to 20 mg per day albumin and the remainder other proteins, often of tubular origin [7]. Albumin excretion during normal pregnancy appears to be unchanged but total protein excretion is increased across all trimesters, with an upper limit of excretion around 300 mg per day. The mechanisms of this increased excretion are unclear but appear to relate to increased porosity [14] rather than to substantial changes in glomerular hemodynamics.

Recent evidence has shown that production of soluble fms-like tyrosine kinase-1 (sFLT), a protein which inhibits vascular growth by binding circulating vascular endothelial growth factor (VEGF), is increased from the placenta of pregnancies complicated by pre-eclampsia and that this production may predate the clinical appearance of the disorder [39]. It is clear from animal experiments that sFLT reduces the levels of VEGF, resulting in disrupted glomerular endothelial cells, loss of endothelial cell fenestrations in the glomerulus and significant proteinuria [40]. To date, no such studies have been undertaken in women with primary renal disease during their pregnancy but it is possible that such women who develop superimposed pre-eclampsia have resultant changes in glomerular structure and renal function as a result of sFLT and perhaps other angiogenic factors such as endoglin.

As mentioned above, there has been a shift in nephrology practice outside pregnancy to measure urinary protein excretion as the spot urine protein/creatinine ratio instead of 24-hour urinary protein excretion. Urinalysis alone is a poor predictor of protein excretion in pregnancy [16,41,42] and use of spot protein/creatinine ratio in pregnancy has become a popular and reasonably reliable method of determining whether protein excretion is abnormal, i.e. above 300 mg per day, most often needed to diagnose the presence of pre-eclampsia. There have been no studies to date testing whether serial spot protein/creatinine ratio during pregnancy in a woman with renal disease is a reliable method of predicting changes in 24-hour urinary protein excretion in that woman. Whilst it is likely that this would be the case, 24-hour urine protein excretion remains the gold standard for assessing true changes in protein excretion during pregnancy within

an individual woman. A reasonable practical approach given both the cumbersome nature of 24-hour urine testing and the evolving literature on protein/creatinine ratios in pregnancy is to measure 24-hour urinary protein and creatinine excretion at the original visit and determine the protein/creatinine ratio at that stage. Subsequent protein/creatinine ratios will give a guide to that woman's protein excretion, though it needs to be acknowledged that this is a guide only. Urine protein/creatinine ratios, when calculated using protein and creatinine measured in mg/dL, have a correlation to the protein excretion in g/day (i.e. an approximate protein/creatinine ratio of 0.4 mg/mg very roughly correlates with 0.4 g of protein in 24). This relationship between protein/creatinine ratio and 24-hour urine protein is by no means linear, however, and the spot urine protein/creatinine ratio is best used to see if the patient has crossed the threshold from normal to abnormal rather than to quantitate abnormal proteinuria.

Even where there is a true change in protein excretion during pregnancy in women with underlying renal disease, there are very few therapeutic options available apart from ensuring blood pressure control. ACE inhibitors and angiotensin 2 receptor antagonists or aldosterone antagonists cannot be used during pregnancy, though diltiazem may have a small benefit [43]. Therefore, there is no great imperative to keep measuring 24-hour urinary protein excretion in these women. Some advocate increased protein excretion as a marker of superimposed pre-eclampsia in women with underlying renal disease though no studies have been able to confirm this and protein excretion may increase in such women, due to appropriate increases in glomerular filtration, progression of the underlying primary renal disease or suboptimal blood pressure control. In other words, an increase in urinary protein excretion should highlight the need for the clinician to look for other features of pre-eclampsia but by itself is not sufficient to make a diagnosis of superimposed pre-eclampsia. Moreover, increasing proteinuria alone should not be used as an indicator for delivery [44].

The most common cause of nephrotic syndrome during pregnancy is pre-eclampsia but nephrotic syndrome is also a problem for women with underlying primary glomerular disease during pregnancy. Serum albumin normally falls during pregnancy, partly due to volume expansion but values below 30 g/L should raise suspicion of the development of nephrotic syndrome. A spot urine protein/creatinine ratio above 230 mg/mmol (or 2.6 if creatinine and protein are measured in mg/dL) signifies a strong likelihood that protein excretion is above 3 g per day [45] and 24-hour urinary protein and creatinine should then be measured to confirm this. Women with nephrotic syndrome will generally have edema. However, this is a a very nonspecific sign during pregnancy as it accompanies two-thirds of normal pregnancies. There is also little point in measuring serum cholesterol, usually a component of the nephrotic syndrome, as this is often increased during a normal pregnancy.

In pre-eclampsia without underlying chronic renal disease, a retrospective study found that proteinuria above 5 g or even 10 g per day was not associated with any worse maternal outcome than those with lesser degrees of proteinuria, but was associated with earlier onset of pre-eclampsia, earlier gestational age at delivery and higher rates of neonatal complications due to prematurity [46]. Nevertheless, confirmation of true nephrotic syndrome is important as it allows recognition of the other aspects of this syndrome that may accompany the heavy proteinuria and be important to the pregnancy. These include loss of vitamin D-binding protein, transferrin, immunoglobulins, antithrombin (also accompanied by increased hepatic synthesis of other clotting factors) and a propensity for intravascular volume contraction in severe cases. The net results of these changes include calcium deficiency, iron deficiency, increased likelihood of infection, thrombosis, reduced uteroplacental blood flow with fetal growth restriction or death [47] and sometimes reduced renal blood flow with worsening renal function. Treatment requires oral calcium, vitamin D and iron supplementation and subcutaneous prophylactic dose heparin for thrombosis prevention as well as ensuring adequate fetal growth and amniotic fluid by ultrasound and reassessment of maternal serum creatinine on a regular basis. Low molecular weight heparin is suitable provided GFR is near normal, i.e. above 60 mL/min, and unfractionated heparin may be used for patients whose GFR falls below this range. When nephrotic syndrome occurs early in pregnancy and low molecular weight heparin is commenced, at that point we add vitamin D for prophylaxis against subsequent osteoporosis though there are as yet no controlled trials to test the benefit of this practice.

Follow-up of proteinuria after pregnancy is important and ACE inhibitors or angiotensin 2 antagonists should be commenced soon after delivery for their antiproteinuric effect. Enalapril and captopril are both deemed compatible with breastfeeding by the American Academy of Pediatrics.

The primary underlying renal disease and its peculiar problems

It is integral to proper antenatal care of women with underlying renal disease to consider the nuances of their underlying primary disorder. The most common renal diseases predating pregnancy in this age group are primary glomerulonephritis (usually IgA nephropathy or focal segmental glomerulosclerosis (FGS or FSGS)), reflux nephropathy and diabetic nephropathy. Clinical features of the former three conditions outside pregnancy are reviewed in Table 7.5. Given the wide range of causes of renal disease, this section will focus only on a few of the more common conditions and those with particular pregnancy-related concerns.

Most patients with IgA nephropathy in pregnancy do well and the risks of pregnancy correlate with the presence of proteinuria, hypertension and renal insufficiency and not the underlying diagnostic cause. Long-term follow-up of childhood IgA nephropathy showed that later pregnancy was complicated by hypertension in half the cases and prematurity in one-third [48] but again, these outcomes are not peculiar to this form of nephropathy. IgA nephropathy should be managed as for other chronic renal diseases during pregnancy, namely good control of blood pressure as the primary issue. Some cases are familial and if such a history is obtained, the pregnant woman should be informed to have her child screened with a urinalysis in the first few years of life. Macroscopic haematuria is no more likely during pregnancy unless there is intervening respiratory or gastrointestinal tract infection.

The outcome of diabetic nephropathy depends upon the usual factors of pre-existing renal insufficiency and control of hypertension with the added issue of potential congenital abnormalities if blood sugar was not adequately controlled at the time of conception. Reece et al. [49] reviewed the outcomes of these pregnancies in 1998 and found high rates of prematurity, cesarean sections and pre-eclampsia with about 15% progressing rapidly to endstage renal disease. Miodovnik et al. [50] concluded from a study of 182 insulin-dependent diabetics that pregnancy did not increase the risk of subsequent nephropathy nor accelerate progression of pre-existing nephropathy. Whilst early diabetic nephropathy (albuminuria alone) did not correlate with increased perinatal risk, both prematurity and superimposed pre-eclampsia rates were higher than in type 1 diabetics without early nephropathy. All pregnancy risks were greater in those with overt nephropathy, though patient numbers were small [51]. Whilst not of proven benefit, it seems likely that meticulous control of both blood sugar and blood pressure during pregnancy in women with early or overt diabetic nephropathy is the key management strategy to ensuring not only good pregnancy outcomes but preservation of renal function postpartum. Ideally, these women should be switched to ACE inhibitors after delivery to prevent progression of diabetic nephropathy, with both captopril and enalapril being considered safe for breastfeeding.

Whilst overall not a common cause of endstage renal failure, lupus nephritis is a disorder with a large preponderance towards women and is another renal disease not uncommonly encountered by obstetricians. In general, women with SLE should have quiescent disease at conception to offer the best chance of a successful pregnancy outcome [52]. Activity of the disease during pregnancy is probably related to activity at conception [53]. Those with active disease at conception have a higher likelihood of developing acute lupus nephritis during pregnancy which is then associated with high fetal risk [19]. Ideally, women with SLE should be in remission for about 12 months preconception and taking prednisolone/prednisone in doses below 20 mg per day. Hydroxychloroquine should be continued as it is relatively safe to use during pregnancy. An acute renal flare, evidenced by increasing proteinuria, active urine sediment and rising creatinine, should be treated by increasing doses of prednisolone/prednisone with consideration of the introduction of azathioprine. Others prefer to undertake renal biopsy at this point in order to confirm the histologic changes before introducing this immunosuppression. Either approach is reasonable. Cyclophosphamide is generally contraindicated in pregnancy but has been used successfully in a few cases of lupus nephritis.

The outcome of pregnancies in women with reflux nephropathy also appears dependent upon the level of pre-existing renal function and control of blood pressure [23]. Approximately one in four may develop pre-eclampsia and about 40% of offspring have vesicoureteric reflux [54]. These women are more predisposed to urinary tract infection throughout pregnancy, as are women who have had corrected vesicoureteral reflux (VUR) in childhood [55]. Significant urinary tract infection can be associated with premature labor or spontaneous rupture of membranes and is therefore an important feature of these cases. For this reason, frequent urine culture should be obtained throughout pregnancy in women with underlying reflux nephropathy. In other respects, management is the same as for other chronic renal diseases, namely good control of blood pressure and monitoring of GFR.

Inherited renal disorders are likely to have been diagnosed prior to the pregnancy and the specific implications of this for the offspring will have been discussed. The most common such renal disorder is adult polycystic kidney disease with an autosomal dominant inheritance; IgA nephropathy and reflux nephropathy are not inherited by specific mendelian traits but tend to co-segregate within families and the pregnant woman needs to be aware of this. While still uncommon, disorders such as Alport's syndrome and familial hyperuricemic nephropathy [56] occur in this age group and appropriate counseling needs to be provided before and during pregnancy.

Clinical assessment and management of volume homeostasis

Adequate intravascular volume is essential to preservation of GFR, and therefore a good pregnancy outcome for mother and baby, regardless of the underlying renal disorder. However, it is particularly difficult to assess maternal volume homeostasis clinically during pregnancy. Typical clinical signs used in nonpregnant women, e.g. edema, are of little value in assessing volume homeostasis during pregnancy. For this reason, the hematocrit should be measured in women with underlying chronic renal disease as part of the full blood count at the initial first-trimester visit, along with serum albumin. Both measures should fall slightly as pregnancy progresses. A rise in either value strongly suggests intravascular volume contraction though there is no discriminant value above which we can be certain that volume depletion is definite [57]. Conversely, a significant fall in either value does not necessarily mean excessive volume expansion because the hematocrit depends on other factors, such as the ability

to maintain adequate red cell production, and serum albumin may fall in patients with nephrotic syndrome who in turn may have reduced intravascular volume.

In practice, even if volume excess has occurred then provided there is no respiratory compromise and blood pressure can be controlled, this is a more favorable situation to preserve maternal renal function and fetal growth than is volume depletion.

There are no controlled trials to show that intravascular volume expansion with intravenous fluids is of benefit or risk in women with underlying renal disease during pregnancy. Studies in pre-eclamptic women have shown no convincing benefit or adverse outcomes [58] though analyses of women having pulmonary edema in association with pre-eclampsia generally point towards overvigorous intravascular fluid replacement. Therefore, when there is concern about fetal growth or deteriorating GFR in women with chronic renal disease, it is prudent to check the change in hematocrit and albumin from baseline. If these suggest reduced intravascular volume, a trial of intravenous normal saline of no more than 1 L under observation in hospital is a reasonable clinical approach, though this recommendation is based on first principles alone.

Appropriate use of medications for treatment of renal disease in pregnancy

As discussed above, control of blood pressure is essential to successful pregnancy outcome in women with underlying renal disease. Antihypertensives to avoid include diuretics, in view of their propensity to induce volume contraction, ACE inhibitors and angiotensin receptor antagonists [59], in view of their fetal risks, and atenolol which has been associated with fetal growth restriction [60].

Cephalosporins, amoxicillin, trimethoprim and nitrofurantoin are safe to use for treatment of urine infection during pregnancy, though trimethoprim can induce hyperkalemia in some women. Gentamicin may be used to treat gram-negative infections in pregnancy despite reports of eighth cranial nerve damage in fetuses exposed to streptomycin or kanamycin. It is the editors' practice to use gentamicin routinely to treat pyelonephritis in pregnancy but the authors prefer that it be reserved for more severe cases of pyelonephritis with sepsis. Quinolones are best avoided though more human pregnancy safety data are available.

Recombinant erythropoietin is routinely advocated to correct anemia during pregnancy in women with chronic renal impairment but it is important to remember that this may worsen blood pressure control [61] and more frequent blood pressure measurement is needed in these women.

Several immunosuppressive drugs are considered safe in the transplant patient [62] and women with lupus nephritis or other connective tissue disorders may also require immunosuppressant drugs during pregnancy. In general, prednisolone, azathioprine, cyclosporine and hydroxychloroquine are safe to use; tacrolimus has been associated with neonatal hyperkalemia [63] but recent data suggest it is probably safe overall [21]; mycophenolate is associated with embryotoxic effects and cyclophosphamide with congenital abnormalities. However, cyclophosphamide has been used successfully in occasional cases of *de novo* lupus nephritis occurring in pregnancy [64].

The PARIS collaboration has built on earlier work [65] and confirmed that aspirin is of benefit in preventing pre-eclampsia though an average of 56 women require treatment to prevent one case of pre-eclampsia but with no improvement in perinatal outcome [66]. Few studies have examined the prophylactic benefit of aspirin in women with underlying renal disease. However, these studies suggest that aspirin is of benefit in reducing superimposed pre-eclampsia and perinatal death with the need to treat a smaller number of women to gain benefit. Aspirin appears to reduce the likelihood of developing pre-eclampsia in women with underlying chronic renal disease, the number needed to treat being between nine and 57 for prevention of pre-eclampsia but 42–357 to prevent perinatal death [67]. The PARIS analysis found that aspirin reduced superimposed pre-eclampsia in women with underlying renal disease (relative risk (RR) 0.63, 95% CI 0.38–1.06) but only 450 women were included in this analysis [66].

The effects of low doses of aspirin (up to 300 mg per day) on renal function are quite minimal and generally this is a safe approach, particularly for women who have had early-onset severe pre-eclampsia and/or fetal loss in their previous pregnancy.

Identification of superimposed pre-eclampsia

Pre-eclampsia is a placental disorder of unknown etiology that has several predisposing risk factors, one of which is chronic renal disease. There appears to be a genetic predisposition and possibly an altered maternal immune adaptation to the pregnancy with resultant changes in oxidative stress, exaggerated inflammatory response of pregnancy and more recently recognized changes in angiogenic factors. The maternal organ systems mostly affected are the kidney, liver and brain with accompanying systemic hypertension and sometimes thrombocytopenia. Fetal blood flow and/or oxygen and nutrient transfer lead to fetal growth restriction and in some cases intrauterine fetal death. The maternal renal effects include a reduction in renal blood flow, increased sodium and uric acid reabsorption, reduced circulating renin and aldosterone concentrations, proteinuria and impaired GFR [68]. Women who begin pregnancy with impaired renal function have an increased risk of developing pre-eclampsia.

It is readily apparent that the development of superimposed pre-eclampsia in a woman with underlying renal impairment will lead to a worsening of renal function, exaggerated hypertension and proteinuria with risks of nephrotic syndrome, short-term and long-term risks to maternal renal function as well as increased risks for fetal growth restriction, prematurity and perinatal mortality. However, it is very difficult to diagnose superimposed pre-eclampsia in a woman who begins her pregnancy with renal impairment and/or proteinuria. An increase in blood pressure, decline in GFR or increasing protein excretion can all be due to progression of the underlying renal disorder rather than superimposed pre-eclampsia and as yet there is no diagnostic test to distinguish between these two scenarios. However, when these features are accompanied by neurologic symptoms such as hyper-reflexia with clonus or by abnormal liver transaminases or new-onset thrombocytopenia (except in SLE where this may be an autoimmune phenomenon), then it is highly likely that superimposed pre-eclampsia has developed.

Plasma uric acid is commonly measured as a potential marker of pre-eclampsia. Uric acid undergoes reabsorption in the proximal tubule and secretion followed by postsecretory reabsorption and its excretion therefore can be influenced at several points along the nephron. Elevated plasma urate may be in itself pathogenic [69] or else a marker of renal vasoconstriction. Pre-eclamptic women receiving probenecid had lower serum uric acid and creatinine (but no difference in creatinine clearance) and higher platelet counts than women in a control group but pregnancy outcomes were similar in this small study [70]. Consequently, serial measurement of uric acid in women with chronic renal disease is not likely to be of much help in clinical management.

In many ways the distinction between worsening renal disease and superimposed pre-eclampsia can be an academic one as clinicians managing the woman with underlying renal disease should be vigilant for these changes in all cases, leading to increased surveillance not only of the mother but also of fetal well-being (see below). The indications for delivery in women with superimposed pre-eclampsia are broadly the same as those that would prompt these writers to recommend delivery for a woman with progressive underlying renal disease, i.e. inability to control blood pressure, deteriorating GFR with no reversible component, neurologic abnormalities, progressively deteriorating thrombocytopenia, increasing liver transaminases or failure of fetal growth. In rare cases after 20 weeks gestation but prior to 30–34 weeks gestation, a renal biopsy may need to be considered to distinguish between worsening primary renal disease and superimposed pre-eclampsia but in our experience, this is rarely necessary and when performed may not always provide a definitive distinction.

Assessment of fetal well-being

Traditional assessment of fetal well-being has depended upon fetal morphology scan at 18–20 weeks gestation followed by regular ultrasounds to assess fetal growth and amniotic fluid index as well as Doppler studies of umbilical artery blood flow. While there are no data to recommend for or against its use in patients with renal disease, regular fetal nonstress testing is commonly employed, beginning at 32–34 weeks gestation in women with significant renal disease. The role of fetal testing in medical disorders in pregnancy is reviewed for the nonobstetric reader in Chapter 49.

Renal biopsy in pregnancy

It is rare to require renal biopsy in pregnancy. Situations where this may be necessary because the information would significantly impact on the pregnancy outcome for mother and baby are:

• *de novo* onset of nephrotic range proteinuria or unexplained impaired GFR [71] with abnormal urine sediment prior to fetal viability, i.e. before 24 weeks gestation
• rapidly declining GFR without any apparent reversible cause prior to fetal viability in women with underlying primary glomerulonephritis where a clinical decision to use immunosuppression would be accepted
• acute renal failure with active urine sediment prior to fetal viability where the clinician and the pregnant woman would be prepared to use modalities such as immunosuppression, plasma exchange or dialysis
• deteriorating GFR without obvious cause in a woman with a kidney transplant, in order to exclude acute rejection
• declining GFR or increasing proteinuria in a woman with lupus nephritis or SLE without previously known nephritis [72] where the clinician is prepared to use immunosuppression on the basis of the biopsy findings.

One Japanese group [73] biopsied 86 women who had had pre-eclampsia or heavy proteinuria without hypertension during pregnancy. They found IgA nephropathy in 19 of 86 (22%) women, 10 of whom had proteinuria without hypertension and eight had antepartum hematuria, i.e. these patients could reasonably have been expected to have underlying renal disease in any case. Reiter *et al.* [74] noted that provided careful attention was paid to urinalysis and serum creatinine during hypertensive pregnancies, the likelihood of finding underlying chronic renal disease post partum was small, though this was not a renal biopsy study.

Summary

• Women with renal insufficiency should be managed by a team comprising both a high-risk obstetrician and a renal or obstetric medicine physician. The complexity of these patients is greatly served by the involvement of an experienced midwife or nurse. Their care should preferably occur in a high-risk pregnancy clinic or day assessment unit.
• Glomerular filtration rate should still be measured using serum creatinine in pregnancy. Proteinuria should be assessed by following changes in spot urine protein/creatinine ratio after establishing the relationship between the patient's urine protein/creatinine ratio and an initial 24-hour urine collection

for protein. Blood pressure should be assessed, preferably by sphygmomanometry or else a validated automated blood pressure recorder.
• The primary issues during pregnancy are control of maternal hypertension, regular assessment of GFR, keeping a careful watch for features of emerging pre-eclampsia and regular assessment of fetal well-being. All of this allows for optimal timing of delivery.
• Women with renal insufficiency should receive low-dose aspirin ($\leq$150 mg) for the prevention of pre-eclampsia or perinatal death if there is no obvious contraindication and should receive subcutaneous heparin if nephrotic syndrome (>3 g protein/24 h) develops.
• The main determinants of a successful pregnancy outcome are the pre-pregnancy degree of proteinuria, the presence of hypertension and GFR. This should be the focus when counseling women about their pregnancy risks.

Urinary tract infection

Overt urine infection is no more common during pregnancy than outside it, but develops more readily into potentially serious pyelonephritis; for this reason urinary tract infection during pregnancy is generally of greater consequence than in the nonpregnant state. Urinary tract infection (UTI) is usually designated as simple (uncomplicated) or complicated, the latter including diabetics, those with structural abnormalities of the urinary tract, immunosuppressed and the pregnant woman.

Definitions

The presence of bacteria in the urine ($>10^5$/mL) without symptoms or signs is called asymptomatic bacteriuria. Bacteriuria may occur with or without pyuria, the presence of white cells generally indicating tissue inflammation and therefore cystitis, while the presence of epithelial cells points to a "contaminated" sample. Generally, cystitis will present with frequency, dysuria, nocturia, offensive urine or urgency, with one or many of these symptoms present. Where there is microbiologically proven UTI and symptoms of flank pain, nausea, vomiting, fever and sweating or associated loin tenderness, acute pyelonephritis is likely.

Although asymptomatic bacteriuria is not generally treated outside pregnancy, asymptomatic bacteriuria during pregnancy is associated with preterm labor, growth restriction and perinatal mortality [75]. It should therefore be considered a potentially serious complication of pregnancy and managed aggressively, with careful follow-up.

Epidemiology

The reported prevalence of UTI during pregnancy ranges from 2% to 20% [76]. It often occurs during the first trimester, and more frequently in multiparous women and diabetics. Commonly, this condition presents as asymptomatic bacteriuria (2–10% pregnancies) or symptomatic cystitis and less commonly pyelonephritis.

Pathophysiology

Ascending urinary infection (as opposed to blood-borne) is the typical route in the nonpregnant woman due to the short length of the urethra and its proximity to the perineum and bowel organisms. It is likely that the route of infection is similar in the pregnant woman, with most infections presenting as asymptomatic bacteriuria or cystitis, suggesting ascending infection. In the normal nongravid woman, asymptomatic bacteriuria rarely progresses to cystitis. In pregnancy, however, there is a much greater chance of overt infection developing, with rates of pyelonephritis complicating asymptomatic bacteriuria reported as high as 40% [77]. This dictates the importance of treating asymptomatic bacteriuria in pregnant women, which reduces this risk to below 10%.

It is likely that the dilation of the upper urinary tract (and some associated urinary stasis), and possibly the presence of VUR, predispose the pregnant woman to upper tract infection.

Etiology

The organisms causing UTI in pregnancy are the same as those outside pregnancy. *E. coli* causes approximately 90% of infections, with a number of other gram-negative organisms as well as gram-positive streptococci responsible for other infections.

Diagnosis

Standard antenatal care should include culture of a mid-stream specimen of urine early in the pregnancy. Other screening tests are not comparable in sensitivity or specificity in the detection of asymptomatic bacteriuria. Usually a single culture at the booking visit in the first or second trimester is sufficient to exclude asymptomatic bacteriuria in low-risk women. In those with abnormalities of urinary tract structure, with diabetes or other systemic disease, further cultures may be useful. Women who have threatened premature labor should have further urine cultures.

It is not uncommon for women to develop lower urinary tract symptoms in the absence of infection during pregnancy (discussed above). Flank pain and hematuria suggest kidney stone disease, and in the absence of infection should be investigated in the first instance by ultrasound. The presence of hydronephrosis of pregnancy, and the relatively poor sensitivity of kidney stones to ultrasound, sometimes necessitates the use of noncontrast helical CT scanning to exclude calculi. However, the majority of ureteral calculi will be identifiable

on abdominal ultrasound [78]. Transvaginal ultrasounds may be helpful in identifying distal ureteral stones not seen on renal and pelvic ultrasound. The possibility of thromboembolic disease (most commonly pulmonary embolism but including renal artery or vein or ovarian vein thrombosis) should be considered in women presenting with flank pain in the absence of infection, particularly where there is a pleuritic component. Low back pain is common in pregnancy but flank tenderness is not.

Management of UTI in pregnancy

Recurrent UTI prior to pregnancy

Women who begin pregnancy with a history of recurrent cystitis should have their urine cultured monthly. For those with a predictable history of postcoital cystitis, postcoital single-dose cephalexin (250 mg) or nitrofurantoin (50 mg) can significantly reduce the likelihood of infection [79]. Similarly, it is reasonable to examine the urine on more than one occasion for women with complicated urinary tracts or with diabetes. Any woman who has recurrent infection should undergo ultrasound of the urinary tract to exclude structural pathology.

Bacteriuria in pregnancy

Treatment of asymptomatic bacteriuria has been proven beneficial in a number of randomized controlled studies, recently reviewed by Smaill & Vazquez [80], with 3 days of antibiotics being recommended for treating and eradicating bacteriuria. Amoxicillin resistance is relatively common, and this drug may now be ineffective in empiric therapy. We favor the use of cephalexin, amoxicillin-clavulanic acid or nitrofurantoin. Table 7.7 lists useful regimens.

Women who have been treated for bacteriuria must have a follow-up mid-stream urine culture 1–2 weeks after the antibiotic course is complete, to ensure eradication. They should then have their urine cultured monthly until delivery, looking for recurrence.

Cystitis in pregnancy (see Table 7.7)

Acute cystitis in pregnancy is common, affecting 2% of pregnant women. As with asymptomatic bacteriuria, treatment reduces the complications of premature delivery and pyelonephritis. The confirmatory bacterial count ($>10^3$/mL) is lower than for asymptomatic bacteriuria, because the presence of symptoms and pyuria increases the overall likelihood of true positive diagnosis.

Treatment of this condition requires 3–7 days oral antibiotics, in the absence of other systemic symptoms and loin pain. Efficacy of the various regimes have not been proven to be different.

Table 7.7 Antibiotic regimens for treatment of urinary tract infections in pregnancy*

Drug	Dosage	Timing	Duration
Acute cystitis			
Amoxicillin (because of increasing resistance to amoxicillin sensitivities of causative organism must be verified)	500 mg	Twice a day (or 250 mg three times a day)	3–7 days
Nitrofurantoin	100 mg	Twice a day	3–7 days
Cephalexin	500 mg	Twice/three times a day	3–7 days
Amoxicillin-clavulanic acid	500 mg	Twice a day (or 250 mg three times a day)	7 days
Cefpodoxime	100 mg	Twice a day	7 days
Asymptomatic bacteriuria			
Cephalexin	500 mg	Three times a day	3 days
Amoxicillin	500 mg	Three times a day	3 days
Amoxicillin-clavulanic acid	500 mg	Three times a day	3 days
Nitrofurantoin	50 mg	Four times a day	3 days
Fosfomycin	3 g	Single dose	
Recurrent bacteriuria or cystitis			
Cephalexin	250–500 mg night-time (or postcoital)		
Nitrofurantoin	50–100 mg night-time (or postcoital)		
Amoxicillin	250 mg night-time (or postcoital)		
Pyelonephritis (initial IV therapy for patients with normal renal function)			
Ceftriaxone	1 g daily		
Ampicillin (with gentamicin)	1 g q6h		
Gentamicin	3 mg/kg daily		
Ticarcillin	3.2 g q8h		
Piperacillin	4 g q8h		
Aztreonam	1 g q8–12h		
Piperacillin-tazobactam	3.375 g q6h		
Ticarcillin-clavulanate	3.1 g q6h		
Meropenem	1 g q8h		

*Local bacteriologic patterns and sensitivity results should influence which antibiotics are used.

As above, a urine culture should be performed 2 weeks after cessation of antibiotics to ensure eradication of infection.

Recurrent bacteriuria or cystitis during pregnancy

Prophylactic antibiotics should be given to women with recurrent bacteriuria or infection. The choice of antibiotic should be determined by the sensitivities of the organism. Usually a low-dose daily treatment is sufficient to prevent infection, but sometimes breakthrough infections occur, which should again be treated with a 7-day course of antibiotics. Night-time amoxicillin (250 mg), cephalexin (250 mg) or nitrofurantoin (50–100 mg) are reasonable options.

Pyelonephritis

This condition has been examined in a large prospective study [81]. The incidence of pyelonephritis was 1.4%. Pyelonephritis is usually uncomplicated but can cause bacteremia, anemia, respiratory insufficiency, renal impairment and premature labor. Rarely, the infection can cause local severe complications, particularly if untreated or if there are underlying structural problems. For example, pelviureteric junction stenosis may completely occlude in the presence of acute infection, predisposing to pyonephroma and perinephric abcess formation, though this is rare.

Pyelonephritis should be managed initially in hospital with intravenous fluids to support hydration, intravenous antibiotics and general supportive measures. Although blood and urine cultures may add little to the management, they are useful in defining antibiotic sensitivities and in confirming diagnosis. Culture-negative pyelonephritis may occur if prior treatment for cystitis has been received. Empiric antibiotics should include a first or third-generation cephalosporin (e.g. ceftriaxone 1g daily) and gentamicin may be added if this proves unsuccessful. The various regimens are probably similar in efficacy. Pregnant women should continue treatment following discharge for a further 10–14 days. Table 7.7 includes acceptable regimens. The risk of recurrence of pyelonephritis in pregnancy is 6–8% and therefore these patients should be placed on one of the preventive regimens of antibiotics listed in Table 7.7 for the remainder of their pregnancy.

Summary

• Asymptomatic bacteriuria is no more common in pregnancy but it requires antibiotic treatment and vigilant follow-up as it is associated with preterm labor, fetal morbidity and mortality.
• Pyelonephritis should usually be managed as an inpatient, followed up by a total 10–14 day course of oral antibiotics followed by suppresive antibiotics until delivered.
• All infections require a follow-up urine culture 1–2 weeks after the antibiotic course to exclude recurrence.

Acute renal failure

Acute renal failure (ARF), now termed acute kidney injury (AKI) can be defined as a sudden reduction in renal function resulting in accumulation of waste products of metabolism, retention of sodium and water and acid–base disturbances. It is prudent to use a sensitive definition of AKI (e.g. a rise in serum creatinine above the normal range) rather than a more serious endpoint (e.g. the requirement for dialysis) as the former will identify women whose disease is in the early stages and therefore potentially reversible.

Oliguria versus anuria

It is common to observe oliguria in women with pre-eclampsia. Generally, this indicates worsening disease with renal vasoconstriction but it may be a normal renal response to intravascular volume depletion. In the presence of rising serum creatinine, oliguria is an indication for delivery. In the early postpartum period, oliguria is often observed after pre-eclampsia, and does not necessarily warrant a change in management, but rather an assessment of the woman's volume status.

Anuria, on the other hand, is never normal and apart from the case of a blocked indwelling urethral catheter, indicates serious renal disease. The differential diagnosis generally includes renal artery or venous occlusion, urinary tract obstruction, crescentic glomerulonephritis, acute cortical necrosis or occasionally severe acute tubular necrosis. It should be managed as an emergency.

Renal biopsy

Renal biopsy is usually not necessary for diagnosis of AKI in pregnancy, as other features of history, examination and results of investigations will usually allow a diagnosis to be made. However, occasionally the development of a renal parenchymal disease causing AKI without other clinical clues may necessitate renal biopsy. The other indication for renal biopsy in this setting is to answer the question "Are the kidneys likely to recover?" in the woman who may have developed cortical necrosis.

Renal biopsy carries a small risk (about 1%) of major bleeding using modern techniques outside pregnancy. Older literature suggested a higher rate of complications than this in pregnancy but today the rate of complications following a renal biopsy is probably not greater during pregnancy. Although the literature is sparse on this topic, the recommendations have been to consider a renal biopsy in the setting of serious AKI before 32 weeks where the cause is not apparent. After 32 weeks, if a renal biopsy is considered necessary, delivery should be undertaken first.

Epidemiology

The incidence of AKI in pregnancy has fallen markedly in the developed world because of the reduction in septic abortions and attention to modern antenatal care which allows earlier identification and treatment of pre-eclampsia, and in later pregnancy better management of hypovolemia and hemorrhage. Severe renal failure is now rare in developed countries, reported as <0.005% of pregnancies. However, in developing countries AKI in pregnancy contributes to a significant proportion of overall AKI (approximately 10% in several reports from India) and mortality rates remain high [82]. Mild non-oliguric AKI is not uncommon, particularly in the setting of pre-eclampsia, where an increase in serum creatinine >90 μmol/L (1.2 mg/dL) indicates reduction in GFR.

Some causes of AKI in pregnancy are listed in Table 7.8. They can be classified according to the usual clinical process of: pre-renal, intrarenal (or parenchymal) and postrenal (obstructive) causes. The physiologic adaptations of normal pregnancy that lead to volume expansion presumably protect against pre-renal insults, such as mild dehydration unless there is associated vasodilation such as occurs in sepsis. However, acute volume depletion, such as in postpartum hemorrhage, has the propensity to lead to severe oliguric renal failure and even cortical necrosis.

General course of AKI outside pregnancy

Depending on the definition used, AKI may carry a high mortality rate, particularly in the setting of multiorgan failure. Oliguric renal failure requiring dialysis still has a mortality rate of 50%, and milder nonoliguric renal failure 20%. Most who survive AKI will recover renal function, but sometimes there is some irreversible loss of renal function, leaving the patient with chronic kidney disease, and its consequences.

Clinical presentations

In the setting of a severe systemic illness such as sepsis, the woman will often develop oliguria initially, accompanied by a rise in serum urea and creatinine concentrations, then hyperkalemia and metabolic acidosis if more severe. Microangiopathic diseases (thrombotic thrombocytopenic purpura (TTP), hemolytic uremic syndrome (HUS) or HELLP syndrome) are accompanied by thrombocytopenia and hemolytic anemia with red blood cell fragments visible on blood film. In septicemia, fever, anemia, thrombocytopenia, abnormal liver function, leukocytosis, an elevated serum lactate and hypoxia are common features. In pre-eclampsia, features of severe disease including

Table 7.8 Causes of acute renal failure (acute kidney injury) in pregnancy

	Mechanism	Common causes
Pre-renal		
Hypovolaemia	Reduced renal perfusion leading to abrupt decline in GFR	Antepartum and postpartum hemorrhage Severe vomiting +/− diarrhea
Sepsis	Reduced perfusion due to shift of fluid from intravascular to extravascular space Vasodilation leading to hypotension and reduced perfusion	Septic abortion Gram-negative sepsis, including pyelonephritis
Renal (parenchymal)		
Microangiopathy	Platelet-fibrin thrombi obstructing microvasculature "Endotheliosis"	HELLP syndrome/pre-eclampsia TTP-HUS syndrome
Acute tubular necrosis	Toxic or ischemic insult to renal tubulointerstitium	Pre-eclampsia AFLP Sepsis Drugs such as aminoglycosides Any pre-renal cause
Glomerulonephritis	Inflammatory/vasculitic disorder of kidneys	SLE Crescentic glomerulonephritis
Obstructive		
Acute hydroureter	Obstruction to ureters due to extrinsic compression and endogenous relaxation	Gravid uterus, ligamentous impingement, smooth muscle relaxation (rare)
Kidney stones	Bilateral ureteric obstruction	Calcium oxalate calculi

AFLP, acute fatty liver of pregnancy; GFR, glomerular filtration rate; HELLP, hemolysis, elevated liver enzymes, low platelets; SLE, systemic lupus erythematosus; TTP-HUS, thrombotic thrombocytopenic purpura - hemolytic uremic syndrome.

thrombocytopenia, elevated liver transaminases, proteinuria and cerebrovascular involvement are often (but not always) seen before acute oliguric renal failure develops.

Nonoliguric renal failure is usually mild and insidious. A rise in serum urea and creatinine without other obvious clinical features may be first signs of a potentially serious problem. This often occurs in the context of a pre-eclamptic woman under expectant management, a woman with pre-existing chronic renal disease in her third trimester, and occasionally in the woman with flank pain and hydroureter with functional obstruction or a kidney stone causing true obstruction.

The most important issue to be addressed when acute kidney injury develops is to establish the cause. Once this is achieved, a decision can be made on whether it is potentially reversible and pregnancy can be allowed to continue, or whether delivery is required.

Initial investigations should include serum creatinine, urea and electrolytes, full blood count and blood film, urinalysis, urine microscopy and culture, renal ultrasound, and a urine Na and creatinine. A urine sodium of <20 mmol/L is suggestive of a pre-renal cause of ARF. A better predictor, however, is the fractional excretion of sodium (FE Na) which is calculated using the following formula:

$$FE\ Na = [(Urine\ Na \times plasma\ Cr)/(plasma\ Na \times urine\ Cr)] \times 100$$

A FE Na value below 1% is suggestive of a pre-renal cause (with greater likelihood of reversibility) while a value above 1% is suggestive of a renal cause.

Timing of delivery

Timing of delivery may be critical to maternal as well as fetal outcome. If the renal failure is due to the pregnancy and is progressive (e.g. pre-eclampsia) then delivery is indicated. If the renal disease is stimulated by but not solely due to the pregnancy (e.g. TTP/HUS), then early delivery may not benefit the neonate or the mother.

If renal failure progresses, dialysis may be required and in this situation there is a high risk of fetal death and maternal morbidity. Acute cortical necrosis is a serious renal outcome which includes renal cortical infarction, often leading to permanent dialysis requirement. Cortical necrosis may complicate any oliguric renal failure, but the microangiopathic diseases (TTP, HUS and HELLP) are well-recognized causes.

Specific syndromes

Acute renal failure due to pre-eclampsia

This is probably the most common cause of acute renal failure in pregnancy in developed countries. It usually occurs in severe disease, where multiple organ involvement is present.

The only known treatment which reverses organ dysfunction in pre-eclampsia is delivery. If renal function is deteriorating rapidly, delivery is the required treatment. In this setting it is useful to try volume expansion first though we give no more than 500 mL of colloid over 4 hours and delivery is effected if there is no response. Most organ dysfunction following pre-eclampsia is completely reversible, but subtle abnormalities such as slightly reduced GFR, proteinuria or hypertension may remain.

Where renal function is mildly abnormal but not deteriorating, close monitoring of general maternal and fetal welfare is reasonable, particularly before 32 weeks gestation. The additional presence of heavy proteinuria or severe hypertension confers a worse prognosis and likelihood of fetal distress and growth restriction, and in this circumstance delivery is indicated.

Acute renal failure due to acute fatty liver of pregnancy

This potentially fatal condition is fortunately uncommon (about 1/7000 pregnancies from a large series in the USA) [83]. Previously considered rare and fatal, it is more readily diagnosed now, presumably because of earlier recognition. Generally, the presentation is with nausea, vomiting and malaise but may include pruritus and jaundice. Laboratory tests show raised transaminases, hyperbilirubinemia, coagulopathy, leukocytosis and renal failure. The mechanism of acute renal failure is not known but is likely to be multifactorial, with intravascular volume depletion, hyperbilirubinemia, coagulation cascade activation, diabetes insipidus and pancreatitis often co-existing and contributing to maternal disease.

Once the diagnosis is made, delivery is generally indicated and renal function is unlikely to return to normal until after delivery. During this period, supportive care of the mother, correction of metabolic, coagulation, hemodynamic and respiratory perturbations, avoidance of hepatotoxins (e.g. paracetamol) and nephrotoxins (e.g. gentamicin) and aggressive treatment of any sepsis should be instituted.

Acute renal failure due to the TTP/HUS complex

These two conditions were previously considered separate entities but fulfill criteria for extremes of a range of conditions. The underlying pathophysiology is the formation of platelet-fibrin thrombi which circulate, causing obstruction to microvasculature and organ damage. It should be noted that these conditions are not examples of vasculitis but rather diseases characterized by damage to endothelium with subsequent thrombosis and organ hypoperfusion, some cases characterized by the presence of circulating multimeric forms of von Willebrand factor.

In both conditions, the microangiopathy results in hemolytic anemia and consumptive thrombocytopenia. In TTP, the classic diagnosis includes a pentad of features: fever, thrombocytopenia, microangiopathic hemolysis, neurologic disturbance and renal involvement. In HUS, the microangiopathic process affects the kidneys more substantially, causing significant renal failure often requiring dialysis. In adults, a distinction between the two conditions is academic, as some women will develop neither neurologic symptoms nor renal disease but some develop both. Both conditions are managed with plasmapheresis and it has become common to use the term TTP/HUS complex to describe this condition.

Pregnancy certainly precipitates TTP/HUS, usually in the third trimester or post partum, but fortunately it remains a rare condition, affecting approximately 1/25,000 pregnancies [84], approximately 50% of cases occurring antenatally and 50% postnatally [85]. Ten to 25% of all TTP/HUS cases occur in pregnancy and it may be difficult to differentiate TTP/HUS from pre-eclampsia, which also may cause thrombotic microangiopathy. Although there is no clear distinguishing feature between the two illnesses, it has been noted by some clinicians that the hemolysis associated with pre-eclampsia (as assessed by the stability of the hemoglobin, the level of lactate dehydrogenase (LDH) and the number of fragmented red blood cells or schistocytes on a blood smear) tends to be mild in comparison to the more frank hemolysis seen in TTP/HUS. Whether pre-eclampsia initiates a TTP-like illness, which in some women progresses to a more serious ongoing disease, is unknown. It is therefore imperative to carefully assess the pregnant woman who has features which suggest pre-eclampsia and TTP, because usually pre-eclampsia/HELLP syndrome will be reversible with delivery and supportive care. In fact, it is probable that failure for spontaneous recovery to occur after delivery defines a group of women with ongoing microangiopathy who have TTP/HUS rather than pre-eclampsia.

Interestingly, pregnant women with HIV seem to be particularly susceptible to the development of TTP, with case descriptions in the second trimester and in successive pregnancies [86,87].

Treatment of this condition requires early recognition, particularly exclusion of pre-eclampsia/HELLP as a cause. If thrombotic microangiopathy develops in the first half of pregnancy, TTP should be strongly considered as the diagnosis because pre-eclampsia/HELLP is more likely to occur after 25 weeks gestation. Once diagnosed, treatment depends on gestation. If the fetus is viable, it should be delivered, as a high rate of fetal death has been described accompanying this condition.

Plasma therapy should be initiated as soon as possible once the diagnosis is made. Plasma exchange (initially 30 mL/kg/day) has been demonstrated safe and effective in pregnancy. If this resource is not available, plasma infusion using fresh frozen plasma should be initiated. Treatment should commence daily until platelet count and hemolytic parameters stabilize and improve, at which time thrice weekly treatment is reasonable. Glucocorticoids have also been used in this condition, though evidence of efficacy is lacking.

Dialysis treatment is indicated if severe acute renal failure or endstage renal failure develops. The long-term consequences include chronic kidney disease, possible endstage renal disease requiring dialysis or transplantation and a risk of recurrence in subsequent pregnancies. Although the risk of relapse outside pregnancy is about 30–60%, the risk of recurrence in pregnancy is considered low unless the disease is congenital or associated with chronic viral infection.

Renal calculi in pregnancy

Pregnancy is a state of hyperfiltration, hypercalciuria and urinary stasis, increasing supersaturation of calcium salts, yet in the past renal calculus disease was typically not reported as more common in pregnancy than in the nonpregnant state, with a rate of about 1/1500 pregnancies [88]. In 2003, however, a large series from Indianapolis reported an incidence of 1/244 pregnancies [89] which accords more with clinical observation. Protection of the pregnant woman against stone disease has previously been explained by the simultaneous increase in endogenous inhibitors of stone formation, one recent study identifying thiosulfaturia, a known inhibitor of stone formation, parallelling hypercalciuria during gestation and returning to normal post partum [90].

Most women will present with flank pain (89%) or macroscopic hematuria (95%). Renal colic usually develops as a consequence of a ureteric stone but is sometimes due to ureteric "obstruction" without a stone being identified. In occasional women this may be a functional intermittent obstruction of the ureter whilst in others it reflects the inability of ultrasound to detect calculi in some cases. The presence of microscopic or macroscopic hematuria accompanying this pain increases the suspicion for a kidney stone.

The investigation of choice outside pregnancy is noncontrast helical CT scan of the abdomen, which identifies calcium-containing and noncalcium-containing stones with high sensitivity. While the fetal radiation represented by this study is well within what has been deemed to be an acceptable exposure in pregnancy, there is a cultural discomfort with this test as a first-line investigation in pregnancy on the part of both patients and clinicians. Renal and pelvic ultrasound is therefore the most common investigation for renal colic in pregnancy. Unfortunately, this modality visualizes the ureter poorly (unless dilated) and accordingly the sensitivity and specificity for stone diagnosis are poor (in the order of 30–60%) [91]. Performance of the test may be improved in dedicated centers with extensive experience. Identification of stones may also be improved by use of transvaginal ultrasound to look for stones in the distal ureter if the renal and pelvic ultrasound is negative. Combining ultrasound with a plain X-ray of the abdomen approached the diagnostic reliability of helical CT scan in one study of nonpregnant patients and should be considered in situations where urolithiasis is suspected but not visible on ultrasound alone [78]. Another option is to do a limited ("single-shot") intravenous pyelogram (IVP) (which has excellent sensitivity and minimal radiation exposure associated with it [92]) or ureteroscopy (where available). Finally, MRI can be used to identify urolithiasis in pregnancy if necessary. In our experience it is unusual to have to consider extensive investigations such as these.

Management

In the presence of a renal calculus, definitive management of the stone can at most times be left until after delivery, because conservative therapy with admission, rest, analgesia and hydration will result in spontaneous passage of a stone in two out of three cases and avoid the small risks associated with anesthesia and the potential requirement for ionizing radiation with scanning. However, infection must be excluded and, if present, becomes an indication for nephrostomy decompression of an obstructed system. A stone obstructing the ureter may be managed by percutaneous drainage or by the placement of a ureteric stent and if there is evidence of renal insufficiency, should not be delayed. Shock-wave lithotripsy has not been shown to be safe and may potentially be deleterious to fetal hearing [91]. If a surgical procedure is necessary, ureteroscopy with YAG (yttrium-aluminum-garnet) laser lithotripsy has been effectively used and is considered relatively safe [93].

Dialysis in pregnancy

Perhaps one area where there has been significant advance in the outcome of pregnant women with renal disease is that of dialysis. Traditionally, pregnancy in a woman undergoing hemodialysis or peritoneal dialysis was thought to be futile. We are now in an era where the outcome of such pregnancies realistically offers a one in two chance of fetal survival, albeit with about 80% chance of prematurity [94,95]. Reasons for this improved outlook include realization outside pregnancy that general health and long-term outcomes are better with more intensive dialysis and translation of this observation to the pregnant woman, improved modalities of dialysis, including nocturnal hemodialysis to allow improved dialysis clearances with greater hemodynamic stability, and advances in neonatal care allowing survival for more premature and growth-restricted fetuses.

Estimates of likely fertility in women of childbearing age undergoing dialysis are cumulatively around one in 20 across the duration of their dialysis [95,96] though probably only 0.3–1.4% in any prevalence study [97]. A practical point arising from these observations is that all women of childbearing age on any form of dialysis need to be counseled about adequate contraception due to the fairly poor outcomes of these pregnancies overall.

There are more reports relating to women becoming pregnant whilst already on maintenance chronic dialysis than in those for whom dialysis was initiated once pregnancy occurred in advanced chronic kidney disease. In either case, the available evidence which we give to these women to advise them of likely outcomes is based upon collected data and it is not possible to stratify outcomes according to whether dialysis was initiated after pregnancy or before.

One probable factor relevant to greater likelihood of successful pregnancy is that of residual renal function, though again current studies are unable to discern the impact of this on the pregnancy outcome.

There are increasing reports of successful pregnancy outcomes, generally including intensified hemodialysis or peritoneal dialysis schedules [96–103]. Attention has been drawn to the need to increase phosphate in dialysis fluids [104] and to the successful treatment of anemia with erythropoietin [95]. Attention has also been drawn, through one fatal case experience, to the fact that methotrexate, commonly used now for the management of ectopic pregnancy, should never be used for this purpose in patients on dialysis of any type or for that matter in patients with CKD [105].

Just why intensive dialysis has been associated with improved pregnancy outcomes is unknown but recent observations that the placental hormone PAPP-A is associated with vascular disease and oxidative stress in dialysis patients [106] may provide one link, though it is not yet entirely clear to what extent PAPP-A is removed via dialysis.

The broad recommendations for hemodialysis during pregnancy include:
• a minimum 20 hours per week dialysis
• maintenance of serum calcium with additional oral calcium and vitamin D and increased calcium dialysate, monitored with frequent calcium measures as occasionally placental production of vitamin D-like substances may lead to increased serum calcium
• increased folic acid supplementation, generally 4 mg daily
• less aggressive use of alkali treatment to maintain serum bicarbonate in the usual pregnancy range of 18–22 mmol/L
• intravenous iron as required to ensure adequate iron stores, generally a serum ferritin above 200 and iron saturation above 20%
• erythropoietin at generally higher doses than needed pre-pregnancy to maintain hemoglobin around 100–110 g/L (10–11 g/dL), with increased surveillance of blood pressure
• dialysis heparin requirements are often increased due to the hypercoagulable state of pregnancy; this is not the situation for every pregnant woman and is assessed in practical terms by assessing dialysis adequacy and dialyser clotting.

There is little information concerning specific requirements of women on peritoneal dialysis during pregnancy. It is now generally agreed that there is no need to switch from peritoneal dialysis to hemodialysis even as the uterus enlarges. Dialysis adequacy can be maintained throughout pregnancy, though complications such as hemoperitoneum have been observed and the major risk is that of peritonitis with the attendant risk of premature labor or premature rupture of membranes.

Other issues not specific to dialysis but absolutely necessary in order to have a successful pregnancy outcome in this population include the following:

• control of maternal blood pressure, generally to 110–140/80–90 mmHg. This is difficult to achieve in many cases. Firstly, despite minimal or even lack of renal function there still appears to be volume expansion in women on maintenance hemodialysis who become pregnant, as evidenced by their anemia and fall in serum albumin. As in the general dialysis population, volume expansion undoubtedly plays a key role in their hypertension but it is extremely difficult to assess the volume status of the pregnant woman on dialysis. Traditional measures such as weight gain (an expected normal event in pregnancy) and edema are of little use, and falling hemoglobin or albumin may be multifactorial and not only due to volume expansion. In truth, our clinical capacity to assess the pregnant woman's volume status is such that we can only detect extremes, i.e. significant volume overload with chest crepitations and raised JVP or else significant volume contraction with hypotension. The latter has the most significant adverse outcome for the pregnancy, due to presumed reduction to uteroplacental blood flow. There are new means of assessing volume status in dialysis patients, such as ultrasound measurement of inferior vena cava diameter, but these have not been assessed in pregnancy and no normative data exist
• detection of any degree of sepsis, which in turn precipitates premature labor or premature rupture of membranes. Dialysis patients in general have a degree of immunosuppression and the managing clinician needs to be vigilant for any signs of infection during the pregnancy and commence antibiotics rapidly. For those with residual renal function, repeated urine cultures are justified even in the absence of urinary symptoms, to detect and treat asymptomatic bacteriuria
• there are ongoing trials concerning the potential benefit of progesterone or its metabolites for the prevention of preterm labor, though not specifically in dialysis patients. Reports of changes in serum progesterone during dialysis vary widely, from significant reduction to an increase [95].

A key question is when to initiate dialysis in women who have advanced kidney disease but are not yet on dialysis at the time of conception. There is no formal study of this issue though it has become generally accepted to commence dialysis at an estimated GFR of 20 mL/min or a blood urea above 20 mmol/L (56 mg/dL) [5]. Similarly, for women already on dialysis we aim for predialysis urea below 15 mmol/L (42 mg/dL) and urea reduction ratio (a widely used measure of dialysis adequacy calculated with the following formula: URR = (predialysis BUN − postdialysis BUN)/predialysis BUN×100%) above 65%. None of these recommendations is based upon sound scientific research but they are in line with those observed by nephrologists to have increased dialysis delivery and improved pregnancy outcomes.

It is apparent that for a pregnant woman on dialysis to have a successful pregnancy, she needs at least weekly surveillance from her clinicians to assess all the above factors. Fetal monitoring includes at least 4-weekly, and possibly

2-weekly, ultrasounds (for growth and amniotic fluid index) from the time of fetal viability, i.e. usually around 24 weeks gestation. At 32–34 weeks gestation, many centers would add twice-weekly nonstress testing.

Renal transplantation in pregnancy

Successful renal transplantation is an excellent way of restoring fertility in women with endstage renal failure. At the start of this century there was already a generally favorable view towards pregnancy in women who had undergone successful renal transplantation. This was based largely upon data from Davison, most of those women receiving azathioprine and prednisone, with extensive observations in over 3000 pregnancies from 2000 women [107]. A general summary of the view at this time was that about 15% of these pregnancies miscarried spontaneously and of those going past the first trimester, successful pregnancy outcome occurred in over 90% of cases, provided that hypertension or a decline in renal function had not occurred before 28 weeks gestation, in which case successful pregnancy outcome was reduced to about 70%. Not surprisingly, similar outcomes were observed according to the preconception GFR, women with creatinine less than 125 μmol/L (1.4 mg/dL) having a 96% successful pregnancy whilst those with higher serum creatinine had a 75% successful pregnancy. More importantly, and in keeping with the data discussed above for women with chronic renal disease from any origin, long-term decline in renal function occurred significantly more often (27%) in those with preconception creatinine above 125 μmol/L (1.4 mg/dL). This observation also pointed to the fact that pregnancy *per se* was unlikely to affect the course of the renal transplant but rather the transplant function preconception was the determining factor.

Even with these relatively good outcomes, at least 30% of cases developed significant hypertension as the pregnancy progressed (sometimes from superimposed pre-eclampsia), fetal growth restriction occurred in almost 40% of cases and preterm delivery in as many as two-thirds, with attendant long-term risks of prematurity.

The US National Transplantation Pregnancy Registry (NTPR) [108] was established in 1991 and reported in 2004 on the outcomes of 1451 pregnancies, 1125 from women who had received kidney alone transplants. This included women taking cyclosporine, cyclosporine microemulsion and tacrolimus. Mean serum creatinine before pregnancy was excellent in all groups, approximately 125 μmol/L (1.4 mg/dL). Spontaneous abortion rates ranged from 12% to 24%, 40–50% of surviving pregnancies were of low birthweight and around 50% were premature. Graft loss within 2 years ranged from 4% to 13%. Newborn complication rates were similar across all groups, with approximately 4% of babies having a birth defect.

Twenty-four pregnancies were reported in women taking either mycophenolate or sirolimus, 12 of which resulted in spontaneous abortion, raising potential concerns about pregnancy in women taking these agents.

Importantly, this review analyzed the outcomes of pregnancies fathered by male transplant recipients and concluded that mean gestational age and mean birthweight are similar to those of the general population.

A case–control study of pregnant renal allograft recipients found that graft and patient survival were similar in those with and without any pregnancy at a mean of 7 years follow-up [109], also found in a 15-year follow-up study [110]. This same group observed a postpregnancy increase in creatinine associated with cyclosporine use, also observed in the NTPR publication, possibly because cyclosporine doses were increased during pregnancy as plasma levels fell, presumably due to the associated plasma volume expansion of pregnancy. It remains controversial whether cyclosporine or tacrolimus doses should be increased during pregnancy. Assuming stable preconception cyclosporine or tacrolimus blood level, it is not our practice to make dose adjustments unless there are extreme deviations from the baseline level during pregnancy.

A further analysis from the NTPR data showed that the outcomes of women who were transplanted for SLE and then became pregnant were similar to outcomes of pregnancy in women transplanted for other reasons [111].

A number of other recent publications have generally confirmed the high likelihood of a live baby but also fetal growth restriction and prematurity in renal transplant recipients [112–116].

The issues of concern in managing the pregnant woman with a renal transplant should be considered in terms of both mother and baby. The outcomes for the mother and her renal function are generally the same as for any woman with pre-existing chronic renal disease, discussed above. Specific maternal concerns are:

- transplant rejection, occurring in less than one in 20 cases, characterized by a rising serum creatinine, generally non-oliguric and requiring renal biopsy to confirm a true diagnosis
- increased risk of infection (22–34%), particularly urinary tract infection but also CMV infection with attendant maternal and fetal risks. The consequences of any infection can include premature labor and preterm rupture of membranes
- gestational diabetes, present in 3–12% of pregnancies, no more common in tacrolimus-treated women than in those receiving cyclosporine
- hypertension, either accelerated from pre-existing hypertension or *de novo* during pregnancy, present in 58–72% of cases [108]
- need for cesarean section in approximately half of cases
- as discussed above, long-term graft loss is similar in women undergoing pregnancy as in matched women with a renal transplant who did not undergo pregnancy.

The concerns for the baby can be summarized as follows:
- spontaneous miscarriage of about one in 5–10 cases
- prematurity in half of cases
- fetal growth restriction in half of cases
- birth defects, probably no more common than in the general population [62]
- long-term consequences of prematurity, though most babies have normal postnatal growth and development [117,118].

Data from the NTPR report make it clear that we do not really know what recommendations to make regarding breastfeeding for women taking immunosuppressive agents. The transfer of cyclosporine, tacrolimus, corticosteroids and azathioprine into breast milk appears to be low but there are no data for mycophenolate and sirolimus. Only about 25–30 reports of breastfeeding in renal transplant patients have been documented, none with any known adverse effects to date. The decision to proceed is an individual one, informing the woman that effects on the baby remain largely unknown but particularly in premature and growth-restricted babies, breastfeeding may have considerable advantages.

At the present time the most reasonable recommendations regarding pregnancy in women with a renal transplant are as follows:
- graft function should be stable, with at least a 1-year interval from the time of transplant
- the best pregnancy outcome will occur if serum creatinine is less than 125 μmol/L (<1.4 mg/dL), proteinuria is less than 1 g per day and blood pressure below 140/90 mmHg. Therefore, it is sometimes prudent to delay pregnancy whilst using ACE inhibitors to control blood pressure and reduce proteinuria, then switching to other drugs which are safe to use for treatment of hypertension during pregnancy such as oxprenolol, methyldopa or prazosin
- there should be no evidence of sepsis and in particular urinary tract infections should be eradicated before pregnancy; prophylactic antibiotics are indicated for women who have had recurrent urine infections since their transplant, in order to prevent pregnancy complications such as spontaneous rupture of membranes and allograft dysfunction
- cyclosporine or tacrolimus blood levels should be stable: we do not recommend dose adjustments during pregnancy unless there are extreme variations from these stable levels
- diabetes should be assessed for and controlled in advance of a pregnancy
- the pregnant woman should be seen alternately by her nephrologist and obstetrician so that 2-weekly visits are undertaken up until 24 weeks gestation, i.e. fetal viability, and thereafter weekly visits. Fetal growth needs to be assessed by ultrasound at least 2–4 weekly, and possibly more often, from 24 weeks gestation. Fetal nonstress testing may be added once or twice after 32–24 weeks gestation as an additional measure of fetal well-being
- both the transplant recipient and her partner need to be made fully aware of potential risks. Although the pregnancy outcomes are in general favorable, this is not always the case and the impact of fetal death or graft loss is enormous.

Anesthetic management of parturients with renal impairment

Obstetric patients with impaired renal function may require anesthetic intervention antentally for incidental or related surgery, e.g. renal biopsy They are more likely to require anesthetic intervention peripartum and are at increased risk of perioperative complications.

Antenatal anesthetic management

Although there is a great difference between the normovolemic parturient with mild or moderate stable renal impairment, with controlled hypertension, and the patient with endstage renal failure on dialysis, it is essential that all patients with significant renal impairment are assessed antenatally by an experienced anesthesiologist familiar with the management of obstetric patients with renal disease. A detailed plan of management should be drawn up antenatally, covering all possible clinical scenarios and including contact details for senior obstetric, medical and anesthetic personnel knowledgeable about the case.

The antepartum evaluation by an anesthesiologist should include a history, examination and investigations directed at establishing the severity of the multisystem effects of renal impairment that directly impact on anesthetic risks (Table 7.9). These are likely to be particularly severe in the diabetic patient who should be considered particularly vulnerable.

Depending on the severity of the renal impairment, cardiac function should be assessed, using echocardiography. In patients with long-standing renal disease and a poor functional status, consideration should be given to whether stress testing is indicated since these patients are at high risk of ischemic heart disease as they age.

The aim of any anesthetic intervention is to protect renal function and to maintain both placental and renal blood flow and GFR, by avoiding sudden changes in blood pressure. The avoidance of aortocaval compression is crucial in these patients and the supine position should be avoided from the second trimester.

Intrapartum anaesthetic management

Because renal impairment is associated with delayed gastric emptying and patients are at increased risk of requiring surgical delivery, a nil by mouth policy in labor with allowance for modest amounts of clear liquids seems prudent, although modifications on a case-by-case basis are warranted. In addition, H2 blockers and metoclopramide during labor are indicated.

Table 7.9 Pathologic features affecting anesthetic management in chronic renal failure

Abnormality	Anesthetic management
Cardiovascular	
Hypertension	Maintain normotension with goal BP ~130/80. Labetalol, hydralazine are preferred intravenous agents in pregnancy
Fluid retention	Maintain euvolemia – avoid both fluid overload (which can cause pulmonary edema) and hypovolemia (which can harm both the fetus and the maternal kidney)
Cardiac dysfunction (e.g. pericarditis/ischemic heart disease/ hypertensive heart disease/cardiomyopathy)	Consider preoperative EKG, echocardiogram (and in some cases stress testing if prolonged history of renal insufficiency) Role of invasive monitoring is limited but may be used at some centers in patients with both severe renal and cardiac disease
Pulmonary	
Immunosuppression	Consider preoperative CXR if any evidence of respiratory infection
Propensity for pulmonary edema	Maintain euvolemia – avoid both fluid overload and hypovolemia
Metabolic	
Acidosis, K↑, Mg↑, Na↓, Ca↓, Glu↓	Obtain preoperative urine, electrolytes, magnesium, calcium and glucose Avoid suxamethonium if K >5.5 mEq/L Consider preoperative dialysis
Decreased protein binding of drugs	Reduce doses of induction agents/opioids
Hematologic	
Anemia Abnormal platelet function Thrombocytopenia	Ask about any bleeding history. Obtain preoperative complete blood count, coagulation screen, type and screen
Immunosuppression	Use careful aseptic technique for all invasive procedures
Neurologic	
Autonomic neuropathy (especially in patients with diabetic nephropathy)	Regional anesthesia may cause hypotension if patient hypovolemic – ensure euvolemia
Peripheral neuropathy	Document before administering a regional block
Gastrointestinal	
Delayed gastric emptying	Ranitidine/metoclopramide
Increased acidity	Rapid sequence induction

CXR, chest X-ray; EKG, electrocardiogram.

On admission, there should be baseline evaluation of blood pressure and blood sample for creatinine, urea, electrolytes, full blood count, coagulation profile and type and screen should be obtained. Although there are no additional contraindications to regional blockade specific to the patient with renal impairment, there is an increased incidence of coagulation either from the renal insufficiency itself (e.g. platelet function abnormalities) or the underlying disease (e.g. thrombocytopenia associated with SLE) that may preclude regional anesthesia.

Regional analgesia in labor has the benefits of renal vasodilation, improved uteroplacental flow and effective analgesia, reducing maternal catecholamine levels. It can aid control of blood pressure in severe pre-eclampsia [119]. Because a degree of immunosuppression is associated with chronic renal failure, particular attention must be paid to aseptic technique for insertion of neuraxial blockade.

Maintainance of euvolemia (and avoidance of hypotension) is important to preserve both existing renal function and placental perfusion and therefore patients should have adequate fluid replacement in labor and an assessment of volume status with appropriate interventions prior to initiation of regional blockade. At the same time, pregnant women, especially those with superimposed pre-eclampsia, are vulnerable to pulmonary edema from fluid overload. Fluid preloading should therefore only be used if there are clinical indications of pre-existing hypovolemia as it is ineffective in maintaining blood pressure during regional blockade [120]. The use of low-dose combinations of local anesthetics with opioids is preferred as it allows a smooth onset of analgesia for labor [121] with less risk of hypotension.

Women with renal disease are at increased risk of pre-eclampsia and regional anesthesia is now recognized to be the technique of choice for cesarean section in severe pre-eclampsia, in the absence of contraindications [122]. Spinal as opposed to epidural anesthesia is not associated with more hemodynamic instability and produces more reliable anesthesia [123]. Regional anesthesia has also been used for renal transplantation and therefore has a proven track record for use in patients with endstage renal disease [124]. Central venous pressure monitoring may be helpful but is rarely essential as clinical assessment of volume status is generally adequate [125]. Fluid preloading should be minimized and hemodynamic stability maintained through careful titration of a vasoconstrictor. Some experts recommend avoiding ephedrine in patients with renal impairment because of a possible increased risk of central nervous system toxicity but this is not widely agreed upon [126]. The use of the alternative agent phenylephrine is associated with higher umbilical artery pH and smaller base deficit in elective patients but this advantage is not found in patients having nonelective cesarean sections [127].

Theoretically, the hyperdynamic circulation associated with chronic renal failure should result the faster clearance of local anesthetics and therefore reduced duration of action. A study by Orko, however, comparing nonpregnant patients with and without renal impairment found that spinal blockade developed more quickly and the eventual height of the block was higher in those with impaired renal function [128].

If general anesthesia is required, a rapid sequence induction is mandatory to protect the airway. Doses of induction agents (thiopentone or propofol) may need to be reduced [129]. In the presence of hyperkalemia (>5.5 mEq/L), the depolarizing muscle relaxant suxamethonium should not be used as it causes an increase in potassium plasma concentration of 0.5–0.7 mEq/L, which may precipitate arrhythmias [130]. Rocuronium 0.6 mg/kg can be used as an alternative, although its effect may be prolonged and should be monitored with peripheral nerve stimulation.

Neuromuscular blockade may be continued with atracurium, the metabolism of which is independent of renal function. If required, potentially nephrotoxic drugs such as the aminoglycosides should be given in divided doses. All inhalational anesthetics are myocardial depressants and cause vasodilation. The newer agents (e.g. sevoflurane or desflurane) have not been found to produce fluoride ions in concentrations that are potentially nephrotoxic.

Postpartum analgesia is complicated by the relative contraindication of nonsteroidal anti-inflammatory analgesics. Opioid sensitivity is increased and thus caution may be warranted in dose selection.

The patient undergoing dialysis

The patient on dialysis is likely to have many of the multisystem effects of chronic renal failure and requires preoperative in-depth assessment of pulmonary, cardiovascular, neurologic and gastrointestinal systems. Although not a contraindication, peripheral neuropathy should be documented prior to regional blockade for medicolegal purposes. Arteriovenous fistulae should be carefully protected during surgery and blood pressure cuffs applied to the contralateral side. The uremic effects on platelet function are reversed by dialysis which should be carried out within 12–24 hours of surgery. Residual heparinization should be sought. Fluid balance may be particularly hard to ascertain due to changes associated with pregnancy and invasive monitoring is usually indicated.

The patient with renal transplant

In the absence of hypertension or impaired renal function, anesthetic management does not differ from that of the healthy parturient. Blood flow to both the transplanted kidney and the fetus must be protected by avoidance of aortocaval compression and tight control of systemic blood pressure. Strict asepsis during placement of intravascular cannulae and regional blocks is essential due to immunosuppressive regimes that need to be continued throughout pregnancy. Patients receiving steroid therapy may require supplementary doses for labor and surgery. Plasma glucose concentrations should be monitored following an institutionally specific protocol.

Acute renal failure

The management will depend on the cause. If pre-eclampsia is the cause, pulmonary edema poses the most significant risk and fluid should be limited to what is necessary to achieve a normal circulating volume. If the cause is pre-renal, fluid replacement may be necessary. In rare cases, invasive monitoring (either a central venous pressure line or less commonly a pulmonary artery catheter) may be necessary to guide replacement. If time allows, dialysis prior to delivery or labor may be indicated. If general anesthesia is contemplated, chest X-ray should be performed to exclude pneumothorax in patients who have had central venous catheters inserted, prior to positive pressure ventilation. Regional anesthesia may be used in the absence of coagulopathy, hypovolemia or systemic sepsis. Techniques that minimize hemodynamic instability during establishment of the block include epidural or sequential combined spinal-epidural anesthesia. Where there is concern about intravascular volume, single-shot spinal should probably be avoided, as it is associated with the most rapid and profound sympathetic blockade.

Models of antenatal care for women with renal disease

Women with underlying renal disease in pregnancy are best managed jointly by an obstetrician and renal or obstetric medicine physician. It is imperative that the obstetrician has an understanding of maternal renal disease in pregnancy and that the physician has an understanding of the possible fetal issues which may occur. Ideally these women are managed through a high-risk pregnancy clinic.

An appropriate schedule of visits for these "at-risk" pregnancies is as follows.

• Two-weekly visits from 12 weeks gestation, alternating between obstetrician and nephrologist, up until 24–28 weeks.

• Thereafter, weekly visits (alternating as above) so that the pregnant woman is seen weekly until delivery.

• Following delivery, routine obstetric review at 6 weeks post partum is required but nephrology review should occur within the first 4 weeks as impairment of renal function may occur even after delivery in women with underlying renal disease.

Appropriate testing of renal function in such women is as follows.

• Initial visit at 12 weeks gestation – full blood count (Hb, hematocrit, platelet count), serum creatinine and electrolytes, liver function, mid-stream urine culture and 24-hour urinary protein and creatinine if proteinuria is apparent on dipstick testing. Protein/creatinine ratio can be calculated from the 24-hour urine collection and used as a baseline. Additional fetal surveillance options are reviewed in Chapter 49.

• Women with baseline normal GFR do not require further blood tests until around 24 weeks gestation; those with abnormal GFR at baseline require a full blood count, serum creatinine and electrolytes, liver function and spot urinary protein/creatinine ratio 4 weekly with blood pressure and urinalysis at every visit.

• Mid-stream urine culture should be repeated routinely at approximately 24, 28 and 32–34 weeks gestation.

• Fetal assessment in those with impaired GFR and/or heavy proteinuria should include ultrasound for uterine artery pulsatility index at 20 weeks then for fetal growth, blood flow and amniotic fluid index monthly from 24 weeks gestation.

Whilst these pregnancies are certainly high risk compared with the normal pregnant woman, it is important for clinicians and midwives to remember that provided a diligent approach is taken, such as that recommended above, then the final pregnancy outcome in most cases is successful for both mother and baby. For this reason it is important that the clinicians managing the pregnant woman with underlying renal disease take a positive approach to her pregnancy, at all times emphasizing the need for diligence and assessment for potential complications, but highlighting that the end result in most cases will be good, in turn helping to relieve some of the stress that accompanies pregnancy for these women.

References

1. Davison JM, Dunlop W. Renal hemodynamics and tubular function in normal human pregnancy. Kidney Int 1980; 18:152–61.
2. Burge HJ, Middleton WD, McClennan BL, Hildebolt CF. Ureteral jets in healthy subjects and in patients with unilateral ureteral calculi: comparison with color Doppler ultrasound. Radiology 1991;180:437–40.
3. Baker SM, Middleton WD. Color Doppler sonography of ureteral jets in normal volunteers: importance of the relative specific gravity of urine in the ureter and bladder. Am J Roentgenol 1992;159:773–5.
4. Brown MA. Urinary tract dilation in pregnancy. Am J Obstet Gynecol 1991;164:641–3.
5. Lindheimer MD, Greenfeld JP, Davison JM. Renal disorders. In: Barron WM, Lindheimer MD (eds) Medical disorders in pregnancy. Mosby, St Louis, 2000: 39–70.
6. Conrad K, Lindheimer M. Renal and cardiovascular alterations. In: Lindheimer M (ed) Chesley's hypertensive disorders in pregnancy. Appleton and Lange, Stamford, CT, 1999: 263–326.
7. Roberts M, Lindheimer MD, Davison JM. Altered glomerular permselectivity to neutral dextrans and heteroporous membrane modelling in human pregnancy. Am J Physiol 1996;270: F338–F343.
8. Gallery EDM, Brown MA. Volume homeostasis in normal and hypertensive human pregnancy. Baillière's Clin Obstet Gynaecol 1987;1:835–51.
9. Davison JM, Sheills EA, Philips PR, et al. Serial evaluation of vasopressin release and thirst in human pregnancy. Role of human chorionic gonadotrophin in the osmoregulatory changes of gestation. J Clin Invest 1988;81:798–806.
10. Brown MA, Sinosich MJ, Saunders DM, Gallery EDM. Potassium regulation and progesterone aldosterone interrelationships in human pregnancy: a prospective study. Am J Obstet Gynecol 1986;155:349–53.
11. Akbari A, Wilkes P, Lindheimer M, Lepage N, Filler G. Reference intervals for anion gap and strong ion difference in pregnancy: a pilot study. Hypertens Pregnancy 2007;26:111–19.
12. Brown MA, Wang M-X, Buddle ML, et al. Albumin excretory rate in normal and hypertensive pregnancy. Clin Sci 1994;86:251–5.
13. Davison JM, Sheills EA, Barron WM, et al. Changes in the metabolic clearance of vasopressin and in plasma vasopressinase throughout human pregnancy. J Clin Invest 1989;83: 1313–18.
14. Milne JE, Lindheimer MD, Davison JM. Glomerular heteroporous membrane modelling in third trimester and postpartum before and during amino acid infusion. Am J Physiol Renal Physiol 2002;282:F170–5.
15. Higby K, Suiter CR, Phelps JY, Siler-Khodr T, Langer O. Normal values of urinary albumin and total protein excretion during pregnancy. Am J Obstet Gynecol 1994;171:984–9.
16. Saudan PJ, Brown MA, Farrell T, Shaw L. Improved methods of assessing proteinuria in hypertensive pregnancy. Br J Obstet Gynecol 1997;104:1159–64.
17. Brown MA, Holt JL, Mangos GJ, Murray N, Curtis J, Homer C. Microscopic haematuria in pregnancy: relevance to pregnancy outcome. Am J Kidney Dis 2005;45:667–73.
18. Lindheimer MD, Davison JM, Katz AI. The kidney and hypertension in pregnancy: twenty exciting years. Semin Nephrol 2001;21:173–89.
19. Jungers P, Chauveau D. Pregnancy in renal disease. Kidney Int 1997;52:871–85.
20. Jones DC. Pregnancy complicated by chronic renal disease. Clin Perinatol 1997;24:483–96.
21. Hou S. Pregnancy in chronic renal insufficiency and end stage renal disease. Am J Kidney Dis 1999;33:235–52.
22. Jungers P, Chauveau D, Choukroun G, et al. Pregnancy in women with impaired renal function. Clin Nephrol 1997;47:281–8.
23. Jungers P, Houillier P, Chauveau D, et al. Pregnancy in women with reflux nephropathy. Kidney Int 1996;50:593–9.

24. Jones DC, Hayslett JP. Outcome of pregnancy in women with moderate or severe renal insufficiency. N Engl J Med 1996;335:226–32.

25. Lindheimer MD, Katz AS. Kidney function and disease in pregnancy. Lea and Febiger, Philadelphia, 1977: 146–87.

26. Holley JL, Bernardini J, Quadric KH, Greenberg A, Laifer SA. Pregnancy outcomes in a prospective matched control study of pregnancy and renal disease. Clin Nephrol 1996;45:77–82.

27. Lindheimer MD, Katz AI. Gestation in women with kidney disease: prognosis and management. Baillière's Clin Obstet Gynaecol 1994;8:387–404.

28. Ramin SM, Vidaeff AC, Yeomans ER, Gilstrap LC. Chronic renal disease in pregnancy. Obstet Gynecol 2006;108:1531–9.

29. Imbasciati E, Gregorino G, Cabiddu G, et al. Pregnancy in CKD stages 3 to 5: fetal and maternal outcomes. Am J Kidney Dis 2007;49:753–62.

30. Bar J, Orvieto, R, Shalav Y, et al. Pregnancy outcome in women with primary renal disease. Isr Med Assoc J 2000;2:178–81.

31. Chakravarty EF, Colon I, Langen ES, et al. Factors that predict prematurity and preeclampsia in pregnancies that are complicated by systemic lupus erythematosus. Am J Obstet Gynecol 2005;192:1897–904.

32. Brown MA, Buddle ML, Farrell TJ, Davis G, Jones M. Randomised trial of management of hypertensive pregnancies by Korotkoff phase IV or phase V. Lancet 1998;352:777–81.

33. Cooper WO, Hernandez-Diaz S, Arbogast PG, et al. Major congenital malformations after first-trimester exposure to ACE inhibitors. N Engl J Med 2006;354:2443–51.

34. Serreau R, Luton D, Macher MA, Delezoide AL, Garel C, Jacqz-Aigrain E. Developmental toxicity of the angiotensin II type 1 receptor antagonists during human pregnancy: a report of 10 cases. Br J Obstet Gynaecol 2005;112:710–12.

35. Galdo T, Gonzalez F, Espinoza M, et al. Impact of pregnancy on the function of transplanted kidneys. Transplant Proc 2005;37:1577–9.

36. Akbari A, Lepage N, Keely E, et al. Cystatin C and beta trace protein as markers of renal function in pregnancy. Br J Obstet Gynaecol 2005;112:575–8.

37. Levey AS, Bosch JP, Lewis, JB, Greene T, Rogers N, Roth D. A more accurate method to estimate glomerular filtration rate from serum creatinine: a new prediction equation. Modification of Diet in Renal Disease Study Group. Ann Intern Med 1999;130:461–70.

38. Cockcroft DW, Gault MH. Prediction of creatinine clearance from serum creatinine. Nephron 1976;16:31–41.

39. Levine RJ, Lam C, Qian C, et al, CPEP Study Group. Soluble endoglin and other circulating antiangiogenic factors in preeclampsia. N Engl J Med 2006;355:992–1005.

40. Baumwell S, Karumanchi SA. Pre-eclampsia: clinical manifestations and molecular mechanisms. Nephron 2007;106:c72–81.

41. Gangaram R, Ojwang PJ, Moodley J, Maharaj D. The accuracy of urine dipsticks as a screening test for proteiuria in hypertensive disorders of pregnancy. Hypertens Pregnancy 2005;24:117–23.

42. Phelan LK, Brown MA, Davis GK, Mangos G. A Prospective study of the impact of automated dipstick urinalysis on the diagnosis of pre-eclampsia. Hypertens Pregnancy 2004;23:135–42.

43. Khandelwal M, Kumanova M, Gaughan JP, Reece EA. Role of diltiazem in pregnant women with chronic renal disease. J Matern-Fetal Neonat Med 2002;12:408–12.

44. Airoldi J, Weinstein L. Clinical significance of proteinuria in pregnancy. Obstet Gynecol Surv 2007;62:117–24.

45. Lane C, Brown M, Dunsmuir W, Kelly J, Mangos G. Can spot urine protein/creatinine ratio replace 24 h urine protein in usual clinical nephrology? Nephrology 2006;11:245–9.

46. Newman MG, Robichaux AG, Stedman CM, et al. Perinatal outcomes in preeclampsia that is complicated by massive proteinuria. Am J Obstet Gynecol 2003;188:264–8.

47. Basgul A, Kavak ZN, Sezen D, Basgul A, Gokaslan H, Cakalagaoglu F. A rare case of early onset nephrotic syndrome in pregnancy. Clin Exp Obstet Gynecol 2006;33:127–8.

48. Ronkainen J, Ala-Houhala M, Autio-Harmainen H, et al. Long-term outcome 19 years after childhood IgA nephritis: a retrospective cohort study. Pediatr Nephrol 2006;21:1266–73.

49. Reece EA, Leguizamon G, Homko C. Pregnancy performance and outcomes associated with diabetic nephropathy. Am J Perinatol 1998;15:413.

50. Miodovnik M, Rosenn BM, Khoury JC, Grigsby JL, Siddiqi TA. Does pregnancy increase the risk for development and progression of diabetic nephropathy? Am J Obstet Gynecol 1996;174:1180–9.

51. Ekbom P, Damm P, Feldt-Rasmussen B, Feldt-Rasmussen U, Molvig J, Mathiesen ER. Pregnancy outcome in type I diabetic women with microalbuminuria. Diabetes Care 2001;24:1739–44.

52. Germain S, Nelson-Piercy C. Lupus nephritis and renal disease in pregnancy. Lupus 2006;15:148–55.

53. Yasmeen S, Wilkins EE, Field NT, Sheikh RA, Gilbert WM. Pregnancy outcomes in women with systemic lupus erythematosus. J Matern-Fetal Med 2001;10:91–6.

54. North RA, Taylor RS, Gunn TR. Pregnancy outcome in women with reflux nephropathy and the inheritance of vesico-ureteric reflux. Aust NZ J Obstet Gynecol 2000;40:280–5.

55. Mor Y, Leibovitch I, Zalts R, Lotan D, Jonas P, Ramon J. Analysis of the long-term outcome of surgically corrected vesico-ureteric reflux. BJU Int 2003;92:97–100.

56. Simmonds HA, Cameron JS, Goldsmith DJ, Fairbanks LD, Raman GV. Familial juvenile hyperuricaemic nephropathy is not a rare genetic metabolic purine disease in Britain. Nucleotides Nucleic Acids 2006;25:1071–5.

57. Brown MA, Zammit VC, Mitar DM. Extracellular fluid volumes in pregnancy-induced hypertension. J Hypertens 1992;10:61–8.

58. Duley L, Williams J, Henderson-Smart DJ. Plasma volume expansion for treatment of pre-eclampsia. Cochrane Database of Systematic Reviews, 1999;4:CD001805.

59. Bass JK, Faix RG. Gestational therapy with an angiotensin II receptor antagonist and transient renal failure in a premature infant. Am J Perinatol 2006;23:313–17.

60. Podymow T, August P. Hypertension in pregnancy. Adv Chronic Kidney Dis 2007;14:178–90.

61. Kashiwagi M, Breymann C, Huch R, Huch A. Hypertension in a pregnancy with renal anemia after recombinant human erythropoietin (rhEPO) therapy. Arch Gynecol Obstet 2002;267:54–6.

62. Bar J, Stahl B, Hod M, Wittenberg C, Pardo J, Merlob P. Is immunosuppression therapy in renal allograft recipients teratogenic? A single-center experience. Am J Med Genet 2003;116:31–6.

63. Jain A, Venkataramanan R, Fung JJ, et al. Pregnancy after liver transplantation under tacrolimus. Transplantation 1997; 64:559–65.

64. Kart Koseoglu H, Yucel AE, Kunefeci G, Ozdemir FN, Duran H. Cyclophosphamide therapy in a serious case of lupus nephritis during pregnancy. Lupus 2001;10:818–20.

65. Duley L, Henderson-Smart DJ, Knight M, King J. Antiplatelet agents for preventing pre-eclampsia and its complications. Cochrane Database of Systematic Reviews, 2003;1:CD004659.

66. Askie LM, Duley L, Henderson-Smart DJ, Stewart LA, on behalf of the PARIS Collaborative Group. Antiplatelet agents for prevention of pre-eclampsia: a meta-analysis of individual patient data. Lancet 2007;369:1791–8.

67. Coomarasamy A, Honest H, Papaioannou S, Gee H, Khan KS. Aspirin for prevention of pre-eclampsia in women with historical risk factors: a systematic review. Obstet Gynecol 2003; 101:1319–32.

68. Brown MA, Whitworth JA. The kidney in hypertensive pregnancies – victim and villain. Am J Kidney Dis 1992;20:427–42.

69. Kang DH, Finch J, Nakagawa T, et al. Uric acid, endothelial dysfunction and pre-eclampsia: searching for a pathogenetic link. J Hypertens 2004;22:229–35.

70. Schackis RC. Hyperuricaemia and preeclampsia: is there a pathogenic link? Med Hypotheses 2004;63:239–44.

71. Chen HH, Lin HC, Yeh JC, Chen CP. Renal biopsy in pregnancies complicated by undetermined renal disease. Acta Obstet Gynecol Scand 2001;80:888–93.

72. Krane NK, Thakur V, Wood H, Meleg-Smith S. Evaluation of lupus nephritis during pregnancy by renal biopsy. Am J Nephrol 1995;15:186–91.

73. Murakami S, Saitoh M, Kubo T, Koyama T, Kobayashi M. Renal disease in women with severe pre-eclampsia or gestational proteinuria. Obstet Gynecol 2001;96:945–9.

74. Reiter L, Brown MA, Whitworth JA. Hypertension in pregnancy: the incidence of underlying renal disease and essential hypertension. Am J Kidney Dis 1994;24:883–7.

75. Patterson TF. Andriole VT. Detection, significance, and therapy of bacteriuria in pregnancy. Update in the managed health care era. Infect Dis ClinNorth Am 1997;11:593–608.

76. Vazquez JC, Villar J. Treatments for symptomatic urinary tract infections during pregnancy. Cochrane Database of Systematic Reviews, 2003;4:CD002256.

77. Sweet RL. Bacteriuria and pyelonephritis during pregnancy. Semin Perinatol 1977;1:25–40.

78. Catalano O, Nunziata A, Altei F, Siani A. Suspected ureteral colic: primary helical CT versus selective helical CT after unenhanced radiography and sonography. Am J Roentgenol 2002;178(2):379–87.

79. Pfau A. Sacks TG. Effective prophylaxis for recurrent urinary tract infections during pregnancy. Clin Infect Dis 1992;14:810–14.

80. Smaill F, Vazquez JC. Antibiotics for asymptomatic bacteriuria in pregnancy. Cochrane Database of Systematic Reviews, 2007;2: CD000490.

81. Hill JB, Sheffield JS, McIntire DD, Wendel GD Jr. Acute pyelonephritis in pregnancy. Obstet Gynecol 2005;105:18–23.

82. Jayakumar M, Prabahar MR, Fernando EM, Manorajan R, Venkatraman R, Balaraman V. Epidemiologic trend changes in acute renal failure – a tertiary center experience from South India. Renal Failure 2006 28:405–10.

83. Castro MA, Fassett MJ, Reynolds TB, Shaw KJ, Goodwin TM. Reversible peripartum liver failure: a new perspective on the diagnosis, treatment, and cause of acute fatty liver of pregnancy, based on 28 consecutive cases. Am J Obstet Gynecol 1999;181:389–95.

84. Dashe JS, Ramin SM, Cunningham FG. The long-term consequences of thrombotic microangiopathy (thrombotic thrombocytopenic purpura and hemolytic uremic syndrome) in pregnancy. Obstet Gynecol 1998;91(5 Pt 1):662–8.

85. George JN. The association of pregnancy with thrombotic thrombocytopenic purpura-hemolytic uremic syndrome. Cur Opin Hematol 2003;10:339–44.

86. Ranzini AC, Chavez MR, Ghigliotty B, Porcelli M. Thrombotic thrombocytopenic purpura and human immunodeficiency virus complicating pregnancy. Obstet Gynecol 2002;100:1133–6.

87. Robertson C, Wiselka MJ. Thrombotic thrombocytopenic purpura occurring in consecutive pregnancies in an HIV-infected patient. Int J STD AIDS 2007;18:142–3.

88. Drago JR, Rohner TJ Jr, Chez RA. Management of urinary calculi in pregnancy. Urology 1982;20:578–81.

89. Lewis DF, Robichaux AG 3rd, Jaekle RK, Marcum NG, Stedman CM. Urolithiasis in pregnancy. Diagnosis, management and pregnancy outcome. J Reprod Med 2003;48:28–32.

90. Yatzidis H. Gestational urinary hyperthiosulfaturia protects hypercalciuric normal pregnant women from nephrolithiasis. Int Urol Nephrol 2004;36:445–9.

91. McAleer SJ, Loughlin KR. Nephrolithiasis and pregnancy. Curr Opin Urol 2004;14:123–7.

92. Butler EL, Cox SM, Eberts EG, Cunningham FG. Symptomatic nephrolithiasis complicating pregnancy. Obstet Gynecol 2000;96(5 Pt 1):753–6.

93. Watterson JD, Girvan AR, Beiko DT, et al. Ureteroscopy and holmium:YAG laser lithotripsy: an emerging definitive management strategy for symptomatic ureteral calculi in pregnancy. Urology 2002;60:383–7.

94. Hou S. Historical perspective of pregnancy in chronic kidney disease. Adv Chronic Kidney Dis 2007;14:116–18.

95. Hou S. Pregnancy in dialysis patients: where do we go from here? Semin Dialysis 2003;16:376–8.

96. Holley JL, Reddy SS. Pregnancy in dialysis patients: a review of outcomes, complications, and management. Semin Dialysis 2003;16:384–8.

97. Malik GH, Al-Harbi A, Al-Mohaya S, et al. Pregnancy in patients on dialysis – experience at a referral center. J Assoc Physicians India 2005;53:937–41.

98. Bamberg C, Diekmann F, Haase M, et al. Pregnancy on intensified hemodialysis: fetal surveillance and perinatal outcome. Fetal Diagn Ther 2007;22:289–93.

99. Tan LK, Kanagalingam D, Tan HK, Choong HL. Obstetric outcomes in women with end-stage renal failure requiring renal dialysis. Int J Gynaecol Obstet 2006;94:17–22.

100. Haase M, Morgera S, Bamberg C, et al. A systematic approach to managing pregnant dialysis patients – the importance of an intensified haemodiafiltration protocol. Nephrol Dialysis Transplant 2005;20:2537–42.

101. Smith WT, Darbara S, Kwan M, O'Reilly-Green C, Devita MV. Pregnancy in peritoneal dialysis: a case report and review of adequacy and outcomes. Int Urol Nephrol 2005;37:145–51.

102. Erolu D, Lembet A, Ozdemir FN, et al. Pregnancy during hemodialysis: perinatal outcome in our cases. Transplant Proceed 2004;36:53–5.

103. Shemin D. Dialysis in pregnant women with chronic kidney disease. Semin Dialysis 2003;16:379–83.

104. Hussain S, Savin V, Piering W, Tomasi J, Blumenthal S. Phosphorus-enriched hemodialysis during pregnancy: two case reports. Hemodialysis Int 2005 9:147–52.

105. Kelly H, Harvey D, Moll S. A cautionary tale: fatal outcome of methotrexate therapy given for management of ectopic pregnancy. Obstet Gynecol 2006;107:1171.

106. Coskun A, Bicik Z, Duran S, et al. Pregnancy-associated plasma protein A in dialysis patients. Clin Chem Lab Med 2007;45:63–6.

107. Davison JM. Pregnancy in renal allograft recipients: problems, prognosis and practicalities. Baillière's Clin Obstet Gynaecol 1994;8:501–25.

108. Armenti VT, Radomski JS, Moritz MJ, et al. Report from the National Transplantation Pregnancy Registry (NTPR): outcomes of pregnancy after transplantation. Clin Transpl 2005;69–83.

109. Fischer T, Neumayer HH, Fischer R, et al. Effect of pregnancy on long-term kidney function in renal transplant recipients treated with cyclosporine and with azathioprine. Am J Transplant 2005;5:2732–9.

110. Rahamimov R, Ben-Haroush A, Wittenberg C, *et al.* Pregnancy in renal transplant recipients: long-term effect on patient and graft survival. A single-centre experience. Transplantation 2006;81:660–4.

111. McGrory CH, McCloskey LJ. DeHoratius RJ, Dunn SR, Moritz MJ, Armenti VT. Pregnancy outcomes in female renal recipients: a comparison of systemic lupus erythematosus with other diagnoses. Am J Transplant 2003;3:35–42.

112. Cruz Lemini MC, Ibarguengoitia Ochoa F, Vilanueva Gonzalez MA. Perinatal outcome following renal transplantation. Int J Gynaecol Obstet 2007;96:76–9.

113. Ghanem ME, El-Beghdadi LA, Badawy AM, Bakr MA, Sobhe, MA, Ghoneim MA. Pregnancy outcome after renal allograft transplantation: 15 years experience. Eur J Obstet Gynecol Reprod Biol 2005;121:178–81.

114. Al-Khader AA, Al-Ghamdi, Basri N, *et al.* Pregnancies in renal transplant recipients – with a focus on the maternal issues. Ann Transplant 2004;9:62–4.

115. Keitel E, Bruno RM, Durate M, *et al.* Pregnancy outcome after renal transplantation. Transplant Proc 2004;36:870–1.

116. Thompson BC, Kingdon EJ, Tuck SM, Fernando ON, Sweny P. Pregnancy in renal transplant recipients: the Royal Free Hospital experience. Q J Med 2003;96:837–44.

117. Sgro MD, Barozzino T, Mirghani HM, *et al.* Pregnancy outcome post renal transplantation. Teratology 2002;65: 5–9.

118. Willis FR, Findlay CA, Gorrie MJ, Watson MA, Wilkinson AG, Beattie TJ. Children of renal transplant recipient mothers. J Paediatr Child Health 2000;36: 230–5.

119. Jouppila P, Jouppila R, Hollmen A, *et al.* Lumbar epidural analgesia to improve intervillous blood flow during labor in severe preeclamsia. Obstet Gynecol 1982;59:158.

120. Zamora JE, Rosaeg OP, Lindsay MP, Crossan ML. Haemodynamic consequences and uterine contractions following 0.5 or 1.0 litre crystalloid infusions before obstetric epidural analgesia. Can J Anaes 1996;43:347.

121. Shennan A, Cooke V, Lloyd-Jones F, MorganB, de Swiet M. Blood pressure changes iduring labour and whilst ambulating with combined spinal epidural analgesia. Br J Obstet Gynaecol 1995;102:192.

122. Dyer RA, Els I, Farbas J, *et al.* Prospective randomized trial comparing general and spinal anaesthesia for cesarean delivery in preeclamptic patients with nonreassuring fetal heart trace. Anesthesiology 2003;99:561.

123. Sharwood-Smith G, Clark V, Watson E. Regional anaesthesia for caesarean section in severe preeclampsia: spinal anaesthesia is the preferred choice. Int J Obstet Anesth 1999;8:85.

124. Rabey PG, Anaesthesia for renal transplantation. Br J Anaesth 2001:1:24–27.

125. Dyer RA, Piercy JL, Reed AR, *et al.* Hemodynamic changes associated with spinal anesthesia for caesarean delivery in severe preeclampsia. Anesthesiology 2008;108:773.

126. British National Formulary #54 BMJ RPS Publishing. Germany 2007.

127. Ngan Kee WD, Khaw KS, Lau TK, *et al.* Randomised double-blinded comparison of phenylephrine vs ephedrine for maintaining blood pressure during spinal anaesthesia for non-elective caesarean section. Anaesthesia 2008;63:1319.

128. Orko R, Pitkanen M, Rosenberg PH. Subarachnoid anaesthesia with 0.75% bupivacaine in patients with chronic renal failure. Br J Anaesth 1986;58:605.

129. Hand CW. Buprenorphine in patients with renal impairment: single and continuous dosing with special reference to metabolites. Br J Anaesth 1990:64:276.

130. Miller RD, Way WL, Hamilton WK, Layzer RB. Succinylcholine-induced hyperkalaemia in patients with renal failure. Anesthesiology 1972;36:138.

8

Rheumatologic disorders in pregnancy

Megan E. B. Clowse[1], *Michelle Petri*[2] *and Andra H. James*[3]

[1]Division of Rheumatology and Immunology, Duke University Medical Center,
Durham, NC, USA
[2]Division of Rheumatology, Johns Hopkins University School of Medicine, Baltimore,
MD, USA
[3]Division of Maternal-Fetal Medicine, Department of Obstetrics and Gynecology,
Duke University Medical Center, Durham, NC, USA

Introduction

The rheumatologic diseases are a diverse group of ailments that are unified by their pathophysiology. Each is driven by a deregulated immune system that results in autoimmunity. The majority of rheumatologic diseases affect women more often than men, though the cause for this inequity is not clear. Many autoimmune diseases are diagnosed during the reproductive years. As our therapies for these diseases have improved in recent decades, more women with rheumatologic disease desire pregnancy. Fortunately, most pregnancies in women with rheumatologic disease are successful and result in the births of healthy babies to healthy mothers. However, many women will have a worsening of disease activity during pregnancy, prompted by the hormonal and immunologic shifts in pregnancy and compounded by the avoidance of some medications during this period. For optimal care, these women require careful monitoring by both a high-risk obstetrician and a rheumatologist throughout pregnancy.

Inflammatory arthritis

Epidemiology

Inflammatory arthritis is a general term that encompasses women with rheumatoid arthritis (RA), juvenile idiopathic arthritis (JIA), psoriatic arthritis (PsA) and ankylosing spondylitis (AS). The hallmark of each of these diseases is chronic autoreactive inflammation within joints. RA, which affects an estimated 1% of the female population, is the most common form of inflammatory arthritis. The prevalence is 2.5-fold higher in women than in men, and the peak incidence

is between the ages of 30 and 50 [1]. JIA first presents in children under age 16, but half of these patients will have persistent joint inflammation as adults. There are an estimated 35,000–50,000 cases of adult JIA in the United States [1]. PsA affects about 0.1% of the US population, and occurs in about 5–10% of all patients with psoriasis. Men and women are affected equally. The peak incidence is between 30 and 55 years of age [1]. AS is fivefold more common in men than women, but may be present in up to 1% of all Caucasians. The prevalence of AS reflects the prevalence of the genetic marker HLA-B27, which is present in the vast majority of patients with this disease [1].

Etiology/pathophysiology

Though the initial trigger for each of these diseases is unknown, once tolerance has been broken, joint inflammation appears to be a self-propagating process. The inflammatory process is accompanied by an influx of inflammatory cytokines, including tumor necrosis factor (TNF)-alpha, interleukin (IL)-1 and IL-6. These cytokines prompt changes in the differentiation of osteoclasts, chondrocytes and collagen. These changes induce the growth of the joint pannus (granulation tissue in the joint), which leads to the swelling that can be seen clinically. It also leads to joint destruction, which can be observed as erosions surrounding a joint on X-ray. Eventually, the destruction results in a distortion of the joint mechanics, loss of range of motion and disability.

Diagnosis

Inflammatory arthritis is diagnosed clinically based on the patient's history and physical examination. Patients will report significant morning stiffness that lasts usually an hour or more and improves with heat, such as a hot shower, and movement. The pain in the joints can be severe and is accompanied by swelling and warmth. Joints will also have limited range of

de Swiet's Medical Disorders in Obstetric Practice, 5th edition.
Edited by R. O. Powrie, M. F. Greene, W. Camann. © 2010 Blackwell Publishing.

motion either from pain secondary to inflammation or from alteration in joint structure. The location of the inflammation helps to identify the specific type of arthritis (Table 8.1).

Laboratory tests can also help to clarify the diagnosis. Patients with inflammatory arthritis will often have an elevated erythrocyte sedimentation rate (ESR) or C-reactive protein (CRP). During pregnancy, the ESR is often elevated regardless of inflammatory disease, so is not useful for monitoring or diagnosing disease. The CRP is not as well studied, but may be more reliable in pregnancy.

The autoantibodies associated with rheumatoid arthritis are the rheumatoid factor (RF) and the cyclic citrulinated peptide (CCP) antibody. The RF is present in 75–80% of RA patients at some point, but can also be positive for reasons other than RA. A positive RF in the absence of significant joint pain and swelling probably does not indicate rheumatoid arthritis (Box 8.1). The CCP antibody is a more recently discovered marker for RA. A little more than half of all patients with RA have the CCP antibody, but only 10% of tests are falsely elevated. Over 95% of patients with both a positive RF and positive CCP antibody will be diagnosed with RA [2].

Inflammatory arthritis in pregnancy

Rheumatoid arthritis is the best studied inflammatory arthritis in pregnancy. Most reports demonstrate an improvement in joint inflammation during pregnancy. A report of 140 women with RA found that by the third trimester, two-thirds had significant improvement in symptoms. Within 1 month post partum, however, two-thirds of women had relapsed and by 6 months, over three-quarters had worsened joint activity [3]. A recent study of 78 pregnancies in women with RA found a more modest improvement in disease activity.

Box 8.1 Causes of a positive rheumatoid factor

Autoimmune disease	• Rheumatoid arthritis
	• Cryoglobulinemia
	• Sjögren's syndrome
	• Sarcoidosis
	• Systemic lupus erythematosus
Infections	• Subacute bacterial endocarditis
	• Tuberculosis
	• Syphilis
	• Lyme disease
	• Cytomegalovirus (CMV)
	• Epstein–Barr virus (EBV)
	• Influenza
	• Hepatitis C
Malignancy	• Multiple myeloma
	• Metastatic malignancy
	• Hematologic malignancy

Only 11% had major improvement, 37% had moderate improvement, while 45% had either no improvement or worsened [4]. Women with JIA tend to improve, similar to women with RA [5].

Carrying a pregnancy does not worsen the long-term severity of RA. In fact, one study found that women who had a pregnancy during the course of RA had fewer joint abnormalities on X-ray and had better physical functioning than women who had not been pregnant [6]. This study may be biased as women with more severe RA may avoid

Table 8.1 Inflammatory arthritis: distinctions between the types of arthritis

Type of arthritis	Prevalence	Joints affected	Extra-articular disease
Rheumatoid arthritis (RA)	1% of female population M:F ratio 1:2.5 Peak incidence: 30–50 years old	Small joints of the hands and wrists, but not DIP joints Typically bilateral Also the elbows, shoulders, knees, ankles, feet, and neck (C1–2) Does not affect the lumbar spine	Lung fibrosis Rheumatoid nodules
Juvenile idiopathic arthritis (JIA)	0.1% of children Half of children will have persistent disease as adults	Variable: may act like RA, AS, or PsA	Uveitis Systemic form: fevers, rashes, liver disease
Psoriatic arthritis (PsA)	0.1% of population 5–10% of patients with psoriasis Peak incidence: 30–55 years old	Small joints of the hands/feet, especially the DIP joints Rare "sausage digits" Any other joints, including lumbar spine	Psoriasis Nail pitting and onycholysis
Ankylosing spondylitis (AS)	0.5% of population M:F ratio is 5:1 Average age of onset: 26 years	Sacroiliac joints Lumbar spine, then extends into thoracic and cervical spine Enthesitis of tendons and ligaments	Iritis Inflammatory bowel disease

DIP, distal interphalangeal.

pregnancy, but the results are reassuring that pregnancy does not worsen the condition.

Women with AS may have increased pain and stiffness during pregnancy. Though the data are scarce for these pregnancies, it appears that women with AS may have more pain than women with RA during pregnancy [7,8]. PsA is also rarely studied in pregnancy. However, small studies show improvement in symptoms in many women [5].

Few fetal complications have been reported in women with inflammatory arthritis, but the rate of preterm birth may be increased in this population. In a nationwide study of RA pregnancies, about one-quarter of pregnancies were born preterm (prior to 37 weeks gestation), compared to 5% of healthy controls [9]. The risk of spontaneous pregnancy loss, however, is not significantly increased in this population. Infant birth weight may be lower among women with RA [10]. Women with active RA who required prednisone during pregnancy had, on average, 400 g smaller babies than healthy women [9,11]. Women with RA do have an increased risk for hypertension and pre-eclampsia in pregnancy, though the risk is more modest than in other rheumatologic diseases [10,12].

Systemic lupus erythematosus

Systemic lupus erythematosus (SLE) is an autoimmune disease that primarily affects women in their childbearing years. SLE affects about 0.05% of the population, but the incidence is threefold higher among African American women [13]. The peak incidence is between 15 and 40 years old with a female to male ratio of 9 to 1.

Systemic lupus erythematosus is diagnosed through a combination of signs, symptoms and laboratory findings. According to the criteria developed by the American College of Rheumatology (ACR), a woman must have at least four of 11 criteria to be labeled as lupus (Box 8.2) [14]. Over 95% of women with SLE will have a positive antinuclear antibody (ANA) finding. Other antibodies, including the dsDNA, Ro/SSA, La/SSB, RNP and Smith antibodies, are not required for an SLE diagnosis, but are helpful when present. A woman with some symptoms of SLE, but not enough to fulfill the ACR criteria, may be given the label of undifferentiated connective tissue disease (UCTD). In most cases, UCTD is a milder illness with only a small subset of patients progressing to full SLE in the following years [15]. We recommend consultation with a rheumatologist to establish a lupus diagnosis.

The course of SLE, both during and outside pregnancy, can be unpredictable. Some women will have significant fatigue and arthralgias, without internal organ damage. Others may have a fulminant course with rapid progression to endstage renal disease. Close monitoring by a rheumatologist is very important to evaluate lupus and direct treatment.

Systemic lupus erythematosus can present with myriad of symptoms, many of which are nonspecific (Table 8.2).

Box 8.2 ACR revised classification criteria for SLE. A patient must have at least 4/11 to be labeled with SLE. The ANA will be positive in over 95% of women with SLE

- Malar rash
- Discoid lupus
- Photosensitive rash
- Mouth ulcers
- Arthritis
- Serositis (≥1):
  - pericarditis
  - pleurisy
- Nephritis (≥1):
  - Proteinuria ≥3+ or ≥0.5 g per 24 h
  - Cellular casts in urine
- CNS lupus (≥1):
  - seizures
  - psychosis
- Hematologic abnormalities (≥1):
  - Leukopenia/lymphopenia
  - Hemolytic anemia
  - Thrombocytopenia
- Other antibodies (≥1):
  - anti-dsDNA antibody
  - Sm (Smith) antibody
  - anticardiolipin antibodies
  - lupus anticoagulant
- Positive ANA

ANA, antinuclear antibody; CNS, central nervous system; SLE, systemic lupus erythematosus.

The most common symptoms include fatigue, arthralgias, especially in the small joints of the hands, rashes, low-grade fevers, Raynaud's phenomenon and hair loss.

Laboratory findings in lupus

The ANA is the classic autoantibody associated with SLE. It is present in over 95% of patients with SLE, but can also be found in up to 25% of the general population and patients with other autoimmune disease [16]. Therefore, finding a positive ANA, even at a high titer, does not clinch a diagnosis of SLE. Though the ANA titer may fluctuate over time, this fluctuation has no relationship to disease activity or likelihood of an SLE diagnosis. Therefore, once a high-titer ANA has been identified (i.e. ≥1:320), there is no reason to repeat this laboratory test. Similarly, a rising ANA titer should not be a cause for alarm.

Table 8.2 Signs and symptoms of active lupus

System	Frequency*	Sign/symptom	Details
Joints	83%	Inflammatory arthritis	Swollen, tender, painful joints. Morning stiffness. Particularly the small joints of the hands, wrists, and knees
Dermatology	60%	Raynaud's phenomenon	Finger tips turn white and purple from lack of blood flow in the cold or under stress
	58%	Malar rash (butterfly)	Red, raised, photosensitive rash over the cheeks and bridge of the nose, sparing the nasolabial folds
	50%	Mouth ulcers	On upper palate, tongue, buccal mucosa. Also in the nose. Usually painless
	24%	Alopecia	Diffuse without scarring or patchy from discoid scars. "Lupus frizz" with alopecia and hair breakage at the temples
	12%	Discoid lupus	Scarring, nonpainful rash. When on the scalp, will cause permanent alopecia
	15%	Vasculitis	Palpable purpura, splinter hemorrhages under nails, or tender red nodules on fingers
	7%	Subacute cutaneous lupus erythematosus (SCLE)	Red, annular rash with clearing in middle, or psoriaform pattern. Nonscarring. Usually photosensitive
Hematology	60%	Leukopenia	Lymphopenia
	19%	Thrombocytopenia	Immune mediated, can be moderate to severe
	9%	Hemolytic anemia	Direct Coombs test positive
Renal	42%	Lupus nephritis	Proteinuria (>500 mg/24-h urine), RBC/WBC in urine with casts (active sediment). Rising creatinine in severe cases
Neurology	30%	Psychiatric disorders	Depression, anxiety, psychosis
	30%	Organic brain syndrome	Change in consciousness
	18%	Seizures	Focal or generalized
	10%	Stroke	Abrupt onset of neurologic deficit from a brain lesion
	Rare	Transverse myelitis	Abrupt onset of numbness and weakness at a distinct spinal cord level
	Rare	Peripheral neuropathy	Diffuse or a single nerve
Pulmonary	34%	Pleurisy	Chest pain that worsens with inspiration. Fluid on CT scan or chest X-ray
Cardiac	26%	Pericarditis	Substernal chest pain worsened with inspiration, lying flat, often better with bending forward. Pericardial effusion on echocardiogram. ST elevation of EKG
Muscles	3%	Myositis	Weakness of proximal muscles. Elevated CK and/or aldolase

* Frequency: an estimate of the incidence of each SLE sign or symptom at any time during the course of SLE [54,55].
CK, creatine kinase; EKG, electrocardiogram; SLE, systemic lupus erythematosus.

The ANA is a nonspecific antibody that can be further classified by the specific antigen that it targets. These specific targets include the other antibodies used to define SLE and other connective tissue diseases (Table 8.3). The double-stranded DNA and Sm antibodies are unique to lupus, and the vast majority of patients with these antibodies will carry this diagnosis. The dsDNA antibody titer can fluctuate with disease activity, and therefore it is frequently monitored in patients with SLE. The Sm, Ro, La and RNP antibodies do not fluctuate in a meaningful way. Once these have been identified as positive, they need not be re-evaluated. The Ro and La antibodies are important in pregnancy because they can cause neonatal lupus. For this reason, we recommend checking these antibodies at the onset of pregnancy, even if previously negative, to help guide neonatal evaluation (see neonatal SLE discussion below).

A significant minority of women with SLE will have hematologic abnormalities. Thrombocytopenia, prompted by antiplatelet antibodies, can drive platelets to dangerously low levels. A mild chronic anemia is fairly common, but Coombs positive hemolytic anemia can also occur. Many women with SLE will have a mild lymphopenia and leukopenia. This low white blood cell count is rarely a sign of true immunosuppression.

Lupus nephritis is a common, and potentially devastating, component of SLE. Over half of all women with SLE will develop nephritis at some point, but fortunately many cases are mild. Lupus nephritis is best identified through the urinalysis. The urine will have elevated protein (>500 mg/24-h collection) and an "active sediment," meaning increased red and white blood cells and, potentially, cellular casts. Early on, lupus nephritis is asymptomatic, so routine urinalysis is important. However, symptoms such as severe edema from low albumin or signs of uremia may be presentations of more severe disease.

Differential diagnosis

As the symptoms, signs and laboratory testing for SLE can be nonspecific, the differential diagnosis is wide. For women with a positive ANA, other connective tissue diseases must be considered (see Table 8.3). Hematologic abnormalities and

Table 8.3 The connective tissue diseases

	Autoantibodies[*]	Most common symptoms	Severe symptoms that can complicate pregnancy
Systemic lupus erythematosus	• ANA • dsDNA antibody • Smith (Sm) • RNP • Ro/SSA, La/SSB[**]	• Joint pain • Fatigue • Rash • Chest pain • Alopecia	• Lupus nephritis • CNS disease • Thrombosis • Vasculitis
Sjogren's syndrome	• ANA • Ro/SSA[**] • La/SSB[**] • Rheumatoid factor	• Dry eyes • Dry mouth	• Lung and heart disease
Scleroderma (SSc)	• ANA • Anti-centromere • SCL-70	• Tight skin on hands and elsewhere • Severe Raynaud's • GERD	• Pulmonary hypertension • Interstitial lung disease • Scleroderma renal crisis
Dermatomyositis polymyositis	• Anti-Jo1	• Proximal muscle weakness • Rash on face and chest	• Interstitial lung disease
Undifferentiated connective tissue disease (UCTD)	• ANA • Various	• Fatigue • Arthralgias	

[*]Antibodies most characteristic for each connective tissue disease. A patient may have some, none or all of these antibodies.
[**]Ro and SSA identify the same antibody. La and SSB identify the same antibody.
CNS, central nervous system; GERD, gastroesophageal reflux disease.

lymphadenopathy may indicate a malignancy. Alternative causes for nephritis must be considered and a renal biopsy is indicated in most women with significant persistent proteinuria or worsening renal function.

Lupus during pregnancy

Most women with SLE will have some disease activity during pregnancy. Fortunately, however, in the vast majority of patients this activity will be mild, predominantly arthritis and cutaneous disease. A minority of women (up to 30%) will have more significant disease activity [17]. Lupus can flare at any time during pregnancy, including in the weeks post partum. The factors that best predict quiet lupus in pregnancy are:
• quiet lupus activity in the 6 months prior to conception
• few severe flares in the years prior to pregnancy
• continuation of hydroxychloroquine (Plaquenil) through pregnancy.

Fetal complications in SLE pregnancies

The overall pregnancy loss rate is higher among women with SLE. One study of women with SLE compared to their sisters and friends found that the pregnancy loss rate was 2–3-fold higher with SLE [18]. A population-based study of women with SLE found that the pregnancy loss rate prior to an SLE diagnosis was 15.2% and after an SLE diagnosis was 23.4%, both higher than the 8.3% loss rate in the general population.

This is a lower estimate of miscarriage in the general population than is seen in most studies but does suggest an increased risk among women who either have or are developing SLE [19]. Cohort studies of SLE pregnancies demonstrate that the miscarriage rate (<20 weeks gestation) may be similar to the general population, but the stillbirth rate is significantly elevated. In the Hopkins lupus cohort, 8% of all pregnancies resulted in a stillbirth [18]. Risk factors for pregnancy loss are increased lupus activity and antiphospholipid syndrome (APS). Women with first-trimester activity, measured by thrombocytopenia, proteinuria or physician assessment, are at a threefold increased risk for pregnancy loss. Women with uncontrolled first-trimester hypertension are also at an increased risk for pregnancy loss [20].

On average, 33% of lupus pregnancies will result in a preterm birth [21]. Fortunately, most of these will be delivered after 28 weeks. Some deliveries are induced due to the health of the mother or fetus. However, most are spontaneous deliveries precipitated by preterm rupture of membranes or preterm labor [21]. Risk factors for preterm birth include increased lupus activity just prior to or during pregnancy, APS, use of high-dose corticosteroids, low complement and hypertension [17,21,22].

Systemic lupus erythematosus is associated with poor placentation. Placentas have more infarcts and perivillous inflammation, resulting in slowed growth among some infants [23]. In the Hopkins lupus cohort, over 20% of infants were below the 10th percentile of weight for gestational age [18].

Pre-eclampsia and SLE

Pre-eclampsia may be diagnosed in up to one-quarter of SLE pregnancies. The combination of hypertension and proteinuria in a woman with SLE, however, cannot automatically be assumed to be pre-eclampsia. Lupus nephritis, one of the most severe manifestations of SLE, presents in the same manner (Table 8.4). The presence of other SLE symptoms, such as fevers, rashes or arthritis, may assist in the diagnosis of an SLE flare. Treatment for lupus nephritis includes high-dose corticosteroids and immunosuppression. If left untreated, lupus nephritis can progress to renal failure and require dialysis support.

Antiphospholipid syndrome

The antiphospholipid syndrome (APS) is an autoantibody-mediated abnormality. It manifests in two main ways: with thrombosis and with pregnancy morbidity (Table 8.5). More than half of women with APS will not have another autoimmune disease [24]. APS occurs in an estimated 15% of women with SLE, but can also occur in women without other autoimmune disease [25]. Women with APS may also have livedo reticularis (lace-like purplish discoloration of the lower extremities), thrombocytopenia and aseptic vegetations on their heart valves (known as nonbacterial thrombotic endocarditis (NBTE), marantic or Libman–Sacks endocarditis).

In the absence of prior thrombosis or pregnancy morbidity, positive laboratory markers for APS do not increase pregnancy risk. In the Hopkins lupus cohort, 52% of the women with SLE who became pregnant had at least one positive anticardiolipin antibody or lupus anticoagulant test. Of those with positive tests but without the clinical components of APS, 12% of pregnancies resulted in a loss, comparable to the rate of 15% in women with negative antibodies. Women who fulfilled both the laboratory and clinical criteria, however, had a 40% pregnancy loss rate (P < 0.05) [20].

For women with positive laboratory findings but with no prior thrombosis or pregnancy morbidity, we recommend either no therapy or low-dose aspirin throughout pregnancy. For women who do not completely fulfill the pregnancy morbidity criteria, but who have suffered one or two early losses, the decision is more difficult. We offer low-dose aspirin, but a reasonable number of women in this situation will have pregnancy success without medical therapy. For patients with three consecutive losses or one morphologically normal loss after 10 weeks gestation, we offer low-dose aspirin in combination with prophylactic doses of a heparin although the data supporting this practice are not as rigorous as is often believed. Please refer to Chapter 4 on thrombophilia for further information on the treatment of APS in pregnancy.

Table 8.4 Factors that distinguish between pre-eclampsia and SLE activity

	Pre-eclampsia	SLE activity
Risk factors		
First pregnancy	Increases risk	No impact
Pre-eclampsia in prior pregnancy	Increases risk	No impact
Multifetal gestation	Increases risk	Unknown impact
History of lupus nephritis	Increases risk	Increases risk
Timing in pregnancy	Always after 20 weeks, usually after 30 weeks gestation	Anytime in pregnancy
Laboratory tests		
Active urine sediment (WBC, RBC, casts)	Usually negative	Positive
Coombs test	Usually negative	May be positive
Antiplatelet antibody	Usually negative	May be positive
Complement (C3 and C4)	Usually normal	May be low
Anti-dsDNA antibody	Usually negative	May be positive
Serum uric acid	Over 5.5 mg/dL	No change
Urine calcium	Low	Normal
PlGF*	Low	Unknown
sFlt-1*	High	Unknown
Physical findings		
Dermatologic disease	Not present	May be present
Arthritis	Not present	May be present
Serositis	Not present	May be present

*sFlt-1 and PlGF are currently under development and are not available outside research laboratories.
PlGF, placental growth factor; RBC, red blood cells; sFlt-1, soluble FMS-like tyrosine kinase 1; WBC, white blood cells.
Reproduced with permission from Clowse ME. Lupus activity in pregnancy. Rheum Dis Clin North Am 2007;33(2):237–52.

Table 8.5 Diagnosis of APS. To confirm a diagnosis of APS, a woman must fulfill the laboratory criteria and fulfill either the vascular or pregnancy criteria

Criteria	Comments
Laboratory criteria	• Anticardiolipin antibody (IgG or IgM), medium to high titer • Anti beta-2 glycoprotein 1 antibody (IgG or IgM), medium to high titer • Lupus anticoagulant (prolonged PTT with and without mixing studies) Must have at least one of these studies positive twice, 12 weeks apart
Vascular thrombosis	• At least one thrombosis in any location: arterial, venous or small vessel Confirmed by Doppler of biopsy showing vessel thrombosis without inflammation within the vessel wall
Pregnancy morbidity	• At least one pregnancy loss ≥10 weeks gestation with normal morphology • Three or more consecutive spontaneous abortions prior to 10 weeks gestation without another cause for the loss • At least one preterm birth (≤34 weeks) because of eclampsia, severe pre-eclampsia or placental insufficiency

PTT, partial thromboplastin time.

Scleroderma

Scleroderma, also known as systemic sclerosis (SSc), is an autoimmune disease that primarily damages the skin and blood vessels. Scleroderma is a rare disease that affects 20–75 per 100,000 people. It primarily affects women and has a peak occurrence between 35 and 65 years of age. Most women with SSc will have severe Raynaud's phenomenon, sometimes resulting in digital infarctions and digital amputations. Most will also have severe tightening of the skin, starting on the fingers and in some covering the majority of the body. Severe gastroesophageal reflux and stomach dismotility are also common. Joint pain is common, usually caused by the tightened skin but sometimes due to joint inflammation.

A subset of patients will develop severe cardiopulmonary disease, which is the leading cause of death for these patients. Interstitial lung disease is diagnosed with pulmonary function tests and chest computed tomography (CT) scans. Pulmonary hypertension is diagnosed with elevated pulmonary pressures on echocardiogram or cardiac catheterization.

The diagnosis of SSc is based on skin changes, other symptoms and laboratory findings. The ANA will be positive in up to 90% of patients with SSc. The centromere pattern to the ANA or the anti-Scl-70 antibody are both highly specific for SSc, but they are only found in half of all SSc patients [26].

Conventional wisdom, confirmed by multiple case reports, predicts poor maternal and pregnancy outcomes for women with scleroderma. However, the one prospective study of such pregnancies describes surprisingly positive outcomes [27]. Between 1987 and 1997, 91 pregnancies in women with scleroderma were followed at the University of Pittsburgh. Of these, 12% had an elective abortion, 14% had a miscarriage, and 1% ended with a neonatal death. Compared to a control group of healthy women, only the elective abortion rate was elevated. One-quarter of the women with SSc had preterm birth (defined in this study as delivery before 38 weeks gestation), with half of these deliveries between weeks

36 and 38, though this rate was 2.7-fold higher than in the control group. No term baby weighed less than 2500 g.

Scleroderma renal crisis, which manifests with hypertension and rapidly progressive renal failure, can also be life-threatening. The combination of proteinuria, rising creatinine and hypertension is easy to confuse with severe pre-eclampsia. Though angiotensin-converting enzyme (ACE) inhibitors are generally avoided during pregnancy, they may be required to save the life and renal function of the mother.

Scleroderma does not appear to be exacerbated by pregnancy. In the prospective study, 63% of the pregnancies had no change in scleroderma symptoms, 20% had an improvement in symptoms, and 17% had a worsening of symptoms. Post partum, one-third of women experienced worsened symptoms, but most noticed no change [28].

Some women with SSc have interstitial lung disease and/or pulmonary hypertension, which can complicate pregnancy and delivery. Therefore patients with known scleroderma lung or uninvestigated dyspnea should have an evaluation of lung function (typically pulmonary function testing with a test for diffusing capacity of the lung for carbon monoxide (DLCO)) and consideration of some testing for evidence of pulmonary hypertension such as an echocardiogram. Pulmonary hypertension of any etiology is associated with a very poor prognosis during pregnancy and significant risk for maternal mortality. Please refer to Chapters 1 and 5 for details about the management of these conditions in pregnancy.

Vasculitis

Vasculitis, defined as inflammation within the walls of blood vessels, can present in several ways based on the size of vessel involved (Table 8.6). Most patients with vasculitis, irrespective of the size of vessel or final diagnosis, present with fatigue, weight loss and low-grade fevers from systemic inflammation. These patients may also have elevated inflammatory markers (ESR and CRP), as well as anemia of chronic disease.

Table 8.6 Types of vasculitis and their main symptoms

	Small vessel vasculitis	Medium vessel vasculitis	Large vessel vasculitis
Examples of vasculitis	• Henoch–Schönlein purpura • Cryoglobulinemia • Wegener's granulomatosis • Behçet's disease	• Polyarteritis nodosum	• Takayasu's arteritis
Manifestations (vary by disease)	• Palpable purpura • Gut ischemia • Glomerulonephritis • Mouth ulcers • Genital ulcers	• Livedo reticularis • Gut ischemia • Mononeuritis multiplex	• Occlusion of aorta and major vessels • Arm claudication • Stroke • Abdominal angina

All forms of vasculitis are rare, and therefore evidence-based data on their behavior in pregnancy are not available. There are, however, several case series on Wegener's granulomatosis, an antineutrophil cytoplasmic antibody (ANCA)-associated vasculitis that affects the lungs, sinuses, upper airways, and kidneys. In women with active vasculitis at the time of conception, pregnancy and maternal outcomes may be particularly poor. There are not enough data to determine whether vasculitis improves or worsens in pregnancy, but documented relapse has occurred in some women during pregnancy [29]. Treatment of vasculitis in pregnancy is best accomplished with corticosteroids, azathioprine and intravenous immunoglobulin (IVIg) (see Table 8.11).

Takayasu's arteritis is a vasculitis manifesting with inflammation in the aorta and its great vessels which leads to proximal occlusion and/or aneurysms. Takayasu's is rare, but is most common among women of reproductive age. Pregnancy outcomes among these women are poor, particularly if the abdominal aorta is actively inflamed. Due to vasoconstriction of the renal arteries, many women with Takayasu's arteritis will have severe hypertension, which may worsen in pregnancy. Of 24 pregnancies in women with Takayasu's arteritis, 20% resulted in a pregnancy loss, 30% had intrauterine growth restriction, and 25% resulted in preterm birth [30].

Neonatal lupus

When maternal anti-Ro/SSA antibodies cross the placenta to the fetus, they may cause neonatal lupus. The most severe manifestation of neonatal lupus is congenital heart block (CHB). CHB develops during the second trimester when maternal Ro/SSA and La/SSB antibodies promote inflammation and damage in the atrioventricular (AV) node of the fetus. CHB will occur in 1–2% of fetuses in women with positive Ro/SSA and/or La/SSB antibodies, though the risk may be elevated in women with thyroid disease [31]. A woman who has had a prior infant with CHB has an 18% risk of CHB in each subsequent pregnancy [32].

More commonly, neonatal lupus manifests as a rash on the infant within the first 3–6 months of life. This rash worsens with sun exposure and appears to be similar to the subacute cutaneous lupus erythematosus rash seen in adults with lupus. Once the maternal Ro/SSA and La/SSB antibodies are cleared by the baby, the rash resolves completely and does not leave scars. Children with neonatal lupus do not appear to be at an increased risk for autoimmune disease in future years [33].

A smaller percentage of infants will have elevated liver function tests or cytopenias at birth due to maternal antibodies. In most cases, the liver disease will follow a benign course; however, rare cases of severe liver failure during gestation or in the neonatal period do occur [34].

Not all women with Ro/SSA and La/SSB antibodies have overt autoimmune disease. Only 18% of mothers who deliver a baby with immune-mediated CHB have SLE. Over one-third of women are asymptomatic, with the antibodies identified after the birth of a baby with CHB. Of these asymptomatic women, less than half will develop an autoimmune disease in the coming years. Sjogren's syndrome is present in 22%, and undifferentiated rheumatic syndromes are present in 15% of mothers of babies with CHB [35].

Prophylactic treatment with corticosteroids is not recommended for women with Ro/SSA and/or La/SSB antibodies. Given the low incidence of CHB, the adverse effects of chronic corticosteroids throughout pregnancy outweigh the benefits. In addition, the routine use of prednisone, which does not cross the placenta well, has not been shown to prevent or reverse CHB. Therefore, prophylactic therapy for women with a prior affected infant is also not recommended.

We do recommend periodic fetal echocardiographic evaluation for women with Ro/SSA and/or La/SSB antibodies beginning at 16 weeks gestation. The goal of this screening is to identify a fetus with first- or second-degree block, which may be amenable to therapy. If incomplete block is found, therapy with dexamethasone 4 mg per day or betamethasone is recommended based on several case reports of regression of heart block in infants treated *in utero* [36–38]. Once complete heart block occurs in the fetus, it is irreversible. Of the babies born with CHB, about 10% will not survive the neonatal period [39]. Another 60% will require the placement of a pacemaker in the first years of life and the vast majority will be require a pacemaker by adulthood

[35,40]. A small percentage of children with CHB will develop cardiomyopathy, despite the use of a pacemaker, and ultimately require heart transplant.

Management of rheumatic diseases in pregnancy

Antenatal care

Preferably prior to pregnancy, but at least at the first clinic visit during pregnancy, the risks of pregnancy to the fetus and mother should be discussed fully (Table 8.7). To identify pregnancies at particular risk, a full battery of laboratory tests should also be obtained (Table 8.8). Some tests, including the complement, dsDNA, blood counts and urinalysis, should be monitored throughout pregnancy to identify SLE activity as early as possible. Women with SLE, vasculitis, APS or other significant illness also require more intensive ultrasound evaluations. The Duke protocol includes serial nonstress tests in the third trimester weekly from 28 weeks and twice weekly from 32 weeks gestation to identify any fetus at risk for intrauterine demise (Table 8.9). Women with stable inflammatory arthritis or connective tissue disease may not require such intensive evaluation throughout pregnancy, but this assessment must be made on a case-by-case basis.

Medications

The treatment of rheumatic disease during pregnancy is a constant push and pull between the risks and benefits to the mother and the baby. Research shows, however, that maintaining control of the inflammatory process is important to the health of both the mother and the baby. For this reason, we generally tolerate some risk from medications if they will prevent or treat disease activity (Tables 8.10, 8.11).

We recommend that women taking hydroxychloroquine (Plaquenil) prior to pregnancy continue on this medication. It appears to be safe during pregnancy and the cessation of it at the time of conception has been shown to exacerbate lupus activity [41]. Women who require azathioprine (Imuran) to control SLE or vasculitis should continue it during pregnancy, as well. The very low risk of fetal complications is outweighed by the risk to mother and baby if the disease flares during pregnancy. While there has been increasing successful use of anti-TNF-alpha inhibitors in pregnancy for a wide range of indications [42], a recent report suggesting an increased risk of congenital anomalies with these agents has caused some concern at the time of this writing [43].

Low to moderate doses of prednisone are fairly safe during pregnancy as very little drug crosses the placenta, although chronic administration at doses in excess of 30 mg/day is associated with an increased risk for premature rupture of the fetal membranes and premature birth [44]. On the other hand, fluorinated glucocorticoids, including dexamethasone and betamethasone, easily cross the placenta [40]. These should be reserved for treatment of the fetus, such as in the treatment of neonatal lupus, but should be avoided when used to treat the mother. Chapter 47 reviews the use of glucocorticoids in pregnancy.

Breastfeeding

Medications required by women with autoimmune disease may be contraindicated due to adverse effects on the fetus (Table 8.12). It is important to note that medications that are considered to be compatible with breastfeeding are hydroxychloroquine, ibuprofen and low to moderately dosed glucocorticoids. Anti-TNF-alpha biologics are also considered to be compatible with breastfeeding and infliximab appears not to enter breast milk at all [45]. Women who require chronic high-dose prednisone, cyclophosphamide and methotrexate should not nurse. The data on

Table 8.7 Preconception counseling risks to the fetus and the mother

	Inflammatory arthritis	SLE
Risk to the fetus	• Miscarriage rate similar to the population • IUGR increased risk if arthritis active in pregnancy • Preterm birth in up to 25% of patients	• Pregnancy loss rate may be higher than in general population, especially if SLE active prior to or early in pregnancy • IUGR may be increased • Preterm birth in a third of patients, particularly if SLE is active prior to or during pregnancy
Risk to the mother	• Slight increased risk for hypertension, perhaps for pre-eclampsia • Does not worsen long-term condition of arthritis or disability • No known increase in maternal mortality • Many patients have decrease in joint pain and inflammation during pregnancy	• Pre-eclampsia in one-fifth of pregnancies • Low risk for long-term damage from pregnancy • Maternal mortality 20-fold higher than general population, but not higher than mortality risk for nonpregnant SLE patients • Increases the risk of SLE flare. Most flares are mild to moderate

IUGR, intrauterine growth restriction; SLE, systemic lupus erythematosus.

Table 8.8 Laboratory testing for women with connective tissue disease

	Preconception or 1st visit	Monthly through pregnancy	Explanation
ANA	X		If previously positive, no need to recheck
Ro/SSA and La/SSB	X		If previously positive, no need to recheck. If previously negative, recheck now
Antiphospholipid antibodies	X		Anticardiolipin antibodies, anti-beta-2 glycoprotein 1 antibodies, and the lupus anticoagulant
Anti-dsDNA antibody	X	X*	Monitor at each visit: rising level may predict a lupus flare
Complement levels: C3 and C4	X	X*	Monitor at each visit: falling levels may predict a lupus flare
Complete blood count: • hematocrit • white blood count • platelet count	X	X	Monitor at each visit for: • hemolytic anemia • lymphopenia • thrombocytopenia
Kidney function: • serum creatinine • urine protein	X	X	Monitor at each visit to find early lupus nephritis. If elevated, obtain a 24-hour urine protein

*Recommended for women with SLE only.
ANA, antinuclear antibody; SLE, systemic lupus erythematosus.

Table 8.9 Ultrasound monitoring for women with rheumatologic disease: the Duke protocol

Testing	Timing
Ultrasound for dates	As early as possible
Ultrasound for anatomy	16–18 weeks
Fetal echocardiogram	Weekly or every other week for women with Ro/SSA and/or La/SSB antibodies
Ultrasound for fetal growth	Monthly for women at higher risk
Antepartum testing (such as nonstress test)	Weekly from week 28–32 Twice weekly from week 32 to delivery

mycophenolate mofetil and leflunomide are too limited (and somewhat concerning) to support their use in nursing mothers. Azathioprine, while probably safe for breastfeeding, should be used with caution until the published experience is more extensive [46].

Some reports show an increase in rheumatoid arthritis activity in women during lactation. One study of 137 women with RA demonstrated increased joint pain 6 months post partum in women who were breastfeeding for the first time compared to women who did not breastfeed or had breastfed before [47]. The hypothesized cause for this phenomenon is a genetic sensitivity to inflammatory changes associated with elevated prolactin, with women who had problems nursing their first baby opting not to nurse subsequent infants [48]. However, a population-based study showed that a longer duration of breastfeeding decreased a woman's subsequent risk for developing RA [49]. We recommend allowing a woman with RA to attempt breastfeeding. If joint inflammation becomes intolerable, however, the cessation of lactation may improve her symptoms.

Women with SLE may be allowed to breastfeed if contraindicated medications are not required. There may be an association between elevated prolactin levels and increased lupus activity, though this has not been confirmed in clinical studies [50]. One population-based study found that the longer the duration of breastfeeding, the lower the risk for SLE in future years [51].

Delivery

At Duke University, we recommend induction of delivery at 39 weeks gestation in women at high risk for complications because after this point, the risk of stillbirth begins to increase [52,53].

The majority of women with rheumatologic disease will be able to deliver vaginally. The main exception may be women with significant hip pathology from arthritis or avascular necrosis who are unable to position appropriately. The cesarean section rate for women with RA, APS and SLE is higher than in the general population, likely because these pregnancies are more complicated [10]. In particular, there may be placental insufficiency leading to nonreassuring fetal heart rate patterns during labor in women with SLE or APS [23].

The use of stress dose corticosteroids at the time of delivery for women on chronic steroids is poorly studied. Chapter 47 provides a review of this topic and a recommendation for how to manage this important issue. Patients with significant rheumatologic cervical spine disease should be considered for cervical spine X-rays prior to delivery to ensure there is no atlanto-occipital or atlantoaxial instability that will put the patient at risk if endotracheal intubation is required for general anesthesia with delivery.

Table 8.10 Medications to prevent and treat lupus activity in pregnancy

Treatment	FDA classification*	Recommendation for use in pregnancy
Acetaminophen	A	As needed for pain control
NSAID**	B First and second trimesters	As needed for pain control in the latter first and second trimester only.
	D Third trimester	Discontinue in third trimester
Anti-TNF-alpha inhibitors+	B	As needed for moderate to severe inflammatory arthritis. Consider discontinuation when pregnancy identified
Sulfasalazine	B	Continue if taking prior to pregnancy. Controls mild to severe inflammatory arthritis
Prednisone and prednisolone	B	As needed to control inflammatory symptoms
Dexamethasone and betamethasone	C	Not for treatment of inflammation. As needed to treat the fetus
Hydroxychloroquine (Plaquenil)	C	Continue if taking prior to pregnancy. Controls mild symptoms of arthritis and SLE
Intravenous immunoglobulin (IVIg)	C	As needed to control severe inflammatory signs and symptoms
Mycophenolate mofetil (Cellcept)	D	Discontinue prior to pregnancy. Consider switch to azathioprine
Azathioprine (Imuran)	D	Continue if taking prior to pregnancy. Controls moderate to severe symptoms of SLE and vasculitis
Cyclophosphamide (Cytoxan)	D	Avoid if possible. Use only to treat life-threatening SLE or vasculitis
Methotrexate	X	Do not use – discontinue 3 months prior to pregnancy
Leflunomide (Arava)	X	Do not use – discontinue at least 3 months prior to pregnancy. Check serum level prior to conception, treat with cholestyramine if elevated

*FDA pregnancy risk categories:
A: no risk in controlled clinic trials of humans
B: human data reassuring or when absent, animal studies show no risk
C: human data are lacking and animal studies show risk or are not done
D: positive evidence of risk but the benefit may outweigh the risks
X: contraindicated in pregnancy.
**NSAID: nonsteroidal anti-inflammatory drugs, including high-dose aspirin, ibuprofen, naproxen, celecoxib and others.
+TNF-alpha inhibitors: biologic therapy for inflammatory arthritis, includes etanercept (Enbrel), infliximab (Remicade) and adalimumab (Humira).
SLE, systemic lupus erythematosus.

Table 8.11 Basic algorithm for the treatment of rheumatic diseases in pregnancy

Degree of disease activity	Inflammatory arthritis	SLE or vasculitis
No activity	• None required	• None required
		• Continue hydroxychloroquine
Mild activity	• Acetaminophen	• Acetaminophen
	• NSAID in the second trimester	• NSAID in the second trimester
	• Low-dose prednisone (<10 mg per day)	• Low-dose prednisone (<10 mg per day)
	• Hydroxychloroquine	• Hydroxychloroquine
Moderate activity	• Moderate-dose prednisone (10–20 mg per day)	• Moderate-dose prednisone (10–40 mg per day)
	• Hydroxychloroquine	• Hydroxychloroquine
	• Sulfasalazine	• Azathioprine
Severe activity	• High–dose prednisone (20–60 mg per day)	• High-dose prednisone (60 mg)
	• Sulfasalazine	• Pulse-dose prednisolone (1000 mg IV for 3 days)
	• TNF-alpha inhibitors	• Azathioprine
		• Cyclosporine
		• IVIg
		• Cyclophosphamide in second or third trimester (may prompt fetal loss)
		• Delivery of pregnancy

NSAID, nonsteroidal anti-inflammatory drugs; SLE, systemic lupus erythematosus.

Table 8.12 Safety of rheumatologic medications during breastfeeding

Treatment	Relative infant dose*	Nursing recommendation	AAP**
Acetaminophen	6.4%	Considered safe	Low risk
Anti-TNF-alpha inhibitors	0%	Considered safe. The molecule is too large to enter the milk. It is not orally bio-available	Not reviewed
Azathioprine	0.25%	No reported problems, but caution is advised	Not reviewed
Cyclophosphamide	Unknown	Contraindicated: leukopenia in infants	Contraindicated
Glucocorticoids (prednisone)	2%	Low dose considered safe. Chronic high dose theoretically may cause infant growth delay. If possible, avoid nursing for 4 h after dose	Low risk
Hydroxychloroquine	2.9%	Considered safe	Low risk
Intravenous immunoglobulin (IVIg)	Unknown	Unstudied but probably safe as little IgG crosses into breast milk	Not reviewed
Leflunomide	Unknown	Contraindicated, but no data	Not reviewed
Methotrexate	0.12%	Contraindicated due to long half-life in infant tissues	Contraindicated
Mycophenolate mofetil	Unknown	Contraindicated	Not reviewed
NSAID:			
Ibuprofen	0.5%	Considered safe	Low risk
Naproxen	3.3%	Avoid chronic use, long half-life	Low risk
Celecoxib	0.3%	Considered safe	Not reviewed
Sulfasalazine	0.35%	Fairly safe. One report of infant with allergic reaction. Very low risk for kernicterus	With caution
Cyclosporine	Unknown		Contraindicated

*Relative infant dose: the dose that the infant would receive by consuming 150 mL of breast milk per day (mg/kg/day) divided by the dose that the mother takes (mg/kg/day).
**The American Academy of Pediatrics (AAP) guidelines for the use of medications in nursing mothers. Low risk: medication is usually compatible with breastfeeding. With caution: some nursing infants may have complications from the medication. Contraindicated: may have an adverse effect on the nursing infant. Not reviewed: medication was not reviewed by the AAP.

Table 8.13 Anesthesia and perioperative concerns in the rheumatic patient

Issue	Patients at risk	Recommendations
Cervical spine arthritis	• C1–C2 disease with instability of atlantoaxial joint in up to 50% of women with RA	Caution during intubation
Spinal anesthesia	• High risk if thrombocytopenia or on anticoagulants	Evaluate prior to treatment
Laryngeal disease	• RA can affect the cricoarytenoid joint • Wegener's granulomatosis can cause subglottic stenosis	Evaluate prior to treatment
Limited lung function	Restricted lung disease from: • interstitial lung disease • abnormalities of costovertebral joints • pleural effusions	Evaluate prior to treatment
Fever	• Increased risk for infection if on corticosteroids or other immunosuppressants	Treat fevers with broad-spectrum antibiotics
Thrombosis	• SLE and APS increase risk for thrombosis • Immobility from joint pain	Prophylaxis with low-dose anticoagulants or mechanical interventions
Coagulopathy or thrombocytopenia	• SLE and APS can lower the platelet count On anticoagulants	Avoid spinal anesthesia until coagulopathy and thrombocytopenia are reversed
Stress dose corticosteroids	• On ≥20 mg prednisone per day or Cushingoid	Consider stress dose glucocorticoids prior to and after delivery (see Chapter 47)
Wound healing	• Limited by corticosteroids, azathioprine, and other immunosuppressants	Evaluate wounds carefully

APS, antiphospholipid syndrome; RA, rheumatoid arthritis; SLE, systemic lupus erythematosus.

Post partum, women are at fivefold increased risk for thrombosis, most commonly deep vein thrombosis. Women with SLE or APS are already at high risk for this complication, putting them at particular risk after delivery. For this reason, consideration should be given to thromboprophylaxis. It would not be unreasonable to initiate low-dose anticoagulation in a woman with SLE, particularly if she has been ill and a prolonged hospitalization is anticipated. Women on prophylactic heparin therapy for APS should continue on anticoagulation for 6 weeks post partum. Women with inflammatory arthritis who have limited mobility due to arthritis pain and disability also should be considered for thromboprophylaxis post partum.

Some women with rheumatic disease will have specific needs during delivery (Table 8.13). Consideration should be given to the joint changes in the cervical spine or hips in women with inflammatory arthritis. Some women with vasculitis or connective tissue disease may have upper or lower airway disease, putting them at higher risk from general anesthesia. Other women may have coagulopathy from medications or thrombocytopenia from disease that increase the risk for spinal anesthesia. Finally, many of the medications used to treat women with rheumatologic disease will impair wound healing, so extra care should be taken in wound treatment.

Conclusion

Fortunately, the majority of pregnancies in women with rheumatologic disease will result in healthy babies. These women will require additional attention during pregnancy, however, to ensure that their disease is well controlled and the fetus is safe. We recommend a close partnership between the rheumatology and obstetric teams to care for these women in a multidisciplinary manner.

References

1. Klippel JH, Crofford LJ, Stone JH, Weyand CM (eds). Primer on the rheumatic diseases, 12th edn. Arthritis Foundations, Atlanta, GA, 2001.
2. Bas S, Genevay S, Meyer O, Gabay C. Anti-cyclic citrullinated peptide antibodies, IgM and IgA rheumatoid factors in the diagnosis and prognosis of rheumatoid arthritis. Rheumatology (Oxford) 2003;42(5):677–80.
3. Barrett JH, Brennan P, Fiddler M, Silman AJ. Does rheumatoid arthritis remit during pregnancy and relapse postpartum? Results from a nationwide study in the United Kingdom performed prospectively from late pregnancy. Arthritis Rheum 1999;42(6):1219–27.
4. de Man YA, Dolhain RJ, van de Geijn FE, Willemsen SP, Hazes JM. Disease activity of rheumatoid arthritis during pregnancy: results from a nationwide prospective study Arthritis Rheum 2008;59(9):1241–8.
5. Ostensen M. The effect of pregnancy on ankylosing spondylitis, psoriatic arthritis, and juvenile rheumatoid arthritis. Am J Reprod Immunol 1992;28(3–4):235–7.
6. Drossaers-Bakker KW, Zwinderman AH, van Zeben D, Breedveld FC, Hazes JM. Pregnancy and oral contraceptive use do not significantly influence outcome in long term rheumatoid arthritis. Ann Rheum Dis 2002;61(5):405–8.
7. Ostensen M, Fuhrer L, Mathieu R, Seitz M, Villiger PM. A prospective study of pregnant patients with rheumatoid arthritis and ankylosing spondylitis using validated clinical instruments. Ann Rheum Dis 2004;63(10):1212–17.
8. Forger F, Ostensen M, Schumacher A, Villiger PM. Impact of pregnancy on health related quality of life evaluated prospectively in pregnant women with rheumatic diseases by the SF-36 health survey. Ann Rheum Dis 2005;64(10):1494–9.
9. Chambers CD, Johnson DL, Jones KL. Pregnancy outcome in women exposed to anti-TNF-alpha medications: the OTIS rheumatoid arthritis in pregnancy study. Arthritis Rheum 2005;52(9 (suppl)):abstract #1224.
10. Chakravarty EF, Nelson L, Krishnan E. Obstetric hospitalizations in the United States for women with systemic lupus erythematosus and rheumatoid arthritis. Arthritis Rheum 2006;54(3):899–907.
11. deMan YA, van der Heide H, Dolhain RJEM, de Groot CJM, Steeger EAP, Hazes JM. Disease activity and prednisone use influences birth weight in rheumatoid arthritis pregnancies. Arthritis Rheum 2006;54(9 (suppl)):abstract #1319.
12. Wolfberg AJ, Lee-Parritz A, Peller AJ, Lieberman ES. Association of rheumatologic disease with preeclampsia. Obstet Gynecol 2004;103(6):1190–3.
13. Petri M. Epidemiology of systemic lupus erythematosus. Best Pract Res Clin Rheumatol 2002;16(5):847–58.
14. Tan EM, Cohen AS, Fries JF, Masi AT, McShane DJ, Rothfield NF, et al. The 1982 revised criteria for the classification of systemic lupus erythematosus. Arthritis Rheum 1982;25(11):1271–7.
15. Williams HJ, Alarcon GS, Joks R, Steen VD, Bulpitt K, Clegg DO, et al. Early undifferentiated connective tissue disease (CTD). VI. An inception cohort after 10 years: disease remissions and changes in diagnoses in well established and undifferentiated CTD. J Rheumatol 1999;26(4):816–25.
16. Wandstrat AE, Carr-Johnson F, Branch V, Gray H, Fairhurst AM, Reimold A, et al. Autoantibody profiling to identify individuals at risk for systemic lupus erythematosus. J Autoimmun 2006;27(3):153–60.
17. Clowse ME, Magder LS, Witter F, Petri M. The impact of increased lupus activity on obstetric outcomes. Arthritis Rheum 2005;52(2):514–21.
18. Petri M, Allbritton J. Fetal outcome of lupus pregnancy: a retrospective case-control study of the Hopkins lupus cohort. J Rheumatol 1993;20(4):650–6.
19. Hardy CJ, Palmer BP, Morton SJ, Muir KR, Powell RJ. Pregnancy outcome and family size in systemic lupus erythematosus: a case-control study. Rheumatology (Oxford) 1999;38(6):559–63.
20. Clowse ME, Magder LS, Witter F, Petri M. Early risk factors for pregnancy loss in lupus. Obstet Gynecol 2006;107(2 Pt 1): 293–9.
21. Clark CA, Spitzer KA, Nadler JN, Laskin CA. Preterm deliveries in women with systemic lupus erythematosus. J Rheumatol 2003;30(10):2127–32.
22. Chakravarty EF, Colon I, Langen ES, Nix DA, El-Sayed YY, Genovese MC, et al. Factors that predict prematurity and preeclampsia in pregnancies that are complicated by systemic lupus erythematosus. Am J Obstet Gynecol 2005;192(6):1897–904.

23. Magid MS, Kaplan C, Sammaritano LR, Peterson M, Druzin ML, Lockshin MD. Placental pathology in systemic lupus erythematosus: a prospective study. Am J Obstet Gynecol 1998;179(1):226–34.

24. Cervera R, Piette JC, Font J, Khamashta MA, Shoenfeld Y, Camps MT, et al. Antiphospholipid syndrome: clinical and immunologic manifestations and patterns of disease expression in a cohort of 1,000 patients. Arthritis Rheum 2002;46(4):1019–27.

25. Perez-Vazquez ME, Villa AR, Drenkard C, Cabiedes J, Alarcon-Segovia D. Influence of disease duration, continued followup and further antiphospholipid testing on the frequency and classification category of antiphospholipid syndrome in a cohort of patients with systemic lupus erythematosus. J Rheumatol 1993;20(3):437–42.

26. Ward MM. Laboratory testing for systemic rheumatic diseases. Postgrad Med 1998;103(2):93–100.

27. Steen VD. Pregnancy in women with systemic sclerosis. Obstet Gynecol 1999;94(1):15–20.

28. Steen VD, Medsger TA Jr. Fertility and pregnancy outcome in women with systemic sclerosis. Arthritis Rheum 1999;42(4):763–8.

29. Auzary C, Huong DT, Wechsler B, Vauthier-Brouzes D, Piette JC. Pregnancy in patients with Wegener's granulomatosis: report of five cases in three women. Ann Rheum Dis 2000;59(10):800–4.

30. Sharma BK, Jain S, Vasishta K. Outcome of pregnancy in Takayasu arteritis. Int J Cardiol 2000;75(suppl 1):S159–62.

31. Spence D, Hornberger L, Hamilton R, Silverman ED. Increased risk of complete congenital heart block in infants born to women with hypothyroidism and anti-Ro and/or anti-La antibodies. J Rheumatol 2006;33(1):167–70.

32. Buyon JP, Clancy RM. Neonatal lupus syndromes. Curr Opin Rheumatol 2003;15(5):535–41.

33. Martin V, Lee LA, Askanase AD, Katholi M, Buyon JP. Long-term followup of children with neonatal lupus and their unaffected siblings. Arthritis Rheum 2002;46(9):2377–83.

34. Evans N, Gaskin K. Liver disease in association with neonatal lupus erythematosus. J Paediatr Child Health 1993;29(6):478–80.

35. Buyon JP, Clancy RM. Neonatal lupus: review of proposed pathogenesis and clinical data from the US-based Research Registry for Neonatal Lupus. Autoimmunity 2003;36(1):41–50.

36. Vesel S, Mazic U, Blejec T, Podnar T. First-degree heart block in the fetus of an anti-SSA/Ro-positive mother: reversal after a short course of dexamethasone treatment. Arthritis Rheum 2004;50(7):2223–6.

37. Breur JM, Visser GH, Kruize AA, Stoutenbeek P, Meijboom EJ. Treatment of fetal heart block with maternal steroid therapy: case report and review of the literature. Ultrasound Obstet Gynecol 2004;24(4):467–72.

38. Saleeb S, Copel J, Friedman D, Buyon JP. Comparison of treatment with fluorinated glucocorticoids to the natural history of autoantibody-associated congenital heart block: retrospective review of the research registry for neonatal lupus. Arthritis Rheum 1999;42(11):2335–45.

39. Eronen M, Miettinen A, Walle TK, Chan EK, Julkunen H. Relationship of maternal autoimmune response to clinical manifestations in children with congenital complete heart block. Acta Paediatr 2004;93(6):803–9.

40. Costedoat-Chalumeau N, Georgin-Lavialle S, Amoura Z, Piette JC. Anti-SSA/Ro and anti-SSB/La antibody-mediated congenital heart block. Lupus 2005;14(9):660–4.

41. Clowse ME, Magder L, Witter F, Petri M. Hydroxychloroquine in lupus pregnancy. Arthritis Rheum 2006;54(11):3640–7.

42. O'Donnell S, O'Morain C. Review article: use of antitumour necrosis factor therapy in inflammatory bowel disease during pregnancy and conception. Aliment Pharmacol Ther 2008;27(10):885–94.

43. Carter JD, Ladhani A, Ricca LR, Valeriano J, Vasey FB. A safety assessment of tumor necrosis factor antagonists during pregnancy: a review of the food and drug administration database. J Rheumatol 2009;36(3):635–41.

44. Cowchock FS, Reece EA, Balaban D, Branch DW, Plouffe L. Repeated fetal losses associated with antiphospholipid antibodies: a collaborative randomized trial comparing prednisone with low-dose heparin treatment. Am J Obstet Gynecol 1992;166(5):1318–23.

45. Kane S, Ford J, Cohen R, Wagner C. Absence of infliximab in infants and breast milk from nursing mothers receiving therapy for Crohn's disease before and after delivery. J Clin Gastroenterol 2009;43(7):613–616.

46. Hale TW. Medications and mother's milk, 12th edn. Hale Publishing, Amarillo, TX, 2006.

47. Barrett JH, Brennan P, Fiddler M, Silman A. Breast-feeding and postpartum relapse in women with rheumatoid and inflammatory arthritis. Arthritis Rheum 2000;43(5):1010–15.

48. Brennan P, Ollier B, Worthington J, Hajeer A, Silman A. Are both genetic and reproductive associations with rheumatoid arthritis linked to prolactin? Lancet 1996;348(9020):106–9.

49. Karlson EW, Mandl LA, Hankinson SE, Grodstein F. Do breast-feeding and other reproductive factors influence future risk of rheumatoid arthritis? Results from the Nurses' Health Study. Arthritis Rheum 2004;50(11):3458–67.

50. Grimaldi CM. Sex and systemic lupus erythematosus: the role of the sex hormones estrogen and prolactin on the regulation of autoreactive B cells. Curr Opin Rheumatol 2006;18(5):456–61.

51. Cooper GS, Dooley MA, Treadwell EL, St Clair EW, Gilkeson GS. Hormonal and reproductive risk factors for development of systemic lupus erythematosus: results of a population-based, case-control study. Arthritis Rheum 2002;46(7):1830–9.

52. Smith GC. Life-table analysis of the risk of perinatal death at term and post term in singleton pregnancies. Am J Obstet Gynecol 2001;184(3):489–96.

53. Minakami H, Kimura H, Honma Y, Tamada T, Sato I. When is the optimal time for delivery? Purely from the fetuses' perspective. Gynecol Obstet Invest 1995;40(3):174–8.

54. Blanco FJ, Gomez-Reino JJ, de la Mata J, Corrales A, Rodriguez-Valverde V, Rosas JC, et al. Survival analysis of 306 European Spanish patients with systemic lupus erythematosus. Lupus 1998;7(3):159–63.

55. Doria A, Iaccarino L, Ghirardello A, Zampieri S, Arienti S, Sarzi-Puttini P, et al. Long-term prognosis and causes of death in systemic lupus erythematosus. Am J Med 2006;119(8):700–6.

9

Disorders of the liver, biliary system and exocrine pancreas in pregnancy

Sailesh Kumar[1], Mrinalini Balki[2] and Catherine Williamson[3] (with Eliana Castillo[4,6] and Deborah M. Money[5,6] contributing to the section on viral hepatitis)

[1]Centre for Fetal and Maternal Medicine, Queen Charlotte's and Chelsea Hospital, Imperial College London, London, UK

[2]Department of Anesthesia, Mount Sinai Hospital, Toronto, Ontario, Canada

[3]Institute of Reproductive and Developmental Biology, Imperial College London, London, UK

[4]Department of Medicine, University of British Columbia, Vancouver, BC, Canada

[5]Department of Obstetrics and Gynecology, University of British Columbia, Vancouver, BC, Canada

[6]Women's Health Research Institute, British Columbia Women's Hospital, Vancouver, BC, Canada

Normal liver physiology in pregnancy

Outside pregnancy, the liver receives up to 25–35% of the cardiac output [1] and this surprisingly does not change significantly during pregnancy. The size of the liver does not increase during pregnancy and it is indeed more difficult to palpate as pregnancy progresses due to its posterosuperior displacement by the enlarging uterus. A palpably enlarged liver is therefore abnormal in pregnancy and may indicate congestion, infiltration or malignancy.

Metabolic, synthetic, and excretory functions of the liver are affected by the increased levels of estrogen and progesterone in pregnancy [2]. The serum albumin concentration decreases during pregnancy and reaches a nadir towards term secondary to the increased plasma volume. Abnormal liver function tests occur in 3–5% of pregnancies with many potential causes. Table 9.1 summarizes the changes in liver function occurring during pregnancy.

The most significant changes are the decreased liver transaminase (alanine aminotransferase (ALT) and aspartate aminotransferase (AST)) levels to 25% pre-pregnancy levels by the third trimester. Alkaline phosphatase levels can increase up to four times [3] and do not indicate an obstructive

problem within the hepatobiliary tree. The rise is caused by leakage of placental alkaline phosphatase into the maternal circulation and increased maternal bone turnover. Alkaline phosphatase levels may remain elevated for up to 6 weeks post partum. Plasma cholesterol levels increase by 50% by the third trimester with triglyceride levels increasing 2–3-fold from nonpregnant values [4].

Normal pregnancy in a healthy woman is frequently associated with the appearance of both spider nevi (vascular skin lesions with a central arteriole feeding outwardly radiating thin-walled blood vessels) and palmar erythema. These findings are also seen in patients with chronic liver disease but are not of clinical significance in the context of pregnancy.

Table 9.1 Liver function tests in pregnancy

Test	Result
Bilirubin	Unchanged or slightly decreased
Aspartate transaminase (AST)	Unchanged initially but 25% decrease by third trimester
Alanine transaminase (ALT)	Unchanged initially but 25% decrease by third trimester
Gamma-glutamate transaminase (GGT)	Unchanged or slightly decreased
Alkaline phosphatase	2–4-fold increase in the third trimester
Cholesterol	Twofold increase
Triglycerides	2–3-fold increase
Globulin	Increase in alpha and beta globulins

de Swiet's Medical Disorders in Obstetric Practice, 5th edition. Edited by R. O. Powrie, M. F. Greene, W. Camann. © 2010 Blackwell Publishing.

Maternal hyperbilirubinemia and the fetus

Excretion of fetal bilirubin occurs through transplacental transfer into the maternal circulation although the volume of fetal bilirubin is small enough that maternal serum levels of bilirubin are not significantly changed from the normal range for nonpregnant patients. Fetal bilirubin is then conjugated in the maternal liver before being excreted into bile. Elevated levels of unconjugated bilirubin and its metabolites seen in maternal liver failure do not appear to have a deleterious effect on the long-term neurodevelopmental status of the offspring [5,6]. This is in marked contrast to neonatal hyperbilirubinemia in hemolytic disease of the newborn which can result in bilirubin deposition in the brainstem, causing kernicterus [7].

Viral hepatitis and pregnancy

Hepatitis A virus

Hepatitis A virus (HAV) infection usually results in a self-limited icteric illness in adults and an asymptomatic infection in children but, unlike hepatitis B or C, does not cause chronic infections. It is not an important cause of maternal or neonatal morbidity, yet it can be transmitted from mother to child. HAV vaccine is highly effective and vaccination during pregnancy is appropriate for women who may be at high risk for exposure (e.g. ongoing exposure to clotting factor concentrates, occupational exposure to HAV or unavoidable travel to countries with high endemicity of hepatitis).

Virology

Hepatitis A virus is a small nonenveloped RNA virus, similar to other enteroviruses; the lack of lipid envelope makes it relatively heat and acid resistant, so it can remain infectious in the environment for weeks. Humans are the only important reservoir and there is only one known serotype.

Epidemiology

Hepatitis A virus is found worldwide but the prevalence is directly related to sanitary conditions. Infections are acquired early in life in highly endemic areas of the world (parts of Africa, Asia, Central and South America) whereas in low endemic areas (Canada, USA, Western Europe and other developed countries), most adults remain susceptible. Targeted use of HAV vaccine during childhood in some developed countries has dramatically decreased the number of infections in all ages, as children likely were an important reservoir for transmission in the community [8]. Risk factors for infection include attendance at childcare centers, travel to high or intermediate prevalence areas, men who have sex with men and use of illicit drugs [9]. The incidence of acute disease in pregnancy was less than 1:1000 prior to introduction of HAV vaccine in the mid 1990s, but updated estimates are lacking.

Pathogenesis

Person-to-person transmission by the fecal–oral route is the primary means of HAV acquisition [10], usually through ingestion of contaminated foods and person-to-person contact. Once ingested, HAV replicates in the small bowel and the liver, is then excreted to the bile, and then shed in the stool in high quantities. There is a short-lived period of viremia and peak infectivity occurs during the 2 weeks before the onset of symptoms. At this time there is jaundice and liver enzyme elevation. HAV is not directly cytopathic to the liver.

Pathogenesis of mother-to-child transmission

Mother-to-child transmission of HAV is very rare. Only two cases of intrauterine transmission following maternal infection in the first trimester have been reported and resulted in fetal meconium peritonitis [11,12]. Maternal infection in the third trimester of pregnancy may result in asymptomatic neonatal infection and/or self-limited neonatal cholestasis [13–15]. Breastfeeding is not implicated in transmission [15].

Clinical presentation

Acute HAV infection in pregnancy has the same clinical presentation and prognosis as that in the nonpregnant adult; pregnant women do not appear to be more susceptible to this disease. The average incubation period lasts 2–7 weeks (mean of 4); it is followed by a mild illness consisting of fever, chills, anorexia, nausea and vomiting and then by the onset of dark urine, pale stools, jaundice and hepatomegaly. Transaminases are classically elevated by 10–100 times the normal range. Most symptoms and signs resolve within 3 weeks.

Complications include cholestasis in about 7% of patients [16] (i.e. prolonged jaundice, pruritus and fever), prolonged and relapsing disease present in 10–15% of cases, fulminant hepatitis in less than 1% of cases, and death. Mortality rate is low at 0.4% [17]. Chronic hepatitis A infection, as can be seen with hepatitis B and C, does not occur.

Other obstetric considerations

Hepatitis A virus is not a recognized teratogenic agent. In a recent retrospective report, acute HAV in the second half of pregnancy was associated with premature contractions and premature rupture of membranes [18].

Diagnosis

Diagnosis requires laboratory confirmation, as clinical presentation can be indistinguishable from other acute viral hepatitis.

Anti-HAV IgM is the test of choice to diagnose acute infection given that it remains positive for 3–6 months only. Total anti-HAV antibodies are not clinically useful to diagnose acute infection because anti-HAV IgG persists for life.

Treatment and prevention

Treatment is supportive (see general treatment in HBV section).

Currently licensed HAV vaccines are inactivated killed virus vaccines. They are very effective at preventing infection and their risk to the developing fetus is expected to be very low. Therefore, vaccination during pregnancy is appropriate for women who may be at high risk for exposure, including chronic liver disease, ongoing exposure to clotting factor concentrates, occupational exposure to HAV or unavoidable travel to countries with high endemicity of hepatitis A. Patients visiting endemic areas should receive one dose of HAV vaccine at least 2 weeks before traveling, and a booster dose 6–12 months after the initial vaccination [19]. Equally important for any person traveling in areas with endemic hepatitis A is avoidance of uncooked fresh vegetables and shellfish, and access to clean water.

Prevention of maternal illness after a known exposure to HAV
Passive immunization with immunoglobulin within 2 weeks of exposure to HAV is effective in preventing 80–90% of HAV cases, and immunoglobulin use is safe in pregnancy [19].

Prevention of neonatal infection
Immunoglobulin at a dose of 0.02 mg/kg is recommended to prevent neonatal infection if maternal illness develops 2 weeks before or 1 week following delivery.

Infection control
Hospitalized patients with HAV do not require isolation or contact precautions unless incontinent. Frequent hand washing should be enough to prevent spread in the hospital setting.

Hepatitis B virus

Hepatitis B virus (HBV) accounts for close to 350 million chronic infections worldwide [20] and for an estimated 1 million deaths each year due to cirrhosis and hepatocellular carcinoma. Thirty to fifty percent of HBV chronic infections are acquired through the mother-to-child route, as acquisition in the neonatal period poses the highest risk for developing chronic HBV infection. Fortunately, HBV vaccination programs have dramatically reduced the occurrence of chronic HBV infection and its complications; in addition, most infections transmitted from mother to child can be prevented by timely recognition of maternal infection and neonatal active and passive immunization.

Virology

Hepatitis B virus is a small, double-stranded DNA hepatotropic virus, meaning that this virus primarily infects liver cells but does not directly kill them. Any cellular damage associated with the virus appears to be immune related. Its lipid envelope has a unique antigenic protein called hepatitis B surface antigen (HBsAg), which is overproduced and hence found free in the blood of infected patients. The inner core contains the genome, a polymerase, an inner nucleocapsid "core" antigen (HBcAg), essential for virus packaging, and the e antigen (HBeAg), which is related to infectivity. HBV cannot be cultured, so diagnosis relies on rapid virus detection (i.e. viral load) or serology. There are eight recognized serotypes, with distinctive rates of progression to chronic infection and cirrhosis, and different prevalence by geographic location.

Epidemiology

Hepatitis B virus infection is found worldwide, but the prevalence of chronic infection ranges widely from 0.1–2% in so-called low-prevalence areas like North America, Western Europe, Australia, and New Zealand to 10–20% in high-prevalence areas like South East Asia, China, and sub-Saharan Africa. Japan, Central Asia, the Middle East, Central America, and South America are intermediate-prevalence areas. Mode of transmission clearly differs among these geographic areas; mother-to-child transmission predominates in high-prevalence areas, whereas horizontal transmission, particularly in early childhood, accounts for most cases of chronic HBV infection in intermediate-prevalence areas. Unprotected sexual intercourse and intravenous drug use in adults are the major routes of spread in low-prevalence areas.

In the United States, acute hepatitis B occurs in approximately 1 in 1000 pregnancies. Prevalence of HBsAg among pregnant women in an urban setting has been reported as 5.79% for Asian Americans, 0.97% for African Americans, 0.6% of whites and 0.14% for Hispanics [21].

Transmission

Hepatitis B virus can be transmitted transplacentally, perinatally, by sexual contact, by parenteral inoculation (IV drug use or exposure to blood products) and by close person-to-person contact presumably by open cuts and sores, especially among children in highly endemic areas. Blood contains the highest concentrations of virus, but other body fluids (semen, saliva, cervical secretions) and leukocytes also contain high viral titers. Although breast milk from chronically HBV-infected mothers is known to contain the virus [22,23], breastfeeding does not seem to increase the risk of transmission to the neonate above that already posed by pregnancy and delivery [24]. In addition, appropriate neonatal immunoprophylaxis has been shown to eliminate any theoretical risk of transmission through this route [25].

General course outside pregnancy

The natural history of hepatitis B is variable and still not completely understood. After initial infection, there is a 30–180-day incubation period followed by 30–90 days of acute hepatits. Only one-third of adults experience symptoms of acute hepatitis, while the majority (65%) have subclinical disease. Symptomatic acute hepatitis B syndrome presents no differently from other acute viral and nonviral hepatic diseases (including HELLP syndrome or acute fatty liver of pregnancy) and consists of malaise, fatigue, anorexia, nausea, vomiting, right upper quadrant discomfort, jaundice and tender hepatomegaly. The risk of developing symptomatic icteric hepatitis is inversely proportional to age, ranging from 0% among neonates to 80% of adults [26]. The diagnosis is usually made serologically with the demonstration of HBsAg, HBeAg or HBV DNA in maternal blood. Liver enzymes (AST and ALT) are elevated in both symptomatic and asymptomatic patients, although transaminase levels are rarely greater than 2000 IU/L. ALT is characteristically higher than AST. Figures 9.1 and 9.2 and Table 9.2 review the typical progression of serologic testing in acute and chronic hepatitis B.

Over 90% of immunocompetent adult patients clear the infection and experience complete resolution after acute illness. Between 0.1% and 0.5% of patients with acute hepatitis B will develop a poorly understood acute fulminant hepatitis believed to be due to massive immune-mediated cell lysis of

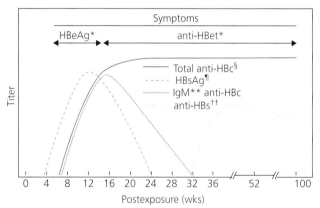

* Hepatitis B e antigen.
† Antibody to HBeAg.
§ Antibody to hepatitis B core antigen.
¶ Hepatitis B surface antigen.
** Immunoglobulin M.
†† Antibody to HBsAg.

Figure 9.1 Serologic findings over time in a patient with acute hepatitis B.

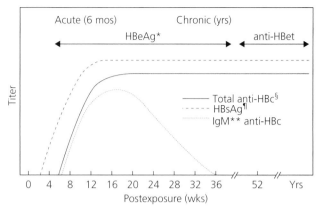

* Hepatitis B e antigen.
† Antibody to HBeAg.
§ Antibody to hepatitis B core antigen.
¶ Hepatitis B surface antigen.
** Immunoglobulin M.

Figure 9.2 Serologic findings over time in a patient with chronic hepatitis B.

Table 9.2 Interpretation of hepatitis B serology

Tests	Results	Interpretation
HBsAg	Negative	Susceptible
Anti-HBc	Negative	
Anti-HBs	Negative	
HBsAg	Negative	Immune due to natural infection
Anti-HBc	Positive	
Anti-HBs	Positive	
HBsAg	Negative	Immune due to hepatitis B vaccination
Anti-HBc	Negative	
Anti-HBs	Positive	
HBsAg	Positive	Acutely infected
Anti-HBc	Positive	
IgM anti-HBc	Positive	
Anti-HBs	Negative	
HBsAg	Positive	Chronically infected
Anti-HBc	Positive	
IgM anti-HBc	Negative	
Anti-HBs	Negative	
HBsAg	Negative	Interpretation unclear: four possibilities:
Anti-HBc	Positive	1. resolved infection (most common)
Anti-HBs	Negative	2. false-positive anti-HBc and therefore susceptible
		3. "low level" chronic infection
		4. resolving acute infection

• HBsAg is the hepatitic B surface antigen and its presence indicates that the person is infectious.
• Anti-HBc is the IgG antibody to hepatitis B core antigen and appears early on with acute hepatitis B infection and stays for life. Its presence indicates infection with hepatitis B without a specific time frame.
• IgM anti-HBc is the IgM antibody to hepatitis B core antigen and is presence indicates acute infection with hepatitis B within the past 6 months.
• Anti-HBs is the IgG antibody to hepatitis B surface antigen and is presence indicates recovery from (or vaccination for) hepatitis B infection.

Adapted from: A comprehensive immunization strategy to eliminate hepatitis B virus transmission in the US: recommendations from the Advisory Committee on Immunization Practices. Part 1. Immunization of infants, children and adolescents. MMWR 2005;54:RR-16.

infected hepatocytes [27]. Another 5% of all infected adults (2% of women and 7% of men) will not "clear" the virus and develop chronic hepatitis B. Chronic infection is defined as persistence of HBsAg for more than 6 months or HBsAg without anti-Hbc IgM. Rates of chronicity are higher in newborns (90%) and children (30%) and in immune-deficient individuals. Some of the variation in outcome of HBV infection may relate to the genetic heterogeneity of the virus. Eight genotypes of HBV have been described, genotype A being most common in the United States and Northern Europe, B and C in Asia, and D in Mediterranean countries and the Middle East. Chronic infection with HBV genotype C appears to have a poorer prognosis and greater likelihood of cirrhosis and hepatocellular carcinoma (HCC) than genotype B [28–30].

The transition from acute to chronic infection represents a failure of immune clearance of virus-infected cells and is characterized by the persistence of high levels of HBV DNA and HBeAg in serum. The course of chronic hepatitis B is highly variable. Typical chronic hepatitis B is marked by the presence of HBeAg and high levels of HBV DNA with variable elevations in ALT and histologic activity. Patients are generally asymptomatic but may experience mild "flu-like" symptoms, arthralgia, malaise, anorexia, vomiting or occasionally a skin rash. The main long-term risks of chronic hepatitis B include hepatocellular carcinoma and cirrhosis with liver failure.

Approach to patients with possible chronic hepatitis B outside pregnancy

Patients who are HBsAg positive (without IgM antibodies to hepatitis B core antigen to suggest that the patient has an acute hepatitis B infection) should undergo an evaluation for chronic hepatitis B. This includes full liver function testing (AST, ALT, bilirubin, alkaline phosphatase, albumin, international normalized ratio (INR)) and testing for HBeAg, HBeAb and hepatitis B viral load (HBV DNA by polymerase chain reaction (PCR)). Patients should also be tested for hepatitis C and HIV, both of which are transmitted in a similar manner to hepatitis B and have implications for treatment of chronic hepatitis B. It is important to be aware that normal liver function testing on one occasion does not preclude chronic hepatitis. These patients should be sent, with these results, to a clinician who routinely cares for patients with chronic hepatitis B. Decisions will then be made as to whether the patient warrants observation, liver biopsy and/or treatment based on a wide range of clinical criteria. In some patients, treatment decisions may need to be deferred while the patient is followed over time to determine if they have an inactive carrier state or if they will clear the virus on their own.

Two major types of antiviral treatment are currently used. These include interferon alpha (IFN-alphia or PEG-IFN-alpha) and nucleoside or nucleotide analogs such as lamivudine.

Outside pregnancy the major goal of treatment for hepatitis B is to prevent progression of the disease to cirrhosis, end-stage liver disease or hepatocellular carcinoma. Suppression of HBV replication can reduce histologic chronic active hepatitis and therefore the subsequent risk of cirrhosis and hepatocellular carcinoma. Extrahepatic manifestations of hepatitis B such as glomerulonephritis or polyarteritis nodosa also require treatment. If the disease has not progressed to cirrhosis, then prevention of progression to advanced fibrosis or cirrhosis is desirable. If cirrhosis has developed then preventing decompensation or hepatocellular carcinoma or death is important. The endpoints of treatment have not been clearly defined and differ in HBeAg-positive versus -negative disease. Improvement can be defined if HBV replication is suppressed to $<1\times10^4$ copies/mL (2000 IU/mL), with an accompanying improvement in serum ALT and hepatic inflammation. Newer agents are capable of suppressing most patients to fewer than 1×10^3 copies/mL (200 IU/mL) or even to levels undetectable by current PCR assays (i.e. <200 copies/mL (50 IU/mL)).

Hepatitis B in pregnancy

Screening and vaccination

All pregnant women should be screened for HBV infection at their first prenatal visit by determination of their HBsAg status [31,32]. If the initial HBSAg is negative but the patient has an ongoing high risk of infection (countries with high prevalence, intravenous drug use, multiple sexual partners, multiple transfusions, immunosuppressed patients, bisexual, hepatitis B-positive partner, healthcare workers, etc.), then patients should be screened again in late pregnancy. The aim of prenatal screening is to identify infected women whose babies can then be offered neonatal immunoprophylaxis. Women at high risk for acquiring hepatitis B infection who are HBsAg negative and have not been vaccinated for hepatitis B should be tested for anti-HBsAg. If they show no immunity to hepatitis B, advice should be given regarding risk factor modification and the patient should be offered hepatitis B vaccine, generally after the first trimester. The vaccine is not a live virus and has not been associated with adverse effects in pregnancy but because of limited published data about its use in pregnancy (even in the first trimester), its use in pregnancy is generally recommended only for pregnant women at ongoing risk for hepatitis B virus infection, including occupational risks (e.g. healthcare worker), lifestyle risks (e.g. history of intravenous drug use, sexually transmitted diseases, more than one sexual partner in the preceding 6 months), co-morbidities that place the patient at risk of acquiring hepatitis B (e.g. hemophilia and hemodialysis) and environmental risks (e.g. prison inmates, refugees, international travelers).

Approach to the HBsAg-positive patient in pregnancy

The most common problem that obstetricians will encounter in screening for hepatitis B is an asymptomatic pregnant woman found to be hepatitis B surface antigen positive at the time of her first prenatal visit. The question then arises as to whether this represents a chronic carrier state or an acute infection. If there is no history of recent exposure or any symptoms of acute hepatitis, most of these cases will represent a chronic carrier state. When there is uncertainty about whether the patient has acute or chronic hepatitis B, IgM antibodies against hepatitis B core antigen can be obtained. These antibodies should be elevated in acute hepatitis B but not in chronic hepatitis B. For patients with both acute and chronic hepatitis B in pregnancy, it is important to plan for neonatal prophylaxis. For patients with chronic hepatitis B infection, it is also important to have the mother fully assessed as to whether she herself will require treatment after delivery. This assessment is best carried out by a practitioner who routinely cares for patients with chronic hepatitis B.

Patients should be informed that there is no evidence that pregnancy alters the clinical course of either acute or chronic hepatitis B. Acute or chronic infection with HBV is also not a cause of congenital malformations [33], nor of pregnancy loss or stillbirth.

Evidence for the efficacy of antiviral therapy for chronic HBV during pregnancy is very limited and its use is generally deferred until after pregnancy. Lamivudine has been used to treat HBV in pregnancy among chronically infected [34] or highly viremic women [35] and is reported to decrease mother-to-child transmission and delayed active hepatitis in mothers, but there are no data from randomized trials to routinely recommend its use at this time. It is unlikely that delays in treatment for the duration of gestation will have significant adverse effects on long-term prognosis for most patients and proper postpartum prophylaxis for the newborn is highly effective at preventing mother-to-child transmission of hepatitis B.

Pathogenesis of mother-to-child transmission

Hepatitis B virus mother-to-child transmission happens by two different mechanisms: *in utero* infection (transplacental) and direct inoculation during delivery, also called perinatal.

Perinatal transmission of HBV is the most frequent route of transmission to the newborn, as the fetus is exposed to infected blood and other fluids present in the birth canal, and can result from both maternal chronic HBV infection or acute maternal HBV infection in the third trimester.

Maternal HBV replicative status determines the mother's infectivity, i.e. her risk of transmission to the infant. In the absence of HBV active and passive neonatal immunization, the risk of transmission for infants born to a "highly infectious" mother, e.g. HBsAg positive plus HbeAg positive and HBV DNA positive, is 85–90%, whereas the risk for an infant born to a "less infectious" mother, e.g. HBsAg positive but HbeAg negative, is only 10–32% [36,37].

Transplacental HBV transmission is very unusual except in the setting of acute HBV infection during the third trimester, when infection of placental capillaries transmits HBV to the fetus. HBV placental infection propagates from cell to cell, starting in the decidual cells, proceeding then to the fetal villous capillary endothelial cells and eventually reaching the fetal circulation. It is not interrupted by neonatal hepatitis B vaccination and may account for the small percentage of infants who are not protected by hepatitis B immunoglobulin.

Children born to mothers who are HBsAg positive at delivery, either from chronic hepatitis B infection or from acute HBV in the last trimester of pregnancy, should receive active (i.e. HBV vaccine) and passive (i.e. hepatitis B immune globulin – HBIG) immunization as follows:
- HBV vaccine: first dose given within 12 hours of birth and the second and third doses at 1 and 6–12 months of age.
- HBIG (0.06 mL/kg) once shortly after birth.

This regimen has an overall efficacy of 95% [36,37] but the efficacy is lower for mothers with very high HBV viral load [38]. There is no evidence that cesarean section prevents maternal–infant transmission, and thus routine cesarean section is not recommended.

Breastfeeding should be encouraged in women with hepatitis B, irrespective of viral load. While HBV is found in breast milk, transmission by breast milk appears to be rare and the administration of HBV vaccinations and/or immunoglobulin should further decrease any theoretical risks. However, it is our practice to advise temporary suspension of breastfeeding if a woman develops cracked nipples or mastitis.

Acute HBV during pregnancy: general treatment considerations

Treatment of acute hepatitis B infection during pregnancy is primarily supportive. Acute hepatitis often presents with nausea, vomiting, and anorexia so volume depletion is common and may result in decreased uterine blood flow and preterm uterine activity. Hospitalization may be needed to ensure adequate volume resuscitation and to monitor for preterm labor.

In general, no antiviral treatment is indicated as up to 95% of adults will recover spontaneously, but nucleoside analogs (lamivudine, telbivudine or entecavir) are recommended for the 0.5–1.5% of patients who progress to fulminant hepatitis B and those with protracted, severe acute HBV [39].

Maternal exposure to HBV during pregnancy

As with the nonpregnant patient, susceptible patients exposed to HBV should receive HBIG and start the hepatitis B vaccine series. Patients who become pregnant while receiving the vaccine series must be encouraged to complete the series. Due to the common mode of transmission, HIV testing is recommended for all documented hepatitis and all exposures to hepatitis B or C.

Hepatitis C virus

Hepatitis C virus (HCV) has the particular ability to establish chronic infections, leading to cirrhosis and hepatocellular carcinoma; it is the leading cause of liver transplant in North America. Although regarded as a blood-borne infection among adults, mother-to-child transmission is the leading cause of hepatitis C infection among infants and children, and more so if there is maternal HIV-HCV co-infection. Currently, HCV infection is not preventable by vaccine and antiviral therapies have shown only limited response rates.

Virology

Hepatitis C virus is an RNA virus of the Flaviviridae family. There are six recognized genotypes worldwide but each genotype includes thousands of subtypes, also called quasispecies, as a result of its high propensity to mutate. Envelope proteins express hypervariable regions that undergo high mutation rates under the pressure of host antibodies and its RNA polymerase lacks the ability of "self-correction" which among other viral factors account for the HCV's ability to establish chronic infections and for some of the difficulties faced in developing an effective vaccine.

The overall seroprevalence of HCV infection among pregnant women in Europe and North America ranges from about 0.2% to 4.3%; two-thirds of these women have detectable serum levels of HCV RNA and close to 30% will develop overt liver cirrhosis [40,41]. History of substance abuse appears to be the most common risk factor for chronic HCV infection in pregnancy in Europe and North America [42].

Pathogenesis

Hepatitis C virus infection is most efficiently acquired from parenteral inoculation (i.e. IV drug use or exposure to blood products). Acquisition from percutaneous exposure (medical procedures in resource-poor settings or tattooing) as well as sexual contact has been documented, but is less efficient [42]. Mother-to-child transmission (MTCT) is the most common route of infection among infants and children.

Hepatitis C virus preferentially infects and replicates in hepatocytes but is not directly cytopathic to them. HCV RNA viremia is detected in plasma within days of exposure, but peaks in the first 8–12 weeks of infection and then fluctuates if chronic infection occurs. Liver enzymes (ALT in particular) rise within 4 weeks of infection. Although antibodies are detectable 2–4 weeks following infection, the lack of a vigorous T-lymphocyte response and the virus's tendency to mutate result in a high rate of chronic infection.

Pathogenesis of MTCT

Most recently reported rates of transmission from infected mothers (mostly chronic infections) range between 3.6% and 6.2% [43,44]. The predominant mechanism has traditionally been thought to be intrapartum (perinatal) but debate exists about whether a greater proportion happens *in utero* [45]. Breastfeeding is not an established mechanism of transmission despite the fact that HCV can be found in breast milk [46,47].

The risk factors that increase the risk of mother-to-child HCV transmission include HCV viremia (i.e. detectable HCV RNA in maternal blood), maternal HIV-HCV co-infection (which increases transmission rate up to three times) [48], rupture of membranes for greater than 6 hours prior to delivery [44,46], and intrapartum exposure to maternal blood (i.e. perineal lacerations) [49]. Given that level of HCV viral load has inconsistently been reported as an independent risk factor for transmission, it should not be used alone to counsel women on risk of transmission. Neonatal factors have also been implicated in the pathogenesis of MTCT; HLA-DR13-positive neonates seem to be less likely to acquire HCV infection from their mothers, which may be related to a better infant immune response [50].

Clinical presentation

The clinical course and presentation of acute HCV infection in pregnancy do not differ from age-matched nonpregnant adults. Following an incubation period of 7 weeks, acute hepatitis C may cause malaise, nausea, and right upper quadrant pain, followed by dark urine and jaundice. However, more than 75% of acute HCV infections do not develop jaundice and do not have documentation of the laboratory abnormalities typically associated with acute viral hepatitis (i.e. acute ALT increments to >10 times the upper limit of normal). The rate of spontaneous clearance of infection after acute HCV is estimated to be 20–25%. Host factors associated with spontaneous clearance include age <40 years, female sex, and presence of jaundice. Extrahepatic manifestations are not prominent in acute but are seen in chronic HCV infection, and include essential mixed cryoglobulinemia, membranoproliferative glomerulonephritis, and porphyria cutanea tarda. HCV chronic infection leads to hepatic fibrosis; cirrhosis and hepatocellular carcinoma may develop 30–40 years after infection.

Other obstetric considerations

Hepatitis C virus infection during pregnancy is not a recognized cause of congenital malformations, pregnancy loss or stillbirth [51].

Diagnosis

Universal prenatal screening for HCV infection is not recommended at present. Prenatal testing should be guided by evidence of any risk factors for HCV infection including maternal history of intravenous drug use, HIV or HBV infection, solid organ transplant or transfusion recipient before 1992, hemodialysis, piercing and increased transaminases. HCV infection is also found more commonly in women with intrahepatic cholestasis of pregnancy. Anti-HCV antibodies are the test of choice for screening. Positive anti-HCV antibodies do not imply recovery from infection or lack of contagiousness, so they must be followed by serum HCV RNA identification which, if present, defines active infections. HCV viremia is known to fluctuate during the course of chronic infection but one determination during pregnancy is likely to be sufficient for diagnosis and counseling of pregnant women. Transmission of HCV is extremely unlikely from a HCV antibody-positive and HCV RNA-negative mother.

Infants born to HCV-infected mothers should have anti-HCV antibodies done at age >16 months (when maternal antibodies should have disappeared from the infant's serum) or nucleic acid testing on two occasions between ages 2 and 6 months [47]. Definitive antibody testing of the infant is delayed until >16 months of age because it may take this long for a infant to develop its own antibody response to infection, given that maternal antibodies to HCV may persist in the infant circulation for 2–3 months. Some authors even recommend delaying anti-HCV antibody determination to beyond the age of 18 months as cases of late seroconversion have been reported.

Treatment

Antiviral treatment of HCV infection is contraindicated during pregnancy [52]. The drugs currently available to treat HCV infection include ribavirin, which is a known teratogen, and interferon-alpha.

Prevention of MTCT

Internal fetal monitoring and prolonged labor after rupture of membranes in HCV-infected pregnant women should be avoided [47] but many questions remain regarding management of labor, including the best mode of delivery. No randomized controlled trials of planned cesarean section to decrease MTCT of HCV have been conducted; data from cohort studies (with methodologic weaknesses and hence potential for bias) have not provided evidence that planned cesarean section prevents or reduces the incidence of MTCT of HCV [53]. At the time of writing, active infection with hepatitis C is not considered to be an indication for cesarean delivery or a contraindication to breastfeeding. Currently there is no available vaccine but the higher frequency of spontaneous clearance and shortened duration of reinfection in persons with prior immunity to HCV provide a rationale for vaccine development.

Hepatitis E

Hepatitis E virus (HEV) causes an acute, usually self-limiting hepatitis, common in tropical Asia, Africa and Mexico but rarely seen in industrialized countries. It can lead to fulminant hepatitis, which happens more frequently among pregnant women than any other subgroup. It is a major cause of water-borne epidemics associated with poor sanitary conditions.

Virology

Hepatitis E virus belongs to its own genus (*Hepevirus*) and family (Hepeviridae). Its RNA genome is enclosed within a capsid that is composed of one or possibly two proteins but many questions remain on its antigenicity.

Epidemiology

It is the most common cause of sporadic and epidemic hepatitis among adults in Asia and the second most important cause among adults (after HBV) in the Middle East and North Africa [54]. Attack rates during outbreaks range from 1% to 15%. Peak incidence occurs between ages 15–40 years.

Pathogenesis

Reported epidemics have been mostly water-borne, especially during rainy season or flooding in endemic areas. Once ingested, the virus first appears in the liver, followed by viremia and subsequent shedding in the stool. Liver injury coincides with ALT elevation and appearance of anti-HEV IgM, which argues for immune-mediated liver injury. The mechanisms behind its aggressive course during pregnancy are not understood [55].

Pathogenesis of MTCT

Transplacental transmission of HEV has been documented by specific HEV IgM in cord blood and virus isolation by PCR, in up to 33% of neonates born to women infected in the third trimester [56], resulting in neonatal massive hepatic necrosis and death. Nonetheless, other infants have recovered from *in utero* infection [57].

Clinical presentation

The incubation period ranges between 2 and 10 weeks. Clinical presentation varies from asymptomatic infection common among children to anicteric, icteric and fulminant hepatitis. Jaundice, flu-like symptoms, fever, chills, anorexia, nausea, and abdominal pain are usually self-limited and resolve within 4 weeks. ALT is markedly elevated and may precede the onset of symptoms by 10 days. HEV infection does not cause chronic hepatitis, cirrhosis or hepatocellular carcinoma.

Pregnant women during the second and third trimesters are more susceptible to infection by HEV and progression to fulminant hepatic failure [57]. Mortality rates as high as 26.9% have been reported recently [56] in addition to high rates of preterm deliveries. There is no evidence for associated developmental anomalies. Available data suggest that breastfeeding does not increase MTCT [58].

Diagnosis

Specific anti-HEV IgM and IgG can document maternal and neonatal infections. Such testing may only be available in reference laboratories in areas where hepatitis E is not endemic. Molecular techniques for HEV RNA detection in stool and blood are not yet standardized for commercial use. The virus is difficult to grow on cell cultures.

Treatment

Treatment during pregnancy is supportive. There are no data on antiviral therapy for human infections.

Prevention

Postexposure prophylaxis with immunoglobulin does not reduce disease incidence [59].

Autoimmune hepatitis

Autoimmune hepatitis (AIH) is a disorder of unknown etiology that most commonly occurs in women of childbearing age [60]. As AIH is often diagnosed in young women, a considerable number of affected women will want to conceive. Older studies reported reduced fertility rates due to oligomenorrhea secondary to impaired function of the hypothalamopituitary gonadal axis. However, with immunosuppressive treatment, the disease usually improves and menstruation returns.

Diagnosis

Autoimmune hepatitis is classified according to the pattern of autoantibodies that are raised. The different subgroups are associated with different HLA serotypes. HLA-DR3 seropositivity occurs more commonly in early-onset, severe disease, i.e. the form of disease that is most commonly seen in young women.

Epidemiology

Autoimmune hepatitis occurs more commonly in women than men. However, it may affect children and adults of any age and individuals of either gender. The classification of autoimmune hepatitis is shown in Table 9.3. All disease types affect individuals from a variety of ethnic groups. Patients with progressive disease can develop cirrhosis, and hepatocellular carcinoma may also occur.

Etiology/pathophysiology

Autoimmune hepatitis has a complex etiology with genetic and environmental components. HLA-DR3 and -DR4 are the main loci that have been shown to influence susceptibility to the disease. In susceptible individuals, AIH may be triggered by additional environmental events. It has been proposed that the disease can be precipitated by viral infections, e.g. measles, hepatitis, cytomegalovirus and Epstein–Barr virus, or drugs, e.g. methyldopa, diclofenac or nitrofurantoin.

The autoimmune process in AIH is driven by T-cell-mediated responses and T-helper 1 (Th1) cells. Therefore it has been proposed that the shift from a Th1 to Th2-driven immune response in pregnancy may explain the remission of AIH that is often seen in pregnant women.

Table 9.3 Classification of autoimmune hepatitis

	Typical antibodies	Clinical features
Type 1 (classic)	Most commonly: antinuclear antibodies (ANA) anti-smooth muscle antibodies (SMA) anti-actin antibodies May also see: antimitochondrial atypical perinuclear antineutrophilic cytoplasmic antibodies pANCA Antisoluble liver/liver pancreas (anti-SLA/LP)	• Presents in all age groups with marked female preponderance • Variable severity and presentation • More commonly responds to treatment
Type 2	Anti-liver kidney microsome 1 antibodies (anti-LKM-1) Anti-liver cytosol-1 antibodies (anti-LC-1)	• Presents more commonly in childhood and early adulthood • Higher female preponderance than type 1 • Usually more advanced at the time of presentation • Less frequently responds to treatment • Cirrhosis and hepatocellular carcinoma more common as long-term complications

General course outside pregnancy

The clinical presentation of AIH is variable. Presenting features range from nonspecific symptoms of malaise to fulminant hepatic failure. Common presenting symptoms include fatigue, arthralgia, nausea, anorexia and pruritus. A recent Italian multicenter study reported that older patients more commonly have an acute presentation [61]. There may be signs of liver disease including jaundice, hepatomegaly and splenomegaly. Biochemical abnormalities include raised liver transaminases, bilirubin, and a prolonged prothrombin time. A sizeable proportion of cases will have cirrhosis at the time of diagnosis. However, even in individuals without apparent chronic disease at the time of diagnosis, the liver biopsy often shows features of cirrhosis, consistent with the insidious presentation of AIH. Disease complications include cirrhosis, ascites and esophageal varices and approximately 10% of patients will require liver transplantation within 10 years. In some studies, but not all, this is more likely in patients with cirrhosis at the time of presentation. However, in the majority of patients remission can be induced with the use of immunosuppressive treatment. Affected individuals may also have co-existing autoimmune disease, most commonly type 1 diabetes or thyroid disease.

Clinical presentation in pregnancy

Symptoms

Approximately 6% of AIH cases present in pregnancy [61]. The presenting features are the same as outside pregnancy. One case presented with pre-eclampsia in addition to a *de novo* diagnosis of AIH [62], indicating the importance of considering other diagnoses when women present with marked hepatic impairment in association with pre-eclampsia. There are two reports of women newly diagnosed in pregnancy who presented with fulminant hepatic failure [62,63].

Signs

Most women with AIH in pregnancy will not have signs of hepatic dysfunction. However, some will have cirrhosis, hepatomegaly and/or splenomegaly.

Laboratory tests

It is important to measure liver function tests and autoantibodies of relevance to liver disease (see Table 9.3) and it may be warranted in some cases to test for those that are found in association with adverse pregnancy outcome (anti-Ro/SSA, anti-La/SSB and anticardiolipin antibodies). In women with abnormal liver function tests, it is important to also measure the prothrombin time and a blood glucose level. A full blood count may reveal thrombocytopenia in women with hypersplenism. Thyroid dysfunction and type 1 diabetes are the most common autoimmune conditions that co-exist with AIH [61] and therefore it is advisable to screen specifically for these disorders.

Diagnostic testing

In addition to laboratory tests, women with AIH should have an abdominal ultrasound to visualise the liver, spleen and, if possible, portal venous circulation. Magnetic resonance imaging (MRI) is often also useful to establish whether a woman with AIH has portosystemic varices.

Differential diagnosis

If a woman with AIH develops hepatic impairment in pregnancy, it is most likely to be caused by a flare in the disease and should be managed as such unless there is evidence to the contrary. The differential diagnosis includes viral infection, a drug reaction, pre-eclampsia or cholestasis.

Management

Preconception counseling

A Swedish survey of 63 pregnancies in 35 women with AIH revealed that 48% did not consult their doctor before becoming pregnant [64]. It is therefore important for hepatologists and fertility specialists to refer affected women for preconception counseling. In particular, women should be advised to continue their immunosuppressive treatment. In addition, they should be screened to establish whether they have gastroesophageal varices as banding should be considered before conception.

Potential fetal complications

Table 9.4 summarizes the rates of adverse fetal events seen in pregnancies where the mother has AIH.

In a retrospective German survey of 42 pregnancies complicated by AIH in four centers, 26% had an adverse pregnancy outcome [63]. The principal causes were spontaneous early fetal loss and preterm labor. The authors identified seropositivity for antibodies to Ro/SSA as a risk factor for adverse pregnancy outcome with an odds ratio of 27 (95% confidence interval (CI) 2–369). In other studies, preterm labor is the main cause of adverse fetal outcomes, including the relatively high perinatal mortality rate. There is no evidence that immunosuppressive therapy with azathioprine is associated with adverse pregnancy outcome [63]. To date, no studies have shown an increased congenital abnormality rate in AIH, regardless of whether women are treated with immunosuppressive agents.

Table 9.4 Fetal outcome in pregnancies complicated by AIH

Study	Number of pregnancies (cases)	Fetal loss <24 weeks of gestation (%)	Congenital malformations (%)	Stillbirths or perinatal deaths (%)	Preterm delivery	Cesarean section rate
Werner et al. 2007 [64]	63 (35)	NS (15.4% miscarriage rate)	2 (3)	1 (2)	NS	16% (6.5% in controls)
Floreani et al. 2006 [61]	10 (10)	2 (20)	0	0	NS	0
Schramm et al. 2006[63]	42 (22)	7 (17)	0†	3 (7)**	7 (17)	NS
Candia et al. 2005 [65]*	101 (58)	12 (NS)	2 (2)	PMR 4%	5/95 (5)	11 (11)

NS, not stated or not apparent from the text of the paper.
†One child had Edwards syndrome.
*This study included all previous cases in the literature, including some specifically mentioned in the text [62,66].
**Three perinatal deaths secondary to preterm delivery, one neonate also had congenital heart block.

Table 9.5 Maternal complications in AIH

Study	Number of pregnancies (cases)	Overall flare rate (%)	Antenatal flare (%)	Postpartum flare (%)	Pre-eclampsia/ eclampsia (%)	Maternal death or transplantation	Other
Werner et al. 2007	63 (35)	NS	6 (10)	18 (29)	NS	0	
Floreani et al. 2006	10 (10)	NS	NS	(30)	NS	0	
Schramm et al. 2006	42 (22)	NS	9 (21)	22 (52)	0	2**	73% remission at conception
Candia et al. 2005*	101 (58)	47 (47)	35 (35)	12 (12)	16 (16)	3***	

*This study included all previous cases in the literature, including some specifically mentioned in the text [62,66].
**One maternal death, one de novo presentation in a woman who developed fulminant hepatic failure and required transplantation.
***Two maternal deaths, one related to GI bleed 6 months post partum.

Potential maternal complications

The maternal complications of AIH are summarized in Table 9.5. It is clear that disease flares are relatively common in pregnancy. However, flares during pregnancy are less common in the more recent case series. The oldest study in the table summarized the rate of flares in 101 pregnancies complicated by AIH reported between 1996 and 2004. In this series there were 47 flares, the majority of which (35) occurred prior to delivery and there were 12 in the postpartum period [65]. The more recent studies report lower rates of antepartum flare and a higher frequency of postpartum flares [61,63,64]. Flares in pregnancy may be less common in these studies because women are less likely to stop their immunosuppressive treatment now that there are better safety data for the use of prednisolone, prednisone and azathioprine in pregnancy. Also the diagnosis of AIH was not as certain in the older series, so some cases may have had an exacerbation of a different disease pathology during pregnancy. These data indicate that it is advisable for women with AIH to continue taking glucocorticoids and azathioprine during pregnancy. In the more recent studies postpartum flares are more common. Women should be aware of this and should report symptoms suggestive of a flare as soon as they occur. Doctors caring for women with AIH should also consider increasing the dose of immunosuppressive therapy in the third trimester or immediately after delivery.

A subgroup of women with AIH have cirrhosis when they conceive. In some series, there is no difference in maternal outcome in women with cirrhosis [64]. Disease activity at the time of conception also does not appear to predict whether a woman will have a flare [63].

In a retrospective German case series that included 42 pregnancies in 22 patients, there was one maternal death and one woman required transplantation following presentation and diagnosis of AIH in pregnancy and subsequent development of fulminant hepatic failure [63]. In a British study of 35 pregnancies in 18 AIH patients, there was one maternal death in a woman who had pulmonary hypertension secondary to microthrombi and another woman died 6 months post partum from a gastroesophageal variceal bleed [62]. Two additional women died within 3 years of pregnancy in the British study.

Antenatal care

Early

Medications

Most women with AIH are treated with prednisolone and azathioprine, although cyclosporine and tacrolimus may also be used. These drugs should be continued, as should other immunosuppressive drugs if they are required to maintain remission of the disease. Flares should be treated with corticosteroids and often also respond to an increased dose of other immunosuppressive medication. Most flares will respond well to medical treatment.

If azathioprine is used for the first time in pregnancy it is important to measure the activity of maternal enzymes that metabolize thiopurines, e.g. thiopurine S-methyltransferase (TPMT), to help identify those woman at most risk for azathioprine-related bone marrow suppression and hepatotoxicity. Women with gastroesophageal varices can be treated with propranolol to reduce the risk of variceal bleeding. Proton pump antagonists or H2 antagonists should also be considered to reduce gastric acid production.

Nonmedications

Women with AIH should be advised to inform the medical team if they have any symptoms suggestive of a flare. Women with portal hypertension should be managed by a multidisciplinary team. They should be educated about the appearance of melena, and if they have any symptoms suggestive of gastrointestinal bleeding they should go immediately to a hospital where massive gastrointestinal hemorrhage is regularly managed.

Close to term

Women should be informed of the risk of having a flare in the postpartum period and consideration should be given to augmentation of immunosuppressive treatment to reduce the chance of a subsequent flare.

Labor and delivery

In some series there is a higher cesarean section rate in women with AIH compared to controls [64]. However, women with uncomplicated disease who have not had a flare should be able to have a normal labor and delivery. If a woman with AIH has portal hypertension, it is advisable to avoid pushing in the second stage of labor. However, providing there are no abnormalities of clotting or platelets, it is feasible to have a normal delivery with an assisted second stage.

Postpartum period

Adjustments to treatment

If immunosuppressive therapy has been increased at the end of pregnancy, this should be maintained for 4–6 months after delivery. Women with AIH should be followed by a hepatologist at this time and treatment should subsequently be adjusted according to disease severity.

Long-term health concerns

Most women with AIH are treated effectively with immunosuppressive therapy. However, the condition can be complicated by progressive liver damage, cirrhosis and hepatic failure. There is no evidence that pregnancy worsens the course of AIH.

Advice for subsequent pregnancies

There are no studies that indicate that the prognosis worsens (or improves) in subsequent pregnancies. If a woman with AIH wants a subsequent pregnancy, it is advisable to conceive whilst in remission.

Issues related to medications and lactation

Azathioprine and prednisolone/prednisone enter breast milk in low concentrations. Given the potential maternal risk from stopping treatment, women should continue taking their medication and may be reassured that there are no data documenting adverse fetal effects from exposure to thiopurine metabolites in breast milk.

Contraceptive recommendations

Providing they have well-controlled disease, women with AIH can use any form of contraception. If hepatic impairment is present, estrogen-containing contraceptives are usually discouraged.

Conclusions

Women with AIH can have disease flares in pregnancy and in the puerperium, and therefore should be discouraged from stopping immunosuppressive treatment. Indeed, there is an argument for increasing their treatment dose close to term.

Intrahepatic cholestasis of pregnancy

Intrahepatic cholestasis of pregnancy (ICP), also known as obstetric cholestasis, most commonly presents in the third trimester with maternal pruritus and liver dysfunction. It causes transient maternal cholestasis that resolves after delivery and is associated with fetal complications, including spontaneous preterm labor and in rare cases third-trimester intrauterine death.

Epidemiology

Intrahepatic cholestasis of pregnancy affects 0.5–1.5% of pregnancies in Europeans and is more common in women of South Asian and South American origin. Most affected women are asymptomatic outside pregnancy, although up to 20% of cases have pruritus in the second half of the menstrual cycle or if they take estrogen-containing contraceptives.

Etiology/pathophysiology

The condition has a complex etiology with genetic and endocrine components. Evidence for genetic factors includes sibling studies that report a 20-fold increase in risk for first-degree relatives, pedigree studies that demonstrate sex-limited autosomal dominant inheritance in a subgroup of cases and reports of heterozygous mutations in genes that encode biliary transporters or receptors. It is likely that these genetic abnormalities cause women to be predisposed to the cholestatic effects of reproductive hormones.

Raised serum levels of reproductive hormones are thought to play a role in the etiology of ICP because the condition is more common in twin pregnancies in which estrogen levels are higher, and because women with a history of cholestasis may develop pruritus and abnormal liver function when given exogenous estrogens. The condition also occurs more commonly following the administration of progesterone to prevent preterm labor. There is also accumulating evidence that reproductive hormones and/or their metabolites influence the expression and function of hepatic bile acid transporters.

The pathogenesis of the fetal complications of ICP is likely to relate to raised fetal serum bile acids, but the precise mechanisms are not clearly understood. Three studies have demonstrated that ICP cases with higher maternal serum bile acid levels (>40 μmol/L in two studies) more commonly have pregnancies complicated by meconium=stained liquor (amniotic fluid), cardiotocograph (CTG, also known as nonstress tests (NST)) abnormalities and fetal asphyxial events [67–69], and the largest study also demonstrated that patients with higher bile acids have higher rates of spontaneous preterm labor [69]. The majority of stillborn infants are of appropriate weight and the evidence to date suggests that the intrauterine death is a sudden event. Several studies have shown an abnormal fetal heart rate or arrhythmia in pregnancies complicated by ICP, and *in vitro* experiments using neonatal heart cells indicate that they are susceptible to bile acid-induced arrhythmia [70].

Clinical presentation

Symptoms and signs

Cholestasis usually presents with generalized pruritus in the second half of pregnancy. This is often first experienced on the palms and soles, and is not associated with a specific rash. The diagnosis is confirmed if abnormal liver function tests and/or raised serum bile acids are found. The pruritus may precede the biochemical abnormalities by several weeks and therefore liver function tests and serum bile acids should be repeated after a week or two if initially normal in women in whom the diagnosis is suspected. Apart from pruritus, affected women may complain of dark urine and pale stools. However, only a small proportion of cases (≤5%) have jaundice.

Laboratory and diagnostic testing

There is no consensus about whether the most reliable diagnostic test is the demonstration of raised serum transaminases or raised serum bile acids, and therefore many units use both. However, serum bile acids are useful to predict women at higher risk of fetal complications [67–69]. Very few affected women have a raised bilirubin.

Abdominal ultrasound may demonstrate gallstones. However, these may not be the cause of the cholestasis as at least three genes that are thought to be mutated in ICP are also mutated in people with cholesterol gallstones. Hepatitis C infection is more common in women with ICP than in the general obstetric population. It is therefore advisable to screen for hepatitis C as affected women may be referred to a hepatologist for subsequent surveillance and treatment after delivery.

Differential diagnosis

Intrahepatic cholestasis of pregnancy is a diagnosis of exclusion as cholestasis may occur as a consequence of other liver diseases. In addition to performing an abdominal ultrasound and hepatitis screening in all cases, clinicians should be alert to the possibility that women presenting with pruritus and hepatic impairment may rarely also subsequently develop other liver diseases or that over time an alternative diagnosis may become apparent. In particular, pruritus and hepatic impairment occasionally occur in women who subsequently develop (or are recognized to have) acute fatty liver of pregnancy or severe pre-eclampsia. If symptoms and biochemical abnormalities do not resolve within several weeks of delivery, women should also be screened for autoimmune and metabolic liver disease.

Management

A woman complaining of pruritus without a rash in pregnancy should have liver function tests performed. If the itch persists despite normal liver function tests, they should be repeated as cholestasis is often progressive throughout gestation. If possible, serum bile acids should also be checked as a small proportion of cases have isolated hypercholanemia. In addition, a recent study demonstrated that once the serum total bile acids rise above a threshold of 40 μmol/L (i.e. 1.634 mg/dL) there is a 1–2% increase in these fetal complications with each rise of 1 μmol/L (0.571 mg/dL) in the serum bile acid level [69].

Once the diagnosis of ICP has been made, the important considerations are whether to treat with drugs, what is the right strategy for fetal surveillance and what is the ideal timing of delivery. Ursodeoxycholic acid (UDCA) is the only drug that has consistently been shown to improve the maternal symptoms and biochemical features of ICP. There have been several reports of the efficacy of UDCA in ICP, but there have been very few randomized controlled trials. The largest trial randomized 130 women to UDCA, dexamethasone or placebo and demonstrated significant reductions in ALT and bilirubin in the UDCA group only. In a subgroup of cases with serum bile acids ≥40 μmol/L (1.634 mg/dL), UDCA also caused significant reductions in pruritus and serum bile acid levels [71]. UDCA is usually started at a dose of 500 mg twice a day (15 mg/kg/day divided into twice-daily doses) and may be increased further in increments of 500 mg daily (500 mg three times a day and then 1 g twice a day if necessary). The authors have rarely seen a clinical response at doses >2 g per day.

A variety of other drugs have been proposed as treatments for ICP, including dexamethasone, S-adenosyl methionine (SAMe), cholestyramine and guar gum, but the evidence for their efficacy is less consistent than the existing data that support the use of UDCA [72]. Aqueous cream with menthol may improve the symptoms of ICP although it does not affect the disease process. At many centers patients with ICP are given vitamin K (typically 2.5–10 mg orally daily) because of the theoretical risk that cholestasis may be associated with vitamin K malabsorption and thereby a coagulopathy. There are, however, few data to support (or refute) the need for or efficacy of this commonly recommended practice.

There are no treatments that have been shown to reduce fetal risks in ICP, although no studies performed to date have had sufficient power to answer this question. However, it is likely that treatments that reduce maternal bile acids may reduce fetal risks, given the data that implicate bile acids in ICP-related spontaneous preterm delivery, fetal asphyxial events and meconium-stained amniotic fluid [67–69].

Many obstetric units review women with ICP several times per week for fetal assessment by CTG and/or biophysical profile. If the mechanism of fetal death involves bile salt-induced fetal arrhythmias without any placental insufficiency, it may be that such monitoring will not be effective in preventing ICP-associated fetal loss. While there is no guarantee that this approach will prevent subsequent fetal complications,

there are a few reports of abnormal CTG traces having been identified and emergency cesarean section being performed as a consequence. Also many women with ICP find this strategy reassuring.

There is debate about the best time to deliver women with ICP. A review of case series that used a strategy of delivery at 37 weeks gestation compared to those that did not indicates that induction of labor at this stage of pregnancy may protect against fetal death (Table 9.6). These data are consistent with a survey of cases recruited by a patient group in the UK in which the majority of intrauterine deaths occurred after 37 weeks of gestation [73]. While it has to be acknowledged that no studies have been powered to answer the question of whether induction of labor between 37 and 38 weeks of gestation protects against the fetal complications of ICP, the existing data indicate that this is a sensible management strategy. Also, at 37–38 weeks of gestation the risks of respiratory distress drop considerably compared to those reported at 35 or 36 weeks gestation [74]. Many women with ICP have induction of labor, and this has raised concerns about increasing rates of cesarean delivery in this group. No studies have addressed this issue specifically. However, an Italian study that reported a management protocol that included induction of labor at 37 weeks of gestation or earlier if there were unresponsive liver function tests or fetal distress also reported the rates of operative delivery in ICP cases in whom labor was induced. For the 206 women managed using this protocol, the cesarean delivery rate was similar to that of controls (15% vs 16% respectively) [75].

Symptoms and signs of ICP resolve rapidly after delivery and treatment can be stopped within 1–2 days in the majority of cases.

Preconception counseling

If a woman has a previous history of ICP, she has a high probability (90%) of recurrence in subsequent pregnancies [73]. This is reduced if the previous affected pregnancy was a multiple pregnancy and subsequent pregnancies are not.

Table 9.6 Summary of the major studies of fetal outcome in ICP

	No. of cases	IUD and/ or NND(%)	Meconium-stained liquor (%)	Preterm labor (%)	Planned delivery <37–38/40**
1964–69	87	9	–	54	No
1965–79	56	11	27	36	No
Post-1969	91	3	–	–	Yes
1988	83	4	45	44	Yes
1994	320	2	25	12	Yes
1990–96	91	0	15	14.3	Yes
1999–01	70	0	14	6	Yes

NND, neonatal death; IUD, intrauterine death rate as a percentage of all births. **i.e. in the majority of cases in the study.

It is advisable to ensure that baseline liver function tests and serum bile acids are normal, and to determine the hepatitis C status before the woman conceives. It is also sensible to establish whether she has asymptomatic gallstones and to enquire about gastrointestinal symptoms, drug reactions and a family history of cholestasis.

Conclusions

Intrahepatic cholestasis of pregnancy is a relatively common condition that occurs in pregnancy as a consequence of the cholestatic effect of raised estrogen and progesterone in genetically susceptible women. Maternal liver biochemistry should be monitored and one study has reported that serum bile acids >40 μmol/L (1.634 mg/dL) are associated with increased rates of spontaneous preterm labor, fetal asphyxial events and meconium-stained amniotic fluid. Most women respond to treatment with UDCA and at present the available data suggest that delivery at 37–38 weeks of gestation is likely to be of benefit for women with raised serum bile acids.

Wilson's disease

Wilson's disease is a rare autosomal recessive disease that is caused by accumulation of copper in various tissues of the body, and principally in the liver and brain. This results in cirrhosis, liver failure, neurologic and psychiatric symptoms. Treatment is focused on reduction of absorption of copper and on enhanced excretion. Fertility is commonly reduced in women with suboptimally treated disease, and they can have amenorrhea, irregular menses and increased miscarriage rates. However, maternal and fetal outcomes are generally good if Wilson's disease is adequately treated.

Diagnosis

The presenting features of Wilson's disease are very variable. Hepatic impairment is a common presenting feature, particularly in children. Neurologic and psychiatric symptoms are not uncommon, and these include tremor, ataxia and dysphagia. Women may also present with menstrual irregularity, infertility or miscarriage. A characteristic sign seen in affected individuals is Kayser–Fleischer rings, caused by deposition of copper in Descemet's membrane, and visualized as a brown discoloration around the cornea.

There is no single diagnostic test for Wilson's disease. Individuals with unexplained elevated liver transaminases, neuropsychiatric symptoms or Kayser–Fleischer rings should be investigated. Affected individuals usually have low serum levels of copper and ceruloplasmin, and raised urinary copper. Liver biopsy and slit-lamp examination are also of value.

Epidemiology and etiology

Wilson's disease affects approximately 1 in 30,000 people worldwide. It is caused by mutations in the *ATP7B* gene that encodes an ATPase that effluxes copper. In the liver this causes copper to be transported into bile across the hepatocyte canalicular membrane. Mutations in *ATP7B* result in the accumulation of copper in hepatocytes, neurons and other cells. There is a wide spectrum of *ATP7B* mutations, and most are only reported in one or a few families [76]. The clinical phenotype of Wilson's disease is variable, even in individuals with the same mutation, and modifier genes are thought to influence the clinical presentation in individual cases.

General course outside pregnancy

In Wilson's disease the aims of treatment are firstly to enhance efflux of copper from the body and secondly to reduce absorption from the intestine. Drugs that enhance copper efflux are the copper chelators; penicillamine (typically titrated up to a dose of 1000–1500 mg/day in 2–4 divided doses for intial treatment and then at 750–1000 mg/day in two doses for maintenance treatment), trientine (the same dosing as penicillamine) and ammonium tetrathiomolybdate (not available for human use in the US at the time of writing). There is more clinical experience with the first two drugs, both of which bind copper and enhance its urinary excretion. Penicillamine can cause vitamin B6 deficiency and supplements of this vitamin should be taken in conjunction with penicillamine treatment. Individuals who are allergic to penicillin may also have reactions to the drug. Trientine is slightly less toxic than penicillamine, but it can cause iron deficiency. Tetrathiomolybdate is currently being evaluated in clinical trials and is thought to be a promising treatment as it promotes copper efflux and reduces intestinal absorption. Zinc acts on intestinal cells to prevent copper absorption. As zinc therapy is less toxic, treatment regimens may comprise initial treatment with a copper chelator followed by zinc therapy (or combined therapy) to maintain remission of hepatic copper levels. Drug therapy should be continued indefinitely as cessation of treatment results in recurrence of disease, and progression of Wilson's disease commonly results in deterioration and hepatic failure. Some patients do not respond to treatment, and in these cases liver transplantation is indicated.

Preconception counseling

Women with Wilson's disease should be encouraged to continue their treatment in pregnancy. This is particularly important as there are reports of hemolysis, hepatic deterioration and death in women who have stopped D-penicillamine treatment in an attempt to avoid teratogenicity [77].

Antenatal care

Early

Medications

If a woman with Wilson's disease is stable on treatment, she should be advised to continue her current medication. The three principal treatments used for Wilson's disease are D-penicillamine, trientine and zinc.

The use of D-penicillamine is associated with teratogenicity in animals and humans. The principal concerns for humans are a cutis laxa ("loose skin") syndrome, micrognathia ("small jaw") and low-set ears. Trientine has been reported to cause teratogenicity in animal studies. Despite these concerns there are encouraging data on pregnancy outcome following the use of these chelating agents as maintenance therapy for Wilson's disease. This may be because the dose used for maintenance therapy in Wilson's disease is lower than that used to treat cystinuria, and from which the data on teratogenicity were derived. There is more experience of the use of D-penicillamine to treat Wilson's disease in pregnancy and a summary of the current literature reported good outcomes in 144 of 153 pregnancies in 111 women [78]. The adverse outcomes were three therapeutic abortions, one miscarriage, one premature delivery, two cases of cutis laxa, one of cleft lip and palate and one case of mannosidosis (a lysosomal storage disease associated with a wide range of abnormalities). The same author reported 19 good outcomes in 22 pregnancies in 17 women treated with trientine. The adverse outcomes were a therapeutic abortion, one miscarriage and one case of isochromosome X.

Zinc has also been continued as a maintenance therapy for pregnant women with Wilson's disease. A report of the outcome of 26 pregnancies in 19 women reported two congenital abnormalities (7.7%): one was a heart defect requiring surgery at 6 months of age and one baby was born with microcephaly and died soon after birth. All other babies were reported as normal [79].

Taken together, these data indicate that maintenance therapy with D-penicillamine, trientine or zinc should be continued in pregnancy. The congenital abnormalities associated with the chelating agents are thought to be related to fetal copper deficiency rather than a direct effect of the drugs. Therefore some authors have advocated aiming for relatively low doses of these agents during pregnancy, providing the maternal disease is controlled. They advocate a drop from the maintenance dose of 750–1000 mg total per day in the first two trimesters to a 500 mg total per day in the third trimester. It should be remembered that the chelating agents also reduce serum levels of iron and zinc and therefore they should not be given at the same time as iron supplements. Pyridoxine (vitamin B6) supplements (typically 25 mg daily) should also be given as penicillamine inactivates pyridoxine.

Close to term

There is no specific monitoring required for pregnancies in women with Wilson's disease in the third trimester.

Labor and delivery

Labor and delivery should be managed in the same way as in an uncomplicated pregnancy. Newborn babies of women with Wilson's disease have normal copper and ceruloplasmin levels, even if the mother has not complied well with treatment. If the mother has a known *ATP7B* mutation, cord blood can be taken for mutation screening.

Postpartum period

Issues related to medications and lactation

Breastfeeding is not contraindicated in women with Wilson's disease and most experts would support the continued use of penicillamine, trientine and/or zinc in mothers who are lactating. Concentrations of zinc and copper are reduced in breast milk, but no adverse consequences have been reported in their babies.

Contraceptive recommendations

There are no specific forms of contraception that are contraindicated for women with Wilson's disease.

Conclusions

Most women with Wilson's disease have uneventful pregnancy outcomes providing they continue maintenance therapy with chelating agents and/or zinc. Penicillamine or trientine may cause congenital abnormalities as a consequence of fetal copper deficiency, and therefore a reduction in the dose of these chelating agents may be considered if the maternal disease is well controlled. However, the drugs should not be stopped as this may result in deterioration and hepatic failure.

Hemochromatosis

In order to supply sufficient iron for hemoglobin synthesis in developing erythrocytes, about 20 mg of iron is required daily by the bone marrow. Healthy adults typically have 35 mg/kg (women) to 45 mg/kg (men) total body iron. The major source of iron for erythrocyte precursors is plasma iron-transferrin (Fe-Tf). Plasma iron levels are maintained in a relatively constant range (10–30 μmol/L) by balancing the inflow of iron into plasma with the outflow. The inflow is determined by the release of iron from macrophages recycling old red blood cells, release of iron from the liver stores and absorption of iron from the diet. The largest flux, about 20 mg/day, is from iron-recycling macrophages, whereas dietary absorption accounts for only 1–2 mg iron/day and mainly compensates for the small iron losses due to desquamation of cells and minor blood loss. Hereditary hemochromatosis (HH) is an iron overload disorder that is most commonly due to mutations in the HFE gene (also known as the hemochromatosis gene). Mutation of the HFE gene (genetic HH) increases duodenal absorption of iron, leading to iron overload (biochemical HH) and organ damage (clinical HH). The predominant HFE mutation is C282Y. The other common HFE mutation is H63D.

Epidemiology

About 0.4% of people of white, northern European ancestry are homozygous for C282Y, and 75% of these people will develop iron overload. A smaller proportion will develop liver disease (30% of men and 7% of women) or diabetes (2–5%). People who are heterozygous for C282Y do not have a greater risk of clinical HH than noncarriers. Over 85% of patients with clinical HH are homozygous for C282Y. HH can also occur in compound heterozygotes C282Y/H63D or more rarely in homozygotes for H63D. Clinical HH is 2–10 times more common in men than in women as women are somewhat protected from the condition by regular menstrual blood loss.

Clinical presentation and diagnosis

Early iron overload is usually asymptomatic, but chronic iron overload can damage several organ systems, resulting in clinical HH. End-organ damage can cause hepatic cirrhosis and hepatocellular carcinoma, dilated cardiomyopathy or cardiac conduction disturbances, pancreatic dysfunction (including diabetes), hypogonadism, noninflammatory osteo-arthritis and skin bronzing. Common presenting symptoms that may lead to the clinical diagnosis of HH include fatigue, arthralgia, and loss of libido. Diagnosis of hemochromatosis requires clinical suspicion, biochemical testing, and genetic confirmation. Liver enzymes, transferrin saturation, and ferritin concentration should be measured. Raised transferrin saturation and ferritin levels warrant genetic testing for mutations of the HFE gene. Patients homozygous for C282Y with elevated transferrin saturation and ferritin have the diagnosis confirmed.

General management outside pregnancy

Patients with a new diagnosis of HH should be carefully evaluated for the presence of associated organ damage and have the appropriate disease-specific interventions initiated. Management of HH includes both therapy for iron overload and treatment of any secondary diabetes, cardiomyopathy, hypogonadism and cirrhosis. Therapy for iron overload may reverse some but not all of these complications and the best prognosis will be in patients who have their disease identified early.

Initial therapy for iron overload is normally done with serial phlebotomy, typically 0.5–1 unit of blood per week until either the patient's blood shows evidence of iron deficiency anemia or until the serum ferritin and transferrin saturation normalize. Once this is achieved, most patients can be managed with maintenance phlebotomy (typically 500 mL every 2–4 months) with the goal of keeping the ferritin in the normal range. Iron chelation therapy with desferoxamine is almost never used because of the safety and efficacy of phlebotomy.

Management in pregnancy

Most patients known to have HH in pregnancy will have had the diagnosis made and treatment initiated prior to pregnancy and maintenance phlebotomies can be continued as necessary although the increased demands of the fetus for iron may obviate the need for them. As an acute phase reactant, ferritin may normally rise in pregnancy and mild elevations during pregnancy should be interpreted with caution.

The risks of pregnancy for women with HH are those of any associated organ dysfunction. Iron overload of itself has not been associated with adverse obstetric outcomes or fetal effects. Infertility will be an issue in patients with hypogonadism. Poor glycemic control at the time of conception or during the pregnancy can be asscociated with congenital anomalies and other adverse obstetric outcomes. Women with HH-associated cardiomyopathy may be at increased risk of complications such as heart failure and arrhythmias during pregnancy due to the increased cardiac work associated with gestation. Coagulopathies and portal hypertension associated with cirrhosis may put the patient at risk of obstetric or gastroesophageal variceal bleeding. There are no HH-specific management strategies for these complications and the general management of each of these conditions is discussed elsewhere in this textbook in the chapter dealing with the specific system affected.

Biliary disease

The term biliary disease describes a spectrum of diseases that are caused by abnormalities in bile composition, biliary tract anatomy or function. They include common conditions such as cholesterol gallstones and the rarer disorders primary biliary cirrhosis, primary sclerosing cholangitis and biliary atresia. Cholestasis may also be associated with abnormalities in bile composition, and intrahepatic cholestasis of pregnancy (ICP) may occur as a consequence of abnormal hepatic bile homeostasis. ICP has been described in detail earlier in the chapter.

Gallstones and cholescystitis

Diagnosis

Gallstones may be asymptomatic or diagnosed as a consequence of biliary pain. This is usually described as a constant pain that occurs in the epigastric region, may radiate to the back and can last for several hours. If a stone causes obstruction, acute cholecystitis may occur, and this classically causes jaundice, right upper quadrant pain and fever. If gallstones are suspected, liver function tests and an abdominal ultrasound scan should be performed. This allows visualization of the majority of stones with a diameter of ≥1 mm.

Epidemiology and etiology

There are two types of gallstone. The majority of stones (85%) are composed of cholesterol. Bile is principally composed of cholesterol, phospholipids and bile salts. Cholesterol crystals can form when the ratio of the biliary constituents is altered, and this will result in the formation of cholesterol gallstones. Cholesterol gallstones are more commonly found in individuals who live in developed countries, are obese, eat a high-calorie diet, are in middle life, are women and in those taking estrogenic therapies. They also occur more commonly in pregnancy. Pigment stones, composed of bilirubin and calcium, comprise the remaining 15% of gallstones and occur more commonly in patients with chronic hemolysis or cirrhosis.

General course outside pregnancy

The majority of individuals with gallstones are asymptomatic (80%) and rarely have complications. The annual risk for developing abdominal pain in this group of patients is 1.5%. Providing they remain asymptomatic, most clinicians will not treat these patients. In contrast, patients with symptomatic gallstones have a 50% chance of having recurrent biliary colic and are usually offered treatment. There are medical therapies available but many patients are treated surgically, most commonly with laparoscopic cholecystectomy.

Clinical presentation

Cholesterol gallstones occur more commonly in pregnancy. There have been several prospective studies of the prevalence of gallstones or biliary sludge in pregnancy and the puerperium. A US study of 3254 women revealed either sludge or gallstones in 5% of women by the second trimester, 8% by the third trimester and 10% by 4–6 weeks post partum. In this study Body Mass Index was a strong predictor of gallstone disease [80]. These figures are similar to those quoted in European populations. Gallstones are more common in Chile and a study of 980 women from this country revealed that 12% had gallstones in the early puerperium, compared with 1% of nulliparous healthy volunteers [81].

Symptoms

Gallstones in pregnant women are commonly asymptomatic, although 28% of cases with stones in the Chilean study complained of biliary pain. They may co-exist with ICP, and this is likely to be because both conditions have shared genetic predisposing factors. Women with acute cholecystitis complain of right upper quadrant pain that commonly radiates to the back. This may be associated with nausea, vomiting, pyrexia and weight loss.

Management

Asymptomatic gallstones should not be treated in pregnancy. Women should be advised to seek urgent medical help if they develop symptoms consistent with acute cholecystitis and the management should be the same as in the nonpregnant patient. Women should be given intravenous fluids, feeding should be stopped and they should receive antibiotic treatment. If imaging is required, ultrasound examination will commonly confirm stones within the gallbladder but it is less useful for demonstrating gallstones in the common bile duct. If necessary, a technetium-99 HIDA scan (hepatic iminodiacetic acid scan, also known as cholescintigraphy) may be used because of its increased sensitivity for indentifying acute cholecystitis. This test is associated with minimal radiation exposure for the fetus and should be performed when needed in pregnancy.

A recent study compared the medical and surgical management of symptomatic cholelithiasis in 63 pregnant women. No major complications were observed in the 10 cases that were treated surgically. In the 53 cases that were treated medically, there was symptomatic relapse in 38% and two had premature delivery [82]. This study suggests that surgical management should be considered during pregnancy. There are data to support the use of laparoscopic cholecystectomy, as when this was compared with open cholecystectomy in retrospective survey of the literature it was associated with lower rates of spontaneous abortion in the first trimester and premature delivery in the third trimester. There is some debate about the best time to perform surgery. The second trimester (when miscarriage and preterm labor are less likely) is the optimal time to perform a cholecystectomy with regard to fetal outcome. Also in the third trimester uterine enlargement may result in mechanical problems. However, surgery must be performed in any trimester if there is large duct obstruction as this will reduce the chance of pancreatitis and cholangitis.

Postpartum period

Gallstones and biliary sludge that have been identified in pregnant women may resolve following pregnancy, so repeat assessment should be performed prior to making decisions about the need for surgery.

Conclusions

Cholesterol gallstones are relatively common in pregnant women. They are asymptomatic in the majority of cases and in this group do not need any specific management plan. If a woman has symptoms of cholecystitis, surgery is a feasible option and there should be detailed consideration of the associated risks and benefits by a multidisciplinary team.

Primary biliary cirrhosis, primary sclerosing cholangitis and biliary atresia

There are limited data about each of these biliary disorders in pregnancy. They all present with cholestasis and may occur in women of reproductive age. The available data about each condition will be summarized briefly.

Primary biliary cirrhosis

Epidemiology and etiology

Primary biliary cirrhosis is a chronic cholestatic disorder that most commonly affects postmenopausal women. However, it may present in women of childbearing age and there have been reports of the condition in pregnancy. Primary biliary cirrhosis affects approximately 1 in 700 women in developed countries. The condition has a complex etiology with genetic and autoimmune components. Almost all affected individuals have antimitochondrial antibodies.

General course outside pregnancy

The most common presenting symptoms are fatigue and pruritus. Approximately 20% of cases complain of abdominal discomfort. A similar proportion of individuals with primary biliary cirrhosis are diagnosed by chance following routine blood tests. Many women with primary biliary cirrhosis do not have any clinical signs, particularly in the early stages of the disease. However, over 50% of cases have the sicca syndrome (dry eyes and dry mouth). At later stages of disease the most common examination findings are hepatomegaly, splenomegaly, xanthylasmata, jaundice and hyperpigmentation. Most women who are asymptomatic at the time of presentation will have clinical symptoms of cholestasis within 5 years. Once they are symptomatic, affected individuals develop progressive hepatic damage. Therefore, the focus of treatment is to prevent progression. The most commonly used drug is UDCA and women who have a biochemical response to UDCA after a year of treatment have a similar survival rate to controls. Women who do not respond to UDCA may be treated with immunosuppressive agents, glucocorticoids and bile acid sequestrants.

Management in pregnancy

Untreated primary biliary cirrhosis is associated with reduced fertility and this may partly explain the small number of

reported cases in pregnant women. The maternal and fetal outcomes of pregnancies in women with primary biliary cirrhosis have improved in recent series compared to older reports, and this is likely related to the use of UDCA. A study that reviewed 14 cases prior to 1996 reported deterioration of liver function in six pregnancies [83]. Only two cases had treatment, one with UDCA and one with dexamethasone. In this series there were four stillbirths or early miscarriages. A more recent series reported good maternal and fetal outcomes for nine pregnancies in six women who had been treated with UDCA for at least a year before conception [84]. All cases stopped UDCA treatment in the first trimester without deterioration in symptoms or liver function. However, despite an uncomplicated maternal course during pregnancy, all cases had deterioration in their liver function tests in the postpartum period, although all but one returned to baseline levels by 12 months after delivery. In this series there were no fetal losses, nor any cases of preterm birth, intrauterine growth restriction or other pregnancy complications.

Although no cases in this series had deterioration in liver function following cessation of UDCA in the first trimester, there is a case report of worsening liver function following cessation of UDCA that resolved when it was restarted in the first trimester, and the authors are aware of similar cases. Therefore it is advisable to evaluate the treatment needs of each patient on a case-by-case basis. Many experts would offer the option of continuing UDCA throughout the pregnancy, while others, in the context of very limited (but all favorable) first-trimester safety data for UDCA, recommend its use only after the first trimester. Published data on the use of UDCA in breastfeeding are limited, but it is unlikely that this highly protein-bound molecule would enter the breast milk in significant quantities and the authors would support the use of this agent in breastfeeding mothers with primary biliary cirrhosis.

Primary sclerosing cholangitis

Epidemiology and etiology

Primary sclerosing cholangitis (PSC) is a rare chronic cholestatic disease of the liver and bile ducts characterized by progressive inflammation, fibrosis, and stricturing of the intrahepatic and extrahepatic bile ducts. It occurs more commonly in men than women and usually presents before the age of 40. Therefore affected women may become pregnant and some new diagnoses occur in pregnant women with cholestasis. Up to 90% of patients with PSC will also have evidence of ulcerative colitis.

General course outside pregnancy

Patients with PSC are often asymptomatic and present only with incidentally found abnormal liver function tests or may present with fatigue, pruritus, fever, chills, night sweats and abdominal pain. The condition is often progressive, leading to cirrhosis, portal hypertension and liver failure. The most effective drug to treat symptoms and to cause biochemical improvement is UDCA. However, this does not prevent deterioration and therefore liver transplantation is often required. Without transplantation, the median time from diagnosis to death is 5–7 years. While this has improved with the use of liver transplantation, the condition may recur following transplant surgery. Approximately 10–15% of cases develop cholangiocarcinoma.

Management in pregnancy

There have been very few cases reported in pregnancy. One study reported 13 pregnancies in 10 patients with primary sclerosing cholangitis, four of whom had liver cirrhosis while six had mild liver disease [85]. Three cases were diagnosed while pregnant or just after delivery. The most common maternal symptoms in pregnancy were pruritus and abdominal pain. The liver function tests did not deteriorate during pregnancy in any cases, although the serum bile acid levels are not reported. There were good fetal outcomes in all cases, although severe pruritus resulted in delivery in two cases – one elective cesarean section at 30 weeks and an induction of labor at 38 weeks gestation. No cases were treated with UDCA in this study. The majority (70%) of cases had co-existent inflammatory bowel disease and two cases had an exacerbation of their bowel disease during or soon after pregnancy.

There have been a small number of case reports of women with PSC in pregnancy with differing maternal outcomes ranging from development of a new dominant stricture that required stenting soon after delivery to an uncomplicated course. It is not clear from the current literature whether UDCA is of value in the management of maternal cholestasis in pregnant women with PSC. However, it is likely to be of benefit in some cases given that it improves symptoms and biochemistry in nonpregnant cases and it is effective in many women with intrahepatic cholestasis of pregnancy.

In two case reports, the fetal serum bile acids were markedly raised [86,87]. In one report there was fetal bradycardia and in the other there was meconium-stained amniotic fluid.

However, both infants were well after delivery. The maternal serum bile acids were not reported in either study so the cause of the fetal hypercholanemia is not clear.

These reports suggest that there may be a role for managing these patients by following serum bile acids, treating with UDCA and considering early delivery as we do for ICP but at this point, no clear recommendations can be made as to the role of any of these interventions in patients with PSC.

Biliary atresia

Epidemiology and tiology

Biliary atresia is a rare disorder that affects approximately 1 in 15,000 newborns. It is characterized by abnormal development or obliteration of the biliary tree that results in obstruction to bile flow. It presents with severe cholestasis in the neonatal period and is usually surgically corrected with the Kasai procedure, an operation in which a small segment of intestine is used to replace the damaged bile ducts.

General course outside pregnancy

The majority of infants are jaundice free after the Kasai procedure, but many have recurrence of symptoms before they reach adulthood. The most common symptoms are ascending cholangitis, portal hypertension, often with gastrointestinal bleeding, and cirrhosis. As a consequence, most affected individuals will have had a liver transplant by the age of 20.

Management in pregnancy

Table 9.7 summarizes the maternal outcome of the 30 ongoing pregnancies in 22 women with biliary atresia that are reported in two retrospective series from Japan [88,89]. The maternal outcome is better in women who are asymptomatic before conception. Women with cholangitis before pregnancy were more likely to have another episode during pregnancy, and those with pre-existing portal hypertension were more likely to have a gastrointestinal bleed.

In one series maternal deterioration was common after delivery. In particular, 38% of women had deterioration of

Table 9.7 Maternal outcome of pregnancies in women with biliary atresia

Pre-pregnancy clinical features	No. patients	No. pregnancies	Cholangitis in pregnancy	GI bleed in pregnancy	Liver dysfunction in pregnancy	Other hepatic problem in pregnancy	Healthy during pregnancy
No C, no PH	8	10	1	–	2	–	7
C only, no PH	5	8	2	1	–	–	5
No C, PH only	7	10	1	3	1	2	3
C and PH	2	2	–	–	2	–	0
Total	22	30	4	4	5	2	15

C, cholangitis; PH, portal hypertension; GI, gastrointestinal.
Data from Shimaoka *et al.* [88] and Sasaki *et al.* [89].

liver function (one required subsequent liver transplantation) and 25% had ascending cholangitis [88].

In the two series from Japan, there were no congenital abnormalities reported in association with maternal biliary atresia and the majority of babies were normally grown and born at term. However, four intrauterine fetal deaths were reported; one was attributed to hemorrhagic shock after massive gastrointestinal hemorrhage and one related to severe atopic dermatitis [88]. The other intrauterine deaths were unexplained, although they did occur in women with portal hypertension, one of whom also had cholangitis. The deaths occurred in the third trimester and the authors speculated that they may have been related to raised maternal serum bile acid levels [89]. However, this could not be confirmed as the maternal blood was not tested in either case.

Budd–Chiari syndrome

Epidemiology and etiology

Budd–Chiari syndrome is a rare condition caused by occlusion of the hepatic veins or the terminal portion of the inferior vena cava (IVC). Although the syndrome name refers to any obstruction of the hepatic veins or distal IVC, most cases are related to obstruction from thrombosis. It occurs more commonly in women and in individuals with acquired or hereditary thrombophilias. In one series 15% of cases were associated with pregnancy [90] and it has also been reported in association with oral contraceptive use.

General course outside pregnancy

Budd–Chiari syndrome may present acutely with obstruction of major hepatic veins or chronically with involvement of smaller interlobular veins. The clinical features depend upon the rate of onset and pattern of venous obstruction. The most common presentation is with progressive development of ascites over months with tender hepatomegaly at later stages. However, some patients present more acutely with more rapid onset of ascites, abdominal pain and jaundice (in approximately 50%) over several weeks. A small proportion may also have rapid onset of hepatic failure. Diagnosis can be achieved through pulsed-wave Doppler imaging, demonstrating direction and amplitude of flow. Percutaneous hepatic venous catheterization will show elevated hepatic vein pressures, venous occlusion, and collateral circulation. MRI can also aid in diagnosis.

Patients with a patent portal vein and without obstruction of the IVC should have a portocaval shunt. These can be placed with either a transjugular approach or surgically, depending on the degree of obstruction and the local expertise. Alternative shunting procedures (e.g. mesocaval shunt) may be used if the portal vein is not patent and the IVC is blocked or severely compressed. Patients with thrombosis are generally anticoagulated if the risk of bleeding is small, but while the anticoagulant may help prevent propagation and recurrence, it is less likely to reopen obstructed hepatic veins. Liver transplant should be considered in patients in whom hepatic failure persists because of failed shunt procedures or if there is marked fibrosis or cirrhosis.

Management in pregnancy

There are reports of pregnancy in women with a new diagnosis of Budd–Chiari syndrome in pregnancy and in cases of pre-existing disease. Clinically the disorder presents in the same way as outside pregnancy with ascites, abdominal pain and distension. Women who develop acute major venous obstruction can deteriorate rapidly, with portal hypertension, variceal bleeding, and fulminant hepatic failure. Liver enzymes are usually modestly elevated and there is a more marked rise in alkaline phosphatase than is normally seen in pregnancy. Portocaval shunting may improve portal hypertension and ascites, although many pregnant woman are not surgically stable enough to undergo this procedure. These procedures have been primarily accomplished in postpartum cases. There are reports of successful pregnancies after transjugular intrahepatic portosystemic shunting [91] and mesocaval shunting [92] and these options should be considered in pregnancy if they would be offered to a nonpregnant patient. Patients with Budd–Chiari syndrome should be investigated for underlying thrombophilias and thromboprophylaxis should be used during the present and likely subsequent pregnancies.

Cirrhosis and portal hypertension

The most common cause of portal hypertension is liver cirrhosis. However, noncirrhotic portal hypertension can be seen in patients without liver disease and causes include veno-occlusive disease (Budd–Chiari syndrome), noncirrhotic portal fibrosis, infection and extrahepatic obstruction. The management of cirrhotic and noncirrhotic portal hypertension will be discussed. Both are associated with increased rates of pregnancy complications although the etiology of the portal hypertension influences both maternal and fetal outcomes.

Cirrhosis and liver failure

Epidemiology and etiology

The most common causes of cirrhosis in the Western world are alcoholic liver disease and chronic viral hepatitis. Other causes of cirrhosis are shown in Box 9.1. The etiology of fibrosis seen in cirrhotic livers is complex and largely unknown, but central to the process is inflammation and subsequent repair. Local

Box 9.1 Causes of cirrhosis

Autoimmune
- Autoimmune hepatitis

Viral / infectious
- Hepatitis B & C
- Schistosomiasis

Metabolic
- Hereditary hemochromatosis
- Alcohol
- Wilson's disease
- Drugs

Cholestatic
- Primary biliary sclerosis
- Primary sclerosing cholangitis
- Biliary atresia

Vascular
- Sarcoidosis
- Cystic fibrosis
- Right heart failure
- Budd–Chiari syndrome

and distal inflammatory cells are recruited, and tissue fibroblasts (mainly hepatic stellate cells) are activated into extracellular matrix-secreting myofibroblasts. Disruption of normal liver architecture and obstruction to hepatic blood flow occur, leading to further impairment in liver synthetic and metabolic functions as well as portal hypertension.

General course outside pregnancy

Cirrhosis represents a clinical spectrum, ranging from asymptomatic liver disease to hepatic decompensation. Physical findings can include spider telangiectasias, palmar erythema, jaundice, ascites, muscle wasting, edema and fetor hepaticus. Complications include esophageal variceal bleeding, ascites, hepatic encephalopathy, hepatorenal syndrome, hepatopulmonary syndrome, portopulmonary hypertension, and hepatocellular carcinoma (see review by Dong & Saab [93]). The complications of cirrhosis and liver failure are considered below.

Hepatic encephalopathy

Hepatic encephalopathy can manifest with symptoms ranging from impaired memory and attention to confusion and coma. Its pathogenesis is multifactorial: derangements in neurotransmitter pathways, cerebral blood flow modulation, and systemic inflammatory responses have all been implicated. The diagnosis of hepatic encephalopathy is based largely on clinical suspicion in a patient with known cirrhosis. Altered sleep

patterns, slurred speech, asterixis (hands make a flapping motion if held out and dorsiflexed), hyper-reflexia, nystagmus, inappropriate behavior, disorientation and confusion are all suggestive of the diagnosis in a patient with known hepatic failure. Ammonia levels, while commonly used to assist in the diagnosis of hepatic encephalopathy, are neither sensitive nor specific for the condition. Upper gastrointestinal bleeding, hypovolemia, hypoglycemia, hypokalemic metabolic alkalosis, infection, constipation, hypoxia or excessive use of sedatives can precipitate an acute episode. Treatment can include removal or treatment of the precipitating cause, lactulose (titrated to achieve three soft stools per day) and, if these are ineffective, the use of nonabsorbable antibiotics such as neomycin or rifaximin. Liver transplantation dramatically improves the clinical status, although minimal symptoms may persist due to irreversible brain damage.

Metabolic and endocrine dysfunction

Hyperglycemia may result from portal to systemic shunting, which decreases the efficiency of postprandial glucose extraction from portal blood by hepatocytes. Conversely, hepatocyte destruction and impaired glycogenolysis and gluconeogenesis can cause hypoglycemia. Protein synthesis is impaired, which negatively impacts the regulation of oncotic pressure (albumin), blood pressure (angiotensinogen), growth (insulin-like growth factor 1), and metabolism (sex hormone- and thyroid hormone-binding proteins). Protein deamination and transamination in the urea cycle are disrupted, leading to accumulation of toxins, such as ammonia. Cholestasis results in impaired dietary absorption of lipids and fat-soluble vitamins. Jaundice and pruritus may also be present. Decreased hepatic clearance of unbound sex hormones and increased peripheral aromatization of androgens to estrogens may result in pituitary and gonadal suppression.

Electrolyte disturbances

Hyponatremia (serum sodium <135 mmol/L) is an independent predictor of mortality in patients with cirrhosis. A recent large study demonstrated that the degree of hyponatremia correlated with refractory ascites, hepatic encephalopathy, spontaneous bacterial peritonitis, and hepatorenal syndrome [94]. Hyponatremia results from increased secretion of antidiuretic hormone secondary to the reduced intravascular volume, leading to decreased renal perfusion and stimulation of the renin-angiotensin-aldosterone system [95]. Rapid correction of the hyponatremia using hypertonic saline can, however, cause central pontine myelinolysis.

Hematologic abnormalities

Microcytic anemia may result from iron deficiency due to deficiencies in ferritin and transferrin production. Macrocytic anemia due to folate and vitamin B12 deficiencies can also occur. Decreased lipid synthesis may cause red blood cell membrane abnormalities, contributing to hemolytic anemia. Thrombocytopenia may result from impaired liver production of thrombopoietin or increased destruction due to hypersplenism from splenic vein engorgement.

Vitamin K-dependent clotting factors II, VII, IX, and X are produced in the liver, and deficiencies in these factors are reflected in prolongation of the prothrombin time and INR. Levels of anticoagulant proteins (protein C, S, and antithrombin) are also reduced, paradoxically rendering these patients also at risk for thrombosis.

Impaired excretory function

The liver is vital for clearance of endogenous toxins such as ammonia and bile acids. It is also a major site for detoxification of drugs. The effects of nonsteroidal anti-inflammatory drugs, acetaminophen and other medications, particularly those which are metabolized by the cytochrome P450 system (such as benzodiazepines, warfarin, morphine), may be exaggerated or can cause direct hepatic damage and should be monitored carefully.

Gastrointestinal varices

Esophageal varices are present in 30% of patients with compensated cirrhosis and 60% of patients with decompensated cirrhosis [96]. Varices are a direct consequence of portal hypertension, and patients with portal pressures greater than 10 mmHg are at risk. Each episode of hemorrhage carries a 20% mortality rate [97] and untreated patients have a 70% rebleeding risk within 1 year [98].

Ascites

Ascites from cirrhosis develops as a direct consequence of portal hypertension. As sinusoidal pressures rise, hepatic lymph production increases. When lymphatic drainage mechanisms are overwhelmed, excess lymph collects in the peritoneal cavity, thus causing ascites [99]. A right-sided pleural effusion can also complicate ascites.

Sepsis

Spontaneous bacterial peritonitis (SBP) is seen in up to 30% of patients with ascites [100]. It should be considered whenever a patient with known ascites develops signs of infection, abdominal pain and/or changes in mental status. The diagnosis is confirmed by performing paracentesis and finding both a positive fluid culture and greater than 250 neutrophils/mm^3 fluid. Following an initial episode of peritonitis, antibiotic prophylaxis is recommended, because the 1-year recurrence rate is 55% and 1-year survival is <50% [101]. Spontaneous bacterial peritonitis is associated with the development of hepatorenal syndrome in about 30% of patients [100].

Hepatorenal syndrome

Hepatorenal syndrome (HRS) is a late complication resulting from progressive hepatic failure. It is characterized by renal vasoconstriction in response to low renal perfusion secondary to the decreased circulating volume. The annual incidence of HRS in patients with cirrhosis and ascites is around 8% [102]. HRS is classified as either type 1 or 2. Type 1 HRS is a progressive condition with a doubling of serum creatinine to a level >2.5 mg/dL in less than 2 weeks. Frequently it has a precipitating factor such as severe bacterial infection (often peritonitis), gastrointestinal hemorrhage, major surgery or acute hepatitis superimposed on cirrhosis. Without treatment, patients with type 1 HRS have a median survival of 2 weeks.

Type 2 HRS is characterized by a moderate and steady decline in renal function with creatinine >1.5 mg/dL. The dominant feature in type 2 HRS is refractory ascites, and median survival is 6 months [102]. Patients with type 2 HRS are predisposed to developing type 1 HRS after a precipitating event. The only definitive treatment for HRS is liver transplantation.

Pulmonary consequences of portal hypertension

Two distinct pulmonary vascular disorders can occur: portopulmonary hypertension (POPH) and hepatopulmonary syndrome (HPS). Portopulmonary hypertension is seen in 0.5–5% of patients with cirrhosis and/or portal hypertension and presents in similar ways to patients with pulmonary hypertension from other causes (chest pain, syncope, dyspnea on exertion, cardiomegaly) [103]. HPS is defined as a defect in arterial oxygenation induced by intrapulmonary vascular dilations. This entity is seen in 8–17% of patients with cirrhosis, and median survival is 11 months [104]. Patients typically present with progressive dyspnea, platypnea (increased dyspnea in the sitting position that is relieved by lying down), and cyanosis. No medical treatment is available for HPS except for symptomatic measures such as long-term oxygen therapy. Liver transplantation is the only cure [103].

Hepatocellular carcinoma

The yearly risk of developing hepatocellular carcinoma is 1.4% in patients with compensated cirrhosis and 4% in patients with decompensated cirrhosis [105]. Frequent screening with abdominal imaging (ultrasound, computed tomography or MRI) is advantageous since lesions found early may be amenable to treatment.

Management in pregnancy

Cirrhosis is associated with reduced fertility and oligomenorrhea, so pregnancy is relatively rare. However, there are sufficient cases reported in the literature to evaluate the risks associated with the condition in pregnant women and their pregnancies.

Women with cirrhosis have an increased rate of fetal loss, stillbirth and neonatal death [106,107]. The women themselves are also at risk. In an early series of 95 pregnancies in 78 women, there was no significant deterioration in liver function in two-thirds of cases [107a]. In the other cases the maternal complications included bleeding from esophageal varices, anemia, postpartum hemorrhage and pre-eclampsia. The most important complication is variceal bleeding. It is essential that the potential risks of this complication are explained to the pregnant woman with cirrhosis, ideally prior to pregnancy. Indeed, the death rate in pregnant women with cirrhosis has been quoted as 10–18%, with most cases complicated by esophageal variceal bleeding [108]. Women at highest risk are those with a history of gastrointestinal bleeding prior to pregnancy. The risk of bleeding is thought to increase as pregnancy advances because of increasing circulating blood volume, raised portal pressure, and vena cava compression resulting in enhanced flow through the azygos venous system. This increased risk likely continues in the early postpartum period when the involution of the uterus and reabsorption of pregnancy-associated peripheral edema can lead to significant fluid shifts. Beta-blockers (usually propranolol or nadolol) are used to help prevent variceal bleeding in nonpregnant patients and these agents should be continued during pregnancy. It is believed that women who have undergone previous portocaval decompression procedures are less likely to bleed in pregnancy although the procedure carries an increased risk of hepatic encephalopathy and is therefore usually not done unless there has been failure of medical management.

Variceal bleeding is a medical emergency and should, if at all possible, be managed by a team and in a setting that regularly cares for patients with this complication. Early identification of the possibility of variceal bleeding and prompt notification of the appropriate medical team are essential to these patients' survival. In addition to restoring blood volume through rapid transfusion, management of acute bleeding varices typically includes prophylactic antibiotics, endoscopy with sclerotherapy (typically) or band ligation (less commonly) and consideration of the use of intravenous octreotide. Terlipressin should not be used in pregnancy because of concerning animal data. Sclerotherapy may be superior to portosystemic shunting at reducing recurrent bleeding episodes and therefore shunting is typically not done as a first-line intervention.

In a study of 11 women with cirrhosis during pregnancy, four of six with documented varices experienced gastrointestinal hemorrhage requiring endoscopic sclerotherapy [108]. Five of these women had significant coagulation disorders as well. In the entire series, there were six growth-retarded infants, three preterm deliveries, and one neonatal death. Portal decompression surgery has been accomplished during pregnancy; however, it has clearly become a second-line approach to endoscopic sclerotherapy.

Another feared complication associated with portal hypertension is the development of splenic artery aneurysm. Pulsed-wave Doppler and CT imaging may be helpful in establishing the diagnosis and many of these aneurysms are identified incidentally on imaging studies done for other reasons. Elective laparoscopic surgery with ligation should be strongly considered before pregnancy because rupture carries with it an enormous risk of maternal and fetal death. Rupture of a previously undiagnosed splenic artery aneurysm is a rare but life-threatening diagnosis that should be considered in any patient with portal hypertension who presents with sudden onset of abdominal pain and signs of hypovolemia without evidence of variceal or obstetric bleeding. Splenic artery aneurysm rupture has also been described in otherwise healthy pregnant women.

While it is essential to consider the risk of variceal bleeding, most women with cirrhosis will have uncomplicated pregnancies. The pregnancy should be managed and delivery should take place in a tertiary center with facilities for endoscopic control of bleeding varices. Medications (sedatives, diuretics, etc.) used during the pregnancy should be carefully monitored because of the possibility of precipitating liver failure. If varices have been documented, it is preferable to avoid excessive straining at the time of delivery and therefore the second stage of labor should be shortened with forceps or Ventouse delivery. Cesarean delivery should only be performed for obstetric indications as abdominal surgery in patients with cirrhosis may be complicated by bleeding, massive fluid shifts, poor wound healing, infection, and encephalopathy.

It is important to be aware that the metabolism and pharmacokinetics of anesthetic agents will be altered in women with cirrhosis and women may be at increased risk of bleeding. Coagulation parameters and a platelet count should be checked prior to delivery and consideration given to correcting significant abnormalities peripartum with vitamin K, fresh-frozen plasma and/or platelets.

Noncirrhotic portal hypertension

Management in pregnancy

Noncirrhotic portal hypertension is most commonly caused by noncirrhotic portal fibrosis, Budd–Chiari syndrome or extrahepatic portal venous obstruction, and affected women are more likely to be of childbearing age than are women with cirrhosis. Affected women rarely have abnormal liver function and their fertility rates are the same as controls [109,110].

There are varied reports on the fetal risks associated with noncirrhotic portal hypertension. An Indian series of 116 pregnancies in 44 patients [109] and a US series of 38 cases [111] both reported fetal loss rates of 7–8%. Two other series that only included women with extrahepatic portal venous obstruction reported fetal loss rates of 23–28%

[108,112] and this may relate to the different etiology of portal hypertension in this group.

The frequency of variceal bleeding in pregnant women with noncirrhotic portal hypertension is lower if they have had treatment for esophageal varices prior to pregnancy, e.g. by endoscopic injection sclerotherapy or a decompression operation. In an Indian study of 50 pregnancies in 27 women, the rate of bleeding in 35 pregnancies in which the disease was diagnosed and treated prior to conception was 8.6%, compared to a rate of 93% in 15 pregnancies in which disease was diagnosed during pregnancy [110]. In women with bleeding varices during pregnancy, treatment with sclerotherapy is considered a reasonable and appropriate intervention [109]. For prevention of rebleeding, it is advisable to use beta-blocker therapy in addition to sclerotherapy.

In summary, the overall prognosis for women with noncirrhotic portal hypertension in pregnancy is better than in those with cirrhosis, particularly if the disease was diagnosed and treated prior to conception.

Liver transplantation

Transplantation is generally considered after the first episode of decompensated cirrhosis or in those who have impending complications (profound alterations in liver function with INR over 1.7) [113]. Most transplant centers recommend that pregnancy be deferred at least 1 year following transplantation. This is because, after the first post-transplant year, viral prophylaxis treatment has generally been completed, the dose of immunosuppressive agents is reduced, and the overall risk of rejection is felt to be low [114]. It is also recommended that no episodes of rejection should have occurred in the year before conception [115].

Overall, the outcomes of pregnancies in liver transplant recipients appear to be favorable. The livebirth rate is fairly consistent across most studies, at greater than 70%. Outcomes appear to be improved in patients who delay pregnancy at least 1 year after transplant. Although the rates of maternal complications, particularly hypertensive disorders, are increased in pregnancy, there is no increase in rates of organ loss. Rejection episodes that do occur can be managed by the usual interventions, including liver biopsy and alterations in the immunosuppressive regimen.

Pregnancy does not appear to increase maternal mortality. Neonatal outcome data are also good without significant adverse effects due to exposure to immunosuppressants. The high preterm delivery rate is significant, and the incidence of low birthweight is similarly high. Table 9.8 [116] summarizes the maternal and perinatal outcomes for pregnancies following liver transplantation. There is a 3% incidence of congenital malformations and the maternal death rate is 5.5% over a 2-year period following delivery [116].

Table 9.8 Pregnancy outcomes following liver transplantation [116]

Outcome	Typical result
Livebirth	78%
Hypertension	28%
Pre-eclampsia	26%
Reversible liver dysfunction	27%
Rejection	20%
Infection	10%
Mean gestational age	37 weeks
Preterm delivery	31%
Mean birthweight	2612g
Low birthweight (<2500 g)	23%
Cesarean section	43%
Perinatal death	4%

Acute fatty liver of pregnancy

Acute fatty liver of pregnancy (AFLP) is a sudden severe illness occurring almost exclusively in the third trimester, in which microvesicular fatty infiltration results in encephalopathy and hepatic failure.

Epidemiology

Acute fatty liver of pregnancy is a rare condition that is estimated to affect 1 in 7000–16,000 pregnancies [117,118]. It is associated with microvesicular fatty infiltration of the liver, hepatic failure, and encephalopathy. It has been suggested that acute fatty liver of pregnancy is more common in nulliparous women (40–50%), as well as in those with multiple pregnancy [119]. It carries significant perinatal and maternal mortality and requires early diagnosis and intervention to prevent maternal and fetal death.

Etiology

In some cases the etiology of AFLP involves abnormalities in mitochondrial fatty acid oxidation [119]. Beta-oxidation of fatty acids in hepatic mitochondria is a complex process requiring several essential enzymes: mitochondrial trifunctional protein and its alpha-subunit, long-chain 3-hydroxyacyl-CoA dehydrogenase (LCHAD), are the two enzymes of this metabolic process, whose autosomally inherited genetic mutations are most closely associated with AFLP, especially the G1548C mutation of LCHAD [120].

Maternal liver disease (either HELLP syndrome or AFLP) is more common in women who carry this mutation [121]. LCHAD deficiency has been identified in about 20% of babies of mothers with AFLP. Maternal heterozygosity for LCHAD deficiency reduces the maternal capacity to oxidize long-chain fatty acids in both liver and placenta and this, together with the metabolic stress of pregnancy and fetal homozygosity for LCHAD deficiency, causes accumulation in the maternal circulation of potentially hepatotoxic LCHAD metabolites [122]. There are reports of maternal liver disease associated with defects of other enzymes involved in fatty acid oxidation, but the role of these other enzymes in causing AFLP remains unclear.

Clinical presentation

The patient typically presents with a 1–2-week history of malaise, anorexia, nausea, vomiting, mid-epigastric or right upper quadrant pain, headache or jaundice. Some patients may have a low-grade fever. Other findings include hypertension, occasionally proteinuria and ascites, and bleeding from severe coagulopathy. There is overlap between AFLP and pre-eclampsia/HELLP syndrome.

Lethargy, agitation, confusion, and even coma may be present. Symptoms of preterm labor or, more rarely, lack of fetal movements may be the presenting complaint in some patients. In 15–20% of cases these symptoms may be absent. In some cases, the first onset of signs or symptoms may be in the postpartum period.

Laboratory features

The full blood count usually reveals hemoconcentration, leukocytosis and a low platelet count. Fibrinogen levels are low, the prothrombin time is prolonged and antithrombin levels are low. These abnormalities are related to reduced production by the liver. Disseminated intravascular coagulopathy (DIC) may be present. Metabolic acidosis with elevated creatinine and uric acid levels may be present. Hypoglycemia is common. Liver enzymes such as AST and ALT vary from near-normal to 1000 U/L, and they are usually 300–500 U/L. In some cases an apparently mild elevation in aminotransferases may be misleading as this can occur as a consequence of severe hepatic necrosis and is caused by an inability of hepatocytes to synthesize these enzymes. The alkaline phosphatase and bilirubin are elevated and the increase in bilirubin is mainly of the conjugated form, with levels usually exceeding 5 mg/dL. Ammonia levels are also increased, particularly in the late stage of the disease. Amylase and lipase values may be elevated in the presence of concomitant pancreatitis. In some patients, polydipsia and polyuria may develop due to excessive clearance of vasopressin (antidiuretic hormone (ADH)) by placental vasopressinase that is not adequately cleared by the diseased liver.

Liver ultrasound may show decreased echogenicity of the parenchyma but is generally less sensitive than CT and MRI. CT scan of the liver can show decreased or diffuse attenuation in the liver. However, none of these techniques is sufficiently sensitive to exclude a diagnosis of AFLP.

Although liver biopsy is the gold standard for confirming the diagnosis, it is rarely used in clinical practice. Liver histology shows swollen, pale hepatocytes with central nuclei. The diagnosis can be made only on a frozen section liver biopsy with special stains for fat such as oil red. The diagnosis is usually made on the basis of clinical and laboratory findings. The main differential diagnosis is often HELLP syndrome and the two conditions can be very difficult to distinguish. Encephalopathy, marked jaundice or hypoglycemia, however, are features that are highly suggestive of AFLP. Other differential diagnoses include severe atypical cholestasis of pregnancy, Budd–Chiari syndrome, adult-onset Reye's syndrome, and drug-induced hepatic toxicity (acetaminophen overdose, tetracycline-induced toxicity, anticonvulsant drug hypersensitivity, and methyldopa hepatitis).

Management

Early recognition and diagnosis with immediate delivery (following stabilization of the mother) and intensive supportive care are essential for both maternal and fetal survival. The patient should be admitted to allow maternal stabilization, fetal monitoring, and confirmation of diagnosis. Cesarean section is commonly performed as this is the most rapid mode of delivery, although vaginal delivery is not contraindicated and is likely to be associated with less bleeding. Induction of labor with an attempt for vaginal delivery within 24 hours is a reasonable approach. Because of the associated coagulopathy, epidural or spinal analgesia is contraindicated. The use of pudendal block should be avoided because of the risk of bleeding and hematoma formation. Caution should be exercised to avoid vaginal trauma and lacerations during vaginal delivery. In the case of cesarean delivery, the patient should receive general anesthesia. Prophylactic antibiotics are recommended.

Aminotransferase levels and encephalopathy will usually improve within 2–3 days following delivery. However, intensive supportive care may be required in the meantime. In some cases, however, deterioration in liver function tests and coagulopathy may continue for about 1 week. If liver failure develops (encephalopathy, hypoglycemia, coagulopathy) or deterioration continues despite delivery, the patient should be transferred to a liver center. N-acetylcysteine therapy should also be considered. Most patients improve in 1–4 weeks post partum, although a cholestatic phase with rising bilirubin and alkaline phosphatase may persist.

Recovery is usually complete with no signs of chronic liver disease. Maternal mortality ranges between 7% and 18% with slightly higher fetal mortality (9–23%). Sepsis and hemorrhagic complications remain the most life threatening. Liver transplantation has a very limited role because of the reversibility of this disease following delivery but may need to be considered in patients whose clinical course continues to deteriorate. Pancreatitis is a potentially lethal complication of

AFLP and thus all patients with AFLP should undergo serial screening of serum lipase and amylase for several days after the onset of hepatic dysfunction.

Women who are carriers of LCHAD mutation have an increased risk of recurrence of AFLP in 20–70% of pregnancies. All babies of mothers with AFLP should be tested for defects of fatty acid oxidation because presymptomatic diagnosis and appropriate early management will reduce morbidity and mortality in these babies. For mothers with previous AFLP, liver tests, glucose, and carnitine levels and plasma acylcarnitine profile may help identify the obligate carrier to allow closer fetal and maternal monitoring [121].

Pancreatic disease

The pancreas has endocrine and exocrine functions. Disorders of the endocrine pancreas are considered in Chapter 11. The exocrine pancreas secretes trypsin, chymotrypsin, pancreatic amylase, and lipase. The pancreatic disorders that can present in pregnancy include acute pancreatitis and malignancy. Increasing numbers of women are having pancreatic transplants during their reproductive years. Cystic fibrosis can also affect the pancreas and this is considered in Chapter 1.

Acute pancreatitis

Epidemiology and etiology

Acute pancreatitis affects approximately 1 in 10,000 individuals and the frequency of the disorder does not change in pregnancy. The most common cause is gallstones [123]. Rarer causes in pregnancy include hypertriglyceridemia, alcohol, hypercalcemia, viral infection, and drugs, e.g. thiazide diuretics and glucocorticoids.

Clinical presentation and management

Acute pancreatitis presents in pregnant women with the same symptoms as in nonpregnant individuals. It most commonly presents in the second or third trimester with acute, unremitting epigastric pain that may radiate to the back.

A raised serum amylase is the cornerstone of diagnosis and it is often recorded at levels >1000 U/L. Renal clearance of amylase may be increased in pregnancy but amylase will still generally be elevated in pregnant women with acute pancreatitis. Pancreatic lipase and amylase-to-creatinine clearance ratio are alternative markers that may be used when the diagnosis of pancreatitis is suspected but the amylase is not significantly elevated. Patients with acute pancreatitis should have their serum lipids and calcium measured to look for underlying hypertriglyceridemia or hyperparathyroidism. Plasma glucose levels should also be measured.

Management is supportive. Bowel rest and analgesia are essential. Nasogastric drainage is recommended for persistent vomiting or if there is evidence of paralytic ileus. Intravenous fluids are often needed in large volumes (250 cc or more per hour) because of the edema that may accumulate in the injured pancreas. Approximately 10% of cases of acute pancreatitis develop shock and may also have serious pulmonary (pulmonary edema or adult respiratory distress syndrome), cardiac (rarely myocardial infarction), renal (pre-renal renal failure and acute tubular necrosis) or pancreatic complications (necrosis, infection, pseudocysts and fistulas). The majority of these diagnoses should be managed in a medical intensive care setting and not on obstetric units.

The reported maternal and fetal mortality rates in older studies were ≥20%, but this has improved markedly in more recent studies [123,124]. The group that has the highest rates of maternal morbidity and mortality is women with hypertriglyceridemia. In a recent report four out of five cases had complications that included adult respiratory distress syndrome, myocardial infarction and pancreatic pseudocyst [125]. Hypertriglyceridemia can usually be managed with dietary modification. The management of gallstones is discussed earlier in this chapter. Detailed imaging may allow confirmation of the diagnosis. For example, a recent report in which combined magnetic resonance cholangiopancreatography (MRCP) and endoscopic ultrasonography (EUS) were used to evaluate four patients with acute pancreatitis, a biliary cause was confirmed in three cases and anatomic abnormality of the pancreas was demonstrated in the fourth [126].

Women with chronic pancreatitis or recurrent attacks require careful management in pregnancy as they often suffer from malabsorption, requiring enzyme replacement. In addition, gestational diabetes is frequent in these cases. In most, there is a background of alcohol abuse, and their medical care needs to be supplemented by social work and psychologic assistance. Fetal growth restriction may also occur.

Anesthetic concerns in patients with liver disease

Anesthetic management of a parturient during labor and delivery is dictated by the type and severity of liver dysfunction. Mild variations in hepatic function are usually well tolerated by mother and fetus, and do not alter peripartum management, other than requiring close monitoring to ensure that the pre-existing liver function is maintained. However, systemic abnormalities associated with severe acute and chronic liver dysfunction can have profound implications for the outcome of the pregnancy as well as the feasible anesthetic choices for the labor and/or the delivery.

The approach to obstetric anesthesa in the setting of liver disease is summarized in general in Box 9.2 and reviewed

Box 9.2 Anesthesia guidelines for a parturient with liver dysfunction

- Evaluate the extent of hepatic impairment and underlying systemic abnormalities.
- Stabilize and optimize maternal condition before delivery.
- Defer elective operative intervention in the presence of acute hepatitis.
- Exclude or correct coagulopathy before regional block.
- Optimize hepatic blood flow and oxygenation during anesthesia.
- Recognize pharmacokinetic/pharmacodynamic alterations of the anesthetic drugs.
- Avoid hepatotoxic drugs.
- Avoid transmission of viral hepatitis to the healthcare team.
- Monitor for postoperative hepatic dysfunction.

below. Anesthetic concerns related to pregnancy-specific liver disease are reviewed in Table 9.9.

The perioperative risk should be evaluated by assessment of: liver function tests; complete blood count including platelet count; albumin levels; renal function tests; blood glucose, fluid and electrolyte status; coagulation status (INR and partial thromboplasting time (PTT)); and acid–base balance [127]. Assessment should be directed toward optimizing medical treatment and monitoring maternal and fetal condition. Maternal nutrition and volume status should be optimized before the anticipated delivery, and may need to be guided by central venous and peripheral arterial monitoring in cases of significant liver dysfunction. Urine output should be routinely monitored as an indicator of the adequacy of intravascular hydration. Appropriate blood bank arrangements should be made in advance to ensure the blood bank is well informed and ready to supply potentially needed factor replacement, blood and albumin. Patients with acute hepatitis from any cause are at increased risk for hepatic failure and death; hence, when possible, elective operative intervention should be deferred in such patients [128]. Severe coagulopathy and thrombocytopenia may preclude regional anesthesia and necessitate the use of other modes of analgesia for labor pain, and general anesthesia for cesarean section (see below). Specific considerations for pregnancy-related liver disorders are given in Table 9.9.

Regional anesthesia

If the coagulation status allows, consideration should be given to a carefully titrated epidural technique, since it permits better preservation of hepatic blood flow than general or spinal anesthesia [132]. However, epidural and other forms of nerve block are contraindicated in patients with significant thrombocytopenia and other coagulation abnormalities. Ascites and portal hypertension lead to engorged epidural veins, thus increasing the risk of intravascular injection of the local anesthetic and epidural hematoma [133]. A rise in prothrombin time (PT) or INR, particularly if greater than 1.5, is an indicator of a poor prognosis [134] and warrants replacement of clotting factors by administration of vitamin K and fresh-frozen plasma (FFP) prior to delivery. Prophylactic platelet and FFP transfusions are not indicated before a regional block or surgery in the absence of active bleeding if the platelet counts are stable above $80 \times 10^9/L$ (and some experienced anesthetists would say as low as $50 \times 10^9/L$) and the INR is less than 1.5 [135]. If regional anesthesia is used, the volume status should be optimized, and precautions should be taken to avoid hypotension and hypoxia in order to prevent exacerbation of hepatic injury. It is imperative to correct coagulation deficits before removal of the indwelling epidural catheter [136].

General anesthesia

General anesthesia is required for emergency cesarean delivery if there is severe maternal coagulopathy, hemodynamic instability or neurologic deterioration. Pregnant women with ascites and encephalopathy are at higher risk for aspiration and hence should receive a prophylactic H2 receptor antagonist such as ranitidine. Drugs with sole hepatic metabolism, such as cimetidine, are better avoided. In addition to the usual obstetric considerations, the aim of general anesthesia should be to maintain liver and renal blood flow. Parturients with liver dysfunction tolerate hypotension and hypoxia from any cause poorly.

Liver disease may have a significant impact on the pharmacokinetics and pharmacodynamics of anesthetic drugs due to altered protein binding, altered volume of distribution, and reduced metabolism; hence, their judicious administration is advocated [128]. Benzodiazepines may have prolonged effects in these patients and can potentiate hepatic encephalopathy [137]. Inhalational anesthetic agents have a potential to cause hepatotoxicity, although desflurane and sevoflurane may be relatively safe [138,139]. Atracurium or cis-atracurium is the muscle relaxant of choice as it does not rely on hepatic metabolism [140,141]. Opioids should be cautiously administered to provide postoperative analgesia as their clearance is delayed in patients with severe liver disease [142]. Intramuscular injections, acetylsalicylic acid, and nonsteroidal anti-inflammatory drugs should be avoided in patients with severe coagulopathy. Acetaminophen, administered for postdelivery analgesia, can cause hepatotoxicity, even when used at therapeutic dosages, in patients with liver dysfunction [143].

Table 9.9 Anesthetic considerations for liver disorders peculiar to pregnancy

Disorder	Key features of anesthetic concern	Anesthetic implications
Intrahepatic cholestasis of pregnancy (ICP)	Present with pruritus and jaundice, and may develop coagulopathy secondary to vitamin K malabsorption Rapid postpartum resolution occurs	Administer vitamin K, and reverse coagulopathy with fresh-frozen plasma. Regional anesthesia is contraindicated 45if coagulopathy persists The contractile response to oxytocin may be enhanced, leading to uterine hypertonus due to cholic acid-mediated increase in oxytocin receptor expression [129] Prepare for the management of postpartum hemorrhage
Acute fatty liver of pregnancy (AFLP)	Characterized by impaired hepatic metabolic activity, which may progress to liver failure, disseminated intravascular coagulation (DIC) with profound depression of antithrombin level. Other features include anemia, hypoglycemia, metabolic acidosis, sepsis, and renal failure. High maternal mortality if untreated Complete postpartum resolution occurs Expedited delivery is desirable	Provide supportive treatment to optimize and stabilize medical condition. Regularly check biochemical and hemodynamic parameters Obtain good intravenous access for administration of drugs, dextrose, electrolytes, and blood products Treat coagulopathy and prepare for postpartum and gastrointestinal hemorrhage Consider regional anesthesia if there is no contraindication. Remove epidural catheter as soon as possible after delivery, because nadir of platelet count may occur 24–72 h post partum Drugs metabolized primarily by liver may have prolonged duration. Avoid the use of hepatotoxic drugs
Pre-eclampsia and HELLP (hemolysis, elevated liver enzymes, low platelet count) syndrome	Thrombocytopenia, hemolytic anemia, and elevated liver function tests are the hallmarks of HELLP syndrome, a variant of severe pre-eclampsia. The nadir of the platelet count and maximum liver dysfunction can occur 1–2 days post partum [130]	Consider continuous invasive blood pressure monitoring, and concomitant administration of anticonvulsant and antihypertensive drugs Consider dexamethasone in patients with HELLP. It is associated with improved platelet count, liver function values, blood pressure, and urinary output [131] Monitor coagulation parameters serially before administration of regional anesthesia and removal of epidural catheter General anesthesia carries concern about airway issues, especially bleeding and friability, and potential for hypertensive responses during the induction and emergence period
Hepatic rupture	Commonly presents as a triad of pre-eclampsia, right upper quadrant pain, and shock Indication for emergency laparotomy and prompt delivery, often by cesarean section	Aggressive management is essential, with vigorous hemodynamic support and replacement of fluid and blood losses. Invasive monitoring is indicated Laparotomy requires general anesthesia. Use of regional anesthesia is often dictated by the coagulation status
Hyperemesis gravidarum	Presents with severe nausea, vomiting and dehydration. May have minor liver function abnormalities	Correct fluid and electrolyte imbalances Administer optimum pharmacologic antiemetic therapy

Controlled ventilation, inhalational anesthetics, stress response to surgery, persistent low perfusion states, and hypoxemia can decrease liver blood flow in patients with prior hepatic disease and predispose the liver to injury during anesthesia [144]. Perioperative monitoring of patients with severe liver dysfunction should be facilitated in an intensive care setting.

References

1. Robson SC, Mutch E, Boys RJ, Woodhouse KW. Apparent liver blood flow during pregnancy: a serial study using indocyanine green clearanc e. Br J Obstet Gynaecol 1990;97(8):720–4.
2. Van Thiel DH, Gavaler JS. Pregnancy-associated sex steroids and their effects on the liver. Semin Liver Dis 1987;7(1):1–7.
3. Valenzuela GJ, Munson LA, Tarbaux NM, Farley JR. Time-dependent changes in bone, placental, intestinal, and hepatic alkaline phosphatase activities in serum during human pregnancy. Clin Chem 1987;33(10):1801–6.
4. Freund G AD. Clinical biochemistry of pre-eclampsia and related liver diseases of pregnancy: a review. Clin Chem Acta 1990;191:123–51.
5. Waffarn F, Carlisle S, Pena I, Hodgman JE, Bonham D. Fetal exposure to maternal hyperbilirubinemia. Neonatal course and outcome. Am J Dis Child 1982;136(5):416–17.
6. Baker VV, Cefalo RC. Fulminant hepatic failure in the third trimester of pregnancy. A case report. J Reprod Med 1985;30(3):229–31.
7. Kumar S, Regan F. Management of pregnancies with RhD alloimmunisation. BMJ 2005;330(7502):1255–8.
8. Wasley A, Fiore A, Bell BP. Hepatitis A in the era of vaccination. Epidemiol Rev 2006;28:101–11.
9. Bell BP, Anderson DA, Feinstone SM. Hepatitis A virus. In: Mandell GL, Bennett JE, Dolin R (eds) Mandell, Douglas and Bennett's principles and practice of infectious diseases, 6th edn. Churchill Livingstone, Philadelphia, 2005.
10. Bell BP, Shapiro CN, Alter MJ, Moyer LA, Judson FN, Mottram K, et al. The diverse patterns of hepatitis A epidemiology in the United States – implications for vaccination strategies. J Infect Dis 1998;178(6):1579–84.

11. McDuffie RS Jr, Bader T. Fetal meconium peritonitis after maternal hepatitis A. Am J Obstet Gynecol 1999;180(4):1031–2.

12. Leikin E, Lysikiewicz A, Garry D, Tejani N. Intrauterine transmission of hepatitis A virus. Obstet Gynecol 1996;88 (4 Pt 2):690–1.

13. Urganci N, Arapoglu M, Akyildiz B, Nuholu A. Neonatal cholestasis resulting from vertical transmission of hepatitis A infection. Pediatr Infect Dis J 2003;22(4):381–2.

14. Watson JC, Fleming DW, Borella AJ, Olcott ES, Conrad RE, Baron RC. Vertical transmission of hepatitis A resulting in an outbreak in a neonatal intensive care unit. J Infect Dis 1993;167(3):567–71.

15. Renge RL, Dani VS, Chitambar SD, Arankalle VA. Vertical transmission of hepatitis A. Indian J Pediatr 2002;69(6):535–6.

16. Tong M, el-Farra N, Grew M. Clinical manifestations of hepatitis A: recent experience in a community teaching hospital. J Infect Dis 1995;171(suppl 1):S15–S8.

17. Centers for Disease Control and Prevention. Hepatitis Surveillance Report No. 58. US Department of Health and Human Services, Centers for Disease Control and Prevention, Atlanta, GA, 2003.

18. Elinav E, Ben-Dov IZ, Shapira Y, Daudi N, Adler R, Shouval D, et al. Acute hepatitis A infection in pregnancy is associated with high rates of gestational complications and preterm labor. Gastroenterology 2006;130(4):1129–34.

19. Centers for Disease Control and Prevention. Recommended adult immunization schedule – United States, 2002–2003. [Erratum appears in MMWR 2003;52(15):345.] MMWR 2002;51(40):904–8.

20. Kao J-H, Chen D-S. Global control of hepatitis B virus infection. Lancet Infect Dis 2002;2(7):395–403.

21. Euler GL, Wooten KG, Baughman AL, Williams WW. Hepatitis B surface antigen prevalence among pregnant women in urban areas: implications for testing, reporting, and preventing perinatal transmission. Pediatrics 2003;111(5 Part 2):1192–7.

22. Linnemann CC Jr, Goldberg S. Letter: HBAg in breast milk. Lancet 1974;2(7873):155.

23. Boxall EH, Flewett TH, Dane DS, Cameron CH, MacCallum FO, Lee TW. Letter: Hepatitis-B surface antigen in breast milk. Lancet 1974;2(7887):1007–8.

24. Beasley R, Stevens C, Shiao I, Meng H. Evidence against breast-feeding as a mechanism for vertical transmission of hepatitis B. Lancet 1975;2:740–1.

25. Kroger AT, Atkinson WL, Marcuse EK, Pickering LK, Advisory Committee on Immunization Practices, Centers for Disease Control. General recommendations on immunization: recommendations of the Advisory Committee on Immunization Practices (ACIP). [Erratum appears in MMWR 2006;55(48):1303.] MMWR 2006;55(RR-15):1–48.

26. McMahon BJ, Alward WL, Hall DB, Heyward WL, Bender TR, Francis DP, et al. Acute hepatitis B virus infection: relation of age to the clinical expression of disease and subsequent development of the carrier state. J Infect Dis 1985;151(4):599–603.

27. Wright TL, Mamish D, Combs C, Kim M, Donegan E, Ferrell L, et al. Hepatitis B virus and apparent fulminant non-A, non-B hepatitis [see comment]. Lancet 1992;339(8799):952–5.

28. Chu CJ, Keeffe EB, Han SH, Perrillo RP, Min AD, Soldevila-Pico C, et al. Hepatitis B virus genotypes in the United States: results of a nationwide study. Gastroenterology 2003;125(2):444–51.

29. Kao JH, Chen PJ, Lai MY, Chen DS. Hepatitis B genotypes correlate with clinical outcomes in patients with chronic hepatitis B. Gastroenterology 2000;118(3):554–9.

30. Magnius LO, Norder H. Subtypes, genotypes and molecular epidemiology of the hepatitis B virus as reflected by sequence variability of the S-gene. Intervirology 1995;38(1–2):24–34.

31. Mast EE, Weinbaum CM, Fiore AE, Alter MJ, Bell BP, Finelli L, et al. A comprehensive immunization strategy to eliminate transmission of hepatitis B virus infection in the United States: recommendations of the Advisory Committee on Immunization Practices (ACIP) Part II: immunization of adults. MMWR 2006;55(RR–16):1–33; quiz CE1–4.

32. Mast EE, Margolis HS, Fiore AE, Brink EW, Goldstein ST, Wang SA, et al. A comprehensive immunization strategy to eliminate transmission of hepatitis B virus infection in the United States: recommendations of the Advisory Committee on Immunization Practices (ACIP) part 1: immunization of infants, children, and adolescents.[Erratum appears in MMWR 2006;55(6):158–9.] MMWR 2005;54(RR–16):1–31.

33. Okada K, Yamada T, Miyakawa Y, Mayumi M. Hepatitis B surface antigen in the serum of infants after deliver from asymptomatic carrier mothers. J Pediatr 1975;87(3):360–3.

34. Su G-G, Pan K-H, Zhao N-F, Fang S-H, Yang D-H, Zhou Y. Efficacy and safety of lamivudine treatment for chronic hepatitis B in pregnancy. World J Gastroenterol 2004;10(6):910–12.

35. Van Zonneveld M, van Nunen AB, Niesters HGM, de Man RA, Schalm SW, Janssen HLA. Lamivudine treatment during pregnancy to prevent perinatal transmission of hepatitis B virus infection. J Viral Hepat 2003;10(4):294–7.

36. Stevens CE, Taylor PE, Tong MJ, Toy PT, Vyas GN, Nair PV, et al. Yeast-recombinant hepatitis B vaccine. Efficacy with hepatitis B immune globulin in prevention of perinatal hepatitis B virus transmission. JAMA 1987;257(19):2612–16.

37. Stevens CE, Toy PT, Tong MJ, Taylor PE, Vyas GN, Nair PV, et al. Perinatal hepatitis B virus transmission in the United States. Prevention by passive-active immunization. JAMA 1985; 253(12):1740–5.

38. Wong VC, Ip HM, Reesink HW, Lelie PN, Reerink-Brongers EE, Yeung CY, et al. Prevention of the HBsAg carrier state in newborn infants of mothers who are chronic carriers of HBsAg and HBeAg by administration of hepatitis-B vaccine and hepatitis-B immunoglobulin. Double-blind randomised placebo-controlled study. Lancet 1984;1(8383):921–6.

39. Lok ASF, McMahon BJ. Chronic hepatitis B. Hepatology 2007;45(2):507–39.

40. Silverman NS, Jenkin BK, Wu C, McGillen P, Knee G. Hepatitis C virus in pregnancy: seroprevalence and risk factors for infection. Am J Obstet Gynecol 1993;169(3):583–7.

41. Floreani A, Paternoster D, Zappala F, Cusinato R, Bombi G, Grella P, et al. Hepatitis C virus infection in pregnancy [see comment]. Br J Obstet Gynaecol 1996;103(4):325–9.

42. Clarke A, Kulasegaram R. Hepatitis C transmission – where are we now? Int J STD AIDS 2006;17(2):74–80.

43. European Paediatric Hepatitis CVN. A significant sex – but not elective cesarean section – effect on mother-to-child transmission of hepatitis C virus infection [see comment]. J Infect Dis 2005;192(11):1872–9.

44. Mast EE, Hwang L-Y, Seto DSY, Nolte FS, Nainan OV, Wurtzel H, et al. Risk factors for perinatal transmission of hepatitis C virus (HCV) and the natural history of HCV infection acquired in infancy. J Infect Dis 2005;192(11):1880–9.

45. Mok J, Pembrey L, Tovo P, Newell ML, European Paediatric Hepatitis C Virus Network. When does mother to child transmission of hepatitis C virus occur? Arch Dis Child (Fetal Neonat) 2005;90(2):F156–60.

46. European Paediatric Hepatitis C Virus Network, Pembrey L, Tovo P, Newell M. Effects of mode of delivery and infant feeding on the risk of mother-to-child transmission of hepatitis C virus. Br J Obstet Gynaecol 2001;108:371–7.

47. Management of hepatitis C. Available from: http://consensus. nih.gov/2002/2002HepatitisC2002116html.htm.

48. Pappalardo BL. Influence of maternal human immunodeficiency virus (HIV) co-infection on vertical transmission of hepatitis C virus (HCV): a meta-analysis. Int J Epidemiol 2003; 32(5):727–34.

49. Steininger C, Kundi M, Jatzko G, Kiss H, Lischka A, Holzmann H. Increased risk of mother-to-infant transmission of hepatitis C virus by intrapartum infantile exposure to maternal blood. J Infect Dis 2003;187(3):345–51.

50. Bosi I. HLA DR13 and HCV vertical infection. Pediatr Res 2002;51:746–9.

51. Bradley JS. Hepatitis. In: Remington JS, Klein J, Baker C (eds) Infectious diseases of the fetus and newborn infant, 6th edn. Elsevier Saunders, Philadelphia, 2006:823–43.

52. Strader DB, Wright T, Thomas DL, Seeff LB, American Association for the Study of Liver Diseases. Diagnosis, management, and treatment of hepatitis C. Hepatology 2004;39(4):1147–71.

53. McIntyre PG, Tosh K, McGuire W. Caesarean section versus vaginal delivery for preventing mother to infant hepatitis C virus transmission. Cochrane Database of Systematic Reviews, 2006;4:CD005546.

54. Purcell R, Emerson S. Hepatitis E virus. In: Mandell GL, Bennett JE, Dolin R (eds) Mandell, Douglas and Bennett's principles and practice of infectious diseases, 6th edn. Churchill Livingstone, Philadelphia, 2005.

55. Pal R, Aggarwal R, Naik SR, Das V, Das S, Naik S. Immunological alterations in pregnant women with acute hepatitis E. J Gastroenterol Hepatol 2005;20(7):1094–101.

56. Kumar A, Beniwal M, Kar P, Sharma JB, Murthy NS. Hepatitis E in pregnancy. Int J Gynaecol Obstet 2004;85(3):240–4.

57. Singh S, Mohanty A, Joshi YK, Deka D, Mohanty S, Panda SK. Mother-to-child transmission of hepatitis E virus infection. Indian J Pediatr 2003;70(1):37–9.

58. Chibber RM, Usmani MA, Al-Sibai MH. Should HEV infected mothers breast feed? Arch Gynecol Obstet 2004;270(1):15–20.

59. Krawczynski K, Aggarwal R. Hepatitis E. Infect Dis Clin North Am 2000;14(1):669–87.

60. Krawitt EL. Autoimmune hepatitis. N Engl J Med 2006; 354:54–66.

61. Floreani A, Niro G, Rizzotto ER, et al. Type I autoimmune hepatitis: clinical course and outcome in an Italian multicentre study. Aliment Pharmacol Ther 2006;24:1051–17.

62. Heneghan MA, Norris SM, O'Grady JG, et al. Management and outcome of pregnancy in autoimmune hepatitis. Gut 2001;48:97–102.

63. Schramm C, Herkel J, Beuers U, et al. Pregnancy in autoimmune hepatitis: outcome and risk factors. Am J Gastroenterol 2006;101:556–60.

64. Werner M, Bjornsson E, Prytz H, et al. Autoimmune hepatitis among fertile women: strategies during pregnancy and breastfeeding? Scand J Gastroenterol 2007;42:986–91.

65. Candia L, Marquez J, Espinoza LR. Autoimmune hepatitis and pregnancy: a rheumatologist's dilemma. Semin Arth Rheum 2005;35:49–56.

66. Buchel E, van Steenbergen W, Nevens F, et al. Improvement of autoimmune hepatitis during pregnancy followed by flare-up after delivery. Am J Gastroenterol 2002;97:3160–5.

67. Laatikainen T, Tulenheimo A. Maternal serum bile acid levels and fetal distress in cholestasis of pregnancy. Int J Gynaecol Obstet 1984;22:91–4.

68. Laatikainen T, Ikonen E. Serum bile acids in cholestasis of pregnancy. Obstet Gynecol 1977;50:313–18.

69. Glantz A, Marschall HU, Mattsson LA. Intrahepatic cholestasis of pregnancy: relationships between bile acid levels and fetal complication rates. Hepatology 2004;40:467–74.

70. Gorelik J, Shevchuk A, de Swiet M, Lab M, Korchev Y, Williamson C. Comparison of the arrhythmogenic effects of tauro- and glycoconjugates of cholic acid in an in vitro study of rat cardiomyocytes. Br J Obstet Gynaecol 2004;111:867–70.

71. Glantz A, Marschall HU, Lammert F, et al. Intrahepatic cholestasis of pregnancy: a randomized controlled trial comparing dexamethasone and ursodeoxycholic acid. Hepatology 2005;42:1399–405.

72. Geenes VL, Williamson C. Intrahepatic cholestasis of pregnancy. J Gastroenterol 2009; 15(17): 2049–66.

73. Williamson C, Hems LM, Goulis DG, et al. Clinical outcome in a series of cases of obstetric cholestasis identified via a patient support group. Br J Obstet Gynaecol 2004;111:676–81.

74. Morrison JJ, Rennie JM, Milton PJ. Neonatal respiratory morbidity and mode of delivery at term: influence of timing of elective caesarean section. Br J Obstet Gynaecol 1995;102:101–6.

75. Roncaglia N, Arreghini A, Locatelli A, Bellini P, Andreotti C, Ghidini A. Obstetric cholestasis: outcome with active management. Eur J Obstet Gynecol Reprod Biol 2002;100:167–70.

76. De Bie P, Muller P, Wimenga C, Klomp LWJ. Molecular pathogenesis of Wilson and Menkes disease: correlation of mutations with molecular defects and disease phenotypes. J Med Genet 2007;44:673–88.

77. Shimono N, Ishihashi H, Ikematsu H, et al. Fulminant hepatic failure during perinatal period in a pregnant women with Wilson's disease. Gastroenterol Jpn 1991;26:69–73.

78. Sternlieb I. Wilson's disease and pregnancy. Hepatology 2000;31531–2.

79. Brewer GJ, Johnson VD, Dick RD, Hedera P, Fink JK, Kluin KJ. Treatment of Wilson's disease with zinc: XVII: treatment during pregnancy. Hepatology 2000;31:364–70.

80. Ko CW, Beresford SAA, Schulte SJ, Masumoto AM, Lee SP. Incidence, natural history and risk factors for biliary sludge and stones during pregnancy. Hepatology 2005;41:359–65.

81. Valdivieso V, Covarrubias C, Siegel F, Cruz F. Pregnancy and cholelithiasis: pathogenesis and natural course of gallstones diagnosed in early puerperium. Hepatology 1993;17:1–4.

82. Lu EJ, Curet MJ, El-Sayed YY, Kirkwood K. Medical versus surgical management of biliary tract disease in pregnancy. Am J Surg 2004;188:755–9.

83. Goh SK, Gull SE, Alexander GJM. Pregnancy in primary biliary cirrhosis complicated by portal hypertension: report of a case and review of the literature. Br J Obstet Gynecol 2001;108:760–2.

84. Poupon R, Chretien Y, Chazouilleres O, Poupon RE. Pregnancy in women with ursodeoxycholic acid-treated primary biliary cirrhosis. J Hepatol 2005;42:418–23.

85. Janczewska I, Olsson R, Hultcrantz R, Broome U. Pregnancy in patients with primary sclerosing cholangitis. Liver 1996;16:326–30.

86. Landon MB, Soloway RD, Freedman LJ, Gabbe SJ. Primary sclerosing cholangitis and pregnancy. Obset Gynecol 1987; 69:457–60.

87. Nolan DG, Martin LS, Natarajan S, Hume RF. Fetal compromise associated with extreme fetal bile acidemia and maternal primary sclenosing cholangitis. Obstet Gynecol 1994; 84:695–6.

88. Shimaoka S, Ohi R, Saeki M, et al. Problems during and after pregnancy of former biliary atresia patients treated successfully by the Kasai procedure. J Pediatr Surg 2001;36:349–51.

89. Sasaki H, Nio M, Hayashi Y, Ishii T, Sano N, Ohi R. Problems during and after pregnancy in female patients with biliary atresia. J Pediatr Surg 2007;42:1329–32.

90. Khuroo M, Datta D. Budd–Chiari syndrome following pregnancy: report of 16 cases with roentgenologic hemodynamic and histologic studies of the hepatic outflow tract. Am J Med 1980;8:113.

91. Angermayr B, Cejna M, Karnel F, et al. Transjugular intrahepatic portosystemic shunt in Vienna-a decade later. Wen Klin Wochenschr 2004; 116:608-13.

92. Huguet C, Deliere T, Oliver JM, et al. Budd–Chiari syndrome with thrombosis of the inferior vena cava: long-term patency of mesocaval and cavoatrial prosthetic bypass. Surgery 1984;95:108.

93. Dong MH, Saab S. Complications of cirrhosis. Dis Mon 2008;54(7):445–56.

94. Angeli P, Wong F, Watson H, Gines P. Hyponatremia in cirrhosis: results of a patient population survey. Hepatology 2006;44(6):1535–42.

95. Arroyo V, Terra C, Gines P. New treatments of hepatorenal syndrome. Semin Liver Dis 2006;26(3):254–64.

96. D'Amico G, Pagliaro L, Bosch J. The treatment of portal hypertension: a meta-analytic review. Hepatology 1995;22(1):332–54.

97. McCormick PA, O'Keefe C. Improving prognosis following a first variceal haemorrhage over four decades. Gut 2001;49(5):682–5.

98. Graham DY, Smith JL. The course of patients after variceal hemorrhage. Gastroenterology 1981;80(4):800–9.

99. Sandhu BS, Sanyal AJ. Management of ascites in cirrhosis. Clin Liver Dis 2005;9(4):715–32, viii.

100. Rimola A, Garcia-Tsao G, Navasa M, Piddock LJ, Planas R, Bernard B, et al. Diagnosis, treatment and prophylaxis of spontaneous bacterial peritonitis: a consensus document. International Ascites Club. J Hepatol 2000;32(1):142–53.

101. Tito L, Rimola A, Gines P, Llach J, Arroyo V, Rodes J. Recurrence of spontaneous bacterial peritonitis in cirrhosis: frequency and predictive factors. Hepatology 1988;8(1):27–31.

102. Gines A, Escorsell A, Gines P, Salo J, Jimenez W, Inglada L, et al. Incidence, predictive factors, and prognosis of the hepatorenal syndrome in cirrhosis with ascites. Gastroenterology 1993;105(1):229–36.

103. Herve P, Le Pavec J, Sztrymf B, Decante B, Savale L, Sitbon O. Pulmonary vascular abnormalities in cirrhosis. Best Pract Res Clin Gastroenterol 2007;21(1):141–59.

104. Tsai SL, Chen PJ, Lai MY, Yang PM, Sung JL, Huang JH, et al. Acute exacerbations of chronic type B hepatitis are accompanied by increased T cell responses to hepatitis B core and e antigens. Implications for hepatitis B e antigen seroconversion. J Clin Invest 1992;89(1):87–96.

105. Fattovich G, Giustina G, Degos F, Tremolada F, Diodati G, Almasio P, et al. Morbidity and mortality in compensated cirrhosis type C: a retrospective follow-up study of 384 patients. Gastroenterology 1997;112(2):463–72.

106. Britton RC. Pregnancy and esophageal varices. Am J Surg 1982;143(4):421–5.

107. Schreyer P, Caspi E, El-Hindi JM, Eshchar J. Cirrhosis – pregnancy and delivery: a review. Obstet Gynecol Surv 1982;37(5):304–12.

107a. Huchzermeyer H. Pregnancy in patients with liver cirrhosis and chronic hepatitis. Acta Hepatosplenol (Stuttg) 1971;18:294.

108. Pajor A, Lehoczky D. Pregnancy in liver cirrhosis – assessment of maternal and fetal risks in eleven patients and review of management. Gynecol Obstet Invest 1994;38:45.

109. Kocchar R, Kumar S, Goel RC, et al. Pregnancy and its outcome in patients with noncirrhotic portal hypertension. Dig Dis Sci 1999;44:1356–61.

110. Aggarwal N, Sawhney H, Vasishta K, et al. Non-cirrhotic portal hypertension in pregnancy. Int J Gynecol Obstet 2001;72:1–7.

111. Britton RC. Pregnancy and esophageal varices. Am J Surg 1982;143:421–5.

112. Cheng YS. Pregnancy in liver cirrhosis and/or portal hypertension. Am J Obstet Gynecol 1977;128:812.

113. Kamath PS, Kim WR. The model for end-stage liver disease (MELD). Hepatology 2007;45(3):797–805.

114. McKay DB, Josephson MA. Pregnancy in recipients of solid organs – effects on mother and child. N Engl J Med 2006;354(12):1281–93.

115. McKay DB, Josephson MA, Armenti VT, August P, Coscia LA, Davis CL, et al. Reproduction and transplantation: report on the AST Consensus Conference on Reproductive Issues and Transplantation. Am J Transplant 2005;5(7):1592–9.

116. Dei Malatesta MF, Rossi M, Rocca B, Iappelli M, Giorno MP, Berloco P, et al. Pregnancy after liver transplantation: report of 8 new cases and review of the literature. Transpl Immunol 2006;15(4):297–302.

117. Castro MA, Fassett MJ, Reynolds TB, Shaw KJ, Goodwin TM. Reversible peripartum liver failure: a new perspective on the diagnosis, treatment, and cause of acute fatty liver of pregnancy, based on 28 consecutive cases. Am J Obstet Gynecol 1999;181(2):389–95.

118. Reyes H, Sandoval L, Wainstein A, Ribalta J, Donoso S, Smok G, et al. Acute fatty liver of pregnancy: a clinical study of 12 episodes in 11 patients. Gut 1994;35(1):101–6.

119. Sibai BM. Imitators of severe preeclampsia. Obstet Gynecol 2007;109(4):956–66.

120. Shames BD, Fernandez LA, Sollinger HW, Chin LT, d'Alessandro AM, Knechtle SJ, et al. Liver transplantation for HELLP syndrome. Liver Transpl 2005;11(2):224–8.

121. Ibdah JA. Acute fatty liver of pregnancy: an update on pathogenesis and clinical implications. World J Gastroenterol 2006;12(46):7397–404.

122. Ibdah JA, Bennett MJ, Rinaldo P, Zhao Y, Gibson B, Sims HF, et al. A fetal fatty-acid oxidation disorder as a cause of liver disease in pregnant women. N Engl J Med 1999;340(22):1723–31.

123. Hernandez A, Petrov MS, Brooks DC, et al. Acute pancreatitis and pregnancy: a 10-year single center experience. J Gastrointest Surg 2007;11:1623–7.

124. Swisher SG, Hunt KK, Schmit PJ, et al. Management of pancreatitis complicating pregnancy. Am Surg 1994;60:759–62.

125. Crisan LS, Steidl ET, Rivera-Alsina ME. Acute hyperlipidemic pancreatitis in pregnancy. Am J Obstet Gynecol 2008;198:e57–9.

126. Romieu F, Ponchon T, Adura P, et al. Acute pancreatitis in pregnancy: place of the different explorations (magnetic resonance cholangiopancreatography, endoscopic ultrasonography) and their therapeutic consequences. Eur J Obstet Gynecol Reprod Biol 2008;140(1):141–2.

127. Knox TA. Evaluation of abnormal liver function in pregnancy. Semin Perinatol 1998;22:98–103.

128. Gholson CF, Provenza JM, Bacon BR. Hepatologic considerations in patients with parenchymal liver disease undergoing surgery. Am J Gastroenterol 1990;85:487–96.

129. German AM, Kato S, Carvajal JA, Valenzuela GJ, Valdes GL, Glasinovic JC. Bile acids increase response and expression of human myometrial oxytocin receptor. Am J Obstet Gynecol 2003;189:577–82.

130. Martin JN Jr, Blake PG, Perry KG Jr, McCaul JF, Hess LW, Martin RW. The natural history of HELLP syndrome: patterns of disease progression and regression. Am J Obstet Gynecol 1991;164:1500–9.

131. Van Runnard Heimel PJ, Franx A, et al. Corticosteroids, pregnancy, and HELLP syndrome: a review. Obstet Gynecol Surv 2004;60:57–70.

132. Gelman S, Frenette L. Effects of anesthetics on liver blood flow. Baillière's Clin Anaesthesiol 1992;6:729–50.

133. Morisaki H, Doi J, Ochiai R, Takeda J, Fukushima K. Epidural hematoma after epidural anesthesia in a patient with hepatic cirrhosis. Anesth Analg 1995;80:1033–5.

134. Pugh RN, Murray-Lyon IM, Dawson JL, Pietroni MC, Williams R. Transection of the oesophagus for bleeding oesophageal varices. Br J Surg 1973;60:646–9.

135. Roberts WE, Perry KG, Martin JN. The intrapartum platelet count in patients with HELLP (hemolysis, elevated liver enzymes, and low platelets) syndrome: is it predictive of later hemorrhagic complications? Am J Obstet Gynecol 1994;171:799–804.

136. Tsui SL, Yong BH, Ng KF, Yuen TS, Li CC, Chui KY. Delayed epidural catheter removal: the impact of postoperative coagulopathy. Anaesth Intens Care 2004;32:630–6.

137. Branch RA, Morgan MH, James J, Read AE. Intravenous administration of diazepam in patients with chronic liver disease. Gut 1976;17:75–83.

138. Njoku D, Laster MJ, Gong DH, Eager EI 2nd, Reed GF, Martin JL. Biotransformation of halothane, enflurane, isoflurane, and desflurane to trifluoroacetylated liver proteins: association between protein acylation and hepatic injury. Anesth Analg 1997;84:173–8.

139. Kharasch ED. Biotransformation of sevoflurane. Anesth Analg 1995;81:S27.

140. Ward S, Neill EA. Pharmacokinetics of atracurium in acute hepatic failure (with acute renal failure). Br J Anaesth 1983;55:1169–72.

141. De Wolf AM, Freeman JA, Scott VL, Tullock W, Smith DA. Pharmacokinetics and pharmacodynamics of cisatracurium in patients with end-stage liver disease undergoing liver transplantation. Br J Anaesth 1996;76:624–8.

142. Tegeder I, Lotsch J, Geisslinger G. Pharmacokinetics of opioids in liver disease. Clin Pharmacokinet 1999;37:17–40.

143. Yaghi C, Honein K, Boujaoude J, Slim R, Moucari R, Sayegh R. Influence of acetaminophen at therapeutic doses on surrogate markers of severity of acute viral hepatitis. Gastroenterol Clin Biol 2006;30:763–8.

144. Kaufman BS, Roccaforte JD. Anesthesia and the liver. In: Barash PG, Cullen BF, Stoelting RK (eds) Clinical anesthesia, 5th edn. Lippincott Williams and Wilkins, Philadelphia, 2001: 1072–111.

Further reading

Chen DS. From hepatitis to hepatoma: lessons from type B viral hepatitis. Science 1993;262(5132):369–70.

Chisari FV, Ferrari C. Hepatitis B virus immunopathogenesis. Annu Rev Immunol 1995;13:29–60.

Chu CM. Natural history of chronic hepatitis B virus infection in adults with emphasis on the occurrence of cirrhosis and hepatocellular carcinoma. J Gastroenterol Hepatol 2000;15(suppl):E25–30.

Dinsmoor MJ. Hepatitis in the obstetric patient. Infect Dis Clin North Am 1997;11(1):77–91.

Donovan A, Lima CA, Pinkus JL, Pinkus GS, Zon LI, Robine S, et al. The iron exporter ferroportin/Slc40a1 is essential for iron homeostasis. Cell Metab 2005;1(3):191–200.

Doo E, Liang TJ. Molecular anatomy and pathophysiologic implications of drug resistance in hepatitis B virus infection. Gastroenterology 2001;120(4):1000–8.

Dryden KA, Wieland SF, Whitten-Bauer C, Gerin JL, Chisari FV, Yeager M. Native hepatitis B virions and capsids visualized by electron cryomicroscopy. Mol Cell 2006;22(6):843–50.

Guidotti LG, Morris A, Mendez H, Koch R, Silverman RH, Williams BR, et al. Interferon-regulated pathways that control hepatitis B virus replication in transgenic mice. J Virol 2002;76(6):2617–21.

Guidotti LG, Rochford R, Chung J, Shapiro M, Purcell R, Chisari FV. Viral clearance without destruction of infected cells during acute HBV infection. Science 1999;284(5415):825–9.

Lau GK, Yiu HH, Fong DY, Cheng HC, Au WY, Lai LS, et al. Early is superior to deferred preemptive lamivudine therapy for hepatitis B patients undergoing chemotherapy. Gastroenterology 2003;125(6):1742–9.

Le Mire MF, Miller DS, Foster WK, Burrell CJ, Jilbert AR. Covalently closed circular DNA is the predominant form of duck hepatitis B virus DNA that persists following transient infection. J Virol 2005;79(19):12242–52.

Lok AS. Chronic hepatitis B. N Engl J Med 2002;346(22):1682–3.

Lowe RC, Grace ND. Primary prophylaxis of variceal hemorrhage. Clin Liver Dis 2001;5(3):665–76.

Maini MK, Boni C, Lee CK, Larrubia JR, Reignat S, Ogg GS, et al. The role of virus-specific CD8(+) cells in liver damage and viral control during persistent hepatitis B virus infection. J Exp Med 2000;191(8):1269–80.

Nelson-Piercy C, Fayers P, de Swiet M. Randomised, double-blind, placebo-controlled trial of corticosteroids for the treatment of hyperemesis gravidarum. Br J Obstet Gynaecol 2001;108:9–15.

Nemeth E. Iron regulation and erythropoiesis. Curr Opin Hematol 2008;15(3):169–75.

Nemeth E, Tuttle MS, Powelson J, Vaughn MB, Donovan A, Ward DM, et al. Hepcidin regulates cellular iron efflux by binding to ferroportin and inducing its internalization. Science 2004;306(5704):2090–3.

Park CH, Valore EV, Waring AJ, Ganz T. Hepcidin, a urinary antimicrobial peptide synthesized in the liver. J Biol Chem 2001;276(11):7806–10.

Rehermann B, Ferrari C, Pasquinelli C, Chisari FV. The hepatitis B virus persists for decades after patients' recovery from acute viral hepatitis despite active maintenance of a cytotoxic T-lymphocyte response. Nat Med 1996;2(10):1104–8.

Saab S, Nieto JM, Lewis SK, Runyon BA. TIPS versus paracentesis for cirrhotic patients with refractory ascites. Cochrane Database of Systematic Reviews, 2006;4:CD004889.

Safari HR, Fassett MJ, Souter IC, Alsulyman OM, Goodwin TM. The efficacy of methylprednisolone in the treatment of hyperemesis gravidarum: a randomized, double-blind, controlled study. Am J Obstet Gynecol 1998;179:921–4.

Selitsky T, Chandra P, Schiavello HJ. Wernicke's encephalopathy with hyperemesis and ketoacidosis. Obstet Gynecol 2006;107:486–90.

Somberg KA, Riegler JL, LaBerge JM, Doherty-Simor MM, Bachetti P, Roberts JP, et al. Hepatic encephalopathy after transjugular intrahepatic portosystemic shunts: incidence and risk factors. Am J Gastroenterol 1995;90(4):549–55.

Sullivan CA, Johnson CA, Roach H, Martin RW, Stewart DK, Morrison JC. A pilot study of intravenous ondansetron for hyperemesis gravidarum. Am J Obstet Gynecol 1996;174:1565–8.

Thabut D, Bernard-Chabert B. Management of acute bleeding from portal hypertension. Best Pract Res Clin Gastroenterol 2007;21(1):19–29.

Triantos CK, Burroughs AK. Prevention of the development of varices and first portal hypertensive bleeding episode. Best Pract Res Clin Gastroenterol 2007;21(1):31–42.

Trogstad LIS, Stoltenberg C, Magnus P, Skaerven R, Irgens LM. Recurrence risk in hyperemesis gravidarum. Br J Obstet Gynaecol 2005;112:1641–5.

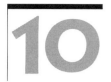

Disorders of the gastrointestinal tract in pregnancy

Niharika Mehta[1], *Sumona Saha*[1], *Edward K.S. Chien*[2], *Silvia Degli Esposti*[1] *with Scott Segal*[3]

[1]Department of Medicine, Warren Alpert Medical School of Brown University, Women & Infants' Hospital of Rhode Island, Providence, RI, USA
[2]Department of Obstetrics and Gynecology, Warren Alpert Medical School of Brown University, Women & Infants' Hospital of Rhode Island, Providence, RI, USA
[3]Department of Anesthesia, Harvard Medical School, Brigham and Women's Hospital, Boston, MA, USA

Physiologic changes in the gastrointestinal system in pregnancy

Gastrointestinal physiology is poorly studied during pregnancy even though gastrointestinal symptoms are the cause of a significant number of patient questions and concerns. Nonspecific symptoms of vomiting, epigastric pain, abdominal cramps, and diarrhea can occur frequently in pregnancy. Motor dysfunction of the gastrointestinal system and increasing uterine size are believed to be contributing factors. These gestational problems are self-limiting and most do not affect maternal or fetal outcome. Their importance in obstetric practice is to differentiate them from the diseases with similar presentation requiring diagnosis and management.

Oral cavity

The oral cavity undergoes a variety of changes during pregnancy. Many of these changes have been attributed to changes in the hormonal milieu. Changes in both salivary gland secretion and connective tissue changes have been described [1]. Pregnancy alters salivary composition, specifically decreasing pH and sodium content while increasing protein content. These changes are thought to be secondary to an increase in circulating estrogens [2]. Estimates of salivary secretion suggest that there is no overall increase in salivary volume.

Connective tissue changes occurring throughout the body during pregnancy can also be seen upon examination of the oral cavity. The most prominent connective tissue findings are gingival hyperplasia that may occur in 30–75% of pregnant women [1]. This presents as increased erythema and edema of the gingival tissue that some refer to as "pregnancy gingivitis." The most prominent sites of occurrence include the marginal and interdental papillae [1]. Pregnancy gingivitis may be more evident due to an exaggerated inflammatory response that occurs in the presence of periodontal disease. Changes in both progesterone and estrogen have been shown to alter the bacterial microflora, increasing the percentage of *Prevotella intermedia* [3]. In addition, changes in microflora are associated with altered secretion of lysosomal enzymes that may enhance tissue destruction and gingival bleeding [4]. Many of these changes regress after completion of pregnancy. Therapeutic interventions for these findings are not generally recommended during pregnancy.

Gastrointestinal motility

Our current understanding of gastrointestinal motility in pregnancy is limited. Esophageal function has been studied mainly in relationship to gastroesophageal reflux which is reported at some point in up to 80% of pregnant women [5]. Lower esophageal sphincter (LES) tone gradually declines during pregnancy and reaches a nadir at 36 weeks, declining by as much as 50% [6]. While progesterone is mainly felt to be responsible for the decrease in LES tone [6], estrogen has not been excluded from the etiology, possibly exerting a priming effect [5]. The increased intra-abdominal pressure produced by the expanding uterus also adds to the decrease in esophageal sphincter tone. Esophageal motility is not altered during pregnancy [7]. The combined effects of these changes increase the likelihood of gastroesophageal reflux.

The effects of pregnancy on gastric emptying are conflicting. Available studies suggest that gastric emptying may be more affected during labor than at other times in gestation. Gastric motility is mediated by a variety of inputs that enhance and delay emptying. The composition of oral intake is responsible for a variety of paracrine signals that modulate gastric motility. Foods high in fat content are known to delay gastric emptying. Studies evaluating clearance of water at various periods during the first through third trimester suggest that gastric emptying is delayed [8]. In contrast, other studies evaluating

de Swiet's Medical Disorders in Obstetric Practice, 5th edition. Edited by R. O. Powrie, M. F. Greene, W. Camann. © 2010 Blackwell Publishing.

a liquid saline meal suggest that more rapid emptying occurs during pregnancy than in nonpregnant individuals [9]. These differences reinforce the role of paracrine signaling in gastric motility. Other studies evaluating the time from ingestion to small bowel entry suggest that gastric motility is delayed mainly in individuals with symptoms of gastroesophageal reflux [8]. Patients who were asymptomatic had gastric emptying times comparable with those of nonpregnant individuals.

Few studies are available evaluating small and large intestinal motility in normal pregnancy, despite the role it might have on the frequently reported symptoms of irritable bowel and constipation in pregnancy. A variety of techniques have been used to evaluate small intestinal transit times with significantly different results. Parry [10], using radiographic examination to evaluate the transit of a rubber balloon filled with mercury, demonstrated small intestine mean transit times of 58 and 52 hours in a group of pregnant and nonpregnant women respectively. Wald [11], in contrast, determined small intestinal transit times to be in the range of 2 hours during the third trimester of pregnancy and only 90 minutes during the postpartum period by measuring exhaled hydrogen after ingestion of the nonabsorbable carbohydrate lactulose. Lawson [12] showed a similar delay in small intestinal transit during pregnancy compared to post partum. In addition, Lawson noted slower rates during the second and third trimesters compared to the first trimester in the handful of patients examined.

In summary, clinical observation and most available studies indicate that gastrointestinal motility during pregnancy is diminished. Studies evaluating the effects of progesterone on smooth muscle activity clearly demonstrate a decrease in contractility and tone, suggesting that the decreased motility most likely has a hormonal basis.

Nausea and emesis

Nausea and vomiting during the first trimester of pregnancy is so frequent that it is caricatured across most cultures as the initial sign of pregnancy. Nausea is reported in up to 80% of women during their first trimester and can persist in a subset of individuals throughout pregnancy. A variety of theories have been proposed to explain these common symptoms. Goodwin [13] has suggested that the symptoms are either a direct chemical stimulus from placental products or are due to resetting of the stimulus threshold in the vestibular or gastrointestinal systems. The evidence to support these theories is presented.

Both human chorionic gonadotropin (HCG) and estrogens have been implicated as the chemical mediators of nausea and emesis during pregnancy. There is temporal association of HCG level with severity of symptoms during normal pregnancy. Also, complicated pregnancies, associated with higher HCG levels, are frequently affected with greater symptomatology. Nausea is common in patients taking oral contraceptive pills with

a similar dose–response relationship. The temporal relationship of estrogens and nausea and vomiting in pregnancy supports this theory.

A change in vestibular or gastrointestinal sensitivity has been another explanation for increased nausea and vomiting in pregnancy. Studies have demonstrated that individuals prone to motion sickness are likely to be more symptomatic with pregnancy [14]. Changes in serum osmolarity have been shown to induce vestibular-mediated nausea and vomiting [15].

Changes in gastric rhythmic activity have more recently been implicated in the causation of nausea in pregnancy. Normal gastric myoelectric activity results in slow wave propagation from the proximal body to the distal antrum at a rate of 3 cycles per minute (cpm). Rhythm disturbance, either increased or decreased slow wave propagation, is associated with nausea. Koch and colleagues demonstrated that women with normal slow wave activity (3 cpm) were less likely to complain of nausea during pregnancy [16]. In contrast, individuals with high or slower rates were more likely to complain of nausea. Jednak [17] demonstrated that protein-dominant meals were associated with decreased symptoms and corrected slow wave dysrhythmias. Carbohydrate- or fat-dominant meals had no effect on symptoms or slow wave dysrhythmias. These studies suggest that meal composition may also affect symptomatology.

Disorders of the oral cavity

Clinical studies have shown that oral tissues are affected by pregnancy and several oral lesions may have an impact on pregnancy outcomes. A few commonly seen oral lesions are discussed below.

Aphthous ulcers

Aphthous ulcers (also known as canker sores) are painful open sores inside the mouth or upper throat caused by a break in the mucous membranes. There is no evidence for an association between aphthous stomatitis and pregnancy; the importance for the obstetric provider is to recognize underlying systemic illnesses that may be associated with recurrent aphthae. Celiac sprue, gluten-sensitive enteropathies, inflammatory bowel disease, vitamin and mineral deficiencies, particularly B vitamins (1, 2, 6 and 12) iron, folic acid and zinc, HIV infection, Behçet's syndrome, neutropenia of any cause may be associated with oral ulcers. Sodium lauryl sulfate, a toothpaste detergent, has also been linked to recurrent aphthous stomatitis (RAS). Herpetiform ulcers have similar appearance and presentation.

Management is generally palliative, with use of topical analgesics; topical or oral corticosteroids may be indicated for severe recalcitrant disease. Identification and treatment of underlying disorders are important, especially with nutritional deficiency as replacement of a deficient vitamin or mineral should result in prompt resolution. Treatment with thalidomide has shown benefit in RAS associated with HIV infection; however, its only FDA-approved uses are for multiple myeloma and erythema nodosum leprosum and its use in pregnancy is clearly contraindicated.

Periodontal disease

Gingivitis in pregnancy has been reported at prevalence rates of 40–100% [18]. The cause of pregnancy-induced gingivitis is likely multifactorial and includes pregnancy-related physiologic vascular and inflammatory changes. Clinically, the gingival tissue appears smooth, swollen, and dark red and bleeds easily. Hyperplasia of interdental papillae may be noted.

Periodontitis is characterized by gingival inflammation with accompanying loss of supportive connective tissues, including alveolar bone. Recent studies have suggested that periodontal inflammation is associated with an increased risk of preterm birth, as well as low birthweight and pre-eclampsia [19–21]. However, in a study involving 823 pregnant women, treatment of periodontitis was not shown to significantly alter rates of preterm birth, low birthweight or fetal growth restriction [22].

Optimal oral hygiene and removal of dental plaque can reduce gingival swelling, erythema and bleeding. Regular exams and cleaning should be continued through pregnancy.

Pyogenic granuloma

Pyogenic granuloma, previously known as epulis gravidarum, is a benign growth on the oral mucosa and can occur in up to 5% of pregnancies. It usually occurs buccally on the upper anterior teeth and is painless. It can be colored from red to pink and may be smooth in surface or lobulated. The lesion can grow rapidly, but is rarely greater than 2 cm in diameter. It resolves spontaneously after delivery. Surgical resection, if needed, should only be done after delivery as recurrence is extremely common when the granuloma is removed during pregnancy.

Gastroesphageal disorders

Gastroesphageal reflux

Background and epidemiology

Gastroesphageal reflux disease (GERD) is common in pregnancy. It is estimated that 30–50% of pregnant women experience heartburn and that in some populations the incidence may be as high as 80% [23]. Reported risk factors for GERD in pregnancy include increasing gestational age, parity, and a history of heartburn [24]. While most pregnant women with GERD experience symptoms for the first time in pregnancy, some may suffer from an exacerbation of pre-existing disease [25]. Most patients have a benign disease course, with only a few experiencing GERD-related complications such as gastrointestinal bleeding or stricture formation. In general, symptoms begin at the end of the first trimester, worsen through the remainder of pregnancy, and then resolve promptly after delivery.

Pathophysiology

The pathogenesis of GERD in pregnancy is likely multifactorial. Decreased sensitivity of the basal LES to hormonal, pharmacologic, and physiologic stimuli may cause gestational GERD [26]. Other proposed mechanisms include decreased esophageal peristalsis, esophageal dysmotility and delayed gastric emptying due to hormonal and mechanical changes [27].

The role of increased intra-abdominal pressures due to the expanding gravid uterus in the development of GERD is controversial. Loss of the intra-abdominal segment of the LES with loss of the normal pressure gradient between the intrathoracic and intra-abdominal segments has been shown in pregnancy and proposed as a possible factor contributing to gestational GERD [27]. However, in one study, nearly 40% of pregnant women without heartburn were also found to have loss of the intra-abdominal LES [28]. In addition, it remains unknown whether the LES can compensate in pregnancy as it does in other states of increased abdominal pressure, such as cirrhosis, wherein LES pressures rise proportionally to increasing intra-abdominal pressure [5,25,29].

Clinical presentation

The presenting symptoms of GERD in pregnancy are similar to those of the general population. Patients complain most frequently of pyrosis (heartburn) and regurgitation. Other reported symptoms include indigestion, epigastric pain, waterbrash (sour taste in the mouth), anorexia and nausea and vomiting [25]. Although symptoms may be intense, complications such as esophagitis, gastrointestinal bleeding, and stricture formation are rare due to the short duration of acid exposure [25,27].

Diagnosis and evaluation

Diagnosis of GERD is based upon symptoms. Radiographic evaluation by upper GI series is avoided in most circumstances due to the risks of radiation exposure to the fetus. Upper endoscopy is generally not necessary but can be considered in refractory cases, severe dysphagia and gastrointestinal bleeding. Odynophagia (painful swallowing) refractory to acid-reducing medications should be evaluated by upper endoscopy because infectious esophagitis (e.g. *Candida* esophagitis) may occur in pregnancy even in immunocompetent hosts [30] and can masquerade as GERD.

Treatment

Treatment of GERD in pregnancy should follow a "step-up" approach. Patients with mild symptoms are often adequately treated with therapeutic lifestyle modifications. These include strict abstinence from tobacco and alcohol. Patients should also avoid late-night meals, recumbency after eating, and trigger foods (e.g. spicy or sour foods, carbonated beverages, coffee). Eating several small meals throughout the day and elevating the head of the bed by 6 inches with blocks (and not simply propping up the upper body with pillows which may actually exacerbate symptoms) may provide additional benefit [5].

For patients who fail conservative measures, antacids are first-line pharmacologic therapy. It is estimated that 30–50% of women take antacids for the control of heartburn symptoms during pregnancy [5]. Aluminum, magnesium, and calcium-based antacids ($Al(OH)_3$, $Mg(OH)_2$, and $CaCO_3$) are all considered safe for the treatment of GERD in pregnancy. However, aluminum-containing antacids can cause constipation, and magnesium-containing antacids can cause diarrhea [31]. Patients on supplemental iron should be advised to not take iron and antacids together in order to maximize iron absorption by an acidic gastric pH. Sodium bicarbonate should not be taken due to the risk of metabolic alkalosis and fluid overload in the mother and fetus [25].

Other first-line agents include the nonabsorbable alginates and sucralfate. Alginic acid (a combination of this with antacids is marketed in the US as Gaviscon®) is considered effective and fast-acting in most pregnant patients [32]. The mucosal protectant sucralfate is also safe in pregnancy and is classified as a category B drug by theUS Food and Drug Administration (FDA) Pregnancy Safety Classification (see Chapter 30 for a summary of this classification system). Sucralfate has been shown in a randomized controlled trial in pregnancy to provide greater relief from heartburn and regurgitation than lifestyle and dietary modifications alone [33].

Metoclopramide, FDA pregnancy category class B, may be useful in the treatment of GERD by increasing LES pressure but its main use in pregnancy is in the treatment of nausea and vomiting. Use of metoclopramide is often limited by its poor tolerability and the risk for irreversible extrapyramidal side effects (tardive dyskinesia: irregular involuntary movements of the face), restlessness, dystonias of neck, eyes or tongue and Parkinson-like rigidity, tremor and paucity of spontaneous movement) [5]. Other common side effects include restlessness, drowsiness and fatigue.

H2 receptor antagonists (H2-RA) form the next tier of therapy. The four H2-RA (ranitidine, cimetidine, famotidine and nizatidine) are FDA category B and considered safe in pregnancy. Surveillance studies of infants exposed to ranitidine and cimetidine during early pregnancy have shown an average congenital malformation rate of 4.4%, a rate nearly identical to that among nonexposed infants [34]. In addition, no increased risks for spontaneous abortions, preterm labor or low birthweight have been reported after first-trimester exposure to H2-RA [35].

Despite the longstanding availability of H2-RA, only ranitidine given twice daily has been shown in a randomized, double-blind trial to be efficacious in pregnancy, making it the preferred H2-RA for gestational GERD [36]. Cimetidine is likely equally effective; however, due to the antiandrogenic effects seen in animals and nonpregnant humans, some authors advise against its use in pregnancy [5]. Nizatidine recently changed classification from FDA category C to category B and is considered safe in pregnancy. However, concerns remain over adverse outcomes in pregnant animals exposed to the drug, making it a less preferred option for many experts [25].

Proton pump inhibitors (PPI) are typically reserved for patients with severe symptoms refractory to lifestyle modification and the older generation medications. Concern over the long-term safety of PPI has limited their use. However, there is now a large amount of data supporting their safety in pregnancy. A meta-analysis found no significant increase in risk for major malformations in women taking PPI during the first trimester [37]. Other studies have found no increased risk of low birthweight or number of preterm deliveries [38]. Four of the five PPI (lansoprazole, rabeprazole, pantoprazole and esomprezole) are FDA category B with only omeprazole carrying a class C rating due to fetal toxicity in animal studies.

Anesthesia considerations during labor and delivery

Anesthetics lower LES pressure and delay gastric emptying. The risk of aspiration of gastric contents during regional and general anesthesia may be particularly high in pregnancy. Pulmonary aspiration during labor or Mendelson's syndrome is a leading cause of obstetric morbidity and mortality due to anesthesia [25]. Due to the serious complications of aspiration, much attention has been given to methods to decrease gastric volume and acidity prior to the administration of anesthesia to prevent lung injury.

Mitigating the effects of aspiration by raising the gastric pH to greater than 2.5 is recommended during labor and delivery [25]. Among the antacids, soluble antacids such as sodium citrate and sodium bicarbonate are preferred over insoluble antacids such as aluminum and magnesium hydroxide, carbonates and trisilicates because they are less likely to cause lung injury if aspirated. Ranitidine and the other H2-RA are also effective in reducing gastric acidity [39]. Prokinetic drugs like metoclopramide may be helpful in decreasing gastric volume by promoting gastric emptying [40]. More recently, omeprazole given orally the evening before surgery has been shown to be safe in obstetric anesthesia and effective in raising gastric pH [41].

Postpartum and lactation considerations

Gastroesophageal reflux disease symptoms typically resolve shortly after delivery but some women may have persistent symptoms. Most medications begun during pregnancy for the treatment of GERD can be continued safely post partum even during lactation. Antacids, sucralfate, and all of the H2-RA except nizatidine are safe for use by breastfeeding women [6]. There are limited safety data concerning PPI use in breastfeeding.

Hyperemesis gravidarum

Hyperemesis gravidarum is discussed in detail in Chapter 48.

Peptic ulcer disease

Background and epidemiology

Estimates from case studies and retrospective series suggest that the incidence of peptic ulcer disease (PUD) is decreased in pregnancy [42]. Older studies from 1939 and 1966 have reported rates of active ulceration as low as 1 in 70,310 hospitalizations of pregnant women and 6 in 23,000 deliveries, respectively [43,44]. However, these studies are limited by their retrospective nature and the fact that they predated flexible endoscopic evaluation. It is likely that PUD is not as uncommon in pregnancy as the literature suggests, but that it is under-recognized. Under-reporting of symptoms by patients and reluctance to perform diagnostic tests by physicians may contribute to this.

Risk factors for PUD in pregnancy are the same as for the general population. They include smoking, nonsteroidal anti-inflammatory drug (NSAID) use, alcoholism, genetic predisposition, gastritis and *H. pylori* infection [42]. Advanced maternal age is a pregnancy-specific risk factor for PUD.

Pathophysiology

Peptic ulcer disease results from the imbalance of complex interactions between defensive and aggressive factors, the most important of which is likely *H. pylori* [45]. *H. pylori*, a motile, urease-producing, gram-negative bacterium, produces inflammation that may lead to ulceration and carcinoma in affected individuals. Host immune factors, genetic predisposition and bacterial virulence likely account for the varied clinical responses to *H. pylori* infection.

Clinical presentation

Patients with PUD in pregnancy typically present with epigastric pain, anorexia, postprandial nausea and vomiting, abdominal distension and eructation [42]. While these symptoms are similar to those of the general population, PUD symptoms have been reported to be milder in pregnancy [46]. Factors which

may account for this include a healthier diet during pregnancy, avoidance of alcohol and cigarette smoking, and increased medical supervision [47].

Patients with PUD and gastrointestinal bleeding present with coffee-grounds emesis, hematemesis or melena. Hematochezia may also be present in the setting of brisk upper gastrointestinal tract bleeding. Patients with perforated PUD may be hypotensive and present with a rigid abdomen from peritonitis.

The differential diagnosis of PUD in pregnancy includes non-ulcer dyspepsia, GERD, nausea and vomiting of pregnancy, hyperemesis gravidarum, pancreatitis, acute cholecystitis, viral hepatitis, appendicitis, and acute fatty liver of pregnancy [42].

Diagnosis

Diagnosis of peptic ulcer disease relies on a high index of suspicion. The physical exam may be normal or may reveal only minimal tenderness despite severe ulceration. Fluoroscopic evaluation of the upper gastrointestinal tract with barium is to be avoided if possible during pregnancy. Abdominal radiographs and computed tomography of the abdomen are also generally avoided; however, they should be performed if there is suspicion for perforation.

Esophagogastroduodenoscopy (EGD) can be performed safely in pregnancy when necessary and is the diagnostic modality of choice. Considerations regarding maternal and fetal monitoring, medication used and hemostasis are necessary prior to performing the procedure (see "Endoscopy in pregnancy and lactation" below).

Management

General treatment guidelines are unaffected by pregnancy. Treatment begins with lifestyle and dietary modification. Conservative measures such as abstinence from smoking and alcohol, avoiding trigger foods and diminishing psychologic stress are recommended. Patients not responding to these measures are advised to take antacids and/or sucralfate. In nonpregnant populations, high-dose antacid therapy has been shown to heal 75% of duodenal ulcers [48].

In patients not responding to antacids, empiric therapy with H2-RA may be tried. Patients who remain symptomatic on H2-RA may be switched to PPI therapy. They should also be strongly considered for diagnostic EGD to rule out complications from PUD such as stricture and gastrointestinal bleeding.

Patients who are found to have active *H. pylori* infection during pregnancy as part of their evaluation for PUD or hyperemesis gravidarum (see section on pathophysiology of hyperemesis gravidarum) can be treated [49]. The most common treatment regimen for nonpregnant patients is a 10–14-day course of twice-daily PPI, amoxicillin, and clarithromycin. For nonpregnant patients who are allergic to penicillin or have resistant infection, "quadruple" therapy with metronidazole, bismuth, tetracycline and high-dose acid suppression by PPI or H2-RA therapy can be used. For pregnant patients who are penicillin tolerant, the usual regimen may be given in pregnancy (amoxicillin is category B and clarithromycin is category C) although concern about the safety of clarithromycin in pregnant animals has led some experts to delay its use until after the first trimester or even until after the pregnancy [50]. However, treatment of penicillin-allergic patients during pregnancy is limted by the teratogenicity of tetracycline (category D) and the possible association of bismuth (category C) with fetal ductus arteriosus closure. Metronidazole (category B) is generally considered safe for use in the second and third trimesters of pregnancy but is less effective in the eradication of *H. pylori* when not used as part of quadruple therapy. Fortunately, most peptic ulcers will readily heal with PPI or H2-RA therapy and *H. pylori* treatment, which will help prevent recurrence, can usually be safely delayed until after delivery.

Disorders of the intestinal tract

Diarrheal illness

Acute diarrhea

Most cases of acute diarrhea are due to infections with viruses and bacteria and are self-limited. Noninfectious etiologies are more likely in patients with chronic symptoms. Table 10.1 represents some common etiologies of acute diarrhea, with a brief outline of clinical features and management of each.

In general, a diagnostic evaluation is only indicated in patients presenting with relatively severe symptoms such as profuse watery diarrhea, hypovolemia, bloody diarrhea, fever, severe abdominal pain, recent use of antibiotics or in an immunocompromised patient. Diagnostic evaluation should likely also occur if diarrhea persists for more than a week and is associated with weight loss. Such an evaluation should include fecal leukocytes and a stool culture and testing for stool ova and parasites, especially in patients with history of exposure to infants, in international travelers or in patients with AIDS. Endoscopy is not indicated very often in acute diarrhea, but should be considered in patients with bloody diarrhea to differentiate infectious causes from inflammatory bowel disease or colonic ischemia.

Recommendations from the Infectious Diseases Society of America with regard to investigation of acute diarrheal illnesses are presented in Table 10.2.

The initial management of patients with acute diarrhea must include hydration and alteration of diet. Antibiotic

therapy is not required in most cases since the illness is usually self-limited. Loperamide may be used for the symptomatic treatment of acute diarrhea, but only when fever is absent or low grade and the stools are not bloody.

Chronic diarrhea

Diarrhea lasting for 3 weeks or more can result from several etiologies including irritable bowel syndrome, lactose intolerance, inflammatory bowel disease, microscopic colitis, malabsorption and chronic infections. Box 10.1 lists some differential diagnoses for chronic diarrhea. Box 10.2 summarizes the investigation of chronic diarrhea. A thorough medical history and physical exam are important and may help to narrow the differential. The minimum laboratory tests indicated in most patients include a complete blood count, electrolytes, thyroid function tests, total protein and albumin and stool occult blood. Most patients will need referral to gastroenterology for endoscopic evaluation, especially if blood is found in the stool.

Celiac disease

Background and epidemiology

Celiac disease is an immune-mediated disease of the small intestine with associated systemic manifestations and complications. It is characterized by intestinal inflammation and loss of absorptive capacities with resulting nutrient, mineral and vitamin deficiency. It is not known whether pregnancy exacerbates the disease; however, due to increased nutritional demands in pregnancy, compromised absorption of nutrients may become evident and unmask underlying disease.

Celiac disease had been considered to be a rare disease, especially in the United States. Due to the recognition of silent and atypical disease, it is now estimated that as many as 1– 3% of the general population in Europe and the United States are affected with celiac disease [51]. Celiac disease has been diagnosed in individuals of all ages and ancestry. Women are more likely to be affected than men with a female-to-male ratio of 2.9:1 [52].

Family history of celiac disease is a strong risk factor for the development of the disease as 10–20% of first-degree relatives of individuals with celiac disease are also affected [53]. Other risk factors include human leukocyte antigen (HLA) class II antigens DQ2 and DQ8 which are expressed in over 95% of patients, early and massive gluten exposure and other autoimmune diseases [54]. Type I diabetes mellitus (DM), in particular, is strongly associated with celiac disease with an estimated 1–10% of type I diabetic patients having celiac disease [55]. Individuals with Down's syndrome, Turner's syndrome, Williams' syndrome, and selective IgA deficiency are also at increased risk [56].

Table 10.1 Common diarrheal agents

Etiologic agent	Comments	Clinical features	Management
Salmonella (*S. enteritidis*, *S. typhimurium*)	Infection associated with ingestion of poultry, eggs and milk. Possible transmission from pet reptiles	Onset of nausea, vomiting, fever, diarrhea, and cramping, usually occurs within 6–72 hours of ingesting contaminated food or water	Nontyphoidal salmonella gastroenteritis is usually self-limited. Fever generally resolves within 48–72 hours, and diarrhea within 4–10 days. Antibiotics (trimethoprim/sulfamethoxazole, amoxicillin, ceftriaxone) are recommended only for severely ill or immunocompromised patients
Campylobactor spp. (*C. jejuni*, *C. coli*)	Infection generally obtained from raw or undercooked poultry. *C. jejuni* infection in pregnancy has been linked to intrauterine fetal infection, stillbirth, and neonatal death. Infection of a newborn during the birth process may lead to neonatal enteritis, bacteremia, and/or meningitis. Late-onset complications of the infection include Guillain–Barré syndrome and reactive arthritis	Average incubation 3 days. Crampy abdominal pain and diarrhea are common, with low- to high-grade fever	Diagnosis established by stool culture. Although diarrhea is self-limiting (about 7 days), treatment with erythromycin or azithromycin in pregnant, severely ill or immunocompromised patients is recommended
Shigella (*S. dysenteriae* 1, *S. flexneri*, *S. sonnei*, and *S. boydii*)	Classic cause of dysentery. As few as 10 organisms can cause clinical disease. Transmission can occur through direct person-to-person spread as well as from contaminated food and water	Typically presents with high fever, abdominal cramps, and bloody, mucoid diarrhea, after 3-day incubation. Although number of stools per day can be huge, stools are of small volume and significant fluid loss is uncommon. Several complications exist, but are relatively rare, including toxic megacolon, intestinal perforation and possible seizures	Illness is usually self-limited, but empiric antibiotic therapy with TMP/SMX or azithromycin while awaiting stool isolates is recommended in severely ill, immunocompromised or malnourished patients. Antibiotic therapy may decrease duration of shedding there by decreasing person-to-person spread
Enterotoxigenic *E. coli* (ETEC)	Most common cause of traveler's diarrhea and food poisoning	Short incubation period. Onset of nausea, diarrhea and rarely vomiting is rapid	Duration of illness is usually less than 48–72 hours. Treatment should primarily focus on rehydration. Loperamide is generally not recommended
Enterohemorrhagic *E. coli* (EHEC)	These organisms differ from other pathogenic *E. coli* by the production of one or more Shiga toxins. The main serotype in the United States is O157: H7 which can cause HUS, particularly in children. Transmission is food borne (undercooked ground beef) or person to person	Onset of bloody diarrhea 3–4 days after exposure	*E. coli* isolates can be screened for the O157:H7 strain by the inability to ferment sorbitol. Treatment is largely supportive. Most authorities recommend against using antibiotics which may increase toxin production and risk of developing HUS
Clostridium difficile	Causative organism of antibiotic-associated colitis. The probability of diarrhea and colitis is greatest with clindamycin but ampicillin is also a frequent cause	The typical presentation is acute watery diarrhea with lower abdominal pain, low-grade fever, and leukocytosis, starting during or shortly after antibiotic administration, typically 5–10 days	The diagnosis is established by bio-assay of stool for *C. difficile* cytotoxins. Sigmoidoscopy or colonoscopy, though not generally necessary, may show evidence of pseudomembranes which is pathognomonic for *C. difficile* infection. Symptomatic patients are treated with oral metronidazole or oral vancomycin
Staphylococcus (*S. aureus*)	Food-borne illness from ingestion of preformed toxin	Nausea, vomiting and abdominal cramps begin with 1–6 hours of ingestion. Fever/diarrhea occur only in a minority of patients	The illness usually lasts for 48–72 hours with a rapid and full recovery
Bacillus (*B. cereus*)	Food-borne illness from ingestion of preformed toxin	Rapid (within 1–6 hours) onset of nausea and profuse vomiting	The disease is usually self-limited, although very rarely associated with acute hepatic necrosis

Table 10.1 (Continued)

Etiologic agent	Comments	Clinical features	Management
Norwalk-like virus	Over one-third of outbreaks of nonbacterial gastroenteritis in the United States have been associated with noroviruses	Acute explosive vomiting and diarrhea	Usually lasts 24–48 hours
Cryptosporidium	One of the most common gastrointestinal parasites in the United States. Transmission occurs via spread from an infected person or animal, or from fecally contaminated food or water source	Can cause asymptomatic infection, mild diarrheal illness or severe enteritis. Patients frequently have associated malaise, nausea and anorexia and crampy abdominal pain	The illness usually resolves without therapy in 10–14 days in immunologically healthy people but is frequently protracted and severe, and can lead to significant wasting in immunocompromised patients. There is no specific treatment. Therapy is supportive. Untreated HIV-infected patients should be initiated on antiretroviral therapy
Giardia	One of the most common gastrointestinal parasites in the United States, responsible for water-borne and food-borne diarrhea, day-care center outbreaks, and diarrhea in international travelers	Up to 60% exposed may remain asymptomatic. Others present with sudden-onset diarrhea, steatorrhea, malaise, abdominal cramps and bloating	Diagnosis is established by stool microscopy and/or immunoassay. Metronidazole and paromomycin are treatments of choice in pregnant women
Entamoeba histolytica	Endemic in the tropics and subtropics, but also occurs in the UK, Europe and North America, especially among immigrants	Subacute onset, usually over 1–3 weeks. Symptoms range from mild diarrhea to severe dysentery. Fever and weight loss can occur. Rare complications include fulminant colitis, bowel perforation, and extraintestinal infection such as liver, lung or brain abscess	Demonstration of cysts or trophozoites in the stool suggests an intestinal amebic infection. Metronidazole is used to treat both intestinal and hepatic amebiasis
Vibrio cholerae	Gram-negative bacteria endemic in developing countries of Africa and Asia. It is also seen with less frequency each year in most other countries. Serotypes 01 and 0139 are the cause of cholera epidemics	Causes profuse watery diarrhea (often 500–1000 cc/h) that can be fatal if untreated. Diarrhea is often associated with vomiting and abdominal pain but fever is not typically part of cholera as the infection is noninvasive. Massive fluid and electrolyte losses can cause renal failure and life-threatening electrolyte disturbances. Diagnosis made by microscopic examination of stool and/or rectal or stool culture. PCR studies and monoclonal antibody-based testing are often done when investigating epidemics. Serologic testing can be used as a confirmatory test but should not delay treatment	Oral rehydration solutions formulated in accordance with present WHO recommendations are the mainstay of treatment. Intravenous fluid and electrolyte repletion will be necessary for more severe cases. Antibiotic treatment is not essential but will shorten length of illness and decrease volume of diarrhea. While fluoroquinolones and tetracyclines are commonly used to treated cholera outside pregnancy, azithromycin (one dose of 1000 mg) or erythromycin (250 mg PO four times a day for 3 days) preferred in pregnancy

Pathogenesis

Celiac disease is the result of an inflammatory cascade incited by dietary gluten proteins in genetically susceptible individuals [57]. Gluten proteins found in wheat, barley and rye cross intercellular tight junctions of enterocytes to reach the lamina propria. There they are degraded into peptides and modified by the enzymatic activity of tissue transglutaminase (tTG). Postmodification of the peptides allows binding to HLA-DQ molecules on antigen-presenting cells. The gluten–HLA-DQ complexes are presented to gluten-reactive CD4 + T-cells and recognized as foreign. This triggers an abnormal mucosal response and induces tissue damage.

Clinical presentation

The clinical presentation of celiac disease varies greatly. In the classic presentation patients are severely symptomatic. Gastrointestinal symptoms such as dyspepsia, upper abdominal pain, chronic diarrhea, steatorrhea and failure to thrive predominate. However, diarrhea and weight loss are uncommon with less than 50% of patients reporting diarrhea at the time of diagnosis and approximately 30% of patients presenting overweight [58]. Atypical presentations in which extraintestinal symptoms predominate are becoming increasingly recognized [59]. These include osteoporosis, iron deficiency anemia, and neurologic disorders [57]. Obstetric and

Table 10.2 Investigations for acute infectious diarrhea in pregnancy

Syndrome	Comments	Testing
Community-acquired or traveler's diarrhea	Often self-resolving without treatment in a few days Investigate especially if fever or blood in stool Fecal leukocytes or lactoferrin may help suggest inflammatory/invasive cause Traveller's diarrhea may be treated empirically with azithromycin 1 g PO×1 dose and investigate only if symptoms persist. Alternative treatment with fluoroquinolones not recommended in pregnancy	Culture or test for: • Salmonella • Shigella • Campylobacter • *E. coli* (STEC) 0157:H7 • *C. difficile* toxin A +/− B • *Vibrio* if seafood or seacoast exposure
Nosocomial diarrhea (onset after 3 days in hospital)	Only consider nosocomial rather than community acquired if onset after 3 days in hospital	Test for: • *C. difficile* toxins A+/− B
Persisitent diarrhea >7 days	Investigate especially if immunocompromised host Fecal leukocytes or lactoferrin may help suggest inflammatory/invasive cause	Test for parasites: • *Giardia* • *Cryptosporidium* • Cryptospora • *Isospora belil* If HIV positive, test for: • Microsporidia • *M. avium* complex • organisms listed for community-acquired diarrhea

Box 10.1 Differential diagnosis of chronic diarrhea

- Osmotic diarrhea (ssmotic laxatives, lactose intolerance, sorbitol or mannitol (in many "sugar-free" foods) ingestion)
- Secretory diarrhea (bacterial toxins, inflammatory bowel disease)
- Disordered motility (irritable bowel syndrome, diabetic neuropathy)
- Endocrine causes (hyperthyroidism, gastrinoma, Addison's disease)
- Fatty diarrhea (Whipple's disease, celiac disease, pancreatic exocrine insufficiency)
- Inflammatory diarrhea (inflammatory bowel disease (IBD), ischemic or radiation colitis, colon cancer, vasculitis)
- Infections (pseudomembranous colitis, tuberculosis, yersiniosis, HSV, CMV, amebiasis and strongyloidosis)
- Laxative abuse

Box 10.2 Suggested evaluation for chronic diarrhea

- History (to differentiate functional from organic cause): duration greater than 1 year, lack of significant weight loss, absence of nocturnal diarrhea and straining with defecation suggest functional cause
- CBC with differential, thyroid function tests, electrolytes, LFT
- Stool analysis: for occult blood, WBC, presence of fat, ova and parasites
- Temporary cessation of lactose-containing foods (when lactose intolerance is suspected). Pregnant women frequently increase their milk product intake and may be unable to accommodate the increased lactose load
- Quantitative stool measurement and analysis for pH, electrolytes and laxatives
- Colonoscopy/sigmoidoscopy and mucosal biopsy
- Radiologic studies: barium follow-through (to evaluate small intestine; this study is rarely warranted in pregnancy), mesenteric angiography (when mesenteric ischemia is suspected), CT scan of the abdomen

gynecologic presentations may also occur in the form of delayed menarche, early menopause, secondary amenorrhea, infertility, recurrent miscarriage, and low birthweight infants [60]. Box 10.3 provides a list of clinical presentations

Box 10.3 Persons who should be tested for celiac disease

- Individuals with gastrointestinal symptoms, including chronic diarrhea, malabsorption, weight loss, and abdominal distension
- Individuals without other explanations for persistent elevations of transaminases, short stature, delayed puberty, iron deficiency anemia, recurrent fetal loss and infertility
- Discuss benefits and risks of screening in asymptomatic, high-risk populations
  - Persons with type 1 diabetes mellitus
  - Persons with other autoimmune endocrinopathies
  - First- and second-degree relatives of persons with celiac disease
  - Persons with Turner's syndrome
  - Persons with Williams' syndrome (a rare congenital condition due to deletions in the genes for elastin and LIM kinase)

Adapted from James SP. National Institutes of Health Consensus Development Statement on Celiac Disease, June 28–30, 2004. Gastroenterology 2005;128(4)(suppl 1): S1–S9.

that should be investigated for celiac disease. Currently, iron deficiency anemia due to both iron malabsorption and occult gastrointestinal bleeding is the most common clinical presentation of celiac disease [61].

Nearly every organ system can be affected by celiac disease as a result of malabsorption of nutrients and both fat-soluble and water-soluble vitamins. Severe extraintestinal manifestations may be seen after years of poorly controlled disease. Some of these findings are short stature, failure to thrive, aphthous stomatitis, hair loss, fractures, dental enamel hypoplasia, chronic fatigue, muscular atrophy, peripheral neuropathy, ataxia and depression [62]. Dermatitis herpetiformis, a pruritic, symmetric papulovesicular rash that is seen on the elbows, knees, buttocks and scalps in patients with celiac disease, is seen exclusively in patients with celiac disease and is nearly pathognomonic for the disease [59].

Diagnosis

Accurate serologic tests are now available for screening for celiac disease. These include antigliadin (AGA) IgA and IgG, antiendomysial (EMA) IgA and antitissue transglutaminase (tTG) IgA. A recent review of the diagnostic accuracy of the serologic tests for celiac disease found EMA and tTG to be superior to AGA [63]. False-negative results of the serologic tests may be seen in patients with selective IgA deficiency and patients on a gluten-free diet at the time of testing. Anti-tTG IgA with total serum IgA are currently recommended in the US as screening tools for celiac disease.

Endoscopy with small bowel biopsy remains the gold standard for the diagnosis of celiac disease [56] and should be performed on all patients having positive serologic tests. It is recommended that multiple biopsies be obtained from the second portion of the duodenum or beyond, due to the histologic patchiness of the disease, in order to increase the diagnostic yield. Histologic confirmation by the presence of intraepithelial lymphocytosis and villous atrophy with associated crypt hyperplasia is necessary for the diagnosis [64]. As with the serologic testing, patients must be on a gluten-containing diet to prevent false-negative biopsies.

The differential diagnosis includes infectious gastroenteritis, bacterial overgrowth, lactose intolerance, anorexia nervosa, ischemic enteritis, tropical sprue, hypogammaglobulinemia, Whipple's disease, intestinal lymphoma and Zollinger–Ellison syndrome [65].

Management

Treatment of celiac disease is a strict gluten-free diet for life. Wheat, rye and barley, all of which contain gluten, must be excluded from the diet. Oats have been shown to be safe but their inclusion in the gluten-free diet remains controversial due to cross-contamination with gluten-containing starches during processing [66]. Due to the complexity of the gluten-free diet and the need for strict adherence, referral to an expert dietitian and to celiac disease advocacy groups is recommended.

Nutrient deficiencies are common in celiac disease. Newly diagnosed patients should be screened for deficiencies of the fat-soluble vitamins (A, D, E and K) and water-soluble vitamins (folate, B6, and B12). Patients should also be screened for iron, calcium, phosphorus and zinc deficiency. Vitamin and mineral supplementation is required in most patients. This includes a multivitamin, calcium (1000–1500 mg/day), vitamin D (400–800 IU/day) and iron, if needed. Caution must be taken not to consume vitamin or mineral preparations that contain gluten.

Bone density scanning to screen for osteoporosis is recommended in all newly diagnosed patients [67]. Screening for other autoimmune disorders such as diabetes mellitus, autoimmune thyroid disorder, and rheumatoid arthritis is not routinely recommended, but may be applied on a case-by-case basis.

Lifelong follow-up of affected individuals is necessary to monitor for dietary compliance and response as patients who are noncompliant or become refractory are at increased risk for malignancy [68]. These malignancies include lymphomas, mostly T-cell type, as well as adenocarcinoma of the small bowel, stomach and esophagus, primary hepatocellular carcinoma and melanoma [69].

Dietary avoidance of gluten leads to symptom improvement in 70% of patients with celiac disease within 2 weeks [70], although based on clinical experience, complete resolution of symptoms can take as long as 6–9 months after initiation of a strict gluten-free diet. Serologic testing can be used to approximate dietary compliance as antibody titers decrease with initiation of the gluten free-diet within 4–6 weeks [71]. In contrast, mucosal recovery with histologic resolution of inflammation may take up to 2 years [72].

Rarely, patients do not respond to nutritional therapy. Abdominal bloating and pain may indicate refractory sprue, concomitant irritable bowel syndrome or bacterial overgrowth. In these refractory cases repeat endoscopy is indicated. Persistent histologic damage, despite dietary compliance, indicates refractory sprue. Intravenous steroids [73], azathioprine [74], cyclosporine [75] and infliximab [76] have been used in these cases in nonpregnant patients with success. Patients with histologic improvement require investigation for other causes of their symptoms.

Prenatal considerations

Infertility is a reported complication of celiac disease [77]. Several European studies have suggested a higher prevalence of celiac disease among infertile women (4–8%) who are otherwise asymptomatic compared with the general population (less than 1%) [78,79]; however, these findings have not been consistent. A recent study from northern California found that only one of 121 (0.8%) women attending an infertility clinic screened positive for celiac disease using tissue transglutaminase and antiendomysial antibody [80], suggesting no difference in the prevalence of celiac disease among women with infertility compared with the general population. Male celiac patients have also been reported to experience infertility secondary to hypogonadism, sexual dysfunction and poor semen quality [81]. Consideration of the diagnosis of celiac disease and testing in those with any possibly associated symptoms is likely warranted in any patient with infertility of recurrent pregnancy losses.

For individuals with known celiac disease, compliance with the gluten-free diet and correction of all vitamin and mineral deficiencies should be achieved before attempting pregnancy.

Pregnancy considerations

Celiac disease should be considered in any pregnant patients presenting with chronic diarrhea, severe iron deficiency, failure to thrive or unexplained abdominal pain. Serologic tests are accurate in pregnancy and confirmatory endoscopy can be performed safely when indicated (see "Endoscopy in pregnancy and lactation" below).

Prompt recognition of *de novo* celiac disease in pregnancy is important because uncontrolled disease carries an increased risk of adverse pregnancy-related events. These include an increased risk for spontaneous abortion, intrauterine growth retardation and low birthweight [82]. These complications are most likely secondary to nutritional deficiency and are preventable with dietary changes and vitamin and mineral replacement. The risk of cesarean section was also found to be moderately higher for women with celiac disease (odds ratio (OR) 1.33, 95% confidence interval (CI) 1.03–1.70) in a British study, possibly due to socio-economic or educational advantages of women with celiac disease [83].

It is recommended that pregnant women with celiac disease be followed by high-risk obstetrics as well as a dietitian with expertise in celiac disease to ensure total adherence to the gluten-free diet. Malabsorption and steatorrhea, the hallmark characteristics of uncontrolled disease, are associated with oxalate kidney stone formation, fat-soluble vitamins deficiency and calcium malabsorption. Thus, pregnant women with celiac disease should be monitored for dietary compliance with serial tTG. Levels of the fat-soluble vitamins (A, D, E, and K) should also be monitored and replacement should be initiated if levels are low.

Inflammatory bowel disease

Background and epidemiology

The inflammatory bowel diseases (IBD) are a group of chronic, idiopathic, inflammatory conditions of the gastrointestinal tract. The term is used most commonly to refer to Crohn's disease (CD) and ulcerative colitis (UC). Other inflammatory bowel diseases are indeterminate colitis and the microscopic colitides: lymphocytic and collagenous colitis. Inflammation leads to ulcerations, loss of absorptive capacity and fibrostenotic areas with intestinal obstruction.

The incidence and prevalence of CD and UC vary greatly with population. Incidence rates are considerably higher in northern and western Europe and in North America compared with Africa, South America and Asia. The incidence is also greater (3–6 times greater) in Jewish populations [84].

It is estimated that the worldwide incidence of UC is 0.5–24.5 per 100,000 persons and the worldwide incidence of CD is 0.1–16 per 100,000 persons [85]. Interestingly, in western, industrialized nations the incidence of UC has remained relatively constant, whereas the incidence of CD rose substantially between the 1960s and 1980s [85,86]. Whether this increase is due to better detection or to environmental and dietary changes leading to a true rise in new cases has yet to be determined. The overall prevalence of UC and CD in western countries is 150–250 per 100,000 persons and 100–200 per 100,000 persons, respectively [87].

The incidence and prevalence of IBD also vary with age. CD and UC are both diseases of young people, with the highest incidence seen between 20 and 40 years of age.

A second, smaller peak is seen in men and women between the sixth and ninth decades of life [88]. Whether this second peak represents a delayed diagnosis, misdiagnosed ischemic colitis or true *de novo* disease has been controversial.

Risk factors for IBD include high socio-economic status and urban environment. Male gender confers a slightly higher risk of UC with a male-to-female ratio of 1.7:1, whereas female gender may confer a small excess risk of CD with a male-to-female ratio between unity and 1:1.2. Smoking is a definite risk factor for CD. It doubles the risk for developing CD and increases the risk of having an aggressive disease course [89]. In contrast, smoking is protective for UC. A meta-analysis found that the risk of developing UC was 60% lower in smokers compared with nonsmokers [90].

The relationship between oral contraceptives and IBD is unclear. Early studies which did not account for tobacco use suggested an increased risk for the development of CD and UC in women using oral contraceptives. A more recent large Italian population-based study also found that women who used oral contraceptives for at least 1 month before the onset of symptoms had a threefold higher risk of CD [91]. However, no significant risk was found for UC and no dose–response relationship was seen. Other case–control studies have found a lack of association between oral contraceptives and both UC and CD [92,93].

The role of diet has been investigated in multiple studies. Associations have been reported for dairy products, fast food, cold drinks and refined sugars and both UC and CD; however, no causal explanation has been found between any specific dietary factor and IBD [94]. NSAID and cyclo-oxygenase-2 inhibitors may precipitate colitis and worsen the disease course of IBD [95]. However, as in the case of diet, no definite risk between NSAID use and the development of IBD has been found.

Appendectomy has been shown to be protective for UC in several studies, especially if appendicitis occurred before age 20 [96]. This protective effect may be due to postoperative changes to the immune system. Several infectious agents, most notably *Mycobacterium paratuberculosis* and measles virus, have been proposed to cause CD [97].

Pathophysiology

The exact pathogenesis of IBD is unknown. It is likely that IBD is due to complex interactions between genetic, immunologic and environmental factors. One theory that has been proposed is based on the inverse relationship between the incidence of IBD and the rates of enteric infection at the population level [98]. Dubbed the "hygiene hypothesis," this theory suggests that early exposure to enteric infections protects against the future development of IBD.

It has long been theorized that genetic factors predispose to the development of IBD. Familial aggregation, ethnic variations in disease frequency and twin studies showing higher disease rates between monozygotic twins than dizygotic twins all suggest a role for genetic factors. Recently, specific susceptibility genes for CD and UC have been identified. The NOD2 gene located on chromosome 16 was the first of such genes [99,100]. Loss-of-function mutations in the NOD2 gene, as detected in some patients with CD, may impair intracellular bacterial sensing and immune response. CD patients who are carriers of NOD2 mutations display a specific phenotype. They are more likely to have small bowel disease as well to have early onset of disease, strictures and fistulas [101]. Other genetic loci that have been linked to IBD include the multidrug resistance 1 (MDR-1) gene on chromosome 7, SLC22A4/5 genes on chromosome 5 and DLG5 gene on chromosome 10.

In addition to genetic and environmental factors, immune dysregulation is also likely to be necessary for the development of IBD. Studies in CD have demonstrated disruptions in mucosal homeostasis with an excessive and persistent T- helper cell type 1 (Th1) immune response in the gut mucosa [102]. This creates a deficiency in regulatory T-cells, allowing patients with CD to react to their own microflora. In contrast, an atypical Th2 response has been described in UC [103].

Further evidence of the important role of the immune system in the pathogenesis of IBD is provided by the marked elevation of tumor necrosis factor (TNF)-alpha, an important mediator of intestinal inflammation, in patients with CD [104]. The central role of TNF in the pathogenesis of IBD is substantiated by the recent development of effective targeted pharmacotherapy using anti-TNF antibodies.

Clinical presentation

Patients with IBD present with a range of symptoms, depending on the extent and severity of the disease. While CD and UC have many overlapping signs and symptoms, substantial differences exist (Table 10.3). In UC, patients generally present with frequent, small-volume diarrhea [105]. Nocturnal stools may also be present. Stools are generally bloody although the amount of blood passed per rectum may vary from scant to copious. Patients may also report tenesmus and fecal urgency due to rectal involvement. Abdominal pain and cramping are also often present. Systemic symptoms such as fever, anorexia, weight loss, fatigue and malaise may be present in individuals with diffuse involvement of the colon (i.e. pancolitis). Patients with severe, diffuse colonic involvement, termed fulminant colitis, may have severe abdominal distension due to toxic megacolon.

Patients with small bowel and colonic CD may also present with diarrhea and abdominal pain. Perianal disease in the form of fissures, abscesses, and fistulas is common in CD and may be present in the absence of other gastrointestinal

Table 10.3 Distinguishing features of ulcerative colitis and Crohn's disease

	Ulcerative colitis	Crohn's disease
Clinical features		
Hematochezia	Common	Rare
Passage of mucus or pus	Common	Rare
Small bowel disease	No (except in backwash ileitis)	Yes
Can affect upper gastrointestinal tract	No	Yes
Abdominal mass	Rare	Sometimes
Extraintestinal manifestations	Common	Common
Small bowel obstruction	Rare	Common
Colonic obstruction	Rare	Common
Fistulas and perianal disease	No	Common
Biochemical features		
Antineutrophil cytoplasmic antibodies	Common	Rare
Anti-*Sacchromyces cervisiae* antibodies	Rare	Common
Pathologic features		
Transmural mucosal inflammation	No	Yes
Distorted crypt architecture	Yes	Uncommon
Cryptitis and crypt abscesses	Yes	Yes
Granulomas	No	Yes (but rarely in mucosal biopsies)
Fistulas and skip lesions	No	Yes

Reproduced with permission from Baumgert, DC, Sandborn, WJ. Inflammatory bowel disease: clinical aspects and established and evolving therapies. Lancet 2007;369:1641.

symptoms [106]. Intestinal obstruction from inflammation and fibrostenotic disease is also common in CD. Patients with esophageal and gastric involvement may report odynophagia, gastroesophageal reflux, dyspepsia, epigastric pain, and chest pain and upper gastrointestinal tract bleeding [107]. They also commonly present with anorexia, weight loss and cachexia.

Extraintestinal manifestations are seen in 20–40% of patients with IBD and may affect nearly every organ system [108]. They may precede the development of gastrointestinal disease. Some manifestations respond to treatment of the underlying bowel disease whereas others do not. Organ systems commonly involved include the skin, joints, and eyes [109]. Extraluminal gastrointestinal organs may also be involved. Dermatologic manifestations include erythema nodosum (reddish painful bumps, generally on the front of the leg below the knees) and pyoderma gangrenosum (deep ulcers with a violaceous border, usually on the legs). Sacroiliitis, ankylosing spondylitis, and peripheral arthritis are frequently encountered rheumatologic manifestations. Patients with ocular involvement may have iritis, uveitis and/or episcleritis. Primary sclerosing cholangitis and bile duct carcinoma are extraluminal gastrointestinal conditions associated with UC.

Diagnosis

The diagnosis of IBD relies on laboratory, radiographic, endoscopic and histologic data. Hematologic abnormalities that may be present include low hemoglobin, high white blood cell count with left shift and high platelet count [110]. C-reactive protein (CRP), a nonspecific marker for inflammation, has been shown to correlate well with disease activity in IBD, especially in CD [111]. CRP has been shown to be a more sensitive marker for detecting IBD compared to the erythrocyte sedimentation rate (ESR), albumin, and complete blood count abnormalities.

Stool examination may be positive for fecal leukocytes in IBD. This is a nonspecific finding and not helpful in the diagnosis of IBD [112]. However, newer fecal markers have emerged that have a higher sensitivity and specificity for IBD. These include fecal lactoferrin, elastase, myeloperoxidase and calprotectin [113]. Their utility as noninvasive markers of intestinal inflammation is the subject of active research. In the future, they may be used to avoid invasive examinations such as colonoscopy which may be particularly helpful during pregnancy.Radiographic imaging plays an important role in the diagnosis of IBD. Plain films are often obtained to rule out toxic megacolon (acute severe colitis with potentially life-threatening dilation of the colon), perforation and obstruction. Air-contrast barium studies are frequently obtained to evaluate for bowel wall thickening, loss of smooth mucosa, ulcers, dilated bowel, strictures, fistulas and perirectal disease [114]. However, their use is limited in pregnancy by high radiation exposure and variations in examiner experience [115]. Computed tomography (CT) is used widely to identify bowel wall thickening, intra-abdominal abscesses and other extraluminal complications of IBD. Over the last decade, bowel ultrasound has become an increasingly accepted mode of evaluating IBD, particularly in Europe. Ultrasound can detect transmural inflammation and determine the anatomic location of CD and its extension within the bowel [116]. Newer cross-sectional imaging techniques, including CT enterography, MRI and MRI enterography are potential future strategies to evaluate intra- and extraluminal changes in IBD.

Despite the development of noninvasive markers of inflammation and novel imaging techniques, endoscopy with biopsy remains the gold standard for the diagnosis of suspected IBD. No endoscopic finding is specific for IBD but the pattern of inflammation can help distinguish UC from CD [117]. UC is characterized by inflammation in the rectum spreading continuously and uniformly to the proximal colon. The extent of colonic involvement is variable, with 50% of patients having disease confined to the rectosigmoid. Disease is generally limited to the colon in UC, although distal small bowel involvement may occur in up to 17% of patients [118]. Termed "backwash" ileitis, this inflammation in the distal terminal ileum is likely due to reflux of colonic contents into the ileum from an incompetent ileocecal valve.

In contrast, CD is characterized by focal intestinal inflammation with segments of complete or relative sparing (i.e. "skip lesions"). One-third of cases of CD involve the small bowel only, while 20% of patients have disease limited to the colon [119]. The majority of remaining cases have ileocolitis. Endoscopic evaluation of the small bowel for CD has been facilitated by the introduction of wireless capsule endoscopy which has been reported to have up to a 70% yield in diagnosing small bowel CD [120].

Pathologic features in IBD include architectural distortion, cryptitis and crypt abscesses. These are nonspecific findings and may be seen in other causes of colitis. Granulomas are a hallmark feature of CD but may be seen in UC as well.

A definitive diagnosis can be made in the majority of cases of chronic IBD but up to 10–15% of adult cases have overlapping features of UC and CD and are deemed indeterminate [121]. In some of these cases, checking the recently characterized IBD-specific antibodies (e.g. ASCA, p-ANCA, omp C, c-Bir 1) may prove helpful but their routine use is still controversial.

The differential diagnosis includes infectious colitis, ischemic colitis, diverticular disease-associated colitis, medication-induced colitis (e.g. NSAID, antineoplastic drugs), radiation colitis/proctitis, and Behçet's disease [119]. Colonic and small bowel neoplasms may also present with inflammatory changes that resemble IBD. Noninflammatory causes of hematochezia which should be ruled out include hemorrhoids and angiodysplasias of the colon and small bowel. Irritable bowel syndrome may share some clinical features of IBD but is easily distinguished from IBD in most cases due to the absence of laboratory, radiographic, endoscopic and histologic findings.

Fertility

As IBD is a disease of young people, often presenting during the childbearing years, fertility is a major concern. In general, infertility rates for women with IBD, which range from 5% to 14%, are no higher than in the normal population [122–124]. Initial epidemiologic data suggested higher infertility rates in women with CD but these data did not account for higher voluntary childlessness rates in IBD patients presumed secondary to self-image and sexual dysfunction common in affected individuals [125].

Fertility may, however, be compromised in women who have undergone surgery for IBD refractory to medical therapy. While resectional surgery does not decrease and may in fact improve fertility in women with Crohn's disease [126, 127], ileal pouch–anal anastomosis (IPAA) after total colectomy is associated with a dramatic decrease in female fertility. IPAA has become an option as treatment for pancolitis poorly controlled by medical therapy or for longstanding UC with dysplastic premalignant features. A Scandinavian study of 237 women who had undergone IPAA found that postoperative births were 49% of expected and only 35% of expected

when *in vitro* fertilization was excluded [128]. A subsequent meta-analysis which included eight studies confirmed that the relative risk of infertility was 48% after IPAA [129]. While some of this effect may be due to the fact that women with severe IBD (and therefore more likely to have tubal disease) are more likely to require an IPAA, this decrease in fertility has also been attributed to tubal dysfunction caused by abnormal adhesion formation after deep pelvic dissection and appears to be permanent. No procedural factors have been identified (e.g. one-step versus two-step procedure) that consistently affect the risk of infertility. Women considering having children and requiring proctocolectomy should be informed of this risk for infertility as deferring reconstruction after completing childbearing may be a preferable approach.

Fertility in women with CD may also be impaired due to active inflammation causing direct or indirect complications [130]. Transmural inflammation from CD can create fistulas from the rectum, proximal colon and ileum to the uterus and ovaries. Disease may also directly extend to the fallopian tubes and ovaries, causing granulomatous salpingitis and oophoritis. Indirectly, CD may decrease fertility by causing anovulatory cycles or amenorrhea or by causing dyspareunia and impairing sexual function.

Regarding fertility in men with IBD, long-term treatment with sulfasalazine has been shown to decrease sperm counts and semen quality. This infertility is temporary and reverses with discontinuation of the drug. Male fertility otherwise does not appear to be affected by IBD [131].

Preconception considerations

Preconception counseling and management are of fundamental importance to insure a successful pregnancy in patients with IBD. Indeed, discussion about reproductive issues should be a routine part of the care of women with IBD of childbearing age. In addition to fertility issues, preconception counseling should include educating the patient and her partner that the optimal time to conceive is during a period of clinical remission as this maximizes the chance of maintaining remission during pregnancy without escalating therapy.

During the preconception period, potentially teratogenic drugs should be discontinued. Sulfasalazine interferes with folic acid metabolism and patients wishing to get pregnant should be switched to one of the newer 5-aminosalicylates or increase their dose of folic acid supplementation to 2 mg/day to counter the effects of sulfasalazine on folic acid metabolism, which could theoretically increase the risk of neural tube defects in the fetus.

Methotrexate and thalidomide are FDA category X and must be discontinued before conception because of their teratogenic and abortifacient properties. The optimum duration of discontinuation before conception is not known but a minimum of 6 months is recommended. In those women who require an immunodulator such as methotrexate to maintain remission, transitioning to azathioprine or 6-mercaptopurine (6-MP) prior to conception may be advised to avoid disease flare in pregnancy.

Nutritional status should be assessed periodically and corrected in all individuals with IBD and certainly in women with IBD considering pregnancy. Vitamin and mineral deficiencies common in IBD include vitamin B12, folic acid, iron, calcium, and the fat-soluble vitamins (A, D, E and K). It is also timely at the preconception visit to discuss the management of IBD in pregnancy and educate patients and their family about the risks and benefits of medical therapy. A frank discussion about the currently available safety data of each medication commonly used to treat IBD is necessary to achieve a satisfactory therapeutic plan. Women should be advised not to discontinue those medications that keep their disease in remission unless they are contraindicated in pregnancy.

Effect of pregnancy on IBD

It is generally accepted that pregnancy does not significantly alter the course of IBD. For women with quiescent disease, the rate of relapse is approximately the same in pregnant versus nonpregnant patients [132,133]. Miller reported a relapse rate of 34% and 27% for women with quiescent UC and CD, respectively, during the 12 months of gestation and puerperium [134]. These are similar to the 1-year relapse rates for women with IBD who are not pregnant.

For women with active disease at conception, the "rule of thirds" is said to apply. Active disease at conception carries a one-third risk of getting better, one-third risk of getting worse, and one-third risk of maintaining the same level of disease activity [135]. Based on this association of active disease at the start of pregnancy with continued or worsening disease activity in almost 70% of women, experts advise delaying pregnancy until the disease is in remission [136].

De novo presentation of IBD in pregnancy occurs, although the exact incidence is unknown. Symptoms suggestive of IBD such as hematochezia, chronic diarrhea, unexplained abdominal pain and weight loss should prompt the work-up of IBD.

In terms of long-term effects of pregnancy on disease course, a recent European cohort study which followed female IBD patients for 10 years did not find any influence of pregnancy on disease phenotype or surgery rates [136].

Effect of IBD on pregnancy

Women with IBD are at increased risk of certain adverse pregnancy outcomes. A meta-analysis of 12 studies found a higher incidence of preterm delivery (<37 weeks) and low birthweight (<2500 g) in patients with IBD [137]. A higher rate of cesarean sections was also found. No significant increase was found in the risk of congenital anomalies, stillbirths or small for gestational age. One population-based cohort study did find a

statistically significantly higher rate of congenital malformations in infants born to mothers with IBD (7.9% vs 1.7%) but this study did not adjust for medical therapy of IBD. Likewise, other studies have not reproduced these results [138].

It is unclear whether a history of prior surgery for IBD increases the complication rate in pregnancy. A recent population-based cohort study found a history of surgery for IBD to be an independent predictor of an adverse pregnancy outcome [139]. Other studies have found no increased risk of pregnancy complications after surgery [140]. The effect of disease severity on pregnancy outcomes is also unclear, with some studies showing worse pregnancy outcomes in women with severe disease and others showing no association between disease severity and pregnancy complications [139]. Careful monitoring by a team of specialists, including maternal and fetal health specialists, is advised through the pregnancy.

The mode of delivery should be dictated by obstetric considerations except when active perianal disease is present in which case cesarean section is advised. Healed perianal disease does not warrant cesarean section. Cesarean section is often advocated in patients with IPAA to avoid trauma to the anal sphincter and future incontinence. However, IPAA does not preclude vaginal delivery as studies have found only transient changes in pouch function with vaginal delivery and no increased risk of incontinence [141].

Data on the risk of developing perianal disease after episiotomy are lacking. Episiotomies are not advised in women with Crohn's disease and active perianal disease [142]. In general, a mediolateral approach is favored over a medial approach in women with IBD who require episiotomy to reduce the risk of extension into the anal sphincter and rectum.

Management

The foremost concern of physicians caring for pregnant patients with IBD should be to maintain remission since active disease has been associated with poor pregnancy outcomes. Medications used to maintain remission should be continued during pregnancy, with certain exceptions, as discontinuation of therapy may lead to disease flare and poor outcome. In cases of moderate to severe IBD and disease flares during pregnancy, treatment should follow the same guidelines as for nonpregnant patients, with the major goal being to achieve prompt remission. The use of sulfasalazine, topical and oral 5'ASA agents, and steroids is generally viewed as "safe" for treatment of IBD in pregnancy. Although less is known about these agents, azathioprine, 6-MP and cyclosporine are generally viewed as justifiable to treat more severe disease during pregnancy. Use of metronidazole (for prolonged periods) and ciprofloxacin is discouraged. Data on the use of anti-TNF agents are evolving although some risk of congenital anomalies may exist with first-trimester use. Specific data about each of these agents are found below under the section on drug safety and summarized in Table 10.4.

Table 10.4 Medications used in the treatment of inflammatory bowel disease

Drug	US FDA pregnancy category	Recommendations for pregnancy	Recommendations for breastfeeding
Adalimumab	B	Limited human data; low risk	No human data; probably compatible
Amoxicillin/clavulinic acid	B	Low risk	Probably compatible
Azathioprine/6- mercaptopurine	D	Data in IBD, transplant literature suggest low risk	No human data; potential toxicity
Balsalazide	B	Low risk	No human data; potential diarrhea
Certolizumab pegol	B	No human data	No human data
Ciprofloxacin	C	Avoid; potential toxicity to cartilage	Limited human data; probably compatible
Corticosteroids	C	Low risk; possible increased risk of cleft palate, adrenal insufficiency, premature rupture of membranes	Compatible
Cyclosporine	C	Low risk	Limited human data; potential toxicity
Fish oil supplements	–	Safe. Possibly beneficial	No human data
Infliximab	B	Low risk	No human data; probably compatible
Mesalazine	B	Low risk	Limited human data; potential diarrhea
Methotrexate	X	Contraindicated: teratogenic	Contraindicated
Metronidazole	B	Given limited efficacy in IBD, risk of cleft palate, would avoid	Limited human data; potential toxicity
Natalizumab	C	No human data	No human data
Olsalazine	C	Low risk	Limited human data; potential diarrhea
Rifaximin	C	Animal teratogen. No human data	No human data; probably compatible
Sulfasalazine	B	Considered safe. Give folate 2 mg daily	Limited human data; potential diarrhea
Tacrolimus	C	Use if mother's health mandates	Limited human data: potential toxicity
Thalidomide	X	Contraindicated: teratogenic	No human data; potential toxicity

Reproduced with permission from Kane S. Caring for women with inflammatory bowel disease. J Gender Specific Med 2001;4(1):54–9.

Women with insufficient weight gain in pregnancy due to active disease may need nutritional support along with pharmacologic therapy. Total parenteral nutrition in women with IBD can be used in pregnancy although it carries a high risk of complications. Pregnant women receiving parenteral nutrition must be followed closely for the development of line-related complications, including infection and thrombosis.

Most cases can be treated with medical therapy; however, cases of severe refractory disease may require surgery. The indications for surgery in pregnancy are the same as for the nonpregnant patient. These include intractable bleeding, intestinal obstruction, megacolon and perforation. In cases of fulminant colitis in the first trimester, Turnbull blow-hole colostomy to achieve colonic decompression and fecal diversion may be safer than total colectomy [143]. Later in pregnancy, patients with fulminant colitis failing medical therapy may do well with colectomy and synchronous delivery.

Monitoring disease activity in pregnancy

Normal physiologic changes in pregnancy complicate the monitoring of disease activity in pregnant women with IBD. Laboratory studies which are used routinely to monitor disease activity such as hemoglobin, white blood cell count, and platelet count [144], as well as serum ferritin [145], sedimentation rate [146] and CRP [147], are all altered by healthy pregnancy, making fluctuations difficult to interpret.

Imaging techniques commonly used to evaluate IBD such as abdominal and pelvic CT and even fluoroscopy may be performed if necessary for maternal health in pregnancy but are generally avoided due to concerns about ionizing radiation to the developing fetus. Ultrasonography and magnetic resonance imaging may be preferred in assessing disease activity and complications.

Endoscopy can be safely performed in pregnancy and may be required to assess disease activity and evaluate patients with refractory symptoms as well as to establish *de novo* diagnoses. Frequent clinical evaluations with careful review of signs and symptoms remain the best indicator of IBD activity in pregnancy (see "Endoscopy in pregnancy and lactation" below).

Drug safety

The use of medications in pregnancy is associated with a great deal of anxiety in patients so extensive education is needed to ensure compliance. Pregnancy data about most of the medications commonly used to treat IBD are summarized below and in Table 10.4.

Sulfasalazine

Sulfasalazine is used both to treat mild to moderately active IBD and to maintain remission. It is broken down in the colon into an anti-inflammatory agent (5'ASA) and an antibiotic one (sulfapyridone). Its efficacy is predominantly from the 5'ASA and its side effects from the sulfa moiety. Because it is broken down into its active components in the colon, it is only effective in treating colonic disease.

Sulfasalazine (category B) has not been shown to increase the risk of fetal malformations. However, it does cross the placenta and can be detected in minimal amounts in breast milk. Because sulfasalazine interferes with folic acid metabolism, patients taking it are advised to take 2 mg/day of supplemental folate before and during pregnancy to lower the risk of neural tube defects [148]. Men taking sulfasalazine may suffer from infertility due to the drug's effect on sperm quantity and quality. This infertility is reversible and men considering conception are advised to discontinue sulfasalazine for 3 months prior to attempting conception.

5-Aminosalicylates

5'ASA are anti-inflammatory medications with similar efficacy to sulfasalazine but fewer side effects. They are used both to treat mild to moderately active disease and to maintain remission. 5'ASA is rapidly absorbed in the jejunum so several formulations have been developed to allow delivery to the distal small bowel and colon These formulations include mesalazine products (marketed in the US as Pentasa, Asacol and Salofalk), dimerized 5'ASA products (such as olsalazine and balsalazine) and enemas and suppositories for the treatment of disease in the distal colon and rectum.

The 5-aminosalicylates (all category B except olsalazine which is category C) are used in mild to moderate CD and UC. A prospective study of pregnant women with IBD receiving a mean daily dose of 2 g of mesalazine did not report any increased risk of fetal malformations [149]. Likewise, a large case series did not show any increased risk of teratogencity [150]. However, placental and breast milk transfer of mesalazine does occur and this carries a potential risk of watery diarrhea in the infant.

Corticosteroids

Medical therapy of active disease in pregnancy often involves the use of corticosteroids and these agents warrant some additional discussion here. Corticosteroids are potent nonspecific anti-inflammatory agents for moderate to severe relapses of UC and CD.

Steroid for IBD may be given topically (in the form of foams and suppositories) or systemically (orally or intravenously). Patients with severe symptoms requiring hospitalization may require intravenous corticosteroids (hydrocortisone 400 mg/day or methylprednisolone 60 mg/day) [151] whereas outpatients may be treated with oral steroids (prednisone 40 mg/day).

There are no standardized weaning protocols for steroids in either pregnant or nonpregnant IBD patients. As disease flares are common when prednisone is tapered below 20 mg/day, one common strategy is to maintain patients on approximately 20 mg/day of prednisone until delivery and to attempt further medication tapering after the puerperium. Pregnant women on corticosteroids are at increased risk of glucose intolerance and may warrant early or additional screening. Stress-dose steroid therapy in peripartum women is advised for mothers on prolonged corticosteroid therapy (see Chapter 47 on stress-dose steroids in pregnancy).

Corticosteroids (category C) cross the placenta easily but it is estimated that 90% of the maternal dose is metabolized within the placenta before reaching the fetus [152]. Case–control studies have reported an increased risk of cleft palates after *in utero* exposure; however, a prospective study of women with IBD taking steroids did not find any increased risk of congenital malformations [153]. Most experts agree that corticosteroids can be used safely for moderate to severe disease [122]. Adrenal suppression is rare in fetuses exposed to corticosteroids, likely due to poor placental transfer, but it has been reported [153,154]. Prednisolone and prednisone are more efficiently metabolized by the placenta than other steroids and may pose a particularly low risk of this complication.

Antibiotics

Antibiotics (usually metronidazole and fluoroquinolones but clarithromycin and the nonsystemic antibiotic rifaximin have also been used) have at best a modest effect on treating active CD of the colon but have no role in the treatment of UC. However, not much is not known about the degree of efficacy or the ideal dose or duration of therapy.

Antibiotic therapy for IBD in pregnancy is generally avoided as safety with prolonged use, as is often required, has not been demonstrated. A prospective controlled study of pregnant women exposed to ciprofloxacin (category C) found a low risk of defects [155]. However, the fluoroquinolones have a high affinity for bone tissue and cartilage and may cause arthropathies in children. Extensive data are lacking but ciprofloxacin is probably compatible with breastfeeding. Metronidazole (category B) has been associated with midline facial defects in pregnancies exposed to metronidazole during the first trimester. Retrospective studies in patients exposed during treatment of *Trichomonas* or bacterial vaginosis have not found increased risk of malformations. Rifaximin (category C) has recently come on the market in the US but has not been adequately studied in pregnancy.

6-Mercaptopurine and azathioprine

The immunomodulators azathioprine and 6-MP act by decreasing intracellular production of purines and thereby decreasing circulating numbers of B- and T-lymphocytes. Azathioprine is a prodrug that is metabolized to 6-MP and both agents have a role in treating active IBD that has been unresponsive to steroids, allowing a reduction in steroid dose in patients requiring long-term steroids to maintain remission, and in treatment of Crohn's fistulas.

The use of 6-MP and azathioprine (both category D) generates a fair amount of anxiety in pregnancy. 6-MP and azathioprine cross the placenta and are detectable in breast milk. However, the fetal liver does not express inosinate pyrophosphorylase, the enzyme needed for thiopurine metabolism, and this appears to be a relative barrier to the effects of azathioprine and its metabolites [156].

A small number of case reports have described human fetal immunosuppression [157] and structural malformations [158,159] in infants exposed to the thiopurines *in utero*. However, these agents have been used widely in the transplant setting with a favorable safety profile in pregnancy [160]. Furthermore, a study of pregnant women with IBD on thiopurines found no increase in prematurity, spontaneous abortion, congenital abnormalities or childhood neoplasia [161]. Based on these data and the frequent need to continue these drugs during pregnancy to maintain remission, discontinuation of the thiopurines before and during pregnancy is not indicated. Careful monitoring of drug metabolite levels with dose reductions as permitted can be considered to further minimize the risks of exposure to the fetus. Women who insist on discontinuing azathioprine or 6-MP before conception should be advised to do so during a period of disease quiescence and at least 3 months prior to conception due to the long half-life of the drugs.

Antitumor necrosis factor agents

The advent of monoclonal immunoglobulin IgG1 antibody to anti-TNF has changed the treatment paradigm of IBD. Three anti-TNF agents are currently FDA approved for the treatment of IBD: infliximab (category B) for CD and UC, adalimumab (category B) for CD, and certolizumab pegol (category B). These agents are primarily indicated for refractory luminal and/or fistulizing disease; however, they are also used for the treatment of extraintestinal manifestations [162]. Postmarketing safety data for infliximab in pregnancy has not reported any increased risk of fetal malformations or miscarriages [163,164]. However, infliximab does cross the placenta and can be detected at high levels in infants exposed to the drug *in utero* [165]. It is postulated that efficient transplacental transfer of IgG antibodies in the third trimester leads to high serum levels of infliximab at birth. Whether this leads to adverse outcomes in the infant is not entirely clear.

Preliminary data do not suggest any immune dysfunction in infants exposed to infliximab *in utero*. However, until long-term data are available, a reasonable practice is to avoid infliximab dosing in the last trimester in order to avoid high levels of fetal exposure and to bridge patients with steroids when necessary until delivery.

Data regarding adalimumab and certolizumab pegol safety in pregnancy are limited but case reports and a small case series have found adalimumab to be safe in pregnancy [166,167]. Studies are under way to assess the safety of biologics in pregnancy.

Anti-$_4$-integrins

Natalizumab (category C), a monoclonal antibody to the cellular adhesion molecule $_4$-integrin, was recently reapproved by the FDA for the treatment of refractory CD. As human safety data in pregnancy are lacking, it is recommended that natalizumab be used in pregnant women only when the potential benefit outweighs the potential risk to the fetus.

Cyclosporine

Cyclosporine is used to treat severe pancolitis or toxic megacolon in UC patients who are unresponsive to steroids and resistant to colectomy. Cyclosporine (category C) use in pregnancy to avoid emergency colectomy has been described [168]. A meta-analysis of 15 studies of pregnancy outcome after cyclosporine exposure found no increased risk of major malformations [169]. Cyclosporine is concentrated at high levels in breast milk and breastfeeding while on cyclosporine is not advised.

Methotrexate

Methotrexate is typically reserved for patients with CD who are resistant to steroids and do not tolerate the immunomodulators 6-MP or azathioprine. Methotrexate (category X) is absolutely contraindicated in pregnancy as it is a known teratogen and abortifacient. It is recommended that methotrexate be discontinued for 3–6 months before conception [122]. This is also true for men who wish to father children, as methotrexate is toxic to sperm.

Thalidomide

Thalidomide (category X) has been shown to be beneficial in the treatment of luminal and fistulizing CD refractory to standard therapy [170]. Its use in pregnancy is contraindicated due to its predictable, severe teratogenic effects.

Lactation

Breastfeeding does not appear to influence disease activity although many women with IBD choose not to breastfeed [167].

Sulfasalazine, mesalazine and corticosteroid use are all compatible with breastfeeding [171]. Due to limited or no data, there are no definite recommendations on lactation and azathioprine, 6-MP and infliximab use. Case reports have shown safety in newborns breastfed by mothers on infliximab and it is likely compatible with breastfeeding [122]. Data collection on metabolite levels in the breast milk of mothers on azathioprine and 6-MP is ongoing.

Microscopic colitis

Background and epidemiology

The microscopic colitides are lymphocytic and collagenous colitis. Both are characterized by chronic diarrhea with normal endoscopic findings and histologically abnormal colonic mucosa. Both diseases predominantly affect middle-aged populations, with a peak incidence occurring between the sixth and seventh decades of life [172]. They predominantly affect women with female-to-male ratios of 4.75:1 and 2.7:1 for collagenous and lymphocytic colitis, respectively. A recently published US population-based cohort study identified 8.6 cases per 100,000 person-years, with the incidence increasing each year of the study [173]. This incidence exceeded that of CD in the population, making it a much more common disease than previously recognized.

Pathogenesis

The pathogenesis of microscopic colitis is unknown. Mechanisms that have been proposed include genetic factors [174], abnormal collagen synthesis in the case of collagenous colitis [175], luminal antigens [176], drug toxicity, autoimmunity [177], and immune dysregulation [178]. Abnormal collagen synthesis with resulting inflammation and fibrosis may cause collagenous colitis. Histologica specimens from affected patients exhibit increased subepithelial collagen with a collagen band width of up to five times normal [179].

Multiple drugs have been linked with microscopic colitis, including NSAID, selective serotonin reuptake inhibitors, statins and bisphosphonates [180]. Causality, however, has been difficult to establish.

Given the strong association between microscopic colitis and autoimmune disease (discussed further below), an autoimmune cause for microscopic colitis has been proposed. Studies have shown a statistically significant increase in ANA positivity [181,182] and serum IgM levels [181] in patients with microscopic colitis; however, no specific autoantibody has been identified. In addition, a recent study did not find any diagnostic relevance between the newer generation of autoantibodies (i.e. ASCA and ANCA) and microscopic colitis [182].

Clinical presentation

Patients with microscopic colitis present with large volumes of watery, nonbloody diarrhea [177]. Other symptoms that may be present are abdominal pain and weight loss. Associated diseases, mainly autoimmune conditions, may be seen in as many as 61% of patients [183]. These include autoimmune thyroid disorder, rheumatoid arthritis, celiac disease and diabetes mellitus.

Diagnosis

The diagnosis of microscopic colitis relies on mucosal biopsies as endoscopy, laboratory and radiographic studies in affected patients are generally normal. Biopsies in lymphocytic colitis reveal lymphocytic infiltration with over 20 lymphocytes per 100 epithelial cells (normal <5 lymphocytes per 100 enterocytes) with a normal subepithelial collagen layer. Biopsies in collagneous colitis show a widened collagen layer of over 10 μm (normal 0–5 μm) [184].

Entities to be considered in the differential diagnosis include acute infectious colitis, eosinophilic inflammation, amyloidosis, UC and CD. Rarely, an interchange between UC or CD and microscopic colitis is seen, raising the question of chance association between the diseases or of the presence of a shared common pathway [185].

Management

Multiple agents have been used to treat microscopic colitis including antidiarrheals, bismuth subsalicylate, 5'ASA, antibiotics, probiotics, steroids, and immunomodulators. However, due to a lack of randomized data, treatment is often based on anecdotal evidence from uncontrolled studies [186].

One algorithm that has been proposed for the treatment of microscopic colitis begins with the elimination of dietary factors or drugs that may cause diarrhea, such as caffeine, alcohol, dairy products and NSAID [187]. Patients who do not respond are often treated with antidiarrheals such as loperamide and diphenoxylate as first-line agents due to their efficacy and low cost. Bismuth subsalicylate is often offered as next-line therapy. A small randomized controlled trial of 14 patients found a clinical and histologic benefit in patients treated for 8 weeks with bismuth subsalicylate compared with placebo [188]. Larger confirmatory studies are lacking.

5-ASA compounds have been used with variable results for treatment of microscopic colitis. Retrospective studies have reported response rates of less than 50% [189]. Antibiotics such as metronidazole and erythromycin have also been shown to have some benefit in retrospective studies but prospective controlled data are not available [177].

The best available data for the treatment of microscopic colitis are for budesonide. However, relapse is common after cessation of treatment. Maintenance therapy with low-dose budesonide (3–6 mg/day) has also been proposed [189]. Patients refractory to budesonide may be candidates for immunodulator therapy with azathioprine, 6-MP or methotrexate. Small, uncontrolled trials have shown benefits with these drugs but side effects are common [190,191]. Subtotal or total colectomy has been reported as a last-line option in severely affected patients who fail medical therapy [192].

Pregnancy considerations

The incidence of microscopic colitis in pregnancy is unknown. Women who present with prolonged diarrhea in pregnancy with no obvious cause identified by history, routine labs, and stool studies should undergo flexible sigmoidoscopy with biopsies to rule out inflammatory bowel disease and microscopic colitis.

Medication considerations in pregnancy for the treatment of microscopic colitis are similar to those for the treatment of IBD (see "Management of IBD"). An additional consideration is that the antidiarrheals loperamide (category B) and diphenoxylate (category C) are considered low risk in pregnancy and can be used with discretion [193]. Bismuth salicylate (category C), however, has been associated with fetal toxicity in animal studies. Its use in pregnancy, especially later in gestation, is not recommended as it may increase the risk of closure or constriction of the fetal ductus arteriosus.

Irritable bowel syndrome

Irritable bowel syndrome (IBS) is a functional bowel disorder in which abdominal pain or discomfort is associated with defecation or changes in bowel habits. It is a common disorder with an estimated prevalence of 10–15% in the general population, with a 2:1 female predominance in North America [194].

Although no specific physiologic mechanism is unique to or characterizes IBS, symptoms are thought to be related to several inter-related factors, including altered gut motility and secretion in response to luminal or environmental factors, dysregulation of the brain–gut axis and enhanced visceral perception and pain [195]. Women with IBS are more likely to have anxiety disorders, depression, and somatization disorders and are more likely to have been sexually or physically abused [196].

Although patients with IBS may present with a wide array of symptoms, the presence of chronic abdominal pain with diarrhea and/or constipation remains the nonspecific yet primary characteristic of IBS. Other gastrointestinal symptoms, including gastroesophageal reflux, dysphagia, early satiety, abdominal bloating and flatulence or belching, nausea, and noncardiac chest pain, are common in patients with IBS. Extraintestinal symptoms include impaired sexual function, dysmenorrhea, dyspareunia, and increased urinary frequency and urgency [197].

Diagnosis is primarily clinical. Several symptom-based diagnostic criteria have been devised to assist in diagnosis. Box 10.4 outlines the Rome III criteria for the diagnosis of IBS.

In a pregnant woman with an established diagnosis of IBS prior to conception, no further investigation is indicated during pregnancy in the absence of alarm features (listed in Box 10.5). For a presumed new-onset case of IBS in pregnancy, a limited number of diagnostic studies can rule out organic illness in the majority of patients. These are listed in Box 10.6. Disorders that may mimic IBS are listed in Table 10.5.

Box 10.4 Diagnostic criteria for IBS (Rome III criteria for the diagnosis of IBS 2006)

Recurrent abdominal pain or discomfort at least 3 days per month in the last 3 months with symptom onset at least 6 months prior to diagnosis, associated with two or more of the following:

- Relieved with defecation
- Onset associated with change in frequency of stool
- Onset associated with change in form (appearance) of stool

Supportive symptoms that are not part of Rome III criteria include:

- abnormal stool frequency ($\leq$3 bowel movements per week or >3 bowel movements per day)
- abnormal stool form (lumpy/hard or loose/watery)
- defecation straining, urgency or a feeling of incomplete bowel movement
- passing mucus and bloating

Box 10.5 Alarm features ("red flags") in a patient with GI complaints

- Hematochezia
- Weight loss greater than 10 pounds
- Abdominal pain that interferes with sleep
- Family history of colon cancer
- Recurring fever
- Anemia
- Chronic severe diarrhea

Box 10.6 Diagnostic tests recommended in IBS

- Complete blood count (to assess anemia, leukocytosis or leukopenia)
- Chemistry panel (to rule out electrolyte abnormality)
- Stool ova and parasites (on three separate stool samples)
- Thyroid studies
- Flexible sigmoidoscopy (for patients greater than 40 years or younger patients with persistent diarrhea)

Table 10.5 Disorders that mimic IBS

Disorder	Remarks
Diarrhea predominant	
Lactose, fructose or sorbitol intolerance	Diagnosis may be supported by history of aggravating factors, lactose tolerance test, or improvement of symptoms with exclusion of inciting substance from diet
Celiac disease	Serologic testing, intestinal biopsy, improvement with gluten-free diet
Constipation predominant	
Pelvic floor dysfunction	Diagnostic tests recommended include colonic transit, anorectal manometry, rectal emptying studies, defecation proctogram

Table 10.6 Treatment of constipation in pregnancy

Laxative	Usual dose
• Bulk-forming laxatives	
Natural (e.g. psyllium)	7 g/d
Synthetic (e.g. methylcellulose)	4–6 g/d
• Emollient laxatives	
Docusate sodium	50–500 mg/day in 1–4 divided doses
• Stimulant laxatives*	
Bisacodyl	30 mg, 10 mg suppository
Cascara Sagrada	2–5 mL
Senna	17–39 mg
• Hyperosmotic guts†	
Polyethylene glycol	8–25 g/day
Lactulose	15–30 mL/day
Sorbitol	15–30 mL/day
Glycerine	3 g suppository
Magnesium hydroxide	800 mg/mL – 15–30 mL/day

*Routine use of stimulating laxatives not recommended in pregnancy due to risk of uterine contractions.
†Usually taken in a single dose at bed time.
There is a risk of lipoid pneumonia with aspiration of liquid paraffin and mineral/castor oil and these agents should generally be avoided in pregnancy.

The treatment of the pregnant woman with IBS ranges from patient education and dietary intervention to medications or psychologic intervention. In the constipation-predominant patient, increasing dietary fiber, fiber supplements or osmotic laxative (when response to fiber is inadequate) are recommended. For diarrheal symptoms, kaolin and pectin can be safely used but may be inadequate for symptomatic relief. Loperamide is usually more effective, but should be used judiciously and infrequently. Cholestyramine may be considered in patients who have had a cholecystectomy or those with postprandial diarrhea. Antispasmodic medications are used for abdominal pain in the nonpregnant population, and may sometimes be necessary in pregnancy. Tricyclic antidepressants (amitriptyline and nortriptyline) have shown benefit in IBS with chronic pain and can be used in pregnancy.

Constipation in pregnancy

Constipation is often considered a common consequence of the physiologic effects of pregnancy. Decreased colonic motility, poor oral intake of food and fluid related to nausea and vomiting, psychologic stress, iron supplements and pressure on the rectosigmoid colon by the gravid uterus may all contribute to the development of constipation in pregnancy. Use of tocolytic drugs such as magnesium or nifedipine has also been reported to interfere with colonic motility [198].

An extensive investigation for evaluation of constipation in pregnancy is rarely required. History should elicit the patient's definition of constipation, dietary habits, pre-existing constipation and medications. Consideration should be given to medical conditions such as hypercalcemia, hypothyroidism and diabetes mellitus that may be associated with constipation. A digital rectal exam may help to rule out fecal impaction and presence of blood in stool. The anal and perineal region should be examined to rule out fissures, ulcerative lesions associated with inflammatory bowel disease and rarely malignancy.

Management should include patient education and reassurance about normal bowel function in pregnancy. Behavior modification to increase physical activity, adequate fluid and fiber intake and scheduled defecation after meals to take advantage of the gastrocolic reflex should be encouraged. Laxatives may be necessary in those patients who do not respond to the general measures listed above. The choices in pregnancy include hydrophilic stool-bulking agents such as methyl cellulose, psyllium and unprocessed bran with a high fluid intake, osmotic laxatives such as lactulose, sorbitol, polyethylene glycol (PEG) and magnesium hydroxide, stool softeners such as docusate sodium, stimulant laxatives such as senna, cascara and bisacodyl. These options are reviewed in Table 10.6.

The Cochrane Database of Systematic Reviews [199] studied randomized controlled trials of treatment of constipation in pregnancy and concluded that fiber supplements increase the frequency of defecation and lead to softer stools (OR 0.18, 95% CI 0.05–0.67). Stimulant laxatives are more effective than bulk-forming laxatives (OR 0.30, 95% CI 0.14–0.61), but may have more side effects. Routine use of stimulant laxatives is not recommended in pregnancy because they may precipitate uterine contractions by inducing smooth muscle contractions [200]. Risk of aspiration leading to lipoid pneumonia exists with oral administration of liquid paraffin and mineral oil. In addition, repeated use may be associated with decreased maternal absorption of fat-soluble vitamins including vitamin K, increasing the risk of neonatal hemorrhage [201]. In the rare patient with pre-existing colonic atonia, constipation can become a serious problem, causing severe impaction and obstructive symptoms. Aggressive treatment is recommended for these patients with high doses of osmotic laxatives and cautious use of enemas.

Anorectal and perineal disorders

Anorectal disease in pregnancy is common, occurring in greater than 13.8 per 1000 livebirths [202]. The most common conditions are hemorrhoids, fissure *in ano* and proctitis. Anorectal injuries from obstetric trauma and episiotomies are also common. These injuries, which include anal ulcers, abscesses, and rectovaginal fistulas, can be the source of great discomfort and embarrassment. Lastly, fecal incontinence, the result of obstetric trauma to the anal sphincter muscles or pudendal nerves, can be an immediate or delayed complication of labor and delivery [203].

Hemorrhoids

Pregnancy and the puerperium are risk factors for the development of symptomatic hemorrhoids [204]. It is thought that modification in the tone and position of the anal sphincter muscles and other pelvic floor structures during pregnancy alters the normal function of the hemorrhoidal cushion and impedes venous return [205]. Other risk factors are chronic constipation due to a low fiber or low fluid diet and diseases associated with increased abdominal pressure.

Patients with hemorrhoids classically present with perianal pruritus or burning, pain, and intermittent rectal bleeding. Mucoid and purulent discharge may occur with secondary inflammation and infection. Prolapse may also occur during a bowel movement, leading to the sensation of incomplete evacuation [206].

External hemorrhoids are apparent by direct visualization on physical exam. Internal hemorrhoids can be diagnosed by anoscopy and possibly by digital rectal exam. Other perianal lesions such as skin tags, fistulas, polyps, tumors should be ruled out before the patient is treated empirically for hemorrhoids. Inflammatory bowel disease is an important differential in any patient with lower GI bleeding and a sigmoidoscopy should be considered in patients with rectal bleeding in pregnancy in which an obvious cause is not visualized on physical exam or anoscopy.

Various local therapies are routinely used for the treatment of hemorrhoids such as Sitz baths, ice, and anesthetic and steroid ointments. Increasing fiber content can also help alleviate symptoms by decreasing straining with bowel movements. Data regarding the efficacy of these treatments in pregnancy are limited [204]. In nonpregnant patients, there is good evidence that laxatives are beneficial in the treatment of symptomatic hemorrhoids [207]. In severely symptomatic patients, hemorrhoidectomy may be considered [208].

Anal fissures

Anal fissures are linear splits or breaches in the long axis of the lower anal canal that are thought to be due to increased tonicity of the internal anal sphincter [209]. Patients with anal fissures present with pain, itching and bleeding of varying severity. It is estimated that up to 15% of women suffer from anal fissures post partum [210]. The pathogenesis of anal fissures in pregnancy is unclear as studies have not shown a correlation between anal canal pressures and the development of fissures, and pressures have in fact been shown to drop in the puerperium.

None of the treatment modalities that are typically used for the treatment of anal fissures has been studied in pregnancy. However, it is generally advised that constipation be treated aggressively with laxatives during pregnancy and the puerperium to avoid development of fissures [211].

Proctitis

The incidence of proctitis in pregnancy is unknown. It typically presents with urgency of defecation, frequent possible bloody small volume stools and tenesmus Causes include *de novo* or flare of known inflammatory bowel disease, infection and ischemia. Infectious pathogens that cause proctitis are typically sexually transmitted [212]. These include herpes simplex virus, gonorrhea, syphilis, *Chlamydia trachomatis* (nonlymphogranuloma venereum), and lymphogranuloma venereum.

The evaluation of proctitis begins with history, physical exam, rectal cultures and stool studies. Proctoscopy and/or sigmoidoscopy is often necessary for accurate diagnosis. Treatment is determined by the underlying cause.

Sphincter injuries

Vaginal childbirth is associated with anal sphincter trauma in 2.2–18% of deliveries [213,214]. Complications may arise immediately or decades after the injury. These complications include perineal pain, dyspareunia, urinary and defecatory dysfunction, and urinary and fecal incontinence. Many do not seek medical attention because of embarrassment. Risk factors for anal sphincter tears are primiparity, macrosomia, midline episiotomy, operative vaginal delivery, epidural analgesia and prolonged second stage of labor [215,216].

Patients should be evaluated for patulous anus, diminished rectal tone, and impacted stool on physical exam [203]. Neurologic exam for the assessment of sensation and normal reflexes (anal wink) should also be performed. Anorectal manometry, endoanal ultrasound and most recently MRI with endoanal coil are used to quantify the degree of sphincter dysfunction and help predict who may benefit from surgery [217–219].

Treatments for sphincter injuries include dietary modification, biofeedback, stool-bulking agents, and antidiarrheals. Patients who do not respond to medical management may require surgical sphincter repair.

Malignancy

Gastric cancer in pregnancy

Gastric cancer, usually a disease of the middle-aged and elderly population, occurs in Japan with a relatively high incidence, where 200–300 pregnant women per year are likely to have gastric cancer [220]. Most of the literature concerning gastric cancer in pregnancy is based upon the Japanese experience. Diagnosis requires endoscopy and treatment is usually surgical, although recent evidence shows improvement in survival with adjuvant chemotherapy. The prognosis for patients diagnosed with gastric cancer in pregnancy is poor, with the majority dying in the first year after diagnosis. Fetal survival has been favorable in studies, particularly when maternal diagnosis of cancer was made in late gestation [221].

Colon cancer in pregnancy

Although colon cancer is the third most common cause of cancer death in women, its occurrence before age 40 is uncommon and incidence in pregnancy is rare. However, when it does occur in pregnancy, its diagnosis can pose a challenge, as presenting signs and symptoms are all too common in normal pregnancy. These include abdominal pain, rectal bleeding, nausea, vomiting, constipation, abdominal distension, fatigue and iron deficiency anemia. In order to make the diagnosis of cancer at an early stage, clinicians must be aware of these potential warning signs and symptoms. Rectal bleeding is a particularly ominous sign and must never be attributed solely to pregnancy without proper evaluation.

The diagnosis of colorectal cancer involves endoscopy with biopsy, abdominal imaging and serum carcinoembryonic antigen (CEA) level. The safety of endosocopic and radiologic procedures in pregnancy is discussed elsewhere. CEA level is useful as a prognostic indicator and to detect recurrences but not as a screening test. It is unaffected by pregnancy. Treatment in the pregnant patient includes surgery, adjuvant chemotherapy and radiation, nutritional support and delivery when indicated or termination based upon maternal choice. Fetal prognosis depends on the pathologic stage of maternal cancer, gestational age at diagnosis and type and timing of therapy. Overall, fetal prognosis from maternal colon cancer is relatively favorable as most cases are diagnosed near term. Maternal prognosis is generally poor, attributable to delayed diagnosis and advanced pathologic stage at diagnosis, with 5-year survival rates reportedly ranging from 0% to 42% [222,223].

Common nonobstetric causes of abdominal pain

Acute abdominal pain from any cause may present coincidentally in pregnancy. Some clinical conditions are more likely to occur in pregnancy. Other conditions are specific to pregnancy. Box 10.7 lists several conditions both obstetric and nonobstetric which may present with abdominal pain. The most common causes of abdominal pain in pregnancy are uterine contractions and constipation. Common surgical conditions causing abdominal pain in the pregnant patient include appendicitis, gallbladder disease and pancreatitis. Some common causes of acute abdomen are described below. Cholecystitis and pancreatitis are discussed in Chapter 9.

Appendicitis

Appendicitis is the most common cause of acute abdomen in pregnancy, occurring with a frequency of 1 in 500–2000 pregnancies. The diagnosis of appendicitis in pregnancy can be challenging because of blunting of the signs and symptoms during pregnancy. Furthermore, with advancing gestation, appendiceal location may change, making the presentation atypical.

The single most reliable symptom in pregnant patients with appendicitis is right lower quadrant pain. Rebound tenderness and guarding are not very specific because of the distension of the abdominal wall muscles and interposition of the uterus between the appendix and the anterior abdominal wall. Likewise, anorexia and vomiting, though common in pregnant women with appendicitis, are neither specific nor sensitive predictors. Pain from a retrocecal appendix may result in flank or back pain, which is often confused with urinary tract infection or pyelonephritis. White blood cell counts as high as $17,000/mm^3$ may be normal in pregnancy. Therefore leukocytosis may not be very helpful in diagnosis. However, a left shift may suggest an infectious etiology and a white blood cell count persistently less than $10,000/mm^3$ may give reassurance.

Graded compression ultrasound is the diagnostic procedure of choice and has a sensitivity of 86% in the nonpregnant population. It has been shown to be accurate in the first and second trimesters but technical difficulties limit its usefulness in the third trimester. Helical CT has the potential advantages of rapidity and safety when compared with standard CT, with fetal radiation exposure limited to 0.3 rads [224]. However, the largest case series looking at this technique in pregnant patients included only seven women. Magnetic resonance imaging is emerging as an excellent modality for excluding appendicitis in pregnant women, with an overall sensitivity of 100% and a specificity of 94% in one study of 51 pregnant patients who were clinically suspected to have appendicitis but had inconclusive ultrasound images [225].

Box 10.7 Obstetric and nonobstetric causes of abdominal pain in pregnancy

Causes of acute abdomen not related to pregnancy

Gastrointestinal:
- Acute appendicitis
- Acute pancreatitis
- Peptic ulcer
- Acute cholecystitis
- Bowel obstruction
- Bowel perforation
- Herniation
- Meckel diverticulitis
- Toxic megacolon
- Pancreatic pseudocyst

Genitourinary:
- Acute cystitis
- Acute pyelonephritis
- Ovarian cyst rupture
- Adnexal torsion
- Ureteral calculus
- Rupture of renal pelvis
- Ureteral obstruction

Vascular:
- Superior mesenteric artery syndrome
- Mesenteric venous thrombosis
- Ruptured visceral artery aneurysm

Other:
- Intraperitoneal hemorrhage
- Splenic rupture
- Abdominal trauma
- Acute intermittent porphyria
- Diabetic ketoacidosis
- Sickle cell disease

Conditions that can present with acute abdomen during pregnancy

- Acute fatty liver of pregnancy
- Rupture of rectus abdominis muscle
- Torsion of the pregnant uterus
- Ruptured ectopic or heterotopic pregnancy
- Septic abortion with peritonitis
- Red degeneration of myoma
- Torsion of pedunculated myoma
- Placental abruption
- Placenta percreta
- HELLP (hemolysis, elevated liver function, and low platelets) syndrome – spontaneous rupture of the liver
- Uterine rupture
- Chorio-amnionitis

Both fetal and maternal mortality from appendicitis have dropped sharply over the past 30 years. However, when perforation occurs, fetal loss may be as high as 35%, in contrast to 1.5% when no perforation has occurred. Appendiceal rupture is twice as likely in the third trimester as in the first and second trimesters. Overall, preterm labor and delivery are not common. Maternal death from appendicitis is a rarity but when it does occur, it is usually associated with significant surgical delay.

If laparoscopic surgery is to be performed in pregnancy, open laparoscopy is recommended to avoid trocar or Veress needle injury to the uterus. In the late second trimester and beyond, laparoscopy becomes technically difficult and an open appendectomy or a vertical midline incision (when diagnosis is doubtful) is advisable. In cases with perforation and diffuse peritonitis, copious irrigation, intraperitoneal drain and broad-spectrum antibiotics, including anaerobic coverage, are recommended. Diagnosis of chorio-amnionitis can be difficult due to generalized peritoneal inflammation and abdominal tenderness. Assessment of amniotic fluid is often avoided in cases of suspected appendiceal rupture due to concern about contamination from passing the needle through an infected peritoneal cavity. Other clinical signs such as fetal tachycardia or a poor biophysical assessment may suggest chorio-amnionitis and justify obtaining an amniocentesis or moving towards delivery rather than appendectomy.

Intestinal obstruction

Bowel obstruction is the third most common cause of acute abdomen during pregnancy and occurs in 1 in 1500–16,000 pregnancies. Adhesions from previous abdominal or pelvic surgery or pelvic inflammatory disease are the most common cause, followed by volvulus (torsion of the bowel, most typically the cecum or sigmoid colon) The incidence of volvulus is greatest at times of rapid uterine size changes, especially between 16 and 20 weeks, when the uterus becomes an intra-abdominal organ, 32 and 36 weeks, as the fetus enters the pelvis, and in the puerperium, when uterine size changes rapidly again. Other causes of bowel obstruction such as intussusception (invagination of part of the intestine into itself), hernia, cancer and diverticulitis are rare. Endometriosis and multiple pregnancies may be predisposing factors. Cecal volvulus and pseudo-obstruction of the colon (Ogilvie's syndrome: dilation of the right hemicolon and cecum in the absence of anatomic obstruction) are recognized complications of cesarean section.

The incidence of bowel obstruction has risen over the years because of an increase in the number of abdominal operations performed that cause adhesions. It is being increasingly recognized as a complication of gastric bypass surgery, particularly when laproscopic technique is utilized [226]. As with appendicitis, the morbidity and mortality of bowel obstruction are related to diagnostic and therapeutic delay. Mortality from bowel obstruction is much higher in pregnancy than in the general population, with dramatic progression of fetal mortality with advancing gestation.

Typical symptoms of bowel obstruction in pregnancy include crampy abdominal pain, obstipation and vomiting. High obstruction is characterized by diffuse, poorly localized upper abdominal cramps that occur frequently, nausea and vomiting. In contrast, colonic obstruction may manifest as low abdominal or perineal pain with longer interval (15–20 minutes) between pain attacks. On physical exam, the abdomen is distended and tender. Fever, leukocytosis and electrolyte abnormalities increase the likelihood of finding intestinal strangulation.

If intestinal obstruction is suspected, upright and flat plain abdominal films should be obtained. Presence of air–fluid levels or progressive bowel dilation in serial films obtained at 4–6-hour intervals are diagnostic. Radiologic studies with use of contrast media should be performed if bowel obstruction is still suspected in the absence of typical findings on plain abdominal films. The significant maternal and fetal mortalities associated with obstruction outweigh the potential risk of fetal radiation exposure. Colonoscopy is especially useful in diagnosis and reduction of colonic volvulus.

Management of bowel obstruction in pregnancy is essentially similar to management in the nonpregnant population. Initial therapy is conservative and includes fluid and electrolyte replacement, nasogastric suction for bowel decompression and enemas. The amount of fluid lost is often underestimated and may result in renal insufficiency, hypovolemia, shock and death. A Foley catheter should be placed to monitor urine output. Close monitoring of maternal oxygenation and fetal status is indicated. Endoscopic decompression may be successful in colonic pseudo-obstruction. Unsuccessful medical treatment or fever, tachycardia and progressive leukocytosis in association with abdominal pain and tenderness warrants early surgical exploration. A midline vertical incision is recommended. If necrotic bowel is identified, segmental resection is indicated. Broad-spectrum antibiotics are recommended preoperatively and before endoscopic intervention in view of the high morbidity and mortality associated with bowel ischemia and infarction.

Intestinal infarction

Intestinal ischemia is caused by decreased mesenteric blood flow which can arise from emboli, arterial or venous thrombi or hypoperfusion. The clinical consequences can be catastrophic, including sepsis, bowel infarction and death, with mortality rates as high as 93%. Diagnosis before intestinal infarction is the single most important factor for improving mortality rate.

Bowel ischemia can occur in the setting of abdominal trauma, infection, sickle cell disease, atrial fibrillation, endocarditis, pancreatitis or malignancy. It has been reported as a complication of cesarean section, in pregnant women with prior gastric bypass surgery and in patients with thrombotic microangiopathy (TTP, HUS or HELLP). Patients with acute mesenteric ischemia have been classically described as having a rapid onset of severe periumbilical abdominal pain, which is often out of proportion to findings on physical examination. Nausea and vomiting are also common. Findings on physical exam may be nonspecific, including mild abdominal distension and/or occult blood in stool, and may be overshadowed by development of acute hypovolemic shock in some patients. Diagnosis depends upon a high clinical suspicion and early performance of CT, angiogram or laparotomy. An elevation in serum lactate can be helpful in suggesting this diagnosis. Management includes fluid resuscitation and correction of underlying risk factors, embolectomy, thrombolytic agents or heparin and/or surgical resection.

Nutrition in pregnancy

Proper nutritional intake is believed to be important for optimal pregnancy outcomes. However, the minimum nutritional requirements to achieve these outcomes are yet to be determined. It is clear that severe caloric restriction (450 cal/day) in late pregnancy, as in the Dutch Famine (1944–45), can result in decreased birthweight [227], but the minimum caloric requirement is unknown. A direct association between maternal weight gain and birthweight has been demonstrated and an increased caloric intake of 340 cal/d during the second trimester, and 450 cal/d in the third trimester, to accommodate the increased energy requirements is recommended [228]. The Institute of Medicine recommendation for weight gain during pregnancy for normal Body Mass Index (BMI)(20–26 kg/m^2) is 11–16 kg. Women starting with a low BMI should gain an extra 2 kg while women starting with increased BMI should reduce their weight gain target by 4–5 kg [229].

Specific nutritional requirements

The exact nutritional requirements during pregnancy are unknown. General recommendations can be made based on total body and placental content at term for some common elements. Calcium is required by the fetus for normal metabolic function and development of the musculoskeletal system. It is estimated that total fetal calcium requirements are 20–30 g for a normally grown fetus. In order to achieve this without resulting in a net maternal loss of calcium stores and bone loss, an estimated daily intake of 1000 mg/d is required. For individuals such as teenagers who are also growing, an additional 300 mg/d may be required to maintain a positive maternal calcium balance.

An estimated 800 mg of iron is needed during gestation to account for fetal and maternal demands. A term fetus and placenta contain approximately 300 mg of iron. The increase in maternal red cell mass accounts for 500 mg of iron. Maternal total iron stores are estimated at 500 mg, therefore a single pregnancy will consume all maternal stores. It is estimated that a daily intake of 30 mg of iron should be sufficient to meet increased demand during pregnancy.

Additional nutrient requirements are unknown although folic acid supplementation prior to pregnancy and during the first trimester can improve pregnancy outcome [230]. Folic acid supplementation of 400 µg per day has been shown to reduce the risk of neural tube defects in the general population. Higher consumption is recommended for individuals at high risk for neural tube defects including those with a family history or those on medications that affect folate metabolism (Table 10.7).

Vitamin D supplementation is also highly recommended during pregnancy to enhance calcium absorption, especially for those with limited sun exposure. Vitamin D deficiency is estimated to be as high as 40% of the population in northern latitudes [228].

Fetal considerations

Gastrointestinal disorders during pregnancy can be associated with nutritional deficiencies that increase the risk of adverse outcomes. Malabsorption syndromes can lead to nutritional deficiencies that affect fetal growth. In pregnancies where nutritional deficiency is likely, an early ultrasound is generally recommended to more accurately define the gestational age. Serial growth measurement by ultrasound examination is also suggested beginning in the third trimester where nutritional deficiencies are most likely to have an impact. Examinations are commonly performed at 2–4-week intervals due to the increased variability of growth in the third trimester. The value of other antenatal testing in the absence of fetal growth restriction is unclear but it may be warranted in specific circumstances. When fetal growth restriction is identified consultation evaluation for other etiologies should be considered. Additional monitoring may be warranted when fetal growth restriction is identified.

Nutritional deficiencies and medication exposure can be associated with an increased risk for fetal malformations. The appropriate screening technique should be considered based on the specific risk. In patients likely to have alterations in folate or folate metabolism, maternal serum alpha-fetoprotein should be discussed and offered. Fetal ultrasound may be warranted when specific anomalies are associated with a given medication. Patients should understand that the background risk for a major congenital malformation is in the range of 2–3% and for minor malformations as high as 8–10%.

Bariatric procedures

The incidence of obesity continues to increase in developed countries throughout the world. Obesity, defined as a BMI of greater than 30 kg/m^2, afflicts almost one-third of adults in the United States and one-fifth of western Europeans. This incidence continues to rise and is currently twice the rate reported three decades ago. Surgical treatment for morbid obesity has become more popular over the past decade, with more than 100,000 procedures being performed in the United States during 2004, a significant increase from less than 14,000 in 1998 [231]. Bariatric procedures can be categorized into three main types: restrictive, restrictive-malabsorptive, and malabsorptive [232]. Each of these categories poses unique risks to women conceiving after undergoing these procedures. This section will be devoted to addressing the risks that are imposed after bariatric surgery.

Maternal obesity in pregnancy is associated with adverse pregnancy outcomes which can be attributed to both obesity and related co-morbidities such as hypertension and diabetes

Table 10.7 Folic acid supplementation before, during and after pregnancy

Period	No risk factors	With additional risk factors
Periconception	400 µg	Family history or prior child with neural tube defect: 4 mg (4000 µg)
Pregnancy	400 µg	Disorder or medication affecting folate metabolism: ≥400 µg
With lactation	≥300 µg	Not applicable

mellitus. Improvement in co-morbid conditions associated with obesity has been widely reported in patients undergoing bariatric procedures, which has been a major impetus for their performance and popularity. Ovulatory dysfunction related to obesity will improve after surgery, thus increasing the likelihood of pregnancy. Contraceptive counseling is therefore an important issue to discuss in reproductive-age women prior to and immediately after bariatric surgery.

Although the surgical literature describes many different approaches to bariatric surgery, three main anatomic alterations are the foundation of all techniques: gastric banding, Roux-en-Y gastric bypass, and biliopancreatic diversion [232] (Figure 10.1). Understanding these three basic surgical procedures and their physiologic effects on nutritional status will help in appropriate monitoring and treatment of the maternal and fetal condition during gestation. To date, a limited number of case series and case–control studies have been reported in pregnant patients who have undergone bariatric procedures. It is expected that more reports will ensue over the next decade as the number of women undergoing these procedures increases.

Gastric banding

Gastric banding procedures continue to gain popularity and have proven efficacy for marked weight reduction. These procedures are commonly performed through a laparoscopic approach that allows for shorter operating times and more rapid postoperative recovery rates. The general procedure involves reducing stomach capacity. This is accomplished by creating a small gastric pouch with volumes of 30–50 mL. This can be performed by stapling and banding the stomach or by placement of a band around the fundus just below the gastroesophageal junction to create an appropriate sized pouch.

A variety of banding devices have been introduced that include adjustable bands allowing for variation of stomach capacity. The adjustable gastric bands can be deflated during pregnancy to allow for greater food intake. Anecdotal evidence indicates that adjustment of these bands often provides symptomatic improvement of generalized nausea during pregnancy.

Of the three basic procedures, gastric banding provides the least alteration in physiology. This procedure does not divert food from the main gastrointestinal absorptive regions. Nutritional deficiencies that may occur are usually corrected by simple oral supplementation. The main alteration is related to limited caloric intake because of the restrictive nature of this procedure. Late postoperative complications include band displacement [233] esophageal dilation, pouch dilation and port infections in those patients with adjustable gastric bands [234]. Band removal or surgical revision is necessary in 3–6% of patients [233,234].

Roux-en-Y

The Roux-en-Y induces weight loss through a combined restrictive and malabsorptive mechanism. The procedure involves creation of a small gastric pouch that is anastomosed to the distal jejunum. While the gastric pouch acts to restrict oral intake, attachment of the pouch to the distal jejunum results in a significant reduction of nutrient absorption. Iron, vitamin B12, calcium, and vitamin D absorption are particularly affected since the duodenum, which is bypassed in the Roux-en-Y technique, plays a major role in the absorption of these nutrients. In addition, reduced gastric acidity impairs the reduction of iron from its ferric form to the readily absorbable ferrous form. Gastric acidity also plays an important role in the release of vitamin B12 from binding proteins allowing absorption.

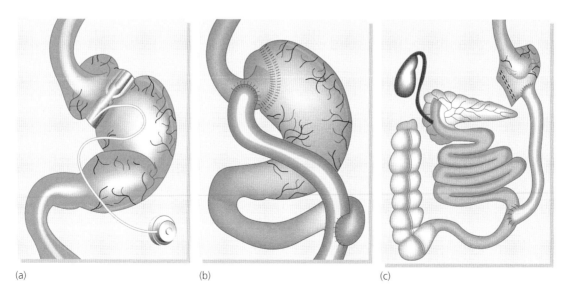

(a)   (b)   (c)

Figure 10.1 (a) Adjustable gastric banding; (b) Roux-en-Y gastric banding; (c) Biliopancreatic diversion.

The Roux-en-Y gastric bypass procedure is effective for weight reduction but is associated with a greater risk of nutrient deficiency than gastric banding procedures. It may be performed in patients who have failed or required reoperation after a gastric banding procedure. Complications of the Roux-en-Y procedure include internal hernias which have also been reported during pregnancy [235]. Patients who have undergone a Roux-en-Y procedure in the past, presenting with abdominal pain during pregnancy, should be evaluated for intestinal obstruction.

Biliopancreatic diversion

This procedure induces weight loss mainly through disruption of nutrient absorption. A portion of the stomach is removed to reduce volume and the duodenum is divided proximal to the common bile duct and anastomosed to the ileum for nutrient absorption. The remaining duodenum and jejunum is then anastomosed to the terminal ileum to allow egress of biliary and pancreatic secretions. As in the Roux-en-Y procedure, physiologic alterations of anatomy in biliopancreatic diversion lead to significant nutritional deficiencies. Besides calcium, iron and vitamin B12 deficiency, interference with the absorption of fat-soluble vitamins A, E, K and greater deficiencies in vitamin D can occur with biliopancreatic diversion procedures. Polyneuropathies and Wernicke–Korsakoff syndrome related to the severe nutritional deficiencies have been reported. Risk of internal hernias exists with this procedure also.

Management

Preconception

Women undergoing bariatric surgery are commonly counseled to avoid pregnancy during the first 12–18 months following their surgical procedure due to the negative energy balance and potential effects of nutritional deficiency during this period. Printen reported on a series of patients during the rapid weight loss period and found no increased incidence in adverse maternal or fetal outcomes [236]. Dao compared patients conceiving during the first year after bariatric surgery to those conceiving after 1 year and also noted no difference in outcomes [237]. Although concern is warranted for adverse fetal effects from nutritional deficiency during the rapid weight loss period after bariatric surgery, pregnancy outcomes do not appear worse if conception occurs shortly after the bariatric procedure.

Nutritional supplementation with multivitamins containing B vitamins, vitamin C, fat-soluble vitamins (A, D, E and K) and minerals is recommended for all women after bariatric surgery although studies demonstrate a high rate of discontinuation. Evaluation and supplementation of the appropriate micronutrients should be based on the type of bariatric procedure performed. Woodard has recommended general supplementation with folic acid (0.5–1.0 mg daily), vitamin B12

(1000–2000 μg sublingually daily), calcium (1200–1500 mg daily), vitamin D (800 IU total daily) and iron (ferrous sulfate 325 mg up to tid). Folic acid deficiency has been associated with an increased risk of open neural tube defects and adequate levels of this vitamin are essential for good pregnancy outcome. Higher doses than 0.5–1.0 mg daily may be recommended based on past obstetric history or other risk factors for folate deficiency. Iron supplementation should be provided in the ferrous form to improve absorption. Calcium citrate is the most readily absorbable form of calcium. Crystalline vitamin B12 is most readily absorbed but its absorption is diminished in the absence of an acidic environment and parenteral supplementation by monthly injections of vitamin B12 (1000 μg intramuscularly once a month) may sometimes be necessary. In patients who have undergone biliopancreatic diversion, ensuring adequate levels of the fat-soluble vitamins is particularly important.

Antenatal

Increased incidence of fetal growth abnormalities has been reported in patients who have undergone bariatric surgery. The incidence of fetal growth restriction has been reported to be greater after bariatric surgery, particularly after biliopancreatic diversion [238]. Fetal macrosomia is commonly associated with maternal obesity and glucose intolerance. It can be challenging to evaluate fetal growth by clinical exam in women who are obese. Serial ultrasound examinations during the third trimester can facilitate this. The utility of antenatal testing such as nonstress tests is unclear in the absence of fetal growth restriction or other complicating conditions.

Obesity is a major risk factor for diabetes mellitus. Bariatric surgery can improve or normalize blood sugar in many individuals. Because of the increased risk of adverse pregnancy outcomes, screening for diabetes mellitus in the first trimester with an oral glucose tolerance test is warranted. In those women who have a normal evaluation, repeat testing in the early third trimester should also be performed. Gestational diabetes screening can be a challenge in individuals who have undergone bariatric surgery. It is generally not recommended for these individuals to consume liquids containing high levels of simple sugars due to the risk of dumping syndrome. Evaluation for diabetes can be performed by obtaining fasting and 2-hour postprandial blood sugar measurements and glycosylated hemoglobin levels. Since gestational diabetes is usually due to insulin resistance, evaluation of postprandial values can be substituted for standard glucose tolerance tests.

Weight gain in the range of 25–35 pounds is often recommended in low-risk uncomplicated pregnancies. In patients who are obese, recommendations are often reduced based on BMI. No clear recommendations are available for women after bariatric surgery. Weight loss is generally not recommended during pregnancy. However, there is no evidence to suggest that continued weight loss in patients with an elevated BMI increases adverse pregnancy outcomes if micronutrient supplementation is adequate.

Small bowel obstructions due to internal hernias have been reported in both pregnant and nonpregnant patients who have undergone Roux-en-Y gastric bypass procedures. Other complications including intussusception, stomal stenosis, gastric band slippage and gastric prolapse and leakage are also possible remote from the initial surgery Delays in diagnosis and intervention may occur because clinicians may incorrectly attribute their patient's symptoms to obstetric or normal pregnancy effects. Early involvement of bariatric surgeons is prudent when a pregnant patient who has undergone gastric bypass surgery presents with nausea, vomiting and/or abdominal pain.

Intrapartum and postpartum factors

Bariatric surgery prior to the ongoing pregnancy does not alter intrapartum risks. The risk for gastric reflux during the intrapartum period after the various bariatric procedures has not yet been studied. Its likelihood may, however, be reduced due to restricted gastric volume and smaller amount of intake.

Breastfeeding is not contraindicated in patients with prior bariatric surgery although nutritional status can affect the nutritional value of breast milk. Failure to thrive and megaloblastic anemia have been reported in breastfed infants.

Contraceptive choices are unchanged in patients who have undergone bariatric surgery. The efficacy of different methods may vary based on maternal weight.

Special considerations in antenatal care, labor and delivery, and puerperal care of patients with stomas

Gastrointestinal and urinary diversions may result in an ostomy that can complicate pregnancy. Pregnancy in patients with a stoma will often require attention based on case series and surveys [239]. The types of complications reported by women with stomas and ongoing pregnancies include problems with the stomal appliance, obstruction, prolapse, peristomal hernia, stomal bleeding, and stomal retraction [239]. Few of these problems required revision during or after pregnancy. The presence of a stoma is not a contraindication to a vaginal delivery. However, the complication that initiated the requirement for a stoma may be a reason to avoid a vaginal delivery and needs to be considered individually.

Stomal therapists should be consulted to assist with patients who have complications with their stomal appliance. The most frequently reported complication related to stomas in pregnancy is a poorly fitting appliance that causes skin irritation. Pregnancy will often induce changes in skin texture and stomal conformation that require changes in adhesive or pouch appliance [240]. As the abdomen increases in size, the stomal shape may change, leading to a poorly fitted pouch. Skin changes due to changes in the hormonal environment can affect appliance adhesion.

Stomal complications requiring intervention occur in the minority of pregnancies but include obstruction, prolapse, peristomal herniation, and stomal retractions in decreasing frequency. In a survey of 54 respondents, obstructive complaints occurred in one-quarter of women, with only one requiring surgery [239]. Obstructions occurred more commonly in the third trimester than at earlier time points and responded to either suction or lavage. Obstructive symptoms also resolved after delivery. Stomal prolapse was the second most frequent complaint and it also usually resolved after delivery. Positional changes with manipulation and supportive clothes often provided palliative therapy during the course of the pregnancy. A peristomal hernia occurring during pregnancy was the complication that most commonly persisted post partum and required surgical correction after delivery in 50% of individuals. There appeared to be no difference in complication rates in individuals having continent pouches compared to other types of stomas.

Endoscopy in pregnancy and lactation

It is estimated that 20,000 women undergo endoscopy during pregnancy each year [241]. Although the safety of endoscopy in pregnancy has not been firmly established, it may be performed if the indication is clear and the risk of not performing the procedure exposes the mother and/or fetus to harm [242]. Accepted indications for endoscopy in pregnancy are summarized in Box 10.8.

Esophagogastroduodenoscopy (EGD), sigmoidoscopy, colonoscopy, percutaneous gastrostomy and endoscopic retrograde cholangiopancreatography (ERCP) may all be safely performed in pregnancy [243–246]. Nevertheless, endoscopy in pregnancy is not without risk and if not properly performed may increase

---

Box 10.8 Indications for endoscopy in pregnancy

- Significant or continued GI bleeding
- Severe or refractory nausea and vomiting or abdominal pain
- Dysphagia or odynophagia
- Strong suspicion of mass in colon
- Severe diarrhea with negative evaluation
- Biliary pancreatitis, choledocholithiasis or cholangitis
- Biliary or pancreatic ductal injury

Reproduced with permission from Qureshi *et al.* [242].

Box 10.9 General guidelines for endoscopy in pregnancy

- Have a strong indication for the procedure, particularly in high-risk pregnancies
- Defer endoscopy to second trimester whenever possible
- Use lowest effective dose of sedative medications
- Use category A or B drugs when possible
- Position patients in left pelvic tilt or left lateral position to avoid vena caval or aortic compression
- Confirm presence of fetal heart tones before giving sedation and at the conclusion of the procedure
- Obtain obstetric support
- Do not perform endoscopy if obstetric complications such as placental abruption, imminent delivery, rupture membranes or eclampsia are present

Reproduced with permission from Qureshi *et al.* [242].

the risk of abortion, stillbirth, low birthweight, congenital abnormality, and neurodevelopmental delay [247]. In cases of placental abruption, imminent delivery, rupture of the membranes or eclampsia, endoscopy should be avoided as the risk of complication increases significantly. As with all invasive procedures in pregnancy, a careful evaluation of the risks and benefits of the procedure with full disclosure to the patient should be carried out in advance (Box 10.9).

Some institutions have adopted protocols for fetal monitoring during surgery in pregnant patients. Continuous fetal heart tone monitoring should be considered after the age of viability when there is a risk for hemodynamic instability. Vital sign monitoring and general observation of the pregnant patient should be continued until the effects of sedation have worn off. Fetal well-being is commonly evaluated prior to discharge in viable pregnancies. It is generally recommended to discuss the patient's obstetric options prior to any procedure in the event of an unexpected complication. Qualified medical personnel should be present to read the tracings if continuous monitoring is performed in the endoscopy suite and to provide obstetric management if needed.

General considerations

Endoscopic procedures (with the exception of flexible sigmoidoscopy) generally require conscious sedation. Most drugs for conscious sedation in nonpregnant patients are

suitable for pregnant patients as well. The most commonly used agents in the US are the combination of a narcotic agent and a benzodiazepine. Previous concerns over an association between benzodiazepines and cleft lip and palate deformities [248,249] were likely confounded, and short-term use of midazolam or diazepam for sedation is safe [250]. Short-acting opioids (fentanyl), morphine or meperidine are also commonly employed [251].

If personnel with advanced airway management skills are available, propofol is an excellent short-acting sedative with minimal side effects which has been used extensively for deep sedation [252].

As the fetus is sensitive to maternal hypoxia and hypotension, care must be taken to avoid maternal oversedation and inappropriate positioning. Supplemental oxygen by nasal cannula should be used in all cases to maintain adequate oxygenation, and continuous pulse oximetry should be performed [252]. In addition, women in the second and third trimesters of pregnancy should avoid lying supine before, during or after endoscopy to prevent compression of the inferior vena cava with resulting hypotension and decreased placental perfusion. Care must be taken to place patients in the left lateral decubitus position and/or place a wedge or pillow under the right hip to create a pelvic tilt that displaces the uterus off the inferior vena cava [242]. Abdominal pressure, if required during colonoscopy, should be directed away from the uterus to avoid uterine trauma [247].

Special considerations: endoscopic retrograde cholangiopancreatography

Endoscopic retrograde cholangiopancreatography (ERCP) may be required in pregnancy. Physiologic changes predispose women to gallstone formation in pregnancy and 0.1% of pregnant women develop symptomatic disease requiring emergency intervention. The indications for ERCP are discussed in Chapter 9. The key consideration in ERCP in pregnancy is to minimize radiation exposure as ionizing radiation poses a significant risk of teratogenesis. Only highly trained endoscopists with experience in endoscopy in the pregnant patient should perform this procedure. The fetus should be shielded with lead placed under the maternal pelvis and possibly over the lower abdomen to minimize fetal radiation exposure [253]. Pulse rather than continuous fluoroscopy should be used and still images should be avoided. Radiation exposure to the uterus should be recorded by placing a dosimeter on the maternal abdomen. The radiation dose to the fetus is taken to be half of the skin dose to account for attenuation by soft tissues between the fetus and skin surface [254]. Biliary sphincterotomy when necessary should be performed with the grounding pad away from the uterus to avoid the conduction of electrical current through the amniotic fluid to the fetus [251].

Lactation considerations

Endoscopy can be performed safely in the lactating mother with minimal risk to the infant if care is taken to avoid rapid breastfeeding after the procedure, depending on the medications received [251]. Fentanyl is found in low levels in breast milk and is therefore compatible with nursing. Meperidine and midazolam are found in higher levels in breast milk [255]. Therefore, it is advised that women receiving meperidine and/or midazolam abstain from nursing for a minimum of 4 hours, to avoid transfer of the drug to the infant through breast milk. Mothers should "pump and dump" during this period and feed with previously stored breast milk or formula.

Anesthetic considerations when caring for women with gatrointestinal disease in pregnancy

Patients undergoing laparoscopic or open surgical procedures will require anesthesia. General considerations for anesthesia in pregnancy are discussed in Chapter 29, but gastrointestinal procedures pose some unique considerations with respect to securing the airway, prevention of pulmonary aspiration of gastric contents, positioning, and protecting the fetus.

Gastrointestinal procedures may pose special airway considerations. Friable mucosa may lead to bleeding during upper endoscopic procedures, potentially compromising the airway. The emergency nature of abdominal surgery in pregnancy (appendectomy, bowel obstruction, gastrointestinal bleeding) adds to the already elevated risk of difficult endotracheal intubation.

Fasted healthy pregnant women do not experience any change in gastric emptying or gastric acid production. Early investigations suggested that pregnancy itself impaired gastric emptying but more recent studies contradict this finding. Using the paracetomol (acetaminophen) absorption methodology, Macfie found no significant differences in gastric emptying between nonpregnant women and pregnant women at any gestation other than a slight change in first-trimester women undergoing termination (which was attributed to anxiety) [256]. Similarly, Whitehead found no changes from nonpregnant women in any trimester or >18 hours post partum [257]. Using ultrasound, Wong found normal gastric emptying of 50 mL of water, and *enhanced* gastric emptying (i.e. below baseline volume) after 300 mL of water in both normal and obese pregnant patients [258,259]. Carp similarly found no solid food in the stomach 4 hours after a standardized meal in nonpregnant or near-term pregnant women, but did observe solid food up to 24 hours after ingestion in *laboring* women [260]. Because of these findings, the American Society of Anesthesiologists recommends fasting prior to elective procedures for 6–8 hours in pregnancy, similar to the

guidelines in nonpregnant women [261]. Women in labor are generally considered to have "full stomachs" regardless of the interval of fasting. In addition, drugs used for sedation, particularly opioids, also retard gastric emptying [262].

Nonetheless, some nonlaboring pregnant women may be at elevated risk of aspiration of gastric contents. First, the expanding uterus displaces the gastroesophogeal junction, decreasing the efficiency of the lower esophageal high pressure zone. Second, many patients with conditions discussed in this chapter will have gastrointestinal pathology which impedes gastric emptying. Third, the position required for many procedures increases the chance of passive regurgitation. In such cases, many anesthesiologists prefer aspiration prophylaxis. Use of a nonparticulate antacid, possibly the use of prokinetic agents (e.g. metoclopramide) or drugs to reduce acid production (H2 blockers, PPI), and the use of cricoid pressure and a cuffed endotracheal tube during induction of general anesthesia are common [263].

Protecting the fetus from the untoward effects of anesthesia is discussed in detail elsewhere. Gastrointestinal procedures produce a few special considerations as well. First, positioning during any procedure should accommodate uterine displacement to avoid vena caval compression. As stated above, endoscopic procedures that are commonly performed in the prone position (e.g. ERCP) may need to be modified to avoid compression of the gravid uterus or else special precautions must be taken to allow prone positioning. Second, many anesthesiologists prefer the use of fetal heart rate monitoring during general anesthesia when the fetus is viable. Most intra-abdominal procedures discussed in this chapter make such monitoring impractical, so meticulous attention to uterine displacement, hemodynamics, oxygenation and ventilation is required [264]. Third, laparoscopic procedures carry some theoretical risks, largely demonstrated in animal models. Anesthetic management for these procedures should include careful attention to maternal acid–base balance and end-tidal CO_2 concentration, use of the minimum sufficient insufflation pressure, and vigilance for signs of intra- and postoperative fetal hypoxia [265].

References

1. Torgerson RR, Marnach ML, Bruce AJ, Rogers RS 3rd. Oral and vulvar changes in pregnancy. Clin Dermatol 2006;24:122–32.
2. Laine MA. Effect of pregnancy on periodontal and dental health. Acta Odontol Scand 2002;60:257–64.
3. Muramatsu Y, Takaesu Y. Oral health status related to subgingival bacterial flora and sex hormones in slaiva during pregnancy. Bull Tokyo Dent Coll 1994;35:139–51.
4. Mahfouz SA, Sherif HA. A study of the lysosomal activity of human gingiva during pregnancy. Egypt Dent J 1985;31:83–92.
5. Richter JE. Review article: the management of heartburn in pregnancy. Aliment Pharmacol Ther 2005;23:749–57.
6. Richter JE. Medical management of patients with esophageal or supraesophageal gastroesophageal reflux disease. Am J Med 2003;115(suppl 3A):179S–187S.

7. Nagler R, Spiro HM. Heartburn in late pregnancy. Manometric studies of esophageal motor function. J Clin Invest 1961;40:954–70.

8. Davison JS, Davison MC, Hay DM. Gastric emptying time in late pregnancy and labour. J Obstet Gynaecol Br Commonw 1970;77:37–41.

9. Hunt JN, Murray FA. Gastric function in pregnancy. J Obstet Gynaecol Br Emp 1958;65:78–83.

10. Parry E, Shields R, Turnbull AC. Transit time in the small intestine in pregnancy. J Obstet Gynaecol Br Commonw 1970;77:900–1.

11. Wald A, van Thiel DH, Hoechstetter L, et al. Effect of pregnancy on gastrointestinal transit. Dig Dis Sci 1982;27:1015–18.

12. Lawson M, Kern F Jr, Everson GT. Gastrointestinal transit time in human pregnancy: prolongation in the second and third trimesters followed by postpartum normalization. Gastroenterology 1985;89:996–9.

13. Goodwin TM. Nausea and vomiting of pregnancy: an obstetric syndrome. Am J Obstet Gynecol 2002;186:S184–9.

14. Whitehead SA, Andrews PLR, Chamberlain GVP. Characteristics of nausea and vomiting in early pregnancy: a survey of 1000 women. J Obstet Gynaecol 1992;12(6):364–9.

15. Kumagami H, Loewenheim H, Beitz E, et al. The effect of antidiuretic hormone on the endolymphatic sac of the inner ear. Pflugers Arch 1998;436:970–5.

16. Koch KL, Stern RM, Vasey M, Botti JJ, Creasy GW, Dwyer A. Gastric dysrhythmias and nausea of pregnancy. Dig Dis Sci 1990;35:961–8.

17. Jednak MA, Shadigian EM, Kim MS, et al. Protein meals reduce nausea and gastric slow wave dysrhythmic activity in first trimester pregnancy. Am J Physiol 1999;277:G855–61.

18. Loe H, Silness J. Periodontal disease in pregnancy. Acta Odontol Scand 1963; 21:533.

19. Boggess KA, Lieff S, Murtha AP, Moss K, Beck J, Offenbacher S. Maternal periodontal disease is associated with an increased risk for preeclampsia. Obstet Gynecol 2003;101:227–31.

20. Goepfert AR, Jeffcoat MK, Andrews WW, et al. Periodontal disease and upper genital tract inflammation in early spontaneous preterm birth. Obstet Gynecol 2004;104:777–83.

21. Offenbacher S, Boggess KA, Murtha AP, et al. Progressive periodontal disease and risk of very preterm delivery. Obstet Gynecol 2006;107:29–36. (Erratum, Obstet Gynecol 2006;107:1171.)

22. Michalowicz BS, Hodges JS, DiAngelis AJ, et al. The Obstetrics and Periodontal Therapy Study. Treatment of periodontal disease and risk of preterm birth. N Engl J Med 2006;355(18)1885–94.

23. Richter JE. Gastroesphageal reflux during pregnancy. Gastroenterol Clin North Am 2003;32:235–61.

24. Marrero JM, Goggin PM, de Caestecker JS, et al. Determinants of pregnancy heartburn. Br J Obstet Gynaecol 1992;99:731–4.

25. Broussard CN, Richter JE. Treating gastro-oesphageal reflux disease during pregnancy and lactation: what are the safest therapy options? Drug Safety 1998;19:325–37.

26. Fisher RS, Robert GS, Grabowoski CJ, et al. Altered lower esophageal sphincter function during early pregnancy. Gastroenterology 1978;74:1233–7.

27. Cappell MS. Clinical presentation, diagnosis, and management of gastroesophageal reflux disease. Med Clin North Am 2005;89:243–91.

28. Nagler R, Spiro HM. Heartburn in late pregnancy: manometric studies of esophageal motor function. J Clin Invest 1961;40:954–70.

29. Van Thiel DH, Wald A. Evidence refuting a role for increasing abdominal pressure in the pathogenesis of heartburn associated with pregnancy. Am J Obstet Gynecol 1981;140:420–2.

30. Kalish RB, Garry D, Figueroa R. Achalasia with Candida esophagitis during pregnancy. Obstet Gynecol 1999;94(5 Pt 2):850.

31. Christopher LA. The role of proton pump inhibitors in the treatment of heartburn during pregnancy. J Am Acad Nurse Pract 2005;17:4–8.

32. Lindow SW, Regnell P, Sykes J, et al. An open-label multicenter study to assess the safety and efficacy of a novel reflux supplement (Gaviscon advance) in the treatment of heartburn in pregnancy. Int J Clin Pract 2003;57:175–9.

33. Ranchet G, Gangemi O, Petrone M. Sucralfate in the treatment of gravid pyrosis. G Ital Obstet Ginecol 1990;12:1–16.

34. Briggs G, Freeman R, Yaffe S (eds). Drugs in pregnancy and lactation: a reference guide to fetal and neonatal medicine, 4th edn. Williams and Wilkins, Baltimore, MD, 1994.

35. Magee LA, Inocencian G, Kambojt R, et al. Safety of first trimester exposure to histamine H2 blockers: a prospective cohort study. Dig Dis Sci 1996;41:1145–9.

36. Larson JD, Patatanian E, Miner PB, et al. Double-blind, placebo-controlled study of ranitidine for gastroesophageal reflux symtpoms during pregnancy. Obstet Gynecol 1997;90:83–7.

37. Nikfar S, Abdollahi M, Moretti ME, et al. Use of proton pump inhibitors during pregnancy and rates of major malformations: a meta-anlysis. Dig Dis Sci 2002;47:1526–9.

38. Nielsen GL, Sorenson HT, Thulstrup AM, et al. The safety of proton pump inhibitors in pregnancy. Aliment Pharmacol Ther 1999;13:1085–9.

39. Rudra A, Mondal M, Acharya A, et al. Anesthesia-related maternal mortality. J Indian Med Assoc 2006;104:312–16.

40. Cohen SE, Jasson J, Talafre ML, et al. Does metoclopramide decrease the volume of gastric contents in patients undergoing cesarean section? Anesthesiology 1984;61:604–7.

41. Moore J, Flynn RJ, Sampaio M, et al. Effect of single-dose omperazole on intragastric acidity and volume during obstetric anesthesia. Anaesthesia 1989;44:559–62.

42. Cappell MS. Gastirc and duodenal ulcers during pregnancy. Gastroenterol Clin North Am 2003;32:263–8.

42. Sandelweiss DJ, Saltzstein HC, Farbmann AA. The relation of sex hormones to peptic ulcer. Am J Dig Dis 1939;6:6–12.

44. Baird RM. Peptic ulceration in pregnancy. Report of a case with perforation. Can Med Assoc J 1966;94:861–2.

45. Modlin IM, Sachs G. Peptic ulcer disease. In: Acid related diseases – biology and treatment, 2nd edn. Lippincott, Williams and Wilkins, Philadelphia, 2004:253–91.

46. Clark DH. Pregnancy and peptic ulcer in women. BMJ 1953;i:1254–7.

47. Crisp WE. Pregnancy complicating peptic ulcer. Postgrad Med 1960;27:445–7.

48. Peterson WL, Sturdevant RA, Frankl HD, et al. Healing of duodenal ulcer with an antacid regimen. N Engl J Med 1977;297:341–5.

49. Mahadevan U, Kane SV. American Gastroenterological Association Institute technical review on the use of gastrointestinal medications in pregnancy. Gastroenterology 2006;131:283–311.

50. Drinkard CR, Shatin D, Clouse J. Postmarketing surveillance of medications and pregnancy outcomes: clarithromycin and birth malformations. Pharmacoepidemiol Drug Saf 2000;9(7):549–56.

51. Rewers M. Epidemiology of celiac disease: what are the prevalence, incidence, and progression of celiac disease? Gastroenterology 2005;128:S47–S51.

52. Green PHR, Stavropoulos SN, Panagi SG, et al. Characteristics of adult celiac disease in the USA: results of a national survey. Am J Gastroenterol 2001;96:126–31.

53. Dube C, Roston A, Sy R, et al. The prevalence of celiac disease in average-risk and at-risk Western European populations: a systematic review. Gastroenterology 2005;128:S57–S67.

54. Schuppan D, Dennis MD, Kelly CP. Celiac disease: epidemiology, pathogenesis, diagnosis, and nutritional management. Nutri Clin Care 2005;8:54–69.

55. Goh C, Banerjee K. Prevalence of coeliac disease in children and adolescents with type 1 diabetes mellitus in a clinic based population. Postgrad Med J 2007;83(976):132–6.

56. National Institutes of Health Consensus Development Conference Statement on Celiac Disease, June 28–30, 2004. Gastroenterology 2005;128:S1–S9.

57. Alaedini A, Green PHR. Narrative review: celiac disease: understanding a complex autoimmune disorder. Ann Intern Med 2005;142:289–98.

58. Dewar DH, Ciclitira PJ. Clinical features and diagnosis of celiac disease. Gastroenterology 2005;128:S19–S24.

59. Harrison MS, Webbi M, Obideen K. Celiac disease: more common than you think. Cleve Clin J Med 2007;74:209–15.

60. Eliakim R, Sherer DM. Celiac disease: fertility and pregnancy. Gynecol Obstet Invest 2001;51(1):3–7.

61. Gheller-Rigoni AI, Yale SH, Abdulkarim AS. Celiac disease: celiac sprue, gluten-sensitive enteropathy. Clin Med Res 2004;2:71–2.

62. Mearin ML. Celiac disease among children and adolescents. Curr Probl Pediatr Adolesc Health Care 2007;37:86–105.

63. Rostom A, Dube C, Cranney A, et al. The diagnostic accuracy of serologic tests for celiac disease: a systematic review. Gastroenterology 2005;128:S38–S46.

64. Cammarota G, Gasbarrini A, Gasbarrini G. No more biopsy in the diagnostic work-up of celiac disease. Gastrointest Endosc 2005;62:119–21.

65. Saha S, Degli-Esposti SD. Celiac disease. In: McGarry K, Tong IL (eds) The 5-minute consult clinical companion to women's health. Lippincott, Williams and Wilkins, Philadelphia, 2007: 56–8.

66. Kupper C. Dietary guidelines and implementation for celiac disease. Gastroenterology 2005;128:S121–S127.

67. Scott EM, Gaywood I, Scott BB. Guidelines for osteoporosis in coeliac disease and inflammatory bowel disease. Gut 2000;46:1–8.

68. Brousse N, Meijer JWR. Malignant complications of celiac disease. Best Pract Res Clin Gastroenterol 2005;19:401–12.

69. Catassi C, Bearzi I, Holmes GKT. Association of celiac disease and intestinal lymphomas and other cancers. Gastroenterology 2005;128:S79–S86.

70. Pink IJ, Creamer B. Response to a gluten-free diet of patients with coeliac syndrome. Lancet 1967;1:300–4.

71. Stategna-Guidetti C, Pulitano R, Grosso S, et al. Serum IgA antiendomysium antibody titres as a marker of intestinal involvement and diet compliance in adult celiac sprue. J Clin Gastroenterol 1993;17:123–7.

72. Grefte JM, Bouman JG, Ground J, et al. Slow and incomplete histological and functional recovery in adult gluten sensitive enteropathy. J Clin Pathol 1988;41:886–91.

73. Lloyd-Still JD, Grand RJ, Khaw KT, et al. The use of corticosteroids in celiac crisis. J Pediatr 1972;81:1074–81.

74. Vaidya A, Bolanos J, Berkelhammer C. Azathioprine in refractory sprue. Am J Gastroenterol 1999;94:219–25.

75. Rolny P, Sigurjonsdottir HA, Remotti H, et al. Role of immunosuppressive therapy in refractory sprue-like disease. Am J Gastroenterol 1999;94:219–55.

76. Gillett HR, Arnott ID, McIntyre M, et al. Successful infliximab treatment for steroid-refractory celiac disease: a case report. Gastroenterology 2002;122:800–5.

77. Green PH, Jabri B. Coeliac disease. Lancet 2003;97:3160–5.

78. Collin P, Vilska S, Heinonen PK, et al. Infertility and coeliac disease. Gut 1996;39:382–4.

79. Meloni GF, Dessole S, Vargiu N, Tomasi PA, Musumeci S. The prevalence of coeliac disease in infertility. Hum Reprod 1999;14(11):2759–61.

80. Jackson JE, Rosen M, McLean T, Moro J, Croughan M, Cedars MI. Prevalence of celiac disease in a cohort of women with unexplained infertility. Fertil Steril 2008;89(4):1002–4.

81. Farthing MJG, Edwards CRW, Rees LH, et al. Male gonadal function in coeliac disease: sexual dysfunction, infertility and semen quality. Gut 1982;23:608–14.

82. Goddard CJR, Gillett HR. Complications of coeliac disease: are all patients at risk? Postgrad Med J 2006;82:705–12.

83. Tata LJ, Card TR, Logan RF, Hubbard RB, Smith CJ, West J. Fertility and pregnancy-related events in women with celiac disease: a population-based cohort study. Gastroenterology 2005;128(4):849–55.

84. Yang H, McElree C, Roth MP, et al. Familial empirical risks for inflammatory bowel disease: differences between Jews and non-Jews. Gut 1993;34:517–24.

85. Lakatos PL. Recent trends in the epidemiology of inflammatory bowel diseases: up or down? World J Gastroenterol 2006;12:6102–8.

86. Farrokhyar F, Swarbrick ET, Irvine EJ. A critical review of epidemiological studies in inflammatory bowel disease. Scand J Gastroenterol 2001;36:2–15.

87. Feagan B, Sy R. Epidemiology of inflammatory bowel disease. In: Lichtenstin GR (ed) The clinician's guide to inflammatory bowel disease. SLACK Incorporated, New Jersey, 2003: 1–8.

88. Robertson DJ, Grimm IS. Inflammatory bowel disease in the elderly. Gastroenterol Clin North Am 2001;30(2):409–26.

89. Johnson GJ, Cosnes J, Mansfield JC. Review article: smoking cessation as primary therapy to modify the course of Crohn's disease. Aliment Pharmacol Ther 2005;21:921–31.

90. Calkins BM. A meta-analysis of the role of smoking in inflammatory bowel disease. Dig Dis Sci 1989;34:1841–54.

91. Corrao G, Tragnone A, Caprilli R, et al. Risk of inflammatory bowel disease attributable to smoking, oral contraception and breastfeeding in Italy: a nationwide case-control study. Int J Epidemiol 1998;27:397–404.

92. Lashner BA, Kane SV, Hanauer SB. Lack of association between oral contraceptive use and ulcerative colitis. Gastroenterology 1990;99:1032–6.

93. Lashner BA, Kane SV, Hanauer SB. Lack of association between oral contraceptive use and Crohn's disease: a community-based matched case-control study. Gastroenterology 1998;97:1442–7.

94. Ekbom A. The changing faces of Crohn's disease and ulcerative colitis. In: Targan SR, Shanahan F, Karp LC, et al. (eds) Inflammatory bowel disease: from bench to bedside, 2nd edn. Springer Science+Business Media, New York, 2003: 5–20.

95. Guslandi M. Exacerbation of inflammatory bowel disease by nonsteroidal anti-inflammatory drugs and cyclooxygenase-2 inhibitors: fact or fiction? World J Gastroenterol 2006;12: 1509–10.

96. Rutgeerts P, d'Haens G, Hiele M, et al. Appendectomy protects against ulcerative colitis. Gastroenterology 1994;106:1251–3.

97. Korzenik JR. Past and current theories of etiology of IBD: toothpaste, worms, and refrigerators. J Clin Gastroenterol 2005;39:S59–65.

98. Green C, Elliot L, Beaudoin C, et al. A population-based ecologic study of inflammatory bowel disease: searching for etiologic clues. Am J Epidemiol 2006;164:615–23.

99. Hugot J, Chamaillard, Zouali H, et al. Association of NOD2 leucine-rich repeat variants with susceptibility to Crohn's disease. Nature 2001;411:599–603.

100. Ogura Y, Bonen D, Inohara N, *et al*. A frameshift mutation in NOD2 associated with susceptibility to Crohn's disease. Nature 2001;411:603–6.

101. Lesage S, Zoulai H, Cezard J, *et al*. CARD15/NOD2 mutational analysis and genotype-phenotype correlation in 612 patients with inflammatory bowel disease. Am J Hum Genet 2002;70:845–57.

102. Kucharzik T, Maaser C, Lugering A, *et al*. Recent understanding of IBD pathogenesis: implications for future therapies. Inflamm Bowel Dis 2006;12:1068–83.

103. Lattine D, Fiasse R. New insights into the cellular immunology of the intestine in relation to the pathophysiology of inflammatory bowel diseases. Acta Gastroenterol Belg 2006;69:393–405.

104. Breese E, Michie C, Nicholls S, *et al*. Tumor necrosis factor alpha-producing cells in the intestinal mucosa of children with inflammatory bowel disease. Gastroenterology 1994;106:1455–66.

105. Legnani P, Korbluth A. Clinical features, course and laboratory findings in ulcerative colitis. In: Lichtenstin GR (ed) The clinician's guide to inflammatory bowel disease. SLACK Incorporated, New Jersey, 2003: 27–39.

106. Brauer B, Korzenik JR. Clinical features, course, and laboratory findings in Crohn's disease. In: Lichtenstin GR (ed) The clinician's guide to inflammatory bowel disease. SLACK Incorporated, New Jersey, 2003:57.

107. Wagtmans MJ, van Hogezand RA, Griffioen G, *et al*. Crohn's disease of the upper gastrointestinal tract. Neth J Med 1997;50: S2–7.

108. Kethu SR. Extraintestinal manifestations of inflammatory bowel disease. J Clin Gastroenterol 2006;40:467–75.

109. Forcione DG, Friedman LS. Extraintestinal manifestations of inflammatory bowel disease. In: Lichtenstin GR (ed) The clinician's guide to inflammatory bowel disease. SLACK Incorporated, New Jersey, 2003: 77–123.

110. Efrat B, Iris G, Wang H. A subgroup of first-degree relatives of crohn's disease patients shows a profile of inflammatory markers in the blood which is more typical of crohn's disease patients than of normal individuals. Mediators Inflamm 2006;2006:747–85.

111. Vermiere S, van Assche G, Rutgeerts P. Laboratory markers in IBD: useful, magic or unnecessary toys? Gut 2006;55:426–31.

112. Beck IT. Laboratory assessment of inflammatory bowel disease. Dig Dis Sci 1987;32:S26–41.

113. Angriman I, Scarpa M, d'Inca R. Enzymes in feces: useful markers of chronic inflammatory bowel disease. Clin Chemica Acta 2007;381(1):63–8.

114. Carucci LR, Levine MS. Radiographic imaging of inflammatory bowel disease. Gastroenterol Clin North Am 2002;31:93–117.

115. Schreyer AG, Seitz J, Feuerbach S, *et al*. Modern imaging using computer tomography and magnetic resonance imaging for inflammatory bowel disease (IBD). Inflamm Bowel Dis 2004;10:45–54.

116. Parente F, Greco S, Molteni M. Imaging inflammatory bowel disease using bowel ultrasound. Eur J Gastroenterol Hepatol 2005;17:283–91.

117. Fefferman DS, Farrell RJ. Endoscopy in inflammatory bowel disease: indications, surveillance, and use in clinical practice. Clin Gastroenterol Hepatol 2006;3:11–24.

118. Haskell H, Andrews CW, Reddy SI, *et al*. Pathologic features and clinical significance of "backwash" ileitis in ulcerative colitis. Am J Surg Pathol 2005;29:1472–81.

119. Moura R. Inflammatory bowel disease. In: McGarry K, Tong IL (eds) The 5-minute clinical consult companion to women's health. Lippincott, Williams and Wilkins, Philadelphia, 2007:158–60.

120. Fireman Z, Mahajna E, Broide E, *et al*. Diagnosing small bowel Crohn's disease with wireless capsule endoscopy. Gut 2003;42:390–2.

121. Guindi M, Riddell RH. Indeterminate colitis. J Clin Pathol 2004;57:1233–44.

122. Mahadevan U. Fertility and pregnancy in the patient with inflammatory bowel disease. Gut 2006;55:1198–206.

123. Baird DO, Narendranathan M, Sandler RS. Increased risk of preterm birth for women with inflammatory bowel disease. Gastroenterology 1990;99:987–94.

124. Hudson M, Flett G, Sinclair TS, *et al*. Fertility and pregnancy in inflammatory bowel disease. Int J Gynaecol Obstet 1997;58:229–37.

125. Mayberry JF, Waterman IT. European survey of fertility and pregnancy in women with Crohn's disease: a case control study by European collaborative group. Gut 1986;27:821–5.

126. Lindhagen T, Bohe M, Ekelund G, Valentin L. Fertility and outcome of pregnancy in patients operated on for Crohn's disease. Int J Colorectal Dis 1986;1(1):25–7.

127. De Dombal FT, Burton IL, Goligher JC. Crohn's disease and pregnancy. BMJ 1972;3(5826):550–3.

128. Olsen KO, Joelsson M, Laurberg S, *et al*. Fertility after ileal pouch-anal anastomosis in women with ulcerative colitis. Br J Surg 1999;86:493–5.

129. Waljee A, Waljee J, Morris AM, Higgins PD. Threefold increased risk of infertility: a meta-analysis of infertility after ileal pouch anal anastomosis in ulcerative colitis. Gut 2006;55(11):1575–80.

130. Feller ER, Ribaudo S, Jackson ND. Gynecologic aspects of Crohn's disease. Am Fam Physician 2001;64:1725–8.

131. Heetun ZS, Byrnes C, Neary P, O'Morain C. Review article: reproduction in the patient with inflammatory bowel disease. Aliment Pharmacol Ther 2007;26(4):513–33.

132. Nielsen OH, Andreasson B, Bondesen S, *et al*. Pregnancy in ulcerative colitis. Scand J Gastroenterol 1983;18:735–42.

133. Nielsen OH, Andreasson B, Bondesen S, *et al*. Pregnancy in Crohn's disease. Scand J Gastroenterol 1984;19:724–32.

134. Miller JP. Inflammatory bowel disease in pregnancy: a review. J R Soc Med 1986;79(4):221–5.

135. Kane SV. Gender issues in inflammatory bowel disease and irritable bowel syndrome. Int J Fertil Womens Med 2002;47:134–42.

136. Riis L, Vind I, Politi P, *et al*. Does pregnancy change the disease course? A study in a European cohort of patients with inflammatory bowel disease. Am J Gastroenterol 2006;101:1539–45.

137. Cornish C, Tan E, Teare J, *et al*. A meta-analysis on the influence of inflammatory bowel disease on pregnancy. Gut 2007;56(6):830–7.

138. Dominitz JA, Young JC, Boyko EJ. Outcomes of infants born to mothers with inflammatory bowel disease: a population-based cohort study. Am J Gastroenterol 2002;97(3):641–8.

139. Mahadevan U, Sandborn WJ, Li DK, Hakimian S, Kane S, Corley DA. Pregnancy outcomes in women with inflammatory bowel disease: a large community-based study from Northern California. Gastroenterology 2007;133(4):1106–12.

140. Ferrero S and Ragni N. Inflammatory bowel disease: management issues during pregnancy. Arch Gynecol Obstet 2004;270:79–85.

141. Hahnloser D, Pemberton JH, Wolff BG, *et al*. Pregnancy and delivery before and after ileal pouch-anal anastomosis for inflammatory bowel disease: immediate and long-term consequences and outcomes. Dis Colon Rect 2004;47:1127–35.

142. Korelitz BI. Inflammatory bowel disease and pregnancy. Gastroenterol Clin North Am 1998;27:213–24.

143. Ooi BS, Remzi FH, Fazio VW. Turnbull-Blowhole colostomy for toxic ulcerative colitis in pregnancy: report of two cases. Dis Colon Rect 2003;46(1):111–15.

144. Milman N, Bergholt T, Byg KE, et al. Reference intervals for haematological variables during normal pregnancy and postpartum in 434 healthy Danish women. Eur J Haematol 2007;79:39–46.

145. Larsson A, Palm M, Hansson LO, et al. Reference values for clinical chemistry tests during normal pregnancy. Br J Obstet Gynaecol 2008;115:874–81.

146. Van den Broe NR, Letsky EA. Pregnancy and erythrocyte sedimentation rate. Br J Obstet Gynaecol 2001;108:1164–7.

147. Belo L. Santos-Silva A, Rocha S, et al. Fluctuations in C-reactive protein concentration and neutrophil activation during normal human pregnancy. Eur J Obstet Gynecol Reprod Biol 2005;123:46–51.

148. Kane S. Inflammatory bowel disease in pregnancy. Gastroenterol Clin North Am 2003;32:323–40.

149. Diav-Citrin O, Park YH, Veerasuntharam G, et al. The safety of mesalamine in human pregnancy: a prospective controlled cohort study. Gastroenterology 1998;114(1):23–8.

150. Mogadam M, Dobbins WO, Korelitz BI, et al. Pregnancy in inflammatory bowel disease: effect of sulfasalazine and corticosteroids on fetal outcome. Obstet Gynecol Surv 1981;36(7):385–6.

151. Carter MJ, Lobo AJ, Travis SP, IBD Section, British Society of Gastroenterology. Guidelines for the management of inflammatory bowel disease in adults. Gut 2004;53(suppl 5):V1–16.

152. Blanford AT, Murphy BE. In vitro metabolism of prednisolone, dexamethasone, betamethasone, and cortisol by the human placenta. Am J Obstet Gynecol 1977;127(3):264–7.

153. Muirhead N, Sabharwal AR, Rieder MJ, Lazarovits AI, Hollomby DJ. The outcome of pregnancy following renal transplantation – the experience of a single center. Transplantation 1992;54:429–32.

154. Anderson GG, Rotchell Y, Kaiser DG. Placental transfer of methylprednisolone following maternal intravenous administration. Am J Obstet Gynecol 1981;140:699–701.

155. Loebstein R, Addis A, Ho E, et al. Pregnancy outcome following gestational exposure to fluoroquinolones: a multicenter prospective controlled study. Antimicrob Agents Chemo Ther 1998;42(6):1336–9.

156. De Boer NK, Jarbandhan SV, de Graaf P, et al. Azathioprine use during pregnancy: unexpected intrauterine exposure to metabolites. Am J Gastroenterol 2006;101:1390–2.

157. Davison JM, Dellagrammatikas H, Parkin JM. Maternal azathioprine therapy and depressed haemopoiesis in the babies of renal allograft patients. Br J Obstet Gynaecol 1985;92(3):233–9.

158. Williamson RA, Karp LE. Azathioprine teratogenicity: review of the literature and case report. Obstet Gynecol 1981;58:247–50.

159. Tallent MB, Simmons RL, Najarian JS. Birth defects in child of male recipient of kidney transplant. JAMA 1970;211:1854–5.

160. McKay DB, Josephson MA. Pregnancy in recipients of solid organs – effects on mother and child. N Engl J Med 2006;354(12):1281–93.

161. Francella A, Dyan A, Bodian C, Rubin P, Chapman M, Present DH. The safety of 6-mercaptopurine for childbearing patients with inflammatory bowel disease: a retrospective cohort study. Gastroenterology 2003;124(1):9–17.

162. Barrie A, Plevy S. Treatment of immune-mediated extraintestinal manifestations of inflammatory bowel disease with infliximab. Gastroenterol Clin North Am 2006;35(4):883–93.

163. Lichtenstein G, Cohen RD, Feagan BG, et al. Safety of infliximab in Crohn's disease: data from the 5000-patient TREAT registry. Gastroenterology 2004;126(suppl):A54.

164. Katz JA, Antoni C, Keenan GF, et al. Outcome of pregnancy in women receiving infliximab for the treatment of Crohn's disase and rheumatoid arthritis. Am J Gastroenterol 2004;99:2385–92.

165. Vasiliauskas EA, Church JA, Silverman N, Barry M, Targan SR, Dubinsky MC. Case report: evidence for transplacental transfer of maternally administered infliximab to the newborn. Clin Gastroenterol Hepatol 2006;4(10):1255–8.

166. Vesga L, Terdiman JP, Mahadevan U. Adalimumab use in pregnancy. Gut 2005;54:890.

167. Kane S, Lemieux N. The role of breastfeeding in postpartum disease activity in women with inflammatory bowel disease. Am J Gastroenterol 2005;100:102–5.

168. Bertschinger P, Himmelmann A, Risti B, Follath F. Cyclosporine treatment of severe ulcerative colitis during pregnancy. Am J Gastroenterol 1995;90(2):330.

169. Bar Oz B, Hackman R, Einarson T, Koren G. Pregnancy outcome after cyclosporine therapy during pregnancy: a meta-analysis. Transplantation 2001;71(8):1051–5.

170. Plamondon S, Ng SC, Kamm MA. Thalidomide in luminal and fistulizing Crohn's disease resistant to standard therapies. Aliment Pharmacol Ther 2007;25(5):557–67.

171. Kroser J, Srinivasen R. Drug therapy of inflammatory bowel disease in fertile women. Am J Gastroenterol 2006;101: S633–S639.

172. Fernandez-Benares F, Salas A, Forne M, et al. Incidence of collagenous and lymphocytic colitis: a 5–year population-based study. Am J Gastroenterol 1999;94:418–23.

173. Pardi DS, Loftus EV Jr, Smyrk TC, et al. The epidemiology of microscopic colitis: a population based study in Olmsted County, Minnesota. Gut 2007;56:504–8.

174. Fernandez-Benares F, Esteve M, Farre C, et al. Predisposing HLA-DQ2 and HLA-DQ8 haplotypes of coeliac disease and associated enteropathy in microscopic colitis. Eur J Gastroenterol Hepatol 2005;17:1333–8.

175. Van den Oord JJ, Geboes K, Desmet VJ. Collagenous colitis: an abnormal collagen table? Two new cases and review of the literature. Am J Gastroenterol 1982;77:377–81.

176. Järnerot G, Tysk C, Bohr J, et al. Collagneous colitis and fecal stream diversion. Gastroenterology 1995;109:449–55.

177. Bohr J, Tysk C, Eriksson S, et al. Collagenous colitis: a retrospective study of clinical presentation and treatment in 163 patients. Gut 1996;39:846–51.

178. Rams H, Rogers AI, Ghandur-Mnaymneh L. Collagenous colitis. Ann Intern Med 1987;106:108–13.

179. Cruz-Correa M, Giardiello FM, Bayless TM. Atypical forms of inflammatory bowel disease: microscopic colitis and pouchitis. Curr Opin Gastroenterol 2000;16:343–8.

180. Fernández-Bañares F, Esteve M, Espinós JC, et al. Drug consumption and the risk of microscopic colitis. Am J Gastroenterol 2007;102:324–30.

181. Bohr J, Tysk C, Yang P, et al. Autoantibodies and immunoglobulins in collagenous colitis. Gut 1996;39:73–6.

182. Holstein A, Burmeister J, Plaschke A, et al. Autoantibody profiles in microscopic colitis. J Gastroenterol Hepatol 2006;21:1016–20.

183. Rubio-Tapia A, Martinez-Salgado J, Garcia-Leiva J, et al. Microscopic colitides: a single center experience in Mexico. Int J Colorectal Dis 2007;22(9):1031–6.

184. Liszka L, Woszczyk D, Pajak J. Histopathological diagnosis of microscopic colitis. J Gastroenterol Hepatol 2006;21:792–7.

185. Nyhlin N, Bohr J, Eriksson S, *et al*. Systemic review: microscopic colitis. Aliment Pharmacol Ther 2006;23:1525–34.

186. Chande N, McDonald JWD, MacDonald JK. Interventions for treating lymphocytic colitis. Cochrane Database of Systematic Reviews, 2007;24:CD006096.

187. Pardi DS. Microscopic colitis: an update. Inflamm Bowel Dis 2004;10:860–70.

188. Fine K, Ogunji F, Lee E, *et al*. Randomized, double-blind, placebo-controlled trial of bismuth subsalicylate for microscopic colitis. Gastroenterology 1999;116:A880.

189. Bohr J, Olesen M, Tysk C, Järnerot G. Budesonide and bismuth in microscopic colitis. Gut 1999;45:A202.

190. Pardi DS, Loftus EV Jr, Tremaine WJ, *et al*. Treatment of refractory microscopic colitis with azathioprine and 6-mercaptopurine. Gastroenterology 2001;120:1483–4.

191. Hillman LC, Ashton C, Chiragakis L, *et al*. Collagenous colitis remission with methotrexate. Gastroenterology 2001;120:A278.

192. Varghese L, Galandiuk S, Tremaine WJ, Burgart LJ. Lymphocytic colitis treated with proctocolectomy and ileal J-pouch-anal anastomosis: report of a case. Dis Colon Rect 2002;45:123–6.

193. Mahadevan U, Kane SV. American Gastroenterological Association Institute technical review on the use of gastrointestinal medications in pregnancy. Gastroenterology 2006;131:283–311.

194. Brandt LJ, Bjorkman D, Fennerty MB, *et al*. Systematic review on the management of irritable bowel syndrome in North America. Am J Gastroenterol 2002;97(11 suppl):S7–26.

195. Official recommendations of the American Gastroenterological Association (AGA) on irritable bowel syndrome. Gastroenterology 2002;123:2105.

196. Philipson EH, Rossi KQ, Isaac RM, Kalhan SC. Glucose, insulin, gastric inhibitory polypeptide, and pancreatic polypeptide responses to polycose during pregnancy. Obstet Gynecol 1992;79:592–6.

197. Whorwell PJ, McCallum M, Creed FH, Roberts CT. Non-colonic features of irritable bowel syndrome. Gut 1986;27(1):37–40.

198. Bonapace ES, Fisher RS. Constipation and diarrhea in pregnancy. Gastroenterol Clin North Am 1998;27:197–211.

199. Jewell DJ, Young G. Interventions for treating constipation in pregnancy. Cochrane Database of Systematic Reviews, 2001;2:CD001142.

200. Lewis J, Weingold AB. Use of gastrointestinal drugs during pregnancy and lactation. Am J Gastroenterol 1985;80:912–23.

201. Gattuso JM, Kamm MA. Adverse effects of drugs used in the management of constipation and diarrhea. Drug Saf 1994;10:47–65.

202. Simmons SC. Anorectal disorders in pregnancy. Proc R Soc Med 1972;65:286.

203. McKee R, Akbari HM. Fecal Incontinence. In: McGarry K, Tong IL (eds) The 5-minute consult clinical companion to women's health. Lippincott, Williams and Wilkins, Philadelphia, 2007:117–19.

204. Quijano CE, Abalos E. Conservative management of symptomatic and/or complicated haemorrhoids in pregnancy and the puerperium. Cochrane Database of Systematic Reviews, 2005;3:CD004077.

205. Pope CE. Anorectal complication of pregnancy. Anatomic and physiologic changes of the anorectum and pelvi-rectum during pregnancy. Am J Surg 1952;84:579.

206. Nisar PJ, Scholefield JH. Managing haemorrhoids. BMJ 2003;327:847–51.

207. Alonso-Coello P, Guyatt G, Heels-Ansdell D, *et al*. Laxatives for the treatment of hemorrhoids. Cochrane Database of Systematic Reviews, 2005;4:CD004649.

208. Saleeby RJ, Rosen L, Stasik JJ, *et al*. Hemorrhoidectomy during pregnancy: risk or relief? Dis Colon Rect 1991;34:260–1.

209. Ayantunde AA, Debrah SA. Current concepts in anal fissures. World J Surg 2006;30:2246–60.

210. Abramowitz L, Battalan A. Epidemiology of anal lesions (fissure and thrombosed external hemorroid) during pregnancy and post-partum. Gynecol Obstet Fertil 2003;31:546–9.

211. Abramowitz L, Sobhani I, Benifla JL, *et al*. Anal fissure and thrombosed external hemorrhoids before and after delivery. Dis Colon Rect 2002;45:650–5.

212. Hamlyn E, Taylor C. Sexually transmitted proctitis. Postgrad Med J 2006;82:733–6.

213. Richter HE, Brumfield CG, Cliver SP, *et al*. Risk factors associated with anal sphincter tear: a comparison of primiparous patients, vaginal birth after cesarean deliveries, and patients with previous vaginal delivery. Am J Obstet Gynecol 2002;187:1194–8.

214. Lowder JL, Burrows LG, Krohn MA. Risk factors for primary and subsequent anal sphincter lacerations: a comparison of cohorts by parity and prior mode of delivery. Am J Obstet Gynecol 2007;196:344.

215. Aukee P, Sundstrom H, Kairaluoma MV. The role of mediolateral episitiomy during labor. Analysis of risk factors for obstetric anal sphincter tears. Acta Obstet Gynecol Scand 2006;85:856–60.

216. Andrews V, Sultan AH, Thakar R. Risk factors for obstetric anal sphincter injury: a prospective study. Birth 2006;33:117–22.

217. Flehsman JW, Dreznik Z, Fry RD. Anal sphincter repair for obstetric injury: manometric evaluation of functional results. Dis Colon Rect 1991;34:1061–7.

218. Nielsen MB, Hauge C, Pedersen JF. Endosonographic evaluation of patients with anal incontinence: findings and influence on surgical management. Am J Roentgenol 1993;160:771–5.

219. Dobben AC, Terra MP, Slors JF, *et al*. External anal sphincter defects in patients with fecal incontinence: comparison of endoanal MR imaging and endoanal US. Radiology 2007;242:463–71.

220. Kurabayashi T, Isii K, Suzuki M, *et al*. Advanced gastric cancer and concomitant pregnancy associated with disseminated intravascular coagulation. Am J Perinatol 2004;21:295–8.

221. Jaspers VK, Gillessen A, Quakernack K. Gastric cancer in pregnancy: do pregnancy, age or female sex alter the prognosis? Case reports and review. Eur J Obstet Gynecol Reprod Biol 1999;87(1):13–22.

222. Nesbitt JC, Moise KJ, Sawyers JL. Colorectal carcinoma in pregnancy. Arch Surg 1985;120:636–40.

223. Bernstein MA, Madoff RD, Caushaj PF. Colon and rectal cancer in pregnancy. Dis Colon Rect 1993;36:172–8.

224. Castro MA, Shipp TD, Castro EE, *et al*. The use of helical computed tomography in pregnancy for diagnosis of acute appendicitis. Am J Obstet Gynecol 2001;184:954–7.

225. Pedrosa I, Levine D, Eyvazzadeh AD, *et al*. MR imaging evaluation of acute appendicitis in pregnancy. Radiology 2006;238(3):891–9.

226. Capella RF, Iannace VA, Capella JF. Bowel obstruction after open and laparoscopic gastric bypass surgery for morbid obesity. J Am Coll Surg 2006;203(3):328–35.

227. Stein Z, Susser M. The Dutch famine, 1944–1945, and the reproductive process. I. Effects of six indices at birth. Pediatr Res 1975;9:70–6.

228. Vause T, Martz P, Richard F, Gramlich L. Nutrition for healthy pregnancy outcomes. Appl Physiol Nutr Metab 2006;31:12–20.

229. Institute of Medicine. Nutrition during pregnancy, National Academies Press, Washington, DC, 1990.

230. Tamura T, Picciano MF. Folate and human reproduction. Am J Clin Nutr 2006;83:993–1016.

231. Santry HP, Gillen DL, Lauderdale DS. Trends in bariatric surgical procedures. JAMA 2005;294:1909–17.

232. Woodard CB. Pregnancy following bariatric surgery. J Perinat Neonatal Nurs 2004;18:329–40.

233. Weiner R, Blanco-Engert R, Weiner S, Matkowitz R, Schaefer L, Pomhoff I. Outcome after laparoscopic adjustable gastric banding – 8 years experience. Obes Surg 2003;13:427–34.

234. Doldi SB, Micheletto G, Lattuada E, Zappa Ma, Bona D, Sonvico U. Adjustable gastric banding: 5–year experience. Obes Surg 2000;10:171–3.

235. Ahmed AR, O'malley W. Internal hernia with Roux loop obstruction during pregnancy after gastric bypass surgery. Obes Surg 2006;16:1246–8.

236. Printen KJ, Scott D. Pregnancy following gastric bypass for the treatment of morbid obesity. Am Surg 1982;48:363–5.

237. Dao T, Kuhn J, Ehmer D, Fisher T, Mccarty T. Pregnancy outcomes after gastric-bypass surgery. Am J Surg 2006;192:762–6.

237. Marceau P, Kaufman D, Biron S, et al. Outcome of pregnancies after biliopancreatic diversion. Obes Surg 2004;14:318–24.

239. Van Horn C, Barrett P. Pregnancy, delivery, and postpartum experiences of fifty-four women with ostomies. J Wound Ostomy Continence Nurs 1997;24:151–62.

240. Solman F. Pregnancy in the woman with a stoma. Midwife Health Visit Community Nurse 1987;23:150–2.

241. Cappell MS. The fetal safety and clinical efficacy of gastrointestinal endoscopy during pregnancy. Gastroenterol Clin North Am 2003;32:123–79.

242. Qureshi WA, Rajan E, Adler DG, et al. ASGE guidelines: guidelines for endoscopy in pregnant and lactating women. Gastrointest Endosc 2005;61:357–62.

243. Siddiqui U, Denise Proctor D. Flexible sigmoidoscopy and colonoscopy during pregnancy. Gastrointest Endosc Clin North Am 2006;16:59–69.

244. Shaheen NJ, Crosby MA, Grimm IS, et al. The use of percutaneous endoscopic gastrostomy in pregnancy. Gastrointest Endosc 1997;46:564–5.

245. Cappell MS, Colon V, Sidhom OA. A study of eight medical centers of the safety and clinical efficacy of esophagogastroduodenoscopy in 83 pregnant females with follow-up of fetal outcome and with comparison to control groups. Am J Gastroenterol 1996;91:348–54.

246. Hogan RB, Ahmad N, Hogan RB III. Video capsule endoscopy detection of jejunal carcinoid in life-threatening hemorrhage, first trimester pregnancy. Gastrointest Endosc 2007;66(1):205–7.

247. Gilinsky, NH, Muthunayagam N. Gastrointestinal endoscopy in pregnant and lactating women: emerging standard of care to guide decision-making. Obstet Gynecol Surv 2006;61:791–9.

248. Laegreid L, Olegård R, Conradi N, Hagberg G, Wahlström J, Abrahamsson L. Congenital malformations and maternal consumption of benzodiazepines: a case-control study. Dev Med Child Neurol 1990;32(5):432–41.

249. Dolovich LR, Addis A, Vaillancourt JM, Power JD, Koren G, Einarson TR. Benzodiazepine use in pregnancy and major malformations or oral cleft: meta-analysis of cohort and case-control studies. BMJ 1998;317(7162):839–43.

250. Koren G, Pastuszak A, Ito S. Drugs in pregnancy. N Engl J Med 1998;338:1128–37.

251. Qureshi WA, Rajan E, Adler DG, et al. ASGE guideline: guidelines for endoscopy in pregnant and lactating women. American Society for Gastrointestinal Endoscopy. Gastrointest Endosc 2005;61(3):357–62.

252. Cappell MS. Sedation and analgesia for gastrointestinal endoscopy during pregnancy. Gastrointest Endosc Clin North Am 2006;16:1–31.

253. Menees S, Elta G. Endoscopic retrograde cholangiopancreatography during pregnancy. Gastrointest Endosc Clin North Am 2006;16(1):41–57.

254. Huda W, Slone R. Radiation protection. In: Huda W, Slone R (eds) Review of radiologic physics, 2nd edn. Lippincott Williams and Wilkins, Philadelphia, 2003: 162–3.

255. Montgomery A, Hale TW, Academy of Breastfeeding Medicine Protocol Committee. ABM Clinical Protocol #15. Anesthesia and analgesia for the breastfeeding mother. Breastfeed Med 2006;1(4): 271–7.

256. Macfie AG, Magides AD, Richmond MN, Reilly CS. Gastric emptying in pregnancy. Br J Anaesth 1991;67:54–7.

257. Whitehead EM, Smith M, Dean Y, O'Sullivan G. An evaluation of gastric emptying times in pregnancy and the puerperium. Anaesthesia 1993;48:53–7.

258. Wong CA, Loffredi M, Ganchiff JN, Zhao J, Wang Z, Avram MJ. Gastric emptying of water in term pregnancy. Anesthesiology 2002;96:1395–400.

259. Wong CA, McCarthy RJ, Fitzgerald PC, Raikoff K, Avram MJ. Gastric emptying of water in obese pregnant women at term. Anesth Analg 2007;105:751–5.

260. Carp H, Jayaram A, Stoll M. Ultrasound examination of the stomach contents of parturients. Anesth Analg 1992;74:683–7.

261. Practice guidelines for obstetric anesthesia: an updated report by the American Society of Anesthesiologists Task Force on Obstetric Anesthesia. Anesthesiology 2007;106:843–63.

262. Nimmo WS, Wilson J, Prescott LF. Narcotic analgesics and delayed gastric emptying during labour. Lancet 1975;1:890–3.

263. Gyte GM, Richens Y. Routine prophylactic drugs in normal labour for reducing gastric aspiration and its effects. Cochrane Database of Systematic Reviews, 2006;3:CD005298.

264. Ni Mhuireachtaigh R, O'Gorman DA. Anesthesia in pregnant patients for nonobstetric surgery. J Clin Anesth 2006;18:60–6.

265. O'Rourke N, Kodali BS. Laparoscopic surgery during pregnancy. Curr Opin Anaesthesiol 2006;19:254–9.

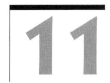

Diabetes mellitus in pregnancy

Michael F. Greene[1], *Caren G. Solomon*[2], *Stephanie L. Lee*[3]
with Robert A. Peterfreund[4]

[1]Vincent Memorial Obstetrics and Gynecology Department, Massachusetts General
Hospital, Boston, MA, USA
[2]Department of Medicine, Brigham and Women's Hospital, Boston, MA, USA
[3]Section of Endocrinology, Diabetes, and Nutrition, Boston Medical Center,
Boston, MA, USA
[4]Harvard Medical School and Massachusetts General Hospital, Boston, MA, USA

Introduction

Elliott Proctor Joslin presented his experience with diabetes in pregnancy in the *Boston Medical and Surgical Journal* in 1915 (7 years prior to the discovery of insulin). He described 10 pregnancies among seven women with three surviving children and four maternal deaths due to diabetic ketoacidosis, pyelonephritis, tuberculosis and a suicide after two failed pregnancies [1]. Following the introduction of insulin, maternal mortality dropped rapidly to 1–2% by the 1950s but perinatal outcome improved much more slowly.

Dr Joslin brought pediatrician Priscilla White to the New England Deaconess Hospital to care for "diabetes in youth." As the girls she followed became pregnant young women, Dr White focused on the complications of pregnancy associated with diabetes, developing the system of classification of diabetes complicating pregnancy that bears her name. The system was intended to both guide physicians in their care of individual patients and facilitate comparisons of outcomes across diabetes centers. Her original classification did not recognize what we now call "gestational diabetes," her "Class A" has been dropped and a class for women with kidney transplants was added later. Although less important now to guide treatment, her classification system is still useful and widely used (Box 11.1). Gestational diabetes is far more common than diabetes antedating pregnancy but the two are the most common and important medical and metabolic complications of pregnancy.

Maternal energy metabolism and the role of insulin

Glucose is central to energy metabolism and is the preferred energy source for most cells. It comes from three sources: ingested food, release from glycogen (glycogenolysis), stored mostly in the liver, and synthesis from smaller molecules (gluconeogenesis) in the liver. Almost all aspects of glucose metabolism and energy homeostasis are controlled by insulin and glucagon. Insulin is released from pancreatic beta cells directly into the portal circulation; thus it reaches the liver in very high concentration but is much more dilute when it reaches peripheral target tissues, including muscle and fat cells. Before it even leaves the pancreas, insulin exerts an important action in suppressing pancreatic alpha cell glucagon production. In the liver, it stimulates glycogen synthesis and suppresses hepatic glucose production by suppressing both glycogenolysis and gluconeogenesis (Figure 11.1). In the periphery the majority of insulin-stimulated glucose uptake is into muscle cells and to a much less extent into adipocytes. Within muscle cells insulin antagonizes protein catabolism, promotes nitrogen retention and protein synthesis and promotes both glycolysis, resulting in energy production, and glycogen synthesis.

Fundamentally different mechanisms control blood glucose levels in the fed and fasting states. The fasting blood glucose level is controlled by the rate of glucose production from the liver, whereas postprandial blood glucose levels are controlled by the rate of disposal of glucose absorbed from the gut into muscle cells.

When carbohydrate calories are plentiful in the fed state, insulin levels are high and the liver contains its normal glycogen stores. In the fasting state, insulin levels fall, glucagon levels rise, and the liver is quickly (over 12–24 hours depending upon caloric demand) depleted of glycogen. Low insulin levels permit muscle protein catabolism, releasing amino

de Swiet's Medical Disorders in Obstetric Practice, 5th edition.
Edited by R. O. Powrie, M. F. Greene, W. Camann. © 2010 Blackwell Publishing.

Box 11.1 Classification of diabetes in pregnancy

Gestational diabetes mellitus noninsulin requiring (GDMNI): abnormal carbohydrate tolerance with onset or first diagnosis during pregnancy, not requiring insulin.

Gestational diabetes mellitus insulin requiring (GDMI): abnormal carbohydrate tolerance with onset or first diagnosis during pregnancy, requiring insulin.

Class A: abnormal carbohydrate tolerance in the nonpregnant state identified prior to the present pregnancy that does not require insulin either prior to or during the pregnancy.

Class B: onset of insulin-requiring diabetes after 20 years of age, with duration of less than 10 years.

Class C: onset of insulin-requiring diabetes between ages 10 and 20 with duration of less than 20 years, or duration 10–20 years regardless of age of onset.

Class D: onset of insulin-requiring diabetes prior to age 10 years, or duration greater than 20 years regardless of age of onset, or insulin-requiring diabetes with chronic hypertension, or insulin-requiring diabetes with benign retinopathy.

Class F: insulin-requiring diabetes with diabetic nephropathy (proteinuria of greater than 500 mg in a 24-hour urine collection).

Class R: insulin-requiring diabetes with proliferative retinopathy.

Class T: insulin-requiring diabetes with renal transplant.

Class H: insulin-requiring diabetes with coronary artery disease.

- Liver
  - ↓ Glycogenolysis
  - ↓ Gluconeogenesis
  - ↓ Ketogenesis
- Adipose
  - ↓ Lipolysis
- Muscle
  - ↓ Protein breakdown

- Liver
  - ↑ Glycogen synthesis
  - ↑ Fat synthesis
- Adipose
  - ↑ Fat synthesis
  - ↑ Glycerol synthesis
- Muscle
  - ↑ Glycogen synthesis
  - ↑ Protein synthesis
  - **↑ Glucose uptake**

Figure 11.1 The major metabolic actions of insulin.

acids (primarily alanine) into the circulation which are taken up in the liver to be used as substrate for gluconeogenesis. That glucose is then sent out into the circulation to meet total body energy needs. As continued muscle catabolism to meet

daily energy needs would ultimately be maladaptive, other mechanisms serve to maintain glucose levels in a more prolonged fasting state. Specifically, four key counter-regulatory hormones, glucagon, cortisol, epinephrine and growth hormone, mobilize fatty acids from triglycerides stored in adipocytes. These fatty acids are transported to the liver where they are converted into ketone bodies (mainly acetoacetate and beta-hydroxybutyrate) which are exported to be used by most tissues, including brain, to help meet total body energy requirements. Within the liver, fatty acid oxidation fuels hepatic gluconeogenesis.

Pregnancy is associated with pancreatic beta cell hyperplasia and increased serum insulin levels in both the fasting and fed states. During pregnancy, fasting glucose levels are 10–15% lower than in the nonpregnant state, while postprandial levels are slightly higher. Early pregnancy is associated with slightly improved insulin sensitivity but as pregnancy progresses, women become increasingly insulin resistant. The insulin resistance is due to the effects of increased levels of several hormones including cortisol, growth hormone and human chorionic somatomammotropin (HCS, also known as human placental lactogen, HPL). Hepatic glycogen stores are reduced in pregnancy and are therefore more rapidly depleted than in the nonpregnant state. During a fast, pregnant women accomplish the switch from the use of hepatic glycogen for daily energy needs to lipolysis and ketone body production quickly and without going through the intermediate stage of protein catabolism and amino acid use for gluconeogenesis described above. This rapid transition from fed physiology to starvation physiology has been termed the "accelerated starvation of pregnancy."

Glucose is transported across the placenta down a concentration gradient by facilitated diffusion in a nonenergy-requiring process. Fetal glucose levels are generally approximately 80% of maternal levels. Amino acids are actively transported across the placenta against a gradient in an energy-requiring process that results in fetal levels of some amino acids that are as much as 140% of maternal serum levels. Mechanisms clearly exist for transport of essential fatty acids, long chain polyunsaturated fatty acids and arachidonic acids across the human placenta but they are not yet fully understood [2].

Gestational diabetes

Gestational diabetes was originally defined by O'Sullivan in a group of pregnant women in Boston in the 1960s as a degree of glucose intolerance greater than two standard deviations from the mean on a 100 g oral glucose tolerance test. By definition, therefore, 2.5% of women were identified as "abnormal." Gestational diabetes is now defined as "glucose intolerance of variable degree with onset or first recognition during pregnancy" [3]. This broad definition inevitably includes some women with undiagnosed type 2 diabetes prior to pregnancy, and a few women who coincidently develop acute type 1 diabetes during pregnancy. The majority of patients diagnosed with gestational diabetes, however, have normal to marginal carbohydrate tolerance prior to pregnancy and are pushed into glucose intolerance by the hormonal changes of advancing gestation that antagonize insulin action.

Since hyperglycemia during pregnancy can increase the risks of both maternal and fetal complications, women should be screened for gestational diabetes, and it should be treated when diagnosed [4]. Few concepts of the dichotomy of "diseased" versus "nondiseased" have evolved as rapidly as the concept for gestational diabetes.

Almost all aspects of the diagnosis and management of gestational diabetes, including whom to screen, how to screen and when to screen, have been controversial. These controversies are not reviewed in detail here but a reasonable consensus representing the recommendations of the American Diabetes Association (ADA) and the American College of Obstetricians and Gynecologists is presented.

Although assessment for risk factors for gestational diabetes mellitus (GDM) should begin at the first prenatal visit, only a minority of women need a biochemical screen for diabetes in early pregnancy. However, there are several historic factors associated with an increased risk for early pregnancy gestational diabetes (Box 11.2). Anyone with any of these risk factors should be screened biochemically as early in pregnancy as possible. Most other patients (and those high-risk patients who pass the early pregnancy screen) should have a biochemical screen at 24–28 weeks gestation. The ADA recommends that all women except those who meet all the criteria for low risk (Box 11.3) should be screened biochemically [5]. Some investigators have reviewed large numbers of women in their practices and found that the ADA criteria eliminate so few women (approximately 10%) from biochemical screening that the difference between universal screening and selective screening on these criteria is trivial [6,7]. Temporal trends in the US, including increasing maternal age, increasing obesity and, especially in major cities, increasing numbers of women in high-risk racial or ethnic groups, will only further reduce the percentage of low-risk women who do not need to be screened. Women who require biochemical screening should be tested at 24–28 weeks gestation. High-risk women (e.g. Body Mass Index (BMI) greater than 30, age greater than 40, with a history of GDM

Box 11.2 Historic risk factors

- "Marked" obesity
- Personal history of GDM
- Strong family history of diabetes
- Glycosuria

Box 11.3 American Diabetes Association 2009 Practice recommendations

Women who meet all these criteria do not need to be screened for gestational diabetes.
1. Are ≤25 years of age
2. Are a normal bodyweight
3. Have no family history (i.e. first-degree relative) of diabetes
4. Have no history of abnormal glucose metabolism
5. Have no history of poor obstetric outcome
6. Are not members of an ethnic/racial group with a high prevalence of diabetes (e.g. Hispanic American, Native American, Asian American, African American, Pacific Islander)

or fetal macrosomia in a prior pregnancy) should be screened as early in pregnancy as possible. Those who pass an early pregnancy screen should be retested at 24–28 weeks.

The precise values to be used for "abnormal" results are still debated. As with any screening test, the value chosen as the threshold for "abnormal" will determine both the sensitivity and specificity of the screen. These test performance characteristics and the prevalence of the "disease" in the population tested determine the positive and negative predictive values of the screen. This principle applies to both the 50 g oral glucose loading test (GLT) used as a screen for an abnormal "diagnostic" 100 g 3 hour oral glucose tolerance test (GTT) and the "diagnostic" 75 g 2 hour or 100 gram GTT as a "screen" for the complications of pregnancy associated with diabetes. A major conceptual advance in recent years has been the demonstration that there is no clear glycemic threshold for the risks of pregnancy complications associated with increasingly poor glucose tolerance, but rather a continuum of risk [8]. Although these observations may lead to the use of lower glycemic values to identify "abnormal" carbohydrate tolerance, on glucose tolerance testing and as treatment goals, it remains to be proven whether changing these thresholds will reduce pregnancy complications and long-term morbidity in the offspring.

Currently the two-stage 50 g 1 hour GLT screen followed by a 100 g 3 hour GTT strategy is used in the US but most of the rest of the world uses a one-stage testing scheme with a standard WHO 75 g 2 hour GTT. Using a threshold GLT value of 130 or 140 mg/dL to proceed to a 100 g 3 hour oral GTT is acceptable. Criteria for normal test results are listed in Table 11.1.

Patients who meet criteria for gestational diabetes should be placed on appropriate diets and have their fasting and 2 hour postprandial capillary blood glucose levels checked regularly. If glucose levels normalize on diet alone, then patients can be

Table 11.1 Diagnosis of GDM with a 100 g or 75 g oral glucose load

Plasma or serum glucose concentration	Plasma glucose concentration			
	Carpenter/Coustan conversion		National Diabetes Data Group conversion	
	mg/dL	mmol/L	mg/dL	mmol/L
100 g glucose load				
Fasting	95	5.3	105	5.8
1 h	180	10.0	190	10.6
2 h	155	8.6	165	9.2
3 h	140	7.8	145	8.0
75 g glucose load				
Fasting	95	5.3	-	-
1 h	180	10.0	-	-
2 h	155	8.6	-	-

Two or more abnormal values are diagnostic for gestational diabetes. The American College of Obstetricians and Gynecologists position is that either set of criteria for the 100 g oral GTT is acceptable and does not recommend the 75 g test. The American Diabetes Association recommends the more stringent Carpenter/Coustan criteria for the 100 g oral GTT and recommends the criteria listed for the 75 g oral GTT though it acknowledges that they are less well validated than the data for the 100 g test.

managed as normal obstetric patients. If the fasting glucose levels are in excess of 95 mg/dL or the 2 hour postprandial levels are greater than 120 mg/dL, then generally the patient should start insulin therapy and be managed as a diabetic patient. The potential role of oral agents in this situation is discussed below.

Effects of diabetes on the fetus and neonate

In 1937, White noted in the *American Journal of Obstetrics and Gynecology* that the three major complications of the neonatal period for infants of diabetic mothers (IDM) were "congenital defects, hypoglycemia and asphyxia" [9]. She regarded congenital defects as "doubtless beyond our therapeutic control" and proceeded to discuss the other two problems in detail. At that time, when the stillbirth rate was 25%, the 9% incidence of congenital malformations aroused less concern. Subsequently the stillbirth rate has fallen by two orders of magnitude, and overall perinatal mortality rate has fallen by one order of magnitude, but the incidence of major congenital malformations is virtually unchanged.

Early pregnancy effects

Congenital malformations

The rates of major congenital malformations in some large reported series of IDM are listed in Table 11.2 in chronologic

Table 11.2 Malformations among infants of diabetic mothers

Location	Reference	N	%
Copenhagen	[10] Pedersen 1964		5.6
Birmingham, UK	[11] Soler 1976	44/585	7.5
Dublin	[12] Drury 1977	34/558	6.1
Los Angeles	[13] Gabbe 1977	19/260	7.3
Boston	[14] Kitzmiller 1978	13/137	9.5
Chicago	[15] Simpson 1983	9/106	8.5
Helsinki	[16] Ylinen 1984	11/142	7.7
Cincinnati	[17] Ballard 1984	19/196	9.7
Dallas	[18] Lucas 1989	8/87	9.2
Stockholm	[19] Hanson 1990	10/491	2.0
France	[20] French Study Group 1991	12/277	4.3
Paris	[21] Tchobroutsky 1991	22/389	5.5
Boston	[22] Greene 1991	32/432	7.4
Nottingham	[23] Gregory 1992	3/139	2.2
Cincinnati	[24] Rosenn 1994	14/163	8.6
Los Angeles	[25] Towner 1995	39/332	11.7
Washington State	[26] Janssen 1996	111/1511	7.2
USA	[27] DCCT 1996	10/194	5.2
Denmark	[28] Nielsen 1997	10/243	4.1
NW England	[29] Hawthorne 1997	42/370	11.3
Northern England	[30] Casson 1997	9/109	8.3
Helsinki	[31] Suhonen 2000	30/709	4.2
NE England	[32] Hawthorne 2000	17/292	5.5
New Zealand	[33] Farrell 2002	27/535	5.0
Denmark	[34] Jensen 2004	61/1215	5.0
South Australia	[35] Sharp 2005	96/946	10.1
Total		746/11,209	6.6

order [10–35]. With the notable exception of a few low rates reported from some series from Europe in the mid-1990s, the incidence of major congenital malformations among IDM remains at 6–9%. Particularly disappointing are the findings of regional surveys from England indicating rates of 8–11% [29,30]. Gabbe observed that the decrease in stillbirth rate and minimal change in rate of major malformations have moved major malformations to first place among all causes of perinatal mortality for IDM, accounting for approximately 50% of the total [36].

The first hint that congenital malformations among IDM might be related to the degree of metabolic control during organogenesis in the first trimester came from Leslie *et al.* [37]. They noted that three out of five diabetic patients in poor metabolic control delivered babies with major congenital malformations. At about that time, measurement of glycosylated hemoglobin became available. Hemoglobin A_{1c} (Hb A_{1c}) is a glycosylated hemoglobin species with a glucose moiety bound to the N terminal valine of the beta globin chain. Its concentration is proportional to the level of blood glucose seen by red blood cells. Its measurement is a useful tool for retrospectively assessing the degree of metabolic control during the previous 8–12 weeks. Miller *et al.* [38] took advantage of these Hb A_{1c} determinations during the first trimester to provide the first reasonably large data set, documenting a relationship between metabolic control and major malformations. They examined Hb A_{1c} values in a series of 116 consecutive patients enrolling for prenatal care prior to 14 weeks. These patients were then rank ordered according to their first-trimester Hb A_{1c} values. The 58 patients in the lower half with better control had a 3.4% incidence of major malformations, while the 58 patients in the upper half with poorer control had a 22.4% incidence of major malformations. This difference was highly statistically significant.

Several years later, much larger series were published from the Joslin Diabetes Center in Boston, again confirming the relationship between first-trimester Hb A_1 levels and risk of major malformation (Table 11.3) and risk of perinatal mortality from major malformations (Table 11.4) [39,40]. Studies that have examined the potential relationship between first-trimester metabolic control and risk for major malformation are summarized in Table 11.5. Not included in the table is the study

of Nielsen et al. [41] because it used a composite outcome measure of spontaneous abortions, induced abortions, and major malformations but it too confirms the relationship between poor first-trimester metabolic control and early adverse pregnancy outcome. All studies have found a relationship except the Diabetes In Early Pregnancy (DIEP) study of the National Institutes of Child Health and Human Development (NICHD) [42]. The DIEP was a multicenter study that enrolled diabetic women either prior to conception or within 21 days of conception. The reason why the DIEP failed to find the relationship between poor control during organogenesis and risk of major malformation was that 86% of the DIEP patients were enrolled prior to conception, with the remaining 14% enrolled within 21 days of conception. This yielded a rather homogeneous group of patients with relatively good metabolic control. Ninety-three percent of their patients had first-trimester glycohemoglobin values less than seven standard deviations above the mean. The best evidence suggests that the risk for major malformations does not begin to rise in a statistically significant manner until Hb A_1 values are well beyond seven standard deviations above the mean [40,41]. Thus, the vast majority of the DIEP study subjects were not at increased risk for major malformations. Not surprisingly, therefore, no increase in risk was found. All the existing data are consistent with the hypothesis that poor metabolic control during organogenesis as evidenced by elevated first-trimester glycohemoglobin values is associated with an increased risk for major congenital malformations among IDM.

Molsted-Pedersen et al. suggested in 1964 that the risk of major malformation might be further increased by the presence of microvascular disease [10]. However, data from the Joslin Diabetes Center have not supported such an association, demonstrating no significant increase in risk of major malformations for patients with nephropathy or proliferative retinopathy, as compared with those without. Moreover, women in the Joslin cohort who delivered nonmalformed liveimbirths actually had diabetes for a significantly longer time prior to pregnancy than women who delivered babies with major malformations (mean 13.4 versus 8.9 years). Because the prevalence of microvascular disease among patients with diabetes increases with increasing duration of illness, this finding further argues against an association between microvascular disease and the risk of major malformations.

Table 11.3 Major malformations and Hb A_1, Joslin Diabetes Center 1984–1992

Hb A_1 Standard deviations above mean	N	%	Risk ratio (95% confidence interval)
<6.10	10/266	3.7	1.0
6.1–9.0	10/193	5.2	1.4 (0.6–3.2)
9.1–12.0	8/97	8.2	2.2 (0.9–5.3)
12.1–15.0	10/31	32.2	8.6 (4.2–17.3)
>15.0	5/12	41.7	11.1 (4.8–25.4)

Table 11.4 Fatal malformations according to first-trimester Hb A_1 level, Joslin Diabetes Center data through 12/31/92

Hb A_1 Standard deviations above mean	Number	%	Risk ratio (95% confidence interval)
<12 SD	9/599	1.5	–
>12 SD	9/43	20.9	13.9 (7.0–27.9)

Table 11.5 Studies of relationship between first-trimester metabolic control and major malformations

Study (ref)	Relationship found
Miller [38]	Yes
Ylinen [16]	Yes
Mills [42]	No
Greene [75]	Yes
Hanson [19]	Yes
Kitzmiller [104]	Yes
French Study Group [20]	Yes
Rosenn [24]	Yes
Towner [25]	Yes
Casson [30]	Yes

Spontaneous abortion

There has been debate as to whether diabetic women have an increased incidence of spontaneous abortion in the first trimester. Early studies suggested that the rate was approximately equal to that in the nondiabetic population [43]. Later studies suggested that the rate was higher than for nondiabetic patients [44,45] but these studies could have been biased by differential ascertainment of miscarriages in diabetic and

Table 11.6 Spontaneous abortions and Hb A$_1$, Joslin Diabetes Center 1984–1992

Hb A$_1$ Standard deviations above mean	N	%	Risk ratio (95% confidence interval)
<6.1	38/304	12	1.0
6.1–9.0	27/220	12	1.0 (0.6–1.6)
9.1–12.0	26/123	21	1.7 (1.1–2.7)
12.1–15.0	14/45	31	2.5 (1.4–4.3)
>15.0	11/23	48	3.8 (2.1–6.8)

nondiabetic women. Wright *et al.* found a 17% first-trimester spontaneous abortion rate among 58 consecutive diabetic pregnancies and demonstrated that the patients who miscarried had significantly higher first-trimester glycohemoglobin levels than those who did not [43]. The DIEP found an increasing risk of spontaneous abortion associated with increasing first-trimester glycosylated hemoglobin levels [46]. The risk of spontaneous abortion in the best controlled diabetic patients was between 10% and 17%. Those patients who entered the first trimester with glycosylated hemoglobin values of more than six standard deviations above the mean for their nondiabetic controls had a twofold increase in risk to about 28%. Data from the Joslin Diabetes Center confirmed the finding of an increasing risk of spontaneous abortion associated with increasing first-trimester Hb A$_1$ values (Table 11.6) [39]. The risk of spontaneous abortion does not rise statistically significantly until greater than nine standard deviations above the mean for the nondiabetic population. This is consistent with the data from the DIEP, but they did not have enough patients at higher glycohemoglobin values to determine whether the risk truly rises at greater than nine standard deviations above the mean or between six and nine.

Defining the phenotype of the diabetic embryopathy

The anomalies found among IDM span the range of the anomalies found in the nondiabetic population. Kucera compiled a series of 7100 IDM from the literature from nine countries spanning 30 years and compared the 340 anomalous fetuses among them to a control group of 7100 anomalous fetuses from 431,000 nondiabetic women from a WHO database [47]. Ten malformations were sixfold more common among the IDM; most strikingly, caudal regression syndrome was 200-fold more common than among offspring of nondiabetic mothers. Kucera considered these "very probably" specific for diabetes.

A case–control study from the Metropolitan Atlanta Congenital Defects Program found an odds ratios of 15 for neural tube defects and 13 for congenital heart disease [48]. A Spanish case–control study found relative frequencies of 66 for defects of the spine and ribs, 53 for caudal dysgenesis,

2.9 for CNS defects and 2.8 for congenital heart disease [49]. A case–control study of congenital heart disease in metropolitan Baltimore and Washington DC found a strong association between both congenital heart disease in general and fatal congenital heart disease and maternal diabetes [50]. A Hungarian case–control study found maternal diabetes to be associated with a prevalence odds ratios of 14.8 for renal agenesis or dysgenesis, 5.0 for multiple anomaly syndromes, and 3.4 for congenital heart disease, but no significant association of maternal diabetes with neural tube defects [51]. In a British cohort study of 609 liveborn IDM, 22 (3.6%) had cardiovascular malformations compared to the 0.74% incidence in 192,000 controls, resulting in an odds ratio of 5.0 [52]. Maternal diabetes, like other environmental teratogens, interacts with genetic factors to result in congenital malformations. Allowing for some geographic and likely genetic differences among study populations, the congenital malformations that emerge as most likely specific to maternal diabetes are renal agenesis/caudal dysgenesis syndrome, congenital heart defects and neural tube defects.

Summary of the relationship between metabolic control and first-trimester events

Synthesis of the available data permits several conclusions. Women with diabetes mellitus who are in good metabolic control in the first trimester do not have a risk for spontaneous abortion higher than the general population, when the control group is comparably recruited and studied. However, women with well-controlled diabetes cannot be glibly reassured that their risk for major malformations is not increased above that for the nondiabetic population. The finding of the DIEP study that even well-controlled diabetic women have an increased risk of major malformations above that for the nondiabetic population seems inescapable. The range of metabolic control over which the risks for abortion and major malformations do not rise is fairly broad. Very poor metabolic control during the first trimester, however, does result in increased risks for both first-trimester spontaneous abortions and major malformations. The mechanism behind the modestly increased risk of major malformations for IDM despite good maternal metabolic control followed by a plateau in risk with fair control and a very high risk with very poor control is not known. Figure 11.2 displays the Joslin Diabetes Center data for spontaneous abortions, major malformations and nonmalformed births graphically by first-trimester Hb A$_1$ values and standardized to 100%, with the actual number of observations in each group at the top of each bar. This makes it very clear that for diabetic women, the risks for spontaneous abortion and major malformation do not increase significantly for Hb A$_1$ values up to nine standard deviations above the nondiabetic mean. However, with very poor metabolic control (Hb A$_1$ values greater than 12 standard deviations above the nondiabetic mean), diabetic women are approximately equally likely to have a spontaneous abortion,

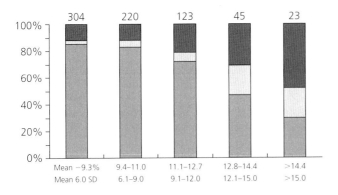

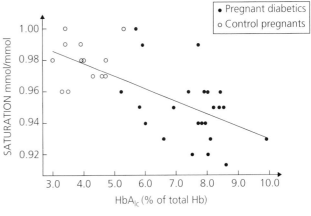

Figure 11.2 Data from the Joslin Diabetes Center, January 1 1984 to December 31 1992, for 715 consecutive pregnancies with first-trimester HbA$_1$ values available. This stacked bar graph demonstrates the relative probabilities of a nonmalformed livebirth, ▦ a major congenital malformation ▢ and a first-trimester spontaneous abortion ■ according to first-trimester HbA$_1$ values and standardized to 100%. Reproduced from Greene [40] with permission from Thieme Medical Publishers.

Figure 11.3 Correlation between Hb A$_{1c}$ and arterial oxygen saturation in diabetic and nondiabetic women. Reproduced from Madsen & Ditzel [53] with permission from Elsevier.

a fetus with a major malformation, and a nonmalformed birth. Although simple hyperglycemia alone does not appear to be the mechanism responsible for teratogenesis, the precise molecular mechanism remains unknown.

Late pregnancy fetal and neonatal effects

Respiratory physiology and fetal demise

Hemoglobin A$_{1c}$ concentrations among diabetic women may be 2–3 times higher than nondiabetic individuals. Beyond being a useful clinical tool for assessing recent metabolic control, the glycosylation of hemoglobin has physiologic implications for oxygen transport. As the percentage of glycosylated hemoglobin rises, the amount of oxygen, molecule for molecule, carried by hemoglobin falls (Figure 11.3) [53]. The avidity with which the oxygen is bound is also changed. The affinity of hemoglobin for oxygen is normally modulated by binding with 2,3-diphosphoglycerate (2,3-DPG) so that in the presence of 2,3-DPG the P$_{50}$ rises (P$_{50}$ is a measure of hemoglobin affinity for oxygen and reflects the partial pressure of oxygen at which hemoglobin achieves 50% saturation). When P$_{50}$ rises, the oxygen is less firmly bound. Hemoglobin A$_{1c}$ changes its P$_{50}$ only minimally in the presence of 2,3-DPG, resulting in an inverse correlation of the P$_{50}$ with the concentration of Hb A$_{1c}$ (Figure 11.4). The displacement of oxygen from native hemoglobin that is facilitated by 2,3-DPG binding is also associated with the acceptance of a proton (H+) by the deoxygenated hemoglobin (the Bohr effect) and thus contributes to the buffering capacity of blood. Hb A$_{1c}$, with its more tightly bound oxygen, releases the oxygen less well at areas of reduced oxygen tension, such as the placental

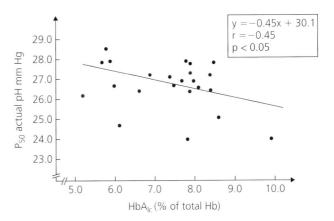

Figure 11.4 Correlation between Hb A$_{1c}$ and P$_{50}$ at actual pH in diabetic women. Reproduced from Madsen & Ditzel [53] with permission from Elsevier.

intervillous space. Diabetic patients who are chronically poorly controlled will have high levels of Hb A$_{1c}$ that will carry less oxygen, release it less well to cross the placenta, and buffer acid less well.

The adverse effects of chronic hyperglycemia on the oxygen-carrying and buffering properties of maternal hemoglobin are exacerbated by fetal hyperinsulinemia. Fetuses of diabetic mothers in poor metabolic control are chronically hyperinsulinemic and develop pancreatic beta cell hyperplasia; fetal hyperinsulinemia is further exacerbated by acute episodes of maternal hyperglycemia. Fetal hyperinsulinemia increases the oxygen requirement of the fetus. Fetal oxygen consumption rises in direct proportion to the insulin concentration, resulting in falls in both venous and arterial oxygen contents (Figure 11.5A,B) [54]. Oxygen supply is unable to keep pace with demand, resulting in fetal hypoxemia reflected in a progressive rise in the arteriovenous oxygen difference between the umbilical artery and vein (Figure 11.5C) and acidosis [54]. These mechanisms, combined with compromise to perfusion of the intervillous space resulting from hypertension and maternal vascular disease, were likely responsible for the late fetal demises that were so common through the 1960s. Over the past 40 years there have been many improvements in the care of pregnant diabetic women, making it impossible to isolate and attribute the reduction in the risk of late fetal demise to any one. It is most likely that improved metabolic control and modern surveillance for fetal well-being are together largely responsible for the dramatic reduction in incidence of stillbirth to rates comparable to the nondiabetic population by the 1990s [55].

Fetal growth

Excessive fetal growth has long been recognized as an important complication of maternal diabetes. According to the expanded Pedersen hypothesis, elevated maternal levels of glucose and possibly other insulin secretagogues like certain amino acids readily cross the placenta, resulting in fetal hyperinsulinemia. Fetal hyperinsulinemia acts as an anabolic stimulus, leading to enhanced accretion of fat, bone and muscle mass. Supporting this hypothesis is the finding that macrosomic fetuses of diabetic women have high C peptide levels and are at increased risk for neonatal hypoglycemia [56].

Early attempts to correlate a variety of indices of glycemic control (e.g. mean daily glucose levels and Hb A_{1c} levels) with fetal growth had limited success. Furthermore, occasional case reports have described the birth of markedly macrosomic infants despite excellent glycemic control by all known parameters. A potential explanation for these apparently conflicting observations was provided by the finding that insulin could cross the placenta from the maternal to the fetal circulation in the form of insulin–anti-insulin antibody complexes [57]. The level of these antigen–antibody complexes was proportional to fetal weight at birth. An increasing body of evidence indicates that there is a relationship between fetal size at birth and maternal glycemia that extends down through the normal, "nondiabetic" range with no "threshold" for excessive growth [8,58,59]. The finding in a UK case series that there was a dramatic reduction in fetal demise, but not in the risk of excess fetal size at birth, with lower glucose levels [55] suggests that the degree of metabolic control needed to minimize the risk for excessive fetal growth is likely to be much more stringent than that needed to reduce the risk of fetal demise. The term "macrosomia" has been used variably to describe fetal weight in absolute terms as greater than 4000 g, or greater than 4500 g, and in relative terms as greater than the 90th centile at any gestational age. Excessive fetal growth is undesirable because it is associated with increased rates for cesarean delivery, birth trauma, stillbirth, neonatal hypertrophic cardiomyopathy and hypoglycemia.

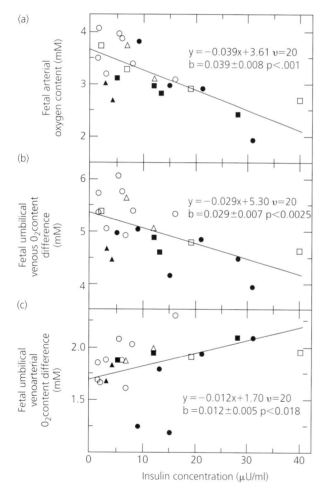

Figure 11.5 The association between fetal plasma insulin concentration and fetal (a) arterial oxygen content, (b) venous oxygen content, and (c) umbilical venoarterial oxygen content difference. Shown in each frame is the regression line as determined by analysis of co-variance. Also shown are the regression equations as well as the slopes with their standard errors and P values. Reproduced from Milley *et al.* [54] with permission from Elsevier.

Fetal lung maturation

It has been recognized for more than 30 years that, after controlling for gestational age, the incidence of respiratory distress syndrome (RDS) among IDM is 5–6-fold higher than the incidence among infants of nondiabetic women [60]. Fetal lung development is an extremely complex process involving hundreds of intercellular signaling events to bring vasculature and airways together and then differentiate the airway epithelium into an efficient respiratory epithelium for gas exchange [61].

The ultimate steps in development of the alveolar epithelium that permit expansion of alveolar spaces with air at birth and that resist collapse are proliferation and maturation of type II pneumocytes that produce surfactant. This process is under endocrine control with glucocorticoids and thyroxin promoting type II pneumocyte proliferation and surfactant production. Both insulin and androgens inhibit surfactant production in mammals [62]. The inhibitory effect of androgens on surfactant production helps to explain the well-known difference between the sexes in respiratory distress syndrome. The inhibitory effect of insulin and the hyperinsulinemia of most fetuses of diabetic mothers help to explain the increased incidence of RDS in IDM. Stillborn male IDM commonly demonstrate Leydig cell hyperplasia in their testes [63]. The cord blood of male IDM demonstrates higher HCG and testosterone concentrations than the cord blood of male infants of nondiabetic mothers [64]. These higher testosterone levels during fetal development further slow fetal lung maturation.

Polycythemia and hyperviscosity syndrome

Polycythemia defined as hematocrit greater than 65% has long been known to be more common among IDM. In a series of 34 IDM paired with 34 infants of nondiabetic women, the rates of polycythemia were 29% and 6%, respectively [65]. However, recent series of IDM born to very well-controlled diabetic women have shown no increase in risk compared to infants of nondiabetic women. The incidence of polycythemia is proportional to fetal insulin levels. Insulin directly stimulates erythroid progenitors in the marrow to make more red cells [66], possibly by cross-reacting with the receptors for insulin-like growth factor 1 (IGF-1) [67]. Elevated levels of insulin also stimulate erythropoiesis indirectly by stimulating elevated levels of erythropoietin (EPO), which stimulates erythropoiesis [68,69]. Insulin also stimulates synthesis of hypoxia-inducible factor 1 (HIF-1) which, under relatively hypoxemic conditions, stimulates synthesis of a number of proteins, including transferrin and IGF-1 receptor protein, further stimulating erythropoiesis [70].

Mild polycythemia may contribute to the increased incidence of hyperbilirubinemia seen in IDM, but severe polycythemia can place the neonate at risk for hyperviscosity syndrome, including ischemia, thrombosis and infarction. This may require treatment by phlebotomy to reduce the hematocrit.

Neonatal hypoglycemia

Chronic stimulation by elevated levels of transplacental glucose and possibly other insulin secretagogues such as branched chain amino acids results in fetal pancreatic beta cell hyperplasia. When the umbilical cord is cut at delivery, the transplacental supply of glucose stops abruptly. As many as one-quarter of all IDM have difficulty downregulating insulin production promptly, resulting in neonatal hypoglycemia (defined as blood glucose less than 40 mg/dL). Not surprisingly, because chronic fetal hyperglycemia causes beta cell hyperplasia and hyperinsulinemia, which in turn cause both macrosomia and neonatal hypoglycemia, macrosomic babies are at greater risk for hypoglycemia than appropriately grown babies. Just as strict metabolic control during pregnancy reduces but does not eliminate macrosomia, the same is true for neonatal hypoglycemia. Before hypoglycemia was recognized as a common problem, it was a frequent cause of neonatal seizures and occasionally death. Modern pediatric care now usually includes routine heel stick capillary blood glucose measurement at about 30 minutes of age and regularly thereafter until stable. Hypoglycemia is treated with glucose feedings or intravenous infusions as necessary. The problem is self-limiting and usually resolves within 48 hours of birth.

Other metabolic abnormalities

Hypocalcemia and hypomagnesemia are both rather common among IDM, each approximately 20–30%, and usually asymptomatic. Routine screening is not recommended, although these conditions should be considered if a baby remains unusually "jittery" despite normal glucose levels. Hyperbilirubinemia occurs with similar frequency in IDM. As noted above, it is more frequent in infants with polycythemia, perhaps due to an increase in red cell fragility and immaturity of conjugation enzyme systems.

Hypertrophic cardiomyopathy

Hypertrophic cardiomyopathy is rarely, if ever, seen among IDM in the absence of macrosomia. It can present along a continuum of severity from frank congestive heart failure to clinical respiratory distress with tachypnea, nasal flaring, grunting, retractions and cyanosis to asymptomatic [71]. Given that many babies discovered to have the echocardiographic signs of hypertrophic cardiomyopathy are asymptomatic, the incidence of the problem varies widely with the frequency with which echocardiograms are done in these babies. The echocardiographic hallmark of the condition is hypertrophy of the interventricular septum and to a much lesser extent the ventricular free walls. The degree of the hypertrophy correlates reasonably well with symptomatology at clinical presentation. Ventricular function is well preserved, although most infants developing congestive failure have some degree of hypertrophic subaortic obstruction. Among infants presenting with respiratory distress, there is frequently evidence of persistent pulmonary hypertension of the newborn. In rare cases, the condition can be lethal in the newborn period but babies who survive generally recover without sequelae and, on echocardiographic follow-up typically remodel their myocardium to normal appearance within 2–12 months [72]. In addition to the almost universal macrosomia in these babies, severe and prolonged hypoglycemia is common, adding to the impression that fetal hyperinsulinemia is etiologic [73]. The more severe end of this spectrum of disease has all but disappeared in recent years, likely due to generally improved metabolic control throughout pregnancy.

Prematurity

There is an increased risk of premature birth among IDM. Mimouni *et al.* reported a 31% incidence of preterm labor among 164 women with insulin-dependent diabetes as compared to a 20% incidence in nondiabetic control women [74]. Of the diabetic women diagnosed with premature labor, 72% actually delivered prematurely for an overall incidence of preterm birth of 22.5%. In a series of 420 pregnancies from the Joslin Diabetes Center, the incidence of preterm birth was 26% compared with a 9.7% rate among 9368 control nondiabetic women [75]. In that series, the single most important cause of preterm birth, 33% of the preterm births, was deliveries indicated due to pre-eclampsia. The other important causes of preterm birth were preterm premature rupture of the membranes 25%, deliveries indicated for nonreassuring fetal evaluation 14%, and spontaneous onset of labor 13%. There was a strong relationship between the presence of diabetic nephropathy and preterm delivery. Among the 59 women entering pregnancy with nephropathy, 39 (66%) developed hypertension during pregnancy and 31 (52%) of the total delivered prematurely. A series of 461 pregnancies among women with pregestational diabetes was reported from the NICHD Maternal Fetal Medicine Unit Network [76]. They too found a statistically significantly higher incidence of preterm birth among their diabetic women, 38%, as compared to 13.9% among 2738 control women. In that study, 42% of the preterm births were spontaneous while 58% were indicated, the majority of those for pre-eclampsia.

Long-term neurodevelopmental outcome

The NIH Collaborative Perinatal Project enrolled more than 50,000 mother/infant pairs with the primary purpose of determining the prenatal causes of cerebral palsy and mental retardation. Diabetic women were matched to nondiabetic controls and their offspring were compared using the Bayley Mental and Motor Development Tests and the Binet IQ Test at 4 years of age [77]. The offspring of diabetic women who experienced acetonuria (acetone is one of the ketones) during pregnancy performed statistically significantly less well on all testing than their nondiabetic controls. These differences were not seen in the offspring of diabetic women who were not acetonuric during pregnancy nor did they find any neurodevelopmental disadvantage among the offspring of diabetic women who experienced more insulin reactions. A second study from that same cohort did not find any developmental disadvantage to the offspring of acetonuric, starved, nondiabetic women who failed to gain weight adequately [78]. These observations suggested that there

was something particularly disadvantageous to the ketosis of poorly controlled diabetes as compared to simple starvation ketosis.

Some years later a cohort study of 89 women with pregestational diabetes, 99 women with gestational diabetes and 35 nondiabetic control women found significant adverse consequences for neurodevelopmental testing results at 2, 3, 4 and 5 years of age related to elevated serum levels of the ketone beta-hydroxybutyrate in the third trimester [79]. There were no significant correlations between intelligence scores and second- or third-trimester fasting plasma glucose levels, Hb A_{1c} levels or hypoglycemic episodes. Continued testing for this cohort at 6–9 years of age confirmed the deleterious neurodevelopmental consequences of late pregnancy elevations of maternal serum beta-hydroxybutyrate levels [80]. Thus there is the strong suggestion that elevated serum levels of ketoacids in diabetic women in late pregnancy are associated with adverse neurodevelopmental consequences for their offspring. Compared to the sons of nondiabetic women, sons of diabetic women were slightly but statistically significantly more likely to be rejected for Danish military service based upon an intelligence test administered to all potential conscripts [81]. A subgroup analysis of the intelligence test scores for those men for whom data were available regarding their mothers' Hb A_{1c} levels during pregnancy showed that the scores for the men whose mothers' Hb A_{1c} values were less than 7% were similar to the sons of the nondiabetic women.

Perinatal mortality

Although major improvements in the care of pregnant diabetic women over the past 80 years have reduced the perinatal mortality rate by an order of magnitude, it still remains higher than that for the offspring of nondiabetic women. Through the 1960s the rate of near-term fetal demise for diabetic women was nearly 10%. This led to the practice of routine delivery at 36–37 weeks resulting in neonatal morbidity and mortality due to hypoglycemia and RDS. During the 1970s, improved metabolic control facilitated by capillary blood glucose monitoring and routine surveillance for fetal well-being using electronic fetal heart rate monitoring and ultrasound reduced the rate of near-term fetal demise. This, coupled with recognition of the toll of neonatal morbidity and mortality of RDS in IDM and development of fetal lung maturity testing, gave obstetricians both the courage and the motivation to continue pregnancies of diabetic women to 39 weeks, dramatically reducing perinatal mortality due to fetal demise and neonatal RDS. By 1978 Gabbe *et al.* observed that 4/9 perinatal mortalities among 322 IDM were due to major congenital malformations, replacing RDS as the main cause of neonatal death in IDM [82].

Twenty-five years later the Confidential Enquiry into Maternal and Child Health for March 2002 through February 2003 in Great Britain found the perinatal mortality rate among IDM to be 32/1000, nearly four times higher than the 8.5/1000 rate for the rest of Great Britain [83]. Consistent with Gabbe's observation, 42% of the 129 perinatal mortalities were due to major congenital malformations. A regional survey in Great Britain 1990–1994 [84], a nationwide survey in Denmark 1993–1999 [85] and a provincial population-based cohort in Nova Scotia 1988–2002 [86] have all reported similar findings. A review of the available studies confirms the impression that the overall risk of perinatal mortality is related to the degree of glycemic control [87].

Risk of diabetes in the offspring

One of the questions most frequently asked by women with diabetes is "Will my child have diabetes?" There are clearly strong hereditary and environmental influences on the development of both type 1 and type 2 diabetes. A major fraction of the risk for type 1 diabetes is strongly associated with the HLA system in a group of genes on chromosome 6p21 and several other chromosome regions [88]. There are undoubtedly also environmental influences, however, including the possibility that a variety of viral infections could serve as triggers in genetically susceptible individuals. The risk of insulin-dependent diabetes by 20 years of age is inherited asymmetrically from mother (1.3%) and father (6.1%) [89]. Furthermore, the risk is inversely related to maternal age at delivery, being approximately 3% for diabetic women under age 25 and 1% over age 25 [90]. The inheritance pattern for type 2 diabetes has been more difficult to discern, with strong associations discovered on genome-wide association studies (GWAS) for mutations in many sites, some of which are in unsuspected genes and outside coding regions [91,92]. The importance of classic clinical risk factors such as a family history of the disease, increased BMI, elevated liver enzymes, current smoking status, and reduced measures of insulin production and action was emphasized by the fact that they were more strongly predictive of the disease than variants in 11 alleles known to be risk factors from GWAS [93]. Some of the variant alleles are associated with impaired beta cell function rather than insulin resistance [94]. Another clue to the mechanisms involved is that the risk for gestational diabetes, as a proxy for type 2 diabetes or pre-pregnancy type 2 diabetes, is inherited asymmetrically from mother and father. Among 232 women with either GDM or type 2 diabetes, 11% had a mother with diabetes while only 5% had a father with diabetes and for the women with two diabetic parents, there was no greater risk of diabetes than with a diabetic mother alone [95]. This suggests a possible epigenetic mechanism to the inheritance.

Medical management

Pre-pregnancy care

The main purpose of pre-pregnancy care is to identify any maternal conditions that might pose a risk to mother or fetus

during a pregnancy. Once identified, the woman should be counseled about the potential risks presented and she should be treated as necessary.

Women presenting for pre-pregnancy care and counseling should have a complete history taken with special attention paid to:
- age of onset and duration of diabetes
- assessment of type (1 or 2) of diabetes
- history of diabetic ketoacidosis and precipitating circumstances
- history of severe hypoglycemia, hypoglycemic seizures and ability to reliably perceive hypoglycemia
- retinopathy, proliferative retinopathy and laser photocoagulation therapy for retinopathy
- proteinuria and nephropathy
- hypertension
- neuropathy including symptoms suggestive of gastroparesis
- cardiovascular disease.

A complete physical examination should be sure to include assessments of BMI (height and weight), blood pressure and thyroid examination. A dilated retinal examination should be considered based upon duration of diabetes, time elapsed since last examination, and history of retinopathy on prior examinations.

Laboratory evaluations should include blood for Hb A_{1c}, hematocrit/hemoglobin, thyroid-stimulating hormone (TSH), blood urea nitrogen (BUN) and creatinine. Urine should be checked for the presence of albumin and, if found, should be quantified with either a 24-hour collection or spot micro-albumin to creatinine ratio or protein to creatinine ratio. If significant proteinuria is found, a serum albumin concentration should be done.

Current recommendations of the American Diabetes Association suggest screening for depression, anxiety, stress and eating disorders. They also recommend discontinuing all oral agents and initiation of insulin therapy to optimize metabolic control prior to conception. Counseling should include discussions of the risks for all the potential fetal and neonatal complications discussed above. Women should be prepared for the fact that prenatal care will require frequent visits, meticulous metabolic control, including multiple capillary blood glucose determinations daily, and routine surveillance for fetal well-being. Women should be advised that retinopathy may develop or progress during pregnancy. If proteinuria is present, the patient should be advised that it will likely increase during pregnancy and is associated with both simple pedal edema and superimposed pre-eclampsia. The most important interventions to minimize the risk for progression of both retinopathy and nephropathy are to control both blood glucose and blood pressure.

Contraception

It is most important that diabetic women plan their pregnancies to enter pregnancy in good metabolic control to minimize the risk for complications of pregnancy associated with inadequate control in the first trimester. All the contraceptive methods available to nondiabetic women can be used by diabetic women, paying attention to the contraindications that pertain to any woman. Natural family planning and barrier methods are safe for all but their effective use requires considerable motivation and their effectiveness in practice is less than that for intrauterine devices (IUD) and hormonal methods. For many years, IUD were avoided in diabetic women due to fear of an excessive rate of infection. However, devices containing both copper and levonorgestrel seem equally safe and effective in diabetic and nondiabetic women and they should be offered as a reasonable option [96,97]. As is true for all women, the doses of hormones in combined estrogen progestin oral contraceptives should be kept as low as possible. Modern low-dose combined preparations have negligible effects on glucose control and atherogenic lipid profiles in diabetic women in good metabolic control [98]. To minimize theoretical risks, the American College of Obstetricians and Gynecologists recommends that hormonal contraception be reserved for diabetic women who are otherwise healthy, young (under age 35), nonsmokers, without hypertension, retinopathy, nephropathy or other evidence of vascular disease [99]. There is insufficient information regarding the use of either the contraceptive ring or patch to recommend their use in diabetic women. These same principles apply to postpartum diabetic women.

Prevention of early pregnancy adverse events

In a review of reported series, Mills *et al.* pointed out that most of the malformations among IDM arise from abnormal development before the seventh week of gestation [100]. Thus, if these anomalies are preventable, any effective intervention must be made very early in pregnancy. This would be so early in pregnancy that most women would not ordinarily have seen their obstetricians for the first visit; many may not have even recognized their pregnancies yet. Recognition of the relationship between first-trimester metabolic control and risk for major malformations has led to several programs designed to reduce them. In view of the very early gestational age at which most major malformations arise, and the time necessary for adjustments in diet, insulin dosage and exercise to improve metabolic control, it is clear that such efforts must begin prior to conception. Both observational and interventional studies have found that compared to diabetic women who do not obtain preconception care, those who do obtain preconception care are less likely to smoke, are less likely to have unplanned pregnancies, enter prenatal care earlier and have lower glycohemoglobin levels at entry to care. They are also less likely to have babies with major congenital malformations (Table 11.7) [101–105]. No randomized controlled trials of preconception care have been done.

Whereas a reasonable explanation for these findings is that preconception care improves early pregnancy glycemic

Table 11.7 Trials of preconception care for women with diabetes mellitus. Incidence of major malformations

Study (ref)	Attenders	Nonattenders
Fuhrmann *et al.* 1983 [101]	1/128 (0.8%)	22/292 (7.5%)
Damm *et al.* 1989 [102]	2/193 (1.0%)	5/61 (8.2%)
Steel *et al.* 1990 [103]	2/143 (1.4%)	10/96 (10.4%)
Kitzmiller *et al.* 1991 [104]	1/84 (1.2%)	12/110 (10.9%)
Willhoite *et al.* 1993 [105]	1/62 (1.6%)	8/123 (6.5%)

control, and that early control improves outcomes, it is possible that other important differences in healthcare or lifestyle between women who do and do not obtain preconception care may contribute to the difference in malformation rates between these groups. Women who seek (or comply with) preconception care may also pay more attention to their health in other respects, and might have good glycemic control regardless of whether they receive such care [106]. We may be devoting expensive and scarce healthcare resources to those persons who need them least. While the possibility has not yet been formally excluded that there are other important differences in healthcare or lifestyle that contribute to the difference in malformation rates between diabetic women who do and do not obtain preconception care, it seems clear that the major determinant of the risk is first-trimester blood glucose control. Although these criticisms cannot be easily dismissed, a randomized trial testing the impact of tight versus poor glycemic control early in pregnancy would not be ethical, given current knowledge, and preconception care should routinely be encouraged.

Principles of treatment in preparation for and during pregnancy

Maintenance of euglycemia

No single medical or obstetric intervention has been as important in improving the outcome for diabetic women and their offspring as improved metabolic control. As pregnancy progresses through the second trimester, placental production of HPL, which antagonizes the action of insulin, rises. This causes a dramatic increase in insulin requirements to levels as high as 150–200% of those prior to pregnancy. Insulin requirements generally peak around 36 weeks and decrease slightly toward term as fetal glucose consumption becomes substantial. Trying to adjust to constantly changing insulin requirements during pregnancy can be difficult and frustrating for a patient. Just when she thinks she has the right dose, it changes. Patients should be seen frequently during pregnancy, preferably by a multidisciplinary team, including a dietician, a diabetes nurse educator, an internist or medical endocrinologist, and an obstetrician familiar with the care of diabetes in pregnancy, to help them with their glycemic control.

Figure 11.6 illustrates the major changes in maternal daily glucose and insulin concentration profiles associated with pregnancy. During pregnancy, fasting glucose levels are somewhat lower, while postprandial glycemic excursions are higher and wider than in nonpregnant women [107]. These changes in postprandial glucose concentrations occur despite levels of insulin higher than in the nonpregnant state. Despite the insulin resistance of pregnancy, nondiabetic women normally control their blood glucose concentrations around the clock within a very narrow range (Figure 11.7) [59]. Appreciation of what are truly "normal" blood glucose concentrations and recognition that minor elevations throughout the second and third trimesters are associated with undesirable fetal consequences [8] will undoubtedly lead to official recommendations for stricter metabolic control in management of pregnant diabetic women.

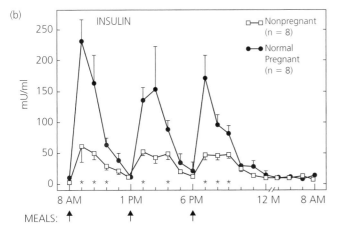
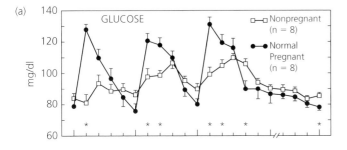

Figure 11.6 The effect of normal late pregnancy on the diurnal changes in plasma glucose and insulin concentration. Asterisks indicate values during pregnancy that are significantly elevated compared to nonpregnant values. Reproduced from Phelps *et al.* [107] with permission from Elsevier.

Diet

In preparation for pregnancy, a proper diet should provide all necessary macro- and micronutrients, minimize cholesterol, saturated fat and trans fat intake, promote euglycemia, and encourage an appropriate body weight (BMI 20–24.9). Thus an appropriate diet would encourage weight gain for underweight women (BMI less than 20) and weight loss for overweight (BMI 25–29.9) and obese women (BMI 30 or more). An appropriate daily distribution of dietary calories is approximately 40–50% of total calories from carbohydrate, 15–20% from protein (0.8 g protein/kg bodyweight) and the remainder from fat. Diabetic women should be encouraged to consume as many of their carbohydrate calories as possible as complex carbohydrates and maintain a fiber intake of 28 g/day by consumption of whole grains, fruits and vegetables [108].

Dietary therapy during pregnancy should adhere to the principles above for nonpregnant women and promote adequate but not excessive weight gain. Appropriate total caloric intake is determined by pre-pregnancy BMI and physical activity level during pregnancy. Most pregnant women should consume a diet that provides 30 kcal/kg of current bodyweight per day, including about 175 g/day of digestible carbohydrate. An occupation or lifestyle that includes more exercise will require more calories. There is some debate as

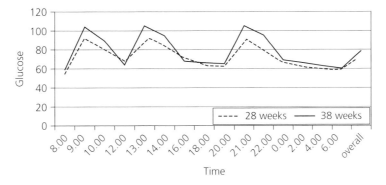

Figure 11.7 Daily blood glucose values at 28 and 38 weeks gestation in nondiabetic pregnancies. Data from Parretti *et al.* [59].

to whether the amount of dietary protein should be increased during pregnancy, but the American Diabetes Association recommends a modest increase to 1.1 g/kg/day. Women who start pregnancy underweight should consume approximately 35 kcal/kg/day and women who are overweight or obese can safely reduce their total caloric intake by as much as 30% to help control weight gain and promote euglycemia.

Insulin therapy

Two human insulins (regular and NPH) and several semi-synthetic human insulin analogues are now available, including rapid, intermediate and long-acting types (see Table 11.8 and Figure 11.8 for their pharmacologic characteristics) [109]. The semi-synthetic human insulin analogues are the result of genetic engineering to replace one or more amino acids in the human insulin molecule to alter the pharmacologic profile of insulin action. They are produced in microorganisms by recombinant DNA technology. All are injectable alone or in combinations with other varieties. Insulin glargine should not be mixed in the same syringe with other types of insulins.

There has been considerable discussion regarding the best insulin regimen for achieving optimal glycemic control in

pregnancy. The majority of patients will achieve adequate control with a conventional regimen of multiple bolus injections of rapid-acting insulin prior to meals and one or more bolus injections of intermediate or long-acting insulin daily. Continuous subcutaneous insulin infusion (CSII) via pump is an expensive, labor-intensive alternative method of insulin therapy that requires a motivated patient. Pump infusion sets are expensive and pumps can malfunction. A systematic review and meta-analysis of randomized trials of standard versus CSII pump therapy during pregnancy was unable to identify any maternal or fetal benefits to CSII pump therapy [110]. Among the rapid-acting insulin analogues, there is little experience to date with the use of insulin glulisine, but reassuring data with both aspart and lispro [111–115]. Less reported experience with insulin glargine, and some theoretical concerns about its use in pregnancy [116], have prompted the American Diabetes Association [108] to suggest using only NPH as a longer acting insulin in pregnancy, but a recently reported, though relatively small series of 115 insulin glargine-treated pregnancies was reassuring [117].

Oral agents

Oral hypoglycemic agents have been avoided during pregnancy due to fears of both potential induction of congenital malformations with first-trimester exposure and neonatal hypoglycemia with exposure later in pregnancy. In a randomized controlled trial among 400 patients with gestational diabetes, hyperglycemia after the first trimester was treated with glyburide, a sulfonylurea with minimal transplacental passage in 200 patients, and compared with insulin in the other 200. Glyburide with the addition of insulin in only 4% of patients achieved metabolic control and short-term complication rates comparable to those with insulin treatment [118]. Metformin has become increasingly popular for treatment of type 2 diabetes and infertility associated with insulin

Table 11.8 Duration of action of standard insulins and insulin analogues

Insulin	Onset of action	Peak action	Effective duration
Standard			
Regular	30–60 min	2–3 h	8–10 h
NPH	2–4 h	4–10 h	12–18 h
Analogues			
Lispro, aspart, glulisine	5–15 min	30–90 min	4–6 h
Glargine	2–4 h	No peak	20–24 h
Detemir	2–4 h	No peak	6–24 h

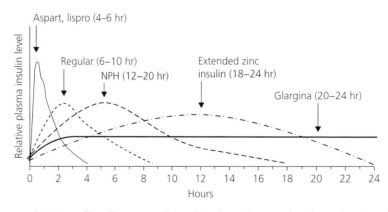

Figure 11.8 Approximate pharmacokinetic profiles of human insulin and insulin analogues. The relative duration of action of the various forms of insulin is shown. The duration will vary widely both between and within persons. Reproduced from Hirsch [109] with permission from the Massachusetts Medical Society.

resistance [119]. This results in many women conceiving on metformin and needing to address the question of whether they should continue the medication during pregnancy. Data published on nearly 400 first-trimester metformin exposures are reassuring that it is not teratogenic [120–122]. A recently reported randomized trial in 751women with gestational diabetes compared metformin to insulin treatment [123]. Although nearly half of the metformin-treated women required the addition of insulin therapy to achieve adequate metabolic control, there were no significant differences in maternal or perinatal outcomes between the two groups. Not surprisingly, the patients generally preferred taking pills to injections.

At this time, insulin must still be considered the most appropriate choice for treating diabetes in pregnancy, but there is enough reassuring information regarding the use of glyburide and metformin for gestational diabetes to suggest that those drugs are reasonable options for women who are unable or unwilling to take insulin.

Blood glucose monitoring

Monitoring the results of treatment is more important than the precise regimen according to which insulin is administered. Any serious effort at achieving euglycemia must include self-monitoring of capillary blood glucose. It is very unusual to have a patient who cannot be taught to test her own capillary blood glucose level. We ask patients to test their glucose levels four times daily: fasting and 2 hours after each meal. The patients are given forms to record their glucose values and they are reviewed at regularly scheduled visits. The American Diabetes Association recommends fasting values below 95 mg/dL and 2-hour postprandial values of 120 mg/dL or less. We obtain a Hb A_{1c} determination at the first prenatal visit and monthly thereafter.

Avoidance of hypoglycemia

Compared with the nonpregnant state, normal pregnancy is associated with a fall in fasting blood glucose levels but a rise in postprandial glucose levels. The net result of these changes is a modest rise in mean daily blood glucose levels throughout later pregnancy [59]. Early pregnancy is frequently associated with some degree of anorexia, nausea, and vomiting. In diabetic women taking a fixed daily dose of insulin, these changes often result in an increased frequency of insulin reactions in early pregnancy. Intensively treated nonpregnant diabetic patients often have a diminished awareness of and response to hypoglycemia. Diamond *et al.* assessed the response to hypoglycemia in nine intensively treated pregnant diabetic women and seven nonpregnant nondiabetic age-matched women using a hypoglycemic insulin clamp technique. They found that the counter-regulatory responses of glucagon, epinephrine, and growth hormone:

• did not begin to rise until lower levels of blood glucose were reached
• rose more slowly
• did not reach the same maximum levels of response in the diabetic pregnant women as compared with the control subjects [124].

This may be exacerbated in patients with long-standing diabetes with some degree of autonomic neuropathy. One must be vigilant about the possibility of hypoglycemia in diabetic parturients undergoing cesarean section. This is particularly true if the patient has been placed nil by mouth (NPO) prior to surgery and is under general anesthesia.

The elevated progesterone levels of pregnancy have been reported in some studies to be associated with delayed gastric emptying. In women with some degree of gastroparesis before pregnancy, this effect can be exacerbated. Delayed and unpredictable gastric emptying can make glycemic control, which depends on insulin injections timed to anticipate gastric emptying, difficult and result in wide swings in postprandial glucose values. At its worst in late pregnancy, it can lead to frequent vomiting, poor weight gain, and frequent hypoglycemia. Frequent vomiting of undigested meals 2–3 hours after eating is characteristic in these cases. Metoclopramide therapy may be quite helpful for these patients. Severe hypoglycemia in the latter half of pregnancy may be associated with a modest degree of fetal bradycardia, as low as 100 beats/min. This bradycardia reverses slowly as maternal blood glucose levels return to normal, with no obvious adverse consequences to the fetus.

Diabetic women and the people with whom they live should be educated to recognize the symptoms and signs of hypoglycemia, including sudden or rapid onset of hunger, tremulousness, diaphoresis, tachycardia, tingling of the lower jaw, confusion, belligerence or combativeness, sleepiness or loss of consciousness and seizures. They should also be instructed on its treatment, including the importance of not trying to force feed someone who is semi-conscious. Patients should be given a prescription for glucagon to be kept in the refrigerator and they and their families should be instructed in the appropriate use of the drug. Patients should be advised that its use may cause nausea and vomiting.

Avoidance of ketonemia

Chronic ketonemia during pregnancy is undesirable, as discussed above, because it is associated with poorer neurodevelopmental outcome among the offspring of diabetic women. As recommended by the American Diabetes Association, we do not ask our patients to routinely check their urine for ketones but we do recommend checking under two specific situations. If a woman reports that she is constantly hungry on her prescribed diet, especially if she is losing weight or failing to gain weight appropriately, then we ask her to check her urine for ketones in the morning. If she is euglycemic under these circumstances, then she is not getting enough calories to meet her needs and her diet should be adjusted appropriately to eliminate the ketonuria. The other circumstance under which it is most important to check for ketonuria is if the patient is hyperglycemic (above 200 mg/dL or 11.1 mmol/L), especially if associated with an acute illness, nausea and/or vomiting. If a patient reports hyperglycemia and ketonuria, she should be evaluated promptly as this must be assumed to be diabetic ketoacidosis until proven otherwise.

Retinopathy

The prevalence of diabetic retinopathy is strongly related to the duration of the disease. After 20 years of diabetes, virtually 100% of type 1 patients and 60% of type 2 patients will have some degree of retinopathy [125]. Diabetic retinopathy can be subdivided into nonproliferative (benign) disease and proliferative retinopathy. After 20 years of diabetes, 50% of type 1 patients but only 10% of type 2 patients will have proliferative retinopathy. In the absence of effective treatment, progression of proliferative retinopathy is associated with risk for severe visual loss. The most important intervention to prevent development and progression of proliferative retinopathy is strict control of blood glucose levels. Initiation of strict control can result in sudden transient worsening of retinal disease but that effect resolves after approximately 12–18 months so that after 18 months less well-controlled patients will progress more rapidly [126,127]. The long-term benefits of strict control outweigh the early short-term worsening [128].

Pregnancy is associated with progression of diabetic retinopathy and the degree of severity of the progression is related to both pre-existing retinopathy and degree of metabolic control [129–131]. The observed progression could be due to improved control with pregnancy or an effect of the pregnancy itself. Although rare patients with particularly active and advanced retinopathy when entering pregnancy may experience some permanent decrease in visual acuity, generally diabetic women suffer no net loss of visual acuity in the long term as the result of having been pregnant [128,129]. Women with retinopathy should be seen regularly during pregnancy by an ophthalmologist familiar with retinal disease.

Nephropathy and hypertension

Diabetic nephropathy is a chronic disease defined as albuminuria in excess of 300 mg/day. Early in the course of the disease, there can be an increase in creatinine clearance (hyperfiltration phase) but the long-term prognosis of the disease inevitably is fall in creatinine clearance, development of hypertension and ultimately renal failure. The lifetime risk for this complication can be minimized and delayed with strict glycemic metabolic control and control of hypertension [132,133]. While angiotensin-converting enzyme inhibitors (ACEI) and angiotensin receptor blockers (ARB) are specifically recommended for diabetic patients outside pregnancy, with the goal of slowing progression of renal disease, these agents are contraindicated in pregnancy. Late pregnancy exposures have been associated with renal dysfunction and death in the fetus, and first-trimester exposure to ACEI is teratogenic [134,135]. These agents should be discontinued prior to conception.

The prevalence of nephropathy among diabetic pregnant women is as high as 14% in series from academic centers and nephropathy is strongly associated with increased perinatal morbidity [75]. Women who enter pregnancy with nephropathy are more likely to develop pre-eclampsia, deliver prematurely, and have growth-restricted infants, while they are less likely to have macrosomic infants [136]. Just as elevated albumin excretion rates below the rate needed to make the diagnosis of nephropathy are strongly associated with progression to frank nephropathy [137], proteinuria early in pregnancy at levels below those necessary to make the diagnosis of pre-eclampsia are associated with an elevated risk of pre-eclampsia later in pregnancy [138].

Diabetic women who enter pregnancy with hypertension with or without nephropathy are at high risk (30–60%) of developing pre-eclampsia. Blood pressure should be controlled with beta-blockers (metoprolol, atenolol or labetalol) and calcium channel blockers. Although there is some concern that beta-blockers may blunt patients' recognition of and response to hypoglycemia, this has not been a major problem in our experience. Virtually all women with diabetic nephropathy will experience a gradual rise in their proteinuria as pregnancy progresses, with return to pre-pregnancy levels 6–8 weeks post partum. Thus, diagnosis of pre-eclampsia in women who enter pregnancy with pre-existing hypertension and albuminuria in excess of 300 mg/day can be difficult and may seem arbitrary. However, development of pre-eclampsia in these women is usually characterized by a dramatic rise over a short period of time (a week) in blood pressure and proteinuria, occasionally accompanied by hemolysis, elevated liver enzymes or thrombocytopenia. Prophylactic low-dose aspirin therapy did not improve perinatal outcome in diabetic patients in the largest randomized controlled trial to date [139]. A meta-analysis of all trials of antiplatelet agents among all types of patients treated found a 10% reduction in a composite measure of "serious adverse outcome" though no reduction in perinatal mortality or intrauterine growth restriction (IUGR) [140]. These patients must be monitored very carefully throughout the second and third trimesters for the development of escalating hypertension and adequate fetal growth.

Early pregnancy

Routine prenatal care should begin as early in pregnancy as possible with continued emphasis on meticulous blood glucose control. It is particularly important to be confident of the gestational age in a diabetic pregnancy so an ultrasound examination should be done early in pregnancy if the menstrual history is not reliable. Fetal evaluation should include an ultrasound examination for major congenital malformations at approximately 18 weeks gestation. A maternal serum alpha-fetoprotein screen is frequently obtained to help screen for neural tube defects, but an ultrasound examination in competent hands performs better as a diagnostic test for major congenital malformations [22].

Third trimester

The marked reduction in the incidence of unexpected near-term demise in recent years [55], while largely attributable to vastly improved metabolic control, may be at least partly attributable to routine assessment of fetal well-being. The nonstress test (NST) has been the standard, with the oxytocin challenge test (OCT) or contraction stress test (CST) used to evaluate nonreactive NST results in diabetic parturients. We routinely begin weekly NST at 32 weeks and perform them twice weekly from 36 weeks until delivery. Although some authors have reported an unacceptable incidence of loss using this scheme, this has not been our experience. It has been proposed that the biophysical profile (BPP) and Doppler umbilical artery flow velocity analysis be integrated into the care of these patients. The BPP is helpful, but given the tendency to polyhydramnios in diabetes, an adequate amniotic fluid volume does not have the same reassurance value that it would have in a nondiabetic patient. The value of Doppler remains to be proven. The NST is inexpensive to perform, relatively fast and reliable.

Delivery

Timing of delivery

As discussed above, it has been known for some time that the lungs of IDM mature less rapidly than those of the offspring of nondiabetic women. Bringing more patients closer to term prior to elective delivery is most important. Before electively delivering a diabetic woman at less than 39 weeks gestation, fetal lung maturity should be assessed. The commercially available fluorescence polarization assay for fetal lung maturity is quick, reproducible, and a reliable predictor of maturity in IDM [141,142]. It has largely replaced other fetal lung maturity assays.

Route of delivery

The decline in perinatal mortality due to late demise and RDS has permitted attention to focus on remaining sources of morbidity and mortality. Chief among these are macrosomia and its associated high incidences of operative delivery and birth trauma. Although the risks for shoulder dystocia and subsequent birth injury increase with increasing birthweight in the general population, these risks are magnified among IDM [143–145]. It has been suggested that this may be due to the body habitus of the IDM with unusually broad shoulders in relation to the head size [146]. Some have proposed elective cesarean delivery for fetuses estimated to be macrosomic by ultrasound examination late in pregnancy [147]. The limits of ultrasound examination to accurately predict macrosomia, the low incidence of permanent injury resulting from traumatic delivery, and the expense and morbidity associated with cesarean delivery make such a proposal controversial [148]. A program in diabetic women to systematically estimate fetal weight sonographically late in pregnancy and deliver fetuses estimated to weigh more than 4250 g by cesarean delivery reduced the shoulder dystocia rate from 2.4% to 1.1% while raising the cesarean delivery rate from 21% to 25% [149]. Recognizing the controversial nature of this issue, the American College of Obstetricians and Gynecologists has stated that "prophylactic cesarean delivery may be considered for suspected fetal macrosomia with estimated fetal weights ... greater than 4500 g in women with diabetes" [150].

The major challenges in managing the late third trimester of diabetic women are to:
• minimize fetal exposure to risk of late intrauterine demise
• minimize intrapartum fetal hypoxemia and acidosis and recognize and treat it promptly if it occurs
• minimize the risks of traumatic birth injury, RDS, and other sources of neonatal morbidity and mortality
• minimize the cesarean section rate
• attempt to meet the parents' expectations for the birthing experience to the greatest possible extent.

Management of diabetes during labor

As discussed above, fetal oxygenation and acid–base balance are critically dependent upon both chronic and acute maternal blood glucose levels. During labor, periodic uterine contractions raise intrauterine pressure above maternal spiral arterial perfusion pressure, briefly shutting off placental intervillous flow during each contraction. A normally oxygenated fetus with good placental respiratory reserve has no difficulty tolerating this challenge to oxygenation. However, in a pregnancy complicated by maternal vascular disease limiting blood supply or excessive fetal size demanding unusually large amounts of oxygen, the ability of the fetus to remain adequately oxygenated with a normal pH can be threatened. It is therefore important to maintain euglycemia throughout labor.

The work of labor keeps insulin requirements relatively low. A woman scheduled for induction of labor should be asked to take approximately one-third to one-half of her usual dose of intermediate or long-acting insulin. An intravenous line should be started with a liter of normal saline. A liter of 5% glucose in half-normal saline should be "piggy-backed" into the main line on an infusion pump. The main line should be shut off and the glucose should be run at 125 mL/h. This will give the mother a limited amount of glucose during labor and avoid a large bolus of glucose should the main line be opened wide to give the mother a large bolus for volume expansion. Maternal capillary blood glucose should be checked hourly during labor and a continuous intravenous insulin infusion started if her blood glucose rises above 120 mg/dL. Solutions containing glucose should never be used for a volume expansion infusion prior to regional anesthesia because they will cause acute maternal hyperglycemia (Figure 11.9) and decrease fetal pH (Table 11.9) [151].

Anesthetic management

The anesthesiologist confronts several forms of diabetes mellitus (DM) in the cohort of obstetric patients. Safe and effective obstetric anesthesia management of these patients depends on appreciating the similarities and differences between DM type 1, DM type 2 and GDM, as well as the

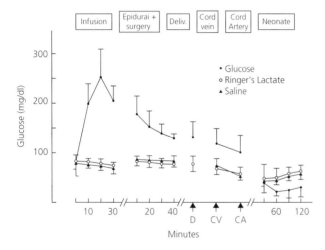

Figure 11.9 Changes in plasma glucose concentration in the mother and infant after administration of 1 L of 5% dextrose in water, Ringer's lactate or normal saline over 20–30 minutes as prehydration prior to administration of epidural anesthesia. D, at delivery; CV, cord vein; CA, cord artery. Data are presented as mean ± standard deviation. Reproduced from Philipson *et al.* [151] with permission from Elsevier.

Table 11.9 Effects of maternal glucose infusion at delivery on maternal and fetal pH values

	Glucose infusion	Lactated Ringer's	Normal saline
Maternal vein	7.36	7.36	7.37
Umbilical cord vein	7.31	7.35	7.34
Umbilical cord artery	7.21	7.27	7.27

Reproduced with permission from Philipson *et al.* [151].

severity of the individual patient's end-organ complications of diabetes. Anesthetic management of the diabetic patient has been reviewed [152–154]. The anesthesiologist works closely with the responsible obstetric team when caring for a patient with DM; timely communication and data sharing assume great importance.

The four most important pieces of information for the anesthesia clinician about an individual diabetic patient are:
• the type of DM
• the current level of blood glucose
• the nature of medical therapy, including the time and dose of the drugs most recently administered to control the disease
• the nature and severity of end-organ consequences resulting from the diabetic condition.

Type of diabetes

Women with type 1 diabetes have an absolute requirement for exogenous insulin to avoid the potentially lethal consequence of diabetic ketoacidosis (DKA), even in the setting of low glucose levels [153,155]. If unaware of a patient's diagnosis of DM 1, the anesthesiologist might make a significant clinical error to withhold insulin therapy if the glucose level is low or near normal. It is important to recognize that diabetic ketoacidosis may present with low or near normal blood sugars [156,157], underscoring the importance of knowing the correct diagnosis.

Corticosteroids administered to promote fetal lung maturation and beta-adrenergic agonists used for tocolysis act as counter-regulatory agents. Therapy with these drugs predisposes to the development of DKA. In addition, labor, vaginal delivery, and cesarean delivery all represent stressors potentially precipitating DKA [158]. During cesarean delivery, the anesthesiologist must exercise particular vigilance to maintain insulin therapy at doses appropriate to prevent or treat DKA while avoiding hypoglycemia. This may entail concomitant provision of a carbohydrate source and insulin therapy with frequent monitoring of blood glucose levels.

In general, anesthetized patients in the operating room should receive regular insulin by continuous intravenous infusion, with intravenous (IV) bolus doses of regular insulin as needed to treat elevated glucose levels or the metabolic derangements of DKA. The onset of insulin action is relatively slow (15–30 minutes after subcutaneous administration). In addition, uptake of insulin administered subcutaneously may be unpredictable due to circulatory changes associated with anesthesia, the use of vasoconstrictors or tissue edema. Insulin therapy promotes potassium uptake by muscle and liver cells, so blood levels of this electrolyte may fall. On the other hand, discontinuation of insulin can lead to significant hyperkalemia [159]. Appropriate electrolyte monitoring will guide therapy.

If there is evidence that a patient has developed DKA during the course of labor and/or delivery, the anesthesia provider needs to appreciate the potential effects of fluid balance, acid–base, and electrolyte abnormalities on the associated anesthetic. For example, a patient in DKA will likely be depleted in total body and intravascular volume. This would have significant implications for maintaining blood pressure stability with neuraxial analgesia or anesthesia. The action of a local anesthetic may be hampered by acidosis because the protonated (hydrophilic) form of the local anesthetic molecule is less likely to cross the cell membrane to reach its site of action on the sodium channel.

Patients with DM 2 are prone to hyperglycemic, hyperosmolar syndrome (HHS). Like DKA in the patient with DM 1, this state of decompensated DM 2 is also associated with profound fluid and electrolyte disturbance. Abnormalities in fluid balance must be corrected immediately as dehydration will reduce perfusion of the uterus and placenta. Acid–base disturbances are less pronounced in HHS than they are in DKA. Ketoacidosis is not a hallmark of the condition. However, there may be some overlap in the clinical presentations and initial resuscitative treatment of DKA and HHS [154].

Of note, the prevalence of DM 2 is increasing in young populations, often in association with obesity [160]. Consequently, the anesthesiologist caring for a patient with DM 2 often encounters other challenges of obesity such as difficult IV access, hypertension, a difficult airway, obstructive sleep apnea, and anatomic barriers to neuraxial analgesia or anesthesia.

Current blood glucose level

In the diabetic patient, blood glucose levels will vary with the counter-regulatory effect of stress hormones, the availability of a carbohydrate source, and the dose and timing of therapy. Labor is a form of exercise and has a glucose-lowering effect [161]. Long-acting oral or injected agents may precipitate hypoglycemia in the patient without a source of carbohydrate. While transient, acute hyperglycemia is unlikely to cause long-lasting harm, hypoglycemia can rapidly produce permanent damage, chiefly due to neuroglycopenia. Of considerable importance is that the anesthetic, particularly a general anesthetic, may mask the autonomic manifestations of hypoglycemia. Moreover, some patients, especially those with excellent glucose control, exhibit the phenomenon of "hypoglycemic unawareness" in which the subjective recognition and autonomic manifestations of even profound hypoglycemia are blunted or absent [162]. Knowledge of the historic level of glucose control and the current level of blood glucose will allow the anesthesiologist to make informed management decisions.

Current medical therapy

Knowledge of the type of recent medical therapy, and the dose and timing of that therapy, will enable the anesthesia provider to assess the risk for abnormal glucose levels and act accordingly. Some oral agents (e.g. the sulfonylureas) have long half-lives, in excess of 12–24 hours [154]; the fasting patient without a source of carbohydrate may be at particular risk for hypoglycemia. Other oral agents, such as insulin sensitizers (e.g. metformin) or the GLP-1 antagonists (sitagliptin), have no theoretical risk of hypoglycemia when used in single-agent therapy, even with prolonged fasting. Furthermore, although some insulin preparations are "peakless" (e.g. glargine, detemir), others exhibit a time-dependent maximum effect, which may coincide with a fasting interval, thereby rendering a patient at risk for hypoglycemia [109]. There is controversy about the risk of lactic acidosis in metformin-treated patients [163–165]. One approach is to withhold metformin for 24–48 hours in advance of elective procedures (e.g. scheduled cesarean delivery, scheduled cerclage placement). In circumstances where it is not feasible to withhold metformin, the anesthesia provider should consider the possibility of lactic acidosis resulting from metformin therapy if evidence of metabolic derangements emerges. Anesthesiologists should become familiar with the newer DM therapies based on the gut peptides GLP-1 and amylin [166], even though these novel medications are not yet commonly used in obstetric patients.

End-organ disease

Diabetes mellitus has multiple potential end-organ consequences which may impact the anesthetic; the nature and severity of these will vary. Patients with GDM are less likely to suffer from major end-organ consequences at the time of their obstetric management due to their relative youth and also to the transient nature of their glucose disorder. However, patients with long-standing, severe, or poorly controlled DM 1 or DM 2 may have profound end-organ consequences, including organ failure in the reproductive years. With obesity-associated DM increasingly detected in relatively young people [160], it is likely that anesthesiologists will encounter obstetric patients with advanced pathophysiology.

Even in patients without evidence of macrovascular (e.g. coronary artery) atherosclerotic disease, pregnant patients with DM may exhibit alterations of left ventricular (LV) function. In a study comparing healthy pregnant women, pregnant women with diabetes mellitus, and healthy controls, an echocardiographic study found that pregnant women developed a restrictive LV filling pattern and a temporary decrease in LV systolic function [167]. Pregnant patients with diabetes developed these changes earlier than healthy pregnant patients, placing them at risk for more hemodynamic complications. Consequently, shifts in preload resulting from neuraxial blockade or blood loss have potentially greater significance in the diabetic parturient compared to the healthy woman at the time of delivery.

Diabetic neuropathy can retard gastric motility in patients already at an enhanced risk of aspiration due to the effects of advanced pregnancy and the gravid uterus on stomach emptying. Although anesthesiologists commonly administer metoclopramide to promote gastric emptying in the diabetic patient, this practice may provide only a limited benefit. Jellish et al. found minimal gastric volumes in fasted patients with diabetes scheduled for elective surgery, and metoclopramide was effective primarily in patients with histories of poor glucose control [168]. These findings may not necessarily apply to the typical obstetric circumstance where fasting in preparation for labor, or for instrumented or cesarean delivery, is impossible.

Diabetic neuropathy can blunt autonomic responses to volume depletion (as during the obligate blood loss of cesarean delivery) or vasodilation as a consequence of neuraxial anesthesia. This may compromise hemodynamic stability. It is at least theoretically possible that patients suffering from diabetic neuropathy may be more prone to injury from regional anesthesia or from positioning or pelvic trauma during delivery although few or no firm clinical data support this [169].

Another manifestation of diabetic polyneuropathy is impaired motor nerve fiber function. Studies of vecuronium neuromuscular blockade and reversal of blockade with neostigmine suggest prolonged return to full strength [170–172]. Although many obstetric patients with diabetes who experience anesthesia would receive a neuraxial technique, general endotracheal anesthesia with a muscle relaxant may be indicated (coagulopathy, abnormal spine anatomy) or become necessary (inadequate spinal or epidural anesthesia). Consequently, the anesthesia provider should anticipate possible prolonged motor weakness in patients with diabetes and evidence of neuropathy.

Nephropathy will impact monitoring and management of fluid balance, electrolytes (particularly potassium and magnesium), and the clearance of certain drugs. One example is the active metabolite of morphine, morphine-6-glucuronide, which can accumulate in renal failure [173]. Other analgesics exhibit altered pharmacokinetics when renal function is compromised [174]. The kidney compromised at baseline by microvascular or macrovascular disease may also be at enhanced risk from low perfusion states including hemorrhagic hypotension or ischemia, or hypotension following neuraxial analgesia and anesthesia.

In addition to the usual degree of hemodynamic fragility associated with severe pre-eclampsia, patients with nephropathy and significant proteinuria may have low serum albumin levels and very low colloid oncotic pressures. This makes these patients particularly vulnerable to pulmonary edema if they are vigorously volume loaded in preparation for regional anesthesia.

Stiff joints result from soft tissue effects of advanced DM, perhaps more commonly in the setting of DM 1 although also seen in DM 2. The consequence of greatest relevance to the anesthesiologist is potential compromise of the ability to manage the airway if the cervical spine or temporomandibular joint range of motion becomes limited [175]. Joint mobility reduction, as assessed by the ability to approximate the hands, "prayer sign" [176], or create a palm print [177], has been described as a predictor of the difficulty of intubation. In a comparison of 75 diabetic patients with 112 nondiabetic patients undergoing kidney transplants, patients with diabetes had a greater than 10-fold increase in the prevalence of difficult laryngoscopy [178]. However, Warner et al. report little problem managing the airways of patients with end-stage DM [179]. Only 2% of 725 patients in their retrospective study were identified as having difficult laryngoscopies; they report that advanced airway techniques were not required to accomplish endotracheal intubation.

Pulmonary dysfunction manifest as compromised oxygenation is an underappreciated consequence of advanced DM [180–182]. The pathophysiologic basis may be pulmonary microvascular disease [183]. Patients at advanced stages of pregnancy, and also during labor and delivery, have increased oxygen demands yet are prone to atelectasis with limitations on respiratory reserve. For example, the induction of general endotracheal anesthesia in the term pregnant patient is often associated with rapid and profound oxygen desaturation despite adequate preoxygenation. Although not well studied or reported, it is at least theoretically possible that a pregnant patient whose respiratory reserve is compromised by advanced DM will exhibit profound and refractory hypoxemia under general anesthesia.

Vascular occlusive disease affecting the carotid and coronary arteries places the patient with advanced diabetes at risk for brain or cardiac ischemia, particularly in settings with compromised perfusion (anemia, hypotension) or enhanced oxygen demand (seizures, tachycardia). Situations with supply/demand mismatch may be encountered in complicated obstetric cases with abnormal placentation (e.g. abruption, previa, accreta), a ruptured uterus or uterine atony with hemorrhage.

Of less immediate consequence to the anesthesia provider in the intrapartum or peripartum period are retinopathy and immune suppression. However, the anesthesia provider needs to consider the enhanced possibility of epidural or other CNS infection when patients present with fever, back pain, headache or neurological deficit following delivery associated with neuraxial analgesia/anesthesia. Such infections require prompt and aggressive therapy to avoid long-term morbidity.

In summary, the obstetric patient with advanced DM poses a number of challenges to the anesthesia provider. Working closely with the obstetric team, the anesthesia provider must appreciate the impact of the specific diabetic diagnosis, the importance of glucose monitoring and diabetic therapy, and the potential impact on anesthetic management of end-organ consequences of DM to safely and effectively provide anesthetic care for the mother and baby.

Postpartum care

Immediately post partum, maternal insulin requirements drop precipitously. Most women diagnosed with gestational diabetes will need no insulin immediately following delivery. Women with pregestational diabetes will usually see their insulin requirements drop below their requirements immediately prior to pregnancy, only to rise slowly over 5–7 days back to their pre-pregnancy levels. Insulin prescription should be cautious on the first postpartum day because it is very easy to induce severe hypoglycemia, especially in a woman who has delivered by cesarean and may have minimal oral intake. Colloid oncotic pressure is lowered during pregnancy for all women, is further depressed by pre-eclampsia and falls even further immediately post partum, contributing with large intravenous fluid infusions during labor to extensive third-space fluid loss and peripheral edema. Women with diabetic nephropathy may have very low levels of serum albumin, further depressing their colloid oncotic pressure and combining with their renal dysfunction to make it very difficult for them to mobilize and excrete a large extravascular fluid burden. These women can easily get into difficulty with pulmonary edema post partum. Furosemide is very helpful in this situation. The hypertension associated with pre-eclampsia may take several weeks to resolve, requiring frequent dose adjustments of antihypertensive medications to prevent hypotension.

Women with gestational diabetes should be screened for type 2 diabetes with a standard WHO 75 g oral GTT 8–12 weeks post partum. Many women with gestational diabetes will develop it in a subsequent pregnancy and type 2 diabetes in the years ahead. The importance of weight loss and exercise in preventing type 2 diabetes should be emphasized to these patients and a fasting glucose obtained every 3 years.

The principles of contraceptive counseling and practice for women with diabetes are discussed above under preconception counseling.

Diabetic ketoacidosis

Diabetic ketoacidosis is a major threat for fetal mortality and morbidity in diabetic women with the loss rate reported as high as 50%. Although severe maternal complications such as acute respiratory distress syndrome (ARDS), acute renal failure, cerebral edema and coma may occur, maternal mortality with modern management has become so rare that the rate is impossible to estimate accurately [184,185].

Pathophysiology

Diabetic ketoacidosis occurs in the presence of a relative or absolute deficiency of insulin and a relative or absolute increase in the major counter-regulatory hormone, glucagon. The state of combined hypoinsulinemia and hyperglucagonemia is associated with increased hepatic glucose production and decreased peripheral glucose utilization, causing severe hyperglycemia. As the process escalates, beta-adrenergic stimulation, through endogenous epinephrine release due to stress, inhibits insulin-induced glucose transport into peripheral tissues. Both insulin deficiency indirectly and beta stimulation directly increase glucagon secretion. The combined results of hypoinsulinemia and hyperglucagonemia are increased hepatic glucose production and decreased peripheral glucose utilization which produce hyperglycemia [186]. The majority of the hepatic glucose production is from gluconeogenesis using amino acids derived from protein catabolism. The resulting hyperglycemia causes an osmotic diuresis and dehydration characteristic of DKA. Both hypoinsulinemia and beta stimulation activate lipolysis in adipose tissue, releasing free fatty acids into the circulation. These travel to the liver where they would simply be re-esterified into triglycerides under normal hormonal circumstances. Hyperglucagonemia, however, which prevails during starvation or uncontrolled diabetes, activates the beta-oxidative enzymes in the liver, which metabolize free fatty acids to ketone bodies. Although at high concentrations of acetoacetate and beta-hydroxybutyrate, there is some suppression of peripheral ketone body utilization, it is mainly their overproduction which is responsible for the hyperketonemia. These ketone bodies are fixed acids which drive down the pH and bicarbonate ion concentration, while accounting almost exclusively for the increased anion gap. The decrease in maternal pH stimulates the woman's respiratory center, causing hyperventilation.

The causes of the water and electrolyte disturbances are complex and result in total body depletion of water, sodium, potassium, chloride, magnesium, phosphate and bicarbonate. Hyperglycemia causes an osmotic diuresis with loss of large amounts of water. The increased osmotic pressure and loss of volume from the intravascular space draws water from the intracellular space, reducing the serum sodium concentration. Catabolism of muscle protein releases intracellular potassium while hypoinsulinemia inhibits the sodium-potassium exchange pump in muscle cell membranes, limiting potassium uptake. Stimulated by hypovolemia, the kidneys retain sodium while wasting potassium into the urine. Vomiting associated with DKA results in further loss of water and electrolytes. Severe loss of maternal fluid volume will decrease cardiac output, blood pressure and tissue perfusion and may ultimately lead to cardiovascular collapse and shock.

Effect on the fetus

All the major metabolic derangements suffered by the mother are due to abnormalities in concentrations in small molecules that freely cross the placenta and they are therefore shared by the fetus. Maternal DKA is frequently associated with the development of nonreassuring fetal heart rate patterns [187].

Presentation and diagnosis

The classic clinical presentation of DKA includes anorexia, nausea, vomiting, polyuria, tachycardia, and abdominal pain or muscle cramps. If sufficiently severe at presentation, the picture could include Kussmaul hyperventilation (deep, labored breathing from acidosis), and signs of volume depletion such as hypotension and oliguria. There may also be an alteration in mental status from lethargy to coma. Body temperature is normal to reduced. The "fruity" odor of ketones may be noticeable on the patient's breath. If DKA is suspected on the basis of clinical signs and symptoms, the urine should first be tested for glucose and ketones. If neither is present, then the diagnosis is very unlikely. If they are present, then blood should be studied. In a nonpregnant person, a blood glucose value of less than 250 mg/dL (13.9 mmol/L) would make the diagnosis of DKA very unlikely. Pregnant women, however, are well known to develop DKA at relatively low blood glucose values (200–250 mg/dL or 11.1–13.9 mmol/L). Although total body sodium and potassium are profoundly depleted, the serum sodium concentration is usually low-normal and the serum potassium normal to slightly elevated. The serum bicarbonate is, by definition, less than 15 mEq/L (15 mmol/L). Although the ketone bodies acetoacetate and beta-hydroxybutyrate are not usually measured clinically, their presence in excess can be inferred from a large anion gap. The anion gap is calculated by the difference between the sodium serum level and the sum of the serum bicarbonate and chloride levels. Although assays vary among laboratories, a normal anion gap is generally 7–13. Serum osmolarity is usually greater than 300 mosmol/L (300 mmol/L). The hematocrit is usually elevated due to hemoconcentration and there is a leukocytosis which can be very dramatic. The arterial pH will be less than 7.30, by definition, and the PCO_2 will be low (<28 mmHg in pregnancy).

In a patient known to have type 1 diabetes, the diagnosis is usually obvious. Occasionally, a diabetic patient experiencing protracted nausea and vomiting due to morning sickness in early pregnancy or gastroenteritis later in pregnancy can present a confusing picture with ketonuria, which can be mistaken for simple starvation ketosis. In this setting hyperglycemia should alert the clinician to the possibility of DKA. Patients with clear type 2 noninsulin requiring diabetes or gestational diabetes may develop DKA during pregnancy [188]. DKA cannot be ruled out just because the patient is not known to have type 1 diabetes. Rarely, patients not previously known to have diabetes of any sort may present with DKA in pregnancy. The differential diagnosis includes alcoholic ketoacidosis, which occurs in chronic alcoholics, usually following a binge. It is frequently associated with pancreatitis and usually the blood glucose is less than 150 mg/dL (8.3 mmol/L). Occasionally, these patients are hypoglycemic.

Precipitating factors

An attempt should be made to find a cause in every case of DKA. Frequently, the cause is simply inadequate insulin therapy in the face of an otherwise minor illness. Patients may reduce or omit their insulin doses with gastroenteritis because they are concerned about the possibility of an insulin reaction due to anorexia, nausea and vomiting. This is a matter of patient education regarding the appropriate therapy for "sick days." A careful history and physical examination with appropriate laboratory studies should be done to search for a significant bacterial infection, e.g. pyelonephritis or pneumonia. As mentioned above, leukocytosis is present due simply to DKA, but a fever should suggest the possibility of an infection. Patients using continuous subcutaneous insulin infusion pumps receive only short-acting insulin. If the pump malfunctions and stops infusing, the patient becomes hypoinsulinemic very quickly because she has no reservoir of longer acting insulin. She may develop DKA very rapidly. Tocolytic therapy with beta-sympathomimetic agents with or without concomitant glucocorticoid therapy can also precipitate DKA [189,190]. Every attempt should be made to avoid beta-sympathomimetic agents in women with diabetes.

Treatment

Volume replacement

Volume replacement and insulin therapy are the two most urgent concerns in treating DKA. The average water volume deficit in established DKA is 3.5–7 L or 5–10% of bodyweight, and the average sodium deficit is 350–600 mEq. Most patients will be deficient in water in excess of their sodium deficit and will therefore require some free water in addition to normal saline. Although ultimately some free water will be necessary, the initial resuscitation should be with isotonic saline because it will restore the circulating volume more quickly and lead to a less rapid fall in osmolarity. It is hypothesized that too rapid a fall in intravascular osmolarity may lead to intracellular swelling and cerebral edema in young patients.

Volume replacement management should include placement of two intravenous lines, one for rapid fluid infusion and a second for insulin therapy. A Foley catheter should be placed early in the resuscitation to accurately monitor urine output. Initial treatment should be with normal saline at a rate of 15–20 mL/kg/h, 400 mL/m²/h or approximately 1 L/h for the first 2 hours of the resuscitation. This will rapidly replete the intravascular volume, improving general tissue perfusion and insulin delivery, permit excretion of glucose in the urine, and slow potassium wasting in the urine. Fluid therapy should be reduced in the third and subsequent hours to 7.5 mL/kg/h according to the clinical situation and urine output. As the blood glucose level comes down to 250 mg/dL (13.9 mmol/L), the intravenous fluid solution should be changed to 5% glucose in water or half-normal saline. This will prevent hypoglycemia and provide substrate to suppress lipolysis and ketogenesis. This also serves to supply free water which is needed to help prevent or correct the hyperchloremic acidosis which would otherwise develop. Bicarbonate is only indicated if the maternal pH is less than 7.10. Serum potassium concentrations should be measured frequently because potassium may need to be replaced due to excessive losses. Potassium replacement should not be initiated, however, until adequate urine output has been established. Intravenous fluids should be continued until all nausea and vomiting have resolved, bowel sounds are present, and the patient is able to tolerate adequate quantities of fluids by mouth.

Management of a patient with severe DKA does require a setting in which the patient can be closely monitored with a 1/1 nurse/patient ratio.

Insulin therapy

Insulin replacement therapy should begin as early in the resuscitation as possible because DKA will not resolve without it. Although it may be administered either intramuscularly or subcutaneously, insulin is best administered intravenously in this circumstance [191]. Poor tissue perfusion will result in delayed and erratic absorption from IM and SC sites, initially delaying response and later leading to more hypoglycemia. Intravenous therapy should begin with a 10 unit bolus followed immediately with a continuous infusion of 5–10 units per hour. All therapy during this initial resuscitation should be with rapid-acting insulin. Insulin tends to bind to plastic intravenous tubing so several milliliters of insulin solution should be run through the IV tubing and discarded to coat its walls with insulin so that the patient receives the full dose of insulin immediately without loss to the tubing.

All patients in DKA are insulin resistant, but these doses of insulin are usually adequate to overcome the resistance and reverse the DKA [192]. If, however the patient does not show improvement in both the hyperglycemia and anion gap within 2 hours of initiating therapy, then very severe insulin resistance is present. In this case, a 20 unit IV bolus should be given and the infusion rate doubled to 20 units per hour. This should be adequate to saturate all insulin receptors and lead to a physiologic response. There is no risk to an excessively large IV bolus of insulin because it has no effect beyond saturating all receptors and has a short half-life. For this reason, and because the severely resistant patient cannot be anticipated, some have suggested that all patients should be initially treated with a much larger initial IV insulin bolus.

Hyperglycemia and acidosis will resolve much more quickly than the ketonemia and ketonuria. Intravenous insulin therapy should be continued with IV glucose after the blood glucose level has been normalized until the acidosis is resolved. Some authors suggest that IV insulin therapy should be continued until ketonuria has resolved. Resolution of the ketonuria, however, may take 24–48 hours which is long after the patient is otherwise apparently recovered and stable. The transition back to routine subcutaneous rapid-acting and intermediate or long-acting insulin should overlap the IV insulin.

Potassium replacement

Although the serum potassium level at presentation in DKA is often high, the mean total body potassium deficit is 200–400 mEq. Insulin therapy in the presence of hyperglycemia will drive potassium from the intravascular to the intracellular space. Intravenous potassium replacement should begin 2–4 hours into the resuscitation as the serum potassium level falls toward the normal range and urine production is demonstrated. Occasionally, patients will present with a low or normal serum potassium in which case replacement should begin at a rate of 30–40 mEq/h. In the rare circumstance where a patient presents with a very low serum potassium, insulin administration should be delayed briefly until 40 mEq of potassium can be infused. Failure to do this could result in a rapid fall in serum levels upon initiation of insulin with the precipitation of a severe cardiac dysrhythmia. Inclusion of an electrocardiogram as part of the initial evaluation of a patient in DKA will help to rapidly estimate the serum potassium level. Lead II is particularly helpful, with high, peaked T waves and a broadened QRS complex indicating hyperkalemia. Hypokalemia is evidenced by low T waves and the appearance of U waves.

Bicarbonate and phosphate therapy

It is intuitively appealing to want to treat acidosis with bicarbonate, but such therapy has not been shown to be helpful and is not routinely used. Theoretical potential advantages to bicarbonate administration include a more rapid correction of the extracellular acidosis, minimization of the hyperchloremic acidosis, reduction of cardiac irritability and increasing the responsiveness of the vascular system to pressors. Despite the lack of documented efficacy for bicarbonate administration, all authors recommend its use in the case of "severe" acidosis [193]. The definition of "severe" varies, but is generally below pH 7.00. If bicarbonate is given, it should be as an IV infusion of 1–2 mEq/kg over 2 hours and discontinued when the pH reaches 7.20.

Phosphate is depleted in DKA and serum levels are usually low due to decreased intake, enhanced catabolism and urinary loss. Hypophosphatemia can deplete serum levels of 2,3-diphosphoglycerate and result in a shift of the hemoglobin-oxygen disassociation curve toward more avid oxygen binding and poorer oxygen delivery to tissues. Severe hypophosphatemia (<2 mEq/L or 0.64 mmol/L) can cause rhabdomyolysis. For these reasons, phosphate replacement would seem desirable [194]. Furthermore, replacing some of the potassium as phosphate rather than chloride can help to minimize the hyperchloremia. On the other hand, administration of too much phosphate intravenously can cause hypocalcemia. Phosphate is rapidly replaced from dietary sources as soon as the patient starts eating, and its acute IV replacement has not been shown to improve outcome in any measurable way. The necessity of its acute IV replacement, therefore, is controversial. If potassium phosphate is used, it should not exceed 90 mEq in 24 hours to avoid hypocalcemia and serum calcium levels should be followed.

General notes on managing the resuscitation

Successful management of DKA does not require an intensive care unit but it does require a setting where the patient can be monitored very frequently with a 1/1 nurse/patient ratio. A labor and delivery suite is perfectly suitable. Initial evaluation of the patient should include a routine history and detailed inquiry into the possible cause for DKA. The usual vital signs, physical examination and documentation of fetal viability or well-being should also include the patient's mental status [195]. The initial laboratory evaluation should include a complete blood count, blood type and irregular antibody screen, serum electrolytes, glucose, BUN, creatinine, calcium, phosphate, urine ketones, and cultures of blood, urine and other sites as appropriate. As mentioned above, a Foley catheter and two intravenous lines should be started. A 12-lead EKG and an initial arterial blood pH should be obtained.

As soon as the diagnosis of DKA is made and the necessity for an intensive resuscitation is recognized, a flow sheet (paper or electronic) should be established at the patient's beside on which should be recorded all vital signs, laboratory data, urine output, fluid, insulin and other medical therapies and mental status, if appropriate. Capillary blood glucose determinations should be done hourly at the bedside to help guide the resuscitation. It is not particularly helpful to follow ketonuria or ketonemia. Attention should rather be directed to correcting the hyperglycemia and anion gap and progress in the resuscitation assessed upon these measures.

The patient should be kept NPO until all nausea and vomiting have resolved and bowel sounds are heard. The first dose of subcutaneous regular and intermediate-acting insulin should be given prior to discontinuing the intravenous insulin infusion. The search for the cause of the DKA episode should be completed and appropriate therapy or education instituted to prevent recurrence. Although DKA is a metabolic emergency, it is largely preventable and treatable, and very rarely results in maternal mortality.

Management of the fetus

Electronic monitoring of the fetal heart rate during maternal DKA is frequently associated with the development of nonreassuring fetal heart rate patterns. Although the pressure to perform a cesarean delivery to extricate a fetus from a situation where there is a nonreassuring or even "ominous" fetal heart rate pattern may be difficult to resist, this could be a dangerous procedure for an unstable mother. Furthermore, these patterns do resolve with treatment of the maternal metabolic disorder without obvious sequelae to the surviving neonate [197]. Reports in the literature are anecdotal because there is not a sufficient volume of these cases to perform a meaningful treatment trial. Most authors recommend vigorous treatment of the maternal metabolic disorder with the fetus *in utero*, reserving cesarean delivery for mothers in stable condition whose fetuses still seem compromised.

Conclusion

Obstetric care for women with diabetes mellitus has made enormous strides in the nearly 90 years since the discovery of insulin in 1922. The maternal mortality rate has fallen by three orders of magnitude and the perinatal mortality rate by two orders of magnitude, but challenges remain. Obesity and with it type 2 diabetes are reaching epidemic proportions, resulting in ever increasing numbers of women with diabetes in pregnancy. It is also becoming increasingly clear that most of the complications of pregnancy that are known to occur with greater frequencies among diabetic women are sensitive to the degree of metabolic control, and that the gradient of risk may not have an obvious threshold, with the continuum of risk extending down into the "euglycemic" range. Minimizing the risks for major congenital malformations and first-trimester spontaneous abortions requires only "good" control, while minimizing the risks for near-term fetal demise, excessive fetal growth and pre-eclampsia will likely require nearly perfect control.

References

1. Joslin EP. Pregnancy and diabetes mellitus. Boston Med Surg J 1915;173:841.
2. Duttaroy AK. Transport of fatty acids across the human placenta: a review. Prog Lipid Res 2009;48(1):52–61.
3. American College of Obstetricians and Gynecologists Committee on Practice Bulletins. Clinical management guidelines: gestational diabetes. ACOG Practice Bulletin No 30. Obstet Gynecol 2001;98:525.
4. Crowther CA, Hiller JE, Moss JR, *et al.* Effect of treatment of gestational diabetes mellitus on pregnancy outcomes. N Engl J Med 2005;352:2477–86.
5. American Diabetes Association. Diagnosis and classification of diabetes mellitus. Diabetes Care 2009;32(S1):S62–S67.
6. Danilenko–Dixon DR, van Winter JT, Nelson RL, Ogburn PL. Universal versus selective gestational diabetes screening: application of 1997 American Diabetes Association recommendations. Am J Obstet Gynecol 1999;181:798–802.
7. Williams CB, Iqbal S, Zawacki CM, Yu D, Brown MB, Herman WH. Effect of selective screening for gestational diabetes. Diabetes Care 1999;22:418–21.

8. HAPO Study Cooperative Research Group. Hyperglycemia and adverse pregnancy outcomes. N Engl J Med 2008;358:1991–2002.

9. White P. Diabetes complicating pregnancy. Am J Obstet Gynecol 1937;33:380–5.

10. Molsted-Pedersen LM, Tygstrup I, Pedersen J. Congenital malformations in newborn infants of diabetic women. Correlation with maternal diabetic vascular complications. Lancet 1964;i:1124–6.

11. Soler NG, Walsh CH, Malins JM. Congenital malformations in infants of diabetic mothers. Q J Med 1976;178:303–13.

12. Drury MI, Greene AT, Stronge JM. Pregnancy complicated by clinical diabetes mellitus: a study of 600 pregnancies. Obstet Gynecol 1977;49:519–22.

13. Gabbe SG, Mestman JH, Freeman RK, et al. Management and outcome of pregnancy in diabetes mellitus, classes B to R. Am J Obstet Gynecol 1977;129:723–32.

14. Kitzmiller JL, Cloherty JP, Younger DM, et al. Diabetic pregnancy and perinatal morbidity. Am J Obstet Gynecol 1978;131:560–80.

15. Simpson JL, Elias S, Martin AO, et al. Diabetes in pregnancy, Northwestern University series (1977–1981). Am J Obstet Gynecol 1983;146:263–70.

16. Ylinen K, Aula P, Stenman U-H, et al. Risk of minor and major fetal malformations in diabetics with high haemoglobin A_{1c} values in early pregnancy. BMJ 1984;289:345–6.

17. Ballard JL, Holroyde J, Tsang RC, et al. High malformation rates and decreased mortality in infants of diabetic mothers managed after the first trimester of pregnancy (1956–1978). Am J Obstet Gynecol 1984;148:1111–18.

18. Lucas MJ, Leveno KJ, Williams ML, et al. Early pregnancy glycosylated hemoglobin, severity of diabetes, and fetal malformations. Am J Obstet Gynecol 1989;161:426–31.

19. Hanson U, Persson B, Thunell S. Relationship between haemoglobin A_{1c} in early type 1 (insulin-dependent) diabetic pregnancy and the occurrence of spontaneous abortion and fetal malformation in Sweden. Diabetologia 1990;33:100–4.

20. Gestation and Diabetes in France Study Group. Multicenter survey of diabetic pregnancy in France. Diabetes Care 1991;14:994–1000.

21. Tchobroutsky C, Vray MM, Altman JJ. Risk/benefit ratio of changing late obstetrical strategies in the management of insulin-dependent diabetic pregnancies. A comparison between 1971–1977 and 1978–1985 periods in 389 pregnancies. Diabet Metab 1991;17:287–94.

22. Greene MF, Benacerraf BR. Prenatal diagnosis in diabetic gravidas: utility of ultrasound and maternal serum, alpha-fetoprotein screening. Obstet Gynecol 1991;77:520–4.

23. Gregory R, Scott AR, Mohajer M, et al. Diabetic pregnancy 1977–1990: have we reached a plateau? J R Coll Physicians Lond 1992;26:162–6.

24. Rosenn B, Miodovnik M, Combs CA, et al. Glycemic thresholds for spontaneous abortion and congenital malformations in insulin-dependent diabetes mellitus. Obstet Gynecol 1994;84:515–20.

25. Towner D, Kjos SL, Leung SL, et al. Congenital malformations in pregnancies complicated by NIDDM. Diabetes Care 1995;18:1446–51.

26. Janssen PA, Rothman I, Schwartz SM. Congenital malformations in newborns of women with established and gestational diabetes in Washington State, 1984–1991. Paediatr Perinat Epidemiol 1996;10:52–63.

27. Diabetes Control and Complications Trial Research Group. Pregnancy outcomes in the diabetes control and complications trial. Am J Obstet Gynecol 1996;174:1343–53.

28. Nielsen GL, Sørensen HT, Nielsen PH, et al. Glycosylated hemoglobin as predictor of adverse fetal outcome in type 1 diabetic pregnancies. Acta Diabetol 1997;34:217–22.

29. Hawthorne G, Robson S, Ryall EA, et al. Prospective population based survey of outcome of pregnancy in diabetic women: results of the northern diabetic pregnancy audit, 1994. BMJ 1997;315:279–81.

30. Casson IF, Clarke CA, Howard CV, et al. Outcomes of pregnancy in insulin dependent diabetic women: results of a five year population cohort study. BMJ 1997;315:275–8.

31. Suhonen L, Hiilesmaa V, Teramo K. Glycaemic control during early pregnancy and fetal malformations in women with Type I diabetes mellitus. Diabetologia 2000;43:79–82.

32. Hawthorne G, Irgens LM, Lie RT. Outcome of pregnancy in diabetic women in northeast England and in Norway, 1994–1997. BMJ 2000;321:730–1.

33. Farrell T, Neale L, Cundy T. Congenital anomalies in the offspring of women with Type I, Type 2 and gestational diabetes. Diabet Med 2002;19:322–6.

34. Jensen DM, Damm P, Moelsted-Pedersen L, et al. Outcomes in Type I diabetic pregnancies: a nationwide population-based study. Diabetes Care 2004;27:2819.

35. Sharpe PB, Chan A, Haan EA, Hiller JE. Maternal diabetes and congenital anomalies in South Australia 1986–2000: a population-based cohort study. Birth Defects Res (A) 2005;73:605–11.

36. Gabbe SG. Congenital malformations in infants of diabetic mothers. Obstet Gynecol Surv 1977;32:125–32.

37. Leslie RDG, John PN, Pyke DA, et al. Haemoglobin A_1 in diabetic pregnancy. Lancet 1978;ii:958–9.

38. Miller E, Hare JW, Cloherty JP, et al. Elevated maternal hemoglobin A_{1c} in early pregnancy and major congenital anomalies in infants of diabetic mothers. N Engl J Med 1981;304:1331–4.

39. Greene MF, Hare JW, Cloherty JP, et al. First-trimester hemoglobin A_1 and risk for major malformation and spontaneous abortion in diabetic pregnancy. Teratology 1989;39:225–31.

40. Greene MF. Spontaneous abortions and major malformations in women with diabetes mellitus. Semin Reprod Endocrinol 1999;17:127–36.

41. Nielsen GL, Møller M, Sorensen HT. HbA_{1c} in early diabetic pregnancy and pregnancy outcomes. Diabetes Care 2006;29:2612–16.

42. Mills JL, Knopp RH, Simpson JL, et al. Lack of relation of increased malformation rates in infants of diabetic mothers to glycemic control during organogenesis. N Engl J Med 1988;318:671–6.

43. Wright AD, Pollock A, Nicholson HO, et al. Spontaneous abortion and diabetes mellitus. Postgrad Med J 1983;59:295–8.

44. Miodovnik M, Lavin JP, Knowles HC, et al. Spontaneous abortion among insulin-dependent diabetic women. Am J Obstet Gynecol 1984;150:372–6.

45. Sutherland HW, Pritchard CW. Increased incidence of spontaneous abortion in pregnancies complicated by maternal diabetes mellitus. Am J Obstet Gynecol 1986;155:135–8.

46. Mills JL, Simpson JL, Driscoll SG, et al. Incidence of spontaneous abortion among normal women and insulin-dependent diabetic women whose pregnancies were identified within 21 days of conception. N Engl J Med 1988;319:1617–23.

47. Kucera J. Rate and type of congenital anomalies among offspring of diabetic women. J Reprod Med 1971;7:61–70.

48. Becerra JE. Diabetes mellitus during pregnancy and the risks for specific birth defects: a population-based case-control study. Pediatrics 1991;25:1–9.

49. Martinez-Frías ML. Epidemiological analysis of outcomes of pregnancy in diabetic mothers: identification of the most characteristic and most frequent congenital anomalies. Am J Med Genet 1994;51:108–13.

50. Loffredo CA, Wilson PD, Ferencz C. Maternal diabetes: an independent risk factor for major cardiovascular malformations with increased mortality of affected infants. Teratology 2001;64:98–106.

51. Nielsen GL, Nørgard B, Puho E, Rothman KJ, Sørensen HT, Czeizel AE. Risk of specific congenital abnormalities in offspring of women with diabetes. Diabet Med 2005;22:693–6.

52. Wren C, Birrell G, Hawthorne G. Cardiovascular malformations in infants of diabetic mothers. Heart 2003;89:1217–20.

53. Madsen H, Ditzel J. Changes in red blood cell oxygen transport in diabetic pregnancy. Am J Obstet Gynecol 1982;143:421.

54. Milley JR, Rosenberg AA, Philipps AF, Molteni RA, Jones MD, Simmons MA, The effect of insulin on ovine fetal oxygen extraction. Am J Obstet Gynecol 1984;149:673–8.

55. Johnstone FD, Lindsay RS, Steel J. Type 1 diabetes and pregnancy. Trends in birth weight over 40 years at a single clinic. Obstet Gynecol 2006;107:1297–302.

56. Sosenko IR, Kitzmiller JL, Loo SW, Blix P, Rubenstein AH, Gabbay KH. The infant of the diabetic mother. N Engl J Med 1988;301:859–62.

57. Menon RK, Cohen RM, Sperling MA, Cutfield WS, Mimouni F, Koury JC. Transplacental passage of insulin in pregnant women with insulin dependent diabetes mellitus. N Engl J Med 1990;323:309–15.

58. Schwartz R, Gruppuso P A, Petzold K, Brambilla D, Hiilesmaa V, Teramo KA. Hyperinsulinemia and macrosomia in the fetus of the diabetic mother. Diabetes Care 1994;17:640–8.

59. Parretti E, Mecacci F, Papini M, et al. Third-trimester maternal glucose levels from diurnal profiles in nondiabetic pregnancies. Diabetes Care 2001;24:1319–23.

60. Robert MF, Neff RK, Hubbell JP, Taeusch HW, Avery MW. Association between maternal diabetes and the respiratory–distress syndrome in the newborn. N Engl J Med 1976;294: 357–60.

61. Maeda Y, Davé V, Whitsett JA. Transcriptional control of lung morphogenesis. Physiol Rev 2007;87(1):219–44.

62. Smith BT, Post M. Fibroblast-pneumonocyte factor. Am J Physiol 1989;257:L174–L178.

63. Driscoll SG, Benirschke K, Curtis GW. Neonatal deaths among infants of diabetic mothers. Postmortem findings in ninety-five infants. Am J Dis Child 1960;100:818–35.

64. Barbieri RL, Saltzman D, Phillippe M, et al. Elevated beta-human chorionic gonadotropin and testosterone in cord serum of male infants of diabetic mothers. J Clin Endocrinol Metab 1985;61:976–9.

65. Mimouni F, Miodovnik M, Siddiqi TA, Butler JB, Holyroyde J, Tsang RC. Neonatal polycythemia in infants of insulin-dependent diabetic mothers. Obstet Gynecol 1986;68:370–2.

66. Perrine SP, Greene MF, Lee PD, Cohen RA, Faller DV. Insulin stimulates cord blood erythroid progenitor growth: evidence for an aetiological role in neonatal polycythaemia. Br J Haematol 1986;64:503–11.

67. Miyagawa S, Kobayashi M, Konishi N, Sato T, Ueda K. Insulin and insulin-like growth factor I support the proliferation of erythroid progenitor cells in bone marrow through the sharing of receptors. Br J Haematol 2000;109:555–62.

68. Widness JA, Susa JB, Garcia JF, et al. Increased erythropiesis and elevated erythropoietin in infants born to diabetic mothers and in hyperinsulinemic rhesus fetuses. J Clin Invest 1981;67:637–42.

69. Widness JA, Teramo KA, Clemons GK, et al. Direct relationship of antepartum glucose control and fetal erythropoietin in human type 1 (insulin-dependent) diabetic pregnancy. Diabetalogia 1990;33:378–83.

70. Treins C, Giorgetti-Peraldi S, Murdaca J, Semenza GL, van Obberghen E. Insulin stimulates hypoxia-inducible factor 1 through a phosphatidylinositol 3-kinase/target of rapamycin-dependent signaling pathway. J Biol Chem 2002;277:27975–81.

71. Mace S, Hirschfeld, SS, Riggs T, Fanaroff AA, Merkatz IR, Franklin W. Echocardiographic abnormalities in infants of diabetic mothers. J Pediatr 1979;95:1013–19.

72. Way GL, Wolfe RR, Esgaghpour E, Bender RL, Jaffe RB, Ruttenberg HD. The natural history of hypertrophic cardiomyopathy in infants of diabetic mothers. J Pediatr 1979;95:1020–5.

73. Breitweser JA, Meyer RA, Sperling MA, Tsang RC, Kaplan S. Cardiac septal hypertrophy in hyperinsulinemic infants. J Pediatr 1980;96:535–9.

74. Mimouni F, Miodovnik M, Siddiqi TA, Berk MA, Wittekind C, Tsang RC. High-spontaneous premature labor rate in insulin-dependent diabetic pregnant women: an association with poor glycemic control and urogenital infection. Obstet Gynecol 1988;72:175–80.

75. Greene MF, Hare JW, Krache M, et al. Prematurity among insulin-requiring diabetic gravid women. Am J Obstet Gynecol 1989;161:106–11.

76. Sibai BM, Caritis SN, Hauth JC, et al. Preterm delivery in women with pregestational diabetes mellitus or chronic hypertension relative to women with uncomplicated pregnancies. Am J Obstet Gynecol 2000;183:1520–4.

77. Churchill JA, Berendes HW, Nemore J. Neuropsychological deficits in children of diabetic mothers. Am J Obstet Gynecol 1969;105:257–68.

78. Naeye RL, Chez RA, Effects of maternal acetonuria and low pregnancy weight gain on children's psychomotor development. Am J Obstet Gynecol 1981;139:189–92.

79. Rizzo T, Metzger BE, Burns WJ, Burns K. Correlations between antepartum maternal metabolism and intelligence of offspring. N Engl J Med 1991;325:911–16.

80. Rizzo TA, Dooley SL, Metzger BE, Cho NH, Ogata ES, Silverman BL. Prenatal and perinatal influences on long-term psychomotor development in offspring of diabetic mothers. Am J Obstet Gynecol 1995;173:1753–8.

81. Nielsen GL, Dethlefsen C, Sorensen HT, Pedersen JF, Molsted-Pedersen L. Cognitive function and army rejection rate in young adult male offspring of women with diabetes. A Danish population-based cohort study. Diabetes Care 2007;30:2827–31.

82. Gabbe SG, Lowensohn RI, Wu P, Guerra G. Current patterns of neonatal morbidity and mortality in infants of diabetic mothers. Diabetes Care 1978;1:335–9.

83. Macintosh MC, Fleming KM, Bailey JA, et al. Perinatal mortality and congenital anomalies in babies of women with type 1 or type 2 diabetes in England, Wales, and Northern Ireland: population based study. BMJ 2006;333(7560):177.

84. Casson IF, Clarke CA, Howard CV, et al. Outcomes of pregnancy in insulin dependent diabetic women: results of a five year population cohort study. BMJ 1997;315:275–8.

85. Jensen DM, Damm P, Moelsted-Pedersen L, et al. Outcomes in type 1 diabetic pregnancies. Diabetes Care 2004;27:2819–28.

86. Yang J, Cummings EA, O'Connell C, Jangaard K. Fetal and neonatal outcomes of diabetic pregnancies. Obstet Gynecol 2006;108:644–50.

87. Inkster ME, Fahey TP, Donnan PT, Leese GP, Mires GJ, Murphy DJ. Poor glycated haemoglobin control and adverse pregnancy outcomes in type I and type 2 diabetes mellitus: systematic review of observational studies. BMC Pregnancy Childbirth 2006;6:30.

88. Rich SS. Genetics of diabetes and its complications. J Am Soc Nephrol 2006;17:353–60.

89. Warram JH, Krolewski AS, Gottlieb MS, Kahn CR. Differences in risk of insulin-dependent diabetes in offspring of diabetic mothers and diabetic fathers. N Engl J Med 1984;311:149–52.

90. Warram JH, Krolewski AS, Kahn CR. Determinants of IDDM and perinatal mortality in children of diabetic mothers. Diabetes 1988;37:1328–34.

91. Diabetes Genetics Initiative Insititute of Harvard and MIT, Lund University, and Novaritis Institutes for BioMedical Research. Genome-wide association analysis identifies loci for type 2 diabetes and triglyceride levels. Science 2007;316: 1331–6.

92. Meigs JB, Shrader P, Sullivan LM, et al. Genotype score in addition to common risk factors for prediction of type 2 diabetes. N Engl J Med 2008;359:2208–18.

93. Lyssenko V, Johnson A, Almgren P, et al. Clinical factors, DNA variants and the development of type 2 diabetes. N Engl J Med 2008;359:2220–32.

94. Florez JC, Jablonski KA, Bayley N, et al. TCF7L2 Polymorphisms and progression to diabetes in the diabetes prevention program. N Engl J Med 2006;355:241–50.

95. McLean M, Chipps D, Cheung NW. Mother to child transmission of diabetes mellitus: does gestational diabetes program type 2 diabetes in the next generation? Diabet Med 2006;23: 1213–15.

96. Kimmerle R, Weiss R, Berger M, Kurz KH. Effectiveness, safety, and acceptability of a copper intrauterine device (CU Safe 300) in type I diabetic women. Diabetes Care 1993;16:1227–30.

97. Rogovskaya S, Rivera R, Grimes DA, et al. Effect of a levonorgestrel intrauterine system on women with type 1 diabetes: a randomized trial. Obstet Gynecol 2005;105:811–15.

98. Petersen KR, Skouby SO, Vedel P, Haaber AB. Hormonal contraception in women with IDDM. Influence on glycometabolic control and lipoprotein metabolism. Diabetes Care 1995;18:800–6.

99. American College of Obstetricians and Gynecologists Committee on Practice Bulletins. Clinical management guidelines: use of hormonal contraception in women with coexisting medical conditions. ACOG Practice Bulletin No 73. Obstet Gynecol 2006;107:1453–72.

100. Mills JL, Baker L, Goldman AS. Malformations in infants of diabetic mothers occur before the seventh gestational week. Implications for treatment. Diabetes 1979;28:292–3.

101. Fuhrmann K, Reiher H, Semmler K, et al. Prevention of congenital malformations in infants of insulin-dependent diabetic mothers. Diabetes Care 1983;6:219–23.

102. Damm P, Molsted Pedersen L. Significant decrease in congenital malformations in newborn infants of an unselected population of diabetic women. Am J Obstet Gynecol 1989;161:1163–7.

103. Steel JM, Johnstone FD, Hepburn DA, et al. Can prepregnancy care of diabetic women reduce the risk of abnormal babies? BMJ 1990;301:1070–4.

104. Kitzmiller JL, Gavin LA, Gin GD, et al. Preconception care of diabetes: glycemic control prevents congenital anomalies. JAMA 1991;265:731–6.

105. Willhoite MB, Bennert HW, Palomaki GE, et al. The impact of preconception counseling on pregnancy outcomes. The experience of the Maine Diabetes in Pregnancy Program. Diabetes Care 1993;16:450–5.

106. Gregory R, Tattersall RB. Are diabetic pre-pregnancy clinics worth while? Lancet 1992;340:656–8.

107. Phelps RL, Metzger BE, Freinkel N. Carbohydrate metabolism in pregnancy. XVII. Diurnal profiles of plasma glucose, insulin, free fatty acids, triglycerides, cholesterol and individual amino acids in late normal pregnancy. Am J Obstet Gynecol 1981;140:730–6.

108. Kitzmiller JL, Block JM, Brown FM, et al. Managing preexisting diabetes for pregnancy. Diabetes Care 2008;31:1060.

109. Hirsch IB. Insulin analogues. N Engl J Med 2005;352:174–83.

110. Mukhopadhyay A, Farrell T, Fraser RB, Ola B. Continuous subcutaneous insulin infusion vs. intensive conventional insulin therapy in pregnancy diabetic women: a systematic review and metaanalysis of randomized, controlled trials. Am J Obstet Gynecol 2007;197(5):447–56.

111. Wyatt JW, Frias JL, Hoymet HE, et al. Congenital anomaly rate in offspring of mothers with diabetes treated with insulin lispro during pregnancy. Diabet Med 2005;22(6):803–7.

112. Di Cianni G, Volpe L, Ghio A. Maternal metabolic control and perinatal outcome in women with gestational diabetes mellitus treated with lispro or aspart insulin. Diabetes Care 2007;30:e11.

113. Mathiesen ER, Kinsley B, Amiel SA, et al. Maternal glycemic control and hypoglycemia in type 1 diabetic pregnancy. A randomized trial of insulin aspart versus human insulin in 322 pregnant women. Diabetes Care 2007;30(4):771–6.

114. Hod M, Damm P, Kaaja R, et al. Fetal and perinatal outcomes in type 1 diabetes pregnancy: a randomized study comparing insulin aspart with human insulin in 322 subjects. Am J Obstet Gynecol 2008;198:186.e1–186.e7.

115. Jovanovic L, Ilic S, Pettitt DJ, et al. Metabolic and immunologic effects of insulin lispro in gestational diabetes. Diabetes Care 1999;22:1422–7.

116. Jovanovic L, Pettitt DJ. Treatment with insulin and its analogs in pregnancies complicated by diabetes. Diabetes Care 2007;30(suppl 2):S220–4.

117. Gallen IW, Jaap A, Rolandt JM, Chirayath HH. Survery of glargine use in 115 pregnant women with type 1 diabetes. Diabet Med 2008;25:165–9.

118. Langer O, Conway DL, Berkus MD, Xenakis MJ, Gonzales O. A comparison of glyburide and insulin in women with gestational diabetes mellitus. N Engl J Med 2000;343:1134–8.

119. Nestler JE. Metformin in the treatment of infertility in polycystic ovarian syndrome: an alternative perspective. Fertil Steril 2008;90(1):14–16.

120. Gilbert C, Valois M, Koren G. Pregnancy outcome after first-trimester exposure to metformin: a meta-analysis. Fertil Steril 2006;86(3):658–63.

121. Glueck CJ, Goldernberg N, Pranikoff J, Loftspring M, Sieve L, Wang P. Height, weight, and motor-social development during the first 18 months of life in 126 infants born to 109 mothers with polycystic ovary syndrome who conceived on continued metformin through pregnancy. Hum Reprod 2004;19:1323–30.

122. Bolton S, Cleary B, Walsh J, Dempsey E, Turner MJ. Continuation of metformin in the first trimester of women with polycystic ovarian syndrome is not associated with increased perinatal morbidity. Eur J Pediatr 2009:168:203–6.

123. Rowan JA, Hague WM, Gao W, Battin MR, Moore P, for the MiG Trial Investigators. Metformin versus insulin for the treatment of gestational diabetes. N Engl J Med 2008;358:2003–15.

124. Diamond M, Reece EA, Caprio S, et al. Impairment of counterregulatory hormone responses to hypoglycemia in pregnant women with insulin-dependent diabetes mellitus. Am J Obstet Gynecol 1992;166:70–7.

125. Klein R, Klein B. Diabetic eye disease. Lancet 1997;350:197–204.

126. Reichard P, Nilsson BY, Rosenqvist U. The effect of long-term intensified insulin treatment on the development of microvascular complications of diabetes mellitus. N Engl J Med 1993;329:304–9.

127. Diabetes Control and Complications Trial Research Group. The effect of intensive treatment of diabetes on the development and progression of long-term complications in insulin-dependent diabetes mellitus. N Engl J Med 1993;329:977–86.

128. Diabetes Control and Complications Research Group. Early worsening of diabetic retinopathy in the Diabetes Control and Complications Trial. Arch Ophthalmol 1998;116:874–6.

129. Klein BE, Moss SE, Klein R. Effect of pregnancy on progression of diabetic retinopathy. Diabetes Care 1990;13:34–40.

130. Chew EY, Mills JL, Metzger BE, et al., Metabolic control and progression of retinopathy. Diabetes Care 1995;18:631–7.

131. Diabetes Control and Complications Trial Research Group. Effect of pregnancy on microvascular complications in the diabetes control and complications trial. Diabetes Care 2000;23:1084–91.

132. Krolewski AS, Laffel LMB, Krolewski M, Quinn M, Warram JH. Glycosylated hemoglobin and the risk of microalbuminuria in patients with insulin-dependent diabetes mellitus. N Engl J Med 1995;332:1251–5.

133. Nielsen FS, Rossing P, Gall MA, Skott P, Smidt UM, Parving HH. Long-term effect of lisinopril and atenolol on kidney function in hypertensive NIDDM subjects with diabetic nephropathy. Diabetes 1997;46:1182–8.

134. Barr M Jr, Cohen MM Jr. ACE inhibitor fetopathy and hypocalvaria: the kidney-skull connection. Teratology 1991;44:485–95.

135. Cooper WO, Hernandez-Diaz S, Arbogast PG, et al. Major congenital malformations after first-trimester exposure to ACE inhibitors. N Engl J Med 2006;354:2443–51.

136. Sibai BM, Caritis S, Hauth J, et al. Risks of preeclampsia and adverse neonatal outcomes among women with pregestational diabetes mellitus. Am J Obstet Gynecol 2000;182:364–9.

137. Mogensen CE, Christensen CK. Predicting diabetic nephropathy in insulin-dependent patients. N Engl J Med 1984;311:89–93.

138. Combs CA, Rosenn B, Kitzmiller JL, Khoury JC, Wheeler BC, Miodovnik M. Early-pregnancy proteinuria in diabetes related to preeclampsia. Obstet Gynecol 1993;82:802–7.

139. Caritis S, Sibai B, Hauth J, et al. Low-dose aspirin to prevent preeclampsia in women at high risk. N Engl J Med 1998;338:701–5.

140. Askie LM, Duley L, Henderson–Smart DJ, Stewart LA. Antiplatelet agents for prevention of pre-eclampsia: a meta-analysis of individual patient data. Lancet 2007;369:1791–8.

141. Livingston EG, Herbert WN, Hage ML, Chapman JF, Stubbs TM. Use of the TDX–FLM assay in evaluating fetal lung maturity in an insulin-dependent diabetic population. Obstet Gynecol 1995;86:826–9.

142. Transasijevic MJ, Winkelman JW, Wybenga DR, Richardson DK, Greene MF. Prediction of fetal lung maturity in infants of diabetic mothers using the FLM s/a and disaturated phosphatidylcholine tests. Am J Clin Pathol 1996;105(1):17–22.

143. McFarland LV, Raskin M, Daling J R, Benedetti TJ. Erb/Duchenne's palsy: a consequence of fetal macrosomia and method of delivery. Obstet Gynecol 1986;68:784–8.

144. Acker DB, Gregory KD, Sachs BP, Friedman EA. Risk factors for Erb-Duchenne palsy. Obstet Gynecol 1988;71:389.

145. Nesbitt TS, Gilbert WM, Herrchen B. Shoulder dystocia and associated risk factors with macrosomic infants born in California. Am J Obstet Gynecol 1998;179:476–80.

146. Modanlou HD, Komatsu G, Dorchester W, Freeman RK, Bosu SK. Large-for-gestational-age neonates: anthropometric reasons for shoulder dystocia. Obstet Gynecol 1982;60:417.

147. Langer O, Berkus M, Huff RW, Samueloff A. Shoulder dystocia: shoulder the fetus weighing ≥ 4000 grams be delivered by cesarean section? Am J Obstet Gynecol 1991;165:831–7.

148. Rouse DJ, Owen J, Goldenberg RL, Cliver SP. The effectiveness and costs of elective cesarean delivery for fetal macrosomia diagnosed by ultrasound. JAMA 1996;276:1480–6.

149. Conway DL, Langer O. Elective delivery of infants with macrosomia in diabetic women: reduced shoulder dystocia versus increased cesarean deliveries. Am J Obstet Gynecol 1998;178:922–5.

150. American College of Obstetricians and Gynecologists Committee on Practice Bulletins. Clinical management guidelines: fetal macrosomia. ACOG Practice Bulletin No 22. American College of Obstetricians and Gynecologists, Washington, DC, 2000.

151. Philipson EH, Kalhan SC, Rihi MM, Pimentel R. Effects of maternal glucose infusion on fetal acid–base status in human pregnancy. Am J Obstet Gynecol 1987;157:866–73.

152. Robertshaw HJ, McAnulty GR, Hall GM. Strategies for managing the diabetic patient. Best Pract Res Clin Anesthesiol 2004;18:631–43.

153. Moitra VK, Meiler SE. The diabetic surgical patient. Curr Opinion Anaesth 2006;19:339–45.

154. Peterfreund RA, Lee SL. Endocrine surgery and intraoperative management of endocrine conditions. In: Longnecker DE, Brown, DL, Newman MF, Zapol WM (eds) Anesthesiology. McGraw-Hill, New York, 2008:1420–49.

155. Sonksen, P, Sonksen J. Insulin understanding its action in health and disease. Br J Anaesth 2000;85:69–79.

156. Chico M, Levine SN, Lewis DF. Normoglycemic diabetic ketoacidosis in pregnancy. J Perinatol 2008;28:310–12

157. Guo RX, Yang LZ, Li LX, Zhao XP. Diabetic ketoacidosis in pregnancy tends to occur at lower blood glucose levels: case-control study and a case report of euglycemic diabetic ketoacidosis in pregnancy. J Obstet Gynaecol Res 2008;34:324–30.

158. Kamalakannan D, Baskar V, Barton DM, Abdu TA. Diabetic ketoacidosis in pregnancy. Postgrad Med J 2008;79:454–7.

159. Groudine SB, Phan B. Significant hyperkalemia after discontinuation of an insulin pump. J Clin Anesth 2005;17:630–2.

160. Bloomgarden ZT. Type 2 diabetes in the young: the evolving epidemic. Diabetes Care 2004;27:998–1010.

161. Jovanovic L. Glucose and insulin requirements during labor and delivery: the case for normoglycemia in pregnancies complicated by diabetes. Endocr Pract 2004;10(suppl 2):40–5.

162. Cryer PE. Diverse causes of hypoglycemia-associated autonomic failure in diabetes. N Engl J Med 2004;350(22):2272–9.

163. Vreven, R, de Kock M. Metformin lactic acidosis and anaesthesia: myth or reality? Acta Anaesthesiol Belg 2005;56:297–302.

164. Stades AM, Heikens JT, Erkelens DW, Holleman F, Hoekstra JB. Metformin and lactic acidosis: cause or coincidence? A review of case reports. J Intern Med 2004;255:179–87.

165. Salpeter S, Greyber E, Pasternak G, Salpeter E. Risk of fatal and nonfatal lactic acidosis with metformin use in type 2 diabetes mellitus. Cochrane Database of Systematic Reviews, 2006;25:1: CD002967.

166. Chen D, Lee SL, Peterfreund RA. New therapeutic agents for diabetes mellitus: implications for anesthetic management. Anesth Analg 2009;108(6):1803–10.

167. Schannwell CM, Schneppenheim M, Perings SM, Zimmermann T, Plehn G, Strauer BE. Alterations of left ventricular function in women with insulin-dependent diabetes mellitus during pregnancy. Diabetologia 2003;46:267–75.

168. Jellish WS, Kartha V, Fluder E, Slogoff S. Effect of metoclopramide on gastric fluid volumes in diabetic patients who have fasted before elective surgery. Anesthesiology 2005;102:904–9.

169. Hebl JR. Neurological complications in regional anesthesia and pain medicine: the patient with pre-exisitng peripheral disease. American Society of Regional Anesthesia and Pain Medicine, Park Ridge, IL, 2005:223–31.

170. Saitoh Y, Kanded K, Hattori H, Nakajima H, Murakawa M. Monitoring of neuromuscular block after administration of vecuronium in patients with diabetes mellitus. Br J Anaesth 2003;90:480–6.

171. Saitoh Y, Hattori H, Sanbe N, Nakajima H, Akatu M, Murakawa M. Reversal of vecuronium with neostigmine in patients with diabetes mellitus. Anaesthesia 2004;59:750–4.

172. Saitoh Y, Hattori H, Sanbe N, Nakajima H, Akatu M, Murakawa M. Delayed recovery of vecuronium neuromuscular block in diabetic patients during sevoflurane anesthesia. Can J Anesth 2005;52:467–73.

173. Davies G, Kingswood C, Street M. Pharmacokinetics of opioids in renal dysfunction. Clin Pharmacokinet 1996;31:410–22.

174. Murphy EJ. Acute pain management pharmacology for the patient with concurrent renal or hepatic disease. Anaesth Intens Care 2005;33:311–22.

175. Reissell E, Orko R, Maunuksela EL, Lindgren L. Predictability of difficult laryngoscopy in patients with long–term diabetes mellitus. Anaesthesia 1990;45:1024–7.

176. Erden V, Basaranoglu G, Delatioglu H, Hamzaoglu NS. Relationship of difficult laryngoscopy to long-term non-insulin-dependent diabetes and hand abnormality using the "prayer sign". Br J Anaesth 2003;91:159–60.

177. Vani V, Kamath SK, Naik LD, The palm print as a sensitive predictor of difficult laryngoscopy in diabetics: a comparison with other evaluation indices. J Postgrad Med 2000;46:75–9.

178. Hogan K, Rusy D, Springman SR. Difficult laryngoscopy and diabetes mellitus. Anesth Analg 1988;67:1162–5.

179. Warner ME, Contreras MG, Warner MA, Schroeder DR, Munn SR, Maxson PM. Diabetes mellitus and difficult laryngoscopy in renal and pancreatic transplant patients. Anesth Analg 1998;86:516–19.

180. Philips B, Baker E. Hyperglycemia and the lung. Br J Anaesth 2003;90:430–3.

181. Tiengo A, Fadini GP, Avogaro A. The metabolic syndrome, diabetes, and lung dysfunction. Diabetes Metab 2008;34:447–54.

182. Kaparianos A, Argyropoulou E, Sampsonas F, Karkoulias K, Tsiamita M, Spiropoulos K. Pulmonary complications in diabetes mellitus. Chron Respir Dis 2008;5:101–8.

183. Hsia CC, Raskin P. Lung function changes related to diabetes mellitus. Diabetes Technol Ther 2007;9:(suppl)1:S73–82.

184. Breidbart S, Singer L, St Louis Y, Saenger P. Adult respiratory distress syndrome in an adolescent with diabetic ketoacidosis. J Pediatr 1987;111:736.

185. Winegard AI, Kern EFO, Simmons DA. Cerebral edema in diabetic ketoacidosis. N Engl J Med 1985;312:1184.

186. Flier JS, Moore MJ. The metabolic derangements and treatment of diabetic ketoacidosis. N Engl J Med 1983;309:159.

187. Rhodes RW, Ogburn Jr PL. Treatment of severe diabetic ketoacidosis in the early third trimester in a patient with fetal distress. J Reprod Med 1984;29:621.

188. Maislos M, Harman-Bohem I, Weitzman S. Diabetic ketoacidosis: a rare complication of gestational diabetes. Diabetes Care 1992;15:968.

189. Thomas DJB, Gill B, Brown P, Stubbs WA. Salbutamol-induced diabetic ketoacidosis. BMJ 1977;2:438.

190. Borberg C, Gillmer MDG, Beard RW, Oakley NW. Metabolic effects of beta-sympathomimetic drugs and dexamethasone in normal and diabetic pregnancy. Br J Obstet Gynaecol 1978;85:184.

191. Fisher JN, Shahshahani MN, Kitabchi AE. Diabetic ketoacidosis: low-dose insulin therapy by various routes. N Engl J Med 1977;297:238.

192. Luzi L, Barrett EJ, Groop LC, et al. Metabolic effects of low-dose insulin therapy on glucose metabolism in diabetic ketoacidosis. Diabetes 1988;37:1470.

193. Morris LR, Murphy MB, Kitabchi AE. Bicarbonate therapy in severe diabetic ketoacidosis. Ann Intern Med 1986;105:836.

194. Keller U, Berger W. Prevention of hypophosphatemia by phosphate infusion during treatment of diabetic ketoacidosis and hyperosmolar coma. Diabetes 1980;29:87.

195. Rosenbloom AL. Intracerebral crises during treatment of diabetic ketoacidosis. Diabetes Care 1990;13:22.

196. Lobue C, Goodlin RC. Treatment of fetal distress during diabetic keto-acidosis. J Reprod Med 1978;20:101.

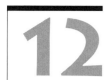

Thyroid disease in pregnancy

Erin Keely[1] and Brian M. Casey[2]

[1]Department of Endocrinology and Metabolism, The Ottawa Hospital, Ottawa, Ontario, Canada
[2]Department of Obstetrics and Gynecology, Division of Maternal-Fetal Medicine, University of Texas Southwestern Medical Center, Dallas, TX, USA

Introduction

The prevalence of thyroid disorders in women of childbearing age and the potential for long-term impact on the offspring exposed to abnormal thyroid hormone levels make it essential that caregivers have a sound approach to identifying and treating abnormal thyroid function during pregnancy. Women may have pre-existing thyroid disease that requires monitoring during pregnancy, have thyroid disease that is not yet diagnosed or treated until after conception, or develop pregnancy-related thyroid dysfunction during or after pregnancy. Thyroid disease may manifest as a change in size of the thyroid gland, a change in level of thyroid hormone or by effects of autoantibodies on the mother or fetus. Interpretation of laboratory test results requires an understanding of the normal physiologic changes in pregnancy in order to prevent mislabeling and avoid inappropriate treatment that may have serious consequences for the developing fetus.

Normal physiologic changes in pregnancy

Pregnancy is associated with significant but reversible changes in maternal thyroid physiology (Table 12.1, Figure 12.1). Thyroid hormone is derived from iodination of tyrosine residues in thyroglobulin to form mono- or di-iodotyrosine which are then coupled to form T4 and T3. The majority of released hormone is T4 and is bound to circulating transport proteins – thyroxine-binding globulin (TBG), thyroxine-binding prealbumin or transthyretin, and albumin. The unbound or free fraction represents 0.04% of total T4 and is the physiologically active hormone or free T4. Thyroid-stimulating hormone (TSH) from the anterior pituitary increases the synthesis and release of thyroid hormone and is the primary regulator of thyroid function.

Table 12.1 Clinical importance of physiologic changes in pregnancy

Physiologic change	Clinical importance
Increased TBG	• Need for increased T4 production • Elevation of total T4 and T3 levels • Interference with free T4 assay accuracy
Placental de-iodination of T4	• Increase in T4 and T3 metabolism • Need for increased T4 production
Increased iodine clearance (renal clearance and fetal transfer)	• Increased need for iodine supplementation • Risk of maternal and fetal hypothyroidism and goiter
Beta-HCG elevation first trimester	• Elevation of free T4 and suppression of TSH • May have mild thyrotoxicosis transiently
Reduction in TSHRAb during pregnancy	• Graves' disease may improve during pregnancy
Postpartum increase in thyroid antibodies	• Exacerbation of Graves' disease • Precipitation of postpartum thyroiditis

HCG, human chorionic gonadotropin; TBG, thyroid-binding globulin; TSH, thyroid-stimulating hormone; TSHRAb, TSH receptor.

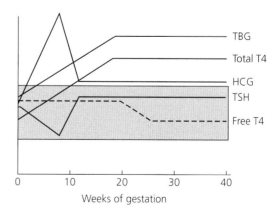

Figure 12.1 Change in thyroid function indices throughout gestation. The shaded area represents the normal range of TBG (thyroid-binding globulin), total T4 (thyroxine), TSH (thyroid-stimulating hormone) and free T4. HCG (human chorionic gonadotropin). Reproduced with permission from Casey [54].

de Swiet's Medical Disorders in Obstetric Practice, 5th edition. Edited by R. O. Powrie, M. F. Greene, W. Camann. © 2010 Blackwell Publishing.

The pregnant woman is required to make 50% more thyroid hormone during pregnancy due to an estrogen-mediated increase in production of TBG [1]. The increased binding of thyroid hormone together with increased metabolism of thyroid hormones by the placenta leads to a greater requirement for thyroid hormone production in order to maintain free T4 levels. Total T4 levels are 150% above the normal non-pregnant reference interval. The increased production of thyroid hormone together with the increased renal clearance and placental transfer of iodine to the fetus in turn results in an increased maternal demand for iodine, an essential building block for thyroid hormone. Women who have borderline iodine deficiency, for example, may be unable to meet this increase in demand, resulting in an overall reduction in thyroid hormone production, a preference for T3 production (the more biologically active form of thyroid hormone, produced from T4 predominantly in extrathyroid tissue), and progression toward hypothyroidism.

Thyroid function studies during pregnancy

Thyroid function tests may be outside the nonpregnant reference range in the normal pregnant woman. Human chorionic gonadotropin (HCG) shares some structural homology with thyrotropin (TSH) and is known to stimulate TSH receptors in thyroid tissue. The rising levels of HCG in the first trimester result in a transient increase in T4 production and subsequent suppression of TSH. It is thus "normal" to have a suppressed TSH and possibly a slightly elevated free T4 during the first trimester. Additionally, there are numerous pregnancy conditions associated with higher than usual HCG levels such as a molar gestation or hyperemesis gravidarum. These conditions may result in an exaggerated stimulation of the thyroid gland and transient first-trimester thyrotoxicosis [2] (see below). Women with twin pregnancies would also be expected to have lower TSH related to the higher HCG in a multiple gestation [3].

The interpretation of thyroid function tests in the second and third trimesters also requires careful consideration because of the known physiologic changes and pitfalls in current assays. TSH will "rebound" to normal nonpregnant levels once HCG returns to a steady state during pregnancy [4]. A majority of studies have demonstrated a subsequent mild decline in free T4 and an increase in TSH after the first trimester and into the third trimester in iodine-replete women. These changes, however, typically remain within the reference range [5]. Importantly, interpretation of the free T4 level and its accuracy is assay dependent and contingent on gestational age and the interference from the progressively increasing TBG level. Free T4 results, and TSH for that matter, should ideally be compared to trimester-specific reference ranges established for specific assays in individual laboratories [6,7]. Some authorities recommend using total

T4 levels, rather than free levels, and adjusting the reference interval by 150% compared to the nonpregnant value [8,9]. However, many clinical labs no longer provide total T4 and T3 resin uptake assays (and the associated calculated free thyroxine index (FT4I)) as they are not recommended outside pregnancy.

Fetal thyroid physiology

Embryogenesis of the fetal thyroid gland is largely complete and begins synthesizing thyroid hormone by 12 weeks of gestation. Fetal TSH is also detected at this age and the negative feedback control of thyroid hormone synthesis evolves by approximately mid-gestation. The thyroid–pituitary axis continues to develop throughout gestation with progressive increases in TSH, total T4, and TBG [10].

Especially relevant is the intimate relationship between maternal and fetal thyroid function during the first half of pregnancy. Any requirement for thyroid hormones prior to 12 weeks gestation is supplied by the mother and it is during this time that thyroid hormones are most important to fetal brain development [11]. While overt maternal thyroid failure during the first half of pregnancy has been associated with several pregnancy complications and intellectual impairment in offspring [12–15], it is less clear whether milder forms of thyroid dysfunction have similar effects on pregnancy and infant outcomes [16]. Significant fetal brain development continues considerably beyond the first trimester, making thyroid hormone also important later in gestation. The mother continues to supply thyroxine as well as iodine for fetal thyroid hormone production throughout pregnancy. The role of maternal thyroxine after fetal thyroid production begins is less clear; however, if there is insufficient placental transfer of iodine, fetal hypothyroidism will result.

Autoimmune thyroid disease

Because of the association of thyroid antibodies with particular obstetric outcomes and the effect of pregnancy on antibody titers, consideration of the autoimmune nature of most thyroid disease is important in the course of the illness during pregnancy and fetal consequences. There are two main types of thyroid antibodies: those that are directed towards cytoplasmic antigens (thyroid peroxidase (TPOAb) and thyroglobulin (TgAb) antibodies) and those directed to the TSH receptor (TSHRAb). According to the NHANES III data, 10–15% of women of childbearing age, not known to have thyroid dysfunction, will be positive for TPOAB [17]. Another recent study of over 17,000 pregnant women screened in the first half of pregnancy indicates that approximately 5% will have TPO antibodies [18].

Thyroid autoimmunity, with normal thyroid function, has been associated with increased miscarriage rates in some, but not all, studies. This increase in miscarriage does not appear to be related to antibody titer or the presence of thyroid dysfunction. It is hypothesized that the increased risk of miscarriage may be due to:
- subtle maternal thyroid dysfunction
- an underlying autoimmune imbalance reflected by the presence of thyroid antibodies which results in rejection of the fetus
- thyroid antibodies which cross the placenta and directly affect the developing fetal thyroid gland, thus increasing early loss
- increased maternal age of women with thyroid autoimmunity [19].

Pregnancy is associated with a decrease in antibody titers due to trophoblast secretion of immunosuppressant factors [20]. For example, the TSH receptor antibodies associated with Graves' disease have been shown to decrease substantially during gestation, resulting in clinical improvement and the ability to discontinue medication in many patients. Conversely, antibody titers will increase post partum and are responsible for flares of Graves' disease in the postpartum period and the development of postpartum thyroiditis (see below) [21,22]. In women who continue to have high titers during pregnancy, passive placental transfer can lead to fetal thyroid disorders after mid-gestation (see below).

Hyperthyroidism

Hyperthyroidism complicates approximately 0.2% of pregnancies [23]. Hyperthyroidism is defined by excessive thyroid hormone production due to an overactive thyroid gland. A woman may be tested because of known thyroid disease, the presence of a goiter, symptoms suggestive of thyrotoxicosis or as part of a routine screening strategy. Based on biochemical tests, individuals might be identified with subclinical (suppressed TSH, normal T4 and T3) or overt (suppressed TSH and elevated T4 and/or T3) hyperthyroidism. In women with a depressed TSH yet a normal free T4, hypermetabolic symptoms may rarely be explained by T3 thyrotoxicosis. The most common cause of pre-existing hyperthyroidism is Graves' disease, an autoimmune hyperthyroidism caused by stimulation of the thyroid gland by thyroid-stimulating hormone receptor antibody (TSHRAb). The differential diagnosis includes toxic solitary thyroid nodule, multiple nodular goiter, exogenous thyroid hormone, amiodarone ingestion, excess iodine intake, and subacute thyroiditis (Box 12.1) [24,25].

Clinical presentation depends on the severity of the thyrotoxicosis and its underlying cause (Box 12.2). Individuals with thyrotoxicosis may present with adrenergic symptoms of stare, lid lag, palpitations, anxiety, nervousness, weight loss, heat intolerance and menstrual irregularity. The thyroid exam may also be helpful when developing a differential diagnosis. For

> **Box 12.1** Causes of thyrotoxicosis in pregnancy
>
> **Intrinsic thyroid disease**
> - Graves' disease
> - Toxic nodule – single or multiple
> - Subacute or silent thyroiditis
>
> **Excessive, exogenous thyroid hormone**
> - Factitious
> - Therapeutic
>
> **Gestational thyrotoxicosis**
> - Hyperemesis
> - Placenta mediated
>   - Hydatidiform mole
>   - Multiple gestations
>   - Hydrops

example, a diffuse, symmetric, soft goiter, which may have an audible bruit, is typical of Graves' disease. A palpable nodule (usually >3 cm) is direct evidence of nodular thyroid disease and generalized thyroid tenderness is consistent with subacute thyroiditis [25]. Associated autoimmune manifestations of hyperthyroidism such as orbitopathy (proptosis, soft tissue periorbital swelling, extraocular muscle dysfunction), pretibial myxedema and clubbing are exclusive to Graves' disease.

Thyroid storm is an acute, life-threatening exacerbation of thyrotoxicosis. The classic findings are fever, tachycardia, tremor, nausea, vomiting, diarrhea, dehydration, and delirium or coma. Thyroid storm is rare in pregnancy and its diagnosis is based entirely on clinical grounds in women with laboratory tests consistent with overt hyperthyroidism. Heart failure due to cardiomyopathy from excessive thyroxine in women with uncontrolled hyperthyroidism is probably more common in pregnant women [26].

Diagnosis during pregnancy

The clinical features of hyperthyroidism can be easily confused with findings or symptoms typical of pregnancy. Suggestive complaints include nervousness, heat intolerance, palpitations, thyromegaly or goiter, failure to gain weight or weight loss, and exophthalmos. Although nausea is common in early pregnancy, the occurrence of hyperemesis gravidarum together with weight loss may also signify overt hyperthyroidism. Thyroid testing may be beneficial in this circumstance but routine testing in women with hyperemesis gravidarum is not recommended. Importantly, one must consider the impact of gestational age on measurement of TSH. It is important to not overdiagnose hyperthyroidism in the first trimester as 10–20% of women will have a suppressed TSH. Subclinical hyperthyroidism (suppressed TSH with normal free T4) has not been shown to adversely affect pregnancy [27].

Box 12.2 Most common causes of thyrotoxicosis in pregnancy

All causes
- Nervousness
- Agitation
- Fatigue
- Tachycardia/palpitations
- Heat intolerance
- Weight loss
- Increased frequency of bowel habits
- Skin/hair/nail changes
  - Skin is soft and moist
  - Onycholysis (separation of the distal nail from its bed)
  - Hair becomes soft, fine and may thin
- Eye signs (distinct from Graves' ophthalmopathy)
  - Lid lag (elicited by having the patient follow your finger as you move it from the top to the bottom of their visual field. Lid lag is present if the upper lid is slow to follow the eye on downward movement and white sclera becomes exposed above the iris)
  - Lid retraction and stare (the white sclera above the iris is visible at rest. The orbit appears prominent but is not actually bulging (proptotic))

Specific to Graves' disease
- Graves' orbitopathy: chemosis (swelling of the conjunctiva), proptosis (exophthalmos or bulging orbit), dysconjugate gaze (double vision on looking to the extremes of the visual field)
- Pretibial myxedema (a skin disorder presenting as bilateral, firm, nonpitting, asymmetric plaques or nodules that are most often confined to the pretibial area but may occur anywhere)
- Thyroid bruit
- Clubbing (individuals without clubbing display a diamond-shaped window at the base of the nail beds when two fingers from opposite hands are opposed dorsally. The distal angle between the two opposed nails should be minimal. In individuals with digital clubbing, the diamond window is obliterated and the distal angle between the nails increases with increasing severity of clubbing)

At present, there is no convincing evidence that subclinical hyperthyroidism should be treated in nonpregnant individuals and treatment during pregnancy is also unwarranted [28]. Indeed, it should be considered contraindicated because maternal antithyroid drugs cross the placenta and may cause fetal thyroid suppression [29].

Box 12.3 Indications for measurement of maternal TSH receptor antibodies in pregnancy

First trimester
- Previous radio-active iodine or thyroidectormy for Graves' disease
- New-onset thyrotoxicosis to differentiate Graves' disease from gestational thyrotoxicosis
- Previous pregnancy complicated by fetal or neonatal hyperthyroidism

Third trimester
- Woman requiring antithyroid drugs for Graves' disease into third trimester

Once a diagnosis of biochemical hyperthyroidism is confirmed in pregnancy by a suppressed TSH and an elevated free T4 and/or freeT3, it is important to determine the cause. A woman may have previously undiagnosed Graves' disease, nodular thyroid disease or a condition unique to pregnancy. Gestational thyrotoxicosis, also referred to as first-trimester thyrotoxicosis or HCG- related thyrotoxicosis, is typically associated with hyperemesis gravidarum. It can also be due to high levels of HCG resulting from molar pregnancy. Both conditions are associated with high HCG levels that lead to TSH receptor stimulation and transient hyperthyroidism. Women with gestational thyrotoxicosis are rarely symptomatic, have minimal thyroid enlargement, and are TSHRAb negative [30]. With expectant management of hyperemesis gravidarum, serum free T4 levels usually normalize in parallel with the decline in HCG concentrations as pregnancy progresses beyond the first trimester. Similar results would be expected with definitive treatment of a molar gestation.

It may be challenging to decide between gestational hyperthyroidism and primary thyroid disease in the first trimester (see Box 12.1). Since radio-active iodine thyroid scanning is prohibited during pregnancy, the clinician must rely more on clinical presentation. If clinical findings are inconclusive, it may be helpful to measure TSHRAb. TSH receptor antibodies are positive in 80% of patients with Graves' disease [31].

Management

The goal of management of thyrotoxicosis is primarily to normalize, but not suppress thyroid hormone levels and to secondarily treat bothersome adrenergic symptoms of hyperthyroidism. Antithyroid drugs cross the placenta and may cause fetal thyroid suppression, so the minimal dose to achieve adequate metabolic control is preferred. Treatment options for nonpregnant women include treatment for 12–24 months with antithyroid medication, radio-active iodine to partially ablate the thyroid gland, and near-total thyroidectomy. The selection of one of these three depends on patient and clinician preferences, plans for pregnancy as well as clinical characteristics such as severity of thyrotoxicosis, size of the thyroid gland, and presence of ophthalmopathy. For example, in cases of toxic thyroid nodules, radio-active iodine is the preferred choice outside pregnancy. The risk of permanent hypothyroidism is less than when treating Graves' disease with radio-active iodine, and antithyroid drugs generally do not result in remission of the hyperthyroidism related to thyroid nodules. Moreover, if symptoms related to compression are present with multinodular goiters or there is a question of malignancy in a nodule, a near-total thyroidectomy may be recommended.

Preconceptional counseling

Pregnancy outcomes

Severe thyrotoxicosis is associated with poor obstetric outcomes, but controlled hyperthyroidism is tolerated well during pregnancy [32,33]. Pregnant women with hyperthyroidism are at increased risk for spontaneous pregnancy loss, congestive heart failure, thyroid storm, preterm birth, pre-eclampsia, fetal growth restriction, and associated increased perinatal morbidity and mortality [32,34]. Fetal risks depend on degree of thyrotoxicosis, underlying cause of the thyrotoxicosis and treatment modality used. In most cases, the perinate of a hyperthyroid mother is euthyroid. Placental transfer of TSHRAb, however, can cause fetal Graves' disease. This manifests as fetal tachycardia, high output cardiac failure, hydrops, craniosynostosis, intrauterine growth restriction (IUGR) and fetal goiter [35,36]. This occurs in approximately 2–10% of offspring of affected women [37]. The risk to offspring is directly related to maternal antibody titer in the third trimester [38]. Fetuses of low-risk mothers, those without detectable serum antibody levels, are rarely identified with goiter and are typically euthyroid at delivery.

Fetal goiter may also result from excessive thio-amide exposure. In this case the fetus is hypothyroid, not hyperthyroid. Current data indicate that thio-amides carry an extremely small risk for causing hypothyroidism in the neonate [39,40] and at least four long-term studies have found no abnormal intellectual and physical development in these children [41].

Chronic exposure to hyperthyroidism from inadequately treated maternal hyperthyroidism may impair maturation of the fetal hypothalamic-pituitary-thyroid axis. This can lead to central congenital hypothyroidism in the infant [42].

Thio-amide drugs

Women who are taking antithyroid medications and desire pregnancy should be counseled regarding the potential risks of the medication, the need for close monitoring during pregnancy, the risk of congenital central hypothyroidism from inadequately treated maternal disease, and the risk of fetal Graves' disease. Approximately 40–60% of women with Graves' disease who are treated with antithyroid medication will have long-term remission [43] and may not require treatment at the time of pregnancy. Those on therapy at the time of conception should know that both propylthio-uracil (PTU) and methimazole are equally effective. Some clinicians prefer PTU because it crosses the placenta less readily than methimazole [39,44,45]. There have been reports of congenital anomalies including aplasia cutis of the scalp and esophageal/choanal atresia with methimazole although a direct causal relationship has not been established [46,47]. If the mother with Graves' disease is taking antithyroid medication, fetal Graves' disease may not be apparent until after delivery. The neonate will clear the antithyroid medication before clearing the maternal antibodies. Such infants may be irritable and tachycardic, feed poorly and exhibit an inability to gain weight within 14 days of life. These are temporary conditions which will resolve as the infant clears the maternal antibodies but should be anticipated and treated to avoid serious sequelae.

Radio-ablative therapy

It has been recommended by the International Commission on Radiological Protection that women avoid pregnancy for a period of at least 6 months after radio-ablative therapy for safety reasons [48]. In general, however, women treated with radio-active iodine should probably be counseled to delay pregnancy for a year due to the high risk of permanent hypothyroidism requiring thyroid hormone replacement or the possibility that a second dose will be necessary due ineffective treatment [25]. There is no evidence of long-term consequences to fertility or obstetric outcomes in women who receive ^{131}I, but it is essential that thyroid function is stable prior to pregnancy [49,50]. Importantly, thyroid function tests in women who have been treated with radio-active iodine or surgery prior to pregnancy will no longer reflect their autoimmune status. Although they are now euthyroid or hypothyroid, antibody titers may remain elevated and cross the placenta. Such women should be counseled regarding the continued risk of fetal Graves' disease and the need for surveillance during the pregnancy.

Antenatal management

Women with gestational thyrotoxicosis do not require thio-amides since the natural course of the illness is to improve in the second trimester. Treatment with beta-blockers should be reserved for symptomatic relief of severe adrenergic symptoms until the free T4 levels are normalized. Women who are on thio-amides prior to pregnancy or those with newly diagnosed toxic nodules or Graves' disease should be continued or started on thio-amides during pregnancy. The dose of thio-amide is empirical. The usual starting dose of PTU is 50–100 mg three times a day and for methimazole 5–20 mg twice daily. Individuals with large goiters and markedly elevated T4 or T3 may require higher doses. The goal of treatment during pregnancy is to maintain free T4 in the upper normal range using the lowest possible dose of thio-amide. Thyroid studies should be repeated every 4 weeks. Dosage should be adjusted based on the free T4 levels as the TSH values will take several more weeks to increase and should not be used to adjust the dose. The dose should be reduced as the T4 level approaches normal. Due to the immunosuppressant effect of pregnancy the TSHRAb titer may decrease substantially during gestation. This may result in improvement in the clinical picture and even the ability to discontinue medication in the second or third trimester in many patients.

The most common side effect of thio-amides is rash. Transient leukopenia occurs in about 10% of pregnant women treated with thio-amides but usually does not require cessation of therapy. In approximately 0.2% of women, agranulocytosis develops suddenly and mandates discontinuation of the drug. Agranulocytosis is not dose related, and because of its acute onset, serial leukocyte counts during therapy have not been helpful in prevention. Therefore, women given thio-amide drugs should discontinue medication immediately if they develop a fever or sore throat until complete evaluation for agranulocytosis can be performed. Migratory arthritis and liver dysfunction may also occur, albeit rarely. Liver function tests should be monitored as clinically indicated. If the woman develops a significant adverse reaction to thio-amides, thyroidectomy must be considered. As suggested earlier, ^{131}I therapy is contraindicated during pregnancy due to the potential for fetal hypothyroidism.

Fetal monitoring

In most cases of maternal hyperthyroidism, the fetus remains euthyroid and does not require monitoring beyond that which is routine for pregnancy. Fetuses of women taking antithyroid drugs during the third trimester or those with a persistent TSHRAb have been shown to be at increased risk for development of a goiter [51]. Specifically, the fetus may develop Graves' disease caused by placental transfer of thyroid-stimulating immunoglobulins and may subsequently develop nonimmune hydrops or fetal demise [35,36]. Conversely, fetal exposure to maternally administered thio-amides may cause goitrous hypothyroidism. Current data, however, indicate that thio-amides carry an extremely small risk for causing hypothyroidism in the perinate [39,40]. Routine maternal antibody testing has been recommended only if the mother has previously undergone ^{131}I ablation or thyroidectomy [52].

Documentation of fetal heart rate at each obstetric visit (looking for fetal tachycardia) and serial ultrasounds every 2–4 weeks in the third trimester (looking for both growth and assessment of fetal thyroid size, although fetal goiter is not always readily demonstrable on routine obstetric ultrsounds) should be considered in all women with hyperthyroidism

but particularly in those taking thio-amide drugs or those with persistently high TSHRAb [9,51,53]. Some experts also recommend routine fetal blood sampling for thyroid indices if maternal thyroid-stimulating antibodies are abnormal or if there is evidence of fetal growth restriction, heart failure or goiter, with or without tachycardia [35]. Because fetal hyper- or hypothyroidism can cause hydrops, growth restriction, goiter or tachycardia, fetal blood sampling seems appropriate if any of these conditions develop and the diagnosis is not certain based on clinical grounds in women being treated for Graves' disease with thio-amides. The routine use of fetal blood sampling in all mothers being treated for hyperthyroidism is discouraged, however, because of an associated 1–2% risk of fetal loss.

Thyroid storm/congestive heart failure

Pregnancy is a potential precipitant of thyroid storm or heart failure, although both are extremely rare. Thyroid storm is a clinical diagnosis of an acute, severe, life-threatening exacerbation of thyrotoxicosis. The classic features are fever, tachycardia with atrial fibrillation, nausea/vomiting, agitation/delirium/coma and high-output cardiac failure. Jaundice and/or abdominal pain can also be present in severe cases. Thyroid storm is an indication for immediate admission, with cardiac monitoring in an intensive care unit. Treatment options include high doses of thio-amides (1 g PTU followed by 200 mg every 4 hours), iodide to inhibit thyroid hormone release (Lugol's solution 10 drops three times daily or SSKI five drops every 6 hours or the iodinated radiocontrast agents ipodate and iopanoic acid 0.5–1.0 g daily (not available in the US)) intravenous dexamethasone (2 mg every 6 hours for four doses) to further block peripheral conversion of T4 to T3, and use of beta-blockers to control tachycardia (one such protocol is propranolol 1 mg/min intravenously until several milligrams have been administered or adequate beta-blockade has been achieved, followed by oral or nasogastric tube administration at a dose of 60–80 mg every 4 hours) [54].

Labor and delivery

The obvious goal of management of maternal hyperthyroidism during pregnancy is to achieve the euthyroid state as soon as possible. As suggested above, uncontrolled thyrotoxicosis will increase the risk of pre-eclampsia and heart failure and may precipitate preterm labor and delivery. Treatment of symptomatic women with hyperthyroidism in labor includes antithyroid medications, beta-blockers if necessary, and supportive care. Simultaneous maternal and fetal thyrotoxicosis during labor is extremely rare [55]. If fetal thyrotoxicosis is suspected in labor, appropriate management includes aggressive treatment of maternal thyrotoxicosis and may include consideration of the best route of delivery if the fetus is identified with a large goiter. Elective cesarean delivery may be suitable to avoid dystocia from an extremely large fetal goiter and for management of the fetal airway.

The *ex utero* intrapartum treatment (EXIT) procedure was developed to manage airway obstruction after fetal surgery and its indications have expanded to include a variety of fetal anomalies including large fetal neck masses. It involves securing the neonatal airway (usually with endotracheal intubation often guided by laryngoscopy or bronchoscopy) while the umbilical cord and maternal-fetal circulation remain intact in the hopes of avoiding difficult emergency intubations in the delivery room. It is usually perfomed with cesarean deliveries but has been described with vaginal deliveries. Fetuses with neck masses large enough to cause airway obstruction are considered candidates for this procedure at centers with the required expertise. Such cases of fetal goiter, however, are rarely encountered.

Postpartum management

The majority of women (~70%) will have a postpartum relapse of their Graves' disease, usually within the first 3 months after delivery, as the natural immunosuppression of pregnancy disappears. Antithyroid therapy often needs to be reintroduced or increased during this time. Most women should have a TSH and free T4 performed approximately 6 weeks post partum. Both PTU and methimazole are excreted in breast milk but PTU is largely protein bound and does not seem to pose a significant risk to the breastfed infant. Methimazole has been found in breastfed infants of treated women in amounts sufficient to cause thyroid dysfunction. However, at low doses (10–20 mg/day) it does not appear to pose a major risk to the nursing infant [56]. The American Academy of Pediatrics considers both compatible with breast feeding [57]. It is not necessary to check infant thyroid indices unless an unusually large dose is being used for the mother. Women should be reminded of the importance of controlled T4 levels prior to the next pregnancy.

Hypothyroidism

Hypothyroidism complicates between 1 and 3 per 1000 pregnancies and may be defined by inadequate thyroid hormone production despite pituitary gland stimulation (primary) or insufficient stimulation of the thyroid by the pituitary or hypothalamus (central hypothyroidism). Women may enter pregnancy with either known hypothyroidism or could be diagnosed during pregnancy. In the developed world, autoimmune destruction of the thyroid gland (Hashimoto's thyroiditis) is the most common cause of hypothyroidism. Globally, however, iodine deficiency is the leading cause of hypothyroidism. As of 1999, approximately 30% of the world's population was estimated to be at risk for iodine

deficiency and 41 million babies would therefore be at risk for associated neurodevelopmental delay each year [58]. Also, based on the National Health and Nutrition Examination Survey (NHANES III) data set, there was a 50% decrease in urinary iodine concentrations in the United States from 1971–1974 to 1988–1994 such that approximately 15% of women of childbearing age are considered moderately iodine deficient compared to 5% in the 1970s [59]. This has lead to widespread interest in increasing iodine supplementation of prenatal vitamins. Other causes of hypothyroidism include radio-ablation of the thyroid for Graves' disease or thyroid nodule, thyroidectomy (partial or near complete for treatment of benign or malignant neoplasm, Graves' disease), and medications (e.g. lithium, amiodarone). Central hypothyroidism is rare in pregnancy.

Hypothyroidism is characterized by vague, nonspecific signs or symptoms that are often insidious in onset. These include fatigue, constipation, cold intolerance, weight gain, carpal tunnel syndrome, hair loss, voice changes, reduced memory, muscle cramps and dry skin. Women who report that any such symptoms have worsened over the previous year are more likely to have overt thyroid disease [60]. The presence or absence of a pathologically enlarged thyroid gland (i.e. goiter) depends on the etiology of hypothyroidism. Women in areas of endemic iodine deficiency or those with Hashimoto's thyroiditis are more likely to have a goiter.

Diagnosis during pregnancy

The diagnosis of clinical hypothyroidism during pregnancy is particularly difficult since many of the signs or symptoms listed above are also common to pregnancy. Additionally, the thyroid gland volume increases during pregnancy because of increased vascularity and pregnancy-induced glandular hyperplasia. This enlargement, though not pathologic, may prompt laboratory evaluation of thyroid function during pregnancy. Serum TSH is more sensitive than free T4 for detecting hypothyroidism and for following effectiveness of replacement therapy. If the TSH is abnormal, then evaluation of free T4 is recommended. This TSH-centered approach to diagnosis may identify women with either overt (elevated TSH and low free T4) or subclinical (elevated TSH, free T4 in normal reference range) hypothyroidism.

The reference range for serum TSH concentrations in nonpregnant individuals is 0.45–4.5 mU/L. However, recent data indicate that more than 95% of normal individuals have a TSH level below 2.5 mU/L and that those with a TSH between 2.5 and 4.5 mU/L have an increased risk of progression to overt disease [61]. This has led some to recommend a decrease in the upper limit of the TSH reference range to 2.5 mIU/L [62]. Others suggest that this change would only increase the diagnosis of subclinical hypothyroidism without clear evidence for a benefit from treatment [63]. Gestational age-specific TSH thresholds are available [3,64].

Also, a more pragmatic single upper TSH threshold of 3.0 mU/L has been validated for the first half of pregnancy [18]. Evaluation of free T4 levels during pregnancy has repeatedly shown that free T4 levels essentially remain in the reference range reported for nonpregnant adults [2,18].

The measurement of antithyroid antibodies (anti-TPO and antithyroglobulin) is generally not necessary in women with Hashimoto's thyroiditis. The presence of antithyroid antibodies may, however, identify a population of women at particular risk for pregnancy complications, postpartum thyroid dysfunction, and progression to symptomatic disease [65,66]. For example, one study revealed that 50% of women identified with TPO antibodies at 16 weeks gestation developed postpartum thyroid dysfunction and one in four of these women developed permanent overt hypothyroidism within 1 year [67]. An association between the risk of miscarriage and autoimmune thyroid disease has also been described [9,68].

Screening for thyroid disease

The majority of reviews and clinical practice guidelines recommend a case-finding approach rather than universal screening for thyroid disease in nonpregnant women less than 50 years of age [9,16,69,70]. High-risk women who should be screened prior to pregnancy include those with a personal history of thyroid disease (hyper- or hypothyroidism, postpartum thyroiditis), a strong family history, known autoimmune disease, presence of a goiter, previous therapeutic neck irradiation, and those taking medications known to cause thyroid disturbance. Reports published during the last decade have stimulated international controversy regarding identification and treatment of pregnant women with mild or subclinical hypothyroidism to improve neurodevelopment of the fetus. The issue of subclinical hypothyroidism remains unsettled but there is agreement among endocrinologists and obstetricians that large, well-designed randomized studies are necessary to identify the optimal approach to diagnosis and treatment of subclinical hypothyroidism in pregnancy and to determine efficacy. Until such studies are completed, aggressive case finding (thyroid function testing for women with symptoms or those at increased risk as defined above) rather than universal screening remains the recommended approach to diagnosis of thyroid disease during pregnancy. TSH testing for hypothyroidism should ideally be done prior to pregnancy because of the difficulties that can be encountered in interpreting thyroid function tests in early pregnancy. If TSH testing has not been done prior to pregnancy and testing for hypothyroidism is indicated, hypothyroidism can be confidently excluded with a normal or suppressed TSH level. However, the finding of a mildly suppressed TSH in the first trimester should be interpreted with caution as although it may represent hyperthyroidism, it most likely is secondary to the physiologic changes in TSH seen in the first trimester and discussed earlier.

Management

Similar to hyperthyroidism, the goal of therapy in pregnant women with hypothyroidism is to return thyroid hormone levels to within the reference range. Levothyroxine sodium is the treatment of choice. Most investigators had concluded that there is minimal transplacental passage of levothyroxine at physiologic serum concentrations because of placental de-iodinase activity. Despite this, it has been shown that a considerable proportion of fetal circulating thyroxine is maternal in origin [7,11]. Some researchers have hypothesized that the placenta produces thyroid hormone-binding proteins which may modify de-iodination and facilitate placental transport [72]. Nevertheless, improved maternal and fetal outcomes have been demonstrated in hypothyroid women adequately treated with exogenous thyroid hormones [73,74]. Management should include discussion of the importance of euthyroidism at the time of conception, risks of hypothyroidism to mother and offspring, and anticipation of medication changes during pregnancy.

Preconceptional counseling

The goal of treatment in women with overt hypothyroidism and considering pregnancy is clinical and biochemical euthyroidism at the time of conception. The majority of clinicians use TSH levels as an indication of adequate replacement and women should delay pregnancy until TSH is normal. Importantly, many women start a multivitamin containing iron or calcium prior to pregnancy. It is important that they do not take their levothyroxine and multivitamins at the same time since iron and calcium may interfere with absorption of thyroxine. As previously suggested, all women should have adequate iodine intake (200 µg/day). Many manufacturers of prenatal vitamins are now adding at least 150 µg of iodine to their preparations.

Pregnancy outcomes

Women with overt hypothyroidism are at increased risk for pregnancy complications such as early pregnancy failure, pre-eclampsia, placental abruption, low birthweight and stillbirth [13,75]. Overt maternal thyroid failure in the first half of pregnancy has also been associated with intellectual impairment in offspring [14,15]. It is less clear whether milder forms of thyroid dysfunction have similar effects on pregnancy and infant outcomes [16]. Treatment of women with overt hypothyroidism has been associated with improved pregnancy outcomes.

Levothyroxine sodium

Levothyroxine sodium is the most widely prescribed treatment for hypothyroidism and is available in a variety of dosages (25–300 µg). Administration of levothyroxine to pregnant women is regarded as safe for both mother and fetus. Some hypothyroid women may be treated with tri-iodothyronine (T3) or dessicated thyroid. It is best if they change to thyroxine (T4) replacement prior to conception since T3 does not cross the placenta.

Although treatment for thyroid dysfunction seems straightforward, only approximately 60% of patients taking thyroid medication for either hypothyroidism or hyperthyroidism are euthyroid according to TSH level [60]. Specifically, up to 25% of individuals on thyroxine therapy are overtreated [61]. Adverse reactions associated with levothyroxine therapy are therefore primarily related to overtreatment and may result in clinical manifestations of hyperthyroidism [76]. Importantly, the maternal implications of overtreatment are probably negligible when the TSH levels are between 0.1 and 0.5 mU/L. Conversely, in a study of infants born to women on thyroxine replacement for hypothyroidism, those infants with free T4 concentrations above the 95th percentile had smaller head circumference and lower birthweight [77]. Furthermore, in a study of cognitive development in children with congenital hypothyroidism, attention deficits and subtle motor problems were more common among infants with the highest free T4 concentration [78]. In the aggregate, these results imply a potential fetal effect of maternal overtreatment.

Other potential considerations in women treated with levothyroxine include transient hair loss during the first few weeks of hormone treatment and decreased bone mineral density. However, a 1994 meta-analysis of 13 studies found no significant evidence of bone loss in premenopausal women compared with controls [79]. Allergy to commonly prescribed thyroxine formulations has not been documented.

Antenatal management

A 2004 study demonstrated that 85% of hypothyroid pregnant women required an increase in thyroid hormone by an average of 47% by 16 weeks gestation [80]. These increased requirements begin as early as 5 weeks gestation and women with a previous thyroidectomy, history of radio-active iodine ablation or those undergoing assisted reproductive techniques like ovarian stimulation may develop significant hypothyroidism if no dose adjustment is made. For these women, proactive increases of 25% at confirmation of pregnancy should reduce the likelihood of significant hypothyroidism in the first trimester until a TSH can be obtained. Patients can be told to take a "double dose" of their levothyroxine on two days out of seven (e.g. Monday and Thursday) until they have a chance to reach their physician for testing and prescription of an appropriate new dose of thyroid replacement. All other women with hypothyroidism should undergo TSH testing at initiation of prenatal care.

A low normal TSH is the goal during pregnancy (<2.5 mU/mL). Importantly, during the first trimester, TSH may be physiologically suppressed and should not necessarily prompt a decrease in dose. Women who are newly diagnosed

during pregnancy should be initiated on 1.0–2.0 µg/kg/day or approximately 100 µg of levothyroxine daily. In otherwise healthy patients there is no need to titrate gradually up to this replacement dose. Thyroid-stimulating hormones should then be measured in 6 weeks and levothyroxine doses adjusted in 25 or 50 µg increments. Once normalized, a TSH should be checked every 6–8 weeks throughout pregnancy to insure adequate replacement. Assessment of free thyroxine levels may also be helpful when monitoring response to treatment and should be done at similar intervals as for TSH. In addition to iron supplements, several drugs can interfere with levothyroxine absorption (e.g. cholestyramine, aluminum hydroxide antacids) or its metabolism (e.g. phenytoin, carbamazepine, and rifampin).

Maternal/fetal monitoring

Maternal and fetal thyroid abnormalities are related. In both, thyroid function depends on adequate iodide intake. Iodine deficiency results in inadequate fetal thyroid hormone throughout gestation, resulting in significant neurodevelopmental delay, deafness, stunted growth and increased risk of neonatal mortality [58]. As previously suggested, pregnant women's iodine intake should be supplemented if necessary. Uncommonly, maternal TSH receptor-blocking antibodies can cross the placenta and also cause fetal thyroid dysfunction. However, the more common thyroid antibodies to thyroid peroxidase and thyroglobulin have little or no effect on fetal thyroid function even though they readily cross the placenta in the third trimester [81]. Therefore, maternal Hashimoto's thyroiditis is not typically associated with abnormalities of fetal thyroid function. Specifically, the prevalence of antibody-induced fetal hypothyroidism in women with Hashimoto's thyroiditis approximates 1 in 180,000 neonates. Cases of fetal hypothyroidism are not typically associated with fetal thyromegaly, so serial ultrasound evaluation of the fetal thyroid is unlikely to provide benefit [82].

Labor and delivery

Women with known hypothyroidism should be both clinically and biochemically euthyroid prior to labor. Obstetric complications include increased risk of stillbirth, preterm delivery, pre-eclampsia and placental abruption [13,64,83]. Mild hypothyroidism has also been associated with an increased risk of breech presentation and low birthweight [77,84]. Physicians caring for hypothyroid women in labor should be aware of the potential for these outcomes. Otherwise, labor and delivery management should routinely be directed by maternal and fetal condition.

Postpartum care

After delivery, levothyroxine therapy should be returned to the prepregnant dose and the TSH should be checked in 6–8 weeks. Breastfeeding is not contraindicated in women treated for hypothyroidism. Levothyroxine is excreted into breast milk but levels are too low to alter thyroid function in the infant or to interfere with neonatal thyroid screening programs [85]. Given that changing weight and age may modify thyroid function, annual monitoring with serum TSH concentration is generally recommended.

Subclinical hypothyroidism

Primarily, two clinical studies have demonstrated modest but significant changes in psychomotor and IQ testing among children exposed to even mild maternal hypothyroidism [86,87]. In one study, children born to women with free T4 levels below the 10th percentile were found to be at increased risk for impaired psychomotor development. Another study retrospectively evaluated children born to 48 untreated women with serum TSH values above the 98th percentile, and found that overall they had diminished school performance, reading recognition, and IQ scores. Importantly, women in the first study had normal TSH levels and women in the second study had low mean serum free thyroxine levels and thus likely had overt hypothyroidism. Taken together, studies of these two different maternal conditions have been interpreted to mean that children born to women with subclinical hypothyroidism are at risk for impaired neurodevelopment.

Pregnancy outcomes have also been evaluated in women with subclinical hypothyroidism and are better than those with clinically overt disease. In a study of over 17,000 women screened prior to mid-pregnancy, 2.3% were found to have subclinical hypothyroidism. These women had significantly higher incidences of preterm birth, placental abruption, and admission of infants to the intensive care nursery [64]. Other studies have also found associations between mild hypothyroidism, variously defined, and untoward pregnancy outcomes such as stillbirth and low birthweight [77,83].

These findings have led many experts to call for routine screening of pregnant women for subclinical or asymptomatic hypothyroidism. Unfortunately, there are currently no large, randomized treatment trials to determine any risks or benefits of detecting and treating subclinical hypothyroidism. Thus widespread prenatal screening for maternal thyroid disorders is not justifiable at this time. There are several ongoing large trials evaluating these issues. For now, recommendations for routine prenatal thyroid screening are premature and treatment of subclinical hypothyroidism should be considered experimental. Perhaps the most important message of these trials at this time is to heighten our awareness of the probable importance of adequate thyroid replacement in pregnancy for patients already being treated for overt hypothyroidism.

Postpartum thyroiditis

Postpartum thyroiditis (PPT) is caused by a rebound in thyroid autoimmunity after delivery, leading to lymphocytic infiltration of the thyroid gland and transient changes in thyroid function. It has important short- and long-term implications for the mother. The likelihood of developing postpartum thyroiditis antedates pregnancy and is related to serum levels of thyroid autoantibodies. Anti-TPO antibodies which detect the main antigen of the thyroid microsomal fraction are present in >90% of women with PPT and are the most useful marker for prediction of the occurrence of postpartum thyroid dysfunction [21]. Women with high antibody titers in early pregnancy are most commonly affected, having a 40–50% chance of developing PPT [88]. Women with type 1 diabetes have a significantly higher incidence, ranging from 18% to 25% due to the high prevalence of TPO antibodies [89,90].

There are two recognized clinical phases of postpartum thyroiditis. The autoimmune destruction of the gland first results in release of stored thyroid hormone into the circulation. This hyperthyroid phase generally occurs between 1 and 4 months after delivery and is self-limiting to 1–2 months. The onset is abrupt, with symptoms of fatigue and palpitations being the most common. A small, painless goiter may be present. Often this phase goes undetected as it may be attributed to the normal postpartum changes. Occasionally these symptoms can be severe enough to interfere with the mother's functioning due to sleep deprivation, nervousness/irritability or palpitations and require treatment with beta-blockers until resolution of the hyperthyroid phase. Antithyroid medications are not beneficial. The hyperthyroid phase must be distinguished from postpartum Graves' disease by an I[123] uptake and scan (low or normal uptake in PPT compared to a diffusely increased uptake consistent with Graves'). However, this requires interruption of the woman's breastfeeding and care of the infant. If the patient is not severely thyrotoxic, repeating the thyroid function tests in 4 weeks will usually help differentiate the two types of thyroid dysfunction. In Graves' disease, hyperthyroidism will persist, whereas in PPT the hyperthyroid phase will spontaneously resolve.

The loss of functioning thyrocytes from the immune destruction results in a hypothyroid phase between 3 and 8 months postpartum (usually at 6 months). Approximately 40–50% of women diagnosed with PPT will experience hypothyroid symptoms alone without the hyperthyroid phase [91–93]. The hypothyroid phase usually lasts much longer (4–6 months) than the hyperthyroid phase. Any woman who presents with hypothyroidism in the first year post partum should not be labeled as having permanent hypothyroidism. This disorder is often unrecognized because women typically present with nonspecific symptoms including fatigue, weight gain, loss of concentration, and possibly depression, which is erroneously ascribed to maternal stresses due to newborn demands.

Although the association of postpartum depression with PPT has not consistently been demonstrated [94–96], women with postpartum depression should be evaluated for hypothyroidism and women with PPT should be carefully questioned about depressive symptoms and treated appropriately. The hypothyroid phase should be treated in women who are symptomatic and in those planning a pregnancy in the near future. It is usually recommended to treat women for ~6 months and then withdraw thyroid hormone, unless pregnancy is being attempted. A TSH should be rechecked in 5–6 weeks after withdrawal of thyroid hormone to be sure there is no permanent hypothyroidism. Patients identified with PPT should be screened regularly since 20–50% of women will develop permanent hypothyroidism within 2–10 years [93,97]. A TSH level should be done annually and prior to conception.

References

1. Burrow GN. Thyroid function and hyperfunction during gestation. Endocrine Rev 1993;14:194–202.
2. Glinoer D, Denayer PH, Lejeune B, et al. Serum levels of intact human chorionic gonadotropin (HCG) and its free alpha and beta subunits in relation to maternal thyroid stimulation during normal pregnancy. J Endocrinol Invest 1993;16:881.
3. Dashe JS, Casey BM, Wells CE, McIntire DD, Byrd EW, Leveno KJ, et al. Thyroid-stimulating hormone in singleton and twin pregnancy: importance of gestational age-specific reference ranges. Obstet Gynecol 2005;106:753–7.
4. Panesar NS, Li CY, Rogers MS. Reference intervals for thyroid hormones in pregnant Chinese women. Ann Clin Biochem 2001;38:329–32.
5. Fantz CR, Dagogo-Jack S, Ladenson JH, Gronswki AM. Thyroid function during pregnancy. Clin Chem 1999;42:2250–8.
6. Sapin R, d'Herbomez M, Schliegner JL. Free thyroxine measured with equilibrium dialysis and nine immunoassays decreases in late pregnancy. Clin Lab 2004;50:581–4.
7. Soldin OP, Tractenberg RE, Hollowell JG, Jonklaas J, Janicic N, Soldin SJ. Trimester-specific changes in maternal thyroid hormone, thyrotropin, and thyroglobulin concentrations during gestation: trends and associations across trimesters in iodine sufficiency. Thyroid 2004;14:1084–90.
8. Demers LM, Spencer CA. Laboratory support for the diagnosis and monitoring of thyroid disease. Laboratory Medicine Practice Guidelines. National Academy of Clinical Biochemistry, Washington, DC, 2002.
9. Abolovich M, Amino N, Barbour La, et al. Management of thyroid dysfunction during pregnancy and postpartum: an Endocrine Society Clinical Practice Guideline. J Clin Endocrinol Metab 2007;92(8 suppl):S1–47.
10. Thorpe-Beeston JG, Nicolaides KH, McGregor AM. Fetal thyroid function. Thyroid 1992;2(3):207–17.
11. Morreale de Escobar G, Obregon MJ, Escobar del Rey F. Is neuropsychological development related to maternal hypothyroidism or to maternal hypothyroxinemia? J Clin Endocrinol Metab 2000;85:3975–87.
12. Davis LE, Leveno KJ, Cunningham FG. Hypothyroidism complicating pregnancy. Obstet Gynecol 1988;72(1):108–12.
13. Leung AS, Millar LK, Koonings PP, Montoro M, Mestman JH. Perinatal outcome in hypothyroid pregnancies. Obstet Gynecol 1993;81(3):349–53.
14. Cao XY, Jiang XM, Dou ZH, Rakeman MA, Zhang ML, O'Donnell K. Timing of vulnerability of the brain to iodine deficiency in endemic cretinism. N Engl J Med 1994;331(26):1739–44.
15. Delange F, de Benoist B, Pretell E, Dunn JT. Iodine deficiency in the world: where do we stand at the turn of the century? Thyroid 2001;11(5):437–47.
16. Surks MI, Ortiz E, Daniels GH, et al. Subclinical thyroid disease. Scientific review and guidelines for diagnosis and management. JAMA 2004:291:228–38.
17. Hollowell JG, Staehling NW, Flanders WD, et al. Serum TSH, T4 and thyroid antibodies in the United States population (1988 to 1994): National Health and Nutrition Examination Survery (NHANES III). J Clin Endocrinol Metab 2002:87:489–99.
18. Casey BM, Dashe JS, Spong CY, McIntire DD, Leveno KJ, Cunningham GF. Perinatal significance of isolated maternal hypothyroxinemia identified in the first half of pregnancy. Obstet Gynecol 2007;109:1129–35.
19. Stagnaro-Green A, Glinoer D. Thyroid autoimmunity and the risk of miscarriage. Thyroid and pregnancy. Best Pract Res Clin Endocrinol Metab 2004:18:167–81.
20. Davies TF, Roti E, Braverman LE, Degroot LJ. Therapeutic controversy. Thyroid controversy-stimulating antibodies. J Clin Endocrinol Metab 1998;83:377–85.
21. Muller AF, Drexhage HA, Berghout A. Postpartum thyroiditis and autoimmune thyroiditis in women of childbearing age: recent insights and consequences for antenatal and postnatal care. Endocrine Rev 2001;22(5):605–30.
22. Lazarus JH, Kokandi A. Thyroid disease in relation to pregnancy: a decade of change. Clin Endocrinol 2000;53:265–78.
23. Mestman JH, Goodwin TM, Montoro MM. Thyroid disorders of pregnancy. Endocrinol Metab Clin North Am 1995;24(1):41–71.
24. Weetman AP. Graves' disease. N Engl J Med 2000;343:1236–47.
25. Cooper DS. Hyperthyroidism. Lancet 2003;363:459–68.
26. Sheffield JS, Cunningham FG. Thyrotoxicosis and heart failure that complicate pregnancy. Am J Obstet Gynecol 2004;190(1):211–17.
27. Casey BM, Dashe JS, Wells CE, McIntire DD, Leveno KJ, Cunningham FG. Subclinical hyperthyrodism and pregnancy outcomes. Obstet Gynecol 2006:107:337–41.
28. Woeber KA. Observations concerning the natural history of subclinical hyperthyroidism. Thyroid 2005;15(7):687–91.
29. Perelman AH, Clemons RD. The fetus in maternal hyperthyroidism. Thyroid 1992;2(3):225–8.
30. Tan JY, Loh KC, Yeo GS, Chee YC. Transient hyperthyroidism of hyperemesis gravidarum. Br J Obstet Gynaecol 2002;109:683–8.
31. Laurberg P, Nygaard B, Glinoer D, Grussendorf M, Orgiazzi J. Guidelines for TSH-receptor antibody measurements in pregnancy: results of an evidence-based symposium organized by the European Thyroid Association. Eur J Endocrinol 1998:139:584–6.
32. Miller LK, Wing Da, Leung AS, Kooonings PP, Montoro MN, Mestman JH. Low birth weight and preeclampsia in pregnancies complicated by hyperthyroidism. Obstet Gynecol 1994;84(6):946–9.
33. Anselmo J, Cao D, Karrison T, Weiss RE, Refetoff S. Fetal loss associated with excess thyroid hormone exposure. JAMA 2004;292:691–5.
34. Davis LE, Lucas MJ, Hankins GD, Roark ML, Cunningham FG. Thyrotoxicosis complicating pregnancy. Am J Obstet Gynecol 1989;160(1):63–70.
35. Nachum Z, Rakover Y, Weiner E, Shaley E. Graves' disease in pregnancy: prospective evaluation of a selective invasive treatment protocol. Am J Obstet Gynecol 2003;189(1):159–65.
36. Stulberg RA, Davies GA. Maternal thyrotoxicosis and fetal nonimune hydrops. Obstet Gynecol 2000;95:1036.
37. Zimmerman D. Fetal and neonatal hyperthyroidism. Thyroid 1999;9(7):727–33.

38. Peleg D, Cada S, Peleg A, Ben-Ami M. The relationship between maternal serum thyroid-stimulating immunoglobulin and fetal and neonatal thyrotoxicosis. Obstet Gynecol 2002;99:1040–3.

39. Momotani N, Noh JY, Ishikawa N, Ito K. Effects of propylthiouracil and methimazole on fetal thyroid status in mothers with Graves' hyperthyroidism. J Clin Endocrinol Metab 1997;82:3633–6.

40. O'Doherty MJ, McElhatton PR, Thomas SH. Treating thyrotoxicosis in pregnant or potentially pregnant women. BMJ 1999;318:5–6.

41. Mestman JH. Hyperthyroidism in pregnancy. Endocrinol Metab Clin North Am 1998;27:127–49.

42. Kempers MJE, van Tijn DA, van Trotsenburg ASP, de Vijlder JJM, Wiedijk BM, Vulsma T. Central congenital hypothyroidism due to gestational hyperthyroidism: detection where prevention failed. J Clin Endocrinol Metab 2003;88:5851–7.

43. Abraham P, Avenell A, Watson WA, Park CM, Bevan JS. Antithyroid drug regimen for treating Graves' hyperthyroidism. Cochrance Database of Systematic Reviews, 2005;4;CD003420.

44. Wing DA, Millar LK, Koonings PP, Montoro MN, Mestman JH. A comparison of propylthiouracil versus methimazole in the treatment of hyperthyroidism in pregnancy. Am J Obstet Gynecol 1994;170:90–5.

45. Diav-Citrin O, Ornoy A. Teratogen update: antithyroid drugs – methimazole, carbimazole, and propylthiouracil. Teratology 2002;65:38–44.

46. Mandel SJ, Cooper DS. The use of antithryoid drugs in pregnancy and lactation. J Clin Endocrinol Metab 2001;86:2354–9.

47. Mestman JH. Hyperthyroidism in pregnancy. Best Pract Res Clin Endocrinol Metab 2004;18:267–88.

48. International Commission on Radiological Protection. Release of nuclear medicine patients after therapy with unsealed sources. Ann ICRP 2004;34(2):1–79.

49. Read CH, Tansy MJ, Menda Y. A 36-year retrospective analysis of the efficacy and safety of radio-active iodine in treating young Graves' patients. J Clin Endocrinol Metab 2004;89:4229–33.

50. Chow SM, Yau S, Lee SH, Leung WM, Law SC. Pregnancy outcome after diagnosis of differentiated thyroid carcinoma: no deleterious effect after radio-active iodine treatment. Int J Radiat Oncol Biol Phys 2004;59:992–1000.

51. Luton D, Le Gac I, Vuillard E, et al. Management of Graves' disease during pregnancy: the key role of fetal thyroid gland monitoring .J Clin Endocrinol Metab 2005;90:6093–8.

52. Kilpatrick S. Umbilical blood sampling in women with thyroid disease in pregnancy: is it necessary? Am J Obstet Gynecol 2003;189:1–2.

53. Cohen O, Pinhas-Hamiel O, Sivan E, Dolitski M, Lipitz S, Achiron R. Serial in utero ultrasonographic measurements of the fetal thyroid: a new complementary tool in the management of maternal hyperthyroidism in pregnancy. Prenat Diagn 2003;23:740–2.

54. Casey BM, Leveno KJ. Thyroid disease in pregnancy. Obstet Gynecol 2006;108:1283–9.

55. Bowman ML, Bergmann M, Smith JF. Intrapartum labetalol for the treatment of maternal and fetal thyrotoxicosis. Thyroid 1998;8(9):795–6.

56. Cooper DS. Antithyroid drugs: to breast feed or not to breast feed. Am J Obstet Gynecol 1987;157:234–5.

57. Committee on Drugs American Academy of Pediatrics. Transfer of drugs and other chemicals into human milk. American Academy of Pediatrics. Pediatrics 2001;108:776–89.

58. Dunn JT, Delange F. Damaged reproduction: the most important consequences of iodine deficiency. J Clin Endocrinol Metab 2001;86:2360–3.

59. Hollowell JG, Staehling NW, Hannon WH, et al. Iodine nutrition in the United States. Trends and public health implications: iodine excretion data from National Health and Nutrition Examination Surveys I and III (1971–1974 and 1988–1994). J Clin Endocrinol Metab 1998;83:3401–8.

60. Canaris GJ, Manowitz NR, Mayor G, Ridgway EC. The Colorado Thyroid Disease Prevalence Study. Arch Intern Med 2000;160(4):526–34.

61. Vanderpump MPJ, Tunbridge WMG, French JM, et al. The incidence of thyroid disorders in the community – a 20-year follow-up of the Whickham Survey. Clin Endocrinol 1995; 43:55–68.

62. Wartofsky L, Dickey RA. The evidence for a narrower thyrotropin reference range is compelling. J Clin Endocrinol Metab 2005;90:5483–8.

63. Surks MI, Gayotri G, Daniels GH. The thyrotropin reference range should remain unchanged. J Clin Endocrinol Metab 2005;90:5489–96.

64. Casey BM, Dashe JS, Wells CE, et al. Subclinical hypothyroidism and pregnancy outcomes. Obstet Gynecol 2005;105:239–45.

65. Stagnaro-Green A, Roman SH, Cobin RH, El Harazy E, Alvarez-Marfany M, Davies TF. Detection of at risk pregnancy by means of highly sensitive assays for thyroid autoantibodies. JAMA 1990;264:1422–5.

66. Glinoer D, Soto MF, Bourdoux P, et al. Pregnancy in patients with mild thyroid abnormalities – maternal and neonatal repercussions. J Clin Endocrinol Metab 1991;73:421–7.

67. Premawardhana LDKE, Parkes AB, Ammari R, Darke JC, Adams H, Lazarus JH. Postpartum thyroiditis and long-term thyroid status: prognostic influence of thyroid peroxidase antibodies and ultrasound echogenicity. J Clin Endocrinol Metab 2000;85:71–5.

68. Prummel MF, Wiersinga WM. Thyroid autoimmunity and miscarriage. Eur J Endocrinol 2004;150:751–5.

69. Helfand M. Screening for subclinical thyroid dysfunction in nonpregnant adults: a summary of the evidence for the U.S. Preventive Services Task Force. Ann Intern Med 2004;140:128–41.

70. Baskin HJ. American Association of Clinical Endocrinologists medical guidelines for clinical practice for the evaluation and treatment of hyperthyroidism and hypothyroidism. Endocrine Pract 2002;8:457–69.

71. Vulsma T, Gons MH, de Vijlder JJ. Maternal-fetal transfer of thyroxine in congenital hypothyroidism due to a total organification defect or thyroid agenesis. N Engl J Med 1989;321:13–16.

72. McKinnon B, Li H, Richard K, Mortimer R. Synthesis of thyroid hormone binding proteins transthyretin and albumin by human trophoblast. J Clin Endocrinol Metab 2005;90(12):6714–20.

73. La Franchi SH, Haddow JE, Hollowell JG. Is thyroid inadequacy during gestation a risk factor for adverse pregnancy and developmental outcomes? Thyroid 2005;15(1):60–71.

74. Matalon S, Sheiner E, Levy A, Mazor M, Wiznitzer A. Relationship of treated maternal hypothyroidism and perinatal outcome. J Reprod Med 2006;51:59–63.

75. Abalovich M, Gutierrez S, Alcaraz G, Maccallini G, Garcia A, Levalle O. Overt and subclinical hypothyroidism complicating pregnancy. Thyroid 2002;12:63–8.

76. Toft AD. Thyroxine therapy. N Engl J Med 1994; 331(3):174–80.

77. Blazer S, Moreh-Waterman Y, Miller-Lotan R, Tamir A, Hochberg Z. Maternal hypothyroidism may affect fetal growth and neonatal thyroid function. Obstet Gynecol 2003;102:232–41.

78. Rovet J, Alvarez M. Thyroid hormone and attention in school-age children with congenital hypothyroidism. J Child Psychol Psychiatry 1996;37(5):579–85.

79. Faber J, Galloe AM. Changes in bone mass during prolonged subclinical hyperthyroidism due to L-thyroxine treatment: a meta-analysis. Eur J Endocrinol 1994;130(4):350–6.

80. Alexander EK, Marquesee E, Lawrence J, Jarolim P, Fischer GA, Laresen PR. Timing and magnitude of increases in levothyroxine requirements during pregnancy in women with hypothyroidism. N Engl J Med 2004;351:241–9.

81. Fisher DA. Fetal thyroid function: diagnosis and management of fetal thyroid disorders. Clin Obstet Gynecol 1997;40(1):16–31.

82. Brown RS, Bellisario RL, Botero D, et al. Incidence of transient congenital hypothyroidism due to maternal thyrotropin receptor-blocking antibodies in over one million babies. J Clin Endocrinol Metab 1996;81:1147–51.

83. Allan WC, Haddo JE, Palomaki GE, et al. Maternal thyroid deficiency and pregnancy complications: implications for population screening. J Med Screen 2000;7:127–30.

84. Pop VJ, Brouwers EP, Wijnen H, Oei G, Essed GG, Vader HL. Low concentrations of maternal thyroxin during early gestation: a risk factor of breech presentation? Br J Obstet Gynaecol 2004;111:925–30.

85. Franklin R, Ogrady C, Carpenter L. Neonatal thyroid function – comparison between breast-fed and bottle-fed infants. J Pediatr 1985;106:124–6.

86. Haddow JE, Palomaki GE, Allan WC, et al. Maternal thyroid deficiency during pregnancy and subsequent neuropsychological development of the child. N Engl J Med 1999;341:549–55.

87. Pop V, Kuipens JL, van Baar Al, et al. Low maternal free T4 concentrations during early pregnancy are associated with impaired psychomotor development in infancy. Clin Endocrinol (Oxf) 1999;50:149–55.

88. Pearce EN, Farwell AP, Braverman LE. Current concepts: thyroiditis. N Engl J Med 2003;348:2646–55.

89. McCanlies E, O'Leary LA, Foley TP, et al. Hashimoto's thyroiditis and insulin-dependent diabetes mellitus: differences among individuals with and without abnormal thyroid function. J Clin Endocrinol Metab 1998;83:1548–51.

90. Gerstein HC. Incidence of postpartum thyroid dysfunction in patients with type 1 diabetes mellitus. Ann Intern Med 1993;118(6):1993.

91. Stagnaro-Green A. Postpartum thyroiditis. Best Pract Res Clin Endocrinol Metab 2004;18(2):303–16.

92. Terry AJ , Hague WM. Postpartum thyroiditis. Semin Perinatol 1998;22(6):497–502.

93. Lucas A, Pizarro E, Granada ML, Salinas I, Foz M, Sanmarti A. Postpartum thyroiditis: epidemiology and clinical evolution in a nonselected population. Thyroid 2000;10(1):71–7.

94. Pop VJ, deRooy HA, Vader HL, van der Heide D, van Son MM, Komproe IH. Microsomal antibodies during gestation in relation to postpartum thyroid dysfunction and depression. Acta Endocrinol 1993;129(1):26–30.

95. Harris B, Othman S, Davies JA, et al. Association of postpartum thyroid dysfunction and thyroid antibodies and depression. BMJ 1992;305(6846):152–6.

96. Kuijpens JL, Vader HL, Drexhage HA, Wiersinga W, van Son MJ, Pop VJ. Thyroid peroxidase antibodies during gestation are a marker for subsequent depression postpartum. Eur J Endocrinol 2001;145(5):579–84.

97. Othman S, Phillips DIW, Parkes AB, et al. A long-term follow-up of postpartum thyroiditis. Clin Endocrinol 1990;32:559–64.

13 Pituitary and adrenal disease in pregnancy

Mark E. Molitch[1] *and Alan Peaceman*[2]

[1]Division of Endocrinology, Metabolism and Molecular Medicine, Northwestern University Feinberg School of Medicine, Chicago, IL USA
[2]Division of Maternal-Fetal Medicine, Department of Obstetrics and Gynecology, Northwestern University Feinberg School of Medicine, Chicago, IL, USA

Anterior pituitary

Anterior pituitary hormone changes in pregnancy

During pregnancy, the normal pituitary gland enlarges considerably, due to the estrogen-stimulated lactotroph hyperplasia [1,2], Prolactin (PRL) levels rise gradually throughout gestation, preparing the breast for lactation [3]. Thus, the finding of hyperprolactinemia in a woman with amenorrhea could well be due to pregnancy and not to pathologic hyperprolactinemia. This lactotroph hyperplasia results in an increase in overall pituitary size as seen on magnetic resonance imaging (MRI) scans, with the peak size occurring in the first few days post partum when gland heights up to 12 mm may be seen [4,6]. Following delivery, there is a rapid involution of the hyperplasia, so that normal pituitary size is found by 6 months post partum (5,6). This stimulatory effect of pregnancy on lactotrophs has important implications for the patient with a prolactinoma who desires pregnancy.

Beginning in the second half of pregnancy, circulating levels of a growth hormone (GH) variant made by the syncytiotrophoblastic epithelium of the placenta increase and pituitary GH secretion decreases [7,8]. The decreased production of normal pituitary GH is likely due to negative feedback effects of insulin-like growth factor 1 (IGF-1), which is stimulated by the placentally produced GH variant [7,8]. In patients with acromegaly who have autonomous GH secretion and become pregnant, both forms of GH persist in the blood [9].

Cortisol levels rise progressively over the course of gestation, resulting in a two- to threefold increase by term [10]. Most of this elevation is due to the estrogen-induced increase in cortisol-binding globulin (CBG) levels [11]. However, the cortisol production rate is increased, resulting in a threefold increase

in the bio-active "free" fraction, urinary free cortisol levels and salivary cortisol levels [10,11]. Adrenocorticotropic hormone (ACTH) levels have been variously reported as being normal, suppressed or elevated early in gestation [10,12]. However, later in the pregnancy, there is a progressive rise, followed by a final surge of ACTH and cortisol levels during labor [10]. ACTH does not cross the placenta but it is also manufactured by the placenta [12]. The amounts of ACTH in maternal serum that are of placental as compared to pituitary origin at various stages of gestation are not known. Corticotropin-releasing hormone (CRH) is also produced by the placenta and is released into maternal plasma [13]. The CRH is bio-active and may release ACTH both from the placenta, in a paracrine fashion, and from the maternal pituitary [13,14]. The role of placental CRH in regulating ACTH and cortisol secretion during pregnancy in humans is still unclear but it may be driving the marked increase in ACTH and cortisol in the third trimester [14].

Thyroid stimulating hormone (TSH) levels fall in the first trimester, in response to the rise in thyroid hormone levels which are stimulated by human chorionic gonadotropin (HCG), but then return to the normal range by the third trimester [15]. In response to placental sex steroid production, both hypothalamic gonadotropin-releasing hormone (GnRH) and pituitary gonadotropin (follicle-stimulating hormone (FSH)/luteinizing hormone (LH)) levels decline in the first trimester of pregnancy, with a blunted gonadotropin response to GnRH [16].

Pituitary tumors

Pituitary adenomas are quite common in women, comprising nearly 6% of intracranial (malignant and nonmalignant) neoplasms [17]. They may cause problems because of oversecretion of hormones by the tumor as well as by causing hypopituitarism, thereby affecting fertility and pregnancy outcome if pregnancy does ensue. In addition, the pregnancy itself alters hormone secretion and pituitary function, complicating the evaluation of patients with pituitary neoplasms. The influence on various

de Swiet's Medical Disorders in Obstetric Practice, 5th edition.
Edited by R. O. Powrie, M. F. Greene, W. Camann. © 2010 Blackwell Publishing.

types of therapy on the developing fetus also affects therapeutic decision making.

Prolactinoma

Hyperprolactinemia is responsible for about one-third of all cases of female infertility [18]. Hyperprolactinemia impairs the hypothalamic–pituitary–ovarian axis at several levels, the primary site of inhibition being at the hypothalamus where it inhibits the pulsatile secretion of GnRH [19]. The differential diagnosis of hyperprolactinemia is extensive [19,20] but this discussion will focus on the patient with a prolactinoma.

For patients with prolactinomas, the choice of therapy may have important consequences for decisions regarding pregnancy. Transsphenoidal surgery is curative in 50–60% of cases and rarely causes hypopituitarism when it is performed on women with microadenomas (tumors <10 mm in diameter). For patients with macroadenomas (tumors ≥10 mm in diameter), surgery cures a much smaller number with a considerably greater risk of causing hypopituitarism, and may therefore affect fertility [21].

Dopamine agonists, including bromocriptine, pergolide (approved for the treatment of Parkinson's disease but not hyperprolactinemia in the US), quinagolide (not approved in the US)

and cabergoline, have become the primary mode of therapy for virtually all patients with prolactinomas [20,21]. Bromocriptine, pergolide and quinagolide can restore ovulatory menses in 70–80% of women and cabergoline can do so in over 90% [20–22].Once ovulatory menses have been established, mechanical contraception is advised until the first two or three cycles have occurred, so that a woman will know when she has missed a menstrual period and the drug can be discontinued after confirmation with a pregnancy test. In this way, these drugs will have been given for only about 3–4 weeks of the gestation. However, because of its long half-life in the body, cabergoline cessation at that point will result in fetal exposure for an additional week or more.

In addition to their efficacy in lowering PRL levels, dopamine agonists often reduce tumor size of PRL-secreting macroadenomas, bromocriptine reducing the size by ≥50% in 50–75% of patients [21,23] and cabergoline achieving such reductions in over 90% of patients in some series [21,24,25].

Effects of pregnancy on prolactinoma growth

The stimulatory effect of the hormonal milieu of pregnancy may result in significant prolactinoma enlargement during gestation (Figure 13.1). Tumor enlargement may also occur

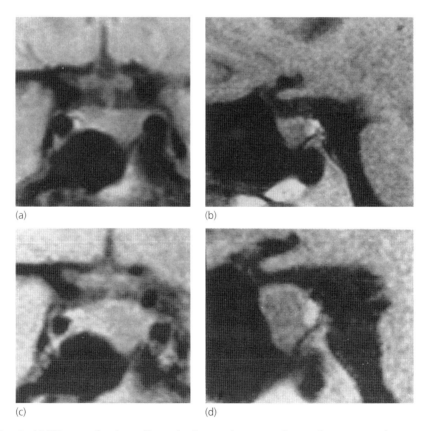

(a) (b) (c) (d)

Figure 13.1 Coronal and sagittal MRI scans of an intrasellar prolactin-secreting macroadenoma in a woman prior to conception (*above*) and at 7 months of gestation (*below*). Note the marked tumor enlargement at the latter point, at which time the patient was complaining of headaches. Reproduced with permission from Molitch ME. Medical treatment of prolactinomas. Endocrinol Metab Clin North Am 1999;28:143–70.

Table 13.1 Effect of pregnancy on prolactinomas

Tumor type	Prior therapy of patients	Number enlargement*	Symptomatic
Microadenomas	None	457	12 (2.6%)
Macroadenomas	None	142	45 (31.7%)
Macroadenomas	Yes	140	7 (5%)

Adapted from Gillam et al. [21].

Table 13.2 Effect of bromocriptine on pregnancies

	Bromocriptine		Normal population
	n	%	%
Pregnancies	6239	100.0	100.0
spontaneous abortion	620	9.9	10–15
terminations	75	1.2	
ectopic	31	0.5	0.5–1.0
hydatidiform moles	11	0.2	0.05–0.7
Deliveries (known duration)	4139	100.0	100.0
at term (>38 weeks)	3620	87.5	85
preterm (<38 weeks)	519	12.5	15
Deliveries (known outcome)	5120	100.0	100.0
single births	5031	9.3	8.7
multiple births	89	1.7	1.3
Babies (known details)	5213	100.0	100.0
normal	5030	96.5	95.0
with major malformations	93	1.8	3–4
with perinatal disorders	90	1.7	>2

*Data from Krupp et al. [33].

because the dopamine agonist that had caused the tumor to shrink has now been discontinued. Data have been compiled from five studies that analyzed the risk of symptomatic tumor enlargement in pregnant women with prolactinomas, divided according to tumor size [26–30] (Table 13.1). For women with microadenomas, only 12 of 457 pregnancies (2.6%) were complicated by symptoms of tumor enlargement (headaches and/or visual disturbances). Surgical intervention was not required in a single case and medical therapy with reinstitution of bromocriptine resolved the symptoms in the five in whom it was tried. In 45 of 142 pregnancies (31%) in women who have not undergone prior surgery or radiotherapy for their macroprolactinomas, there were similar symptoms of tumor enlargement. Of these 45, surgical intervention was undertaken in 12 and medical therapy in 17, leading to resolution of their symptoms. One hundred and forty women with macroadenomas have been identified who have undergone surgery or radiation prior to pregnancy; their risk of tumor enlargement was low (5%). If tumor enlargement occurs, reinstitution of bromocriptine or cabergoline usually is successful in reducing the size of the tumor, but transsphenoidal surgery may be necessary [20,21,31].

Effects of hyperprolactinemia and its treatment on pregnancy

Bromocriptine crosses the placenta [32]. When taken for only the first few weeks of gestation, it has not been associated with any increase in spontaneous abortions, ectopic pregnancies, trophoblastic disease, multiple pregnancies, congenital malformations or perinatal abnormalities (Table 13.2) [33,34]. Long-term follow-up studies of 64 children between the ages of 6 months and 9 years whose mothers took bromocriptine in this fashion have shown no ill effects [35]. Experience is limited to only just over 100 women, however, with the use of bromocriptine throughout gestation, but no abnormalities were noted in the infants, except one with an undescended testicle and one with a talipes deformity [36]. Pergolide has been shown to cross the placenta in mice [37] and limited data suggest that there is an unacceptable risk of congenital malformations [38,39]. Some early publications reported no detrimental effects on pregnancy or fetal development in women who became pregnant during treatment with quinagolide [40]. However, a review of 176 pregnancies reported 24 spontaneous abortions, one ectopic pregnancy, one stillbirth and nine fetal malformations [41].

Therefore, we do not recommend that pergolide or quinagolide be used if pregnancy is desired. In the US, pergolide has recently been withdrawn from use because of its association with cardiac valvular abnormalities.

Cabergoline has been shown to cross the placenta in animal studies, but such data are lacking in humans. Data on exposure of the fetus during the first several weeks of pregnancy have been reported in just over 350 cases and such use has not shown an increased percentage of spontaneous abortion, premature delivery, multiple pregnancy or congenital abnormalities [42–46]. Available data from 107 children whose mothers had taken cabergoline in the first few weeks of gestation and who were followed for 1–72 months showed normal physical and mental development [42].

In conclusion, with respect to using a dopamine agonist to facilitate ovulation and fertility, bromocriptine has the largest safety database and has a proven safety record for pregnancy. Although the database for cabergoline use in pregnancy is much smaller, it does not appear that cabergoline exerts any deleterious effects on pregnant women and the incidence of malformation in their offspring is not greater than in the general population. The safety databases for pergolide and quinagolide are quite limited, but they raise concerns and so these drugs should not be used when fertility is desired. The effects of transsphenoidal surgery during gestation are not known specifically, but would not be expected to be significantly different from the effects of other types of surgery [47] unless hypopituitarism should ensue.

Management of prolactinoma in pregnancy

For patients with microadenomas or intrasellar macroadenomas, bromocriptine or cabergoline therapy is generally preferred to surgery because it is safe for the fetus when discontinued early in gestation and poses only a small risk of tumor enlargement for the mother. Such patients should be assessed each trimester for symptoms such as headaches or visual problems; visual field testing need only be done when clinically indicated. When the tumor is large or extends to the optic chiasm or into the cavernous sinus, the following approaches should be considered: (1) pre-pregnancy surgical debulking; (2) frequent monitoring without dopamine agonist therapy unless symptoms develop; or (3) continuous dopamine agonist therapy. The second option is usually chosen by most clinicians. The safety of continuous dopamine agonist therapy during pregnancy has not been established, but based on the small number of cases cited earlier for bromocriptine, it probably is not harmful. Patients with macroadenomas should be assessed monthly for symptoms of tumor enlargement and visual fields should be tested each trimester. PRL levels, which normally increase in pregnancy, may not rise in women with prolactinomas [48]. Conversely, PRL levels may not always rise with pregnancy-induced tumor enlargement [48]; therefore, periodic measurements of PRL levels are of little benefit and may even be misleading.

When there is evidence of tumor enlargement during pregnancy, dopamine agonist therapy should be reinstituted immediately and the dosage increased as rapidly as tolerated. Such therapy must be monitored closely and transsphenoidal surgery or delivery (if the pregnancy is far enough advanced) should be considered if there is no response to the dopamine agonist [20,21].

Although suckling stimulates PRL secretion in normal women for the first several weeks post partum, there are no data to suggest that breastfeeding can cause tumor growth. Thus, there is no reason to discourage nursing in women with prolactinomas but, of course, dopamine agonist treatment must be withheld during breastfeeding.

In some women, postpartum PRL levels are considerably lower than prepartum levels so that menses may resume spontaneously and resumption of dopamine agonist therapy may not be necessary. Therefore, resumption of dopamine agonist therapy post partum should not be routine.

Acromegaly

Reports of pregnancy in patients with acromegaly are uncommon [49–60], perhaps because 30–40% of such patients have hyperprolactinemia [61]. Correction of hyperprolactinemia with a dopamine agonist may be necessary to permit ovulation and conception in these patients [50,56]. Most patients with acromegaly are treated with surgery as primary therapy and those not cured by surgery are usually treated medically [49]. The primary medical therapy is a somatostatin analog and both octreotide LAR and lanreotide autogelare used [49]. Cabergoline may also be helpful, usually as add-on therapy to a somatostatin analog but occasionally as monotherapy [49].

Diagnosis of acromegaly during pregnancy

Conventional immunoassays for GH cannot distinguish between normal pituitary GH and the placental GH variant [7]. Special immunoassays using antibodies that recognize specific epitopes on the two hormones [7] must be used in this regard. When such specific assays are not available, it may be necessary to wait until after delivery to assess pituitary GH secretion accurately, because the placental variant falls to undetectable levels within 24 hours [7]. However, there are two differences between the secretion of the placental GH variant and the secretion of pituitary GH during acromegaly that may allow a distinction to be made during pregnancy. First, pituitary GH secretion in acromegaly is highly pulsatile, with 13–19 pulses per 24 hours [62], whereas secretion of the pregnancy GH variant is nonpulsatile [9]. Second, in acromegaly, about 70% of patients have a GH response to thyrotropin-releasing hormone (no longer available in the US) [63], whereas the placental GH variant does not respond to this hormone [9].

Effects of pregnancy on tumor size and acromegaly

Only three patients with tumors secreting GH have been reported to have enlargement of their tumors with a resultant visual field defect in one during pregnancy [28,60,64]. However, in one of these three the tumor size had been controlled by somatostatin analogs prior to pregnancy, so how much of the tumor enlargement was due to withdrawal of the somatostatin analog versus the pregnancy cannot be ascertained with certainty [60]. In addition, one patient with acromegaly experienced pituitary apoplexy at 33 weeks [59]. Therefore, patients with acromegaly with macroadenomas should be monitored for symptomatic tumor enlargement in a fashion similar to that for patients with PRL-secreting macroadenomas.

Effects of acromegaly on the pregnancy

Carbohydrate intolerance is present in as many as 50% of patients with acromegaly, and overt diabetes is seen in 10–20% [61]. Insulin resistance secondary to the increased levels of GH may increase the risk of gestational diabetes. There is increased salt retention, and hypertension occurs in 25–35% of patients. In addition, cardiac disease is present in about one-third of patients. There may be a specific cardiomyopathy associated with acromegaly, and coronary artery disease may be increased [61]. Thus, the risks for gestational diabetes, hypertension and heart disease are likely increased in women with acromegaly during pregnancy but there are no specific data to document increased frequencies of these complications.

Management of acromegaly and pregnancy

The considerations regarding the use of bromocriptine and cabergoline in women with prolactinomas also apply to those with acromegaly. For most patients, these drugs should not be continued during pregnancy. Data on the use of somatostatin analogs during pregnancy are limited. Only 14 pregnant patients treated with octreotide, octreotide LAR, and lanreotide have been reported; no malformations were found in their children [57]. Octreotide binds to somatostatin receptors in the placenta [65] and crosses the placenta [66] and therefore can affect developing fetal tissues where somatostatin receptors are widespread, especially in the brain. Because of the limited data documenting safety, we recommend that octreotide and other somatostatin analogs be discontinued if pregnancy is considered and that contraception be used when these drugs are administered. Considering the prolonged nature of the course of most patients with acromegaly, interruption of medical therapy for 9–12 months should not have a particularly adverse effect on the long-term outcome. On the other hand, these drugs can control tumor growth and for enlarging tumors, their reintroduction during pregnancy may be warranted versus operating. Both bromocriptine [58] and octreotide [57] have been started during pregnancy because of tumor enlargement, with successful shrinkage of the tumor and no adverse outcome on the baby being noted.

TSH-secreting tumors

Only three cases of pregnancy occurring in women with TSH-secreting tumors have been reported [67–69]. In one of these cases, octreotide, which had been stopped, had to be reinstituted to control tumor size [67] and in a second, octreotide was continued during pregnancy for tumor size control [68]. The most pressing issue with such tumors is the need to control hyperthyroidism during pregnancy and that can usually be done with standard antithyroid drugs [68]. However, with growing macroadenomas, octreotide may be necessary for tumor size control [67,68] and it is possible that it may be necessary to control the hyperthyroidism if thionamides are ineffective.

Clinically nonfunctioning adenomas

Pregnancy would not expected to influence tumor size in patients with clinically nonfunctioning adenomas (CNFA) and only two cases have been reported in which tumor enlargement during pregnancy resulted in a visual field defect [28,70]. It might be expected that if the normal lactotroph hyperplasia were to occur in a patient with a pre-existing CNFA, this hyperplasia could push up the CNFA to cause chiasmal compression or headaches. In the second case of tumor size increase reported, the patient responded rapidly to bromocriptine treatment, probably due to shrinkage of the lactotroph hyperplasia with decompression of the chiasm and probably with little or no direct effect on the tumor itself [70].

Most CNFA are actually gonadotroph adenomas [71]. Two patients have been reported who had gonadotroph adenomas

secreting intact FSH with a resultant ovarian hyperstimulation syndrome [72,73]; both became pregnant, one after having the FSH hypersecretion controlled by bromocriptine [72] and the second following surgical removal of the tumor [73].

Hypopituitarism

Hypopituitarism may occur because of tumor compression of the hypothalamus and/or pituitary stalk or from prior neurosurgery. Hormone deficits can be partial or complete and loss of gonadotropin secretion is common. Induction of ovulation may be difficult and a variety of techniques have been used, including administration of HCG and FSH (in the past as human menopausal gonadotropin [74–77], pulsatile GnRH [78–80] and in vitro fertilization [81]. In a report of 30 courses of fertility treatment over a total of 164 cycles in 19 women, Hall *et al.* found that two women responded to pulsatile GnRH treatment and the remainder were treated with gonadotropins and HCG, with 98 (68%) of cycles being ovulatory and pregnancy achieved in 18 (11%) cycles [82].

Overton *et al.* reported on 18 pregnancy outcomes occurring in nine women with hypopituitarism who conceived with ovulation induction; two pregnancies were achieved with a GnRH pump and the remainder with gonadotropins and HCG [83]. Of the 14 singletons, there were five (28%) miscarriages, a number thought to be within the expected range; one-half of the livebirths were small for gestational age but there were no congenital malformations [83]. However, of the four sets of twins, two sets miscarried in the first trimester and two sets ended in intrauterine deaths in the second trimester [83]. Ten of the 11 births were by cesarean section, six being emergencies [83]. Post partum, only one woman successfully breastfed [83]. Thus, these authors considered pregnancies in women with hypopituitarism to be high risk [83].

In adult women, the primary hormone replacements to be considered during pregnancy are thyroid and adrenal hormones. Because of the increased thyroxine turnover and increased volume of distribution that occurs during pregnancy, often T4 levels fall and TSH levels rise with a fixed thyroxine dose over the course of gestation [15,84]. The average increase in thyroxine need in these patients is about 0.05 mg/day. Because patients with hypothalamic/pituitary dysfunction may not elevate their TSH levels normally in the face of increased need for thyroxine, it may be reasonable to increase the thyroxine supplementation by 0.025 mg after the first trimester and by an additional 0.025 mg after the second trimester, also following free T4 levels. However, there are no actual data to support this approach.

Because the cortisol production rate is normally increased in pregnancy [10,11,14], the dose of chronic glucocorticoid replacement theoretically ought to be increased during pregnancy. However, this does not seem to be necessary in practice and patients usually can be kept on their standard replacement doses [14]. Hydrocortisone, prednisolone and prednisone can be used. Hydrocortisone is metabolized by the placental enzyme 11-beta-hydroxysteroid dehydrogenase 2, so the fetus is generally protected from any overdose of hydrocortisone; the usual dose is in the range of 12–15 mg/m^2 given in two or three divided doses [14]. Additional glucocorticoids are needed for the stress of labor and delivery, with rapid tapering post partum, and a proposed regimen for doing this is discussed in detail in Chapter 47. Prednisolone does not cross the placenta [85]. Prednisone crosses the placenta in only small amounts [85,86] and suppression of neonatal adrenal function in offspring of women taking prednisone during pregnancy is very uncommon [87]. Glucocorticoids may also pass to the neonate in breast milk, but the amounts (0.14% of maternal blood levels) are not sufficient to alter neonatal adrenal function, even with large maternal doses of prednisone [88].

Adult women with hypopituitarism are being treated with GH replacement in increasing numbers [89]. Although GH was used as an adjunct to fertility treatment with gonadotropins for many years, systematic reviews did not show particular benefit [90] and this treatment has been largely abandoned. On the other hand, there was also little harm. There are few data on the use of GH during pregnancy in hypopituitary individuals and in most series GH therapy has been stopped at conception [91]. As the GH variant, which is biologically active, is produced by the placenta in substantial amounts beginning in the second half of pregnancy and can access the maternal circulation (see above), then at most the mother would be GH deficient only in the first half of pregnancy. When Curran *et al.* analyzed 25 pregnancies that occurred in 16 patients with GH deficiency during which GH therapy was not continued, they found that there was no adverse outcome of omitting GH therapy on either the fetus or mother and concluded that GH replacement therapy during pregnancy is not essential for GH-deficient women [91]. Given the lack of proven benefit of GH treatment during pregnancy and the absence of reassuring safety data, it seems prudent to stop GH treatment during pregnancy.

Sheehan's syndrome

Sheehan's syndrome consists of pituitary necrosis secondary to ischemia occurring within hours of delivery [92,93]. It is usually secondary to hypotension and shock from an obstetric hemorrhage. Pituitary enlargement during pregnancy apparently predisposes to the risk for ischemia with occlusive spasm of the arteries to the anterior pituitary and stalk [92,93]. The degree of ischemia and necrosis dictates the subsequent patient course. It rarely occurs with current obstetric practice [94].

Acute necrosis is suspected in the setting of an obstetric hemorrhage where hypotension and tachycardia persist following adequate replacement of blood products (Table 13.3). In addition, the woman fails to lactate and may have hypoglycemia

Table 13.3 Symptoms and signs of Sheehan's syndrome

Acute form	Chronic form
Hypotension	Light-headedness
Tachycardia	Fatigue
Failure to lactate	Failure to lactate
Hypoglycemia	Persistent amenorrhea
Extreme fatigue	Decreased body hair
Nausea and vomiting	Dry skin
	Loss of libido
	Nausea and vomiting
	Cold intolerance

[92,93,95]. Investigation should include obtaining blood samples for ACTH, cortisol, prolactin, and free thyroxine. The ACTH stimulation test would be normal, as the adrenal cortex would not be atrophied. Free thyroxine levels may prove normal initially, as the hormone has a half-life of 7 days, and an additional sample should be sent after 1 week. Prolactin levels are usually low, although they are generally 5–10-fold elevated in the puerperium.

Treatment with saline and stress doses of corticosteroids should be instituted immediately after drawing the blood tests. If later free thyroxine levels become low, then therapy with levothyroxine is indicated. Additional pituitary testing with subsequent therapy should be delayed until recovery. Diabetes insipidus may also occur secondary to vascular occlusion with atrophy and scarring of the neurohypophysis [96,97].

When milder forms of infarction occur, the diagnosis of Sheehan's syndrome may be delayed for months or years [93,95]. These women generally have a history of amenorrhea, decreased libido, failure to lactate, breast atrophy, loss of pubic and axillary hair, fatigue, and symptoms of secondary adrenal insufficiency with nausea, vomiting, diarrhea, and abdominal pain (see Table 13.3) [93,95]. Usually growth hormone and gonadotropins are lost before ACTH and TSH with pituitary damage; however, some women retain gonadotropin secretion and may have normal menses and fertility [95]. Although some women may have episodes of transient polydipsia and polyuria, many demonstrate impaired urinary concentrating ability and deficient vasopressin secretion [97]. Computed tomography (CT) or MRI scans generally reveal partial or completely empty sellae [98].

Lymphocytic hypophysitis

Lymphocytic hypophysitis is thought to be autoimmune in nature, and is manifested by infiltration and destruction of the parenchyma of the pituitary and infundibulum by lymphocytes and plasma cells [99–101]. It generally occurs during pregnancy or the postpartum period [99,101]. It is associated with symptoms of hypopituitarism or an enlarging mass lesion with headaches and visual field defects, and is suspected based on its timing and lack of association with an obstetric hemorrhage or prior history of menstrual difficulties or infertility.

It is generally associated with mild hyperprolactinemia (<150 ng/mL) and occasionally with diabetes insipidus. On MRI scans, there is usually diffuse enhancement rather than a focal lesion that might indicate a tumor; definitive diagnosis requires a biopsy [99,101]. However, the clinical picture often allows a clinical diagnosis to be made without invasive procedures.

Treatment is generally conservative and involves identification and correction of any pituitary deficits, especially of ACTH secretion which is particularly common in this condition [99,101]. Data indicating that high-dose corticosteroids are of benefit in treating the destructive process are inconclusive. Surgery to debulk but not remove the gland is indicated in the presence of uncontrolled headaches, visual field defects, and progressive enlargement on scan. Spontaneous regression and resumption of partial or normal pituitary function may occur, although most patients progress to chronic panhypopituitarism [99,101–103]. Other autoimmune disorders may also be associated.

Posterior pituitary

The osmostat, the setpoint for plasma osmolality at which arginine vasopressin (AVP) is secreted, is reduced approximately 5–10 mOsm/kg in pregnancy, dropping from about 285 to 275 mOsm/kg. As a result, pregnant women experience thirst and release AVP at lower levels of plasma osmolality than do nonpregnant women [104]. This reset osmostat and altered thirst threshold is possibly due to high levels of HCG [104]. The placenta produces an amino-terminal peptidase, vasopressinase, an enzyme that rapidly inactivates AVP and oxytocin. Vasopressinase levels increase 1000-fold between the fourth and 38th weeks of gestation [105]. AVP consequently has a 4–6-fold increased metabolic clearance rate during gestation [106,107].

The lower osmostat and increased clearance of AVP by vasopressinase in pregnancy alter the nomograms of plasma osmolality and AVP used in the nonpregnant patient. Serum sodium levels may also be lower than those normally expected in patients with diabetes insipidus [107]. Standard water deprivation tests which require 5% weight loss should be avoided during pregnancy as they may cause uterine irritability and alter placental perfusion. Instead, desmopressin (dDAVP) is used to assess urinary concentrating ability over 11 hours, with a value greater than 700 mOsm/kg considered normal [108]. Urinary concentrating ability in the pregnant patient should be determined in the seated position, as the lateral recumbent position inhibits maximal urinary concentration [104,107]. Delivery of the placenta generally results in a return to normal AVP metabolism in 2–3 weeks.

Plasma oxytocin levels increase progressively during pregnancy, with a dramatic increase at term [109,110]. Oxytocin levels rise further during labor and peak in the second stage. Uterine sensitivity to oxytocin increases with a rise in oxytocin receptors in the myometrium. Hypophysectomy does not alter onset of labor, indicating that oxytocin only facilitates labor [111]. Oxytocin levels rise rapidly during suckling [112].

Diabetes insipidus

Three types of diabetes insipidus may occur in pregnancy: central, nephrogenic or transient vasopressin resistant. Polydipsia, polyuria, and dehydration may occur with all three.

Central diabetes insipidus may occur spontaneously in pregnancy with an enlarging pituitary adenoma, with lymphocytic hypophysitis or with the development of other conditions such as histiocytosis X. Diabetes insipidus (DI) usually worsens during gestation [107], likely due to the increased clearance of AVP by placental vasopressinase. Patients with asymptomatic DI may develop symptoms during pregnancy with the lower osmostat for vasopressin release, elevation in vasopressinase levels, and increased AVP clearance [113–116]. Patients with mild disease usually treated with chlorpropamide should discontinue this agent, as it readily crosses the placenta and causes hypoglycemia in the fetus. The AVP analog desmopressin (dDAVP) is resistant to vasopressinase, and provides satisfactory treatment during gestation, although a higher dose may be required [107]. During monitoring of the clinical response, clinicians should remember that normal basal plasma osmolality and sodium concentration are 5 mEq/L lower during pregnancy [116]. No adverse events have been described in the offspring of pregnancies in which dDAVP was used throughout gestation [117,118]. dDAVP transfers minimally into breast milk [107] and is poorly absorbed from the gastrointestinal tract, so its use will not adversely affect an infant's water metabolism.

Transient AVP-resistant forms of DI secondary to placental production of vasopressinase may occur spontaneously in one pregnancy, but not in a subsequent one [119]. Some of these patients may respond to dDAVP therapy. The symptoms resolve within several weeks of delivery [107,116,119].

Acute fatty liver of pregnancy and other disturbances of hepatic function such as hepatitis may be associated with late-onset transient DI of pregnancy in some patients [120]. In some cases, this has been associated with the HELLP syndrome [121]. It is presumed that the hepatic dysfunction is associated with reduced degradation of vasopressinase, further increasing vasopressinase levels and the clearance of AVP. The polyuria may develop either prior to delivery or post partum. Complete resolution of the hepatic abnormalities and DI occurs by the fourth postpartum week.

Diabetes insipidus that develops post partum may be a result of Sheehan's syndrome, particularly in the setting of an obstetric hemorrhage (see above). Transient DI of unknown etiology has been described post partum, lasting only days to weeks [122].

Congenital nephrogenic DI is a rare X-linked disorder caused by a mutation in the vasopressin V2 receptor gene which predominantly affects males. Female carriers of this disease may have significant polyuria during pregnancy. Treatment is with thiazide diuretics [107], which should be used with caution in pregnant women.

In patients with idiopathic DI, oxytocin levels are normal and labor may begin spontaneously and proceed normally [123]. Patients with DI secondary to trauma, infiltrative disease or a neoplasm may have adversely affected oxytocinergic pathways, resulting in poor progression of labor and uterine atony.

Adrenals

In addition to the changes during pregnancy in the hypothalamic–pituitary–adrenal axis outlined previously, numerous changes occur in the renin–angiotensin–aldosterone system as well. Plasma renin activity increases 3–7-fold and plateaus at 20 weeks, despite the increase in plasma volume with pregnancy [124,125]. Angiotensin II levels increase approximately threefold by term, although there is resistance to its pressor effects. Plasma mineralocorticoid levels increase 5–20-fold during gestation [125,126], but aldosterone secretion continues to respond normally to physiologic stimuli such as posture and varies inversely to changes in volume or dietary salt [127]. The increase in aldosterone correlates with the pregnancy increase in glomerular filtration rate (GFR) and in progesterone [128], which competitively inhibits sodium retention and sodium–potassium exchange by aldosterone at the distal renal tubule [129].

Cushing's yndrome

Just over 100 cases of Cushing's syndrome in pregnancy have been reported [130–146]. The distribution of causes of Cushing's syndrome in pregnancy differs markedly from that in the nonpregnant population. Less than 50% of the pregnant patients described had pituitary adenomas, a similar number had adrenal adenomas, and more than 10% had adrenal carcinomas [130–146]. Pregnancies associated with the ectopic ACTH syndrome have been reported only rarely [132,136].

In many cases, the hypercortisolism first became apparent during pregnancy, with improvement after parturition, leading to the speculation that unregulated placental CRH was instrumental in causing this pregnancy-induced exacerbation [131,132,136,142]. Rarely, recurrent Cushing's syndrome may be associated with pregnancy only to completely remit following delivery; the etiology for this has not been found [143,144].

Diagnosis of Cushing's syndrome during pregnancy

Diagnosing Cushing's syndrome during pregnancy may be difficult. Both conditions may be associated with weight gain in a central distribution, fatigue, edema, emotional upset, glucose intolerance, and hypertension. The striae associated with the weight gain and increased abdominal girth are usually pale in normal pregnancy and red or purple in Cushing's syndrome. Hirsutism and acne may point to excessive androgen production. Proximal myopathy and bone fractures point to Cushing's syndrome.

The laboratory evaluation of Cushing's syndrome during pregnancy is not straightforward. Elevated total and free serum cortisol and ACTH levels, and urinary free cortisol excretion are compatible with those of normal pregnancy. The overnight dexamethasone test usually demonstrates inadequate suppression during normal pregnancy [14,133]. The increasing loss of suppressibility over the course of gestation has been attributed to several factors, including the high levels of CBG, tissue refractoriness to glucocorticoids, resetting of the hypothalamic–pituitary axis, antiglucocorticoid actions of progesterone, and placental ACTH and CRH [14]. At least in the latter part of the third trimester, the elevated cortisol levels are not suppressed during the low-dose dexamethasone test but are suppressed during the high-dose test, similar to what is observed in patients with Cushing's disease [14,131]. ACTH levels are normal to elevated in pregnant patients with all forms of Cushing's syndrome [14,130–136]. These "normal" rather than suppressed levels of ACTH in patients with adrenal adenomas may result from the production of ACTH by the placenta or from the nonsuppressible stimulation of pituitary ACTH by placental CRH.

A persistent circadian variation in the elevated levels of total and free serum cortisol during normal pregnancy may be most helpful in distinguishing Cushing's syndrome from the hypercortisolism of pregnancy, because this finding is characteristically absent in all forms of Cushing's syndrome [11,14]. Salivary cortisol measurements may turn out to be useful in this regard but normal limits for midnight levels of salivary cortisol during pregnancy have not yet been standardized [142]. In many cases, MRI scanning of the pituitary (without contrast) or ultrasound of the adrenal may be required, although MR images of the pituitary in patients with Cushing's disease are often nondiagnostic. Little experience has been reported with newer techniques such as CRH stimulation testing or petrosal venous sinus sampling during pregnancy [134,136,137,145]. For the latter technique, catheterization is performed via the direct jugular vein approach rather than the femoral vein approach to minimize fetal irradiation; in these cases, clearly increased central-to-peripheral ACTH gradients were found.

Effects of Cushing's syndrome on the pregnancy

Cushing's syndrome is associated with a pregnancy loss rate of 25% due to spontaneous abortion, stillbirth, and early neonatal death because of extreme prematurity [130–142,145,146]. Premature labor occurs in more than 50% of cases, regardless of etiology [130–142,145,146]. The passage of cortisol across the placenta may rarely result in suppression of the fetal adrenals [138] and the neonate should be tested for this potential problem and given exogenous corticosteroids until the results of the evaluation are known.

Hypertension develops in most mothers with Cushing's and diabetes and myopathy are frequent. Postoperative wound infection and dehiscence are common after cesarean section. The pregnancy appears to induce an amelioration of Cushing's syndrome in some patients, but an exacerbation in others [130–136,142].

Management of Cushing's syndrome during pregnancy

In a review of 136 pregnancies, Lindsay *et al.* found that there were 56 livebirths (76%) when no active treatment was instituted as compared to 50 livebirths (89%) in women in whom treatment was instituted by a gestational age of 20 weeks [145]. Therefore, treatment during pregnancy has been advocated [130,133,145].

Medical therapy for Cushing's syndrome during pregnancy is not very effective [132,133,142,145]. A few case reports have documented the efficacy of metyrapone but hypertension and pre-eclampsia have been reported [145]. Ketoconazole has been used successfully in a few patients after the first trimester, with complications of intrauterine growth retardation but no malformations or other perinatal disorders [139,140]. Use of other drugs has been very limited [142]; because of potential toxicity to the fetus, aminoglutethimide and mitotane should be avoided. Transsphenoidal resection of a pituitary ACTH-secreting adenoma has been carried out successfully in several patients during the second trimester [131,134,137,138,141,142,145]. Adrenal surgery may be performed using a laparoscopic approach. The livebirth rate is approximately 87% after unilateral or bilateral adrenalectomy [145,146]. Although any surgery poses risks for the mother and fetus [47], it appears that with Cushing's syndrome, the risks of not operating are considerably higher than those of proceeding with surgery.

Adrenal insufficiency

The incidence of primary adrenal insufficiency in pregnancy was reported to be 1 in 3000 births from 1976 to 1987 [147]. In developed countries, the most common etiology for primary adrenal insufficiency is autoimmune adrenalitis, which may be associated with autoimmune polyglandular syndrome. Primary adrenal insufficiency from infections (tuberculous or fungal), bilateral metastatic disease, hemorrhage or infarctions is uncommon. Secondary adrenal insufficiency, from pituitary neoplasms or glucocorticoid suppression of the hypothalamic–pituitary–adrenal axis, is more common.

Recognition of adrenal insufficiency may be difficult in the first trimester as many of the clinical features are found in normal pregnancies, including weakness, lightheadedness, syncope, nausea, vomiting, hyponatremia, and increased pigmentation. Addisonian hyperpigmentation may be distinguished

from chloasma of pregnancy by its presence on the mucous membranes, on extensor surfaces, and on nonexposed areas. Weight loss, hypoglycemia, salt craving, hyponatremia more severe than the normal 5 mmol/L decrease of pregnancy or seizures should prompt a clinical evaluation. If unrecognized, adrenal crisis may ensue at times of stress, such as a urinary tract infection or labor [147]. Fetal cortisol production may be protective, shielding the mother from severe adrenal insufficiency until after the birth [148].

The fetoplacental unit largely controls its own steroid milieu, so maternal adrenal insufficiency generally causes no problems with fetal development. Maternal antiadrenal autoantibodies may cross the placenta, but usually not in sufficient quantities to cause fetal or neonatal adrenal insufficiency [149]. Although earlier studies observed intrauterine growth retardation in offspring of women with Addison's disease [150], this observation has not been supported in most subsequent case series. Severe maternal hyponatremia or metabolic acidosis may cause a poor fetal outcome, including death [151]. Association with other autoimmune conditions such as anticardiolipin antibodies may lead to additional risks such as miscarriage [152].

Adrenal insufficiency may be associated with laboratory findings of hyponatremia, hyperkalemia, hypoglycemia, eosinophilia, and lymphocytosis. Early morning plasma cortisol levels of ≤ 3.0 μg/dL (83 nmol/L) confirm adrenal insufficiency [153], while a cortisol >19 μg/dL (525 nmol/L) in the first or early second trimester excludes the diagnosis in a clinically stable patient [153,154]. However, plasma cortisol levels may fall in the normal "nonpregnant" range due to the increase in CBG concentrations in the second and third trimesters, but will not be appropriately elevated for the stage of pregnancy [155]. Appropriate pregnancy-specific cut-offs for diagnosis with the standard cosyntropin (1–24 corticotropin) test using a 250 μg dose have not been established, with plasma cortisol levels 60–80% above nonpregnant responses in normal pregnant women tested in the second and third trimesters in one series [155]. McKenna *et al.* examined the 1 μg low-dose cosyntropin test for diagnosis of secondary adrenal insufficiency in women at 24–34 weeks gestational age, finding high sensitivity of diagnosis using a cut-off of 30 μg/dL (828 nmol/L) [153]. Accuracy of dosing is more difficult with this than with the standard cosyntropin test. The cosyntropin test is less sensitive in detecting early secondary or tertiary forms of adrenal insufficiency. Cortisol and ACTH responses to CRH are blunted in pregnancy [156], making the CRH stimulation test unreliable for differentiating secondary and tertiary adrenal insufficiency in pregnancy. With primary adrenal insufficiency, ACTH levels will be elevated, and a level above 100 pg/mL (22 pmol/L) is consistent with the diagnosis [154]. However, ACTH will not be low with secondary forms because of the placental production of this hormone, which is nevertheless insufficient to maintain normal maternal adrenal function. Adrenal antibodies may assist in confirming autoimmune adrenal insufficiency, as approximately 90% of patients will have 21-hydroxylase antibodies; however, the absence of antibodies does not exclude the diagnosis [157]. Aldosterone to renin ratios are low with elevated plasma renin activity in patients with mineralocorticoid deficiency from adrenal atrophy [158].

In the unstable patient, empiric glucocorticoid therapy of hydrocortisone 75–100 mg IV should be administered pending the results of diagnostic testing. Thereafter, stress doses of 75–100 mg every 6–8 hours during the crisis mimic the maximal cortisol production rates of 200–300 mg/day [159]. Despite the normal increase in plasma cortisol during pregnancy, baseline maternal replacement doses of corticosteroids usually are not different from those required in the nonpregnant state. Higher doses are needed at times of stress, such as during the course of "morning sickness" or during labor and delivery. Patients should be educated in the self-administration of intramuscular hydrocortisone. Stress doses of steroids are generally given during labor with rapid tapering post partum and an approach to doing this is reviewed in Chapter 47 [159]. Mineralocorticoid replacement requirements usually do not change during gestation, though some clinicians have reduced doses of fludrocortisone in the third trimester in an attempt to treat Addisonian patients who develop edema, exacerbation of hypertension, and pre-eclampsia [147,160].

Patients who have received glucocorticoids as anti-inflammatory therapy are presumed to have adrenal axis suppression for at least 1 year following cessation of such therapy [161]. These patients should be treated with stress doses of glucocorticoids during labor and delivery as noted above. They are at risk for postoperative wound infection and dehiscence, as are patients with endogenous Cushing's, and their offspring are at risk for transient adrenal insufficiency.

As noted above (see section on Hypopituitarism), hydrocortisone, prednisone and prednisone may all be used in replacement doses safely during pregnancy and suppression of neonatal adrenal function is uncommon [87]. Glucocorticoid therapy during lactation is also safe, as less than 0.5% of the dose is passed into breast milk [150,162,163].

Congenital adrenal hyperplasia

Congenital adrenal hyperplasia (CAH) is a family of monogenic inherited enzymatic defects of adrenal steroid biosynthesis, with manifestations secondary to an accumulation of precursors proximal to the enzymatic deficiency. The most common form of CAH in the population is 21-hydroxylase (CYP21 gene) deficiency, seen in more than 90% of the CAH cases in pregnancy [164–168]. Untreated classic, severe 21-hydroxylase deficiency is associated with ambiguous genitalia, an inadequate vaginal introitus, and progressive postnatal virilization including precocious adrenarche, advanced somatic development, central precocious puberty, menstrual irregularity, a reduced fertility rate, and possibly salt wasting [165].

The spontaneous abortion rate is twice that in the normal population [169], and congenital anomalies are more frequent. Cephalopelvic disproportion from an android pelvis may occur, sometimes complicated by the previous reconstructive surgery [170,171]. Conception requires adequate glucocorticoid therapy, which then continues at stable rates during gestation, except at labor and delivery when stress doses are needed. Nonclassic (late-onset) 21-hydroxylase deficiency patients present with pubertal and postpubertal hirsutism and menstrual irregularity, and may have improved fertility with glucocorticoid therapy [172].

Fetal risk depends on the carrier status of the father, as the disorder is genetically recessive. Unfortunately, ACTH stimulation testing to measure 17-OH progesterone demonstrates overlap between heterozygotes for CAH and the normal population [173]. Ideally, CYP21 genotyping of the father is performed [167] but if this cannot be done, the mother must be treated as outlined below. Virilization is not seen in the female fetus with nonclassic 21-hydroxylase deficiency [172] but occurs in a fetus with classic 21-hydroxylase deficiency unless fetal adrenal androgen production is adequately suppressed. Dexamethasone most readily crosses the placenta as it is not bound to CBG and is not metabolized by placental 11-beta-hydroxysteroid dehydrogenase. It is commonly used at doses of 20 μg/kg maternal bodyweight per day to a maximum of 1.5 mg daily in three divided doses, beginning at recognition of pregnancy before the 9th week of gestation [167,174,175], though lower doses are recommended by some [176]. Treatment by the 9th week of gestation is very effective in reducing the risk of virilization in the affected female fetus [167]. Maternal plasma and/or urinary estriol levels reflect fetal adrenal synthesis and are monitored to assess efficacy. Maternal cortisol and dehydroepiandrosterone (DHEA-S) will determine maternal adrenal suppression. There is little effect on maternal 17-OH progesterone with therapy. As only 25% of female fetuses are affected in a family with CAH, it is important to discontinue therapy as soon as possible in the male fetus and unaffected female fetus. Chorionic villus sampling at 9–11 weeks gestation may be used for gender determination and direct DNA analysis for the 21-hydroxylase gene CYP21 [164,167,174]. This test is associated with a 1% risk of fetal loss. An alternative is karyotyping and DNA analysis or measuring androstenedione and 17-OH progesterone levels in amniotic fluid at 16–18 weeks of gestation after dexamethasone has been withheld for 5 days [174].

Several series have reported benefits with the use of dexamethasone begun before week 9. New et al. reported that of 27 affected females, dexamethasone treatment resulted in completely normal female genitalia in 11 and 13 with significantly less virilization compared to those who were untreated [177]. Similarly, Forest & Dörr found that of 38 affected girls, 10 were normal, 17 had only slightly virilized genitalia, three had moderate virilization, and eight had more severe virilization [178]. Side effects of dexamethasone therapy are significant, including excessive weight gain, severe striae with scarring, edema, irritability, gestational diabetes mellitus, hypertension, and gastrointestinal intolerance [167,175]. In affected pregnancies, dexamethasone may be lowered to 0.75–1.0 mg/day in the second half of pregnancy to decrease maternal side effects while avoiding fetal virilization [175]. The use of dexamethasone as outlined above is not accepted by all experts in the field, as the long-term benefits and risks of this treatment in large numbers of patients have not been fully assessed.

Primary hyperaldosteronism

Primary hyperaldosteronism rarely has been reported in pregnancy [179–183] and is most often caused by an adrenal adenoma. There are rare reports of glucocorticoid-remediable hyperaldosteronism in pregnancy [184]. The elevated aldosterone levels found in affected patients during pregnancy are similar to those in normal pregnant women, but the plasma renin activity is suppressed [179–182]. Moderate to severe hypertension develops in 85%, proteinuria in 52%, and hypokalemia in 55% of patients [183] and symptoms may include headache, malaise, and muscle cramps [185]. Placental abruption and preterm delivery are also risks [186]. Interestingly, the very high progesterone levels of pregnancy may have an antimineralocorticoid effect at the renal tubules and thus the hypertension and hypokalemia may ameliorate during pregnancy in some women [187].

The physiologic rise in aldosterone during pregnancy overlaps the levels seen in primary aldosteronism, making diagnosis difficult [125,183]. Suppressed renin in the setting of hyperaldosteronism is diagnostic. Salt loading tests may be used to diagnose hyperaldosteronism, but there are potential fetal risks and no normative data [182]. If baseline and suppression testing are equivocal or radiologic scanning does not suggest unilateral disease, patients may be treated medically until delivery to allow more definitive investigations [181].

Spironolactone, the usual nonpregnant therapy, is contraindicated in pregnancy as it crosses the placenta and is a potent antiandrogen which can cause ambiguous genitalia in a male fetus [182]. There is no published experience with the use during pregnancy of eplerenone, the new aldosterone receptor antagonist. Surgical therapy may be delayed until post partum if hypertension can be controlled with agents safe in pregnancy, such as amiloride, methyldopa, labetalol, and calcium channel blockers [181,187,188]. Potassium supplementation may be required, but as noted above, the hypokalemia may ameliorate in pregnancy because of the antikaliuretic effect of progesterone. Both hypertension and hypokalemia may worsen post partum due to removal of the progesterone effect [189,190].

Pheochromocytoma

Exacerbation of hypertension is a typical presentation of pheochromocytoma in nonpregnant patients, but during pregnancy is frequently mistaken for pregnancy-induced hypertension or pre-eclampsia [191]. The prevalence is estimated at 1 in 54,000 pregnancies [192]. As the uterus enlarges and an actively moving fetus compresses the neoplasm, maternal complications such as severe hypertension, hemorrhage into the neoplasm, hemodynamic collapse, myocardial infarction, cardiac arrhythmias, congestive heart failure, and cerebral hemorrhage may occur. Extra-adrenal tumors which occur in 10%, such as in the organ of Zuckerkandl at the aortic bifucation, are particularly prone to hypertensive episodes with changes in position, uterine contractions, fetal movement, and Valsalva maneuvers [193]. Unrecognized pheochromocytoma has been associated with a maternal mortality rate of 50% at induction of general anesthesia or during labor [194,195].

There is minimal placental transfer of catecholamines [196,197], likely due to high placental concentrations of catechol-O-methyltransferase and monoamine oxidase [196, 198]. Adverse fetal effects such as hypoxia are a result of catecholamine-induced uteroplacental vasoconstriction and placental insufficiency [199–201], and of maternal hypertension, hypotension or vascular collapse. Placental abruption may also occur.

The diagnosis of pheochromocytoma requires a high index of suspicion. Preconception screening of families known to have multiple endocrine neoplasia (MEN) type 2, von Hippel–Lindau disease, and neurofibromatosis is important [202–204]. The diagnosis should be considered in pregnant women with severe or paroxysmal hypertension, particularly in the first half of pregnancy or in association with orthostatic hypotension or episodic symptoms of pallor, anxiety, headaches, palpitations, chest pain or diaphoresis. Symptoms may occur or worsen during pregnancy because of the increased vascularity of the tumor and mechanical factors such as pressure from the expanding uterus or fetal movement [200].

Laboratory diagnosis of pheochromocytoma is unchanged from the nonpregnant state as catecholamine metabolism is not altered by pregnancy per se [205].The diagnosis is typically made by testing a 24-hour urine specimen for fractionated metanephrines (metanephrine and normetanephrine) and/or catecholamines (dopamine, epinephrine and norepinephrine). Fractionated free plasma metanephrine testing is a highly sensitive but not specific alternative to urinary testing but is best used in higher risk patients because of the high incidence of false positives when the test is performed in a low-risk population. If possible, methyldopa and labetalol should be discontinued prior to the investigation as these agents may interfere with the quantification of the catecholamines and vanillylmandelic acid (VMA) [206]. Provocative testing should be avoided because of the increased risk of maternal and fetal mortality. Tumor localization with MRI, with high-intensity signals noted on T2-weighted images, provides the best sensitivity without fetal exposure to ionizing radiation. The safety of meta-iodobenzylguanidine and

[^{18}F]-dopamine-labeled positron emission tomography scans has not been studied in pregnancy, but they may be used post partum to assess extra-adrenal disease.

Differentiation from pre-eclampsia is generally simple. The edema, proteinuria, and hyperuricemia found in women with pre-eclampsia are absent in those with pheochromocytomas. Plasma and urinary catecholamines may be modestly elevated in severe pre-eclampsia and other serious pregnancy complications requiring hospitalization, though they remain normal in mild pre-eclampsia or pregnancy-induced hypertension [207]. Catecholamine levels are 2–4 times normal after an eclamptic seizure, however [208].

Initial medical management involves alpha-blockade with phenoxybenzamine, phentolamine, prazosin or labetalol. All of these agents are well tolerated by the fetus, but phenoxybenzamine is considered the preferred agent as it provides long-acting, stable, noncompetitive blockade [200]. Phenoxybenzamine is started at a dose of 10 mg twice daily, with titration until the hypertension is controlled. Placental transfer of phenoxybenzamine occurs [209] but is generally safe [210,211]. However, two neonates of mothers treated with phenoxybenzamine have been reported, with respiratory distress and hypotension requiring ventilatory and inotropic support in the first 72 hours following delivery [212]. If hypertension remains inadequately controlled, metyrosine has also been used successfully to reduce catecholamine synthesis in a pregnancy complicated by malignant pheochromocytoma [213] but may potentially adversely affect the fetus. Beta-blockade is reserved for treating maternal tachycardia or arrhythmias which persist after full alpha-blockade and volume repletion. Beta-blockers may be associated with fetal bradycardia and with intrauterine growth retardation but generally are safe and there is wide experience with their use [205,214]. All these potential fetal risks are small compared to the risk of fetal wastage from unblocked high maternal levels of catecholamines. Hypertensive emergencies should be treated with phentolamine (1–5 mg) or nitroprusside, although the latter should be limited to brief periods of time because of potential fetal cyanide toxicity.

The timing of surgical excision of the neoplasm is controversial and may depend on the success of the medical management and the location of the tumor. As noted above, pressure from the uterus, motion of the fetus, and labor contractions are all stimuli that may cause an acute crisis, particularly in patients with a tumor at the organ of Zuckerkandl. In the first half of pregnancy, surgical excision may proceed once adequate alpha-blockade is established, although there may be a higher risk of fetal loss with first-trimester surgery. In the early second trimester, fetal loss is less likely with surgery and the size of the uterus will not make excision difficult. If the pheochromocytoma is not recognized until the second half of gestation, increasing uterine size makes surgical exploration difficult. Successful laparoscopic excision of a pheochromocytoma has been described in the second trimester of pregnancy [215]. Other options include combined cesarean delivery and tumor resection or delivery followed by tumor resection at a later date. Delivery is generally delayed until the fetus reaches sufficient maturity to reduce neonatal morbidity, providing successful medical management can be instituted.

Although successful vaginal delivery has been reported [217], it has been associated with higher rates of maternal mortality than cesarean section. Labor may result in uncontrolled release of catecholamines secondary to pain and uterine contractions [217]. Severe maternal hypertension may lead to placental ischemia and fetal hypoxia. However, in the well-blocked patient, vaginal delivery may be possible with pain management with epidural anesthesia and employment of techniques of passive descent and instrumental delivery.

There is no available information regarding the impact of maternal use of phenoxybenzamine on the nursing neonate.

References

1. Goluboff LG, Ezrin C. Effect of pregnancy on the somatotroph and the prolactin cell of the human adenohypophysis. J Clin Endocrinol Metab 1969; 29: 1533–8.
2. Scheithauer BW, Sano T, Kovacs KT, Young WF Jr, Ryan N, Randall RV. The pituitary gland in pregnancy. A clinicopathologic and immunohistochemical study of 69 Cases. Mayo Clin Proc 1990; 65: 461–74.
3. Rigg LA, Lein A, Yen SSC. Pattern of increase in circulating prolactin levels during human gestation. Am J Obstet Gynecol 1977; 129: 454–6.
4. Gonzalez JG, Elizondo G, Saldivar D, Nanez H, Todd LE, Villarreal JZ. Pituitary gland growth during normal pregnancy: an in vivo study using magnetic resonance imaging. Am J Med 1988; 85: 217–20.
5. Elster AD, Sanders TG, Vines FS, Chen MYM. Size and shape of the pituitary gland during pregnancy and post partum: measurement with MR imaging. Radiology 1991; 181: 531–5.
6. Dinç H, Esen F, Demirci A, Sari A, Gümele HR. Pituitary dimensions and volume measurements in pregnancy and post partum. MR assessment. Acta Radiol 1998; 39: 64–9.
7. Frankenne F, Closset J, Gomez F, Scippo ML, Smal J, Hennen G. The physiology of growth hormones (GHs) in pregnant women and partial characterization of the placental GH variant. J Clin Endocrinol Metab 1988; 66: 1171–80.
8. Eriksson L, Frankenne F, Eden S, Hennen G, von Schoultz B. Growth hormone 24-h serum profiles during pregnancy lack of pulsatility for the secretion of the placental variant. Br J Obstet Gynaecol 1989; 106: 949–53.
9. Beckers A, Stevenaert A, Foidart J-M, Hennen G, Frankenne F. Placental and pituitary growth hormone secretion during pregnancy in acromegalic women. J Clin Endocrinol Metab 1990; 71: 725–31.
10. Carr BR, Parker CR Jr, Madden JD, MacDonald PC, Porter JC. Maternal plasma adrenocorticotropin and cortisol relationships throughout human pregnancy. Am J Obstet Gynecol 1981; 139: 416–22.
11. Nolten WE, Lindheimer MD, Rueckert PA, Oparil S, Ehrlich EN. Diurnal patterns and regulation of cortisol secretion in pregnancy. J Clin Endocrinol Metab 1980; 51: 466–72.

12. Rees LH, Burke CW, Chard T, Evans SW, Letchworth AT. Possible placental origin of ACTH in normal human pregnancy. Nature 1975; 254: 620–2.

13. Sasaki A, Shinkawa O, Yoshinaga K. Placental corticotropin-releasing hormone may be a stimulator of maternal pituitary adrenocorticotropic hormone secretion in humans. J Clin Invest 1989; 84: 1997–2001.

14. Lindsay JR, Nieman LK. The hypothalamic-pituitary-adrenal axis in pregnancy: challenges in disease detection and treatment. Endocr Rev 2005; 26: 775–99.

15. Glinoer D. The regulation of thyroid function in pregnancy: pathways of endocrine adaptation from physiology to pathology. Endocr Rev 1997; 18: 404–33.

16. Jeppsson S, Rannevik G, Liedholm P, Thorell JI. Basal and LHRH stimulated secretion of FSH during pregnancy. Am J Obstet Gynecol 1977; 127: 32–6.

17. Central Brain Tumor Registry of the United States (CTBRUS). Statistical Report. Primary brain tumors in the US 1997–2001. www.cbrtus.org.

18. Kredentser JV, Hoskins CF, Scott JZ. Hyperprolactinemia: a significant factor in female infertility. Am J Obstet Gynecol 1981; 139: 264–7.

19. Molitch ME. Disorders of prolactin secretion. Endocrinol Metab Clin North Am 2001; 30: 585–610.

20. Casanueva FF, Molitch ME, Schlechte JA, Abs R, Bonert V, Bronstein MD, et al. Guidelines of the Pituitary Society for the diagnosis and management of prolactinomas. Clin Endcrinol 2006; 65: 265–73.

21. Gillam MP, Molitch MP, Lombardi G, Colao A. Advances in the treatment of prolactinomas. Endocr Rev. 2006; 27: 485–534.

22. Webster J, Piscitelli G, Polli A, Ferrari CI, Ismail I, Scanlon MF. A comparison of cabergoline and bromocriptine in the treatment of hyperprolactinemic amenorrhea. N Engl J Med 1994; 331: 904–9.

23. Bevan JS, Webster J, Burke CW, Scanlon MF. Dopamine agonist and pituitary tumor shrinkage. Endocr Rev 1992; 13: 220–40.

24. Biller BMK, Molitch ME, Vance ML, Cannistaro KB, Davis KR, Simons JA, et al. Treatment of prolactin-secreting macroadenomas with the once-weekly dopamine agonist cabergoline. J Clin Endocrinol Metab 1996; 81: 2338–343.

25. Colao A, DiSarno A, Landi ML Scavuzzo F, Cappabianca P, Pivonello R, et al. Macroprolactinoma shrinkage during cabergoline treatment is greater in naïve patients than in patients pretreated with other dopamine agonists: a prospective study of 110 patients. J Clin Endocrinol Metab 2000; 85: 2247–52.

26. Gemzell C, Wang CF. Outcome of pregnancy in women with pituitary adenoma. Fertil Steril 1979; 31: 363–72.

27. Molitch ME. Pregnancy and the hyperprolactinemic woman. N Engl J Med 1985; 312: 1364–70.

28. Kupersmith MJ, Rosenberg C, Kleinberg D. Visual loss in pregnant women with pituitary adenomas. Ann Intern Med 1994; 121: 473–7.

29. Rossi AM, Vilska S, Heinonen PK. Outcome of pregnancies in women with treated or untreated hyperprolactinemia. Eur J Obstet Gynecol Reprod Biol 1995; 63: 143–6.

30. Musolino NRC, Bronstein MD. Prolactinomas and pregnancy. In: Bronstein MD (ed) Pituitary tumors and pregnancy. Kluwer, Norwell, MA, 2001: 91–108.

31. Liu C, Tyrrell JB. Successful treatment of a large macroprolactinoma with cabergoline during pregnancy. Pituitary 2001; 4: 179–85.

32. Bigazzi M, Ronga R, Lancranjan I, Ferraro S, Branconi F, Buzzoni P, et al. A pregnancy in an acromegalic woman during bromocriptine treatment: effects on growth hormone and prolactin in the maternal, fetal, and amniotic compartments. J Clin Endocrinol Metab 1979; 48: 9–12.

33. Krupp P, Monka C, Richter K. The safety aspects of infertility treatments. Presented at the Second World Congress of Gynecology and Obstetrics, Rio de Janeiro, Brazil, 1988, p9.

34. Krupp P, Monka C. Bromocriptine in pregnancy: safety aspects. Klin Wochenschr 1987; 65: 823–7.

35. Raymond JP, Goldstein E, Konopka P, Leleu MF, Merceron RE, Loria Y. Follow-up of children born of bromocriptine-treated mothers. Horm Res 1985; 22: 239–46.

36. Konopka P, Raymond JP, Merceron RE, Seneze J. Continuous administration of bromocriptine in the prevention of neurological complications in pregnant women with prolactinomas. Am J Obstet Gynecol 1983; 146: 935–8.

37. Buelke-Sam J, Byrd RA, Johnson JA, Tizzano JP, Owen NV. Developmental toxicity of the dopamine agonist pergolide mesylate in CD-1 mice. I: Gestational exposure. Neurotoxicol Teratol 1991; 13: 283–95.

38. De Mari M, Zenzola A, Lamberti P. Antiparkinsonian treatment in pregnancy. Mov Disord 2002; 17: 428–9.

39. Acharya V. Review of pregnancy reports in patients on pergolide treatment, July, 2004. Data on file. Eli Lilly & Co.

40. Morange I, Barlier A, Pellegrini I, Brue T, Enjalbert A, Jaquet P. Prolactinomas resistant to bromocriptine: long-term efficacy of quinagolide and outcome of pregnancy. Eur J Endocrinol 1996; 135: 413–20.

41. Webster J. A comparative review of the tolerability profiles of dopamine agonists in the treatment of hyperprolactinaemia and inhibition of lactation. Drug Safety 1996; 14: 228–38.

42. Robert E, Musatti L, Piscitelli G, Ferrari CI. Pregnancy outcome after treatment with the ergot derivative, cabergoline. Reprod Toxicol 1996; 10: 333–7.

43. Data on file, Pharmacia & Upjohn, 1997.

44. Verhelst J, Abs R, Maiter D, van den Bruel A, Vandeweghe M, Velkeniers B, et al. Cabergoline in the treatment of hyperprolactinemia: a study in 455 patients. J Clin Endocrinol Metab 1999; 84: 2518–22.

45. Ricci E, Parazzini F, Motta T, Ferrari CI, Colao A, Clavenna A, et al. Pregnancy outcome after cabergoline treatment in early weeks of gestation. Reprod Toxicol 2002; 16: 791–3.

46. Musolino NRC, Bronstein MD. Prolactinomas and pregnancy. In: Bronstein MD (ed) Pituitary tumors and pregnancy. Kluwer, Norwell, MA, 2001: 91–108.

47. Brodsky JB, Cohen EN, Brown BW Jr, et al. Surgery during pregnancy and fetal outcome. Am J Obstet Gynecol 1980; 138: 1165–7.

48. Divers WA, Yen SSC. Prolactin-producing microadenomas in pregnancy. Obstet Gynecol 1983; 62: 425–9.

49. Melmed S. Acromegaly. N Engl J Med 2006; 355: 2558–73.

50. Herman-Bonert V, Seliverstow M, Melmed S. Pregnancy in acromegaly: successful therapeutic outcome. J Clin Endocrinol Metab 1998; 83: 727–31.

51. Mozas J, Ocón E, López de la Torre M, Suárez AM, Miranda JA, Herruzo AJ. Successful pregnancy in a woman with acromegaly treated with somatostatin analog (octreotide) prior to surgical resection. Int J Gynecol Obstet 1999; 65: 71–3.

52. DeMenis E, Billeci D, Marton E. Uneventful pregnancy in an acromegalic patient treated with slow-release lanreotide: a case report. J Clin Endocrinol Metab 1999; 84: 1489.

53. Hierl T, Ziegler R, Kasperk C. Pregnancy in persistent acromegaly. Clin Endocrinol 2000; 53: 262–3.

54. Neal JM. Successful pregnancy in a woman with acromegaly treated with octreotide. Endocr Pract 2000; 6: 148–50.

55. Fassnacht M, Capeller B, Arlt W, *et al.* Octreotide LAR treatment throughout pregnancy in an acromegalic woman. Clin Endocrinol 2001; 55: 411–15.

56. Bronstein MD, Salgado LR, Musolino NR. Medical management of pituitary adenomas: the special case of management of the pregnant woman. Pituitary 2002; 5: 99–107.

57. Serri O, Lanoie G. Successful pregnancy in a woman with acromegaly treated with octreotide long-acting release. Endocrinologist 2003; 13: 17–19.

58. Hisano M, Sakata M, Watanabe N, Kitagawa M, Murashima A, Yamaguchi K. An acromegalic woman first diagnosed in pregnancy. Arch Gynecol Obstet 2006; 274: 171–3.

59. Atmaca A, Dagdelen S, Erbas T. Follow-up of pregnancy in acromegalic women: different presentations and outcomes. Exp Clin Endocrinol Diabetes 2006; 114: 135–9.

60. Cozzi R, Attanasio R, Barausee M. Pregnancy in acromegaly: a one-center experience. Eur J Endocrinol 2006; 155: 279–84.

61. Molitch ME. Clinical manifestations of acromegaly. Endocrinol Metab Clin North Am 1992; 21: 597–614.

62. Barkan AL, Stred SE, Reno K, Markovs M, Hopwood NJ, Kelch RP, *et al.* Increased growth hormone pulse frequency in acromegaly. J Clin Endocrinol Metab 1989; 69: 1225–33.

63. Chang-DeMoranville BM, Jackson IMD. Diagnosis and endocrine testing in acromegaly. Endocrinol Metab Clin North Am 1992; 21: 649–68.

64. Okada Y, Morimoto I, Ejima K, Yoshida K, Kashimura M, Fujihira T, *et al.* A case of active acromegalic woman with a marked increase in serum insulin-like growth factor-1 levels after delivery. Endocr J 1997; 44: 117–20.

65. Caron P, Buscail L, Beckers A, Estève J-P, Igout A, Hennen G, *et al.* Expression of somatostatin receptor SST4 in human placenta and absence of octreotide effect on human placental growth hormone concentration during pregnancy. J Clin Endocrinol Metab 1997; 82: 3771–6.

66. Caron P, Gerbeau C, Pradayrol L. Maternal-fetal transfer of octreotide. N Engl J Med 1995; 333: 601–2.

67. Caron P, Gerbeau C, Pradayrol L, Simonetta C, Bayard F. Successful pregnancy in an infertile woman with a thyrotropin-secreting macroadenoma treated with the somatostatin analog (octreotide). J Clin Endocrinol Metab 1996; 81: 1164–8.

68. Blackhurst G, Strachan MW, Collie D, Gregor A, Staatham PF, Seckl JER. The treatment of a thyrotropin-secreting pituitary macroadenoma with octreotide in twin pregnancy. Clin Endocrinol 2002; 56: 401–4.

69. Chaiamnuay S, Moster M, Katz MR, Kim YN. Successful management of a pregnant woman with a TSH secreting pituitary adenoma with surgical and medical therapy. Pituitary 2003; 6: 109–13.

70. Masding MG, Lees PD, Gawne-Cain ML, Sandeman DD. Visual field compression by a non-secreting pituitary tumour during pregnancy. J Roy Soc Med 2003; 96: 27–8.

71. Molitch ME. Clinically non-functioning adenomas. In: Bronstein MD (ed) Pituitary tumors and pregnancy. Kluwer, Norwell, MA, 2001: 123–9.

72. Murata Y, Ando H, Nagasaka T, Takahashi I, Saito K, Fukugaki Y, *et al.* Successful pregnancy after bromocriptine therapy in an anovulatory woman complicated with ovarian hyperstimulation caused by follicle-stimulating hormone-producing plurihormonal pituitary microadenoma. J Clin Endocrinol Metab 2003; 88: 1988–93.

73. Sugita T, Seki K, Nagai Y, Saeki N, Yamaura A, Ohigashi S, *et al.* Successful pregnancy and delivery after removal of gonadotrope adenoma secreting follicle-stimulating hormone in a 29-year-old amenorrheic woman. Gynecol Obstet Invest 2005; 59: 138–43.

74. Golan A, Abramov L, Yedwab G, David MP. Pregnancy in panhypopituitarism. Gynecol Obstet Invest 1990; 29: 232–4.

75. Verdu LI, Martin-Caballero C, Garcia-Lopez G, Cueto MJ. Ovulation induction and normal pregnancy after panhypopituitarism due to lymphocytic hypophysitis. Obstet Gynecol 1998; 91: 850–2.

76. Volz J, Heinrich U, Volz-Köster S. Conception and spontaneous delivery after total hypophysectomy. Fertil Steril 2002; 77: 624–5.

77. Kitajima Y, Endo T, Yamazaki K, Hayashi T, Kudo R. Successful twin pregnancy in panhypopituitarism caused by suprasellar germinoma. Obstet Gynecol 2003; 102: 1205–17.

78. Gompel A, Mauvais-Jarvis P. Induction of ovulation with pulsatile GnRH in hypothalamic amenorrhea. Hum Reprod 1988; 3: 473–7.

79. Martin KA, Hall JE, Adams JM, Crowley WF Jr. Comparison of exogenous gonadotropins and pulsatile gonadotropin-releasing hormone for induction of ovulation in hypogonadotropic amenorrhea. J Clin Endocrinol Metab 1993; 77: 125–9.

80. Hall JE, Martin KA, Whitney HA, Landy H, Crowley WF Jr. Potential for fertility with replacement of hypothalamic gonadotropin-releasing hormone in long term female survivors of cranial tumors. J Clin Endocrinol Metab 1994; 79: 1166–72.

81. Suganuma N, Furuhashi M, Ando T, Assada Y, Mori O, Kurauchi O. Successful pregnancy and delivery after in vitro fertilization and embryo transfer in a patient with primary hypopituitarism. Fertil Steril 2000; 73: 1057–8.

82. Hall R, Manski-Nankervis J, Goni N, Davies MC, Conway GS. Fertility outcomes in women with hypopituitarism. Clin Endocrinol 2006; 65: 71–4.

83. Overton CE, Davis CJ, West C, Davies MC, Conway GS. High risk pregnancies in hypopituitary women. Human Reprod 2002; 17: 1464–7.

84. Mandel SJ, Larsen PR, Seely EW, Brent GA. Increased need for thyroxine during pregnancy in women with primary hypothyroidism. N Engl J Med 1990; 323: 91–6.

85. Beitins IZ, Bayard F, Ances IG, Kowarski A, Migeon CJ. The transplacental passage of prednisone and prednisolone in pregnancy near term. J Pediatr 1972; 81: 936–45.

86. Turner ES, Greenberger PA, Patterson R. Management of the pregnant asthmatic patient. Ann Intern Med 1980; 93: 905–18.

87. Kenny FM, Preeyasombat C, Spaulding JS, Migeon CJ. Cortisol production rate: IV. Infants born of steroid-treated mothers and of diabetic mothers. Infants with trisomy syndrome and with anencephaly. Pediatrics 1966; 37: 960–6.

88. McKenzie SA, Selley JA, Agnew JE. Secretion of prednisolone into breast milk. Arch Dis Child 1975; 50: 894–6.

89. Molitch ME, Clemmons DR, Malozowski S, Merriam GR, Shalet SM, Vance ML. Evaluation and treatment of adult growth hormone deficiency: an Endocrine Society Clinical Practice Guideline. J Clin Endocrinol Metab 2006; 91: 1621–34.

90. Homburg R. Growth hormone and fertility – clinical studies. Horm Res 1996; 45: 81–5.

91. Curran AJ, Peacey SR, Shalet SM. Is maternal growth hormone essential for a normal pregnancy? Eur J Endocrinol 1998; 139: 54–8.

92. Sheehan HL, Davis JC. Pituitary necrosis. Br Med Bull 1968; 24: 59–70.

93. Kelestimur F. Sheehan's syndrome. Pituitary 2003; 6: 181–8.

94. Feinberg E, Molitch M, Endres L, Peaceman A. The incidence of Sheehan's syndrome after obstetric hemorrhage. Fertil Steril 2005; 84: 975–9.

95. Ozbey N, Inanc S, Aral F, et al. Clinical and laboratory evaluation of 40 patients with Sheehan's syndrome. Isr J Med Sci 1994; 30: 826–9.

96. Sheehan HL. The neurohypophysis in post-partum hypopituitarism. J Pathol Bacteriol 1963; 85: 145–69.

97. Iwasaki Y, Oiso Y, Yamauchi K, et al. Neurohypophyseal function in post-partum hypopituitarism: impaired plasma vasopressin response to osmotic stimuli. J Clin Endocrinol Metab 1989; 68: 560–5.

98. Bakiri F, Bendib S-E, Maoui R, et al. The sella turcica in Sheehan's syndrome: computerized tomographic study in 54 patients. J Endocrinol Invest 1991; 14: 193–6.

99. Gillam M, Molitch ME. Lymphocytic hypophysitis. In: Bronstein MD (ed) Pituitary tumors and pregnancy. Kluwer, Norwell, MA, 2001: 131–48.

100. Pressman EK, Zeidman SM, Reddy UM, et al. Differentiating lymphocytic adenohypophysitis from pituitary adenoma in the peripartum patient. J Reprod Med 1995; 40: 251–9.

101. Caturegli P, Newschaffer C, Olivi A, Pomper MG, Burger PC, Rose NR. Autoimmune hypophysitis. Endocr Rev 2005; 26: 599–614.

102. Leiba S, Schindel B, Weinstein R, et al. Spontaneous postpartum regression of pituitary mass with return of function. JAMA 1986; 255: 230–2.

103. McGrail KM, Beyerl BD, Black PM, et al. Lymphocytic adenohypophysitis of pregnancy with complete recovery. Neurosurgery 1987; 20: 791–3.

104. Lindheimer MD, Davison JM. Osmoregulation, the secretion of arginine vasopressin and its metabolism during pregnancy. Eur J Endocrinol 1995; 132: 133–43.

105. Davison JM, Shiells EA, Barron WM, et al. Changes in the metabolic clearance of vasopressin and of plasma vasopressinase throughout human pregnancy. J Clin Invest 1989; 83: 1313–18.

106. Barron WM. Water metabolism and vasopressin secretion during pregnancy. Baillière's Clin Obstet Gynaecol 1987; 1: 853–71.

107. Durr JA. Diabetes insipidus in pregnancy. Am J Kidney Dis 1987; 9: 276–83.

108. Huchon DJR, van Zijl JAWM, Campbell-Brown MB, et al. Desmopressin as a test of urinary concentrating ability in pregnancy. J Obstet Gynecol 1982; 2: 206.

109. Dawood MY, Ylikorkala O, Trivedi D, et al. Oxytocin in maternal circulation and amniotic fluid during pregnancy. J Clin Endocrinol Metab 1979; 49: 429–34.

110. Russell JA, Leng G, Douglas AJ. The magnocellular oxytocin system, the fount of maternity: adaptations in pregnancy. Front Neuroendocrinol 2003; 24: 27–61.

111. Gibbens GLD, Chard T. Observations on maternal oxytocin release during human labor. Am J Obstet Gynecol 1976; 126: 243–6.

112. Dawood MY, Khan-Dawood FS, Wahi R, et al. Oxytocin release and plasma anterior pituitary and gonadal hormones in women during lactation. J Clin Endocrinol Metab 1981; 52: 678–83.

113. Soule SG, Monson JP, Jacobs HS. Transient diabetes insipidus in pregnancy – a consequence of enhanced placental clearance of arginine vasopressin. Hum Reprod 1995; 10: 3322–4.

114. Iwasaki Y, Oiso Y, Kondo K, et al. Aggravation of subclinical diabetes insipidus during pregnancy. N Engl J Med 1991; 324: 522–6.

115. Yamamoto T, Ishii T, Yoshioka K, et al. Transient central diabetes insipidus in pregnancy with a peculiar change in signal intensity on T1-weighted magnetic resonance images. Intern Med 2003; 42: 513–16.

116. Barron WM, Cohen LH, Ulland LA, et al. Transient vasopressin-resistant diabetes insipidus of pregnancy. N Engl J Med 1984; 310: 442–4.

117. Källén BAJ, Carlsson SS, Bengtsson BKA. Diabetes insipidus and use of desmopressin (Minirin) during pregnancy. Eur J Endocrinol 1995; 132: 144–6.

118. Ray JG. DDAVP use during pregnancy: an analysis of its safety for mother and child. Obstet Gynecol Surv 1998; 53: 450–5.

119. Brewster UC, Hayslett JP. Diabetes insipidus in the third trimester of pregnancy. Obstet Gyneol 2005; 105: 1173–6.

120. Kennedy S, Hall PM, Seymour AE, Hague WM. Transient diabetes insipidus and acute fatty liver of pregnancy. Br J Obstet Gynaecol 1994; 101: 387–91.

121. Ellidokuz E, Uslan I, Demir S, Cevrioglu S, Tufan G. Transient postpartum diabetes insipidus associated with HELLP syndrome. J Obstet Gynaecol Res 2006; 32: 602–4.

122. Raziel A, Rosenberg T, Schreyer P, et al. Transient postpartum diabetes insipidus. Am J Obstet Gynecol 1991; 164: 616–18.

123. Hawker RW, North WG, Colbert IC, Lang LP. Oxytocin blood levels in two cases of diabetes insipidus. Br J Obstet Gynaecol 1987; 74: 430–1.

124. Brown MA, Wang J, Whitworth JA. The renin-angiotensin-aldosterone system in preeclampsia. Clin Exp Hypertens 1997; 19: 713–26.

125. Wilson M, Morganti AA, Zervoudakis I, et al. Blood pressure, the renin-aldosterone system and sex steroids throughout normal pregnancy. Am J Med 1980; 8: 97–104.

126. Dorr HG, Heller A, Versmold HT, et al. Longitudinal study of progestins, mineralocorticoids, and glucocorticoids throughout human pregnancy. J Clin Endocrinol Metab 1989; 68: 863–8.

127. Boonshaft B, O'Connell JM, Hayes JM, et al. Serum renin activity during normal pregnancy: effect of alterations of posture and sodium intake. J Clin Endocrinol Metab 1968; 28: 1641–8.

128. Jones KM, Lloyd-Jones R, Riondel A, et al. Aldosterone secretion and metabolism in normal men and women and in pregnancy. Acta Endocrinol 1959; 30: 321–42.

129. Ehrlich EN, Lindheimer MD. Effect of administered mineralocorticoids or ACTH in pregnant women. Attenuation of kaliuretic influence of mineralocorticoids during pregnancy. J Clin Invest 1972; 51: 1301–9.

130. Bevan JS, Gough MH, Gillmer MD Burke CW. Cushings syndrome in pregnancy. The timing of definitive treatment. Clin Endocrinol 1987; 27: 225–33.

131. Casson IF, Davis JC, Jeffreys RV, Silas JH, Williams J, Belchetz PE, et al. Successful management of Cushings disease during pregnancy by transsphenoidal adenectomy. Clin Endocrinol 1987; 27: 423–8.

132. Aron DC, Schnall AM, Sheeler LR. Cushing's syndrome and pregnancy. Am J Obstet Gynecol 1990; 162: 244–52.

133. Buescher MA, McClamrock HD, Adashi EY. Cushings syndrome in pregnancy. Obstet Gynecol 1992; 79: 130–7.

134. Ross RJ, Chew SL, Perry L, Erskine K, Medbak S, Afshar F. Diagnosis and selective cure of Cushing's disease during pregnancy by transsphenoidal surgery. Eur J Endocrinol 1995; 132: 722–6.

135. Chico A, Manzanares JM, Halperin I, Martinez de Osaba MJ, Adelantado J, Webb SM. Cushing's disease and pregnancy. Eur J Obstet Gynecol Reprod Biol 1996; 64: 143–6.

136. Guilhaume B, Sanson ML, Billaud L, Bertagna X, Laudat MH, Luton MP. Cushing's syndrome and pregnancy: aetiologies and prognosis in twenty-two patients. Eur J Med 1992; 1: 83–9.

137. Pinette MG, Pan YQ, Oppenheim D, Pinette SG, Blackstone J. Bilateral inferior petrosal sinus corticotropin sampling with corticotropin-releasing hormone stimulation in a pregnant patient

with Cushing's syndrome. Am J Obstet Gynecol 1994; 171: 563–4.

138. Kreines K, DeVaux WD. Neonatal adrenal insufficiency associated with maternal Cushings syndrome. Pediatrics 1971; 47: 516–19.

139. Amado JA, Pesquera C, Gonzalez EM Otero M, Freijanes J, Alvarez A. Successful treatment with ketoconazole of Cushing's syndrome in pregnancy. Postgrad Med J 1990; 66: 221–3.

140. Berwaerts J, Verhelst J, Mahler C, Abs R. Cushing's syndrome in pregnancy treated by ketoconazole: case report and review of the literature. Gynecol Endocrinol 1999; 13: 175–82.

141. Mellor A, Harvey RD, Pobereskin LH, Sneyd JR. Cushing's disease treated by trans-sphenoidal selective adenomectomy in mid-pregnancy. Br J Anaesth 1998; 80: 850–2.

142. Madhun ZT, Aron DC. Cushing's disease in pregnancy. In: Bronstein MD (ed) Pituitary tumors and pregnancy. Kluwe, Norwell, MA, 2001:149–72.

143. Wallace C, Toth EL, Lewanczuk RZ, Siminoski K. Pregnancy-induced Cushing's syndrome in multiple pregnancies. J Clin Endocrinol Metab 1996; 81: 15–21.

144. Hána V, Dokoupilová M, Marek J, Plavka R. Recurrent ACTH-independent Cushing's syndrome in multiple pregnancies and its treatment with metyrapone. Clin Endocrinol 2001; 54: 277–81.

145. Lindsay JR, Jonklaas J, Oldfield EH, Nieman LK. Cushing's syndrome during pregnancy: personal experience and review of the literature. J Clin Endocrinol Metab 2005; 90: 3077–83.

146. Lindsay JR, Nieman LK. Adrenal disorders in pregnancy. Endocrinol Metab Clin North Am 2006; 35: 1–20.

147. Albert E, Dalaker K, Jorde R, Berge LN. Addison's disease and pregnancy. Acta Obstet Gynecol Scand 1989; 68: 185–7.

148. Drucker D, Shumak S, Angel A. Schmidt's syndrome presenting with intrauterine growth retardation and postpartum Addisonian crisis. Am J Obstet Gynecol 1984; 149: 229–30.

149. Gamlen TR, Aynsley-Green A, Irvine WJ, McCallum CJ. Immunological studies in the neonate of a mother with Addison's disease and diabetes mellitus. Clin Exp Immunol 1977; 28: 192–5.

150. O'Shaughnessy RW, Hackett KJ. Maternal Addison's disease and fetal growth retardation: a case report. J Reprod Med 1984; 29: 752–6.

151. Gradden C, Lawrence D, Doyle PM, et al. Uses of error: Addison's disease in pregnancy. Lancet 2001; 357: 1197.

152. Grottolo A, Ferrari V, Mariano M, et al. Primary adrenal insufficiency, circulating lupus anticoagulant and anticardiolipin antibodies in a patient with multiple abortions and recurrent thrombotic episodes. Haematologica 1988; 73: 517–19.

153. McKenna DS, Wittber GM, Nagaraja HN, et al. The effects of repeat doses of antenatal corticosteroids on maternal adrenal function. Am J Obstet Gynecol 2000; 183: 669–73.

154. Grinspoon SK, Biller BM. Clinical review 62: laboratory assessment of adrenal insufficiency. J Clin Endocrinol Metab 1994; 79(4): 923–31.

155. Nolten WE, Lindheimer MD, Oparil S, et al. Desoxycorticosterone in normal pregnancy: I. sequential studies of the secretory patterns of desoxycorticosterone, aldosterone, and cortisol. Am J Obstet Gynecol 1978; 132: 414–20.

156. Schulte HM, Weisner D, Allolio B. The corticotrophin releasing hormone test in late pregnancy: lack of adrenocortiocotrophin and cortisol response. Clin Endocrinol 1990; 33: 99–106.

157. Nigam R, Bhatia E, Miao D, et al. Prevalence of adrenal antibodies in Addison's disease among north Indian Caucasians. Clin Endocrinol 2003; 59: 593–8.

158. Symonds EM, Craven DJ. Plasma renin and aldosterone in pregnancy complicated by adrenal insufficiency. Br J Obstet Gynaecol 1977; 84: 191–6.

159. Ambrosi B, Barbetta L, Morricone L. Diagnosis and management of Addison's disease during pregnancy. J Endocrinol Invest 2003; 26: 698–702.

160. Normington EA, Davies D. Hypertension and oedema complicating pregnancy in Addison's disease. BMJ 1972; 1: 148–9.

161. Schlaghecke R, Kornely E, Santen RT, Ridderskamp P. The effect of long-term glucocorticoid therapy on pituitary-adrenal responses to exogenous corticotropin-releasing hormone. N Engl J Med 1992; 326: 226–30.

162. Kream J, Mulay S, Fukushima DK, et al. Determination of plasma dexamethasone in the mother and the newborn after administration of the hormone in a clinical trial. J Clin Endocrinol Metab 1983; 56: 127–33.

163. Sidhu RK, Hawkins DR. Prescribing in pregnancy: corticosteroids. Clin Obstet Gynaecol 1981; 8: 383–404.

164. Garner PR. Congenital adrenal hyperplasia in pregnancy. Semin Perinatol 1998; 22: 446–56.

165. Speiser PW, White PC. Congenital adrenal hyperplasia. N Engl J Med 2003; 349: 776–88.

166. Forest MG. Recent advances in the diagnosis and management of congenital adrenal hyperplasia due to 21-hydroxylase deficiency. Hum Reprod Update 2004; 10: 469–85.

167. New MI, Carlson A, Obeid J, et al. Prenatal diagnosis for congenital adrenal hyperplasia in 532 pregnancies. J Clin Endocrinol Metab 2001; 86: 5651–7.

168. Premawardhana LDKE, Hughes IA, Read GF, Scanlon MF. Longer term outcome in females with congenital adrenal hyperplasia (CAH): the Cardiff experience. Clin Endocrinol 1997; 46: 327–32.

169. Feldman S, Billaud L, Thalabard J-C, et al. Fertility in women with late onset adrenal hyperplasia due to 21-hydroxylase deficiency. J Clin Endocrinol Metab 1992; 74: 635–9.

170. Klingensmith GJ, Garcia SC, Jones HW, Migeon CJ, Blizzard RM. Glucocorticoid treatment of girls with congenital adrenal hyperplasia: effect of height, sexual maturity, and fertility. J Pediatr 1977; 90: 996–1004.

171. Krone N, Wachter I, Stafanidou M, Roscher AA, Schwarz HP. Mothers with congenital adrenal hyperplasia and their children: outcome of pregnancy, birth and childhood. Clin Endocrinol 2001; 55: 523–9.

172. Azziz R, DeWailly D, Owerbach D. Nonclassic adrenal hyperplasia: current concepts. J Clin Endocrinol Metab 1994; 78: 810–15.

173. New MI, Lorenzen F, Lerner AJ, et al. Genotyping steroid 21-hydroxylase deficiency: hormonal reference data. J Clin Endocrinol Metab 1983; 57: 320–6.

174. Pang A, Pollack MS, Marshall RN, Immken LD. Prenatal treatment of congenital adrenal hyperplasia due to 21-hydroxylase deficiency. N Engl J Med 1990; 322: 111–15.

175. Pang S, Clark AT, Freeman LC, et al. Maternal side effects of prenatal dexamethasone therapy for fetal congenital adrenal hyperplasia. J Clin Endocrinol Metab 1992; 75: 249–53.

176. Coleman MA, Honour JW. Reduced maternal dexamethasone dosage for the prenatal treatment of congenital adrenal hyperplasia. Br J Obstet Gynaecol 2004; 111: 176–8.

177. New MI, Carlson A, Obeid J, Marshall I, Cabrera MS, Goseco A, et al. Update: prenatal diagnosis for congenital adrenal hyperplasia in 595 pregnancies. Endocrinologist 2003; 13: 233–9.

178. Forest MG, Dörr HG. Prenatal therapy in congenital adrenal hyperplasia due to 21-hydroxylase deficiency: retrospective follow-up study of 253 treated pregnancies in 215 families. Endocrinologist 2003; 13: 252–9.

179. Baron F, Sprauve ME, Huddleston JF, Fisher AJ. Diagnosis and surgical treatment of primary aldosteronism in pregnancy: a case report. Obstet Gynecol 1995; 86: 644–5.

180. Solomon CG, Thiet M-P, Moore F Jr, Seely EW. Primary hyperaldosteronism in pregnancy. A case report. J Reprod Med 1996; 41: 255–8.

181. Webb JC, Bayliss P. Pregnancy complicated by primary hyperaldosteronism. South Med J 1997; 90: 243–5.

182. Robar CA, Poremba JA, Pelton JJ, et al. Current diagnosis and management of aldosterone-producing adenomas during pregnancy. Endocrinologist 1998; 8: 403–8.

183. Okawa T, Asano K, Hashimoto T, et al. Diagnosis and management of primary aldosteronism in pregnancy: case report and review of the literature. Am J Perinatol 2002; 19: 31–6.

184. Wyckoff JA, Seely EW, Hurwitz S, et al. Glucocorticoid-remediable aldosteronism and pregnancy. Hypertension 2000; 35: 668–72.

185. Fujiyama S, Mori Y, Matsubara H, et al. Primary aldosteronism with aldosterone-producing adrenal adenoma in a pregnant woman. Intern Med 1999; 38: 36–9.

186. Neerhof MG, Shlossman PA, Poll DS, et al. Idiopathic aldosteronism in pregnancy. Obstet Gynecol 1991; 78: 489–91.

187. Matsumoto J, Miyake H, Isozaki T, et al. Primary aldosteronism in pregnancy. J Nippon Med Sch 2000; 67: 275–9.

188. Deruelle P, Dufour P, Magnenant E, et al. Maternal Bartter's syndrome in pregnancy treated by amiloride. Eur J Obstet Gynecol Reprod Biol 2004; 115: 106–7.

189. Nezu M, Miura Y, Noshiro T, Inoue M. Primary aldosteronism as a cause of severe postpartum hypertension in two women. Am J Obstet Gynecol 2000; 182: 745–6.

190. Murakami T, Ogura EW, Tanaka Y, Yamamoto M. High blood pressure lowered by pregnancy. Lancet 2000; 356: 1980.

191. Freier DT, Thompson NW. Pheochromocytoma and pregnancy: the epitome of high risk. Surgery 1993; 114: 1148–52.

192. Botchan A, Hauser R, Kupfermine M, et al. Pheochromocytoma in pregnancy: case report and review of the literature. Obstet Gynecol Surv 1995; 50: 321–7.

193. Levin N, McTighe A, Abdel-Aziz MIE. Extra-adrenal pheochromocytoma in pregnancy. Maryland State Med J 1983; 32: 377–9.

194. Oishi S, Sato T. Pheochromocytoma in pregnancy: a review of the Japanese literature. Endocr J 1994; 41: 219–25.

195. Lau P, Permezel M, Dawson P, et al. Phaeochromocytoma in pregnancy. Aust NZ J Obstet Gynaecol 1996; 36: 472–6.

196. Saarikoski S. Fate of noradrenaline in the human fetoplacental unit. Acta Physiol Scand 1974; 421(suppl): 1–84.

197. Dahia PLM, Hayashida CY, Strunz C, Abelin N, Toledo SPA. Low cord blood levels of catecholamine from a newborn of a pheochromocytoma patient. Eur J Endocrinol 1994; 130: 217–19.

198. Barzel US, Barlian Z, Runmery G, et al. Pheochromocytoma and pregnancy. Am J Obstet Gynecol 164; 89: 519–21.

199. Bakri YN, Ingemansson SE, Ali A, Parikh S. Pheochromocytoma and pregnancy: report of three cases. Acta Obstet Gynecol Scand 1992; 71: 301–4.

200. Harper MA, Murnaghan GA, Kennedy L, Hadden DR, Atkinson AB. Phaeochromocytoma in pregnancy: five cases and a review of the literature. Br J Obstet Gynaecol 1989; 96: 594–606.

201. Combs CA, Easterling TR, Schmucker BC. Hemodynamic observations during paroxysmal hypertension in a pregnancy with pheochromocytoma. Obstet Gynecol 1989; 74: 439–41.

202. Falterman CJ, Kreisberg R. Pheochromocytoma: clinical diagnosis and management. South Med J 1982; 75: 321–9.

203. Kalff V, Shapiro B, Lloyd R, et al. The spectrum of pheochromocytoma in hypertensive patients with neurofibromatosis. Arch Intern Med 1982; 142: 2092–8.

204. Kothari A, Bethune M, Manwaring J, Astley N, Wallace E. Massive bilateral phaeochromocytomas in association with von Hippel Lindau syndrome in pregnancy. Aust NZ J Obstet Gynaecol 1999; 39: 381–4.

205. Freier DT, Eckhauser FE, Harrison TS. Pheochromocytoma. Arch Surg 1980; 115: 388–91.

206. Sheps SG, Jiang NS, Klee GC. Diagnostic evaluation of pheochromocytoma. Endocrinol Metab Clin North Am 1988; 17: 397–414.

207. Pederson EB, Rasmussen AB, Christensen NJ, et al. Plasma noradrenaline and adrenaline in pre-eclampsia, essential hypertension in pregnancy and normotensive pregnant control subjects. Acta Endocrinol 1982; 99: 594–600.

208. Khatun S, Kanayama N, Hossain B, El Maradny E, Kobayashi T, Jahan S, et al. Increased concentrations of plasma epinephrine and norepinephrine in patients with eclampsia. Eur J Obstet Gynecol Repord Biol 1997; 74: 103–9.

209. Santeiro ML, Stromquist C, Wyble L. Phenoxybenzamine placental transfer during the third trimester. Ann Pharmacother 1996; 30: 1249–51.

210. Lyons CW, Colmorgen GHC. Medical management of pheochromocytoma in pregnancy. Obstet Gynecol 1988; 72: 450–1.

211. Ahlawat SK, Jain S, Kumari S, Varma S, Sharma BK. Pheochromocytoma associated with pregnancy: case report and review of the literature. Obstet Gynecol Surv 1999; 54: 728–37.

212. Aplin SC, Yee KF, Cole MJ. Neonatal effects of long-term maternal phenoxybenzamine therapy. Anesthesiology 2004; 100: 1608–10.

213. Devoe LD, O'Dell BE, Castillo RA, Hadi HA, Searle N. Metastatic pheochromocytoma in pregnancy and fetal biophysical assessment after maternal administration of alpha-adrenergic, beta-adrenergic, and dopamine antagonists. Obstet Gynecol 1986; 68(suppl 3):15S–18S.

214. Chatterjee TK, Parekh U. Phaeochromocytoma in pregnancy. Aust NZ J Obstet Gynaecol 1985; 25: 290–1.

215. Finkenstedt G, Gasser RW, Hofle G, et al. Pheochromocytoma and sub-clinical Cushing's syndrome during pregnancy: diagnosis, medical pre-treatment and cure by laparoscopic unilateral adrenalectomy. J Endocrinol Invest 1999; 22: 551–7.

216. Schenker JG, Granat M. Phaeochromocytoma and pregnancy – an updated appraisal. Aust NZ J Obstet Gynaecol 1982; 22: 1–10.

217. Schenker JG, Chowers I. Pheochromocytoma and pregnancy: review of 89 cases. Obstet Gynecol Surv 1971; 26: 739–47.

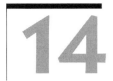

14 Calcium metabolism and diseases of the parathyroid glands during pregnancy

Martin N. Montoro and T. Murphy Goodwin

Departments of Medicine and Obstetrics and Gynecology, Keck School of Medicine, University of Southern California, Los Angeles, CA, USA

Calcium and phosphate homeostasis during pregnancy and lactation

Pregnancy

Pregnancy increases the requirement for many nutrients, including minerals. If exogenous sources are insufficient, the mother's system will be called upon to satisfy the demands. In particular, the maternal calcium storage found in bone mass is available, and therefore potentially vulnerable.

Calcium

Approximately 50% of the total serum calcium is protein bound, and 50% is a free (unbound) ionized fraction. The binding is predominantly to albumin, some to immunoglobulins, and a small fraction to phosphate, citrate, sulfate or other anions. Early in gestation, there is a fall in the total serum calcium which is not considered to be metabolically important, because it is a consequence of a decreased serum albumin level due to hemodilution. The biologic activity of calcium relates to its free (unbound) ionized fraction which remains constant throughout pregnancy [1]. Since the binding is largely to albumin, variations in albumin concentration will alter the total serum calcium level and could lead to misinterpretation unless corrective calculations are performed. In general, the plasma total calcium concentration falls by 0.8 mg/dL (0.02 mmol/L) for every 1.0 g/dL (1 g/L) fall in the plasma concentration of albumin. The formula to determine the corrected total calcium level in the context of a low albumin that is often used is as follows:

> Corrected calcium in conventional (US) units, i.e. mg/dL = measured total calcium in mg/dL + (0.8 × (4.0 − [albumin in g/dL]))

de Swiet's Medical Disorders in Obstetric Practice, 5th edition. Edited by R. O. Powrie, M. F. Greene, W. Camann. © 2010 Blackwell Publishing.

> Corrected calcium in SI units, i.e. mmol/L = measured total calcium in mmol/L + (0.02 × (40 − albumin measured in g/L))

However, these calculations give only a rough estimate of the actual free or ionized calcium, which is the main concern. Since most clinical laboratories now measure ionized calcium readily, it is recommended that ionized calcium be measured directly whenever there is a question of whether a pregnant patient has an abnormal calcium rather than relying on the estimations provided by these or similar formulas.

The total body calcium content is 1000–2000 g, and 99% of the calcium in the body of adult individuals is in the skeleton. About 200–400 mg of calcium are absorbed daily by active transport from the proximal small bowel in the nonpregnant adult. During pregnancy, however, intestinal absorption increases twofold, particularly during the third trimester [2–4]. Increased intestinal calcium absorption is already present at 12 weeks, which is the earliest gestational age that has been studied. It is associated with higher serum levels of 1-alpha-25-dihydroxyvitamin D ($1\alpha,25\text{-}(OH)_2D_3$) as well as increased intestinal expression of the vitamin D-dependent calcium-binding protein calbindin-9K. Prolactin (PRL) and human placental lactogen (HPL) are believed to be other factors contributing to the increased intestinal calcium absorption. Because the increased intestinal calcium absorption starts so early in gestation and well before the peak demands of the third trimester, it is thought that some calcium is stored in the maternal skeleton in anticipation for subsequent demands. The fetus accumulates about 30 g of calcium and 16 g of phosphorus in its own tissues; 80% of the total fetal calcium accumulation takes place in the third trimester, which is when fetal skeletal growth is maximal. At that time, 250–300 mg of calcium are deposited daily into the fetal skeleton. Without an anticipatory rise in calcium absorption, the increased needs would have to be drawn from the maternal skeleton, and some of it probably is. Current research indicates that the major adaptation to the increased calcium demands during pregnancy is the higher intestinal calcium absorption with, perhaps, some contribution from the maternal skeleton [5].

The daily dietary calcium requirement during pregnancy is 1200 mg, which is 400 mg higher than outside pregnancy [6]. Some women do increase their dietary calcium during pregnancy [7], but there is concern that the calcium intake of most women may be less than the recommended 1200 mg/day [6,8].

Under normal circumstances, 98% of calcium filtered by the kidney is reabsorbed, mostly in the proximal tubules. However, in pregnancy the urinary calcium excretion is higher than outside pregnancy and correlates with the increased glomerular filtration rate (GFR) [9]. The increased urinary calcium excretion has also been detected as early as 12 weeks of gestation. Besides the higher GFR of pregnancy, the increased intestinal calcium absorption and the higher calcitonin (CT) levels of pregnancy are believed to be contributing factors favoring renal calcium excretion.

Early in gestation fetal serum calcium concentration is lower than the maternal serum calcium [10] but at term, fetal levels exceed the maternal for both total [10,11] and free ionized calcium [12]. The fetal calcium concentration increases from 5.5 mg/dL (1.37 mmol/L) in early pregnancy to 11 mg/dL (2.75 mmol/L) at term. Therefore calcium is transported across the placenta against a gradient indicating the existence of an active transport mechanism [13]. At present, a parathyroid hormone-related protein (PTHrP) is considered to be the most likely candidate for this role [14]. It may be of placental origin [15] and some may be produced in the mammary glands [16], but the exact source or sources of this peptide or in what proportion each contributes to the maternal circulation have not been conclusively established [17] (see PTHrP section below).

Phosphorus

Of the approximately 600 g of total body phosphorus, 85% is in the skeleton and the remainder is a major intracellular component. In contrast to calcium, about 88% of inorganic phosphate is free and not protein bound. The normal levels in adults are 2.5–4.5 mg/dL (0.81–1.45 mmol/L). Phosphate concentration is labile and may change rapidly by as much as 50% on a given day. There is a normal daily variation with a nadir between 7 and 10 am. Food intake also has a major effect and after eating, plasma phosphate falls because it enters the cells, along with glucose, under the influence of insulin. Therefore, samples for phosphate estimation should be taken early in the morning with the patient fasting.

Phosphate is abundant in normal foods. Its absorption is very efficient, 65% by the small intestine, and it may increase to 85–90% through stimulation by $1\alpha,25\text{-}(OH)_2D_3$. Dietary deprivation, short of actual starvation, does not lead to deficiency. Nevertheless, nonabsorbable antacids, if taken in large amounts, can interfere with phosphate absorption by binding

it in the intestinal lumen. Under normal circumstances, the daily requirement of 500–1000 mg is easily satisfied by gastrointestinal absorption.

The kidney plays a major role in regulating phosphate balance. After glomerular filtration, 80–90% of phosphate is reabsorbed in the proximal tubules. A rise in plasma phosphate is countered by increased renal excretion. Bone uptake and release of phosphate also contribute to homeostasis, but the renal mechanism predominates.

Inorganic phosphorus economy in pregnancy is based upon an increase in its renal tubular reabsorption, and also by enhanced intestinal absorption mediated by $1\alpha,25\text{-}(OH)_2D_3$ [18]. This is important as inorganic phosphorus, no less than calcium, is essential for the growing fetus.

Vitamin D

The healing effect of ultraviolet light on bone lesions caused by rickets was recognized in 1919. Soon afterwards, it was demonstrated that sunlight activates a sterol in the skin that was labeled the "antirachitic agent." This process is the photochemical conversion of 7-dehydrocholesterol to cholecalciferol or vitamin D3 after the skin is exposed to ultraviolet radiation. Although the diet also contributes to the body stores of vitamin D, it does so to a lesser extent and about 90% of circulating vitamin D is skin derived [19]. Absorption from the proximal small intestine is aided by bile salts as it is for other fat-soluble vitamins. Natural dietary sources include fish oils, eggs, and liver. Fortified cereals and dairy products are increasingly being relied upon. Animal sources provide vitamin D3 while plant sources yield vitamin D2 (ergocalciferol). Vitamin D2 is 30% less effective than vitamin D3 in maintaining adequate serum 25-hydroxyvitamin D (25-OHD) levels, and therefore larger doses will have to be administered when vitamin D2 is used instead of vitamin D3 [20,21].

More recently, there has been more reliance on dietary sources due to overall reduced sun exposure as modern lifestyle changes lead to less time spent outdoors, widespread use of sun-blocking creams to reduce the risk of skin cancer, dress style, and residing in latitudes with reduced sunlight. Studies from many countries are reporting a high prevalence of vitamin D deficiency not only in the general population but also in women of childbearing age during pregnancy and lactation [22–24]. There is also a growing consensus that current vitamin D intake is insufficient in populations with reduced exposure to sunlight and increasing concern not only about calcium and bone metabolism but also about preventing other diseases. Interest is accumulating in the many extraskeletal actions of vitamin D, including immune maintenance which might help to prevent autoimmune disorders (multiple sclerosis, systemic lupus erythematosus, rheumatoid arthritis, etc.), certain cancers (breast, colon, ovarian), type 2 diabetes, asthma, and several other chronic conditions as well. Paradoxically, the mounting knowledge about the many potential health benefits of vitamin D, beyond its actions on the skeleton, is occurring at the same time that vitamin D deficiency is becoming more widespread [23,24].

From the skin, cholecalciferol (vitamin D3) is transported bound to a specific vitamin D-binding alpha-globulin, which is synthesized in the liver. Also in the liver, vitamin D3 is hydroxylated, its first metabolic activation step to 25-hydroxycholecalciferol (25-OH vitamin D), which is the dominant form of both the circulating and stored vitamin D. The serum concentration of 25-OH vitamin D is an index of vitamin D nutritional status. However, vitamin D in this form is not metabolically active and for that purpose it has to be converted in the kidneys to the biologically active metabolite. The same alpha-globulin carrier protein transports 25-OH vitamin D to the kidney, the only known site of the 1-alpha-hydroxylase enzyme in the nonpregnant state, although there are extrarenal sites in pregnancy, the placenta in particular [25–27]. Hydroxylation takes place in cells of the proximal convoluted tubule producing $1\alpha,25\text{-}(OH)_2D_3$ which is the most potent vitamin D metabolite. Its serum concentration is 1000 times less than that of 25-OH vitamin D but, in its absence, the syndrome of vitamin D deficiency develops. As it is synthesized in the kidney, secreted into the bloodstream, and exerts its chief effects elsewhere in the body, it could correctly be regarded as a hormone.

The prime function of $1\alpha,25\text{-}(OH)_2D_3$ is to sustain plasma levels of calcium and phosphate which allow mineralization of newly forming bone. Vitamin D acts on at least three target organs: intestine, bone and kidney. Its major function is in the small intestine, where it induces synthesis of brush border calbindin-9K proteins that bind calcium and phosphate, promoting their active transport from the intestinal lumen to the bloodstream. In the absence of vitamin D, the intestinal absorption of these ions decreases almost completely. There is growing evidence to suggest that besides promoting intestinal absorption, skeletal mobilization, and renal tubular reabsorption of calcium, $1\alpha,25\text{-}(OH)_2D_3$ has many other actions. These include an antiproliferative effect on several cell types, such as keratinocytes and certain cancer cells [23,24,28]. An important effect relevant to pregnancy is related to mediation in the immune tolerance needed to maintain gestation [29,30].

The gestational increase in $1\alpha,25\text{-}(OH)_2D_3$ indicates that maternal 1-alpha-hydroxylase enzymatic activity is stimulated. This increase seems to be largely unrelated to parathyroid hormone (PTH) levels which decrease in early pregnancy and increase, but only to the mid-normal range, by term [31–33]. Under these conditions a lower concentration of $1\alpha,25\text{-}(OH)_2D_3$ should be expected. Therefore, other factors must be operating during pregnancy responsible for the upregulation of 1-alpha-hydroxylase activity and the gradual increase of $1\alpha,25\text{-}(OH)_2D_3$ that reaches levels that are twice as high as in nonpregnant women. These other factors include estradiol, PRL, HPL and particularly PTHrP

[14,15,17]. The maternal kidneys are believed to account for most of the increased levels of $1\alpha,25\text{-}(OH)_2D_3$ which persists until delivery. The decidua, placenta and fetal kidneys might contribute small amounts.

Parathyroid hormone

The physiologic function of PTH is to regulate and maintain calcium concentration within narrow limits. Its effects are mediated by intracellular cyclic adenosine monophosphate (cAMP). Any fall in ionized calcium is countered by secretion of PTH. The fall in calcium is checked by the direct effects of PTH on bone and kidney, and its indirect stimulation of intestinal calcium absorption mediated by $1\alpha,25\text{-}(OH)_2D_3$ [34].

In bone, PTH stimulates the activity of osteoclasts and osteoblasts with a predominant effect on bone resorption and calcium and phosphate mobilization. As it stimulates secretion of osteoclast collagenases and similar lytic enzymes, it acts to accomplish metabolic destruction of the bony matrix. This is reflected in increased urinary and plasma hydroxyproline. Remodeling activity is also stimulated, but osteoclast function predominates [35].

In the kidney, PTH inhibits phosphate reabsorption by the proximal tubule. Phosphate released from bone is thereby rapidly excreted with resulting hypophosphatemia and hyperphosphaturia in states of PTH excess. PTH is also the main factor regulating 1-alpha-hydroxylase activity, the enzyme involved in the conversion of 25-(OH) vitamin D to $1\alpha,25\text{-}(OH)_2D_3$ which also takes place in the proximal renal tubules, although during pregnancy this activity might be predominantly exerted by PTHrP rather than by PTH. Therefore, PTH has a major effect on the renal clearance and reabsorption of calcium. If the flood of calcium from bone exceeds the capacity for calcium reabsorption, hypercalciuria ensues. PTH also inhibits proximal tubular reabsorption of bicarbonate, so that states of PTH excess are often accompanied by a mild metabolic acidosis [34].

Initial studies on PTH levels in pregnancy reported contradictory results, with some showing an increase [36,37], no change [9,38] or a decrease [39,40,41]. A previous notion that pregnancy was a state of "mild physiologic hyperparathyroidism" seems to have been an artifact of earlier, less valid measurement methods. Studies measuring the intact PTH molecule by means of a two-site immunoradiometric assay (IRMA) show a decrease to the low-normal range in the first trimester and a gradual increase to the mid-normal range by term [1,4,5,17,18,31–33,42,43].

Parathyroid hormone-related protein

This is a peptide with PTH-like activity first recognized as a protein from some malignant tumors with humoral hypercalcemia. Although different from PTH, it shares enough amino acid sequences in its structure to bind effectively to PTH receptors and to have some of its physiologic actions as well, including the bone-resorbing, phosphaturic and hypocalciuric effects [44,45].

PTHrP levels increase during the late pregnancy stages. The origin of this peptide in pregnancy is probably multifactorial and the proportional amounts contributed by each possible source have not been determined. It is produced by tissues in both the mother and fetus, including the placenta, amnion, decidua, umbilical cord, breasts and fetal parathyroid glands. It may also be involved in embryogenesis, fetal differentiation and growth [46,47], onset of labor [48], milk production [49], maternal–fetal calcium transfer [13,14,50] and protection of the maternal skeleton during pregnancy [51,52]. PTHrP is thought to contribute to the higher $1\alpha,25$-$(OH)_2D_3$ and to the lower PTH levels during pregnancy. The protective effect on the maternal skeleton is thought to be related to a five amino acid fragment in its carboxyl-terminal section [51,52]. Adequate levels of PTHrP might also be protective against premature labor because of its smooth muscle relaxant properties which favor uterine stretching. PTHrP levels fall very rapidly after the rupture of the fetal membranes, thus allowing labor to proceed [48,53].

Calcitonin

Calcitonin is secreted by the parafollicular C cells of the thyroid. Its output is stimulated by a rise in ionized calcium concentration; hypocalcemia, on the other hand, has the opposite effect. The calcium-lowering effect of calcitonin is accompanied by a fall in serum phosphate, and both probably result from a direct inhibition of bone breakdown. Calcitonin also inhibits the bone reabsorption produced by a number of substances, including PTH and vitamin D metabolites. However, in medullary carcinoma of the thyroid, where there is hypersecretion of calcitonin, there are no overt bony changes and no disturbances of calcium or phosphate levels. An intriguing observation has been that of osteopetrosis in the newborn babies of women with medullary thyroid carcinoma, but this may represent genetic linkage of two disorders rather than a calcitonin effect [54]. Calcitonin levels increase during pregnancy and it is possible that, in addition to the amounts secreted by the parafollicular C cells of the thyroid, the placenta and breast tissues may contribute to its circulating levels. The action of CT is antagonistic to that of PTH, but it is not yet known if it might act as a protector of the maternal skeleton during pregnancy. In a mouse animal model lacking CT, increased skeletal mineral content during pregnancy was not impaired [55].

Bone changes during pregnancy

Animal experiments in rodents suggest that there is a net increase of 5–10% in mineral skeletal content during pregnancy. However, studies in humans have not been clear-cut

in this regard. Publications reporting studies on the serum indices of bone formation (bone-specific alkaline phosphatase, osteocalcin, procollagen I and carboxypeptidase) and urine markers of bone resorption (24-hour collection of deoxypyridinoline, hydroxyproline and pyridinoline) indicate that bone formation indices are decreased and bone resorption markers are increased. Based on those results, it has been assumed that there is decreased bone formation and accelerated bone resorption. However, these studies have been criticized because of their failure to account for the effects of the hemodilution as well as the increased GFR of pregnancy on the serum and urine concentration of those markers, among other confounding variables. Therefore they may not be accurate indicators of bone metabolism in pregnant women [17].

One prospective study using X-ray spectrophotometry showed a small but significant loss of mineral from trabecular but not cortical bone during pregnancy [56]. Ultrasonic bone propagation velocity was used in two studies scanning the proximal phalanges of fingers [57] and the os calcis [58,59] which showed a small but significant fall in bone mineral density (BMD) in the third trimester. It has also been noted that women with low calcium intake have significantly lower bone density in the third trimester than women with adequate calcium intake [57].

In a longitudinal study using dual energy X-ray absorptiometry (DEXA) in 10 women from preconception to post partum, BMD decreased 3.5% at the hip and 2% at the lumbar spine but forearm density did not change significantly [60]. Another study [61] also measured DEXA at various sites before, during and after pregnancy. BMD in pelvis and lumbar spine densities fell by 3.2% and 4.6% respectively. In a prospective cohort study of 49 women in Sweden, BMD of the forearm fell by about 1% between 12 weeks gestation and 5 months post partum. In a small study [62] of six women, BMD decreased about 3% in the femoral neck, radius and lumbar spine between 6 weeks before and 6 months after pregnancy when compared to 25 nonpregnant women matched for age, weight, height, calcium intake and activity level.

The studies using ultrasound or DEXA measurements suggest that there may be a small loss of bone mineral content of 1–4% in the pelvis and lumbar spine. However, these reports have not been able to elucidate whether or not there is an increase in BMD earlier in pregnancy in anticipation of the higher third-trimester demands when the calcium transfer to the fetus is most active and as suggested by animal studies. In addition, the postpartum measurements in some of those studies took place some time after delivery and might have measured the bone density losses that occur in the puerperium in lactating women rather than losses that took place exclusively during pregnancy.

Prospective studies using either single or dual-photon absorptiometry have not found significant change in bone density during pregnancy [5].

Changes during lactation

Human milk contains two to three times the maternal serum level of calcium, and it is estimated that between 280 and 400 mg of calcium go into breast milk daily [63]. Women breastfeeding twins might lose up to 1000 mg per day. During the first 6 months after delivery the mean calcium concentration in breast milk is slightly higher than during the succeeding 6 months but calcium loss in breast milk remains significant throughout lactation [64]. Calcium losses during lactation are even greater than in late pregnancy when calcium transfer to the fetus is greatly increased. Studies of skeletal calcium metabolism indicate that there are great demands on the maternal skeleton during lactation and bone loss may be as high as 1–3% per month [65,66].

Calcium and phosphorus

Serum levels of ionized calcium are higher than during pregnancy but do not exceed the upper normal range. Urinary calcium excretion decreases during lactation [67]. Serum phosphorus levels are also higher during lactation due to increased renal tubular reabsorption and increased bone resorption, besides the amounts obtained from the diet.

Vitamin D

The high levels of $1\alpha,25$-$(OH)_2D_3$ decrease rapidly after delivery and remain in the normal range afterwards [68].

Parathyroid hormone

Serum PTH levels are also lower during lactation but increase after weaning, sometimes even above normal. PTH is believed to play an important role in the rapid recovery of bone mass that takes place after weaning and also in the renal conservation of calcium and phosphorus [67,69].

Parathyroid hormone-related protein

The most striking of the hormonal changes observed during lactation is the marked increase in PTHrP levels in breast milk. PTHrP is produced by mammary tissue and appears to regulate calcium transfer into breast milk [70,71]. Prolactin seems to be an important factor regulating mammary PTHrP production in conjunction with local mammary factors [72]. The combination of high PTHrP and prolactin with rapidly decreasing estrogen levels is believed to be the main reason for the skeletal changes in lactating women [73]. It is estimated that lactation causes a 3–10% decline in bone mineral content after breastfeeding for 6 months, as reported by studies measuring serial bone density changes. The loss is greater in trabecular than in cortical bone [7,39,65,66]. Taller women have been reported to have greater bone loss during lactation [7,74]. Additional calcium intake does not seem to prevent bone loss during lactation or accelerate the recovery after weaning. Even in cases of low calcium intake, skeletal recovery after weaning still occurs, although there is concern that in adolescents with habitually low calcium intake, bone recovery may not be sufficient to attain peak bone mass at maturity [75].

In general, bone density is regained rapidly after weaning, and recovery of bone is complete for most women even when there are short intervals in between pregnancies [76,77].

Calcitonin

Calcitonin seems to have an important role during lactation acting as protector of the maternal skeleton against excessive bone resorption during this period of rapid demineralization [78].

Vitamin D deficiency

Diagnosis

Vitamin D deficiency in the general population appears to be more widespread than previously thought. Insufficient amounts of vitamin D alter calcium and phosphorus metabolism and cause diminished mineralization of the collagen matrix, which results in rickets in children and osteomalacia in adults [23]. The many extraskeletal actions of vitamin D have already been described above.

Vitamin D deficiency is generally defined as a 25-hydroxyvitamin D serum level of <20 ng/mL (<50 nmol/L). Levels of 21–29 ng/mL (50–75 nmol/L) point to relative insufficiency and ≥30 ng/mL (>75 nmol/L) are indicative of sufficient amounts. Levels of 150 ng/mL (375 nmol/L) or higher are considered toxic [79,80].

Deficiency of vitamin D has also been reported to occur frequently during pregnancy and lactation [29,81–83]. Vitamin D deficiency *in utero* may cause growth retardation, skeletal deformities, and impaired first-year growth as well as teeth enamel defects and higher risk of fractures later in life. Neonatal hypocalcemia and, rarely, even convulsions from tetany have also been reported [84–86]. Overt clinical osteomalacia with bone fractures in the mother, or delivery of an infant with florid rickets at birth, has been described as presenting features of vitamin D deficiency [87–91], but these are now unusual presentations. More often, the vitamin D deficiency is less severe and usually there are no overt maternal clinical symptoms. However, even in these milder cases the fetus develops in a state of hypovitaminosis D which is likely to have an effect on immune function, fetal and childhood bone development and increased risk of other childhood chronic conditions [23].

Vitamin D insufficiency appears to be common even in otherwise healthy appearing pregnant women [29,81–83,92].

Some women are more likely to have children with complications, and it has been reported that 50% of the newborns of strict vegetarians have hypocalcemia [84,93–95]. Other causes of vitamin D deficiency include reduced skin synthesis because of lack of exposure to sunlight when residing in certain geographical latitudes, from sunscreen use or from wearing clothing that completely covers the skin [96].

Other causes of vitamin D deficiency include the following.

Decreased bio-availability

Decreased bio-availability of vitamin D may occur because of intestinal malabsorption in cases of celiac disease, cystic fibrosis, Whipple's disease, Crohn's disease, intestinal bypass surgery and medications that reduce cholesterol absorption [97]. In obesity vitamin D may remain sequestered in body fat. Obese pregnant women and their neonates have been reported to have increased risk of vitamin D deficiency [98].

Increased catabolism

Long-term use of certain medications including anticonvulsants (e.g. phenytoin, carbamazepine, phenobarbital), glucocorticoids, some anti-AIDS medications, antirejection medications and the antimicrobial agent rifampin can cause vitamin D deficiency by inducing the catabolism of $1\alpha,25$-$(OH)_2D_3$. They do so by activating the steroid and xenobiotic (foreign substances found in the body) receptor known as pregnane X receptor. Pregnane X receptor is a nuclear receptor that senses and responds to the presence of foreign toxic substances by upregulating the expression of proteins involved in their detoxification and clearance [99–104]. This effect can be significant enough to cause osteomalacia.

Decreased synthesis

Vitamin D deficiency may occur in cases of advanced liver disease when there is significant hepatic dysfunction. In these cases there is decreased synthesis of 25-hydroxyvitamin D. With less severe liver dysfunction, vitamin D production is still possible but intestinal malabsorption will occur [96].

In chronic kidney disease there is decreased synthesis of $1\alpha,25$-$(OH)_2D_3$ which may occur with creatinine clearance rates as high as 31–89 mL/min (0.5–1.49 mL/s) but particularly in more severe cases when the GFR decreases to <30 mL/min (<0.5 mL/s). Under these conditions there is hypocalcemia, secondary hypoparathyroidism, and renal bone disease [105]. In hyperphosphatemia there is decreased activity of the enzyme 25-hydroxyvitamin D-1-alpha-hydroxylase caused by increased fibroblast growth factor 23, resulting in lower serum levels of $1\alpha,25$-$(OH)_2D_3$ [106].

Increased urinary loss

Vitamin D deficiency may be seen in cases of nephrotic syndrome with heavy proteinuria when 25-hydroxyvitamin D_3 bound to its alpha-globulin carrier protein is lost in the urine [107].

Hereditary disorders

The various forms of hereditary rickets may affect $1\alpha,25$-$(OH)_2D_3$ either by decreasing its synthesis (pseudovitamin D deficiency rickets or vitamin D-dependent rickets type 1) or by causing partial or complete resistance to its action (vitamin D-resistance rickets or vitamin D-dependent rickets type 2 and vitamin D-dependent rickets type 3). In autosomal dominant hypophosphatemic rickets and X-linked hypophosphatemic rickets, there is decreased 1-alpha-hydroxylase activity resulting in low levels of $1\alpha,25$-$(OH)_2D_3$ [108,109].

Acquired disorders

Acquired causes of osteomalacia include tumors secreting fibroblast growth factor 23 which results in phosphaturia, decreased intestinal absorption of phosphorus, hypophosphatemia and decreased activity of the enzyme 25-dihydroxyvitamin D-1-alpha-hydroxylase. Some lymphomas cause increased macrophage conversion of 25-OHD to $1\alpha,25$-$(OH)_2D_3$ which is the same mechanism by which granulomatous disorders cause disruption of calcium metabolism. Under these conditions the 25-OHD levels are lower and the $1\alpha, 25$-$(OH)_2D_3$ levels are increased. In hyperparathyroidism the excess PTH levels also cause increased metabolism of 25-OHD to $1\alpha,25$-$(OH)_2D_3$ and as a consequence the serum levels of the former decrease and those of the latter will be in the high normal range or elevated. Hyperthyroidism also enhances 25-OHD metabolism, which will reduce its serum levels [106–108,110].

Lactation

Infants who are exclusively breastfed and have no other vitamin D source will develop vitamin D deficiency if there are insufficient amounts in breast milk [79,108,111].

Prevention of vitamin D deficiency

Many recent studies have reported that vitamin D deficiency has become widespread and emphasize that the replacement doses should be higher than those that have been previously recommended [23,24]. However, the optimal vitamin D dosages required to achieve meaningful clinical outcomes are still under investigation. Until more specific and widely accepted recommendations are issued, this topic should be considered to be in a state of transition.

Breastfed infants and children

Human milk does not contain much vitamin D (20 IU/L) in mothers who are vitamin sufficient, and even less in women who are vitamin D deficient. Administering relatively high doses to the mother (e.g. 4000 IU/day) has been reported to allow the transfer of enough vitamin D via breast milk to satisfy the infant's needs [111]. However, administering the vitamin D directly to the infant, rather than relying only on the vitamin D content in breast milk, is considered more effective because of the limited transfer of vitamin D through breast milk. In Canada, current guidelines recommend that all infants and children be given 400 IU of vitamin D3 daily [112]. In the USA, the American Academy of Pediatrics recommends 200 IU of vitamin D3 daily for breastfed infants [113]. However, it has been pointed out that 200 IU/day may not be enough [114] given the accumulating evidence that insufficient vitamin D in childhood is associated with an increased risk of several chronic conditions [23,24].

Pregnant or lactating women

The only vitamin D supplement taken by the majority of US women is the 400 IU contained in the prenatal vitamin preparations. However, vitamin D deficiency is still common by the end of pregnancy even in women who take prenatal vitamins [83]. It is generally agreed that the current recommendations (200–600 IU/day) [115] are not enough and that the requirements may be 1000 IU/day [79] or more [81]. Higher dosages, 4000 IU/day or 60,000 IU/month of vitamin D2, were more effective than lower doses in preventing hypovitaminosis D in lactating women and without reports of toxicity [81,82,111,116].

Reduced skin synthesis

The 1000–2000 IU of vitamin D3/day recommended for pregnant and lactating women might also be sufficient for those lacking exposure to adequate amounts of sunlight [96,117] although doses >2000 IU/day may be more desirable and have been reported to be safe and effective in men and nonpregnant women [118,119].

Decreased bio-availability from malabsorption syndromes

In addition to sensible sunlight or ultraviolet B radiation exposure, the doses recommended for these conditions are up to 10,000 IU of vitamin D3/day. These dosages have been reported to be safe, effective and without evidence of toxicity when taken for as long as 5 months [117,120–122]. An alternative dosing could be 50,000 IU of vitamin D2/week. In obesity, 1000–2000 IU of vitamin D3/day or 50,000 IU of vitamin D2 every 1–2 weeks are the recommended preventive doses to avoid deficiency [96].

Increased catabolism

Patients taking anticonvulsants and other medications that activate the steroid and xenobiotic receptor [98–103], as well as antirejection medications used after transplantation, are recommended to take 50,000 of vitamin D2 every other day or every week.

Liver failure

The dosages recommended for situations of reduced synthesis should be followed for these patients as well. If malabsorption is also present, the recommendations given above should be advised [96,107].

Increased urinary loss: nephrotic syndrome

The recommended doses are 1000–2000 IU/day of vitamin D3 or 50,000 IU of vitamin D2 every 2–4 weeks [96,105,107,123,124].

Chronic kidney disease

Control of serum phosphate is necessary [107]. Vitamin dosing is 1000 IU/day of vitamin D3 or 50,000 IU of vitamin D2 every 2 weeks [105,123]. Once vitamin D sufficiency is obtained (30–60 ng/mL), a vitamin D analog may be needed in the milder renal insufficiency cases (creatinine clearance 31–89 mL/min or 0.4–1.49 mL/s) and generally recommended when the GFR is 30 mL/min (0.5 mL/s) or less. Calcitriol 0.25–1.0 μg once or twice a day is more often used, but other active vitamin D analogs may be utilized as well [123,124].

Hereditary disorders

In X-linked hypophosphatemic rickets and autosomal dominant hypophosphatemic rickets, in order to improve bone mineralization, phosphorus levels need to be brought up to normal. Calcitriol (0.5–1 μg/day) and oral phosphate (1–4 g/day in divided doses) are effective, but close monitoring is needed to avoid renal insufficiency and nephrocalcinosis. Vitamin D-dependent rickets type 1 responds to calcitriol 0.5–1 μg/day, and calcium and phosphorus supplements are generally not needed. In vitamin D-dependent rickets type 2 and 3, there is end-organ resistance to $1\alpha,25\text{-}(OH)_2D_3$. These patients require pharmacologic doses of calcitriol (5–30 μg/day) as well as mineral supplementation. Even so, some patients may have little or no response even to these high calcitriol doses [108,109].

Acquired disorders

Nonpregnant patients with hyperparathyroidism commonly have co-existent vitamin D deficiency, and those with lower vitamin D levels have evidence of more severe hyperparathyroidism, including higher PTH levels, lower phosphorus levels and enhanced bone turnover [125]. Vitamin D compounds reduce PTH secretion [126] and indeed, vitamin D treatment does not exacerbate hypercalcemia. It also successfully decreased PTH levels and bone turnover, although some patients experienced an increase in urinary calcium excretion [127]. Size and weight reduction of parathyroid adenomas did not correlate with vitamin D levels in one study [128], but adenomas were smaller in patients with higher vitamin D levels in another report [129].

In view of this information these patients are advised to take 800–1000 IU of vitamin D3/day or 50,000 IU of vitamin D2 every 2 weeks. However, at present there is no information as to whether hyperparathyroid pregnant women could also benefit from these recommendations. For patients with granulomatous disorders and some lymphomas, the recommended preventive dose of vitamin D_3 is no more than 400 IU/day or 50,000 IU of vitamin D2 every month. The levels of 25-OHD should be kept between 20 and 30 ng/mL because levels greater than this may cause hypercalcemia and hypercalciuria in these patients [23,130].

Parathyroid disease

Primary hyperparathyroidism

Primary hyperparathyroidism is a fairly common disease in the general population. It is reported to be as high as 0.2% per year and $\geq 1\%$ if as yet undiscovered and asymptomatic patients are included [131]. In women of childbearing age the incidence is reported to be 8/100,000 per year. However, less than 150 cases [132,133] have been reported during pregnancy since the first publication in 1931 [134]. It is unclear if hyperparathyroidism is indeed less frequent in pregnant women or if it is under-reported during pregnancy. Bias reporting could also be a factor, because cases with poor outcome or unusual features are more often sent for publication. Since there are no population studies that include pregnant women, the true incidence of hyperparathyroidism in pregnancy remains unknown.

Etiology

A single parathyroid adenoma is the most frequent cause of hyperparathyroidism and affects about 90% of cases; hyperplasia of all glands is present in 8–9%, and carcinoma in 1–2%. Ectopic, malignancy-related, parathyroid hormone production is exceptionally rare in a population of reproductive age women, and only two cases have been reported thus far [135,136].

Hyperparathyroidism may, rarely, be part of an inherited disease with or without other accompanying endocrine abnormalities such as multiple endocrine neoplasia syndromes 1 (i.e. hyperparathyroidism with pituitary and enteropancreatic tumors such as insulinomas or gastrinomas) and 2A (i.e. parathyroid hyperplasia with medullary thyroid cancer, pheochromocytoma and cutaneous lichen amyloidosis). Secondary hyperparathyroidism occurs with renal insufficiency in patients undergoing chronic dialysis or after renal transplation. Overall, the etiology of hyperparathyroidism seems to be similar in pregnant and nonpregnant patients, except for the much lower incidence of malignancy-related cases [137].

Maternal complications

It is commonly stated that most patients with hypercalcemia are asymptomatic, and that this abnormality is usually detected by automated, multichannel analysis of blood sent for other purposes. It is not known if there are hypercalcemic pregnant patients who do well and remain undetected while pregnant. However, among the cases thus far reported during pregnancy, only a relatively small percentage are said to be asymptomatic and the maternal complication rate has been as high as 67% [138]. Reported symptoms include nausea, vomiting and anorexia in 36% (the nausea and vomiting of hypercalcemia may be severe and mistaken for hyperemesis gravidarum [139]) weakness, tiredness and fatigue in 34%, headaches, agitation, emotional lability, inappropriate behavior, confusion, lethargy and even delirium in 26%. Other consequences of hypercalcemia, such as nephrolithiasis, occur in 24–36%, bone disease in 13–19%, urinary tract infections and pyelonephritis in 13%. Pancreatitis is reported in only 1.5% of nonpregnant hyperparathyroid patients and in <1% of normal pregnancies, but it is present in 7–13% of hyperparathyroid pregnant women. Hypertension/pre-eclampsia was reported in 10% of patients in earlier publications [140–145] but more recently found to be as high as 25% [132]. Of interest is that all cases of parathyroid carcinoma thus far reported developed severe pre-eclampsia [146]. Thirst, polyuria, muscle and bone aches and memory loss may also occur. Hypercalcemic crisis has been reported in 8% of patients. Maternal deaths have occurred only in hyperparathyroid women who developed either a hypercalcemic crisis or pancreatitis. With hypercalcemic crisis (i.e. marked elevation of serum calcium, usually >14 mg/dL or >3.5 mmol/L associated with acute signs and symptoms) there was a 30% maternal death and a 40% fetal demise rate [147].

Fetal complications

It has been said that most women with hyperparathyroidism tolerate pregnancy well, and that in fact pregnancy may offer some protection against hypercalcemia because of the low serum albumin and calcium transfer to the fetus. However, a review of the publications to date reveals that hyperparathyroidism in pregnancy is a serious condition associated with a high rate of perinatal morbidity and mortality. Although the identification and publication of cases likely emphasize those patients with adverse outcomes, several literature reviews [140–145,147] have reported a high fetal risk including spontaneous abortion, intrauterine growth restriction, stillbirth, neonatal tetany and neonatal death [148–151]. Even cases with initially mild maternal disease may worsen during pregnancy and require emergency treatment at a less optimal time than elective surgery during the second trimester [152,153]. Even when asymptomatic during pregnancy, the mother's hyperparathyroidism is sometimes diagnosed only after her newborn baby develops hypocalcemic tetany [147–148].

The incidence of fetal complications in untreated maternal hyperparathyroidism has been reported to be as high as 80% [151]. In patients managed conservatively, the complication rate was somewhat lower at 53%, but obviously still unacceptably high. Particularly disturbing was a neonatal death rate of 27–31% [154–156].

Neonatal hypocalcemia occurs because the high levels of maternal calcium inhibit the activity and proper development of the fetal parathyroid glands, and after delivery there is an abrupt halt of the maternal calcium being transported across the placenta. Hypocalcemia more often develops between days 2–14 after delivery, and it can persist for weeks and even months, depending on the severity of the maternal hypercalcemia. In general, neonatal hypocalcemia eventually resolves with appropriate treatment, but permanent neonatal hypoparathyroidism has been described [157–159]. The best results are obtained when calcium supplementation in the newborn is started in a timely manner, otherwise the neonate may suffer severe damage and even death.

Diagnosis

The hallmark of diagnosis is a persistently elevated serum calcium (both total and ionized) and a "normal" (but inappropriate) or elevated level of PTH despite hypercalcemia. Hypercalciuria is usually present. Lower serum levels of phosphorus, magnesium and bicarbonate are usually seen but chloride and citrate are more often elevated. The chloride/phosphorus ratio is >30 in hyperparathyroidism but <30 in hypercalcemia of other etiologies when chloride is measured in mEq/L and phosphate in mg/100 mL. When there is significant bone involvement, the serum alkaline phosphatase of bone origin and urinary hydroxyproline levels will be elevated [131]. Parathyroid carcinoma should be suspected in cases of severe hyperparathyroidism, particularly if there is a palpable neck mass [146].

Localizing parathyroid adenomas before surgery may be very useful. This is particularly relevant during pregnancy because it is likely to result in shorter surgery and anesthesia times. Isotope studies (99m-technetium sestamibi with or without a subtraction 123-thyroid scan with 123-I-iodine) are not usually performed in pregnancy (and certainly the 123-I-iodine portion should not be), but ultrasound is safe and it may successfully locate a parathyroid adenoma. It has been reported to have 69% sensitivity and a 94% specificity [160–162]. Lesions not detected by ultrasound may be identified by computed tomography (CT) or magnetic resonance imaging (MRI) [163]. Magnetic resonance is considered safer during pregnancy although a neck CT with abdominal shielding should pose minimal risk to the fetus.

Treatment

While mild and asymptomatic cases of hyperparathyroidism occurring in patients over the age of 50 who have good bone mass are sometimes managed with observation, surgery is the treatment of choice for hyperparathyroidism occurring in patients under the age of 50 and the only potentially curative treatment available. It should be offered to pregnant women, emphasizing the high cure rate and low risk of complications in the hands of an experienced neck surgeon and anesthesiologist. The most frequently reported complications are laryngeal nerve injury and hypoparathyroidism, but neck exploration has proven to be a relatively safe procedure in pregnancy. In a review of cases published up to 1982, surgery was performed during pregnancy in 16 women and there was only one stillbirth, at 26 weeks. The remaining 27 of the 28 fetal losses described occurred in women who did not have surgery. The 35 cases of neonatal tetany also occurred in newborns of mothers not treated surgically [143]. Other reviews [141,144,151] also concluded that there was a higher risk of fetal and neonatal complications when parathyroidectomy was not performed antenatally. Therefore, for the fetus, maternal parathyroidectomy seems to be the best course of action.

The optimal surgery time is considered to be the second trimester. Patients diagnosed early in pregnancy and who are stable can safely be managed conservatively until the second trimester when surgery is thought to be safer [164]. Surgery in the third trimester has been traditionally avoided because of fear of complications, as reported in one study [140]. However, there have been many cases of successful third-trimester parathyroidectomies [165–171]. Surgery is now considered to be less risky than previously thought. Because of the high risk of fetal complications, not only in untreated mothers but also in those managed conservatively by nonsurgical means, a recent review has suggested that surgical intervention should be offered to all pregnant women regardless of their gestational age [132]. In that review, surgery was performed up to 37 weeks of gestation. It was also noted that there have not been serious complications reported from surgery since 1992, and that many of the surgical complications reported prior to that date were actually complications from the hyperparathyroidism itself rather than the surgical procedure.

Despite our belief that all pregnant women with hyperparathyroidism should undergo parathyroidectomies regardless of symptoms, to date there is no uniform consensus guideline establishing the clinical features of patients for whom this surgery is definitely indicated during pregnancy. Specific guidelines for surgery in hyperparathyroidism outside pregnancy do exist, however [172]. An adaptation of these guidelines has been suggested for hyperparathyroid pregnant women [151] and recommends surgery during pregnancy for patients with hyperparathyroidism who meet any of the following criteria:

- symptoms of hyperparathyroidism
- a serum calcium ≥12 mg/dL (≥3 mmol/L)
- a previous hypercalcemic crisis
- a creatinine clearance reduction of 30% or more
- nephrolithiasis or nephrocalcinosis
- a 24-hour urinary calcium excretion of ≥400 mg
- evidence of bone involvement
- poor compliance with follow-up visits
- patient requests surgery.

However, in the international consensus guidelines (adopted by the US Endocrine Society and other organizations) for hyperparathyroidism in nonpregnant patients, it is stated that all patients younger than 50 years should have surgery [172], and we believe this recommendation should hold in pregnancy as well.

At present, if the hyperparathyroidism is diagnosed in the first trimester and the woman is stable, she can be managed medically and the surgery postponed until the second trimester. We believe that all hyperparathyroid pregnant women should be offered surgery in the second trimester. The risk/benefit ratio appears to favor surgery because of the high risk of fetal complications even in medically treated mothers. It also appears that surgery, even in the third trimester, is safer than medical treatment alone, and the risks of complications from surgery are low in the hands of experienced surgical and anesthesia teams. The reasons for recommending surgery should be discussed with the mother in detail [132].

Hypocalcemia (usually transient) may develop postoperatively, but it is unlikely to occur if there is no bone involvement (osteitis fibrosa cystica), hypomagnesemia or injury to the other parathyroid glands during surgery. The majority of patients, who usually have a single adenoma, no bone involvement and normal renal and gastrointestinal function, experience few or no postoperative difficulties. The possibility of postsurgical hypoparathyroidism should be considered if the serum calcium remains <8 mg/dL, particularly if there is a simultaneous elevation of the serum phosphate level [131].

When surgery is not possible or the patient declines surgical management, it is imperative to maintain adequate hydration and to administer oral phosphates (1.5–2.5 g of inorganic phosphorus per day in divided doses), which are generally safe except in patients with renal insufficiency or hyperphosphatemia [168,173,174]. Nevertheless, these patients should be thoroughly informed of the high risk of neonatal morbidity and mortality despite conservative, nonsurgical management, particularly if the serum calcium level remains ≥12 mg/dL.

Hypercalcemic crisis

This condition needs to be treated aggressively in the same manner as outside pregnancy with saline hydration first (generally at least 3–4 L of 0.9% saline for a fluid balance, that is at least 2 L positive in the first 24 hours) and if fluid overload is a problem, forced diuresis with a loop diuretic afterwards (furosemide 20–40 mg bid) [131,175]. Calcitonin (2–8 IU/kg IM or SQ q6–12 h) does not cross the placenta and has been used safely in pregnant women [176]; it is most useful when administered within the first 24–36 hours, since tachyphylaxis develops rapidly. Among the bisphosphonate compounds, pamidronate is the one most used to treat hypercalcemic emergencies because it is very potent, causing prolonged inhibition of osteoclast-mediated bone resorption without mineralization defects [176]. Animal data are concerning for the safety of this class of agents in pregnancy [151] but the very limited published data on its use in human pregnancies suggest it may have a role in pregnancy for those rare cases of hypercalcemia (and some bone diseases) unresponsive to other agents [136].

Glucocorticoids (typically prednisone 20–50 mg PO bid or its equivalent until calcium stabilizes and then a gradual taper until the minimum dose is reached that controls symptoms of hypercalcemia) are effective in hypercalcemia due to vitamin D intoxication, sarcoidosis and in certain malignancies, but not in hyperparathyroidism [131,176]. Dialysis would be the treatment of choice for severe hypercalcemia complicated by renal failure. Cinacalcet, a calcimimetic drug, lowers PTH levels by selectively increasing the sensitivity of the calcium-sensing receptor to extracellular calcium. It suppresses PTH secretion, and is associated with decreased calcium levels as well. However, it is a category C drug for pregnancy. No anomalies have occurred when administered in high doses to rats and rabbits, although decreased fetal weight was observed. There is no experience about its effects on human pregnancies, and its routine use is not recommended at this time. When administered to lactating rats, it passed into the breast milk with high milk to plasma ratio, and because there are no studies in humans, its use in breastfeeding mothers is discouraged.

Hypoparathyroidism

Etiology

The most common cause of hypoparathyroidism is inadvertent injury, surgical removal of the parathyroid glands or damage to their vascular supply during thyroid or other neck surgeries. Hypoparathyroidism is reported in 0.2–3.5% of cases after thyroid surgery and the frequency varies with the skill and experience of the operating surgeon. Because of improved surgical techniques and more use of nonsurgical treatments of thyroid diseases, mainly hyperthyroidism, acquired hypoparathyroidism is now less prevalent. Idiopathic hypoparathyroidism is infrequently encountered in pregnancy. It may be an isolated disorder or occur in association with agenesis of the thymus (Di George syndrome). It may also be part of a familial autoimmune disorder where antibodies are also directed against adrenal, thyroid, ovarian and gastric tissue, resulting in deficiencies of adrenal, thyroid and ovarian functions and pernicious anemia besides the hypoparathyroidism. These patients usually suffer from mucocutaneous candidiasis, alopecia and vitiligo as well. Another rare hereditary disorder not often seen during pregnancy is pseudohypoparathyroidism. In this condition there is PTH secretion, but the bones and kidneys are unresponsive to its action [177].

Diagnosis

Chronic, untreated hypocalcemia is usually symptomatic, and the symptoms are the same for both acquired and hereditary hypoparathyroidism. The onset of symptoms in the hereditary form is more gradual and, in addition, it may be associated with other developmental defects. Therefore, obtaining a detailed family history is very important. Symptoms of hypocalcemia include perioral and acral (i.e. in the extremities) paresthesias, facial twitching, muscle spasms and carpopedal spasms. Irritability, depression and even psychosis may be seen. When the hypocalcemia is severe, laryngeal spasms and even respiratory arrest and convulsions may occur. Papilledema and increased intracranial pressure have been described in cases of long-standing hypocalcemia. The electrocardiogram will show a prolonged Q-T interval (measured from the beginning of the QRS complex to the end of the T wave and normally <0.45 seconds) and cardiac arrhythmias may ensue. Abdominal cramps and intestinal malabsorption may be seen. Positive Chvostek's (i.e. tapping anterior to the ear elicits ipsilateral facial twitching) and Trousseau's signs (i.e. inflating a blood pressure cuff above the systolic blood pressure elicits characteristic contractions of the hand muscles) will be elicited, but it should be noted that these signs are also positive in 10% of normals. Other signs may include dry, scaly skin, coarse hair and brittle nails. Lenticular cataracts that resolve after normalization of serum calcium have been described. Most patients with pseudohypoparathyroidism will also have developmental abnormalities such as short stature, a round face, brachydactyly and ectopic soft tissue calcifications.

Laboratory testing will reveal hypocalcemia and a "normal," low or undetectable PTH level, hyperphosphatemia and normal renal function. Other useful tests include serum magnesium, as well as assays for vitamin D (both 25-hydroxyvitamin D and $1\alpha,25\text{-}(OH)_2D_3$) in order to be able to diagnose other possible disorders of calcium metabolism

such as hypomagnesemia, chronic renal failure, vitamin D deficiency, rickets or pseudohypoparathyroidism.

Maternal considerations

Before specific treatment was available, maternal morbidity and mortality rates were considerable and pregnancy termination was often recommended. At the present time the prognosis is much better, provided that the maternal serum calcium level is maintained in the normal range. Frequent, at least monthly laboratory determinations are needed because of the narrow therapeutic margin of this form of treatment and the possibility of frequent episodes of either hyper- or hypocalcemia. More frequent determinations will be necessary if hyper- or hypocalcemia develops.

Fetal and neonatal considerations

Severe maternal hypocalcemia has been associated with midtrimester abortion and premature labor, which are attributed to uterine irritability triggered by the low calcium levels [178]. If the mother becomes hypercalcemic, the fetal parathyroid function will be suppressed and the newborn will develop hypocalcemia and even tetany, the same complications as when the mother suffers from hyperparathyroidism. On the other hand, if the mother becomes hypocalcemic, the fetus will experience parathyroid gland hyperplasia, subperiosteal bone resorption, generalized skeletal demineralization and at times even osteitis fibrosa because of calcium mobilization out of the bones [179]. The perinatal mortality is very high if the mother is chronically hypocalcemic, but in the surviving newborns the symptoms will subside in 4–7 months if they are properly treated.

Treatment

Treatment is intended to maintain a serum calcium level within normal limits with oral calcium supplements and vitamin D or its analogs. In the past, 50,000–100,000 units of vitamin D per day, in addition to 1–4 g of calcium per day, was the standard treatment. Maternal therapy with oral vitamin D and calcium will prevent deleterious effects in the fetus [180,181]. During pregnancy, the requirements for vitamin D may increase 2–3-fold, and it will usually be necessary to adjust the dose upward in order to maintain normocalcemia as the pregnancy progresses [182,183]. In modern treatment, vitamin D analogs are usually preferred: either 1-alpha-OHD or more often $1\alpha,25\text{-}(OH)_2D_3$ (calcitriol). They have a shorter half-life (6–8 h), which allows easier titration of the dose.

The safety and successful use of oral $1\alpha,25\text{-}(OH)_2D_3$ in pregnancy have been reported [181]. There have been concerns about using any form of vitamin D because of earlier reports linking high doses of vitamin D with fetal defects [184,185]. However, more recent studies have shown that vitamin D is safe at the doses recommended to maintain maternal eucalcemia [181–183]. There are also reports that even women treated with high doses of vitamin D delivered normally developed newborns [186,187]. At the present time it is believed that the risk of vitamin D teratogenicity is low and that the benefits greatly outweigh the risks if the mother is properly treated. Calcitriol is preferred because of its predictable bio-availability and shorter half-life, which will facilitate dose adjustments. Also, if hypercalcemia develops during the course of treatment, it will be easier and faster to correct. When hypercalcemia develops while using vitamin D instead of its analogs, it may take weeks to correct because vitamin D is stored in the adipose tissue and its biologic effects are long-lasting, in contrast to calcitriol, which has a rapid turnover [188].

The daily dose of calcitriol varies from 0.25 to 3 μg. It is recommended to start with the lower dose and adjust it as needed as pregnancy progresses. Because of its short half-life some patients may need split doses to avoid hypocalcemia, particularly at night [188]. If maternal hypercalcemia develops, the calcitriol is stopped, the patient is hydrated with normal saline solution and a short course of corticosteroids is given (40–60 mg/day of prednisone or equivalent steroid with rapid tapering). Once the hypercalcemia resolves, the doses of calcium and calcitriol are revised to prevent further complications. If hypocalcemia develops, calcium is administered. If tetany and convulsions occur, 1–2 g of calcium gluconate should be given intravenously (which is equivalent to 90–180 mg of elemental calcium), in 50 mL of 5% dextrose over 10–20 minutes. This should be followed by an infusion of calcium gluconate solution. A solution of 1 mg/mL of elemental calcium can be prepared by adding 100 mL of 10% calcium gluconate to 1 L of D5W. It can be started at 50 mL/h with the rate gradually adjusted to maintain a serum calcium concentration in the lower range of normal. Once again, after the acute episode subsides, the daily dosages of oral calcium and calcitriol are readjusted to prevent further recurrences.

In pseudohypoparathyroidism there is end-organ resistance to the action of PTH, resulting in hypocalcemia and renal resistance to the phosphaturic effect of PTH [189]. The implications for pregnancy are the same as in hypoparathyroidism, but the doses of vitamin D and calcium needed are usually lower than in true hypoparathyroidism [190,191]. There are wide individual responses to therapy as well; therefore it is recommended that the optimal dosages be determined for each patient based on the serum calcium levels and urinary calcium excretion.

Lactation

After delivery, hypoparathyroid women may develop hypercalcemia while taking the same dosages of vitamin D or calcitriol that successfully maintained the serum calcium in the normal range during pregnancy. During lactation, hypersensitivity to vitamin D develops. It was thought to result from an effect of prolactin on the 1-alpha-hydroxylase vitamin D enzyme activity, but this effect is now attributed to the production of PTHrP by mammary epithelial cells in lactating women. PTHrP probably stimulates endogenous calcitriol formation [192,193]. Several cases of hypercalcemia developing while breastfeeding have been reported and required the discontinuation of calcitriol and calcium intake [192,194–195]. Hypercalcemia has also been reported in women with massive mammary hyperplasia, even when not taking calcitriol or calcium, and attributed in those particular cases to mammary PTHrP gaining access to the systemic circulation [16,196]. Hypercalcemia while breastfeeding has also been reported in a woman without any parathyroid disease, who was taking large doses of calcium in an effort to avoid osteoporosis during lactation [197]. The authors suggest that lactating women should not exceed the recommended daily calcium dosage. Therefore, it is imperative to closely monitor the serum calcium level after delivery in lactating women with hypoparathyroidism to prevent acute hypercalcemia, which is likely to develop 1–2 weeks after initiation of breastfeeding if the therapy is not readjusted. Some women may remain normocalcemic while lactating even without calcitriol, but the hypocalcemia and the need to resume treatment will reappear quickly after stopping breastfeeding.

The pediatrician should be made aware of the mother's condition and the newborn calcium levels monitored as well. As already mentioned, PTHrP has been detected in human and animal milk. However, PTHrP administered to newborn mice did not influence serum calcium concentration [49,70,71]. Therefore it is probably safe for most of these women to breastfeed, except in cases similar to the few anecdotal reports of maternal hypercalcemia associated with massive mammary hyperplasia or in women taking large amounts of calcium [16,163,164].

Obstetric and perinatal care

For women with no history of a disorder of calcium metabolism, the obstetrician, as the primary care provider, must consider when to suspect such conditions. Pregnant women are not routinely screened for calcium disorders. However, a serum calcium should be checked in patients who present with new onset of otherwise unexplained severe nausea and vomiting. This includes cases of suspected hyperemesis gravidarum [139]. It should also be checked (along with a complete blood count, potassium, creatinine, urinalysis and TSH) as part of the initial investigation of any patient with newly diagnosed hypertension remote from term. Other indications include mental status changes, nephrolithiasis, renal insufficiency, liver disease, HIV/AIDS, pancreatitis, thyrotoxicosis, adrenal insufficiency, tuberculosis, sarcoidosis and other inflammatory disorders, excess intake of vitamin A and vitamin D as well as when taking several other medications such as thiazide diuretics, theophylline, anticonvulsants, lithium, magnesium and phosphate-containing enemas or laxatives. Also in severe hypertension, particularly if a pheochromocytoma is suspected [131]. Nevertheless, hyperparathyroidism will be the cause of hypercalcemia in >70% of the cases in pregnancy.

For women with known disorders of calcium metabolism, the central role of the obstetrician is to allow the patient and endocrinologist to pursue an aggressive treatment strategy. There is a natural reticence to employ complex medical regimens in pregnancy and even more so to consider surgical intervention. Nevertheless, treatment strategies to maintain eucalcemia that are safe for mother and fetus can be designed and it is clear that pregnancy outcomes, particularly in hyperparathyroidism, are much worse with less aggressive treatment.

In primary hyperparathyroidism, one must anticipate the need for surgery at any time in pregnancy, although the second trimester is favored if feasible. It may be necessary for the obstetrician to impress upon the patient, family and in some cases the other consultants that failure to intervene surgically is associated with poor pregnancy outcomes that may include pancreatitis and hypercalcemic crisis in the mother as well as a high rate of fetal or neonatal death. Medical therapy, even when pursued aggressively, is associated with poor outcomes. Surgery can be safely performed, even in the third trimester [132].

Genetic counseling is indicated for patients suspected of having an inherited disorder of calcium metabolism including hereditary rickets, multiple endocrine neoplasia syndromes, idiopathic hypoparathyroidism, familial autoimmune hypoparathyroidism, and peudohypoparathyroidism.

A high rate, 25%, of superimposed pre-eclampsia has been seen in the more recent reports of hyperparathyroidism in pregnancy [132] and it has been reported in all cases of hyperparathyroidism due to parathyroid carcinomas [146]. Therefore, a mid-trimester uterine artery Doppler will be particularly helpful in hyperparathyroidism for prediction of early-onset pre-eclampsia and fetal growth restriction. Low-dose aspirin (<100 mg daily) for pre-eclampsia prevention may be considered as well. Serial ultrasound examinations, every 4–6 weeks, in the second half of pregnancy are indicated for early detection of fetal growth restriction.

There are conflicting data on the effect of calcium on uterine activity. Older reports suggested that maternal hypocalcemia was associated with increased uterine activity, reduced resting potential and spike frequency of the uterine muscle fibers, leading to spontaneous abortion and premature labor [178,198]. A more recent report described failure of labor to progress in a noncompliant hypoparathyroid woman who was hypocalcemic at the time of delivery. The failure to labor was attributed to hypocalcemia. The labor resumed and proceeded normally after the mother's calcium level was normalized with the appropriate therapy [199]. It is clear, on the other hand, that hypercalcemia is associated with increased uterine activity and spontaneous preterm birth. Transvaginal measurement of cervical length may be helpful in assessing the degree of risk, but there are no data to speak directly to these measurements in this specific situation. Antepartum fetal surveillance by 34 weeks gestation is indicated to attempt to identify fetuses at risk for death *in utero*.

Because of the complexity of the maternal–fetal interaction, a neonatal consultation is required. If parathyroid surgery is performed in the third trimester, for example, there might be a benefit of delaying delivery 7–15 days if at all possible. This would allow the fetus time to recover parathyroid function and thus minimize or even prevent neonatal hypocalcemia. Neonatal tetany is a dreaded complication in poorly controlled maternal hyperparathyroidism.

Magnesium and calcium interaction

Maternal effects

Magnesium sulfate is widely used in obstetrics for the treatment of premature labor, pre-eclampsia and eclampsia. Its use as a tocolytic agent has been reported to be generally safe [200]. However, hypocalcemia has been reported in women being treated with short-term magnesium sulfate to suppress premature labor [201–203] and it is very common with long-term use. Magnesium in high doses suppresses PTH levels by affecting the calcium-sensing receptors in the parathyroid glands and the kidneys [204–206].

Prolonged (2–3 weeks or longer) administration of magnesium sulfate may also result in impaired maternal bone mineralization. Urinary calcium loss is the main mechanism causing hypocalcemia in these cases [207] and maternal osteoporosis has indeed been reported after several weeks of magnesium sulfate administration [207–209]. However, such prolonged use of magnesium sulfate is rarely seen in current obstetric practice.

Effect of magnesium sulfate on the fetus and newborn

Hypotonia and respiratory depression that might require intubation and mechanical ventilation have been reported in newborns of mothers treated with magnesium sulfate [210]. The risk was higher when the mother received prolonged (>4 days) therapy [211]. The serum magnesium concentration may not accurately reflect intracellular levels and therefore, cord blood or neonatal serum magnesium levels may be of limited value in assessing the clinical picture except when quite elevated [211,212]. In one report of five mothers treated with intravenous magnesium sulfate initiated in the second trimester and continued for several weeks [213], radiographic abnormalities of rickets were observed in two of the infants (defective ossification of bone and teeth enamel); these were attributed to fetal parathyroid gland suppression by the magnesium. Other reports have described abnormal mineralization of metaphyses as well [214–216]. The interference with bone mineralization occurs because magnesium occupies the osteoid calcium-binding sites and therefore calcification is inhibited [214,215]. The newborns will require several days to eliminate the excess magnesium because their kidneys are still immature [201]. Newborns of mothers treated with magnesium sulfate for longer than 2 days may require ventilation assistance, fluids and electrolytes and at times intravenous calcium to counteract the effect on central nervous system depression and peripheral neuromuscular blockade from magnesium. Intravenous calcium infusion will require careful cardiac monitoring [211].

References

1. Kovacs CS. Calcium and bone metabolism in pregnancy and lactation. J Clin Endocrinol Metab 2001;86:2344–8.
2. Heaney R, Skillman T. Calcium metabolism in normal pregnancy. J Clin Endocrinol Metab 1971;33:661–70.
3. Kent G, Price R, Gutteridge D, et al. The efficiency of intestinal calcium is increased in late pregnancy but not in established lactation. Calcif Tissue Int 1991;48:293–5.
4. Seely EW, Brown EM, DeMaggio DM, et al. A prospective study of calciotropic hormones in pregnancy and postpartum: reciprocal changes in serum intact parathyroid hormone and 1,25-dihydroxyvitamin D. Am J Obstet Gynecol 1997;176:214–17.
5. Kovacs CS, Kronenberg HM. Maternal-fetal calcium and bone metabolism during pregnancy, puerperium and lactation. Endocr Rev 1997;18:832–72.
6. Institute of Medicine. Nutrition during pregnancy, Part II. Nutrient supplements. National Academies Press, Washington, DC, 1990: 258–71.
7. Ritchie LD, Fung EB, Halloran BP, et al. A longitudinal study of calcium homeostasis during human pregnancy and lactation and after resumption of menses. Am J Clin Nutr 1998;67:693–701.
8. Institute of Medicine. Nutrition during lactation. Nutrients supplements. National Academies Press, Washington, DC, 1990: 50–79.
9. Gertner J, Coustan D, Kliger A, et al. Pregnancy as a state of physiologic absorptive hypercalciuria. Am J Med 1986;81:451–6.
10. Moniz DF, Nicolaides K, Bamforth FJ, Rodeck CH. Normal reference ranges for biochemical substances relating to renal, hepatic, and bone function in fetal and maternal plasma throughout pregnancy. J Clin Pathol 1985;38:468–72.
11. Wieland P, Fischer JA, Trechsel U, et al. Perinatal parathyroid hormone, vitamin D metabolites and calcitonin in man. Am J Physiol 1980;239:e385–90.
12. Martinez ME, Sanchez C, Salinas M, et al. Ionic calcium levels during pregnancy, at delivery and in the first hours of life. Scand J Clin Lab Invest 1986;46:27–30.
13. MacIsaac R, Heath J, Rodda C, et al. Role of the fetal parathyroid glands and parathyroid hormone-related protein in the regulation of placental transport of calcium, magnesium and inorganic phosphate. Reprod Fertil Dev 1991;3:447–57.
14. Kovacs CS, Lanske B, Hunzelman JL, et al. Parathyroid hormone-related peptide (PTHrP) regulates fetal-placental calcium transport through a receptor distinct from the PTH/PTHrP receptor. Proc Natl Acad Sci USA 1996;93:15233–8.
15. Bertelloni S, Baroncelli G, Pelletti A, et al. Parathyroid hormone-related protein in healthy pregnant women. Calcif Tissue Int 1994;54:195–7.
16. Khosla S, van Heerden J, Gharib H, et al. Parathyroid hormone-related protein and hypercalcemia secondary to massive mammary hyperplasia (letter)N Engl J Med 1990;322:1157.
17. Kovacs CS, El-Hajj Fuleihan G. Calcium and bone disorders during pregnancy and lactation. Endocrinol Metab Clin North Am 2006;35:21–51.
18. Weiss M, Eisenstein Z, Ramot Y, et al. Renal reabsorption of inorganic phosphorus in pregnancy in relation to the calciotropic hormones. Br J Obstet Gynaecol 1998;105:195–9.
19. Arnaud SB, Matthusen M, Gilkinson JB, Goldsmith RS. Components of 25-hydroxyvitamin D in serum of young children in upper midwestern United States. Am J Clin Nutr 1977;30:1082–6.
20. Armas LAG, Hollis BW, Heaney RP. Vitamin D2 is much less effective than vitamin D3 in humans. J Clin Endocrinol Metab 2004;89:5387–91.
21. Trang HM, Cole DEC, Rubin LA, et al. Evidence that vitamin D3 increases serum 25-hydroxyvitamin D more efficiently than does vitamin D2. Am J Clin Nutr 1998;68:854–8.
22. Thomas MK, Demay MB. Vitamin D deficiency and disorders of vitamin D metabolism. Endocrinol Metab Clin North Am 2000;29:611.
23. Holick MF. Vitamin D deficiency. N Engl J Med 2007;357:266–81.
24. Dawodu A, Wagner CL. Mother-child vitamin D deficiency: an international perspective. Arch Dis Child 2007;92:737–40.
25. Gray TK, Lester GE, Lorenc RS. Evidence for extrarenal 1-hydroxylation of 25-hydroxyvitamin D3 in pregnancy. Science 1979;204:1311–13.
26. Halhai A, Diaz L, Sanchez I, et al. Effects of IGF-I on 1, 25 dihydroxyvitamin D (3) synthesis on human placenta in culture. Mol Hum Reprod 1999;5:771–6.
27. Zerwekh J, Breslau N. Human placental production of 1-alpha, 25-dihydroxyvitamin D3: biochemical characterization and production in normal subjects and patients with pseudohypoparathyroidism. J Clin Endocrinol Metab 1986;62:192–6.
28. Bringhurst FR, Demay MB. Krane SM, Kronenberg HM. Bone and mineral metabolism in health and disease. In: Kasper DL, Braunwald E, Fauci AS, et al. (eds) Harrison's principles of internal medicine, 16th edn. McGraw-Hill, New York, 2005: 2238–49.
29. Hollis BW, Wagner CL. Nutritional vitamin D status during pregnancy: reasons for concern. CMAJ 2006;174:1287–90.
30. Evans KN, Bulmer JN, Kilby MD, Hewison M. Vitamin D and placental-decidual function. J Soc Gynecol Invest 2004; 11(5):263–71.
31. Davis O, Hawkins D, Rubin I, et al. Serum parathyroid hormone (PTH) in pregnant women determined by an immunoradiometric assay for intact PTH. J Clin Endocrinol Metab 1988;67:850–2.
32. Saggese G, Baroncelli G, Bertelloni S, et al. Intact parathyroid hormone levels during pregnancy, in healthy term neonates and in hypocalcemic preterm infants. Acta Pediatr Scand 1991;80:36–41.

33. Seki K, Makimura N, Mitsui C, *et al*. Calcium-regulating hormones and osteocalcin levels during pregnancy: a longitudinal study. Am J Obstet Gynecol 1991;164:1248–52.

34. Habener JF, Rosenblatt M, Potts JT Jr. Parathyroid hormone: biochemical aspects of biosynthesis, secretion, action and metabolism. Physiol Rev 1984;64:985–1053.

35. Tam CS, Heersche JN, Murray TM, *et al*. Parathyroid hormone stimulates the bone apposition rate independently of its resorptive action: differential effects of intermittent and continuous administration. Endocrinology 1982;110:506–12.

36. Pitkin RM, Reynolds W, Williams GA, Hargis GK. Calcium metabolism in normal pregnancy. A longitudinal study. Am J Obstet Gynecol 1979;133:781–91.

37. Allgrove J, Adami S, Manning RM, O'Riordan JL. Cytochemical bioassay of parathyroid hormone in maternal and cord blood. Arch Dis Child 1985;60:110–15.

38. Whitehead M, Lane G, Young O, *et al*. Interrelations of calcium regulating hormones during normal pregnancy. BMJ 1981;283:10–12.

39. Cross NA, Hillman LS, Allen SH, *et al*. Calcium homeostasis and bone metabolism during pregnancy, lactation and post weaning: a longitudinal study. Am J Clin Nutr 1995;61:514–23.

40. Rasmussen N, Frolich A, Horness PJ, *et al*. Serum ionized calcium and intact parathyroid hormone levels during pregnancy and postpartum. Br J Obstet Gynaecol 1990;97:857–9.

41. Okonofua F, Menon RK, Houlder S, *et al*. Calcium, vitamin D and parathyroid hormone relationships in pregnant Caucasian and Asian women and their neonates. Ann Clin Biochem 1987;24:22–8.

42. Dahlman T, Sjoberg HE, Bucht E. Calcium homeostasis in normal pregnancy and puerperium: a longitudinal study. Acta Obstet Gynecol Scand 1994;73:393–8.

43. Gallacher SJ, Fraser WD, Owens OJ, *et al*. Changes in calciotropic hormones and biochemical markers of bone turnover in normal human pregnancy. Eur J Endocrinol 1994;131:369–72.

44. Burtis W, Brady T, Orloff J, *et al*. Immunochemical characterization of circulating parathyroid hormone-related protein in patients with humoral hypercalcemia of cancer. N Engl J Med 1990;322:1106.

45. Kaji H, Sugimoto T, Fukase M, *et al*. Role of dual signal transduction systems in the stimulation of bone resorption by parathyroid hormone-related peptide: the direct involvement of cAMP-dependent protein kinase. Horm Metab Res 1993;25:421–4.

46. Burton P, Moniz C, Quirke P, *et al*. Parathyroid hormone-related peptide: expression in fetal and neonatal development. J Pathol 1992;167:291–6.

47. Moseley M, Hayman J, Danks J, *et al*. Immunochemical detection of parathyroid hormone-related protein in human fetal epithelia. J Clin Endocrinol Metab 1991;73:478–84.

48. Ferguson J, Gorman J, Bruns D, *et al*. Abundant expression of parathyroid hormone-related protein in human amnion and its association with labor. Proc Natl Acad Sci USA 1992;89:8384–8.

49. Bucht E, Carlqvist M, Hedlund B, *et al*. Parathyroid hormone-related peptide in human milk measured by a mid-molecule radioimmunoassay. Metab Clin Exp 1992;41:11–16.

50. Care AD. The placental transfer of calcium. J Dev Physiol 1991;15:253–7.

51. Cornish J, Callon KE, Nicholson GC, Reid IR. Parathyroid hormone-related protein-(107–139) inhibits bone resorption in vivo. Endocrinology 1997;138:1299–304.

52. Fenton A, Kemp B, Kent G, *et al*. A carboxyterminal peptide from the parathyroid hormone-related peptide inhibits bone resorption by osteoclasts. Endocrinology 1991;129:1762–8.

53. Germain A, Attaroglu H, MacDonald P, *et al*. Parathyroid hormone-related protein mRNA in avascular human amnion. J Clin Endocrinol Metab 1992;75:1173–5.

54. Verdy M, Beaulieu R, Demers L. Plasma calcitonin activity in a patient with thyroid medullary carcinoma and her children with osteopetrosis. J Clin Endocrinol 1971;32:216–21.

55. Woodrow JP, Noseworthy CS, Fudge NJ, *et al*. Calcitonin/calcitonin gene-related peptide protect the maternal skeleton from excessive resorption during lactation [abstract], J Bone Miner Res 2003;18 (suppl 2):S37.

56. Lamke B, Brundin J, Moberg P. Changes of bone mineral content during pregnancy and lactation. Acta Obstet Gynecol Scand 1977;56:217–19.

57. Aguado F, Revilla M, Hernandez ER, *et al*. Ultrasonographic bone velocity in pregnancy: a longitudinal study. Am J Obstet Gynecol 1988;178:1016–21.

58. Yamaga A, Taga M, Minaguchi H, Sato K. Changes in bone mass as determined by ultrasound and biochemical markers of bone turnover during pregnancy and puerperium: a longitudinal study. J Clin Endocrinol Metab 1996;81:752–6.

59. Gambacciani M, Spinetti A, Gallo R, Cappagli B, Teti GC, Facchini V. Ultrasonographic bone characteristics during normal pregnancy. Longitudinal and cross-sectional evaluation. Am J Obstet Gynecol 1995;173:890–3.

60. Black AJ, Topping J, Durham B, *et al*. A detailed assessment of alterations in bone turnover, calcium homeostasis, and bone density in normal pregnancy. J Bone Miner Res 2000;15(3): 557–63.

61. Naylor KE, Iqbal P, Fledelius C, *et al*. The effect of pregnancy on bone density and bone turnover. J Bone Miner Res 2000;15(1):129–37.

62. Drinkwater BL, Chesnut CH. Bone density changes during pregnancy and lactation in active women: a longitudinal study. Bone Miner 1991;14:153–60.

63. Feeley RM, Eitenmiller R, Jones JB Jr, Barnhart H. Calcium, phosphorus, and magnesium contents of human milk during early lactation. J Pediatr Gastroenterol Nutr 1983;2:262–7.

64. Jenness R. The composition of human milk. Semin Perinatol 1979;3:225–39.

65. Sowers M. Pregnancy and lactation as risk factors for subsequent bone loss and osteoporosis. J Bone Miner Res 1996;11:1052–60.

66. Kolthoff N, Eiken P, Kristensen B, Nielsen SP. Bone mineral changes during pregnancy and lactation: a longitudinal cohort study. Clin Sci 1998;94:405–12.

67. Retallack RW, Jeffries M, Kent GN, *et al*. Physiological hyperparathyroidism in human lactation. Calcif Tissue Res 1977;22 (suppl):142–6.

68. Gutteridge DH. Serum free 1, 25-dihydroxyvitamin D and the free 1, 25-dihydroxyvitamin D index during pregnancy and lactation. Clin Endocrinol (Oxf) 1990;32:613–22.

69. Kent GN, Price RI, Gutteridge DH, *et al*. Human lactation: forearm trabecular bone loss, increased bone turnover, and renal conservation of calcium and inorganic phosphate with recovery of bone mass following weaning. J Bone Miner Res 1990;5:361–9.

70. Gallacher SJ, Fraser WD, Owens OJ, *et al*. Changes in calciotrophic hormones and biochemical markers of bone turnover in normal human pregnancy. Eur J Endocrinol 1994;131:369–74.

71. Budayr AA, Halloran BP, King JC, *et al*. High levels of a parathyroid hormone-like protein in milk. Proc Natl Acad Sci USA 1989;86:7183–5.

72. Thiede MA. The mRNA encoding a parathyroid hormone-like peptide in mammary tissue in response to elevations in serum prolactin. Mol Endocrinol 1989;3:1443–7.

73. Brommage R, de Luca HF. Regulation of bone mineral loss during lactation. Am J Physiol 1985;248:E182–7.

74. Laskey MA, Prentice A, Hanratty LA, et al. Bone changes after 3 months of lactation: influence of calcium intake, breast-milk output, and vitamin D-receptor genotype. Am J Clin Nutr 1998;67:685–92.

75. Bezerra FF, Mendonca LM, Lobato EC, et al. Bone mass is recovered from lactation to post weaning in adolescent mothers with low calcium intakes. Am J Clin Nutr 2004;80(5):1322–6.

76. Kalkwarf HJ, Specker BL. Bone mineral changes during pregnancy and lactation. Endocrine 2002;17(1):49–53.

77. Ardeshirpour L, Dann P, Adams DJ, et al. Weaning triggers a decrease in receptor activator of nuclear factor-$_k$B ligand expression, widespread osteoclast apoptosis, and rapid recovery of bone mass after lactation in mice. Endocrinology 2007;148:3875–86.

78. Woodrow JP, Sharpe CJ, Fudge NJ, et al. Calcitonin plays a critical role in regulating skeletal mineral metabolism during lactation. Endocrinology 2006;147(9):4010–21.

79. Bischoff-Ferrari HA, Giovanucci E, Willett WC, et al. Estimation of optimal serum concentrations of 25-hydroxyvitamin D for multiple health outcomes. Am J Clin Nutr 2006;84:18–28.

80. Dawson-Hughes B, Heaney RP, Holick MF, et al. Estimates of optimal vitamin D status. Osteoporosis Int 2005;6:713–16.

81. Hollis BW, Wagner CL. Assessment of dietary vitamin D requirements during pregnancy and lactation. Am J Clin Nutr 2004;79:717–26.

82. Lee JM, Smith JR, Philipp BL, et al. Vitamin D deficiency in a healthy group of mothers and newborn infants. Clin Pediatr 2007;46:42–4.

83. Bodnar LM, Simham HN, Powers RW, et al. High prevalence of vitamin D insufficiency in black and white pregnant women residing in the northern United States and their neonates. J Nutr 2007;137:447–52.

84. Heckmatt JZ, Peacock M, Davies AE, et al. Plasma 25-hydroxyvitamin D in pregnant Asian women and their babies. Lancet 1979;ii:546–9.

85. Camadoo L, Tibbott R, Isaza F. Maternal vitamin D deficiency associated with neonatal hypocalcemic convulsions. Nutr J 2007;6:23–5.

86. Purvis RJ, Barrie WJM, MacKay GS, et al. Enamel hypoplasia of the teeth associated with neonatal tetany; a manifestation of maternal vitamin D deficiency. Lancet 1973;ii:811–14.

87. Dandona F, Okonofua F, Clements RV. Osteomalacia presenting as pathological fractures during pregnancy in Asian women of high socioeconomic class. BMJ 1985;290:837–18.

88. Parr JH, Ramsay I. The presentation of osteomalacia in pregnancy. Case report. Br J Obstet Gynaecol 1984;91:816–18.

89. Ford JA, Davidson DC, McIntosh WB, et al. Neonatal rickets in Asian immigrant population. BMJ 1973;iii:211–12.

90. Moncrief MW, Fadahunsi TO. Congenital rickets due to maternal vitamin D deficiency. Arch Dis Child 1974;49:810–11.

91. Park W, Paust H, Kaufmann HJ, et al. Osteomalacia of the mother-rickets of the newborn. Eur J Pediatr 1987;146:292–3.

92. Dawodu A, Agarwal M, Hossain M, et al. Hypovitaminosis D and vitamin D deficiency in exclusively breastfeeding infants and their mothers in summer: a justification for vitamin D supplementation of breastfeeding infants. J Pediatr 2003;142:168–73.

93. Brooke OG, Brown IRF, Bone CD, et al. Vitamin D supplements in pregnant Asian women. Effects on calcium status and fetal growth. BMJ 1980;i:751–4.

94. Dent CE, Gupta MM. Plasma 25-hydroxyvitamin D levels during pregnancy in Caucasians and in vegetarian and non-vegetarian Asians. Lancet 1975;ii:1057–60.

95. Polanska N, Dale RA, Wills MR. Plasma calcium levels in pregnant Asian women. Ann Clin Biochem 1976;13:339–44.

96. Holick MF. High prevalence if vitamin D inadequacy and implications for health. Mayo Clin Proc 2006;81:353–73.

97. Lo CW, Paris PW, Clemens TL, et al. Vitamin D absorption in healthy subjects and in patients with intestinal malabsorption syndromes. Am J Clin Nutr 1985;42:644–9.

98. Bodnar LM, Catov JM, Roberts JM, Simham HN. Prepregnancy obesity predicts poor vitamin D status in mothers and their neonates. J Nutr 2007;137:2437–42.

99. Zhou C, Assem M, Tay JC, et al. Steroid and xenobiotic receptor and vitamin D receptor crosstalk mediates CYP24 expression and drug-induced osteomalacia. J Clin Invest 2006;116:1703–12.

100. Xu Y, Hashizume T, Shuhart MC, et al. Intestinal and hepatic CYP3A4 catalyze hydroxylation of 1 alpha, 25-dihydroxyvitamin D3: implications for drug-induced osteomalacia. Mol Pharmacol 2006;69:56–65.

101. Pack AM, Morrell MJ. Epilepsy and bone health in adults. Epilepsy Behav 2004;5(suppl 2): S24-S29.

102. Shah SC, Sharma RK, Hemangini, et al. Rifampicin induced osteomalacia. Tubercle 1981;62:207–9.

103. Karaaslan Y, Haznedaroglu S, Ozturk M. Osteomalacia associated with carbamazepine/valproate. Ann Pharmacother 2000;34:264–5.

104. Pascussi JM, Robert A, Nguyen M, et al. Possible involvement of pregnane X receptor-enhanced CYP24 expression in drug-induced osteomalacia. J Clin Invest 2005;115:177–86.

105. Holick MF. Vitamin D for health and in chronic kidney disease. Semin Dial 2005;18:266–75.

106. Shimada T, Hasegawa H, Yamazaki Y, et al. FGF-23 is a potent regulator of vitamin D metabolism and phosphate homeostasis. J Bone Miner Res 2004;19:429–35.

107. Dusso AS, Brown AJ, Slatopolsky E. Vitamin D. Am J Physiol Renal Physiol 2005;289:F8-F28.

108. Holick MF. Resurrection of vitamin D deficiency and rickets. J Clin Invest 2006;11:2062–72.

109. Chen H, Hewison M, Hu B, Adams JS. Heterogeneous nuclear ribonucleoprotein (hnRNP) binding to hormone response elements: a cause of vitamin D resistance. Proc Natl Acad Sci USA 2003;100:6109–14.

110. Ward LM, Rauch F, White KE, et al. Resolution of severe, adolescent-onset hypophosphatemic rickets following resection of an FGF-23-producing tumor of the distal ulna. Bone 2004;34:905–11.

111. Hollis BW, Wagner CL. Vitamin D requirements during lactation: high-dose maternal supplementation as therapy to prevent hypovitaminosis D for both, the mother and the nursing infant. Am J Clin Nutr 2004;80(suppl 6):S1752-S1758.

112. Calvo MS, Whiting SJ, Barton CN. Vitamin D fortification in the United States and Canada: current status and data needs. Am J Clin Nutr 2004;80(suppl 6):S1710-S1716.

113. Gartner LM, Greer FR. Section on Breastfeeding and Committee on Nutrition, prevention of rickets and vitamin D deficiency: new guidelines for vitamin D intake. Pediatrics 2003;111:908–10.

114. Vieth R, Bischoff-Ferrari HA, Boucher BJ, et al. The urgent need to recommend an intake of vitamin D that is effective. Am J Clin Nutr 2007;85:649–50.

115. Institute of Medicine. Dietary reference intake for calcium, phosphorus, magnesium, vitamin D and fluoride. National Academies Press, Washington, DC, 1997.

116. Saadi HF, Dawoudu A, Afindi BO, et al. Efficacy of daily and monthly high-dose calciferol in vitamin D deficient nulliparous and lactating women. Am J Clin Nutr 2007;85:1565–71.

117. Glerup H, Mikkelsen S, Poulsen L, *et al*. Commonly recommended daily intake of vitamin D is not sufficient if sunlight exposure is limited. J Intern Med 2000;247:260–8.

118. Vieth R, Chan PCR, MacFarlane GD. Efficacy and safety of vitamin D3 intake exceeding the lowest observed adverse level (LOAEL). Am J Clin Nutr 2001;73:288–94.

119. Heaney RP, Davies KM, Chen TC, *et al*. Human serum 25-hydroxycholecalciferol response to extended oral dosing with cholecalciferol. Am J Clin Nutr 2003;77:204–10.

120. Vieth R. Why the optimal requirements for vitamin D3 is probably much higher than is officially recommended for adults. J Steroid Mol Biol 2004;89:575–9.

121. Koutkia P, Lu Z, Chen TC, *et al*. Treatment of vitamin D deficiency due to Crohn's disease with tanning bed ultraviolet B radiation. Gastroenterology 2001;121:1485–8.

122. Aris RM, Merkel PA, Bachrach LK, *et al*. Guide to bone health and disease in cystic fibrosis. J Clin Endocrinol Metab 2005;90:1888–96.

123. Clinical practice guidelines for bone metabolism and disease in chronic kidney disease. Am J Kidney Dis 2003;42(suppl 3): S1-S201.

124. Brown AJ. Therapeutic uses of vitamin D analogues. Am J Kidney Dis 2001;38(suppl 5):S3-S19.

125. Silverberg SJ, Shane E, Dempster DW, Bilezikian JP. The effects of vitamin D insufficiency in patients with primary hyperparathyroidism. Am J Med 1999;107:561–7.

126. Brown AJ, Ritter CS, Knutson JC, Strugnell SA. The vitamin D prodrugs 1α (OH)D2, 1α(OH)D3 and BCI-210 suppress PTH secretion by bovine parathyroid cells. Nephrol Dial Transplant 2006;21 644–50.

127. Grey A, Lucas J, Horne A, *et al*. Vitamin D repletion in patients with primary hyperparathyroidism and coexistent vitamin D insufficiency. J Clin Endocrinol Metab 2005;90:2122–6.

128. Moosgaard B, Vestergaard P, Heickendorff L, *et al*. Vitamin D status, seasonal variations, parathyroid adenoma weight and bone mineral density in primary hyperparathyroidism. Clin Endocrinol (Oxford) 2005;63:506–13.

129. Rao DS, Honasoge M, Divine GW, *et al*. Effect of vitamin D nutrition on parathyroid adenoma weight: pathogenetic and clinical implications. J Clin Endocrinol Metab 2000;85:1054–8.

130. Adams JS, Hewison M. Hypercalcemia caused by granulomas-forming disorders. In: Favus MJ (ed) Primer on the metabolic bone diseases and disorders of mineral metabolism, 6th edn. American Society for Bone and Mineral Research, Washington, DC, 2006: 200–2.

131. Potts JT Jr. Diseases of the parathyroid gland and other hyper- and hypocalcemic disorders. In: Kasper DL, Braunwald E, Fauci AS, *et al*. (eds) Harrison's principles of internal medicine, 16th edn. McGraw-Hill, New York, 2005: 2249–68.

132. Schnatz PF, Thaxton S. Parathyroidectomy in the third trimester of pregnancy. Obstet Gynecol Surv 2005;60(10):672–82.

133. Haenel LC, Mayfield RK. Primary hyperparathyroidism in a twin pregnancy and review of fetal/maternal calcium homeostasis. Am J Med Sci 2000;319:191–4.

134. Hunter D, Turnbull H. Hyperparathyroidism: generalised osteitis fibrosa with observations upon bones, parathyroid tumors and the normal parathyroid glands. Br J Surg 1931;19:203–6.

135. Usta M, Chammas U, Khalil AM. Renal cell carcinoma with hypercalcemia complicating a pregnancy: case report and review of the literature. Eur J Gynaecol Oncol 1998;19:584–7.

136. Ornoy A, Wajnberg R, Diav-Citrin O. The outcome of pregnancy following pre-pregnancy or early pregnancy alendronate treatment. Reprod Toxicol 2006;22(4):578–9.

137. Kohlmeier L, Marcus R. Calcium disorders of pregnancy. Endocrinol Metab Clin North Am 1995;24:15–39.

138. Kort KC, Schiller HJ, Numann PJ. Hyperparathyroidism and pregnancy. Am J Surg 1999;177:66–8.

139. Gould CS, O'Malley BP, MacVicar J Endocrine hyperemesis – the need for a high index of clinical suspicion. J Obstet Gynaecol 1984;4:191–2.

140. Carella MJ, Gossain W. Hyperparathyroidism and pregnancy. Case report and review. J Gen Intern Med 1992;7:448–53.

141. Krissoffersson A, Dahlgren S, Lithner F, *et al*. Primary hyperparathyroidism in pregnancy. Surgery 1985;97:326–30.

142. Lowe DK, Orwoll ES, McClung MR, *et al*. Hyperparathyroidism in pregnancy. Am J Surg 1983;145:611–14.

143. Shangold MM, Dor N, Welt SI, *et al*. Hyperparathyroidism and pregnancy: a review. Obstet Gynecol Surv 1982;37:217–28.

144. Wilson DT, Martin T, Christensen R, *et al*. Hyperparathyroidism in pregnancy. Case report and review of the literature. Can Med Assoc J 1983;129:986–9.

145. Thomason JL, Sampson MB, Farb HF, Spellacy WN. Pregnancy complicated by concurrent primary hyperparathyroidism and pancreatitis. Obstet Gynecol 1981;57:345–65.

146. Montoro MN, Paler RL, Mestman JH, Goodwin TM. Parathyroid carcinoma during pregnancy. Obstet Gynecol 2000;96(5, suppl 2):841.

147. Ficinski ML, Mestman JH. Primary hyperparathyroidism during pregnancy. Endocr Pract 1996;2:362–7.

148. Ip P. Neonatal convulsion revealing maternal hyperparathyroidism: an unusual case of late neonatal hypoparathyroidism. Arch Gynecol Obstet 2003;268:227–9.

149. Graham EM, Freedman LJ, Forouzan I. Intrauterine growth retardation in a woman with primary hyperparathyroidism. A case report. J Reprod Med 1998;43:451–4.

150. Kaplan EL, Burrington JD, Klementschitsch P, *et al*. Primary hyperparathyroidism, pregnancy, and neonatal hypocalcemia. Surgery 1984;96:717–22.

151. Schnatz PF, Curry SL. Primary hyperparathyroidism in pregnancy: evidence-based management. Obstet Gynecol Surv 2002;57:365–76.

152. Tan HA. Incipient primary hyperparathyroidism in a primigravida. Endocrinologist 2005;15:361–5.

153. Amaya Garcia M, Acosta Feria M, Soto Moreno A, *et al*. Primary hyperparathyroidism in pregnancy. Gynecol Endocrinol 2004;19:111–14.

154. Delmonico FL, Neer RM, Cosimi AB, *et al*. Hyperparathyroidism during pregnancy. Am J Surg 1976;131:328–37.

155. Kelly TR. Primary hyperparathyroidism during pregnancy. Surgery 1991;110:1028–34.

156. Wagner G, Transhol L, Melchior JC. Hyperparathyroidism and pregnancy. Acta Endocrinol 1964;47:549–64.

157. Ludwig GD. Hyperparathyroidism in relation to pregnancy. N Engl J Med 1962;267:637–42.

158. Bruce J, Strong JA. Maternal hyperparathyroidism and parathyroid deficiency in the child. Q J Med 1955;96:307–19.

159. Mitchell TG. Chronic hypoparathyroidism associated with multicystic kidney. Arch Dis Child 1954;29:349–53.

160. Reading CC, Charboneau JW, James EM, *et al*. High-resolution parathyroid sonography. Am J Roentgenol 1982;139:539–46.

161. Sauer M, Steere A, Parsons MT. Hyperparathyroidism in pregnancy with sonographic documentation of a parathyroid adenoma. A case report. J Reprod Med 1985;30:615–17.

162. Van Dalen A, Smit CP, van Vroohoven TJ, *et al*. Minimally invasive surgery for solitary parathyroid adenomas in patients with primary hyperparathyroidism: role of ultrasound with supplemental computed tomography. Radiology 2001;220:631–9.

163. Higgins RV, Hisley JC. Primary hyperparathyroidism during pregnancy: a report of two cases. J Reprod Med 1988;33:726–30.

164. Tollin SR. Course and outcome of pregnancy in a patient with mild, asymptomatic, primary hyperparathyroidism diagnosed before conception. Am J Med Sci 2000;320:144–7.

165. Dorey LG, Gell JW. Primary hyperparathyroidism during the third trimester of pregnancy. Obstet Gynacol 1975;45:469–71.

166. Hsieh Y, Chang C, Tsai H, et al. Primary hyperparathyroidism in pregnancy – report of 3 cases. Arch Gynecol Obstet 1998;261:209–14.

167. Patterson R. Hyperparathyroidism in pregnancy. Obstet Gynecol 1987;70:457–60.

168. Levine G, Tsin D, Risk A. Acute pancreatitis and hyperparathyroidism in pregnancy. Obstet Gynecol 1979;54:246–8.

169. Clark D, Seeds JW, Cefalo RC. Hyperparathyroid crisis and pregnancy. Am J Obstet Gynecol 1981;140:840–2.

170. Negishi H, Kobayashi M, Nishida R, et al. Primary hyperparathyroidism and simultaneous bilateral fracture of the femoral neck during pregnancy. J Trauma Injury Infect Crit Care 2002;52:367–9.

171. JesudasonWV, Murphy J, England RJ. Primary hyperparathyroidism in pregnancy. J Laryngol Otol 2004;118:891–2.

172. Bilezikian JP, Khan AA, Potts JT Jr. Guidelines for the management of asymptomatic primary hyperparathyroidism: summary statement from the third international workshop. J Clin Endocrinol Metab 2009;94(2):335–9.

173. Montoro MN, Collea JV, Mestman JH. Management of hyperparathyroidism in pregnancy with oral phosphate therapy. Obstet Gynecol 1980;65:431–4.

174. Levy HA, Pierucci L, Stroup P. Oral phosphate treatment of hypercalcemia in pregnancy. J Med Soc NJ 1081;78:113–15.

175. Nussbaum SR. Pathophysiology and management of severe hypercalcemia. Endocrinol Metab Clin North Am 1993;22:343–62.

176. Murry JA, Newman WA, Dacus JV. Hyperparathyroidism in pregnancy. Diagnostic dilemma? Obstet Gynecol Surv 1997;52:202–5.

177. Bastepe M, Jüppner H. Pseudohypoparathyroidism: new insights into an old disease. Endocrinol Metab Clin North Am 2000;29:569–89.

178. Eastell R, Edmonds CJ, Chayal RCS, et al. Prolonged hypoparathyroidism presenting eventually as second trimester abortion. BMJ 1985;291:955–6.

179. Thomas AK, McVie R, Levine SN. Disorders of maternal calcium metabolism implicated by abnormal calcium metabolism in the neonate. Am J Perinatol 1999;16(10):515–20.

180. Graham WP, Gordan GS, Loken HF, et al. Effect of pregnancy and of the menstrual cycle on hypoparathyroidism. J Clin Endocrinol Metab 1964;24:512–16.

181. Callies F, Arlt W, Scholz HJ, et al. Management of hypoparathyroidism during pregnancy – report of twelve cases. Eur J Endocrinol 1998;139(3):284–9.

182. Sadeghi-Nejad A, Wolfsdorf JI, Senior B. Hypoparathyroidism and pregnancy: treatment with calcitriol. JAMA 1980;243:254–5.

183. Salle BL, Berthezene F, Glorieux FH, et al. Hypoparathyroidism during pregnancy: treatment with calcitriol. J Clin Endocrinol Metab 1981;52:810–12.

184. Friedman WF, Mills LE. The relationship between vitamin D and the craniofacial and dental anomalies of the supravalvular aortic stenosis syndrome. Pediatrics 1969;43:12–18.

185. Taussig HB. Possible injury to the cardiovascular system from vitamin D. Ann Intern Med 1966;65:1195–200.

186. O'Leary J, Klainer LM, Neuwirth RS. The management of hypoparathyroidism in pregnancy. Am J Obstet Gynecol 1966;15:1103–7.

187. Marx SJ, Swart EG, Hamstra AJ, et al. Normal intrauterine development of the fetus of the fetus of a woman receiving extraordinarily high doses of 1, 25-dihydroxyvitamin D. J Clin Endocrinol Metab 1980;51:1138–42.

188. Levine BS, Singer FR, Bryce GF, et al. Pharmacokinetics and biologic effects of calcitriol in normal humans. J Lab Clin Med 1985;105:239–46.

189. Bastepe M, Jupner H. Pseudohypoparathyroidism and mechanisms of resistance toward multiple hormones: molecular evidence to clinical presentation. J Clin Endocrinol Metab 2003;88(9):4055–8.

190. O'Donnell D, Costa J, Meyers AM. Management of pseudohypoparathyroidism in pregnancy. Case report. Br J Obstet Gynaecol 1985;92:639–41.

191. Glass EJ, Barr DG. Transient neonatal hyperparathyroidism secondary to maternal pseudo-hypoparathyroidism. Arch Dis Child 1981;56:566–8.

192. Mather KJ, Chik CL, Coremblum B. Maintenance of serum calcium by parathyroid hormone-related peptide during lactation in a hypoparathyroid patient. J Clin Endocrinol Metab 1999;84(2):424–7.

193. VanHouten JN, Dann P, Stewart AF, et al. Mammary-specific deletion of parathyroid hormone-related protein preserves bone mass during lactation. J Clin Invest 2003;112(9):1429–36.

194. Caplan RH, Wickus GG. Reduced calcitriol requirements for treating hypoparathyroidism during lactation. A case report. J Reprod Med 1993;38(11):914–18.

195. Shomali ME, Ross DS. Hypercalcemia in a woman with hypoparathyroidism associated with increased parathyroid hormone-related protein during lactation. Endocr Pract 1999;5(4):198–200.

196. Lepre F, Grill V, Ho PW, et al. Hypercalcemia in pregnancy and lactation associated with parathyroid hormone-related protein (letter). N Engl J Med 1993;328:666–7.

197. Caplan RH, Miller CD, Silva PD. Severe hypercalcemia in a lactating woman in association with moderate calcium carbonate supplementation: a case report. J Reprod Med 2004;49(3):214–17.

198. Abe Y. Effects of changing the ionic environment on passive and active membrane properties of pregnant rat uterus. J Physiol 1971;214:173–90.

199. Narang R, Jain V, Kaur J. Hypoparathyroidism. An unusual cause for nonprogress of labor. Endocrinologist 2008;18:11–12.

200. Wilkins IA, Goldberg JD, Phillips RN, et al. Long-term use of magnesium sulfate as a tocolytic agent. Obstet Gynecol 1986;67(suppl 3):38S-40S.

201. Donovan EF, Tsang RC, Steichen JJ, et al. Neonatal hypermagnesemia: effect on parathyroid hormone and calcium homeostasis. J Pediatr 96: 305–310, 1980.

202. Cholst IN, Steinberg SF, Tropper PJ, et al. The influence of hypermagnesemia on serum calcium and parathyroid hormone levels in human subjects. N Engl J Med 1984;310:1221–5.

203. Cruikshank DP, Pitkin RM, Reynolds WA, et al. Effects of magnesium sulfate treatment on perinatal calcium metabolism: maternal and fetal responses. Am J Obstet Gynecol 1979;134:243–9.

204. Brown EM, Pollak M, Seidman CE, et al. Calcium-ion-sensing cell-surface receptors. N Engl J Med 1995;333:234–40.

205. Brown EM, El-Hajj Fuleihan G, Chen CJ, Kifor O. A comparison of the effects of divalent and trivalent cations on parathyroid hormone release, 3′, 5′-cyclic-adenosine monophosphate accumulation, and the levels of inositol phosphates in bovine parathyroid cells. Endocrinology 1990;127:1064–71.

206. Koontz SL, Friedman SA, Schwartz ML. Symptomatic hypocalcemia after tocolytic therapy with magnesium sulfate and nifedipine. Am J Obstet Gynecol 2004;190:1773–6.
207. Smith Jr. LG, Burns PA, Schanler RJ. Calcium homeostasis in pregnant women receiving long-term magnesium sulfate therapy for preterm labor. Am J Obstet Gynecol 1992;167:45–51.
208. Hung JW, Tsai MY, Yang BY, Chen JF. Maternal osteoporosis after prolonged magnesium tocolysis therapy: a case report. Arch Phys Med Rehabil 2005;86:146–9.
209. Levav AL, Chan L, Wapner RJ. Long-term magnesium sulfate tocolysis and maternal osteoporosis in a triplet pregnancy: a case report. Am J Perinatol 1998;15:43–6.
210. Lipsitz PJ, English IC. Hypermagnesemia in the newborn infant. Pediatrics 1967;40:856–62.
211. Lipsitz PJ. The clinical and biochemical effects of excess magnesium in the newborn. Pediatrics 1971;47:501–9.
212. Savory G, Monif GR. Serum calcium levels in cord sera of the progeny of mothers treated with magnesium sulfate for toxemia of pregnancy. Am J Obstet Gynecol 1971;110:556–9.
213. Lamm CI, Norton KI, Murphy RJ, *et al*. Congenital rickets associated with magnesium sulfate infusion for tocolysis. J Pediatr 1988;113:1078–82.
214. Santi MD, Henry GW, Douglas GL. Magnesium sulfate treatment of preterm labor as a cause of abnormal neonatal bone mineralization. J Pediatr Orthop 1994;14:249–53.
215. Cumming WA, Thomas VJ. Hypermagnesemia: a cause of abnormal metaphyses in the neonate. Am J Roentgenol 1989;152:1071–2.
216. Malaeb SN, Rassi AI, Haddad MC, *et al*. Bone mineralization in newborns whose mothers received magnesium sulfate for tocolysis of premature labour. Pediatr Radiol 2004;34:384–6.

15 Neurologic disorders in obstetric practice

Dominic C. Heaney[1], David J. Williams[2], Patrick O'Brien[2] with Chris Elton[3]

[1]UCL Institute of Neurology, University College London and UCL Hospitals NHS Foundation Trust, London, UK
[2]UCL Institute of Women's Health, University College London and UCL Hospitals NHS Foundation Trust, London, UK
[3]Department of Anaesthesia, Leicester Royal Infirmary, Leicester, UK

Introduction

Neurologic conditions are an important cause of morbidity and mortality in pregnant women. In the UK between 2003 and 2005, women with neurologic conditions accounted for 37 out of a total 87 maternal deaths, with stroke (n=24) and epilepsy (n=11) [1] accounting for the majority of deaths from neurologic causes [2]. Several other disabling neurologic conditions, ranging from multiple sclerosis to migraine, present both medical and obstetric challenges to clinicians unfamiliar with their management within the context of pregnancy.

The natural history of key neurologic conditions has been observed during pregnancy, providing a useful basis on which to counsel women and organize services. Less information is available about the safety of neurologic treatments or investigations during pregnancy or obstetric and neonatal outcomes for these women. Therefore many decisions rely on applying key obstetric and neurologic principles to situations where published data are not available.

This chapter outlines neurologic assessment and investigation in pregnancy. The most common and important neurologic presentations – multiple sclerosis, epilepsy, stroke, central nervous system (CNS) tumors and headache – are considered. These disparate conditions allow basic principles of management to be described. Overall, women with pre-existing neurologic conditions or who develop neurologic symptoms during pregnancy rely on good communication between their obstetrician, neurologist, physician and anesthetist to achieve optimal obstetric and neonatal outcome.

Neurologic assessment

History and examination

Neurologic symptoms in pregnancy should be elicited in the usual way with particular emphasis on their onset and progression, and their associated features.

Higher mental function

Neurologic examination should first consider higher mental function. It may be sufficient to establish that the patient is alert and orientated, and that her conversation is normal in both its form and content. But any suspicion of impaired cognitive functioning either at the time of assessment or in the past should lead to assessment of conscious level using a simple instrument such as the Glasgow Coma Scale (Table 15.1) or the more detailed Mini-Mental State Examination (Box 15.1).

Cranial nerves, trunk and limbs

Neurologic examination of the cranial nerves, trunk and limbs can be an involved and lengthy process. Over 150 years, numerous eponymous signs and methods of examination have been described but what follows is a basic neurologic screen, which should be sufficient for an obstetrician to establish most important neurologic findings, which will guide investigation and further referral.

The minimum cranial nerve examination involves consideration of each of the 12 cranial nerves (Table 15.2).

Trunk and limbs

Examination of the trunk and limbs involves examination of their appearance (inspection), tone, strength, co-ordination and sensory perception.

de Swiet's Medical Disorders in Obstetric Practice, 5th edition.
Edited by R. O. Powrie, M. F. Greene, W. Camann. © 2010 Blackwell Publishing.

Table 15.1 Glasgow Coma Scale

	1	2	3	4	5	6
Eyes	Does not open eyes	Opens eyes in response to painful stimuli	Opens eyes in response to voice	Opens eyes spontaneously	N/A	N/A
Verbal	Makes no sounds	Incomprehensible sounds	Utters inappropriate words	Confused, disoriented	Oriented, converses normally	N/A
Motor	Makes no movements	Extension to painful stimuli	Abnormal flexion to painful stimuli	Flexion/ withdrawal to painful stimuli	Localizes painful stimuli	Obeys commands

Box 15.1 Mini-Mental State Exam

The Mini-Mental State Examination (MMSE) is a tool that can be used to objectively assess mental status. It is an 11-question measure that tests five areas of cognitive function: orientation, registration, attention and calculation, recall, and language. The maximum score is 30. A score of 23 or lower is indicative of cognitive impairment. The MMSE takes only 5 minutes to administer and is therefore practical for routine repeated use.

Orientation
5 ( ) What is the (year) (season) (date) (day) (month)?
5 ( ) Where are we (state) (country) (town) (hospital) (floor)?

Registration
3 ( ) Name 3 objects: 1 second to say each. Then ask the patient
all 3 after you have said them. Give 1 point for each correct answer.
Then repeat them until he/she learns all 3. Count trials and record.

Attention and calculation
5 ( ) Serial 7's. 1 point for each correct answer. Stop after 5 answers.
Alternatively spell "world" backward.

Recall
3 ( ) Ask for the 3 objects repeated above. Give 1 point for each correct answer.

Language
2 ( ) Name a pencil and watch.
1 ( ) Repeat the following "No ifs, ands, or buts."
3 ( ) Follow a three-stage command: "Take a paper in your hand, fold it in half, and put it on the floor."
1 ( ) Read and obey the following: CLOSE YOUR EYES.
1 ( ) Write a sentence.
1 ( ) Copy the design shown.

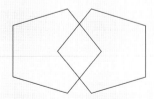

Adapted from: Folstein M Folstein SE, McHugh PR. "Mini-Mental State": a practical method for grading the cognitive state of patients for the clinician. J Psychiatr Res 1975;12(3):189–98.

Table 15.2 Examination of cranial nerves – summary

Cranial nerve	Number	Examination	Comment
Olfactory	1	Formal smell testing (coffee, cloves, peppermint, etc.)	Usually sufficient to ask a patient whether their taste and smell is normal
Optic	2	Visual acuity Visual fields Fundi Pupillary reaction to light and close gaze (accommodation)	It is very important from a medical legal standpoint to document objective assessment of visual acuity in any patient with visual complaints
Oculomotor	3	Eyelid retraction (look for ptosis) Eye movements	Ask if double vision present Verify conjugate gaze to 8 points in visual field (up, down,
Trochlear	4	Eye movements	to the right, left, upper right, lower right, upper left and
Abducens	6	Eye movements	lower left)
Trigeminal	5 (a,b,c)	Sensory (face) Motor (jaw muscles) Afferent portion of corneal reflex (touch tissue to cornea, over iris) and watch for bilateral eyelid closure via CN7	Verify bilateral sensation in upper, middle and lower face and ask patient to bite down while palpating temporomandibular and masseter muscles, then asking them to move jaw from side to side to test pterygoids Any hint that trigeminal function impaired warrants assessment of corneal reflex to establish risk of exposure keratitis
Facial	7	Facial weakness	Ask patient to raise eyebrows, tightly close eyes then bare teeth Preservation of ability to raise eyebrows suggests upper (central nervous system, e.g. stroke) not lower (peripheral nervous system, e.g. Bell's palsy) motor nerve lesion
Vestibulocochlear	8	Hearing/balance	Ask about vertigo Gently rub fingers close to each ear to test hearing
Glossopharyngeal	9	Palate	Listen to quality of voice and examine palatal and uvula
Vagus	10	Various, including recurrent laryngeal nerve	movements – for example when saying "ahh"
Accessory	11	Motor to trapezius and sternocleidomastoid	Ask patient to raise her shoulders and to rotate the head left and right against resistance
Hypoglossal	12	Tongue movements	Assess quality of speech. Ask patient to stick out her tongue and ensure it is midline

Inspection involves looking for atrophy, hypertrophy, spasm or fasciculations of the muscles.

Tone can be examined throughout range of movement in each of the major joints and it may be appropriate to assess truncal tone, either in the sitting or ideally the standing position. In general, increased tone may be the result of a CNS disorder affecting the brain or spinal cord whereas reduced tone (flaccid weakness) is the result of a more peripheral problem.

Power is described by the Medical Research Council (MRC) scale (0–5) at each major joint in flexion, extension and if necessary in abduction and adduction (Box 15.2).

The pattern of any weakness demonstrated is important; for example, metabolic disorders such as thyroid disease or diabetes may cause a more proximal weakness. Neuropathies typically cause a distal weakness.

Co-ordination can be assessed in the upper limbs by examining ability to alternately touch the examiner's outstretched finger and then the patient's own nose. A further examination is for the presence of dysdiadochokinesis, which is assessed by asking the patient to rapidly tap their palm with alternating sides of their fingers, and considering the fluency and speed with which this is achieved. Assessment of lower limb co-ordination involves examination of normal gait, and then tandem (heel to toe) walking.

Sensation should be assessed using a "sharp" stimulus (ideally a "Neurotip", although a broken tongue blade may be used if nothing else is available) and dabbing (rather than stroking) with cotton wool or similar stimulus. Thought

Box 15.2 MRC scale for muscle power

0   No muscle contraction is visible
1   Muscle contraction is visible but there is no movement of the joint
2   Active joint movement is possible with gravity eliminated
3   Movement can overcome gravity but not resistance from the examiner
4   The muscle group can overcome gravity and move against some resistance from the examiner
5   Full and normal power against resistance

should be given to the pattern of sensory loss expected from history and earlier examination. For example, a woman complaining of back pain may have radicular (nerve root) rather than distal ("glove and stocking") sensory loss. Even where there is no obvious loss of sensation to pinprick or soft touch, joint position and vibration sense may be impaired.

Reflexes and plantar responses (reviewed in Boxes 15.3 and 15.4) are an important element of both motor and sensory examination. Brisk reflexes are very common in pregnancy but may indicate hyperarousal or CNS pathology – and the latter is supported if the plantar reflexes are extensor. Clonus (five or more repetitive, rhythmic contractions of a muscle when attempting to hold it in a stretched state) is always abnormal. Reduced or absent reflexes may imply a neuropathy.

Finally, Romberg's test, where the patient is asked to stand with their feet close together and eyes closed, is sensitive to a wide range of neurologic impairments. For example, patients with pathologies as disparate as distal neuropathy, cerebellar disease or generalized weakness may all sway when the test is performed, and this can act as a useful screening check that an abnormality has not been missed in an otherwise normal patient.

Neurologic investigations

Many neurologic investigations pose no risk to the pregnant mother or her fetus. For example, neurophysiologic assessment such as electroencephalography (EEG), nerve

---

Box 15.3 Deep tendon reflexes and the associated spinal cord nerve roots

- Biceps reflex (C5, C6)
- Brachioradialis reflex (C5, C6, C7)
- Triceps reflex (C6, C7, C8)
- Patellar reflex or knee-jerk reflex (L2, L3, L4)
- Ankle jerk reflex (Achilles reflex) (S1, S2)
- Plantar reflex or Babinski reflex (L5, S1, S2)

Box 15.4 The plantar reflex

The lateral side of the sole of the foot is rubbed with a blunt instrument from the heel along the curve to the metatarsal pads of the toes.

A "flexor response" (absent Babinski response), in which the toes curl into themselves, is normal.

An "extensor response" (the Babinski reponse is present), in which the big toe bends up towards the top of the foot and the other toes fan out, is abnormal and is highly suggestive of central nervous system damage.

---

conduction studies and electromyography (EMG) may be uncomfortable but are noninvasive.

Cerebrospinal fluid (CSF) is obtained by lumbar puncture and can show evidence of intrathecal infection, inflammation or the presence of subarachnoid hemorrhage or neoplasia. Lumbar puncture is relatively invasive and standard relative and absolute contraindications should be considered. In particular, lumbar puncture may cause CSF leak and a fall in CSF pressure. Neuroimaging should precede this investigation if raised intracranial pressure is suspected. Interpretation of CSF analysis is reviewed in Chapter 16.

Neuroimaging is often an integral part of patient assessment. Diagnostic imaging in pregnancy is reviewed in Chapter 32 but will be briefly reviewed here. The ionizing radiation associated with computed tomography (CT) neuroimaging leads to obvious concern on the parts of both clinicians and patients when imaging the pregnant woman. However, CT head involves a fetal radiation exposure of less than 0.005 mGy (0.0005 rad) and thus is extremely unlikely to have any fetal effects [3]. Uterine shields are routinely employed and will reduce exposure even further. The advantages that CT imaging of the head offers by way of early diagnosis, particularly when cerebral hemorrhage is suspected, should outweigh any cultural aversion to radiologic imaging in pregnancy.

Magnetic resonance imaging (MRI) of the brain has greater resolution than CT and greater diagnostic flexibility. It does not involve ionizing radiation and thus avoids any issues related to radiation exposure in pregnancy. However, although there is no evidence of fetal harm in humans after 20 years of widespread use of this technology, many guidelines recommend that MRI be delayed to the end of the first trimester when possible. Two other disadvantages of MRI are that performing the scans takes up to 45 minutes and they are more difficult to obtain in a timely manner in most countries as there are fewer MR than CT scanners.

Iodinated contrast agents can be used in pregnancy and lactation but intravenous contrast agents used in MR (e.g. gadolinium) are not [4].

Certain clinical situations may indicate the use of other ionizing radiologic techniques such as digital subtraction angiography. The expected radiation dose depends on the procedure. For example, this may be low with head imaging, but higher for spinal procedures. Clinicians should balance the risks of not fully investigating a patient against potential harm to the fetus.

Multiple sclerosis

Definition and Incidence

Multiple sclerosis (MS) is a disease of the CNS (brain and spinal cord) that is characterized by both neuroinflammation and neurodegeneration (Figure 15.1). Incidence is 3.6 cases per 100,000 person-years (95% confidence interval (CI) 3.0–4.2)

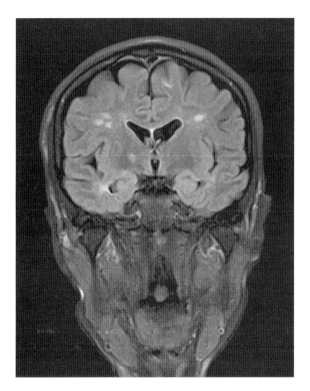

Figure 15.1 MRI scan showing T2 hyperintensities typical of multiple sclerosis.

in women and is higher in northern latitudes, although this trend seems to be reducing [5]. The disease can have many clinical manifestations (with sensory loss in the limbs, visual loss, subacute motor loss, double vision and gait disturbance being most common) and a highly variable pace of progression (relapsing remitting, secondary progressive, primary progressive and progressive relapsing). The median survival from onset of symptoms is 38 years. MS is usually diagnosed between 20 and 50 years of age, and women with MS will therefore become pregnant relatively early in the course of their illness and have correspondingly little associated disability [6]. Nevertheless the issues of symptom management and counseling are relevant at all stages throughout pregnancy.

Preconception advice

Preconception counseling offers the opportunity to discuss the effect that pregnancy may have on MS, the effect that MS-related neurologic impairment may have on pregnancy and delivery, and the use of disease-modifying or symptomatic treatments both in pregnancy and post partum.

Many people with relapsing and remitting MS are treated with disease-modifying drugs (DMD). These include beta-interferons and a synthetic polypeptide, glatiramer acetate. These treatments are administered by subcutaneous or intramuscular injection at least weekly and have been shown to have a modest but significant effect on reducing relapse rate

(approximately 30% per year) and to some extent long-term disability. The safety of these treatments in pregnancy has not been established. The US Food and Drug Administration (FDA) has assigned glatiramer acetate to pregnancy safety category B (i.e. appears to be safe for pregnancy in animal studies but not adequately studied in pregnant humans). It has not been shown to be a teratogen in animal studies and its large molecular weight (4700–11,000) suggests that if it crosses the placenta, it does not do so by simple diffusion. The interferons are US FDA pregnancy safety category C (i.e. human studies are lacking and animal studies are either positive for fetal risk or lacking as well). In high doses, interferons appear to be abortifacients, but not teratogens. Limited human data suggest that interferon-alpha (not used to treat MS) does not cross the placenta or cause congenital anomalies in humans. However, data on interferon-beta products used to treat MS are very limited and suggest it may be an abortifacient [7].

The authors recommend that women should therefore stop treatment with DMD if they are planning to become pregnant or find themselves pregnant. This is less because of any known toxicity of the majority of DMD and more because of the combined considerations of the limited human pregnancy safety data and the fact that many of these agents have only limited efficacy over long periods of time. Although stopping treatment may expose the patient to increased risk of relapse, in absolute terms the risk is relatively low (an "extra" 0.2 relapse/year) [8]. This risk is further modified by the beneficial effect of pregnancy itself (see below). Other experts would offer women with MS the option of continuing agents for which there is reassuring pregnancy data such as glatiramer acetate.

Women with MS may also be taking other drugs, such as antimuscarinics for bladder disorders (e.g. oxybutinin), antispasmodics (e.g. baclofen or diazepam), and antidepressants (e.g. tricyclic antidepressants). All these have low teratogenic potential. Table 15.3 lists some agents used to treat patients with MS and offers some opinions as to which agents might be considered for continued use or introduction during pregnancy.

Rarely, patients with MS or other conditions that cause spasticity have implantable devices delivering an antispasmodic agent, typically intrathecally. These pumps are sited within the abdominal wall, extraperitoneally. They supply a continuous infusion of baclofen through a catheter directly into the CSF in small doses. Several case reports have reported successful obstetric outcomes using these devices [8a].

The inheritance of MS is poorly understood and is likely to involve a complex interaction between genetic and environmental factors. Nevertheless, in general the child of a mother with MS has an approximately 2–3% chance of developing MS, compared with 0.1% prevalence in the general population [10] although the mother should be counseled that should MS occur, symptoms are unlikely to present until their third decade or later. The risk is increased further if both parents are affected.

Table 15.3 Risks and recommendations about the use of agents to treat MS during pregnancy

Drug	US FDA pregnancy category	Symptom the agent is used to treat	Use generally justifiable in pregnancy	Use justifiable in pregnancy in rare circumstances	Use almost never justifiable	Briggs *et al.* fetal risk recommendation [7]	Hale breastfeeding risk [9]
Amantadine	C	Fatigue			✓	Contraindicated – first trimester	L3
Baclofen	C	Muscle spasm	✓			Human data limited, animal data suggest low risk	L2 Approved by the American Academy of Breastfeeding for use with lactation.
Carbamazepine	D	Paroxysmal attacks of motor or sensory phenomena		✓		Known teratogen but may be used if risk outweighed by benefit	L2 Approved by the American Academy of Breastfeeding for use with lactation
Cladribine	D	Disease-modifying drug Lymphocytotoxic chemotherapy agent			✓	Not classified by Briggs *et al.* Human data extremely limited	n/a
Corticosteroids	C	Disease-modifying drug	✓			See Chapter 48	While lower dose steroids are compatible with breastfeeding, it is recommended that women breastfeeding on high-dose pulse methylprednisolone should pump and discard breast milk for between 8 and 24 hours after treatment
Cyclophosphamide	D	Disease-modifying drug Chemotherapy agent			✓	Contraindicated first trimester	L5
Desmopressin	B	Bladder dysfunction	✓			No human data, animal data suggest low risk	L2
Donepezil	C	Cognitive function		✓		No human data, animal data suggest low risk	L3
Glatiramer acetate	B	Disease-modifying drug	✓			Compatible: maternal benefit much greater than embryo/fetal risk	L3
Interferon-beta 1a	C	Disease-modifying drug		✓		No human data, animal data suggest moderate risk	L2
Interferon-beta 1b	C	Disease-modifying drug		✓		No human data, animal data suggest moderate risk	L2
Methotrexate	X	Disease-modifying drug Chemotherapy agent			✓	Contraindicated	L3
Mitoxantrone	D	Disease modifying drug Chemotherapy agent			✓	Contraindicated in first trimester Human data extremely limited	L5

Table 15.3 (Continued)

Drug	US FDA pregnancy category	Symptom the agent is used to treat	Use generally justifiable in pregnancy	Use justifiable in pregnancy in rare circumstances	Use almost never justifiable	Briggs et al. fetal risk recommendation [7]	Hale breastfeeding risk [9]
Natalizumab	C	monoclonal antibody against alpha-4 integrins			✓	Not classified by Briggs et al. Human data extremely limited	L3
Oxybutynin	B	bladder dysfunction	✓			No human data, animal data suggest low risk	L3
Selective serotonin reuptake inhibitors	Varies with agent	depression	✓			See Chapter 21. Sertraline, fluoxetine. probably the preferred agents of this class. Paroxetine should be avoided	Varies with agent. Sertraline probably preferred agent in this class.
Tizanidine	C	spasticity		✓		No human data animal data suggests risk (increased pregnancy loss and retarded development)	L4
Tolterodine	C	bladder dysfunction		✓		No human data, animal data suggest low risk	L3
Tricyclic antidepressants	Varies with agent	Depression	✓			See chapter 21. Nortriptyline and amçitriptyline probably preferred agents	Amitryptiline L2 Nortriptyline L2

US FDA pregnancy classification is reviewed in Chapter 30.
Hale classification for medications in lactation is reviewed in Chapter 31 (L1, safest; L2, safer; L3, moderately safe; L4, possibly hazardous; L5, contraindicated).

Effect of pregnancy on relapse rate

One of the most significant issues to discuss with women who are planning to become pregnant is the likely effect of pregnancy on relapse rate. In the past, the relatively high number of relapses observed post partum led to the false conclusion that pregnancy might lead to a long-term poorer outcome when compared with nonpregnant women. More reassuring advice should now be given, largely through the publication of a large prospective study ("PRegnancy In MS" (PRIMS)), which has continued to monitor enrolled mothers many years after enrolment into the study [11]. This study showed that although risk of relapse post partum was increased for approximately 3 months by a factor of two, this was equally balanced by the observation of significantly fewer relapses during pregnancy. Thus, overall no difference is observed in the long-term disability of women who become pregnant.

Relapse management

Although the risk of relapse is reduced during pregnancy, this effect is less pronounced during the first and second trimesters. Should relapse occur, management is the same as for nonpregnant women. Mild relapses require no treatment, but are likely to warrant assessment by occupational or physiotherapists, as levels of disability may be increased for several weeks. High-dose corticosteroids (for example, a total of 3 g methylprednisolone administered over 3–5 days intravenously or orally) may be used to speed up remission. Steroids present well-known risks including reduced bone density, infection, mood alteration and adverse gastrointestinal effects. Nevertheless, where standard precautions and pretreatment assessment are applied, steroids may avoid the need for hospitalization or reduce considerably the length of stay. The risks of glucocorticoid use for the embryo and fetus are discussed in Chapter 48 but these agents can and should be used when indicated to treat MS during pregnancy.

Occasionally, relapses are severe and progressive. In the nonpregnant woman these may be treated with more aggressive treatment, such as mitoxantrone (a chemotherapeutic agent) or natalizumab (a monoclonal antibody directed against alpha-4-integrin, which reduces white cell traffic into the CNS). These treatments are either clearly teratogenic and embryotoxic or have no evidence to support their safety in pregnancy. Clinicians should consider the advantages and risks to both mother and fetus on a case-by-case basis. Intravenous immunoglobulin [12] or possibly hemodialysis are alternative treatments, which may pose less risk to the fetus, but there is less evidence to suggest their efficacy in reducing MS progression.

Management of other symptoms

Women with MS may suffer from a range of symptoms during pregnancy including fatigue, restless lower limbs and urinary symptoms (see Table 15.3).

Nonpharmacologic advice to improve quality of sleep ("sleep hygiene") should be offered. This includes examination of an individual's sleep routine and the sleeping environment. Women should be encouraged to avoid psychologically stimulating activities in the evenings and pharmacologic stimulants such as caffeine should be minimized. Drug treatments such as amantadine or modafinil, which are sometimes used to reduce MS-related fatigue, cannot be recommended, as there is no evidence to support their safety in pregnancy.

A sense of restlessness in the lower limbs is common in pregnant women, but women with MS may also have a degree of spasticity manifest by painful or irritating spasm. Neurologic examination can be useful to demonstrate spasticity and localize relevant muscle groups. Physiotherapy advice and possibly use of benzodiazepines may be warranted.

Urinary symptoms should be carefully evaluated as impaired bladder emptying in women with MS predisposes to infection. Baclofen to treat bladder spasm is a reasonable option in pregnancy. Vigilance for early signs of urinary tract infections is important for any pregnant woman with bladder dysfunction. Women with pre-existing urinary problems may be concerned that vaginal delivery will exacerbate urinary symptoms post partum and may benefit from some discussion with their obstetrician as to the relationship between mode of delivery and future urinary continence.

Third trimester and delivery

In most cases, third trimester and the peripartum period are no different between populations of women with MS and the normal population. Specifically, obstetric and neonatal outcomes do not differ, with similar rates of induction, instrumentation, cesarean section and infant mortality.

Nevertheless, women with MS may have specific neurologic impairments that affect interpretation of symptoms during pregnancy. For example, women with plaques at T11 or lower will have impaired bladder and bowel function but normal sensation of uterine contractions and pain. Lesions between T6 and T10 will impair perception of uterine contractions and where significant lesions are present above T6, other signs of labor will have to be considered such as worsening lower limb spasticity.

In the past theoretical concerns have been expressed regarding the safety of epidural anesthesia and exacerbation of MS. Evidence from the PRIMS study, however, has been reassuring, demonstrating no significant difference in outcomes between women with and without epidural anesthesia.

Post partum

Women who are more mildly affected by MS are more likely to choose to breastfeed. Breastfeeding does not protect (or cause) a post partum relapse [13]. Women who have been taking DMD before pregnancy balance the benefits of breastfeeding against the risk of relapse without treatment. The agents commonly used to treat MS are classified according to their compatibility with breastfeeding in Table 15.3. Women who defer DMD treatment should be counseled that should they suffer relapse, most centers require good recovery before DMD are restarted, thus producing further delay.

Some centers have advocated prophylactic use of intravenous immunoglobulin post partum to prevent relapses [14]. Activity of disease in the year before pregnancy and in the first trimester to some extent predicts risk of relapse in the 3 months post partum. Nevertheless, a recent authoritative multivariate model predicts that using this information to make a decision about treatment would lead to 50% of women being treated unnecessarily [13] and the current consensus is therefore not to treat.

Stroke

Definition and incidence

Stroke is an acute neurologic impairment that follows interruption of blood supply to a specific part or the brain (Figure 15.2). It is the cause of 700,000 deaths per year in the US, a total of 1 in 15 of all deaths. The causes of stroke in the general population are reviewed in Box 15.5.

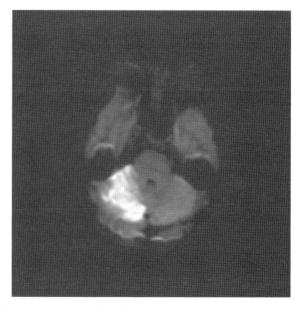

Figure 15.2 Acute stroke affecting the right cerebellum seen on diffusion-weighted MRI.

Box 15.5 Causes of stroke in the nonpregnant population

Ischemic 85%
- Thrombosis
- Arterial
  - Venous
  - Embolism
- Hypoperfusion

Hemorrhagic 15%
- Intracerebral, usually hypertension related
- Subarachnoid hemorrhage, usually related to aneurysms and AVM

Stroke is an uncommon but serious complication of pregnancy. The incidence of stroke in nonpregnant women aged 15–44 has been reported to be as low as 10.7 per 100,000 women-years [15]. Multicenter or long-term observational studies are therefore required to establish incidence in pregnancy. Estimates using such methods produce widely differing rates between 4.3 and 210 strokes per 100,000 deliveries, depending on inclusion criteria, with most studies suggesting an increased risk of stroke associated with pregnancy [16–18]. Most (up to 90%) strokes in these studies occurred at the time of delivery or or in the weeks following [19].

Risk factors for stroke

Physiologic

Progressive physiologic changes occurring throughout pregnancy predispose to stroke, including increasing hypercoagulability, venous stasis and vascular wall changes. The second stage of labor involves episodes of significantly increased intrathoracic pressure (Valsalva) and elevation of cerebral perfusion pressure, which may lead to changes in cerebral blood flow, particularly where cerebral autoregulation or anatomy is disordered [20].

Obstetric

The main obstetric factor associated with an increased risk of stroke is pre-eclampsia, in particular uncontrolled systolic hypertension. This is still the major cause of death due to pre-eclampsia in the UK [1]. Age more than 35 years, black ethnicity, greater parity and multiple gestation are all risk factors for stroke although quantifying this risk is not possible from available data.

Co-morbidity

Women who become pregnant may have co-morbidity that increases their risk of vascular events, including stroke, such as obesity (Body Mass Index (BMI) >30 kg/m^2), diabetes, pre-existing hypertension, renal and heart disease, vasculopathies such as sickle cell disease, vasculitis and pre-existing collagen or atherosclerotic disease. Alcohol, tobacco and cocaine use may cause a vasculopathy or hypertension.

Migraine with aura (see later) also produces excess risk for stroke but this condition is common and stroke in pregnancy is rare, and so caution should be applied when counseling women about this risk factor.

Previous stroke during pregnancy presents a particular dilemma for women considering further pregnancy. Unfortunately, data are lacking although in a follow-up study, 13 of 489 (2.7%) women aged 15–40 who had suffered a stroke had a recurrent event and only two of these occurred during pregnancy [21]. Full ascertainment of vascular risk factors, including CT or MR angiography, is likely to be appropriate to best inform the individual of her likely risk of pregnancy-related recurrent stroke.

Clinical presentation and management of stroke

Presentation and investigation

Stroke presents as in the nonpregnant and clinical features may suggest either infarction or hemorrhage but neuroimaging is required to confirm diagnosis. Stroke should be considered in any woman who presents with any of the symptoms listed in Box 15.6. While an imperfect screen with a specificity of 88% and a sensitivity varying from 66–100%, the Cincinnati Prehospital Stroke Scale may be useful in obstetric patients presenting with headache or other softer neurologic complaints to help decide if a patient warrants prompt complete neurologic assessment and neuroimaging. This screening test is summarized in Box 15.7.

As stated above, most pregnancy-related cerebral infarction occurs in the puerperium [17,23,24] at a time when the mother is often bedbound, still hypercoagulable and may just have had pelvic surgery. Widespread adoption of postpartum thromboprophylaxis in the UK has been associated with a

Box 15.6 Symptoms that warrant consideration of stroke

- Sudden weakness or numbness of face, arm or leg especially if on one side of the body
- Sudden confusion
- Trouble speaking or understanding
- Sudden trouble seeing in one or both eyes without a prior history of migraines
- Sudden trouble walking
- Sudden loss of balance or co-ordination not readily attributable to pregnancy
- Sudden severe headache with no known cause

Box 15.7 Cincinnati Stroke Scale [22]

Facial droop
- Have the patient smile and assess for facial droop
- Normal: both sides of face move equally
- Abnormal: one side of face does not move

Arm drift
- Have the patient hold both arms out and up with palms facing upwards
- Normal: both arms move equally
- Abnormal: one arm drifts compared with the other

Speech
- Have the patient repeat a sentence
- Normal: patient uses correct words with no slurring
- Abnormal: slurred or inappropriate words of mute

If any of these three elements or any other neurologic findings are newly abnormal, the possibility of acute stroke is high and the patient should have urgent imaging and evaluation by a neurologist.

Box 15.8 Guidelines for interventions in acute ischemic stroke

Patients presenting with symptoms of acute stroke to an emergency room should:
- be seen by a provider within 10 minutes with early notification of local "stroke team" of possible stroke patient
- have a neurologic assessment and head CT performed within 25 minutes of presentation
- have the head CT scan read within 45 minutes of presentation to determine whether they are candidates for fibrinolytic therapy
- receive fibrinolytic therapy administered within 60 minutes of presentation to the ER and no longer than 180 minutes since the time of onset of symptoms.

Box 15.9 Additional investigations for patients presenting with possible acute stroke

- Assess airway (can the patient protect her own airway or does she require intubation?), breathing (what is her respiratory rate and oxygenation?) and circulation (are her pulse and blood pressure normal?)
- Obtain secure intravenous access
- Obtain a fingerstick glucose
- Obtain a complete blood count, electrolytes, blood urea nitrogen, creatinine, serum glucose, serum troponin, liver function tests
- Consider urine toxicology screen and blood alcohol level
- Arterial blood gas if oxygen saturation abnormal Obtain an EKG

decrease in the incidence of cerebral infarction due to emboli, but not that due to uncontrolled systolic hypertension [1].

Stroke is a medical emergency. Patients with acute arterial ischemic stroke from embolism or thrombosis can have their long-term outcome greatly improved by the use of thrombolytic therapy within 180 minutes of the onset of symptoms. Therefore all patients with symptoms suggestive of stroke require prompt neuroimaging to determine if they have had an ischemic stroke that may benefit from the use of thrombolytic therapy. Box 15.8 lists the recommended guidelines for timing of interventions for patients presenting with acute ischemic stroke. Box 15.9 reviews the other assessments recommended for patients presenting with possible acute stroke. Patients should be positioned with the head of the bed between 0° and 15° and blood pressure should be treated acutely if greater than 180/105 with labetalol. Aspirin should not be given while investigating an acute stroke. Box 15.10 reviews the contraindications for thrombolytic therapy. The use of thrombolysis should be considered for pregnant and postpartum women with severe acute cerebral nonhemmorhagic infarction if it can administered within 180 minutes of onset of the neurologic deficit [25]. Thrombolysis is well tolerated by the fetus in pregnancy and should not be withheld if the maternal condition is life-threatening. Risks of postpartum uterine or pelvic haemorrhage can be dealt with by local haemostasis or surgery.

The authors and editors would, however, not recommend the use of thrombolytics for acute ischemic stroke in the setting of probable or confirmed pre-eclampsia.

Specific syndromes will be considered below, but in most cases pregnant women who have cerebral infarction should be managed within a multidisciplinary stroke unit. Aspirin is the mainstay of treatment for acute ischemic sroke. Aspirin and the other anitplatelet agents (aspirin with dipyridamole, or clopidogrel) are also the most effective preventive treatment of stroke. Unfractionated or low molecular weight heparin is not recommended for acute stroke or stroke prevention except in the case of stroke from cardioembolism, arterial dissections or large artery intraluminal thrombus [26]. Warfarin is teratogenic and usually avoided in pregnancy.

Box 15.10 Contraindications and cautions to thrombolytic therapy for acute stroke

Contraindications
- Intracranial hemorrhage on CT
- Presentation suggests SAH
- Multilobar infarction on CT
- History of intracranial hemorrhage
- Uncontrolled hypertension (>185/110 when treatment with fibrinolytics to be given)
- Known AVM/neoplasm
- Witnessed seizure at onset of stroke
- Active bleeding/acute bleeding diathesis (platelets <100, PTT elevated, INR >1.7)
- Within 3 months of intracranial or intraspinal surgery/serious head trauma or previous stroke
- Arterial puncture at a noncompressible site in the past 7 days

Cautions: consider whether benefits of thrombolytic therapy outweigh risks
- Minor or clearing stroke
- Within 14 days of major surgery or trauma
- Within 21 days of GI/GU hemorrhage
- Within 3 months of acute MI
- Post MI pericarditis
- Glucose <50 or >400 mg/dL

The differential diagnosis of acute stroke in pregnancy is broad and includes migraine, transient ischemic attacks, head trauma, brain tumor, Todd's palsy (a neurologic deficit following a seizure), systemic infection, functional deficits ("conversion disorders"), and toxic-metabolic disturbances (e.g. hypoglycemia, acute renal failure, hepatic insufficiency, drug intoxication). Perhaps the most challenging and common differential diagnosis for stroke in the obstetric population is migrainous aura. Migrainous auras are typically brief and more likely to be positive (the alteration of a sensory perception) rather than negative (the absence of a perception) (e.g. wavy lines in vision versus no vision or "pins and needles" versus numbness). Migrainous auras are most commonly visual (typically scotoma and/or zig-zag lines) or sensory ("pins and needles") in the perioral region. Less commonly, they are sensory in the upper limbs or difficulties with speech (typically disarticulation with word-finding difficulty or use of wrong words but no difficulty with comprehension). Neurologic symptoms other than these should not be casually attributed to migrainous aura. Visual or sensory symptoms should be one-sided, gradually progress and last between 5 and 60 minutes. If more than one aura symptom

is present, symptoms should occur in succession rather than simultaneously. Importantly, migraine and migrainous aura is by definition a recurring problem and the diagnosis cannot be made on first presentation of symptoms. If there is doubt about whether a patient's symptoms represent stroke/transient ischemic attack or migrainous aura, an evaluation by a neurologist and neuroimaging is advisable [27].

Specific stroke syndromes and their management

Pre-eclampsia and eclampsia

Presentation
Pre-eclampsia is a multisystem disorder affecting 3–5% of pregnancies [28]. Although only a tiny proportion of those affected by pre-eclampsia suffer from stroke, up to 45% of women who have pregnancy-related stroke have pre-eclampsia or eclampsia [17,29]. Uncontrolled systolic hypertension and endothelial dysfunction may lead to hemorrhage or infarction [30]. Disordered cerebral autoregulation may also play a role, especially post partum.

Investigation and management
Investigation and management of pre-eclampsia will be familiar to the obstetrician and are reviewed in Chapter 5. Most cases of stroke in the setting of pre-eclampsia are due to arterial hemorrhage but cases of acute arterial thrombosis also occur. While pre-eclamptic stroke is most likely in the setting of severe hypertension (>180/110), it can occur at blood pressures much lower than this and the acute change in blood pressure may be as important a factor as the absolute number [31]. The only definitive treatment for pre-eclampsia is delivery of the fetus and placenta.

Prompt neuroimaging should occur in pre-eclamptic women with sudden-onset (thunderclap) headache and/or any persistent neurologic deficit. Neurosurgical consultation should be sought if intracerebral blood is found on CT or MRI to guide the need for interventions to decrease intracranial pressure. Blood pressure is typically brought to a level of 160/90 (a mean arterial pressure of 110 mmHg) and not much lower as some degree of hypertension may be needed to maintain cerebral perfusion and prevent ischemia. The presence of an intracerebral hemorrhage will complicate options for obstetric anesthesia and anesthesiologists should be involved early in these cases.

Reversible cerebral vasoconstriction syndromes

Presentation
Reversible cerebral vasoconstriction syndrome (RCVS) is an under-recognized and often misdiagnosed syndrome characterized by a sudden, severe headache at onset seen in association with a neurologic deficit. It is caused by reversible vascular

narrowing involving the circle of Willis and its immediate branches. RCVS can present in conjunction with hypertensive encephalopathy, pre-eclampsia, and reversible posterior leukoencephalopathy, physical exertion or bathing and it can occur in isolation [32]. Women may have had an uncomplicated pregnancy and present a few days after delivery with headache [33], cerebral irritation and neurologic deficit. Investigations demonstrate infarction and/or hemorrhage.

The differential diagnosis includes subarachnoid hemorrhage, migraine, arterial dissection, vasculitis and infection.

Investigation and treatment

Computed tomography, MR or catheter angiography may demonstrate multifocal segmental narrowing of the cerebral vessels, which resolves within 4–6 weeks. Spinal fluid should be normal, and this distinguishes this syndrome from subarachnoid hemorrhage.

Treatment is supportive, although vasodilators and steroids have been used.

Intracranial hemorrhage

Presentation

Most intracranial hemorrhage occurring during an otherwise normal pregnancy is the result of aneurysmal subarachnoid hemorrhage (SAH) and arteriovenous malformation (AVM). Intracranial arterial dissections are a much rarer etiology. Hypertension, smoking, alcohol and family history are all risk factors. The incidence of SAH from aneurysmal rupture is 3–11 per 100,000 pregnancies [17,29] but 50% of all aneurysmal rupture in women below 40 occurs in the context of pregnancy [34]. Cavernoma and other venous anomalies are a very infrequent cause of hemorrhagic stroke.

Presentation of intracranial hemorrhage is the same as in the nonpregnant woman. Symptoms are dominated by the sudden onset of headache, often described as "the worst headache of my life," and this presentation should always prompt consideration of the diagnosis of subarachnoid hemorrhage. Meningeal irritation (due to blood spreading through the CSF), altered consciousness, collapse or vomiting at onset, and the absence of lateralizing neurologic findings are features that are characteristic of SAH but not universal.

Investigation and management

Computed tomography scan is very sensitive for SAH within the first 12 hours after the event but is less sensitive with smaller bleeds and as the days go by after the initial event. Lumbar puncture is recommended in patients with a history suggestive of SAH who have a normal CT scan, especially if more than a day has passed since the onset of their symptoms. The presence of xanthochromia in CSF is highly suggestive of a SAH but will not be present until 2–6 hours after the acute event.

Computed tomography offers advantages compared with MRI in ease of obtaining a study and in the past was viewed as better than MRI at identifying early hemorrhage. However, the use of FLAIR and T2 sequences with MRI may be as good or better than CT at identifying a SAH, and is better than CT at identifying a SAH in the days following the acute event.

Ruptured aneurysmal SAH may be complicated by rebleeding, with an associated mortality rate of 50–70% [35] and so monitoring and management of such patients should have a high priority. Four percent of patients will rebleed within 24 hours of initial bleed, with up to 20% occurring within the first month. Vasospasm, cerebral infarction, hydrocephalus, increased intracranial pressure, seizures and hyponatremia are other possible complications. Medical treatment usually involves intravenous fluids, bed rest, compression stockings, analgesia, laxatives and nimodipine 60 mg 4 hourly [36]. Medical management of SAH should be undertaken at or in close liaison with a neurosurgical center.

Once the diagnosis is established, the etiology for the SAH must be determined with cerebral angiography, CT angiography or MR angiography. While cerebral angiography remains the most sensitive test, it is rapidly being replaced by CT angiography due to the ease of testing and steadily improving technology. All of these tests can be safely performed in pregnant or postpartum women when necessary.

Definitive treatment usually involves endovascular coiling or surgical clipping and the timing of these interventions will be decided by the neurosurgeon. In most cases, treatment during pregnancy is justifiable [34,37–39]. Outside pregnancy, coiling is felt to produce better overall outcomes than clipping [40]. In pregnancy, the risks of periprocedure use of radiation, postprocedure anticoagulation, and postcoiling rupture in remaining aneurysm tissue are generally readily outweighed by the benefit of effective intervention. At the time of SAH, women with aneurysms may temporarily lack capacity to consider these issues but in any case, detailed discussion between the obstetrician, the neurosurgical team and the family, wherever possible, should occur.

Women who have had a previous aneurysm completely obliterated by clipping or coiling may consider vaginal delivery [41]. Use of epidural anesthesia is advised. Some recommend avoidance of spinal anesthesia in women in whom the aneurysm is not totally obliterated [42], based on the hypothesis that the decrease in intracranial pressure caused by dural tap could cause an increase in transmural pressure across the arterial wall, thus facilitating the rupture of a potential vascular malformation. But anesthetic input is required as this fall in pressure is likely to be preventable.

Treatment of unruptured aneurysm

In general, management of unruptured aneurysms should be the same as in the nonpregnant state. Management of unruptured aneurysm in the nonpregnant individual is guided by the International Study on Unruptured Intracranial Aneurysms (ISUIA) [43]. Although rupture of aneurysm is associated with significant mortality, treatment of aneurysms also carries risk. ISUIA data suggest that the risk of treating certain low-risk aneurysms (small (<7 mm), asymptomatic, stable, anterior artery aneurysms) may be greater than the risk of conservative "watching and waiting." In common with many trials, pregnancy has not specifically been considered. After discussion with the patient, it may be felt appropriate to treat such aneurysms preconceptually or during pregnancy. While there are no data to guide management of patients with untreated aneurysms in labor and delivery, most clinicians would recommend early good pain control, keeping blood pressure less than 140/90 mmHg and limiting the second stage of labor. An untreated aneurysm is not, however, viewed as an indication for cesarean delivery.

Unruptured AVM

Presentation

Arteriovenous malformations are less common than arterial aneurysms but present similarly with acute SAH. Unruptured AVM (Figure 15.3) present a lower bleeding risk than aneurysms, and overall risk of primary hemorrhage occurring during pregnancy is 3.5%, which is similar to the normal population [44]. Individual case reports suggest that pregnancy is not associated with significant changes to AVM [45], although the obstetrician or neurologist should emphasize the paucity of data to guide decisions in this area.

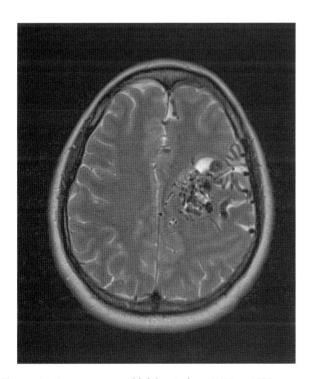

Figure 15.3 Large unruptured left hemisphere AVM on MRI.

Treatment

Arteriovenous malformations are treated with combinations of surgery, endovascular embolization and stereotactic radiosurgery. The decision about treatment is guided by a number of factors including the site and complexity of the lesion.

In most cases, AVM are managed outside pregnancy. Although there is concern that untreated or partially treated AVM may be at risk of hemorrhage from the hemodynamic changes of labor, observed risk of hemorrhage is recognized to be low, particularly where epidural analgesia is used and second stage is assisted [46,47].

Cerebral venous thrombosis

Presentation

Cerebral venous thrombosis (CVT) may account for approximately 20% of strokes during pregnancy [24] and should be considered in any patient complaining of headache and drowsiness, particularly if focal neurologic signs or seizures are present. Its occurrence is now more recognized with the increasing use of MRI and its incidence in pregnancy is estimated to be 11.6 per 100,000 deliveries in the US [48]. Thrombosis of cerebral veins or dural sinuses causes injury to tissue through increased venous pressures and (in the case of dural sinus thrombosis) decreased CSF reabsorption and increased intracranial pressure. The presentation is highly variable and may include headache with or without vomiting, focal deficits, seizures and/or mental status changes. Headache is the most common presentation, with a gradual onset and often localized.

Investigation and management

Presence of papilledema is not a sensitive or specific sign of CVT and diagnosis relies on neuroimaging, which will demonstrate venous distribution infarction with possible hemorrhage. MRI in combination with MR venography is the best test for diagnosing CVT. CT scans can be normal in up to 30% of cases [49].

Even where hemorrhage is evident on imaging, CVT is treated by anticoagulation for 6–12 months. During pregnancy, therapeutic doses of low molecular weight heparin may be used, although evidence for its benefit is lacking [50,51]. Data from nonpregnant patients suggest that 80% of patients have complete recovery and that the rate of recurrence is well under 10% [52].

Paradoxic embolism

Patent foramen ovale (PFO) is an interatrial communication present in approximately 27% of adults, but in up to 50% of young patients presenting with stroke [53]. This abnormal communication may allow right-to-left shunting of venous emboli directly into the arterial circulation or provide a focus of thrombus formation. While case–control studies consistently show a relationship between stroke and PFO, prospective data show a PFO is not associated with an increased risk of first or recurrent stroke. While there is still controversy over this issue, most experts would presently recommend that patients with a single prior stroke, a PFO and no other thrombotic risks should receive only the usual stroke prevention treatments, i.e. antiplatelet agents such as aspirin. Patients with PFO (regardless of whether they have had a stroke) should therefore receive anticoagulation with warfarin or heparin only if they have another indication for anticoagulation. Decisions about the management of patients with recurrent stroke and PFO, or those with a PFO with a single stroke but multiple risk factors for recurrence (thrombophilias, atrial septal aneurysms), should be made in collaboration with cardiology, hematology and (when pregnant or considering pregnancy) a high-risk obstetrician. Options to be discussed include full anticoagulation or surgical closure of the PFO but there is presently little evidence to guide therapy in these situations [26].

Epilepsy

Incidence and resentation

Epilepsy is a common, chronic condition affecting 0.3–0.5% of pregnant women [54]. Seizures may be the presenting symptom of a number of medical conditions in pregnancy, and a small number of women with epilepsy may present with their first seizure during pregnancy. Chapter 45 reviews the approach to the investigation and treatment of new-onset seizures in pregnant women so the focus of this section will be on the management of women with known epilepsy.

Maternal considerations

When any woman with a chronic illness becomes pregnant, care providers must consider the impact of the chronic illness upon potential maternal, fetal, and neonatal complications, and the influence of the pregnancy upon the course of the chronic illness.

Recently, the American Academy of Neurology and the American Epilepsy Society jointly published a series of systematic reviews by an expert panel of the evidence to address many of these issues in women with epilepsy [55–57]. They restricted their analysis to papers published between 1985 and 2005 to reflect modern practice and outcomes. As a general statement, it is fair to say that they found much of the literature available to address many of these issues limited by both methodologic problems and small sample size, resulting in inadequate power. Many studies lacked internal controls of pregnant women without epilepsy or nonpregnant women with epilepsy, and outcome assessments were not blinded to seizure experience. In most of the studies, the vast majority of women with epilepsy were taking antiepileptic drugs so inferences about

women with epilepsy who were not taking antiepileptic drugs were limited. In most studies, there was no way to quantify the effect of seizure frequency on outcomes. The studies were sufficiently heterogeneous in both treatments and outcome measures that formal meta-analysis could not be performed for most outcome measures. Thus many of their conclusions are tentative and qualified, but nonetheless they represent the best assessment of the current state of our knowledge.

Possibly the most important finding of their review was the lack of an obvious increase in most of the maternal complications of pregnancy among women with epilepsy taking antiepileptic drugs. There was no substantial increase in cesarean delivery, although a moderately increased risk could not be ruled out. There was insufficient evidence to either support or refute an increased risk for either pre-eclampsia or pregnancy-induced hypertension among women with epilepsy taking antiepileptic drugs. It is probable that women with epilepsy taking antiepileptic drugs do not have a substantially increased risk of premature contractions or premature labor and delivery. It is possible that women with epilepsy taking antiepileptic drugs who smoke may have a higher risk of premature labor and delivery than women without epilepsy who smoke. Women with epilepsy taking antiepileptic drugs probably do not have a substantially increased risk for bleeding in late pregnancy, though a moderately increased risk could not be excluded. There were not adequate data to either support or refute an increased risk of spontaneous abortion in women with epilepsy taking antiepileptic drugs [55].

In their systematic review, the American Academy of Neurology and the American Epilepsy Society could not find any study that compared the change in seizure frequency among pregnant women with epilepsy to the rate in nonpregnant women with epilepsy; thus there was no "gold standard" comparison group. There was insufficient evidence to determine if pregnancy changes the frequency of seizures in women with epilepsy. Similarly, there was insufficient evidence to support or refute an increased risk for status epilepticus in pregnant women with epilepsy. If women with epilepsy are seizure free for at least 9 months prior to pregnancy, there is an 84–92% probability that they will remain seizure free during pregnancy. Women who suffer more than one generalized seizure per month are at an annual risk of sudden unexpected death in epilepsy (SUDEP) of 1% or higher [58].

Fetal considerations

Few relationships in teratology are as difficult to define as the relationships among epilepsy, the drugs used to treat epilepsy, and the risks for major congenital malformations and poor neurodevelopment in the offspring. Idiopathic epilepsy can result from maldevelopment of the fetal central nervous system, also resulting in impaired cognitive development.

Maldevelopment of the fetal central nervous system could have a genetic etiology that could be passed on to the offspring of women with epilepsy. Grand mal seizures can result in hypoxemia and metabolic acidosis and prolonged duration of poorly controlled temporal lobe epilepsy does seem to result in cognitive decline. This provides credibility to concerns about frequent seizures during pregnancy potentially causing fetal damage.

It is therefore possible that either the genetics of epilepsy or the fetal environmental circumstances of poorly controlled epilepsy could cause fetal malformations or central nervous system maldevelopment, resulting in impaired cognitive development. Thus it has been argued that the adverse fetal outcomes observed among offspring of women with epilepsy taking antiepileptic drugs could be due to the epilepsy *per se* and not the drug treatment. It is difficult to identify large numbers of women with epilepsy who remain untreated throughout pregnancy to compare their rates of fetal complications to those of women without epilepsy to test this hypothesis. Few studies of women with epilepsy taking antiepileptic drugs have included control groups of both women with epilepsy taking no drugs and women without epilepsy. The study with the largest control group of women with epilepsy taking no drugs did not find an increased risk of teratogenesis among controls as compared to women without epilepsy [59]. Similarly, a meta-analysis of this issue has found no evidence for a significant risk of major malformations among women with epilepsy taking no drugs [60].

Despite this evidence, it could still be argued that failure to find the relationship between untreated epilepsy and major malformations or adverse cognitive outcome could be due to the problem of confounding by indication. That argument is that women with epilepsy who remain untreated throughout pregnancy have the mildest degree of disease and are least likely to have affected offspring, while women with severe disease are at highest risk for poor fetal outcome and are most likely to be treated. The only evidence that could definitively put this question to rest would be from a large randomized controlled trial in which women at high risk for seizures were assigned to management with and without antiepileptic drugs. Such a trial would be unethical for maternal reasons and therefore unlikely to ever be done.

Similar issues pertain to the question of the impact of maternal epilepsy and antiepileptic drug therapy on cognitive outcome for the offspring. This relationship is further complicated by the fact that in most studies, the single most important determinant of the IQ of a child is the IQ of his or her mother. Although most persons with epilepsy have intelligence within the normal range, persons with epilepsy, as a group, have reduced cognitive performance compared to healthy subjects matched for age and education.

With this as background, the American Academy of Neurology and the American Epilepsy Society joint statement was very cautious in stating their findings regarding the teratogenicity of antiepileptic drugs [56]. They compared separately the risks of major congenital malformations among the offspring of women with epilepsy taking antiepileptic drugs and the offspring of women with epilepsy not taking antiepileptic drugs. They concluded that, as a group, antiepileptic drugs taken during the first trimester "probably increase" the risk of major congenital malformations. They also concluded that valproic acid monotherapy "possibly" increases the risk of major congenital malformations and that it "probably" increases the risk when used in polytherapy. These conclusions seem overly cautious as the relationship between first-trimester valproic acid exposure and neural tube defects is well documented [61], as is the relationship between multiple antiepileptic drug therapy and malformations [62].

There is growing evidence that both frequent tonic-clonic seizures during pregnancy and fetal exposure to antiepileptic drugs, especially valproic acid, are associated with cognitive impairment in offspring [63,64]. When compared to lamotrigine, phenytoin and carbamazepine, fetal valproic acid exposure is associated with a dose-dependent decrement in IQ (average 9 points) in childhood [65]. This adverse consequence of fetal valproic acid exposure is likely exacerbated by its use in antiepileptic drug polytherapy [56].

Many antiepileptic drugs (AED) interfere with synthesis of the vitamin K-dependent clotting factors II, VII, IX and X directly and by inducing microsomal enzymes that degrade vitamin K. A resultant neonatal coagulation defect has been demonstrated in the laboratory in many neonates, with frank hemorrhage in a small number [66]. More recently, larger studies have not found evidence of increased risk for clinically significant bleeding in neonates exposed to AED *in utero* [67]. The American Academy of Neurology had recommended maternal treatment with vitamin K in late pregnancy to prevent fetal and neonatal coagulopathy as "theoretically useful" [68] but with no evidence that significant amounts of vitamin K cross the placenta or of clinical efficacy of the treatment [69], it has retreated from that recommendation [57].

Preconception counseling

Obstetric and neonatal risks are reduced by "planned" pregnancy with the lowest effective dose of an antiepilepsy drug with folic acid. All issues relating to epilepsy, antiepileptic drugs and pregnancy should be considered, but consultations tend to be dominated by discussion of the teratogenic potential of antiepileptic drugs.

High-dose (4 mg once daily) folic acid has been recommended to all women planning to become pregnant who take AED or at least for those taking AED associated with a high risk of neural tube defects (NTD) such as valproic acid and carbamazepine. This recommendation is based on a British study which showed that this dose of folic acid decreased the risk of recurrent NTD in women who had a previous child with a NTD. The applicability of these data to women on

AED has always been questioned [70] and recent data from a large registry on the outcome of pregnancies in women taking AED have confirmed the findings in animal studies that use of high-dose folic acid does not appear to protect against NTD in patients taking AED [71]. The joint statement of the American Academy of Neurology and the American Epilepsy Society suggests that the standard 0.4 mg daily dietary supplement dose of folic acid recommended for all women planning pregnancy is adequate [57].

Before pregnancy, it can be useful to obtain a serum drug level, even if this has not been done to care for the patients previously, as this may be useful for comparison during pregnancy.

Preconception antiepileptic drug withdrawal

Epilepsy is a heterogeneous condition. Some women who have infrequent and mild seizures arising from a small and contained focus (partial epilepsy) have a low risk of seizure generalization and consideration should be given to complete drug withdrawal.

Other women may have been seizure free for many years on medication. Pre-pregnancy drug withdrawal should be considered for such patients. This generally involves a slow taper and withdrawal of AED for at least 6 months prior to a planned pregnancy. The risk of a recurrent seizure in the first 2 years off medications is 40% (as compared to 20% for patients who remain on medications) [72,73]. Risk of seizure recurrence depends on many variables [74] and in particular the epilepsy syndrome, which must be carefully defined. Idiopathic generalized epilepsy syndromes associated with myoclonus are very likely to recur off medication, even after many years, whereas other types of epilepsy, such as focal epilepsy where there is no known anatomic substrate and where EEG is normal, may be less likely to relapse [75].

There is little information to guide the optimal approach to tapering and discontinuing AED. Withdrawal of AED should occur under the direction of a neurologist and typically is done no faster than over 2–3 months, with one drug being tapered at a time. Women who present having abruptly discontinued their AED for a few weeks should not be considered to have successfully withdrawn from AED therapy and should generally be encouraged to resume medication and have their AED gradually tapered over time. Women desiring a trial of AED withdrawal should be informed that breakthrough seizures will result in possible injury and loss of eligibility to drive. Many regions require a 3-month period seizure free before the patient may resume the right to drive. There are no generally accepted consensus guidelines as to whether patients may drive while tapering AED and the practitioner and patient should look to local licensing requirements as a guide. In practice, very few women opt for a trial of AED tapering and withdrawal prior to pregnancy but the option should be discussed.

Women may ask whether nondrug measures may help reduce the probability of seizure occurrence. General advice can be given. For example, avoidance of certain drug precipitants (for example, alcohol and higher doses of antidepressants) and care with respect to known triggers (such as certain frequencies of flashing light for the small proportion of patients who are photosensitive). Women should avoid excessive sleep deprivation or disturbance where possible. But for a significant majority, the mainstay of treatment is the use of antiepileptic drugs, as this offers the best protection against seizures and their associated morbidity and mortality.

Preconception antiepileptic drug switching

Table 15.4 reviews the commonly prescribed AED and their pregnancy risk categories. Unfortunately, all the presently used AED are either known teratogens or are agents for which the present pregnancy data are too limited to offer a definitive statement on the associated pregnancy risk.

Women should be carefully counseled about the potential adverse effects that antiepileptic drugs may have on the developing fetus and that many of these effects will occur very early in pregnancy so that decisions about AED therapy should be made prior to pregnancy (Box 15.11). When considering the risk of teratogenicity, women should be informed that even without treatment there is a 2–3% risk of having a child with congenital malformation. A number of pregnancy registers in North America, Europe, UK and Australia have monitored pregnancy outcomes in women taking antiepileptic drugs [62]. These registries share in common the fact that only first-trimester exposures are considered, and the greatest focus is on presence of major congenital malformations. Meta-analysis of their findings suggests that the background risk is increased approximately threefold [76]. Women taking two or more drugs have a >10% chance of having a child with congenital malformation. The latter data are particularly difficult to interpret as numbers of affected women are insufficient to determine whether drugs with known low individual risk, such as benzodiazepines, also carry this higher risk in "polytherapy."

The effect of AED on neurodevelopment is less clear and discussed in detail above.

At present, since there is no consensus as to which AED is most or least teratogenic, the AED that controls seizures in a given patient is the one that should be used. When possible, however, the use of valproate or the use of multiple AED should be avoided during pregnancy or in women planning a pregnancy.

Preconception genetic counseling

Some causes of epilepsy are genetically determined. Certain malformations of cortical development, such as subependymal heterotopia, may have predictable genetics [77] although

Table 15.4 Antiepileptic drugs (AED) safety in pregnancy and lactation

	Type of seizure for which this agent is commonly used	Typical side effects suggestive of high maternal serum levels of this medication	US Food and Drug Administration Pregnancy Safety Classification*	TERIS classification**	Briggs Freeman and Yaffe pregnancy classification†	Thomas Hale breastfeeding classification‡	American Academy of Pediatrics (AAP) recommendation for use with breastfeeding§
Valproate[a]	Absence Partial Generalized tonic-clonic Atypical	Tremor	D	Risk, moderate; data quality, good	Human data suggests risk	L2	Usually compatible with breastfeeding.
Lamotrigine[b]	Absence Partial Generalized tonic-clonic Atypical	Dizziness, sleepiness	C	Risk, undetermined; data quality, fair	Human data suggests risk	L3 agent's effect on nursing infants is unknown but there is cause for concern	Not reviewed by the AAP
Levetiracetam	Absence Partial Generalized tonic-clonic Atypical	Sleepiness, fatigue, dizziness, anxiety, agitation	C	Risk, undetermined risk; data quality, limited	Limited human data; animal data suggests risk	L3 usually compatible with breastfeeding	Not reviewed by the AAP
Carbamazepine	Partial Generalized tonic-clonic	Sleepiness, dizziness, blurred or double vision, fatigue, headache	D	Risk, small to moderate; data quality, fair to good	Compatible with use in pregnancy if maternal benefits outweigh fetal risk	L2	Usually compatible with breastfeeding
Topiramate	Generalized tonic-clonic Atypical	Sleepiness, anxiety, agitation fatigue, trouble concentrating, confusion, depression, decreased appetite, language problems, tremor	C	Risk, undetermined; data quality, limited	Limited human data; animal data suggests risk	L3	Not reviewed by the AAP
Zonisamide	Absence Partial Generalized tonic-clonic Atypical	Sleepiness, dizziness, ataxia, trouble concentrating, confusion	C	Risk, undetermined; data quality, limited	Limited human data; animal data suggests high risk	L5	Not reviewed by the AAP
Oxcarbazepine	Partial Generalized tonic-clonic	Sleepiness, headache, dizziness, vertigo, ataxia, double vision	C	Risk, undetermined; data quality, limited	Limited human data; animal data suggests risk	L3	Not reviewed by the AAP
Phenytoin	Partial Generalized tonic-clonic	Confusion, depression, slurred speech, double vision, ataxia, neuropathy	D	Risk of congenital anomalies small to moderate based on fair to good data Risk of fetal hydantoin syndrome small to moderate based on fair to good data Risk of neurobehavioral abnormalities is minimal to small based on fair data	Compatible with use in pregnancy if maternal benefits outweigh fetal risk	L2	Usually compatible with breastfeeding

(Continued on p. 388)

Table 15.4 (Continued)

	Type of seizure for which this agent is commonly used	Typical side effects suggestive of high maternal serum levels of this medication	US Food and Drug Administration Pregnancy Safety Classification*	TERIS classification**	Briggs Freeman and Yaffe pregnancy classification†	Thomas Hale breastfeeding classification‡	American Academy of Pediatrics (AAP) recommendation for use with breastfeeding§
Gabapentin	Partial	Sleepiness, dizziness, ataxia	C	Risk: undetermined; data quality: limited	Limited human data; animal data suggests risk	L2	Not reviewed by the AAP
Pregabalin	Partial	Dizziness, sleepiness, ataxia	C	Not reviewed by TERIS	No human data; animal data suggests moderate risk	L3	Not reviewed by the AAP
Ethosuximide	Absence	Sleep disturbances, sleepiness, hyperactivity	C	Risk: undetermined; data quality: limited	Human data suggests low risk	L4 American Academy of Pediatrics classifies as an agent that is usually compatible with breastfeeding	Not reviewed by the AAP
Clonazepam	Absence Atypical	Sleepiness	D	Risk: undetermined; data quality: limited	Human data suggests low risk	L3	Not reviewed by the AAP

Atypical refers to atypical absence, myoclonic and atonic seizures

*The US FDA pregnancy classification reviewed in Chapter 30.

**TERIS is an online database described in Chapter 30 "Prescribing in Pregnancy". It is distributed by Thomson Micromedex®. In it summarizes available data on the safety of medications in pregnancy and provides a brief aphorism for each medication to summarize both the risk and the quality of data on which that risk assessment is based. The magnitude of teratogenic risk of the child born after exposure during gestation is described using one of the following terms: minimal, small, moderate, high, undetermined or unlikely. The quality and quantity of data on which this risk estimate is based is described using one of the following terms: none, limited, fair, good, excellent. The TERIS authors suggest that risks that are 'minimal' ought not alter decisions regarding continuation or termination of an exposed pregnancy. 'Moderate' or 'high' risks may be considered important enough to influence such decisions, at least in some cases. Similarly, the authors recommend that risk assessments based on evidence that is 'limited' or 'fair' ought to be considered tentative and may change as more information becomes available. Even with 'good' data, only crude estimates of the magnitude of the risk are often possible. Therefore, although this brief summary statement is provided here, the reader is encouraged to look to this resource for a more detailed discussion of the available literature assessing the risk of each medication. TERIS accessed August 10 2009 http://depts.washington,edu/terisweb/teris.htm

†Drugs in Pregnancy and Lactation is a classic textbook that is described in Chapter 30 "Prescribing in Pregnancy". It is edited by Briggs, Freeman and Yaffe and published by Lippincott Williams and Wilkins. It provides an excellent summary of the available data on the safety of drugs in pregnancy and lactation. Only their brief introductory summary statement is provided here and the reader is encouraged to look to this resource for a more detailed discussion of the available literature assessing the risk of each medication. Briggs GG, Freeman RK, Yaffe SJ. Drugs in Pregnancy and Lactation 8ᵗʰ edn. Lippincott Williams and Wilkins, Philadelphia PA, 2008.

‡Medications and Mother's Milk is a handbook described in Chapter 30 "Prescribing in Pregnancy". It is written and published by Thomas Hale. His summary classification for each antiepileptic agent is provided here but the reader is encouraged to look to this resource for a more detailed discussion of the available literature assessing the risk of each medication. A detailed description of the Thomas Hale classification for medications in lactation is reviewed in Chapter 31 but can be summarized as follows: L1- safer; L2-safe; L3- moderately safe; L4-possibly hazardous, L5- contraindicated). Hale TW. Medications and Mother's Milk 13ᵗʰ edn. Hale Publishing, Amarillo Texas, 2008.

§American Academy of Pediatrics Committee on Drugs. Transfer of drugs and other chemicals into human milk. Pediatrics. 2001;108(3):776–89.

ᵃThe risk of both major congenital malformations and neurodevelopmental impairment appears to be increased with valproate as compared to other AED.

ᵇThis agent appears to have an exaggerated increase in its metabolism during pregnancy compared with other AED. This quickly converts back to baseline clearance within the first few weeks postpartum. AED level monitoring and postpartum decrease in dose may be particularly important for this agent.

Box 15.11 Timing of some of the malformations that have been associated with AED

- Neural tube defect: day 28 after conception/~2 weeks after first missed period
- Cleft lip: day 36 after conception/~3 weeks after first missed period
- Ventricular septal defect: day 42 after conception/~4 weeks after first missed period
- Cleft maxillary palate: day 47–70 after conception/~7–10 weeks after first missed period

in most cases inheritance is complex and is best discussed with a clinical geneticist. Idiopathic generalized epilepsies (IGE) have a tendency to occur more frequently in families and it can generally be advised that children of women with IGE have a 4–5% probability of developing a similar epilepsy. Other epilepsies, such as those arising from head injury or CNS infection, are unlikely to be inherited.

First and second trimester

Women with epilepsy should be managed in the normal way throughout the first and second trimesters. Switching or withdrawal of AED in patients with well-controlled epilepsy should rarely, if ever, be done during pregnancy. Hyperemesis may reduce gastric absorption of AED but this problem may be mitigated by changing the timing of dosing or use of antiemetics. A serum alpha-fetoprotein (AFP) is often obtained at approximately 16 weeks as a screen for NTD associated with AED and will be elevated in most but not all cases of open NTD. Ultrasonography at 18–20 weeks is also recommended to screen for NTD, cleft lip, cardiac anomalies and other major fetal abnormalities to guide further investigations and management. An amniocentesis for AFP and acetylcholinesterase (AChE) may be helpful if the serum AFP is elevated but the fetal ultrasound is unable to reliably exclude a NTD. If both AFP and AChE are elevated in the amniotic fluid, the likelihood of a NTD is >99%.

The type and pharmacokinetic profile of AED used should be considered when making decisions as to whether routine monitoring of AED levels should occur in pregnancy. Although AED concentrations tend to fall during pregnancy due to a rising volume of distribution, this may be partially offset by a rise in the proportion of free drug available due to a pregnancy-associated decrease in serum albumin concentration. This is particularly the case for highly protein-bound antiepileptic drugs such as phenytoin, valproate and carbamazepine. Lamotrigine is widely used to treat epilepsy, but presents considerable challenges as both bound and free lamotrigine clearance increase over twofold between the first and third trimester [78]. Many advocate therapeutic drug monitoring, particularly for lamotrigine and perhaps also for levetiracetam and oxcarbazepine, for individual patients to allow drug dose changes and maintenance of serum levels at a constant level [55,79,80]. A reasonable monitoring strategy would be to check total and free plasma levels (with adjustments in dose if the levels are less than therapeutic) early in pregnancy, towards the end of the first trimester, and then at least once each trimester, with any seizure activity and 2 weeks post partum. Potential harm to the fetus of AED is likely proportional to dose and serum levels, even in later pregnancy, and therefore the lowest effective dose of drug should be used. This is judged on clinical features, in particular prodromal symptoms that the woman might recognize as a need for a higher dose of AED.

Third trimester and delivery

Seizure control may deteriorate during the third trimester: pharmacokinetic factors may be relevant, for example, rates of clearance of both bound and free drug increase; women may be more tired and sleep disturbed. Dose increases may be guided by serum drug levels, where the clinician seeks to maintain a target (pre-pregnancy) drug level. Alternatively, clinical markers may be used for those women who have clear clinical markers such as symptoms or signs of drug toxicity (nausea, double vision, gait unsteadiness) or seizure control (auras, "feelings" of seizures). The latter approach is likely to ensure that the minimum dose of AED is used.

Several antiepileptic drugs, including phenytoin and carbamazepine, induce hepatic enzyme systems and cause a reduction in fetal levels of vitamin K-dependent clotting factors. As discussed above, oral water-soluble vitamin K (10 mg once daily) was advocated for women during the last 4 weeks of pregnancy to prevent the incidence of hemorrhagic disease of the newborn, but is not of proven efficacy [57]. Drug interactions of AED with some medications commonly prescribed in pregnancy are reviewed in Chapter 45, Table 45.2.

Most women with epilepsy are concerned that they may suffer a seizure during delivery. Although it is frequently quoted that 3% of women are at risk within 24 hours of delivery [81], this is likely to be attributable to failure to take AED, sleep deprivation or impaired gastric absorption. Clobazam (a benzodiazepine derivative available in much of the world but not the US) 10 mg once or twice daily may be used prophylactically for women felt to be at particular risk.

Postpartum

Antiepileptic drug doses may have been increased during pregnancy, particularly during the last trimester. Within 2 weeks of the birth, maternal plasma volume and metabolism have largely returned to the pre-pregnant state. If AED doses have been adjusted during pregnancy, they should be returned to their original levels during this period. Some advocate use of therapeutic drug monitoring during this period, but this relies on samples being collected in a timely manner and analyzed quickly. One protocol suggests decreasing lamotrigine doses incrementally on days 3, 7 and 10 postpartum to rapidly return to the preconception dose [78]. When available, liquid forms of AED can be helpful in such incremental tapering regimens.

Avoidance of sleep deprivation, while very difficult for a new mother, should be facilitated by the patient's family as sleep deprivation lowers the seizure threshold. Table 45.3 in Chapter 45 provides other recommendations for the care of new mothers with epilepsy.

All antiepileptic drugs are excreted in breast milk, to varying degrees [82]. Neonatal serum levels of AED are affected by the concentration of the AED in the milk, the amount of milk consumed and the ability of the neonate to eliminate the agent, the latter two of which will vary from infant to infant. Most experts would support breastfeeding in women on AED as benefits are likely outweighed by any theoretical risks. The caveats are as follows: to observe for evidence of sedation in infants exposed to sedative AED such as phenobarbital or primidone, use caution with lamotrigine which has high levels in breast milk and may not be readily eliminated in infants, and avoid the use of zonisamide. Although neonates will have been exposed to drug treatment during pregnancy, neural development continues until the second year and beyond. Due to uncertainties regarding the effect of AED on neurodevelopment, it may be wise to wean earlier than 6 months. Women who do not breastfeed initially may risk AED withdrawal symptoms in the child although in practice these are rarely seen.

Central nervous system tumors

Incidence

In general, pregnant woman are at similar risk of neurologic tumours when compared with nonpregnant women [83]. The most common brain tumors seen in this age group are gliomas and meningiomas. While no brain tumor is caused by pregnancy, some tumors such as meningiomas, acoustic neuromas and prolactionomas may show accelerated growth in the hormonal milieu of pregnancy.

Presentation

Brain tumors often present with headache, nausea and vomiting, all of which are commonly seen in pregnant patients. New-onset seizures may also occur. Concern about the safety of imaging may lead to unnecessary delay in diagnosis of women with intracranial or spinal tumors. For example, chronic and progressive back pain in pregnant women should be investigated particularly when associated with symptoms such as sphincter disturbance or neurologic signs.

A number of women have low-grade and indolent tumors, which may be asymptomatic and are simply monitored by their neurologist or neurosurgeon. Counseling such women about the safety of conservative management when considering pregnancy presents considerable challenges as the effect of pregnancy on the natural history of tumors is poorly understood.

A further group will have such tumors identified during pregnancy. Although a "watch and wait" approach is generally advised, careful monitoring to ensure early identification of relevant symptoms is required. Both radiation and/or surgical resection can be safely carried out during pregnancy if the tumor is growing rapidly or is symptomatic.

Treatment

Antenatal diagnosis of more malignant tumors also presents a considerable treatment dilemma as the safety of the mother and fetus may be in conflict. No class 1 or 2 evidence is available to guide management. Use of corticosteroids and AED should be considered if they would be used outside pregnancy. Where the fetus is remote from viability and the hemodynamic changes in the mother have not peaked, the risks of surgery (and in particular intraoperative hemorrhage) are relatively low. It is often preferred to defer treatment until the second trimester as the ionizing radiation associated with radiotherapy, radiosurgery and image-guided surgery are felt to present greater risk to the developing fetus in the first 12 weeks of gestation.

Although there are no data to guide this practice (and it is not the recommendation of the editors of this text), risk of intraoperative hemorrhage is felt by some to be higher after the end of the second trimester and these individuals recommend delay of surgery until term if possible.

Mononeuropathies

Mononeuropathies are seen with increased frequency in pregnancy due to nerve compression both from increased edema in pregnancy and due to trauma at the time of delivery. The common neuropathies in pregnancy are reviewed in Table 15.5.

Myasthenia gravis

Myasthenia gravis (MG) is a chronic autoimmune condition in which autoantibodies block or destroy acetylcholine receptors (AchR antibodies), causing impaired transmission at the neuromuscular junction (NMJ) [89]. This leads to early fatigue of affected skeletal muscles. In those aged under 40 years, myasthenia commonly affects ocular or extraocular muscles only, causing diplopia and ptosis. Generalized MG affects all muscle groups and bulbar myasthenia affects muscles of speech, swallowing and breathing. Smooth and cardiac muscle, found in the uterus and heart respectively,

Table 15.5 Common neuropathies seen in pregnancy and the pueperium

Neuropathy	Neurologic symptoms/signs	Etiology	Treatment
Bell's palsy (facial nerve or cranial nerve VII palsy)	Asymmetric facial droop and unilateral weakness of eye closure Taste on anterior third of tongue may be impaired and there may be an increased sensitivity to noise from the ear on the affected size	Edema of facial nerve In women of reproductive age 17/100,000 versus 57/100,000 in pregnancy. Most cases occur in third trimester or peripartum and in patients with pre-eclampsia [84,85]	Prednisone (1 mg/kg/day for 7 days) may improve recovery which is generally good but may take up to 6 months. Antivirals to not appear to affect recovery [86] If eye does not close at night, it may need to be patched shut with gauze compressed by tape
Meralgia paresthetica (lateral femoral cutaneous nerve palsy)	Burning, numbness of tingling over the upper outer thigh. Symptoms made worse by standing or extending leg. Improve with sitting or lying. May be bilateral	Compression of lateral femoral cutaneous nerve at groin by gravid abdomen and edema	Usually resolves in weeks to months following delivery
Carpal tunnel syndrome	Numbness, tingling or pain of the thumb, index finger and middle fingers. Often awakes patient at night and relieved by shaking hand. Pain may radiate into forearm. Often bilateral	Edema within the carpal tunnel at the wrist causes compression of median nerve Present in 5–10% of pregnant women [87]	Splints that hold wrist in neutral position may help decrease nerve compression. Most cases resolve in months following pregnancy
Obturator nerve palsy	Medial thigh pain and adductor weakness causing a circumducting wide-based gait	During vaginal delivery the nerve is compressed against the lateral wall of the pelvis as it crosses the upper margin of the obturator internus muscle	Most cases resolve in months following pregnancy [88]
Femoral neuropathy	Weakness of quadriceps ("knee buckling") with sparing of thigh adduction, sensory loss overy the anterior thigh and most of the medial thigh	Lithotomy positioning (with sharp flexion of the hip) can compress the nerve at the inguinal ligament. Excessive hip abduction and external rotation can cause additional stretching of the nerve. This is a particular risk when the patient has had an epidural anesthetic during labor because the anesthetic allows prolonged sharp flexion and external rotation that would otherwise be limited by pain and muscular resistance	Usually treated with physical therapy, avoiding hip abduction and external rotation. Knee bracing can be used to prevent buckling of the knee Recovery typically occurs over 3–4 months
Peroneal nerve compression	Foot drop with tenderness and paresthesias of the dorsum of the foot and anterolateral leg. Often not apparent until 24–48 hours post partum	Prolonged squatting, sustained knee flexion or pressure on the fibular head from stirrups or palmar pressure during pushing	Usually self-resolving within 8 weeks. May require short leg brace for a few weeks

are not affected. Myasthenic crisis is a term used to describe weakness associated with MG that is severe enough to require endotracheal intubation or delay extubation following surgery. It is often accompanied by bulbar muscle weakness that causes dysphagia and potentially aspiration.

Like most autoimmune conditions, MG affects women under 40 years more often than men (3:1). Myasthenia is also associated with other autoimmune diseases, in particular hypothyroidism. More than 80% of women who develop MG before 40 years of age also have hyperplasia of the thymus or a thymoma [90]. It is the thymus that is the source of anti-AchR antibodies and the likely origin of the type of autoimmune MG most commonly seen in pregnancy.

It has been estimated that MG affects one pregnancy in 20,000. Most women who become pregnant with MG are aware of their diagnosis before conception. A prior diagnosis of MG makes management during pregnancy easier, as long as the clinician is aware of specific problems [91]. Particular to pregnancy is the concern that maternal anti-AchR autoantibodies cross the placenta and cause fetal or neonatal myasthenia in up to 20% of pregnancies (see below).

Diagnosis

A new diagnosis of MG is suggested by clinical examination when there is early muscle fatigue and weakness.

Most commonly, ocular muscles are affected first and looking upwards and sideways for 30 seconds will induce ptosis or diplopia. Tendon and pupillary reflexes are normal, as is sensation.

Specific tests to confirm a diagnosis of MG include identification of circulating anti-AchR antibodies, which are evident in the majority of cases of generalized MG but in only 50% of those with ocular MG. In the absence of anti-AchR antibodies, another antibody against muscle-specific receptor tyrosine kinase (anti-MuSK ab) may be present.

A diagnostic test involves intravenous administration of a short-acting cholinesterase inhibitor (edrophonium chloride). Within minutes, patients with MG will transiently improve affected muscle strength, especially ocular muscle weakness.

Electrophysiologic tests using repetitive nerve stimulation will identify a decrease in muscle action potential in up to 75% of patients with generalized MG, but fewer with ocular MG [89].

Once a diagnosis of myasthenia has been made, a CT scan/MRI of the thorax should check the size and architecture of the thymus.

Treatment

Myasthenic weakness is induced by strenuous exercise, emotional stress, infection, thyroid disease or drugs. Prompt management involves removal or treatment of the precipitating cause, support with cholinesterase inhibitors and immunosuppression.

Cholinesterase inhibitors

Inhibition of cholinesterase, the enzyme that metabolizes Ach at the NMJ, allows Ach to survive longer in order to improve neurotransmission. Pyridostigmine is an oral cholinesterase inhibitor that lasts 4–6 hours. Although pyridostigmine readily crosses the placenta, it has not been associated with malformations when taken in recommended doses [91]. Overdose of pyridostigmine can lead to excessive Ach depolarization with muscle weakness. The weakness of a cholinergic overdose (crisis) can sometimes be differentiated from the weakness of a myasthenic crisis by the presence of other cholinergic symptoms and signs, such as small pupil (miosis), hypersalivation and bradycardia.

Immunosuppression

Immunosuppression downregulates autoantibody production. Plasmapheresis and IV immunoglobulin are reserved for a quick response in severe cases of MG crisis. Steroids, azathioprine and cyclosporine are all used long term to dampen the autoimmunity in MG. Steroids may initially make myasthenic weakness worse, before improvement. Withdrawal of steroids can also lead to a myasthenic crisis.

Thymectomy

Removal of a thymoma is essential to prevent malignant transformation. However, clinical improvement following thymectomy is frequently observed in those with thymic hyperplasia (nonthymomatous myasthenia) following thymectomy [92]. Thymectomy, especially within 2 years of disease onset, has been reported to induce a response rate of 90% and a 10-year remission rate of 50% [93]. Those with anti-MuSk ab respond less well to thymectomy.

Myasthenia and pregnancy

Before pregnancy, women with MG should consider removal of their thymus. In one series of 135 pregnancies in women with MG, the risk of neonatal MG was halved in mothers who had had a thymectomy although the benefits of thymectomy on maternal or fetal disease may not be apparent for several years after thymectomy has occurred [94].

During pregnancy

Cholinesterase inhibitors, in particular pyridostigmine, are the mainstay of treatment of MG and have been safely used throughout pregnancy for many decades [95]. Dosing may need to be increased during pregnancy, usually by decreasing the interval between dosing first and then, if this is ineffective, increasing the individual doses. Use of long-term immunosuppression to control MG needs additional consideration during pregnancy. While prednisolone, azathioprine and cyclosporine appear to be reasonable choices in pregnancy, mycophenolate use should be avoided due to concerns about fetal safety. Plasmapheresis and intravenous gamma-globulin can be continued or initiated in pregnancy However, whenever possible, pregnancy is best delayed until stable levels of immunosuppression have been established.

Drugs to avoid in pregnant women with myasthenia

Acetylcholine release at the NMJ is inhibited by magnesium sulfate, which can lead to a life-threatening myasthenic crisis [96]. Magnesium sulfate should not therefore be used in the myasthenic patient. Other drugs that may exacerbate or unmask MG and which should therefore be avoided in patients with MG include aminoglycosides, macrolides, calcium channel blockers, beta-blockers, lithium, iodine contrast and statins. Since MG is relatively rarely seen in obstetric patients, the authors find it helpful to guide prescribing physicians by including in the chart of patients with MG a list of medications to avoid. A list of the more common agents known to exacerbate MG is found in Box 15.12.

Regular antenatal checks should consider maternal symptoms and drug use. Regular fetal assessment should consider fetal growth and movements and amniotic fluid levels.

Box 15.12 Agents known to worsen myasthenia gravis

- *Antibiotics*: fluoroquinolones, aminoglycosides, ampicillin, clarithromycin, clindamycin, erythromycin, tetracyclines
- *Antiepileptic drugs*: gabapentin, phenytoin, trimethadione
- *Antipsychotics*: chlorpromazine, lithium, phenothiazines
- *Cardiac drugs*: beta-blockers, bretylium, calcium channel blockers, procainamide propafenone, quinidine Steroids
- *Anesthetic agents*: chlorprocaine, diazepam, ether, halothane, ketamine, lidocaine, neuromuscular blocking agents (e.g. succinylcholine and vecuronium), propanid, procaine
- *Other agents*: anticholinergics, botulinum toxin, carnitine, cholinesterase inhibitors, chloroquine, deferoxamine, diuretics, hydrochloroquine, ipecac syrup, interferon, iodinated contrast agents, magnesium sulfate, methocarbamol, narcotics, oral contraceptive pills, ophthamologic agents (betaxolol, echothiopate, timolol, tropicamide, proparacaine), oxytocin, penicillamine, ritonavir and antiretroviral protease inhibitors, statins, thyroxine

Important concerns for pregnant women with myasthenia gravis include the following.

• *Myasthenic crisis*: acute weakness of respiratory muscles is a life-threatening situation. Prompt ventilatory support, treatment of any precipitating cause and acute immunosuppression, such as plasma exchange or IV immunoglobulin, could be given.
• *Cholinergic crisis*: an overdose of cholinesterase inhibitors can lead to a depolarization block with muscles weakness. This can be differentiated from myasthenic weakness by co-existent muscarinic symptoms – see above.
• *Immunosuppression*: some mothers with MG are controlled with steroids. Sudden withdrawal of steroids can exacerbate a myasthenic crisis. Therefore continued use of immunosuppression during pregnancy is beneficial to the maternal condition and may reduce the risk of neonatal myasthenia.
• *Transplacental passage of IgG AchR autoantibodies*: in up to 20% of all mothers with MG, AchR IgG antibodies cross the placenta, leading to transient fetal or neonatal myasthenia gravis [95]. The risk of neonatal MG is increased if a sibling was previously affected [94,97]. Maternal autoantibodies cause neonatal MG in an otherwise unpredictable manner [98]. A fetus can be affected *in utero*, leading

to polyhydramnios (from decreased fetal swallowing) or arthrogryposis multiplex congenita, a life-threatening condition marked by joint contractures and pulmonary hypoplasia (from reduced fetal movements). During delivery, nonreassuring fetal heart rate patterns are more common in offspring of myasthenic mothers, but weakness will more usually be evident 24 hours after birth. The weakness is usually evident for a few weeks and responds well to treatment with cholinesterase inhibition.
• *Labor*: during pregnancy, the first stage of labor can progress normally, but weakness of skeletal muscles can limit the laboring mother's ability to contribute to the second stage. As gastric absorption is impaired during labor, intravenous or intramuscular cholinesterase inhibition with pyridostigmine should replace pyridostigmine at a dose equivalent to one-thirtieth of the patient's usual oral dose. Parenteral steroids should also be given to patients on chronic oral steroids for the same reason. The physical and emotional stress of labor can trigger a peripartum myasthenic crisis, for which the anesthetist needs to be prepared.
• *Peripartum infection*: any infection can trigger a myasthenic crisis and therefore peripartum wound infection, cystitis or mastitis should be treated promptly to avoid relapse [95].
• *Breastfeeding*: breastfeeding poses no risk to the mother or fetus. Use of pyridostigmine in breastfeeding mothers is generally viewed as acceptable. The use of immunosuppressive agents in lactating mothers is reviewed in Chapter 8 on rheumatologic disease in pregnancy.
• *Long-term outlook due to pregnancy*: women with myasthenia who become pregnant do not have an altered prognosis because of intervening pregnancy [94].

Headache

Headache and pregnancy

Headache is a common complaint in pregnancy, mostly due to relatively benign primary conditions such as tension and migraine. However, new-onset headache can be secondary to serious underlying cerebral pathology.

A useful classification categorizes headache during pregnancy in a way that prioritizes investigations and management [99].
1. Women known to have a primary headache disorder that present with their typical headache.
2. Women known to have a primary headache disorder, but present with a headache that is different from their usual headache.
3. Women not known to have a primary headache disorder presenting with new-onset headache in pregnancy.
Women in group 1 are of less concern than those in groups 2 and 3 and can be managed with the assumption that there is a gestational exacerbation of their pre-existing condition. Women in groups 2 and 3 need neurologic assessment with a

view to investigation for a potential secondary cause for the headache. Ominous associated features that suggest a secondary cause of headache include seizures, altered consciousness and persistent focal neurologic deficits including papilledema that suggests raised intracranial pressure.

The investigation and management of headache are reviewed here and also summarized in Chapter 35.

Primary headaches

Migraine

Migraine is three times more common in women compared with men, in particular affecting older fertile women [100]. Up to one-third of women aged 35–39 years have a migraine each year [101] and women over 40 years are more than twice as likely to have a pregnancy-related migraine compared with women less than 20 years [102].

A hormonal influence on migraine frequency is reinforced by the association between the menstrual cycle and migraines [103]. Migraines are most frequent in the follicular phase of the menstrual cycle when estrogen levels are at their lowest [104]. Post partum, when estrogen levels fall rapidly, migraines return [105]. Breastfeeding has been reported to delay the return of migraines [106]. It is thought that estrogen stimulates the production of serotonin and reduces its degradation, thus improving one element of the complex system of neurotransmitters that leads to migraine [99].

A prospective study of 55,000 pregnancies found that 2% of women had a diagnosis of migraine in the first trimester and almost 80% of these women had an improvement in migraine frequency by the third trimester [107]. In another large population-based study, only 0.2% of pregnant women were admitted to hospital with a severe migraine [102]. The differential diagnosis of a severe migraine, especially when associated with neurologic deficits, leads to concern about investigation, treatment and prognosis in pregnancy.

A classic migraine headache is preceded by aura, often visual, but occasionally associated with smells or other neurologic deficits. The headache is typically unilateral, throbbing and associated with nausea, sensitivity to light, sound and head movement [108]. Untreated, the headache and associated symptoms can last for 2–3 days.

Migraine prophylaxis

The triggers to migraine attacks are heterogeneous. Furthermore, migraineurs respond variably to the same prophylaxis or treatment. In any one clinical trial, some migraineurs will respond well, while others not at all [109]. This makes it difficult to interpret the results of clinical trials that test new treatments for migraine.

The management of migraines in pregnancy relates to both the prevention and treatment of migrainous episodes.

Prophylaxis is indicated if there is one of the following [109,110]:
- more than two disabling headaches per month
- ineffective symptomatic treatment
- use of abortive treatments more than twice a week or
- migraines with neurologic sequelae.

During pregnancy, the safest strategy to prevent migraines is to avoid recognized triggers. Changes in diet or lifestyle may be effective. These include regular meals, stopping smoking and avoiding sleep deprivation. Stress management can also be beneficial with regard to the prevention of migraines.

If avoidance of provocative stimuli is ineffective, a safe first-line agent used by the authors is low-dose aspirin 75 mg daily. If this is ineffective then propranolol 20–40 mg three times daily may be safely added or substituted. Care should be taken not to lower maternal blood pressure and the dose of propranolol should be adjusted accordingly. Tricyclic antidepressants are also effective at preventing migrainous attacks. Amitriptyline has been widely used and well tolerated throughout pregnancy for many years without adverse fetal consequences [109,111].

Methysergide is a semi-synthetic ergot alkaloid derivative of ergometrine used for migraine prophylaxis outside pregnancy, but it is contraindicated in pregnancy due to its vasoconstrictor effects. Anticonvulsants, including topiramate and gabapentin, should be avoided in pregnancy for this indication due to their teratogenic effects in animals and limited data in humans.

Migraine treatment

Current effective treatment of an acute migrainous attack has reduced the need for chronic migraine prophylaxis. In particular, the use of the serotonin 5-HT1 agonist sumatriptan during the first trimester appears to be safe and is often effective [112]. In a registry that collected 516 women exposed to sumatriptan in the first trimester, there were no more congenital birth defects or adverse pregnancy outcomes compared with a general population [112]. There are too few reports of pregnancies exposed to other triptans, or to sumatriptan during the second half of pregnancy, to be as reassuring.

Alternative therapies for an acute migrainous attack during pregnancy include acetaminophen (paracetamol) 1 g four times daily, although this is often insufficient. Nonsteroidal anti-inflammatory drugs (NSAID) can also be used in the first and second trimesters but regular use should be avoided in the third trimester when they increase musculature within the fetal patent ductus arteriosus (PDA) and can cause pulmonary hypertension in the neonate [113]. The association between NSAID and premature closure of the PDA has, however, recently been disputed [114].

For severe attacks, a regime of opioids – codeine, morphine or pethidine (meperidine in the US and Canada) – with antiemetics is often effective. Regular maternal opioid use must be avoided to prevent dependence and neonatal withdrawal. Prochlorperazine, tablets or suppositories, may also improve headache and settle nausea [111]. Vasoactive treatments, including ergotamine and dihydroergotamine, should be avoided during pregnancy as they are teratogenic and reduce utero-placental blood flow.

Migraine in pregnancy is associated with cerebro-cardiovascular disease

A population database of 33,956 women with migraines during pregnancy showed an increased risk of cerebrovascular and cardiovascular events compared with nonmigraineurs [102]. The strongest association was with ischemic stroke (odds ratio 30.7, 95% CI 17.4–34.1). This study could not, however, identify whether migraine preceded or followed ischemic stroke, therefore some migrainous headache must have been caused by the stroke itself. This observation confirms findings outside pregnancy where a history of migraine with aura is strongly associated with a risk of stroke [115].

It is not just cerebrovascular disease that is associated with migraine. Women who had migraine in pregnancy have an odds ratio (OR) for myocardial infarction of 4.9 (95% CI 1.7–14.2), pulmonary embolus (OR 3.1, 95% CI 1.7–5.6) and thrombophilia (OR 3.6, 95% CI 2.1–6.1). Furthermore, women who have migraines have more than a twofold increased risk of pre-eclampsia, relative risk (RR) 2.3 (95% CI 2.1–2.5) compared with nonmigraineurs [102].

Tension type headache

There are many similarities between tension type headaches (TTH) and migraines. Both types of headache are more common in women than men, tend to improve during pregnancy and share a similar imbalance of the neurotransmitter serotonin [99]. Treatment of a TTH during pregnancy with paracetamol or NSAID can be effective. If headaches are frequent and interfering with daily living then prophylaxis with low-dose aspirin may be beneficial.

Cluster headaches

Cluster headaches are more common in men than women, but have been reported in pregnancy. They are characterized by severe lancinating pain that radiates to the face and orbit. The headaches are usually short-lived, lasting just seconds up to 1 hour. There is no prodromal aura, but there are associated autonomic effects associated with activation of the cranial nerves [99].

Small observational studies have not shown any consistent effect of pregnancy on cluster headaches. During pregnancy an attack can be treated with 100% oxygen and subcutaneous or intranasal sumatriptan [116]. Prednisolone or verapamil can be used to prevent attacks.

Secondary headaches

The differential diagnosis for pregnant women with either new-onset headaches or headaches that differ from a previously established pattern and are suggestive of a secondary cause is reviewed in Chapter 35 but includes all of the following.
- Pre-eclampsia, although most pre-eclampsia is not associated with headache. Investigate maternal condition with blood pressure, urinalysis, maternal biochemistry and hematology.
- Postdural puncture headache.
- Posterior reversible encephalopathy syndrome (PRES): bilateral cortical infarction of the parieto-occipital lobes [117]. Investigate using MRI scanning.
- Intracerebral hemorrhage and infarction, usually associated with focal neurologic signs and more common in the first postpartum week [118]. Investigate with MRI scan.
- Cerebral vein thrombosis, associated with focal neurologic findings and more common in women with a past history or family history of venous thrombosis. Investigate with MRI scan.
- Subarachnoid hemorrhage, often preceded by a "thunderclap" (sudden-onset) headache. Investigate with MRI scan.
- Idiopathic intracranial hypertension. Investigate with MRI scan and then lumbar puncture with record of opening pressure.
- Meningitis or encephalitis. Investigate with lumbar puncture and possibly MRI scan.
- Pituitary infarction (Sheehan's syndrome). Investigate with MRI scan and pituitary function tests and electrolytes.

Pregnant women with new-onset headache suggestive of a secondary cause should be investigated promptly, so that timely intervention can stop or reverse underlying pathology. An approach to the investigation of headache in pregnancy is offered in Chapter 35.

Anesthetic considerations for obstetric patients with neurologic disease

Neurologic disease may be incidental to pregnancy or may result from pregnancy and anesthetic interventions. It may be difficult to establish whether postpartum neurologic deficit results from a difficult labor, obstetric intervention or neurologic intervention if pre-existing neurologic deficit has not been documented antenatally.

Ideally, women with significant neurologic disease should be seen by an obstetric anesthesiologist in prenatal consultation, with full access to notes and relevant imaging. Existing neurologic deficit should be documented, and a plan made for analgesia and anesthesia in conjunction with the parturient and obstetric colleagues.

Box 15.13 Some key points about anesthetic management of neurologic disease

- Antepartum consultation with an obstetric anesthesiologist for patients with chronic neurologic illness or significant neurologic deficits is advisable to determine the suitability of regional anesthesia and document baseline deficits prior to undergoing anesthesia.
- Succinylcholine may precipitate life-threatening release of potassium from muscle that has been denervated in the prior 10 days to 6–7 months.
- Patients with neurologic disease may have had painful or unpleasant lumbar punctures in the past and may need reassurance about the generally painless nature of insertion of regional anesthesia catheters.
- Inadvertent dural puncture with an epidural needle (usually 17 or 18G) may lead to rapid changes in CSF pressure which may put patients with mass lesions and increased intracranial pressure at risk for herniation of the cerebellar tonsils.
- Spinal anesthesia is associated with a much smaller hole in the dura mater, due to smaller needles, and is therefore less likely to be associated with postdural puncture headaches.
- Patients with altered epidural space volume or spinal CSF volume may have unpredictable effects from normal doses of local anesthetic drugs.
- Epidural space pathology may inhibit normal distribution and action of anesthetic medications.
- Minimum periods of time should be observed between discontinuation of LMWH and regional blockade (see Chapters 3, 4 and 46 for more information).
- While regional anesthesia may have some disadvantages in the context of certain neurologic disorders, unmodified obstetric general anesthesia may also carry risks due to associated significant rises in systolic blood pressure and intracranial pressure.

Meningitis

Women with a history of meningitis require an antenatal anesthetic assessment. Where possible, records of the incident should be sought. In most cases there will have been a full recovery but there may be sequelae including cranial nerve palsy, hydrocephalus and, in the case of meningococcal meningitis, tissue loss. Women who have had viral meningoencephalitis can usually be treated as normal but women with a history of bacterial meningitis, particularly tuberculous meningitis, may have significantly abnormal epidural anatomy. A history of traumatic lumbar punctures may require counseling before regional anesthetic techniques are accepted.

Meningitis (either bacterial or aseptic) can occur following a spinal or epidural anesthesia and may present with the usual symptoms of headache, photophobia and neck stiffness, which may be confused with postdural puncture headache. The headache of meningitis is typically worse on lying down and is associated with fever and elevated neutrophil count [119,120].

Benign intracranial hypertension
(see also Chapter 35)

Benign intracranial hypertension (BIH) (also known as pseudotumor cerebri) is an increasingly commonly diagnosed condition of raised intracranial pressure that usually affects obese women. There may be frequent headaches, cranial nerve palsy, visual disturbance and sight-threatening papilledema. Lumbar puncture may have been performed as a diagnostic or therapeutic procedure. Occasionally BIH is treated with a CSF systemic shunt and the most common is a lumbar peritoneal shunt. Information regarding the site of this shunt should be obtained prior to regional anesthesia. There is a risk of trauma to the shunt and of loss of local anesthetic from the CSF but there are reports of successful spinal anesthesia in such patients.

Spinal anesthesia is safe in BIH but increased volumes of CSF may make the dose required unpredictable. Combined spinal epidural anesthesia or continuous spinal anesthesia may be useful to titrate the doses of anesthetic drugs.

AV malformation/berry aneurysm

Arteriovenous malformation or berry aneurysm can present in pregnancy or labor as a subarachnoid hemorrhage and this is discussed elsewhere in this chapter. Women who become pregnant with unruptured aneurysms, or with multiple aneurysms, which may have been partially treated, may be at particular risk during labor. Where the risk of rupture is low, labor can be considered with early epidural, blood pressure monitoring and limited or no pushing during the second stage. As an alternative, cesarean section may be required and spinal or epidural anesthesia may be employed. The small predictable CSF leak associated with spinal anesthesia is unlikely to acutely influence risk of aneurysm rupture. If risk of rupture is considered to be high, neurosurgery or therapeutic neuroradiology should be considered prior to delivery [121].

CNS tumors

Women with pre-existing cerebral or spinal tumors represent a heterogeneous group. Liaison between obstetricians, neurosurgeons, neurologists and obstetric anesthesiologists is essential in deciding appropriate management. Predominant features may be epilepsy, raised intracranial pressure, upper or lower motor neuron neurologic deficit and they may have had neurosurgery or radiotherapy in the past. In general, careful epidural analgesia may be used for the laboring patient, although the potential risks of an inadvertent dural puncture should be considered in each patient. Spinal anesthesia may be used for cesarean section. Spinal cord tumors or AV malformations usually preclude regional anesthesia, but in some circumstances this approach may be appropriate in consultation with neurology after a carefully considered review of the patient's recent neuroimaging.

Neurofibromatosis (see also Chapter 20)

In this disease there is proliferation of neural crest tissue in every organ system. There may be cardiovascular involvement (including pheochromocytoma), lung involvement, difficult venous access and airway involvement. Of particular concern to the obstetric anesthesiologist is the presence of cerebral tumors, airway tumors, raised intracranial pressure and spinal tumors, which may be traumatized by regional techniques. As a result, detailed clinical evaluation is required, including examination of recent MRI scans to establish an appropriate anesthetic plan [122].

Epilepsy

There is an increased risk of seizures during pregnancy, labor and the puerperium among women with epilepsy. This may be because of increased psychologic and physiologic stress, pharmacokinetic factors, changes in medication and drug interactions. Routine advice may be to encourage epidural analgesia to avoid stress and hyperventilation, and to avoid meperidine analgesia because the active metabolite normeperidine lowers seizure threshold. Seizures in pregnancy and particularly in labor may be particularly hazardous because of increased oxygen requirement in pregnancy, risk of aspiration, risk of aortocaval compression and airway difficulties.

The differentiation of seizures presenting in labor from other causes of seizure such as drug toxicity, eclampsia or amniotic fluid embolism may be difficult. It is useful to document a patient's "typical seizure" in the clinical notes during prenatal care. Nonetheless, the initial treatment of seizures in pregnancy is the same as it is for any patient, that is assessment and maintenance of airway, breathing, circulation with appropriate administration of antiepileptic drugs. Intravenous administration of benzodiazepines or other hypnotic drugs to a pregnant woman may precipitate apnea, airway obstruction, hypoxia, aspiration and cardiovascular collapse and should be given cautiously with ready availability of an individual experienced in airway management.

Hyperventilation is a common precipitant of epilepsy and good epidural analgesia in labor is thought to decrease the incidence of epilepsy by relieving pain, stress and hyperventilation in labor.

Multiple sclerosis

Pregnant patients with multiple sclerosis present with a wide spectrum of disease. In some cases a firm diagnosis may not have been made. An antenatal anesthetic appointment is important to document pre-existing neurologic deficit and plan labor analgesia and anesthesia. Patients should be reassured that regional analgesia is safe and there is no evidence that sufferers are more at risk of neurologic injury from neuraxial blockade. Some multiple sclerosis sufferers appear to be more sensitive to sedative or opioid drugs. Patients with multiple sclerosis may find the procedure of epidural or spinal anesthesia extremely distressing because of prior experience of lumbar puncture and may find the sudden occurrence of profound sensory and motor block frightening [123].

Guillain–Barré syndrome

It is rare for this syndrome to present in pregnancy. Although it is usually associated with a full recovery, there may be residual neurologic deficit which needs to be documented antenatally prior to administration of regional anesthesia. Regional analgesia and anesthesia do not appear to represent additional risk to patients who have suffered from Guillain–Barré syndrome. As with MS, sudden onset of sensory and motor anesthesia may bring back unpleasant memories and this needs to be discussed with the patient [124,125].

Spinal cord injury

Neurologic features of patients with pre-existing spinal cord injury will depend on the site of the lesion. High cervical lesions may be associated with borderline respiratory function and patients can decompensate in pregnancy because of increased oxygen demand and diaphragmatic splinting. Labor can exacerbate this problem. Patients with high thoracic lesions may develop sympathetic hyper-reflexia in labor (hypertension and bradycardia) and epidural analgesia should be considered to prevent this even if the patient does not experience the pain of labor. If cesarean section is required regional anesthesia is preferable. Succinylcholine use during general anesthesia may precipitate life-threatening hyperkalemia in patients with dennervated muscle.

Kyphoscoliosis

Kyphoscoliosis is a common cause for referral to an obstetric anesthesiologist in the antenatal period. Most cases of scoliosis are idiopathic but there are associations with infection, neurologic disease (spina bifida, neurofibromatosis, polio, myotonic dystrophy), Marfan's syndrome, rheumatoid arthritis and bony disease. There are a number of key questions that need to be asked. Is there evidence of any associated pathology such as cardiac or respiratory involvement (e.g. restrictive lung disease, valvular abnormalities, pulmonary hypertension)? Women with fixed ribs respond poorly to splinting of the diaphragm in pregnancy or following cesarean section. Pulmonary function tests and an echocardiogram may be predictive of difficulties in pregnancy, labor and following anesthesia. Respiratory failure may occur following cesarean section, especially if general anesthesia is used; such cases can often be predicted and facilities for intensive care should be available. Occasionally the bony pelvis is sufficiently distorted to preclude vaginal delivery. Finally the question of whether regional anesthesia is possible and predictable needs to be considered. Insertion of a needle into a vertebral column that is distorted in three dimensions can be extremely difficult. Once inserted into the epidural or subarachnoid space, spread of local anesthetic and subsequent block can be unpredictable and potentially hazardous. In extreme cases spinal catheters have been used to allow more careful titration of local anesthetic to clinical effect. Feasibility and appropriateness of a trial of regional anesthesia in patients with spinal deformities can only be decided on a case-to-case basis.

Surgical correction may have been employed to prevent further distortion and partially correct a deformity. Ideally, antenatal consultation should be obtained to allow assessment of the surgical procedure and imaging obtained to establish the location of the hardware.

Women with pre-existing back pain

Back pain is common in pregnant and nonpregnant women. Women with back pain can be reassured that regional analgesia/anesthesia will not affect the prognosis of their back pain. Mobility in labor should be encouraged and women should be reminded to avoid positions that they know will exacerbate their back pain while in labor. Prolapsed intervertebral disks occasionally interfere with spread of local anesthetic but this is rare unless there is an existing neurologic deficit. Surgery to decompress prolapsed disks usually results in abnormal anatomy and scarring of the epidural space. Where a posterior approach is used, the surgical scar usually indicates the extent of surgery. If possible, the original surgical notes should be examined and the surgeon contacted. Such surgery may interfere with the spread of epidural, but not spinal, drugs.

Myasthenia gravis

This disease has variable features and course in pregnancy. It is characterized by weakness and fatigue as a result of acetylcholine receptor antibodies. Antenatal anesthetic involvement is essential. There may be significant respiratory involvement, problems with swallowing and chronic aspiration. The second stage of labor may be affected. Any drug that produces motor weakness such as magnesium, sedative drugs and general anesthesia (in particular neuromuscular blocking drugs) may produce life-threatening motor weakness. Cautious regional anesthesia may be useful. Ventilation may be required following general anesthesia and deterioration in respiratory function can occur post delivery.

Myotonic dystrophy

This is a multisystem disease characterized by failure of muscle to relax after forceful contraction. It is associated with cardiomyopathy, respiratory muscle involvement and variable cognitive dysfunction. Affected patients may be very sensitive to sedative drugs, particularly opioids. General anesthesia may be extremely hazardous, succinylcholine should not be used because of the danger of precipitating myotonia and hyperkalemia, and postoperative ventilation may be required. Epidural analgesia in labor is useful. Slow extension of combined spinal epidural or continuous spinal anesthesia may be useful for cesarean section. Early consultation with an obstetric anesthesiologist is essential [126].

Spina bifida

This may vary in severity from spina bifida occulta as an incidental finding with no neurologic implications to severe forms of spina bifida cystica with associated neurologic defect and previous surgery. In addition, there may be hydrocephalus with a ventriculoperitoneal shunt, a tethered spinal cord with progressive neurologic deficit, kyphoscoliosis with associated mechanical cardiorespiratory impairment and pelvic distortion. In particular, regional analgesia and anesthesia can be difficult because of previous surgery, kyphoscoliosis, problems with positioning and the presence of a tethered, low spinal cord, which is sensitive to trauma. General anesthesia is usually well tolerated unless kyphoscoliosis is severe. In the absence of distal neurologic symptoms from a tethered cord (and signs and symptoms such as foot deformities, abnormal back pigmentation or urinary symptoms should be sought), patients with spina bifida occulta can be treated as normal. The area affected should be avoided and MRI scans can be useful. In spina bifida cystica, spinal anesthesia should be avoided unless cord tethering has been excluded with MRI [127,128].

Migraine

Pregnant women with migraine represent a heterogeneous group ranging from the classic prodromal visual symptoms with nausea followed by a unilateral headache to atypical migraine with transient neurologic signs. Migraine attacks may be precipitated by pain, stress and starvation. Patients who have more severe forms of migraine such as hemiplegic migraine should be advised to have early epidural analgesia in labor.

Postdural puncture headache

Postdural puncture headache (PDPH) is caused by leakage of CSF following dural puncture. The risk of headache is dependent on the rate of CSF loss, which is dependent on the type of needle used for dural puncture (atraumatic pencilpoint versus sharp Quincke-tipped needles), the size of needle and the number of dural punctures. If rate of CSF production is exceeded by rate of loss then there is a decreased CSF, which classically causes a postural occipitofrontal headache, neck and back stiffness, photophobia, diplopia and altered hearing. The headache is relieved by lying down and abdominal pressure. Symptoms can last from a few days to several weeks. Subdural hematoma has been reported as a complication of PDPH. Conservative treatment consists of analgesia and hydration. Increased caffeine intake (from beverages or as a 300 mg caffeine pill or as 500 mg in 1 L of normal saline given over 1 hour) and bedrest relieve symptoms but do not alter the risk of occurrence or duration of symptoms. Although a number of alternative treatments have been proposed (e.g. sumitriptan or ACTH), they do not appear to be more effective than caffeine and bedrest.

Patients with persistent PDPH should be considered for an epidural blood patch. In this procedure 10–20 mL of the patient's blood is injected into the epidural space. Success rates may be as high as 90–96% and the response may be immediate. Side effects or complications can rarely include low back pain or aseptic meningitis. The epidural blood patch is believed to work by stimulating platelet aggregation and fibrin and increasing CSF pressure.

Postdural puncture headache should not be confused with other causes of postpartum headache. Venous sinus thrombosis, subarachnoid hemorrhage, intracerebral hemorrhage, pre-eclampsia and meningitis (as well as tension and migraine headaches) are all potential causes of postpartum headache and should be considered in any woman with severe or persistent headache after delivery. Women who have had previous PDPH following anesthetic intervention or as part of neurologic or hematologic investigation and treatment may be very wary of epidural or spinal analgesia/anesthesia. Traditionally neurologists and hematologists have been slow to adopt the use of narrow-gauge (e.g. 25–29G), atraumatic spinal needles (e.g. Sprotte, Whitacre, Gertie Marx) as opposed to wide-bore (18–22G) Quincke-tipped needles partly because of the need to sample CSF/cells and measure CSF pressure. In the absence of obvious clinical features such as morbid obesity, a history of tuberculous meningitis and kyphoscoliosis, women who have had a previous dural puncture can be reassured that they are unlikely to develop another and the institutional inadvertent dural puncture rate (normally in the range 0.3–2%) and spinal headache rate (range 0.3–2%) should be quoted [129,130].

Postpartum neurologic deficit

Postpartum neurologic deficit is common following childbirth. This is not surprising when the proximity of lower limb nerves at the pelvic brim in relation to the descending fetal presenting part is considered. Common injuries are discussed earlier in this chapter and include lumbosacral plexus injury, obturator nerve palsy, lateral cutaneous nerve of the thigh injury and common peroneal nerve injury. Innervation of the bladder wall may be injured by prolonged distension of the bladder as well as direct pressure on nerves supplying the skin of the buttocks by prolonged adoption of the sitting or supine position. These injuries usually resolve over the course of a few months.

Neurologic injury associated with regional anesthesia is extremely rare but may be severe and permanent. Neurologic injury causing permanent harm is very much less common in obstetric anesthetic cases than that associated with regional anesthesia for nonpregnant patients. Injury may be due to chemical contamination or mistaken administration of drugs into the CSF or epidural space. In fact, the epidural space is remarkably forgiving and despite the reported inadvertent administration of a multitude of drugs into the epidural space, very few cases of harm have occurred. However, drugs injected into the CSF may cause direct neuronal toxicity, e.g. cauda equina syndrome following the intrathecal administration of lidocaine and arachnoiditis following contamination of local anesthetic with chlorhexidine. Direct trauma to peripheral nerves, nerve roots and the cord itself can occur. In most cases the patient feels pain or paresthesia on insertion of the needle. Neurologic deficit should be investigated and early consultation with a neurologist is invaluable [131].

Epidural abscess and epidural hematoma

Epidural abscess and epidural hematoma present as space-occupying lesions within the epidural space with localized or generalized back pain, urinary retention and progressive neurologic deficit. Epidural abscess may also present more subtly with headache, photophobia, fever and rigors. They are both extremely rare in obstetric practice compared with surgical practice. Coagulopathy (whether therapeutic, congenital or acquired) is considered an absolute contraindication to regional anesthesia although epidural hematoma is extremely rare. In all cases a balance of risks should be considered and in some cases the risk associated with not performing regional blockade and performing a general anesthetic is greater. There are consensus documents which prescribe the safe intervals between therapeutic and prophylactic low molecular weight heparins (LMWH) and the insertion and removal of epidural catheters and spinal needles. Therapeutic LMWH should be stopped for 24 hours prior to regional blockade, prophylactic LMWH should be stopped 10–12 hours before regional blockade and LMWH should be delayed for 2 hours after regional blockade. Routine tests of coagulation, e.g. INR, aPTT and anti-factor Xa levels, are not helpful in establishing the safety of regional blockade following LMWH. If a space-occupying lesion of the epidural space either from a hematoma or an abscess is suspected, arrangement should be made for MRI scan, neurosurgical or orthopedic opinion and urgent evacuation. Prognosis will depend upon the rapidity of definitive treatment [132–134].

Backache following regional anesthesia

Short- and long-term backache is common following childbirth. Prospective controlled trials have found no association with regional anesthesia. Backache is common following childbirth with or without regional anesthesia [135].

Acute complications of regional anesthesia

When local anesthetic drugs are injected into the spinal or epidural space they cause segmental effects on sympathetic and motor nerves in a distribution that is dependent on the extent of spread. As local anesthetic spreads cephalad, increased sympathetic blockade causes sympathetic-mediated vasodilation, hypotension, and bradycardia. Motor blockade can cause intercostal followed by diaphragmatic paralysis. It is unusual to get extensive spread from injection of drugs into the epidural space but if an epidural drug dose is inadvertently injected spinally then this spread can occur and continue to affect the vasomotor and respiratory centers and potentially cause unconsciousness and cardiac arrest. Even if treated immediately, such cardiac arrests may be fatal.

Opioids such as fentanyl, morphine and sufentanil are commonly administered with local anesthetic into the epidural and subarachnoid space and these can cause mild side effects such as pruritus, nausea, vomiting and drowsiness. All opioids can cause respiratory depression and this occasionally can be late onset. In the case of morphine, this can occur up to 12–24 hours after spinal administration, and is more frequent where additional opioids are given by a different route, usually parenteral.

References

1. Lewis G. Saving mothers' lives: reviewing materal deaths to make motherhood safer. Confidential Enquiries into Maternal Health UK, London, 2007.
2. Department of Health, Scottish Executive Health Department. Why Mothers die. Sixth Report of Confidential Enquiries into Maternal Deaths in the UK. RCOG Press, London, 2004.
3. American College of Radiology. ARC practice guideline for imaging pregnant or potentially pregnant adolescents and women with ionizing radiation. American College of Radiology Council, Reston, VA, 2008.
4. Chen M, Coakley F, Kaimal, A, Laros RK Jr. Guidelines for computed tomography and magnetic resonance imaging use during pregnancy and lactation. Obstet Gynecol 2008;112 (2 Pt 1):333–40.
5. Alonso A, Hernan MA. Temporal trends in the incidence of multiple sclerosis: a systematic review. Neurology 2008;71(2):129–35.
6. Hirst C, Swingler R, Compston DA, Ben-Shlomo Y, Robertson NP. Survival and cause of death in multiple sclerosis: a prospective population-based study. J Neurol Neurosurg Psychiatry 2008;79(9):1016–21.
7. Briggs GG, Freeman RK, Yaffe SJ. Drugs in pregnancy and lactation. Lippincott Williams and Wilkins, Philadelphia, 2008.
8. Lee M, O'Brien P. Pregnancy and multiple sclerosis. J Neurol Neurosurg Psychiatry 2008;79(12):1308–11.
8a. Dalton CM, Keenan E, Jarrett L, Buckley L, StevensonVL. The safety of baclofen in pregnancy: intrathecal therapy in multiple sclerosis. Mult Scler 2008;14(4):571–2.
9. Hale TW. Medications and mother's milk, 13th edn. Hale Publishing, Amarillo, TX, 2008.
10. Carton H, Vlietinck R, Debruyne J, et al. Risks of multiple sclerosis in relatives of patients in Flanders, Belgium. J Neurol Neurosurg Psychiatry 1997;62(4):329–33.
11. Confavreux C, Hutchinson M, Hours MM, Cortinovis-Tourniaire P, Moreau T. Rate of pregnancy-related relapse in multiple sclerosis. Pregnancy in Multiple Sclerosis Group. N Engl J Med 1998;339(5):285–91.
12. Confavreux C. Intravenous immunoglobulins, pregnancy and multiple sclerosis. J Neurol 2004;251(9):1138–9.
13. Vukusic S, Hutchinson M, Hours M, et al., Pregnancy In Multiple Sclerosis Group. Pregnancy and multiple sclerosis (the PRIMS study): clinical predictors of post-partum relapse. Brain 2004;127(Pt 6):1353–60.
14. Achiron A, Kishner I, Dolev M, Stern Y, Dulitzky M, Schiff E, Achiron R. Effect of intravenous immunoglobulin treatment on pregnancy and postpartum-related relapses in multiple sclerosis. J Neurol 2004;251(9):1133–7.
15. Petitti DB, Sidney S, Quesenberry CP Jr, Bernstein A. Incidence of stroke and myocardial infarction in women of reproductive age. Stroke 1997;28(2):280–3.
16. Lanska DJ, Kryscio RJ. Stroke and intracranial venous thrombosis during pregnancy and puerperium. Neurology 1998;51(6):1622–8.
17. Kittner SJ, Stern BJ, Feeser BR, et al. Pregnancy and the risk of stroke. N Engl J Med 1996;335(11):768–74.
18. Witlin AG, Mattar F, Sibai BM. Postpartum stroke: a twenty-year experience. Am J Obstet Gynecol 2000;183(1):83–8.
19. James AH, Bushnell CD, Jamison MG, Myers ER. Incidence and risk factors for stroke in pregnancy and the puerperium. Obstet Gynecol 2005;106(3):509–16.
20. Tiecks FP, Lam AM, Matta BF, Strebel S, Douville C, Newell DW. Effects of the valsalva maneuver on cerebral circulation in healthy adults. A transcranial Doppler study. Stroke 1995;26(8):1386–92.
21. Lamy C, Hamon JB, Coste J, Mas JL. Ischemic stroke in young women: risk of recurrence during subsequent pregnancies. French Study Group on Stroke in Pregnancy. Neurology 2000;55(2):269–74.
22. Kothari RU, Pancioli A, Liu T, Brott T, Broderick J. Cincinnati Prehospital Stroke Scale: reproducibility and validity. Ann Emerg Med 1999;33(4):373–8.

23. Jaigobin C, Silver FL. Stroke and pregnancy. Stroke 2000;31(12):2948–51.

24. Jeng JS, Tang SC, Yip PK. Incidence and etiologies of stroke during pregnancy and puerperium as evidenced in Taiwanese women. Cerebrovasc Dis 2004;18(4):290–5.

25. Cronin CA, Weisman CJ, Llinas RH. Stroke treatment: beyond the three-hour window and in the pregnant patient. Ann NY Acad Sci 2008;1142:159–78.

26. Albers GW, Amarenco P, Easton JD, Sacco RL, Teal P, American College of Chest Physicians. Antithrombotic and thrombolytic therapy for ischemic stroke: American College of Chest Physicians Evidence-Based Clinical Practice Guidelines (8th Edition). Chest 2008;133(6 suppl):630S–669S.

27. Cutrer FM, Huerter K. Migraine aura. Neurologist 2007;13(3): 118–25.

28. WHO International Collaborative Study of Hypertensive Disorders of Pregnancy. Geographic variation in the incidence of hypertension in pregnancy. Am J Obstet Gynecol 1998;158:80–83.

29. Sharshar T, Lamy C, Mas JL. Incidence and causes of strokes associated with pregnancy and puerperium. A study in public hospitals of Ile de France. Stroke in Pregnancy Study Group. Stroke 1995;26(6):930–6.

30. Roberts JM. Endothelial dysfunction in preeclampsia. Semin Reprod Endocrinol 1998;16(1):5–15.

31. Martin JN Jr, Thigpen BD, Moore RC, Rose CH, Cushman J, May W. Stroke and severe preeclampsia and eclampsia: a paradigm shift focusing on systolic blood pressure. Obstet Gynecol 2005;105(2):246–54.

32. Ducros A, Boukobza M, Porcher R, Sarov M, Valade D, Bousser MG. The clinical and radiological spectrum of reversible cerebral vasoconstriction syndrome. A prospective series of 67 patients. Brain 2007;130(12):3091–101.

33. Singhal AB, Kimberly WT, Schaefer PW, Hedley-Whyte T. A 36-year-old woman with headache, hypertension, and seizure 2 weeks post partum. N Engl J Med 2009;360:1126–37.

34. Barrett JM, van Hooydonk JE, Boehm FH. Pregnancy-related rupture of arterial aneurysms. Obstet Gynecol Surv 1982;37(9): 557–66.

35. Dias MS. Neurovascular emergencies in pregnancy. ClinObstet Gynecol 1994;37(2):337–54.

36. Pickard JD, Murray GD, Illingworth R, et al. Effect of oral nimodipine on cerebral infarction and outcome after subarachnoid haemorrhage: British Aneurysm Nimodipine Trial. BMJ 1989;298(6674):636–42.

37. Dias MS, Sekhar LN. Intracranial hemorrhage from aneurysms and arteriovenous malformations during pregnancy and the puerperium. Neurosurgery 1990;27(6):855–65.

38. Stoodley MA, Macdonald RL, Weir BK. Pregnancy and intracranial aneurysms. Neurosurg Clin North Am 1998;9(3):549–56.

39. Weir BK, Drake CG. Rapid growth of residual aneurysmal neck during pregnancy. Case report. J Neurosurg 1991;75(5):780–2.

40. Molyneux AJ, Kerr RS, Yu LM, et al. International Subarachnoid Aneurysm Trial (ISAT) of neurosurgical clipping versus endovascular coiling in 2143 patients with ruptured intracranial aneurysms: a randomised comparison of effects on survival, dependency, seizures, rebleeding, subgroups, and aneurysm occlusion. Lancet 2005;366(9488):809–17.

41. Wilson SR, Hirsch NP, Appleby I. Management of subarachnoid haemorrhage in a non-neurosurgical centre. Anaesthesia 2005;60(5):470–85.

42. Eggert SM, Eggers KA. Subarachnoid haemorrhage following spinal anaesthesia in an obstetric patient. Br J Anaesth 2001;86(3):442–4.

43. Wiebers DO. Unruptured intracranial aneurysms: natural history, clinical outcome, and risks of surgical and endovascular treatment. Lancet 2003;362(9378):103–10.

44. Horton, JC, Chambers WA, Lyons SL, Adams RD, Kjellberg RN. Pregnancy and the risk of hemorrhage from cerebral arteriovenous malformations. Neurosurgery 1990;27(6):867–71.

45. Uchide K, Terada S, Akasofu K, Higashi S. Cerebral arteriovenous malformations in a pregnancy with twins: case report. Neurosurgery 1992;31(4):780–2.

46. Viscomi CM, Wilson J, Bernstein I. Anesthetic management of a parturient with an incompletely resected cerebral arteriovenous malformation. Reg Anesth 1997;22(2):192–7.

47. Finnerty JJ, Chisholm CA, Chapple H, Login IS, Pinkerton JV. Cerebral arteriovenous malformation in pregnancy: presentation and neurologic, obstetric, and ethical significance. Am J Obstet Gynecol 1999;181(2):296–303.

48. Lanska DJ, Kryscio RJ. Risk factors for peripartum and postpartum stroke and intracranial venous thrombosis. Stroke 2000;31(6):1274–82.

49. Linn J, Pfefferkorn T, Ivanicova K, et al. Noncontrast CT in deep cerebral venous thrombosis and sinus thrombosis: comparison of its diagnostic value for both entities. Am J Neuroradiol 2009;30(4):728–35.

50. Nagaraja D, Sarma GR. Treatment of cerebral sinus/venous thrombosis. Neurol India 2002;50(2):114–16.

51. de Bruijn SF, de Haan RJ, Stam J, Cerebral Venous Sinus Thrombosis Study Group. Clinical features and prognostic factors of cerebral venous sinus thrombosis in a prospective series of 59 patients. J Neurol Neurosurg Psychiatry 2001;70(1):105–8.

52. Ferro JM, Canhão P, Stam J, Bousser MG, Barinagarrementeria F, ISCVT Investigators. Prognosis of cerebral vein and dural sinus thrombosis: results of the International Study on Cerebral Vein and Dural Sinus Thrombosis (ISCVT). Stroke 2004;35(3):664–70.

53. Overell JR, Bone I, Lees KR. Interatrial septal abnormalities and stroke: a meta-analysis of case-control studies. Neurology 2000;55(8):1172–9.

54. Sander JW. The epidemiology of epilepsy revisited. Curr Opin Neurol 2003;16(2):165–70.

55. Harden CL, Hopp J, Ting et al., American Academy of Neurology, American Epilepsy Society. Management issues for women with epilepsy – focus on pregnancy (an evidence-based review). I. Obstetrical complications and change in seizure frequency: Report of the Quality Standards Subcommittee and Therapeutics and Technology Assessment Subcommittee of the American Academy of Neurology and the American Epilepsy Society. Epilepsia 2009;50(5):1229–36.

56. Harden CL, Meador KJ, Pennell PB, et al., American Academy of Neurology, American Epilepsy Society. Management issues for women with epilepsy – focus on pregnancy (an evidence-based review). II. Teratogenesis and perinatal outcomes: Report of the Quality Standards Subcommittee and Therapeutics and Technology Subcommittee of the American Academy of Neurology and the American Epilepsy Society. Epilepsia 2009;50(5):1237–46.

57. Harden CL, Pennell PB, Koppel BS, et al., American Academy of Neurology, American Epilepsy Society. Management issues for women with epilepsy – focus on pregnancy (an evidence-based review). III. Vitamin K, folic acid, blood levels, and breast-feeding: Report of the Quality Standards Subcommittee and Therapeutics and Technology Assessment Subcommittee of the American Academy of Neurology and the American Epilepsy Society. Epilepsia 2009;50(5):1247–55.

58. Langan Y, Nashef L, Sander JW. Case-control study of SUDEP. Neurology 2005;64(7):1131–3.

59. Holmes LB, Harvey EA, Coull BA, *et al.* The teratogenicity of anticonvulsant drugs. N Engl J Med. 2001;344(15):1132–8.

60. Fried S, Kozer E, Nulman I, Einarson TR, Koren G. Malformation rates in children of women with untreated epilepsy: a meta-analysis. Drug Saf 2004;27(3):197–202.

61. Wyszynski DF, Nambisan M, Surve T, Alsdorf RM, Smith CR, Holmes LB, Antiepileptic Drug Pregnancy Registry. Increased rate of major malformations in offspring exposed to valproate during pregnancy. Neurology 2005;64(6):961–5.

62. Morrow J, Russell A, Guthrie E, *et al.* Malformation risks of antiepileptic drugs in pregnancy: a prospective study from the UK Epilepsy and Pregnancy Register. J Neurol Neurosurg Psychiatry 2006;77(2):193–8.

63. Adab N, Kini U, Vinten U, *et al.* The longer term outcome of children born to mothers with epilepsy. J Neurol Neurosurg Psychiatry 2004;75(11):1575–83.

64. Eriksson K, Viinikainen K, MonkkonenA, *et al.* Children exposed to valproate in utero – population based evaluation of risks and confounding factors for long-term neurocognitive development. Epilepsy Res 2005;65(3):189–200.

65. Meador KJ, Baker GA, Browning N, *et al.*, NEAD Study Group. Cognitive function at 3 years of age after fetal exposure to antiepileptic drugs. N Engl J Med 2009;360(16):1597–605.

66. Mountain KR, Hirsh J, Gallus AS Neonatal coagulation defect due to anticonvulsant drug treatment in pregnancy. Lancet 1970;i:265.

67. Choulika S, Grabowski E, Holmes LB. Is antenatal vitamin K prophylaxis needed for pregnant women taking anticonvulsants? Am J Obstet Gynecol 2004;190(4):882–3.

68. Practice parameter: management issues for women with epilepsy (summary statement). Report of the Quality Standards Subcommittee of the American Academy of Neurology. Neurology 1998;51(4):944–8.

69. Kaaja E, Kaaja R, Matila R, Hiilesmaa V. Enzyme-inducing antiepileptic drugs in pregnancy and the risk of bleeding in the neonate. Neurology 2002;58(4):549–53.

70. MRC Vitamin Study Research Group. Prevention of neural tube defects: the results of the Medical Research Council Vitamin Study Group. Lancet 1991;338:131–7.

71. Morrow J, Hunt SJ, Russell AJ, *et al.* Folic acid use and major congenital malformations in offspring of women with epilepsy. A prospective study from the UK Epilepsy and Pregnancy Register. J Neurol Neurosurg Psychiatry 2009;80(5):506–11.

72. Medical Research Council Antiepileptic Drug Withdrawal Study Group. Randomised study of antiepileptic drug withdrawal in patients in remission. Lancet 1991;337(8751):1175–80.

73. Specchio LM, Tramacere L, La Neve A, Beghi E. Discontinuing antiepileptic drugs in patients who are seizure free on monotherapy. J Neurol Neurosurg Psychiatry 2002;72(1):22–5.

74. Chadwick D. The discontinuation of AED therapy. In: Pedley TA, Meldrum BS (eds) Recent advances in epilepsy. Churchill Livingstone, Edinburgh, 1985.

75. Chadwick D. Starting and stopping treatment for seizures and epilepsy. Epilepsia 2006;47(suppl 1):58–61.

76. Meador K, Reynolds MW, Crean S, Fahrbach K, Probst C. Pregnancy outcomes in women with epilepsy: a systematic review and meta-analysis of published pregnancy registries and cohorts. Epilepsy Res 2008;81(1):1–13.

77. Raymond A, Fish D, Stevens J, *et al.* Subependymal heterotopia: a distinct neuronal migration disorder associated with epilepsy. J Neurol Neurosurg Psychiatry 1994;57(10):1195–202.

78. Pennell P, Peng L, Newport DJ, *et al.* Lamotrigine in pregnancy: clearance, therapeutic drug monitoring, and seizure frequency. Neurology 2008;70(22 Pt 2):2130–6.

79. Tomson T, Hiilesmaa V. Epilepsy in pregnancy. BMJ 2007;335(7623):769–73.

80. Tomson T, Palm R, Källén K, *et al.* Pharmacokinetics of levetiracetam during pregnancy, delivery, in the neonatal period, and lactation. Epilepsia 2007;48(6):1111–16.

81. O'Brien MD, Gilmour-White SK. Management of epilepsy in women. Postgrad Med J 2005;81(955):278–85.

82. Sabers A, Ohman I, Christensen J, Tomson T. Oral contraceptives reduce lamotrigine plasma levels. Neurology 2003; 61(4):570–1.

83. Roelvink NC, Kamphorst W, van Alphen HA, Rao BR. Pregnancy-related primary brain and spinal tumors. Arch Neurol 1987;44(2):209–15.

84. Shmorgun D, Chan WS, Ray JG. Association between Bell's palsy in pregnancy and pre-eclampsia. QJM 2002;95(6):359–62.

85. Cohen Y, Lavie O, Granovsky-Grisaru S, Aboulafia Y, Diamant YZ. Bell palsy complicating pregnancy: a review. Obstet Gynecol Surv 2000;55(3):184–8.

86. Engström M, Berg T, Stjernquist-Desatnik A, *et al.* Prednisolone and valaciclovir in Bell's palsy: a randomised, double-blind, placebo-controlled, multicentre trial. Lancet Neurol 2008;7(11):993–1000.

87. Baumann F, Karlikaya G, Yuksel G, Citci B, Kose G, Tireli H. The subclinical incidence of CTS in pregnancy: assessment of median nerve impairment in asymptomatic pregnant women. Neurol Neurophysiol Neurosci 2007;2:3.

88. Nogajski JH, Shnier RC, Zagami AS. Postpartum obturator neuropathy. Neurology 2004;63(12):2450–1.

89. Meriggioli MN, Sanders DB. Autoimmune myasthenia gravis: emerging clinical and biological heterogeneity. Lancet Neurol 2009;8:475–90.

90. Leite MI, Jones M, Strobel P, *et al.* Myasthenia gravis thymus: complement vulnerability of epithelial and myoid cells, complement attack on them, and correlations with autoantibody status. Am J Pathol 2007;171:893–905.

91. Ferrero S, Pretta S, Nicoletti A, *et al.* Myasthenia gravis: management issues during pregnancy. Eur J Obstet Gynecol Reprod Biol 2005;121:129–38.

92. Soleimani A, Moayyeri A, Akhondzadeh S, *et al.* Frequency of myasthenic crisis in relation to thymectomy ingeneralised myasthenia gravis. BMC Neurol 2004;4:12.

93. Pompeo E, Tacconi F, Massa R, *et al.* Long-term outcome of thoracoscopic extended thymectomy for nonthymomatous myasthenia gravis. Eur J Cardiothorac Surg 2009;36(1):164–9.

94. Hoff JM, Daltveit AK, Gilhus NE. Myasthenia gravis in pregnancy and birth: identifying risk factors, optimising care. Eur J Neurol 2007;14:38–43.

95. Djelmis J, Sostarko M, Mayr D, *et al.* Myasthenia gravis in pregnancy: report on 69 cases. Eur J Obstet Gynecol Reprod Biol 2002;104:21–5.

96. Muecksch JN, Stevens WA. Undiagnosed myasthenia gravis masquerading as eclampsia. Int J Obstet Anesth 2007;16:379–82.

97. Hoff JM, Daltveit AK, Gilhus NE. Arthrogryposis muliplex congenita – a rare fetal condition caused by maternal myasthenia gravis. Acta Neurol Scand 2006;183(suppl):26–7.

98. Gveric-Ahmetasevic S, Colic A, Elvedji-Gasparovic V, *et al.* Can neonatal myasethnia gravis be predicted? J Perinat Med 2008;36:503–6.

99. Rukmini M, Bushnell CD. Headache and pregnancy. Neurologist 2008;14:108–19.

100. Lipton RB, Stewart WF, Diamond S, Diamond ML, Reed M. Prevalence and burden of migraine in the United States: data from the American Migraine study II. Headache 2001;41:646–57.

101. Launer LJ, Terwindt G, Ferrari M. The prevalence and characteristics of migraine in a population-based cohort: the GEM study. Neurology 1999;53:537–42.

102. Bushnell CD, Jamison M, James AH. Migraines during pregnancy linked to stroke and vascular diseases: US population based case-control study. BMJ 2009;338:664.

103. Brandes JL. The influence of estrogen on migraine: a systematic review. JAMA 2006;295:1824–30.

104. Somerville B. The role of estradiol withdrawal in the etiology of menstrual migraine. Neurology 1972;22:355–65.

105. Marcus DA, Scharff L, Turk D. Longitudinal prospective study of headache during pregnancy and postpartum. Headache 1999;39:625–32.

106. Wall VR. Breastfeeding and migraine headaches. J Hum Lact 1992;8:209–12.

107. Chen TC, Leviton A. Headache recurrence in pregnant women with migraine. Headache 1994;34:107–10.

108. Lipton RB, Bigal ME, Steiner TJ, Silberstein SD, Olesen J. Classification of primary headaches. Neurology 2004; 63(3):427–35.

109. Clavel AL Jr. Migraine prevention. The choices continue to grow. BMJ 2001;78–9.

110. Silberstein SD. Preventive migraine treatment. Neurol Clin 2009;27(2):429–43.

111. Goadsby PJ, Goldberg J, Silberstein SD. Migraine in pregnancy. BMJ 2008;336:1502–4.

112. Evans EW, Lorber KC. Use of 5-HT1 agonists in pregnancy. Ann Pharmacother 2008;42(4):543–9.

113. Koren G, Florescu A, Costei AM, Boskovic R, Moreti ME. Nonsteroidal anti-inflammatory drugs during third trimester and the risk of premature closure of the ductus arteriosus: a meta-analysis. Ann Pharmacother 2006;40:824–9.

114. Savage AH, Anderson BL, Simhan HN. The safety of prolonged indomethacin therapy. Am J Perinatol 2007;24:207–13.

115. Etminan M, Takkouche B, Caamano I, Samii A. Risks of ischaemic stroke in people with migraine: systematic review and meta-analysis of observational studies. BMJ 2005;330(7482):63.

116. Jurgens TP, Schaefer C, May A. Treatment of cluster headache in pregnancy and lactation. Cephalalgia 2009;29:391–400.

117. Finocchi V, Bozzao A, Bonamini M, et al. Magnetic resonance imaging in posterior reversible encephalopathy syndrome: report of three cases and review of the literature. Arch Gynecol Obstet 2005;271:79–85.

118. Skidmore FM, Williams LS, Fradkin KD, Alonso RJ, Biller J. Presentation, etiology and outcome of stroke in pregnancy and puerperium. J Stroke Cerebrovasc Dis 2001;10:1–10. 119. May AE, Fombon S, Francis S. UK registry of high-risk obstetric anesthesia: report on neurological disease. Int J Obstet Anesth 2008;17(1):31–6.

119. Moen V, Irestedt L. Neurological complications following central neuraxial blockades in obstetrics. Curr Opin Anaesthesiol 2008;21(3):275–80.

120. Reynolds F. Infection as a complication of neuraxial blockade. Int J Obstet Anesth 2005;14(3):183–8.

121. Duggan T, Simpson A. An unusual intracranial aneurysm presenting in pregnancy. Int J Obstet Anesth 2008:17(2):194–5.

122. Spiegel JE, Hapgood A, Hess PE. Epidural anesthesia in a parturient with neurofibromatosis type 2 undergoing cesarean section. Int J Obstet Anesth 2005:14(4):336–9.

123. Drake E, Drake M, Bird J, Russell R. Obstetric regional blocks for women with multiple sclerosis: a survey of UK experience. Int J Obstet Anesth 2006;15(2):115–23.

124. Alici HA, Cesur M, Erdem AF, Gursac M. Repeated use of epidural anesthesia for caesarean delivery in a patient with Guillain-Barré syndrome. Int J Obstet Anesth 2005; 14(3):269.

125. Brooks H, Christian AS, May AE. Pregnancy, anesthesia and Guillain–Barré syndrome. Anaesthesia 2000;55:894–8.

126. Boyle R. Antenatal and preoperative genetic and clinical assessment in myotonic dystrophy. Anaesth Intens Care 1999;27(3):301–6.

127. McGrady EM, Davis AG. Spina bifida occulta and epidural anesthesia Anaesthesia 1988;43(10):867–9.

128. Tidmarsh M, May AE. Epidural anaesthesia and neural tube defects. Int J Obstet Anesth 1998;7(2):111–14.

129. Van de Velde M, Schepers R, Berends N, Vandermeersch E, de Buck F. Ten years of experience with accidental dural puncture and post-dural puncture headache in a tertiary obstetric anesthesia department. Int J Obstet Anesth 2008;17(4): 329–35.

130. Zeidan A , Farhat O, Maaliki H, Baraka A. Does postdural puncture headache left untreated lead to subdural hematoma? Case report and review of the literature. Int J Obstet Anesth 2006;15(1):50–8.

131. Cook TM, Counsell D, Wildsmith JA Major complications of central neuraxial block: report on the Third National Audit Project of the Royal College of Anaesthetists. Br J Anaesth 2009;102(2):179–90.

132. Grewal S, Hocking G, Wildsmith JAW. Epidural abscess. Br J Anaesth 2006;96:292–302.

133. Meikle J, Bird S, Nightingale JJ, White N. Detection and management of epidural haematomas related to anaesthesia in the UK: a national survey of current practice.. Br J Anaesth 2008;101:400–4.

134. Moen V, Dahlgren N, Irestedt L. Severe neurological complications after central neuraxial blockades in Sweden 1990–1999. Anesthesiology 2004;101:950–9.

135. Howell CJ, Dean T, Lucking L, Dziedzic K, Jones PW, Johanson RB. Randomised study of long term outcome after epidural versus non-epidural analgesia during labour. BMJ 2002;325(7360):357.

16 Nonviral infectious diseases in pregnancy

Brenna Anderson[1], Melissa Gaitanis[2] with Daniel I. Sessler[3]

[1]Department of Obstetrics and Gynecology, Warren Alpert Medical School of Brown University, Providence, RI, USA

[2]Department of Medicine/Infectious Diseases, Warren Alpert Medical School of Brown University, Providence, RI, USA

[3]Department of Outcomes Research, Cleveland Clinic, Cleveland, OH, USA

Fever and host immune response in pregnancy

The pregnant woman may be exposed to any of the common causes of infection. Women in labor and during the puerperium are particularly susceptible to serious infection of the genitourinary tract. In addition, breast and wound infections may occur. Puerperal sepsis (childbed fever) rightly remains the most feared complication of childbirth, still with a significant mortality and morbidity. Box 16.1 summarizes the nonviral causes of fever complicating pregnancy and the puerperium.

The notion that pregnant women become globally immunosuppressed during pregnancy is inconsistent with evolution and the overall favorable survival of the human fetus. Some authors have noted alterations in maternal innate and cellular immunity during pregnancy, as decreased T-cell function and decreased NK-cell function [1–3]. However, scientists have not noted a trend towards either suppression or enhancement of maternal systemic immune function during pregnancy [4].

Fever is a nonspecific indicator of disease, whether infective or noninfective in origin. Fever is also analogous with other nonspecific indicators of an acute inflammatory state such as the erythrocyte sedimentation rate (ESR) or serum C-reactive protein (CRP) level. Irrespective of race or climate, the body temperature normally lies within the range 37.0–37.5°C, with diurnal variation such that evening temperatures are from 0.5–1.0°C higher than the morning level. Oral and axillary temperatures are approximately 0.5°C and 1.0°C lower than the core temperature. Persistent elevation of core temperature above these levels defines fever or pyrexia.

Central control of thermal regulation resides in the hypothalamus. Products of tissue injury, however caused, termed endogenous pyrogens, appear to mediate disturbance of thermoregulation. In infective causes of fever, bacterial products such as endotoxin are the cause of cell injury, resulting in the release of endogenous pyrogens from granulocytes, monocytes and fixed macrophages. The resulting fever may be characterized by rises followed by precipitous falls with sweating and peripheral dilation of blood vessels. Increased muscle activity may lead to rigors, resulting in peripheral vasoconstriction and the cold clammy skin that is the hallmark of severe septicemia, particularly with gram-negative organisms.

Fever also has implications for pregnancy in terms of development of the normal fetus. Growing evidence associates intrauterine exposure to hyperthermia and inflammation with adverse neurologic outcomes [5]. In term infants intrapartum fever has been associated with a risk of cerebral palsy,

---

Box 16.1 Nonviral infective causes of fever in pregnancy and the puerperium

Clinical diagnoses

- Endometritis
- Pelvic abscess
- Chorio-amnionitis
- Thrombophlebitis
- Intraperitoneal abscess
- Amniotic fluid embolus
- Mastitis and breast abscess
- Wound infection
- Infective endocarditis

Specific organisms

- Disseminated gonococcal infection
- Syphilis
- Listeriosis
- Tuberculosis
- Severe infection consequent on HIV

---

de Swiet's Medical Disorders in Obstetric Practice, 5th edition.
Edited by R. O. Powrie, M. F. Greene, W. Camann. © 2010 Blackwell Publishing.

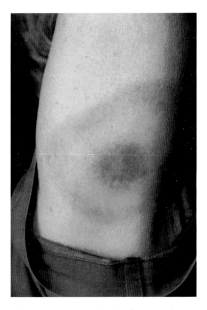

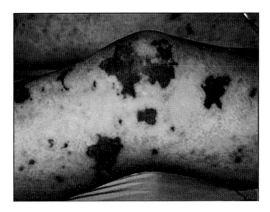

Plate 16.1 Erythema migrans rash of early Lyme disease. From www2.massgeneral.org/rai/index.asp?page=diseases_conditions& subpage=lyme

Plate 16.2 Purpura fulminans in association with meningococcal septicemia. From www.nlm.nih.gov/medlineplus/ency/article/000608. htm. Copyright information at www.nlm.nih.gov/medlineplus/ency-clopedia.html

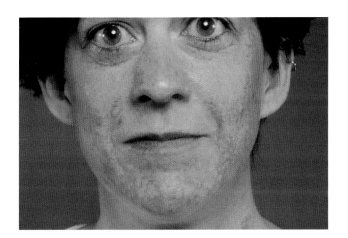

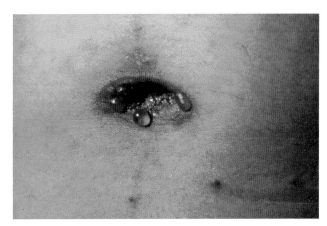

Plate 20.1 Melasma (the "mask of pregnancy").

Plate 20.2 Pemphigoid gestationis.

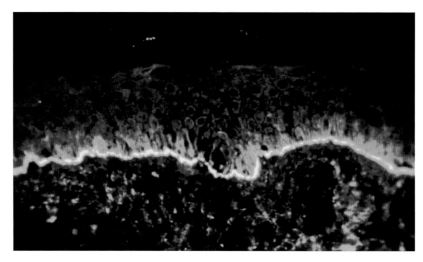

Plate 20.3 Pemphigoid gestationis immunofluorescence. Immunofluorescence staining of pemphigoid gestationis reveals a characteristic linear band of C3 and/or IgG attached to bullous pemphigoid antigen 2 (BPAG2), an antigen in the basement membrane zone of the skin that is important for epidermal–dermal adhesion.

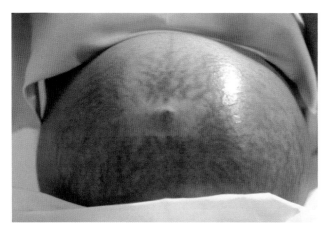

Plate 20.4 Polymorphous eruption of pregnancy (PEP) also known as pruritic urticarial plaques and papules of pregnancy (PUPPP).

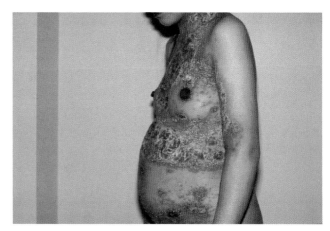

Plate 20.5 Pustular psoriasis.

neonatal hypoxic encephalopathy, and seizures. Studies have examined limiting the effects of inflammation and fever on the neonatal brain by giving acetaminophen, steroids and antibiotics, and other neuroprotective agents during planned vaginal deliveries [5,6].

The investigation of fever in pregnancy requires attention not only to the specific infections of pregnancy, but also to the common causes in the community. Therefore, the need for careful history taking cannot be overemphasized. Questions must include symptoms, chronology, recent travel, eating habits, pets and contacts with others with fever. Careful examination of the whole patient is necessary, with particular attention paid to the genitourinary tract, skin rashes, palpable masses and heart murmurs. Investigation should be relevant and thorough, and include genital swabs, urine (with microscopy), and blood cultures (generally two sets drawn from two different sites to help discern the difference between bacteremia and skin contamination). Serum for antibody tests can be obtained to confirm an etiologic diagnosis of specific infections. Two sets of antibodies (IgG and IgM) are usually drawn, "acute" and "convalescent" serum, and are most helpful in confirming a diagnosis when drawn 4–6 weeks apart.

Genital infections in pregnancy

Normal flora and vaginal discharge

Among women of reproductive age, the vaginal flora is a complex ecosystem of aerobic and anaerobic gram-positive and gram-negative bacteria co-existing in close symbiosis. Under the influence of estrogen, the vaginal epithelium contains glycogen, which favors colonization by large gram-positive rods, *Lactobacillus* spp, which metabolize glycogen to form lactic acid [7]. The resulting pH of less than 4.5 suppresses the growth of potential pathogens, assisted by the production of hydrogen peroxide by lactobacilli. Other bacteria commonly present in large numbers (approximately 10^7/mL vaginal fluid) include anaerobic and nonbeta-hemolytic streptococci, diphtheroids (*Corynebacterium* spp) and coagulase-negative staphylococci [8]. Common commensal organisms that are potentially pathogenic include *Candida* spp, beta-hemolytic streptococci (Lancefield Group B, *Streptococcus agalactiae* is found in 5–30% of normal vaginas, and less commonly Group A *Streptococcus pyogenes*), *Staphylococcus aureus* and *Actinomyces* spp. Mycoplasmas are also frequent commensals, with *Ureaplasma urealyticum* present in over 50% of sexually active women [9,10]. Other organisms, for example coliforms, anaerobic gram-negative rods and *Gardnerella vaginalis*, are often present in low numbers.

Abnormal vaginal discharge is a common problem in both the nonpregnant and pregnant woman. Its particular importance in pregnancy reflects the effect on both outcome and the puerperium. The infective causes of abnormal discharge

Table 16.1 Characterization of vaginal discharge

Condition	pH	Discharge characteristics	Microscope slide preparation	Microscopic appearance
Normal flora	<4.5	Normal odor and volume	Saline	Epithelial cells with distinct borders, many lactobacilli, few white blood cells per high-power field
T. vaginalis	>4.5	Green, frothy	Saline	Motile trichomonads, many white blood cells per high-power field
Bacterial vaginosis	>4.5	Gray, watery, malodorous +amine odor with KOH	Saline	>20% clue cells, decreased lactobacilli
Candidal infections	<4.5	Thick, white, curdlike	KOH	Hyphae, +/− budding yeast, increased white blood cells

KOH, potassium hydroxide.

include viral (herpes simplex), protozoal (*Trichomonas vaginalis*), fungal (*Candida* spp) and bacterial infections. Bacterial causes are cervical infection by *Neisseria gonorrhoeae* and/or *Chlamydia trachomatis*, and the altered state of microbial flora that characterizes bacterial vaginosis. The characteristics differentiating the common causes of vaginal discharge are shown in Table 16.1.

Bacterial vaginosis

Bacterial vaginosis (BV) can be symptomatic or asymptomatic. When symptomatic, it presents as a grayish watery discharge with an odor. Diagnosis can be made clinically using Amsel's criteria or by gram stain (see Table 16.2) [11]. BV is an alteration of the normal vaginal flora with consequent overgrowth of pathogenic bacteria. *G. vaginalis* culture or polymerase chain reaction (PCR) is not useful in the diagnosis of BV, given the frequency of *G. vaginalis* in normal flora. In the past BV has been dismissed as a minor irritation but it is associated with significant adverse pregnancy outcomes. It is a risk factor for premature rupture of membranes with or without labor, preterm labor with intact membranes, chorio-amnionitis, and postpartum endometritis [12–14].

The underlying cause of BV is not understood. The consequence is a fall in the absolute number of hydrogen peroxide-producing lactobacilli, leading to a rise in pH and an increase in the absolute number of *G. vaginalis*, anaerobic gram-negative rods (*Bacteroides* spp, *Prevotella* spp and

Table 16.2 Criteria for diagnosis of bacterial vaginosis

Amsel criteria: three out of four of the following criteria should be present:	Gram stain criteria (Nugent score)
• A white/gray homogenous discharge • A vaginal discharge pH of >4.5 • A positive amine test (drop of 10% potassium hydroxide added to drop of discharge on a slide produces fishy odor) • Microscopy demonstrates clue cells	0–3: Normal flora 4–7: Intermediate flora 8–10: Bacterial vaginosis

---

Box 16.2 Regimens for bacterial vaginosis therapy

- Metronidazole 500 mg orally twice a day for 7 days
- Metronidazole gel, 0.75%, one full applicator (5 g) intravaginally, once a day for 5 days
- Clindamycin cream, 2%, one full applicator (5 g) intravaginally at bedtime for 7 days

Adapted from CDC [34].

Porphyromonas spp), *Mobiluncus* spp and *Mycoplasma hominis*. The metabolic activity of *Mobiluncus* spp leads to a release of trimethylamine, producing the foul fishy odor. Exfoliation of vaginal epithelial cells with their adherent *G. vaginalis* results in the characteristic "clue cells" seen on microscopy of the vaginal discharge [7,8]. An association between pregnancy, BV and human immunodeficiency virus (HIV) infection has also been reported [15].

There is conflicting evidence about the effect of treatment of BV on outcomes. There are several acceptable treatment regimens. When taking oral metronidazole, patients must avoid alcohol, which produces a disulfiram-like reaction with nausea and vomiting. Current recommendations regarding appropriate treatment for symptomatic bacterial vaginosis in pregnancy are listed in Box 16.2. There are several randomized trials that support the treatment of asymptomatic bacterial vaginosis among women at high risk for preterm birth, particularly when screened early in pregnancy [16–18]. Treatment of asymptomatic bacterial vaginosis in low-risk pregnant women is not currently recommended [19].

Trichomonas vaginalis infection

Trichomonas vaginalis is a sexually transmitted flagellated protozoan. It is the most common pathogenic protozoan of humans in industrialized countries. It causes a purulent vaginitis and can be accompanied by vulvar and cervical lesions, abdominal pain, dyspareunia, and dysuria. It can be diagnosed

by wet mount microscopy, which has high specificity but low sensitivity [20–22]. A systematic review of diagnostic tools for *T. vaginalis* found that PCR and culture have the highest sensitivities and specificities of the various tests available [23].

Trichomonas vaginalis has long been associated with premature rupture of membranes [24,25]. It is also associated with an increased risk of HIV seroconversion in areas of high HIV prevalence [26]. In 1997, the Vaginal Infections and Prematurity Study Group reported a significant increase in low birthweight and preterm delivery [27]. A subsequent prospective randomized trial conducted by the Maternal Fetal Medicine Units Network of the National Institute of Heath has since reported failure of metronidazole to prevent preterm delivery in asymptomatic women infected with *T. vaginalis* [28]. This trial was stopped early because of an increased risk of preterm birth in the metronidazole group. Of note, the trial used a larger dose of metronidazole than that recommended by the Centers for Disease Control (CDC) for treatment of trichomoniasis in pregnancy. For this reason, screening for asymptomatic trichomoniasis in pregnancy is not recommended. The regimen for treatment of trichomoniasis in pregnancy recommended by the CDC is a single oral dose of 2 g of metronidazole.

Candida infection

Candida is a common vaginal commensal. It is estimated that some 75% of all women will have at least one episode of *Candida* vaginitis [29]. Asymptomatic carriage in pregnancy occurs in 30–40%, compared with 10–20% of nonpregnant women. *Candida* vaginitis in pregnancy is not associated with adverse outcome [30]. The vaginal discharge is usually white, curdlike, and odorless and associated with intense itching. The vaginal pH is normal or reduced, in contrast to trichomoniasis or BV. It can generally be diagnosed by wet mount with KOH but certain species are more easily detected with the use of yeast culture. Several species of *Candida* may be present, but *C. albicans* predominates (>90%). Treatment is no more difficult than in the nonpregnant woman, but the choice of agent is restricted. Topical nystatin and topical imidazoles (e.g. clotrimazole, econazole, miconazole) for 7 days are safe and effective. The orally active drugs flucytosine and the triazole fluconazole have not been adequately studied in pregnancy.

Neisseria gonorrhoeae infection

The overall prevalence of genital tract infection with *N. gonorrhoeae* in pregnancy is approximately 1% [31]. The vast majority of these infections are asymptomatic. Infection in pregnancy is associated with premature rupture of membranes and preterm delivery [32,33]. Disseminated gonococcal infection (DGI) is possible in pregnancy and classically presents with oligoarthritis involving the hands, feet and elbows.

Fever and skin rash make up the two other parts of the classic triad. The amniotic infection syndrome is a complication of *N. gonorrhoeae* specific to pregnancy. It is associated with maternal fever, premature rupture of membranes, premature delivery, neonatal infection, and high infant morbidity and mortality. An important consequence of untreated maternal gonococcal infection to the neonate is gonococcal ophthalmia neonatorum. Disseminated infection with arthritis and meningitis occurs, but is rare. Since most infants now receive erythromycin ophthalmic ointment at birth, ophthalmic infection occurs less frequently as well.

Current recommendations include screening by cervical swab for all pregnant women with increased risk (patients under the age of 25, with new or multiple sexual partners, a history of sexually transmitted infections or who are members of a population at increased risk). If using a culture-based diagnostic method, gonococcus does not travel well and a suitable transport medium should be used (e.g. Stuart's), even for a short transfer. Alternatively, the specimen should be direct plated on to an antibiotic-screened enriched medium (e.g. Thayer Martin), and transported in a candle extinction jar or commercial system to ensure enhanced levels of carbon dioxide in the culture atmosphere. Nucleic acid amplification tests are now becoming the standard diagnostic tool and are widely available. Culture methods should still be used for tests of the pharynx or rectum because of the potential for cross-reactivity with nongonococcal *Neisseria* from nongenital sites.

The recommended treatment for uncomplicated *N. gonorrhoeae* in pregnancy is one of the following: a single dose of ceftriaxone 125 mg IM or cefixime 400 mg PO or if unable to tolerate cephalosporins, then spectinomycin 2 g IM [34]. Fluoroquinolones and tetracyclines should be avoided in pregnancy. None of the above regimens is adequate to treat concurrent chlamydial infection, which is likely in women with gonococcal infection (see below).

Chlamydia trachomatis infection

Chlamydia trachomatis is the most common bacterial cause of sexually transmitted infection. The median prevalence among young women attending prenatal clinics is 8%, ranging from 2.8% to 16.9% [35]. *Chlamydia trachomatis* is also the most common cause of secondary infertility, consequent upon an attack of overt or covert pelvic inflammatory disease (PID). The risk of ectopic pregnancy is increased by 7–10 times following chlamydial PID. As is the case with *N. gonorrhoeae*, most infected women will be asymptomatic. Risk factors for infection in pregnancy include young age, recent partner change, multiple partners and being unmarried. The routine screening of all pregnant women is recommended by the US CDC, and by the authors and editors. Other bodies have different recommendations. The American College of Obstetricians and Gynecologists (ACOG) recommends testing

only in women with a new or more than one sexual partner and those under the age of 25 or with a history of a sexually transmitted infection. The UK National Insitute for Health and Clinical Excellence (NICE) does not recommend routine *Chlamydia* screening in pregnancy but that women under the age of 25 be given details of their local National Chlamydia Screening Program.

The effect of chlamydial infection on the pregnancy *per se* is not well understood. The role of chlamydial infection in fetal wastage is not proven. *Chlamydia trachomatis* has been associated with premature rupture of membranes, prematurity and perinatal death in some studies [36,37] but not in others [38]. A serologic study by Gencay & Koskinieme found an association between raised maternal antichlamydial IgM and increased incidence of chorio-amnionitis, prematurity and perinatal mortality [39].

True congenital infection of the fetus has not been described. However, acquisition of the organism during vaginal birth is common. Up to 70% of babies born to infected mothers will become colonized. In 30–40% this will manifest as conjunctivitis, and in 10–20% as a characteristic pneumonitis. Infection of the vagina, rectum and pharynx may also occur, but may be delayed for up to 7 months, and persist for over 2 years [40]. Chlamydial ophthalmia neonatorum is more common than gonococcal, and is clinically indistinguishable. Up to 50% of babies with gonococcal conjunctivitis will have concurrent chlamydial infection. The common practice of prophylaxis with erythromycin ointment prevents infection in most cases. Chlamydial pneumonitis presents between 3 weeks and 3 months of birth, and is characterized by dyspnea and staccato cough [41].

The diagnosis of chlamydial infection has been revolutionized by the introduction of nucleic acid amplification (NAA) technology, for example PCR and ligase chain reaction (LCR) [42]. Chlamydial NAA can be carried out as a noninvasive test on urine samples from women. It is important that the test manufacturer's instructions concerning obtaining and transporting specimens are followed closely, and that the testing protocol has been agreed with the diagnostic laboratory.

Because doxycycline is contraindicated in pregnancy, oral azithromycin is the current treatment of choice [43]. The recommended dose is a single oral dose of 1 g azithromycin. Amoxicillin provides alternative therapy in pregnancy, 500 mg three times daily for 7 days. Erythromycin is an alternative drug but is considered to have a decreased efficacy rate, probably related to noncompliance from the gastrointestinal side effects it causes [34].

Mycoplasma infection

Although *M. hominis* isolated from a case of bartholinitis was the first human *Mycoplasma* isolate, the role of the genital mycoplasmas in disease is ill defined. As noted above, both *M. hominis* and *U. urealyticum* are normal constituents of the genital tract flora. They have been associated with acute chorio-amnionitis, but whether their role is causal remains unclear. There is an apparent association with low birthweight, but this finding is clouded by the association of BV *per se* with this condition [44–46]. A randomized treatment trial failed to show any improvement in outcome with treatment of *U. urealyticum* [44].

Mycoplasma hominis can be isolated from blood using conventional blood culture medium, and blood agar incubated micro-aerophilically with 10% CO_2. *Ureaplasma urealyticum* is best isolated using a specific *Mycoplasma* medium. Based on the evidence that treatment does not improve outcome, there is no justification for routine screening for mycoplasmas during pregnancy.

Mycoplasmas are classically sensitive to tetracyclines, but these drugs should not be used during pregnancy or lactation. *Ureaplasma urealyticum* is sensitive to erythromycin and other macrolides, but is resistant to clindamycin, whereas *M. hominis* is resistant to erythromycin and sensitive to clindamycin. This important difference should be borne in mind when a patient with postpartum pyrexia due to presumed endometritis fails to respond to either erythromycin or clindamycin.

Syphilis

Syphilis is a sexually transmitted systemic infection, caused by the spirochete *Treponema pallidum*. Syphilis has the potential for significant illness in mothers but infection in pregnancy can be disastrous for the fetus. Between 70% and 100% of pregnant women with untreated early syphilis will transmit infection to the fetus, and in up to one-third of cases this will result in stillbirth. The prevalence of primary and secondary syphilis has been climbing since reaching an all-time low in the year 2000. Congenital syphilis, however, continues to decline, likely due to continued prenatal screening and treatment [47]. Maternal symptoms are often mild or nonexistent, and the longer the woman has had untreated syphilis before the first pregnancy, the less likely *in utero* death will occur, and the more likely a congenitally syphilitic live child will be born. The longer the duration of untreated illness, and the more pregnancies, the less likely that a subsequent fetus will be infected.

The primary lesion is the ulcer or chancer at the site of inoculation, which may be extragenital. The lesion heals in 6–8 weeks and is followed by the secondary phase of systemic spread. Signs include a rash on the palms and feet, patchy alopecia, cervical lymphadenopathy, and flat warty lesions termed condylomata lata. However, symptoms and signs may be transient or absent. The disease then enters the latent phase, divided into early (the first year) and late, when the disease is relatively quiescent. Subsequently, after several years, the cardiologic and neurologic manifestations of tertiary syphilis may develop in up to one-third of untreated

Table 16.3 Stages and phases of syphilis

Stage	Phase	Symptoms
Primary		Painless chancer
Secondary		Spirochetemia, rash on palms and soles, condyloma lata
Latent	Early <1 year	Asymptomatic
	Late >1 year	Asymptomatic
Tertiary		Cardiologic and neurologic symptoms in up to 1/3 of untreated people

patients. See Table 16.3 for the stages and phases of syphilis. Central nervous system involvement can occur in any stage of syphilis. A patient who has clinical evidence of neurologic involvement with known syphilis (e.g. cognitive dysfunction, motor or sensory deficits, ophthalmic or auditory symptoms, cranial nerve palsies, and symptoms or signs of meningitis) should have a cerebrospinal fluid examination.

Screening for syphilis remains mandatory during pregnancy, because of the importance of identifying infected women early in pregnancy and the availability of effective therapy. Screening is generally carried out either using a nonspecific reagin test such as the rapid plasma reagin test (RPR) or venereal disease research laboratory test (VDRL), or a treponemal specific test such as the *Treponema pallidum* hemagglutination test (TPHA) or *T. pallidum* particle agglutination test (TPPA). A positive test with any of these requires confirmation by another unrelated test (reagin or specific), and an adsorbed fluorescent treponemal antigen test (FTA-Abs). The latter test should also be carried out if early syphilis is suspected, for example in the presence of a genital ulcer, because it may become positive early in the disease before the other tests (Table 16.4). A biologic false positive (BFP) can occur with the reagin tests, where other

Table 16.4 Test characteristics of syphilis by stage

	Reagin tests (e.g. VDRL, RPR)	Specific tests (e.g. TPHA, TPPA)	FTA-Abs
Early primary syphilis	Negative	Negative	Positive
Late primary syphilis	Positive	Positive	Positive
Secondary syphilis	Strong positive	Strong positive	Positive
Latent syphilis	Positive	Positive	Positive
Treated syphilis	Positive, lower titer	Positive	Positive
Yaws, pinta (treated or untreated)	Positive	Positive	Positive
Biologic false positive	Positive	Negative	Negative

VDRL, Venereal Disease Research Laboratory; RPR, rapid plasma reagin; TPHA, *Treponema pallidum* hemagglutination test; TPPA, *Treponema pallidum* particle agglutination test; FTA-Abs, absorbed treponemal antigen test.

unrelated conditions such as acute viral infection, collagen vascular diseases and even pregnancy itself may give a positive reaction. Screening tests generally remain positive for life, even in patients adequately treated in the past for syphilis or other treponemal infection. If active syphilis cannot be excluded, then the woman must receive an adequate course of therapy.

Treatment in pregnancy can successfully decrease the risk of fetal infection. Parenteral penicillin G is the treatment of choice and the regimen should be directed at the maternal stage of disease (Box 16.3) [34]. There is no adequate alternative therapy for women who are allergic to penicillin [48]. Such women should undergo a desensitization protocol and be treated with penicillin [49,50]. This is typically done with administration of sequentially less dilute doses of oral penicillin VK given every 15 minutes and then followed within 30 minutes by a full therapeutic dose by the desired route. It is a potentially life-threatening procedure that requires careful preparation and the ready availability of an experienced resuscitative team.

Box 16.3 Syphilis therapy in pregnancy

Primary and secondary syphilis	Benzathine penicillin G 2.4 million units IM in a single dose
Early latent syphilis	Benzathine penicillin G 2.4 million units IM in a single dose
Late latent syphilis	Benzathine penicillin G 7.2 million units total, administered as 3 doses of 2.4 million units IM each at 1-week intervals
Tertiary syphilis	Benzathine penicillin G 7.2 million units total, administered as 3 doses of 2.4 million units IM each at 1-week intervals
Neurosyphilis	Aqueous crystalline penicillin G 18–24 million units per day, administered as 3–4 million units IV every 4 hours or continuous infusion, for 10–14 days

Adapted from CDC [34].

As in the nonpregnant state, patients being treated for syphilis should be warned of the possibility of a Jarisch–Herxheimer reaction (an immune reaction to the release of toxins into the body as spirochetal bacteria die), manifesting as an acute febrile response with rigors within 24 hours of starting treatment. Fetal distress and premature labor have been reported [43].

Nongenital infections in pregnancy

Listeriosis

Listeria monocytogenes is a small gram-positive rod, morphologically resembling a diphtheroid. The organism is ubiquitous in nature, with a wide range of temperature tolerance. It is frequently found in soil, and survives and multiplies at 4°C. Contaminated food will not be protected in a domestic refrigerator, and the organism will survive inadequate pasteurization.

There are about 16 serotypes of *L. monocytogenes*, but only a few are associated with human infection, usually types 4b, 1/2a and 1/2b [51]. The incidence of listeriosis in pregnant women is 12/100,000, 17 times the incidence in the general population [52]. Most patients with perinatal listeriosis are otherwise healthy, but some predisposing conditions include corticosteroid use, diabetes mellitus, autoimmune diseases or HIV infection. Cellular immunity is the primary line of defense against this infection. Animal studies support a role for a depressed cell-mediated immunity increasing sensitivity to listerial infection during pregnancy [53].

Infection in pregnancy is characterized by a biphasic febrile illness. The first stage is usually only considered retrospectively, consisting of nonspecific symptoms such as headache, malaise, backache and abdominal or loin pain, pharyngitis and conjunctivitis – essentially "flu"-like symptoms. The patient may or may not receive antibiotics that by chance are active against *L. monocytogenes*, and recover. The second attack occurs within 10–15 days of premature delivery, and may reflect reinfection from the contaminated placenta. In about one-third of cases maternal pyrexia in labor will have occurred. Maternal disease can be severe, leading to respiratory distress. However, meningitis (a feature of adult disease) is unusual in pregnancy.

Infants infected during pregnancy are ill at birth or within hours, whereas infants infected at birth will develop late-onset disease 5–7 days later. Predominant features include respiratory distress, bradycardia or apnea, cyanosis, hepatosplenomegaly and jaundice. Neonatal listeriosis can also present with meningitis, as noted in one case series [54]. In one-third of babies a papular rash is found. The cardinal feature of infection is miliary necrosis of the tissues, best seen as white nodules on the cut surface of the placenta or abscesses on the maternal surface [55].

When suspected, listeriosis during pregnancy can be diagnosed by vaginal/cervical swab, stool, urine, culture of amniotic fluid or maternal blood. Maternal blood cultures have been noted to be positive in more than one-third of cases, and are an important part of the diagnostic work-up of a pregnant patient with flu-like symptoms [54,56]. When clinical suspicion is raised, culture for listeriosis should include a tube that is incubated at 4°C in order to maximize the potential for recovery of *L. monocytogenes*.

Listeria monocytogenes is sensitive to a number of antibiotics *in vitro*. What is unusual about its sensitivities, however, is that while it is sensitive to penicillins, it is generally resistant to cephalosporins and so it is often not "covered" by many standard antibiotic regimens used to treat infection in obstetrics and gynecology. Optimal therapy is with ampicillin or amoxicillin plus gentamicin depending on severity. Second-line therapy is trimethoprim/sulfamethoxazole (TMP/SMX). If there is a history of penicillin allergy reported, allergy testing or desensitization should be considered. Treatment should be prolonged for 1 week after resolution of fever.

Emphasis is on prevention, and all pregnant women should be counseled on the importance of food hygiene (cook meats thoroughly and store and handle raw meat separately from other foods) and the potential risks of unpasteurized foods (soft cheeses) and ready-to-eat meats, paté and refrigerated smoked seafood.

Toxoplasmosis

Toxoplasma gondii is an obligate intracellular protozoan parasite that is worldwide in distribution. Infection is benign in immunocompetent persons and often individuals are asymptomatic. Some persons may develop a febrile illness with cervical lymphadenopathy. Untreated, the condition is self-limiting as the parasitemia subsides and the organisms become dormant in the tissues, commonly brain, heart and skeletal muscle. They may remain viable for the life of the host, and become reactivated should immunosuppression occur, such as following infection with HIV. This infection also has important implications for the pregnant host. Unfortunate timing may result in primary infection during pregnancy with transmission to the fetus, resulting in serious congenital sequelae.

Three life forms of *T. gondii* occur and are reviewed in Figure 16.1: the oocyst, the tachyzoite, and the bradyzoite. The oocyst is the product of the sexual cycle in the small intestine of cats. Sporulation of the oocyst is required for its infectivity and occurs after its excretion into the environment. Sporulation is more rapid at higher temperatures. The soil becomes an environmental reservoir, for the cysts remain viable for up to 18 months in moist soil. The tachyzoite form is invasive and is seen during acute infection. They can infect nearly all mammalian cells. Bradyzoites are found in tissues as cysts and are slow growing. Most persist in tissues for life.

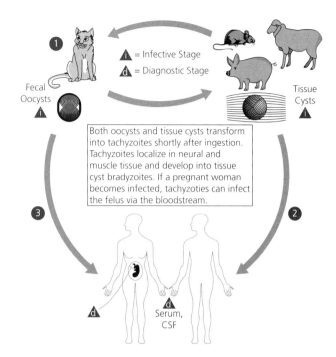

Figure 16.1 Life cycle of *Toxoplasma gondii*. Members of the cat family (Felidae) are the only known definitive hosts for the sexual stages of *T. gondii* and thus are the main reservoirs of infection. Cats become infected with *T. gondii* by carnivorism. After tissue cysts or oocysts are ingested by the cat, viable organisms are released and invade epithelial cells of the small intestine where they undergo an asexual followed by a sexual cycle and then form oocysts, which are excreted. The unsporulated oocyst takes 1–5 days after excretion to sporulate (become infective). Although cats shed oocysts for only 1–2 weeks, large numbers may be shed. Oocysts can survive in the environment for several months and are remarkably resistant to disinfectants, freezing, and drying, but are killed by heating to 70°C for 10 minutes. Human infection may be acquired in several ways: (1) ingestion of undercooked infected meat containing *Toxoplasma* cysts; (2) ingestion of the oocyst from fecally contaminated hands or food; (3) organ transplantation or blood transfusion; (4) transplacental transmission; (5) accidental inoculation of tachyzoites. The parasites form tissue cysts, most commonly in skeletal muscle, myocardium, and brain; these cysts may remain throughout the life of the host. From CDC www.dpd.cdc.gov/dpdx.

Cysts containing bradyzoites are commonly found in three distinct areas: myocardium, skeletal muscle, and brain. Tissue cysts are resistant to digestive juices, so they transmit infection well in raw or undercooked meat.

The predominant mode of transmission is eating infected, undercooked meat. As many as 25% of lamb and 25% of pork samples have been shown to contain tissue cysts [57]. Cysts have been rarely isolated from beef, eggs, and unpasteurized milk. Maternal transmission occurs in several ways:
• ingestion of oocysts due to not washing hands after handling soil or cat litter
• consumption of oocysts due to contaminated food or water

- ingestion of bradyzoites/tachyzoites from the consumption of meat or meat products
- blood transfusion of tachyzoites
- inhalation of oocysts from dust.

Maternal infection is frequently unnoticed or presents as a self-limiting nonspecific illness. Women may present with nontender lymphadenopathy (involving the bilateral posterior cervical nodes), fatigue, fever, headache, malaise, and myalgia. The clinical scenario may be confused with mononucleosis, influenza or an alternative nonspecific viral illness. Estimates of maternal infection are unreliable, and observed rates are much lower than expected rates. A sample US survey from 1988–1994 showed *Toxoplasma* IgG seroprevalence to be 15% among women aged 15–44 years [58]. The prevalence of toxoplasmosis infection in pregnant women has previously ranged from 10% in the United Kingdom and Norway to around 55% in France and Greece [59]. Screening programs, although not popular in the US, have been conducted in European countries such as France and Norway. A screening program in Norway examined 35,940 pregnant women with serology and amniotic fluid for PCR. Forty-seven women (0.17%) showed evidence of primary infection during pregnancy [60].

Fetal infection results from placental infection and transmission of parasites following a primary maternal infection accompanied by parasitemia. The effect on the fetus depends on the time of maternal primary infection in relation to gestation. The earlier the infection, the lower the chance of fetal infection, but the more likely severe involvement (Table 16.5) [61]. An estimated 400–4000 cases of congenital toxoplasmosis occur in the US each year [62].

Establishment of infection in the placenta may lead to congenital infection. Severe early infection may lead to abortion or stillbirth. The classic triad of intracranial calcification, hydrocephalus and chorioretinitis is the most extreme form, but is not common. The majority (>90%) of infants are asymptomatic at birth. Manifestations of the disease are numerous, including encephalitis, epilepsy, mental and growth retardation, jaundice, hepatosplenomegaly, thrombocytopenia and skin rashes.

Testing for toxoplasmosis is far from straightforward. Preconception testing establishes those who have previously been infected, and will not therefore have an infected child, or those susceptible who can be counseled concerning contact with cats, uncooked food and general hygiene. The problem surrounds the interpretation of tests performed during pregnancy. The *Toxoplasma* latex agglutination test should not be used, as it is prone to false-positive as well as false-negative results. In pregnancy, serum should always be sent to a *Toxoplasma* reference laboratory for determination of specific anti-*Toxoplasma* IgM. The presence of IgM-positive serum indicates recent infection, but the problem is to determine how recent, in order to guide the clinician and patient regarding the probability of severe congenital infection. A reference laboratory can help narrow down the time of infection with tests such as the IgG avidity test, the Sabin–Feldman dye test, IgM enzyme-linked immunosorbent assay (ELISA), and the differential agglutination (AC/HS) test [63]. The only certain way of positively identifying acute infection is the demonstration of seroconversion. In acute infection, IgG and IgM antibodies generally rise within 1–2 weeks of infection. IgM antibodies have been reported to persist for up to 18 months post infection. A negative IgM with a positive IgG result indicates infection at least 1 year previously. A positive IgM result may indicate more recent infection or may be a false-positive reaction. In 1997 the FDA distributed an advisory to US physicians on how to interpret commercial test results (Table 16.6). Controversy continues over whether antenatal screening should be routine. However, the imprecision of the currently available tests and the relatively low incidence of congenital disease in the US would suggest that the extra uncertainty and anxiety would not justify any possible benefit.

If acute infection of the mother is likely, then ultrasound and amniocentesis should be considered to determine whether congenital infection is established. Amniotic fluid can be sent for PCR testing and has proven to be more sensitive and safer than fetal blood sampling. Ideally, the amniocentesis is performed in the second trimester and at least 4 weeks after acute maternal infection. Although not without risk, the result is important because it may influence the choice of anti-infective drugs and whether to continue with pregnancy. Ultrasound has also been helpful in identifying fetal abnormalities associated with congenital toxoplasmosis. In one study notable findings included ventricular dilation, intracranial densities, increased placental thickness and/or hyperdensity, intrahepatic densities, hepatomegaly, ascites, and pericardial and/or pleural effusion [64]. Ultrasound becomes more sensitive as the pregnancy progresses, and serial ultrasounds are usually suggested.

Mothers thought to be suffering from acute *Toxoplasma* infection who either do not seek termination or in whom termination is not indicated require antimicrobial therapy for the duration of the pregnancy. The drug of choice is the macrolide spiramycin, which can safely be given throughout pregnancy. Spiramycin concentrates in the placenta and is thought to prevent vertical transmission. To determine if the fetus should be treated, PCR of the amniotic fluid is performed in the second

Table 16.5 Transmission of toxoplasmosis in pregnancy

Time of maternal infection	Fetal infection rate (%)	Severe disease at birth (%)	Ocular sequelae (%)
Preconception	Unknown	Unknown	–
First trimester	25	75	45–65
Second trimester	50	55	45–65
Third trimester	65	<5	45–65

Adapted from Holliman [61].

Table 16.6 Guide to general interpretation of *T. gondii* serology results obtained with commercial assays (FDA 1997)

IgG results	IgM results	Interpretation for humans (except infants)	Action
Negative	Negative	No serologic evidence of infection	Stop
Negative	Equivocal	Possible early acute infection or false-positive IgM reaction	Obtain new specimen for IgG and IgM testing. If results for second specimen remain the same, patient is probably not infected
Negative	Positive	Possible acute infection or false-positive IgM result	Obtain new specimen for IgG and IgM testing. If results for second specimen remain the same, IgM reaction probably false positive
Equivocal	Negative	Indeterminate	Obtain new specimen for testing or retest this specimen for IgG in a different assay
Equivocal	Equivocal	Indeterminate	Obtain new specimen for both IgG and IgM testing
Equivocal	Positive	Possible acute infection	Obtain new specimen for IgG and IgM testing. If results for the second specimen remain the same or if IgG becomes positive, both specimens should be sent to a reference laboratory
Positive	Negative	Infected with *Toxoplasma* for >1 year	Stop
Positive	Equivocal	Infected with *Toxoplasma* for probably >1 year or false-positive IgM reaction	Obtain new specimen for IgM testing. If results with second specimen remain the same, both specimens should be sent to a reference laboratory
Positive	Positive	Possible recent infection within the last 12 months or false-positive IgM reaction	Send the specimen to a reference laboratory

trimester. If the PCR is negative, spiramycin is continued. If the PCR is positive, concern for congenital infection is warranted and the recommendation is to give sulfadiazine and pyrimethamine (or courses of pyrimethamine/sulfadiazine alternating every 3 weeks) until delivery. Side effects of bone marrow and renal toxicity should be monitored when giving sulfadiazine and pyrimethamine. Folinic acid 10–25 mg daily is added to this regimen to prevent bone marrow suppression. It should be noted that although some studies indicate a reduction in congenital infection with these regimens, an individual patient data meta-analysis found "weak evidence for an association between early treatment and reduced risk of congenital toxoplasmosis" [65], and there are no double-blind placebo-controlled trials reported.

Malaria

Plasmodium infection should be considered in any patient with fever and/or jaundice who lives in or has recently traveled through Africa, South East Asia, India or South America. Pregnant women have an increased incidence of infection, and when the infection does occur, it is more likely to be severe and associated with a higher level of parasitemia. This may in part be due to immunologic changes in pregnancy. However, there is also evidence that malarial parasites in pregnant women can express a variant surface antigen on infected red blood cells that facilitates binding to chondroitin sulfate A in the placenta [66,67]. The ability for the malarial parasite to infect the placenta contributes directly to the increased morbidity and mortality seen with pregnancy-associated malaria [68,69,70]. The life cycle of *Plasmodium* species is reviewed in Figure 16.2.

Systemic effects of malaria in pregnancy in patients without prior infection are often pronounced, the most severe including hemolytic anemia, thrombocytopenia, hypoglycemia, respiratory failure and lactic acidosis. Hepatorenal syndrome is often the cause of death. For patients who live in endemic areas and therefore have some partial immunity, the clinical presentation may be much less severe and even asymptomatic. Malaria may infect the placenta, leading to maternal anemia, spontaneous abortion, stillbirth and low birthweight. Malaria parasites may cross the placenta, particularly in nonimmune mothers, leading to congenital malaria. Immune primigravidae are prone to relapse in the second trimester [71,72]. The placenta of patients treated for malaria in pregnancy should always be examined histologically for the presence of parasites. If these are present, the neonate is at risk and should be given a course of antimalarial therapy.

Treatment depends on the local area, the dominant *Plasmodium* type and pattern of drug resistance. In theory, chloroquine would be the treatment of choice for severe infestation with *Plasmodium falciparum* in chloroquine-sensitive areas, and its use in pregnancy is supported by most authorities. It is clearly not a major teratogen although there may be some infrequent fetal effects [72–74].

For chloroquine-resistant *P. falciparum*, a combination of oral quinine sulfate and clindamycin is used. While there are old reports of congenital anomalies in infants who survived high-dose quinine used as an abortifacient, the applicability of this information to its use as an antimalarial agent is doubtful. At the doses used to treat malaria, it is clearly not a major teratogen. In a collaborative perinatal study of 106 women exposed to quinine in early pregnancy, there was no increase in frequency of congenital malformation [75]. It use

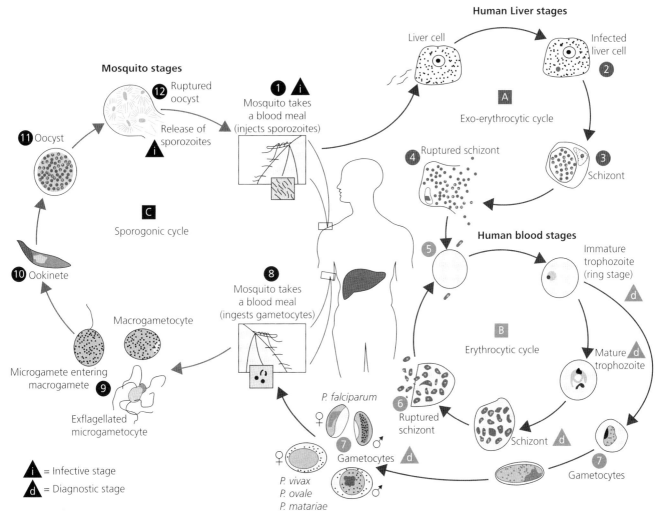

Figure 16.2 Life cycle of malaria. The malaria parasite life cycle involves two hosts. During a blood meal, a malaria-infected female *Anopheles* mosquito inoculates sporozoites into the human host. Sporozoites infect liver cells and mature into schizonts, which rupture and release merozoites. (Of note, in *P. vivax* and *P. ovale* a dormant stage (hypnozoites) can persist in the liver and cause relapses by invading the bloodstream weeks or even years later.) After this initial replication in the liver (exo-erythrocytic schizogony), the parasites undergo asexual multiplication in the erythrocytes (erythrocytic schizogony). Merozoites infect red blood cells. The ring stage trophozoites mature into schizonts, which rupture, releasing merozoites. Some parasites differentiate into sexual erythrocytic stages (gametocytes). Blood stage parasites are responsible for the clinical manifestations of the disease. The gametocytes, male (microgametocytes) and female (macrogametocytes), are ingested by an *Anopheles* mosquito during a blood meal. The parasites' multiplication in the mosquito is known as the sporogonic cycle. While in the mosquito's mid-gut, the microgametes penetrate the macrogametes, generating zygotes. The zygotes in turn become motile and elongated (ookinetes) which invade the mid-gut wall of the mosquito where they develop into oocysts. The oocysts grow, rupture, and release sporozoites, which make their way to the mosquito's salivary glands. Inoculation of the sporozoites into a new human host perpetuates the malaria life cycle. From CDC www.dpd.cdc.gov/dpdx.

in pregnancy has the added benefit of preventing premature contractions and fever in late pregnancy but it is not likely to be a tocolytic [76]. However, pregnant patients on quinine should have their glucose monitored as quinine-induced hyperinsulinemia has been reported in up to 50% of pregnant women with severe *falciparum* infection late in pregnancy and quinine has caused fatal hypoglycemia [76,77]. If 50% dextrose is not effective in restoring euglycemia in such cases, somatostatin analogues such as SMS 201–995 that inhibit insulin release are the treatment of choice for quinine-induced hypoglycemia and they may be the only effective therapy [78].

Other alternatives for chloroquine-resistant malaria include tetracyclines and atovaqone/proguanil (Malarone®). Doxycycline is generally contraindicated in pregnant women but can be used in combination with quinine when patients do not tolerate or have severe side effects to the alternative clindamycin. Treatment benefits need to be weighed against risks of discoloration and dysplasia of the teeth and inhibition of bone growth. The relatively newly approved combination drug Malarone is considered category C in pregnancy as there have been no well-controlled studies in pregnant patients but the data that exist suggest that its use is justifiable when other options are unavailable or ineffective [79]. The same can be said of the older drug mefloquine.

For sensitive *P. vivax* and *P. ovale*, chloroquine is given. Primaquine phosphate should be avoided during pregnancy. This drug may be passed transplacentally to a glucose-6-phosphate dehydrogenase (G6PD)-deficient fetus and cause hemolytic anemia *in utero*. After finishing the treatment dose of chloroquine, prophylactic chloroquine (300 mg once a week) is given for the remainder of the pregnancy. After delivery, primaquine phosphate is administered to eradicate the parasite from the liver [79].

Patients with clinical signs and symptoms of severe malaria should be treated with intravenous therapy. Signs of severe malaria include parasitemia >5%, severe normocytic anemia, organ failure (including pulmonary edema), altered conciousness, oliguria, servere jaundice, and hypoglycemia. Quinidine gluconate is administered presumptively for *P. falciparum*, even if forms of *P. vivax*, *P. ovale* or *P. malariae* are seen on smear, in case of mixed infection or missed diagnosis. Clindamycin should be combined with therapy, as in milder cases as described above. The World Health Organization (WHO) recommends the use of artesunate or artemether over quinidine in the context of severe malaria in pregnancy despite the limited pregnancy data on this agent. Regardless of the treatment regimen, persons with severe malaria should be admitted to an intensive care unit for monitoring of hypotension, arrhythmia, hypoglycemia, and urine output.

Travel to a malaria-endemic area should ideally be deferred in pregnancy. If travel is necessary or if the patient lives in an endemic area, prevention strategies are essential. The woman should avoid mosquitoes by staying in screened areas as much as possible, especially in the evening and night, sleeping under mosquito netting treated with permethrin, wearing clothing that covers skin, and using insect repellant. Chemoprophylaxis should also be employed.

Pregnant women traveling to areas where chloroquine-resistant *P. falciparum* has not been reported may take chloroquine prophylaxis (chloroquine phosphate 500 mg once weekly beginning 2 weeks prior to travel and continuing for 4 weeks after returning). For areas with chloroquine-resistant *P. falciparum* mefloquine (250 mg once weekly beginning 2 weeks prior to travel and continuing for 4 weeks after returning) is currently the only medication recommended for malaria chemoprophylaxis during pregnancy. A Thai study examining stillbirth and exposure to mefloquine suggested that mefloquine use in pregnancy was associated with a small increased risk of stillbirth [80]. However, a large randomized controlled trial showed no difference in the stillbirth rate between women who were treated with mefloquine or

chloroquine prior to starting prophylaxis [81]. Atovaquone/proguanil is another antimalarial prophylactic agent for chloroquine-resistant areas and is often better tolerated than mefloquine. It is not currently recommended for the prevention of malaria in gravid women, however, because of limited clinical data regarding its use in pregnancy.

Women living in endemic areas may benefit from weekly chloroquine or intermittent preventive therapy (IPT). One such regimen is the administration of sulfadoxine-pyrimethamine two times after a woman first feels fetal movement.

Patterns of resistance to antimalarials change so rapidly that expert advice should always be sought regarding treatment and prophylaxis. The crucial importance of compliance must be stressed and advice must be given on the avoidance of mosquito bites. From 1985 through 2002, 11,896 cases of malaria among US civilians were reported to the CDC. Of these, 6961 (59%) were acquired in sub-Saharan Africa, 2237 (19%) in Asia, 1672 (14%) in the Caribbean and Central and South America, and 822 (7%) in other parts of the world. During this period, 76 fatal malaria infections occurred among US civilians; 71 (93%) were caused by *P. falciparum*, of which 52 (73%) were acquired in sub-Saharan Africa [82]. Recommendations which remain current and updated can be found on the WHO and CDC websites (www.who.int/malaria and www.cdc.gov/malaria).

Lyme disease

Since 1977, Lyme disease has grown in importance as an emerging pathogen. In 2005, 23,305 cases of Lyme disease were reported in the United States, yielding a national average of 7.9 cases for every 100,000 persons. In the 10 states where Lyme disease is most common, the average was 31.6 cases for every 100,000 persons [83].

The highest incidences of Lyme in Europe are found in the Baltic states and Sweden in the north, and in Austria, the Czech Republic, Germany, Slovenia and central Europe [84].

Lyme disease is a tick-borne infection caused by the spirochete *Borrelia burgdorferi* and is transmitted by Ixodes ticks. The species *I. scapularis* and *I. pacificus* transmit Lyme within the US while *I. ricinus* and *I. persulcatus* are the dominant species within Europe.

Clinically, Lyme occurs in three stages. In early localized disease, or erythema migrans (EM), examination of the skin reveals an expanding red annular lesion with a clear center which usually appears between 4 days and 3 weeks after the tick bite (Plate 16.1). Dissemination is characteristic of the second stage and is characterized by neurologic or cardiac findings: meningitis, cranial nerve palsies (7th causing a unilateral facial droop; 3rd causing a unilateral ptosis, double vision if the eyelid is opened and inability to elevate, depress and adduct the affected eye; and 6th causing double vision with inability to abduct the affected eye), peripheral radiculopathies, and first- or second-degree AV block. The third stage, or late Lyme, manifests as chronic arthritis and/or neurologic problems.

Lyme disease is a clinical diagnosis that may be confirmed by serologic tests. Laboratory tests may be negative at early stages. The ELISA is used as the initial test and is expressed as a ratio of optical density values. The ELISA test is associated with sensitivities of 68–84% and specificities of 83–100% depending on the clinical kit used [85]. The ELISA has a high false-positive rate and should only be ordered if there is clinical suspicion for Lyme. Positive and equivocal ELISA results should be confirmed with the Western blot analysis. Western blot detects antibodies to individual components of the organism itself, such as the outer surface proteins and heat shock proteins.

There are criteria for interpreting Western blot results. Early antibodies, IgM, to *B. burgdorferi* appear 2–4 weeks after the EM rash and decline to low levels after 4–6 months. Antibodies to IgG appear after 6–8 weeks and peak at 4–6 months and remain elevated. These IgG antibodies may persist long after the initial disease and may be present even after treatment.

Lyme disease in pregnancy may cause anxiety in the patient as well as the treating clinician. As it is a spirochete, there are concerns that the natural history of the disease in pregnancy would have similar outcomes to that of syphilis. The absence of consistent congenital findings after neonatal exposure to Lyme and of inflammatory findings associated with fetal tissue spirochetes has argued against a specific "congenital Lyme disease syndrome."

From the early 1980s to the present, there has been much investigation of the impact of Lyme disease on pregnancy, including postmortem pathologic examination of affected pregnancies and retrospective studies on pregnant women exposed to Lyme in various trimesters. The effect of Lyme disease in pregnancy was initially questioned in case reports and small series. Transplacental transmission of *B. burgdorferi* has been documented via pathologic examination of the placenta [86–88]. Third-trimester fetal death was observed in two cases after the mother had developed first-trimester Lyme but had not been treated with antibiotics. Adverse outcomes associated with pregnancy have been associated with short-term, 7-day antibiotic use due to EM in the first trimester [89]. Markowitz *et al.* retrospectively studied the effect of Lyme disease on pregnancy outcome between 1976 and 1984, and 19 women were evaluated. Thirteen received appropriate antibiotic therapy for Lyme disease. Of the 19 pregnancies, five had adverse outcomes, including syndactyly, cortical blindness, intrauterine fetal death, prematurity, and rash in the newborn. Adverse outcomes occurred in cases with infection during each of the trimesters. None of the infants with adverse outcomes had infection with *B. burgdorferi*. *B. burgdorferi* could not be implicated directly in any of the adverse outcomes, but the authors felt that further evaluation of Lyme disease in pregnancy was warranted [90].

Several larger studies have not found an association of negative effects on the fetus when the mother receives appropriate antibiotic treatment. In a prospective study of 2000 prenatal patients, exposure to Lyme during pregnancy treated appropriately was not associated with stillbirth, prematurity or congenital malforations [91]. A prospective European study evaluated women who were treated for early Lyme (presenting with EM) during pregnancy. One hundred and five women were followed and 93 delivered a healthy infant at term. Nearly all were treated with 14 days of antibiotics. The authors could not implicate causality of the adverse outcomes to Lyme as the incidence of preterm labor and congenital anomalies was not higher than the general obstetric population [92]. One retrospective study looked at children in a Lyme-endemic area to determine if there was a risk of congenital cardiac disease after maternal Lyme exposure; 1957 children with cardiac anomalies were matched to 2750 control subjects. It was determined that if a woman had been bitten by a tick or had Lyme disease diagnosed and treated during or before her pregnancy, she was not at increased risk for giving birth to a child with a congenital heart anomaly [93]. A survey of pediatric neurologists yielded no reports of cases of congenital Lyme disease, although the outcomes were limited to neurologic disorders [94].

In conclusion, exposure to Lyme during pregnancy treated appropriately is not clearly associated with stillbirth, prematurity or congenital malformations, but one cannot rule out that Lyme infection during pregnancy may increase the risk of specific defects or that lack of treatment may increase this risk. Also, studies have demonstrated no increased incidence of adverse pregnancy outcome in women who are seropositive at conception. Neither routine serology screening nor empiric treatment of those having positive serology at conception has been shown to be beneficial [95].

According to guidelines published by the Infectious Disease Society of America (IDSA) in 2006, pregnant or lactating women may be treated in a fashion identical to nonpregnant patients with the same disease manifestation, except that doxycycline should be avoided (Table 16.7) [85]. For oral dosing in patients intolerant of amoxicillin or cefuroxime axetil, azithromycin (500 mg orally per day for 7–10 days) or erythromycin (500 mg orally 4 times per day for 14–21 days) may be given. However, macrolides are considered less efficacious and if they are used, patients should be followed closely for resolution of clinical symptoms. In the pregnant patient, using first-line antibiotics such as penicillins and cephalosporins may still be warranted to ensure against transmission of *B. burgdorferi* to the fetus. If a mother has serious penicillin or cephalosporin allergies, desensitization can be pursued. Cranial nerve palsies should be evaluated to determine whether the patient has symptoms of meningitis, and a lumbar puncture is indicated for those in whom there is strong clinical suspicion of CNS involvement.

Meningitis

Meningitis refers to inflammation of the meninges, which surround the brain and spinal cord. Meningitis can be caused by bacterial and viral organisms as well as noninfectious

Table 16.7 Recommended therapy for patients with Lyme disease

Indication	Treatment	Duration, days (range)
Tick bite in the US		
Erythema migrans	Oral[a]	14 (14–21)
Early neurologic disease		
Meningitis or radiculopathy	Parenteral[b]	14 (10–28)
Cranial nerve palsy	Oral[a]	14 (14–21)
Cardiac disease	Parenteral therapy (can be changed to oral for completion of therapy once absence of heart block is confirmed)	14 (14–21)
Borrelial lymphocytoma	Oral[a]	14 (14–21)
Late disease		
Arthritis without neurologic disease	Oral[a]	28
Recurrent arthritis after oral regimen	Oral[a] or parenteral[b]	28
Antibiotic-refractory arthritis	Symptomatic therapy	
Central or peripheral nervous system disease	Parenteral[b]	14 (14–28)
Acrodermatitis chronica atrophans	Oral[a]	21 (14–28)
Post-Lyme disease syndrome	Consider and evaluate other potential causes of symptoms; if none is found, then administer symptomatic therapy	

Adapted from the IDSA guidelines [85].
[a] Amoxicillin 500 mg 3 times per day or cefuroxime axetil 500 mg twice a day.
[b] Ceftriaxone 2 g IV daily.

etiologies. The various causative organisms of meningitis are shown in Box 16.4.

The term "aseptic meningitis" refers to patients who have clinical and laboratory evidence for meningeal inflammation with negative routine bacterial cultures and it is the most common cause of meningitis in adults. About 90% of cases of viral meningitis are caused by members of a group of viruses known as enteroviruses, such as coxsackieviruses and echoviruses. These viruses are more common during summer and fall months. Enteroviruses are very ubiquitous and young children are the primary spreader of these viruses. Pregnant women often have young children at home and may have frequent exposure to enteroviruses. If there is a lack of protective antibody from previous exposure the risk of infection is higher. The various viral causes of meningitis are shown in Box 16.5. An important cause of aseptic meningitis that should always be considered in pregnant women is acute HIV infection, which can be tested for with a HIV viral load and confirmed with subsequent serology.

Streptococcus pneumoniae and *Neisseria meningitidis* are the leading causes of bacterial meningitis in adolescents and adults. In 2002, the rate of invasive pneumococcal disease was 13 cases per 100,000 in the United States, but these disease rates are changing due to the new conjugate vaccine, which is being used in infants and children [96]. Although pregnant women are at risk of invasive disease with *L. monocytogenes* and bacteremia, they rarely present with meningitis [97].

The clinical presentation of infectious meningitis is usually acute. Symptom onset can be over a few hours, as in *N. meningitides*, to over a few days, as in *S. pneumoniae*. Fever,

Box 16.4 Etiologies of meningitis

Infectious etiologies of meningitis in the adult patient include:
1. Bacterial
   S. pneumoniae
   N. meningitidis
   L. monocytogenes
2. Aseptic
   Viruses (enterovirus)
   Mycobacteria (TB)
   Fungi (cryptococcus or coccidioidal)
   Spirochetes (syphilis and Lyme)
   Parasitic (*Angiostrongylus cantonensis*)

Noninfectious etiologies of aseptic meningitis include:
1. Autoimmune phenomenon (lupus, vasculitis)
2. Sarcoid
3. Drug induced (e.g. NSAIDS, trimethoprim/sulfamethoxazole, intravenous immunoglobulins (IVIG))
4. Neoplasm

headache, photophobia, and stiff neck are more typical features. In more clinically advanced cases or the very young, old or immunocompromised, irritability, confusion, and lethargy may be the first clinical signs. Nausea and vomiting can signify meningeal inflammation or increased intracranial pressure. Fluctuating and more subtle symptoms of meningitis can

Box 16.5 Viral causes of aseptic meningitis

Common

- Enterovirus (including coxsackie and echovirus): summer/fall
- Arbovirus: arthropod borne (West Nile)
- Herpes simplex virus (HSV)-2: Mollaret's

Uncommon

- Mumps
- Human herpesvirus-6: immunocompromised
- Lymphocytic choriomeningitis virus

Rare

- HSV-1, varicella zoster virus, cytomegalovirus, Epstein–Barr virus: immunocompromised
- Influenza A and B
- Parainfluenza
- Measles
- Rotavirus
- Coronavirus
- Parvovirus B19
- HIV: acute seroconversion

Box 16.6 Usual laboratory tests performed for meningitis on a CSF specimen

A total of 8–15 mL of CSF is usually collected and is traditionally sent in four sequentially collected tubes for analysis as follows:

Tube #1   Send for assessment of color and clarity, cell count and differential
Tube #2   Send for glucose, protein
Tube #3   Send for gram stain, culture
Tube #4   Send for cell count and differential

Some CSF should be stored in case some additional testing is subsequently required.

Both the first and the fourth tube are sent for cell count to help determine if there is traumatic or bloody tap. A higher red blood cell count in the first tube than is present in the fourth is said to be suggestive of bleeding from the lumbar puncture and not a subarachnoid hemorrhage. Evidence to support this conjecture id lacking and the only sure evidence of subarachnoid blood is xanthochromia (yellowing of the CSF from hemolyzed red blood cells usually beginning 12 hours after an acute subarachnoid bleed).

also present over weeks, months or even years. The etiologies of subacute meningitis are usually *M. tuberculosis*, syphilis, *Cryptococcus*, and even chronic enteroviral infections.

The physical examination can elucidate clues to a possible etiologic diagnosis and can also help with treatment decisions. Neurologic findings on examination can include cranial nerve palsies (IV, V, VII), focal weakness or hemiparesis, and seizures. The rash in fulminant meningococcemia is often not subtle (Plate 16.2), but when it is found early in a more sparse distribution, prompt administration of antibiotics may have a profound effect on morbidity and mortality.

The diagnosis of meningitis is made by examination of the cerebrospinal fluid (CSF) and this should be obtained promptly. A CT scan of the head to rule out raised intracranial pressure needs to be obtained prior to lumbar puncture (LP) only in patients who have one of the following:
- an immunocompromised state
- an abnormal level of consciousness
- a focal neurologic deficit
- papilledema
- new-onset seizure
- known CNS disease.

Typical studies performed on the CSF are reviewed in Box 16.6. Blood cultures should also be obtained as many patients with bacterial meningitis may be bacteremic. Greater than 5–10 white cells in the CSF is abnormal. In viral meningitis, there

is a CSF pleocytosis with lymphocyte predominance. Early in the course of viral meningitis, there may be a neutrophil predominance, which then shifts to lymphocytes. This happens two-thirds of the time with enterovirus [98]. Elevated protein may be seen in bacterial or viral meningitis, but is often markedly elevated in tuberculous meningitis. A low CSF glucose signifies cerebral anaerobic glycolysis with increased glucose utilization and is often seen in bacterial meningitis. In bacterial meningitis, CSF cultures are positive 80% of the time. However, the likelihood of a positive gram stain varies with the causative organism and will occur in 90% of cases of meningitis caused by *S. pneumoniae*, 86% of cases by *H. influenzae*, 75% of cases by *N. meningitidis*, 50% of cases by gram negatives and 30% of cases by *Listeria*. The yield of culture is 20% lower in cases pretreated with antibiotics but treatment of suspected meningitis should proceed even if LP must be delayed [99]. Expected patterns of cerebrospinal fluid are shown in Table 16.8.

Treatment of viral meningitis usually involves supportive care, as intravenous hydration and pain control. Specific antiviral treatment may be required in viruses such as influenza, HIV or herpes simplex virus (HSV). Treatment of suspected bacterial meningitis requires coverage of organisms such as *S. pneumoniae*, *N. meningitidis*, and *L. monocytogenes* in pregnancy. Third-generation cephalosporins are chosen to

Table 16.8 Cerebrospinal fluid examination: typical CSF findings in bacterial versus aseptic meningitis

CSF parameter	Normal	Bacterial meningitis	Aseptic meningitis
Opening pressure	<180 mmH$_2$O	>180 mm H$_2$O	Normal or slightly elevated
Glucose	Usually one-half to two-thirds of the serum glucose level 2–4 hours earlier	<40 mg/dL (<2.2 mmol/L)	>45 mg/dL (>2.5 mmol/L)
Protein	15–45 mg/dL (0.15–0.45 g/L). Traumatic taps will add 1 mg/dL (0.01 g/L) for every 1000 RBC/mm^3 in the CSF	>50 mg/dL (0.5 g/L)	Normal or elevated
White blood cells	<5 per mm^3 (usually 70% lymphocytes and 30% monocytes). Traumatic taps will add 1 WBC for every 500–1000 RBC/mm^3 in the CSF	>10 to <10,000/mm^3	50–2000/mm^3 (lymphocytes)
Gram stain	Negative	Positive in 70–90% untreated cases	Negative

Reproduced with permission from Seehusen DA, Reeves MM, Fomin DA. Cerebrospinal fluid analysis. Am Fam Physician 2003;68:1103–8.
Note: Normal ranges with different laboratories and assays and values should be interpreted in context of local standardized parameters.

treat *Pneumococcus* and *Neisseria*. There are growing concerns, however, about *S. pneumoniae* resistance patterns in the US and Europe. In 2002, 34% of cases were caused by pneumococci nonsusceptible to at least one drug and 17% were due to a strain nonsusceptible to three or more drugs [96]. Vancomycin, despite its less favorable penetration across the blood–brain barrier, is the drug of choice if there is geographic suspicion for highly resistant strains of *Pneumococcus*. It is often combined with ceftriaxone until antibiotic susceptibilities return as ceftriaxone has far better meningeal penetration. For listeriosis, intravenous ampicillin is used in high doses as *Listeria* is not sensitive to cephalosporins. In cases of allergy, trimethoprim/sulfamethoxazole can be used alone or in combination with chloramphenicol. Although chloramphenicol has been associated with neonatal cardiovascular collapse, known as gray baby syndrome, its use remote from term in this indication is justifiable. Meropenem with vancomyin is another alternative in penicillin-allergic patients. Although meropenem is a carbapenem (which as a class of antibiotic may have some cross-reactivity with penicillin allergies), meropenem's particular structure makes this less likely and its use in patients who have not suffered anaphylaxis from penicillins in the past is probably

Box 16.7 Options for empiric therapy of suspected bacterial meningitis in immunocompetent pregnant women

For penicillin-tolerant patients:
Ceftriaxone 2 g IV every 12 hours +
Vanomycin 500–750 mg IV every 6 hours

For penicillin-allergic patients who did not suffer more than a rash with penicillin exposure:
Meropenem 2 g IV every 8 hours +
Vanomycin 500–750 mg IV every 6 hours

For penicillin-allergic patients who suffered anaphylaxis with prior penicillin exposure and who are not expected to deliver in the near future:
TMP/SMX 15–20 mg/kg/day divided as every 6–8 hours +
Chloramphenicol 50 mg/kg/day divided as every 6 hours

Add dexamethasone (0.15 mg/kg IV every 6 hours for 2–4 days) prior to or concomitantly with the first antibiotic dose in patients with suspected pneumococcal meningitis

justifiable. Box 16.7 provides some options for empiric antibiotic therapy of suspected bacterial meningitis.

Historically, the use of steroids in adults with suspected bacterial meningitis has been inconclusive. However, a prospective, randomized trial in 2002 showed that the use of steroids in meningitis lowered unfavorable outcome and death in the steroid treatment group. The benefits were seen in the subgroup of patients with pneumococcal meningitis[100]. The most recent IDSA guidelines for treating bacterial meningitis therefore recommend use of dexamethasone in adults with suspected or proven pneumococcal meningitis. The dose should be 0.15 mg/kg IV q6h for 2–4 days with the first dose administered 10–20 minutes before, or at least concomitant with, the first dose of antimicrobial therapy [101].

Cellulitis

Cellulitis is a term that refers to an acute, spreading soft tissue infection of the skin involving the subcutaneous tissue. It tends to manifest clinically as rapidly spreading edema, erythema, and warmth. It may involve local inflammation with lymphangitis and regional lymph node swelling. Systemic symptoms are generally mild. Cellulitis can, however, manifest as fever, tachycardia, and leukocytosis. Blood cultures are uncommonly positive and are not generally helpful in management. Needle aspirations and skin biopsies are reserved for complicated cases that are associated with a predisposing risk factor or failure of initial therapy.

The infection tends to occur when the protective skin surface has been disrupted. Predisposing factors include edema and obesity. Injury to the skin may occur in pregnancy in the form of injections, surgery or trauma. Beta-hemolytic streptococci are the most common offending organism. However, other potential organisms and their predisposing factors are listed in Table 16.9.

Treatment can often be provided with oral antibiotics active against streptococci. Reasonable agents in pregnancy include dicloxacillin, cephalexin, clindamycin or erythromycin, unless streptococci or staphylococci resistant to these agents are common in the local community. For pregnant women with evidence of systemic effects or with risk factors for development of more severe sequelae, parenteral therapy may be utilized. Intravenous drug regimens include a penicillinase-resistant penicillin such as nafcillin, a first-generation cephalosporin such as cefazolin or, for patients with life-threatening penicillin allergies, clindamycin or vancomycin [102]. Some reasonable regimens are reviewed in Box 16.8. The literature in nonpregnant populations supports the use of a 5-day course of antibiotics [103]. Extending therapy to a 10-day course may be considered on a case-by-case basis depending on severity of infection at presentation and risk factors.

Methicillin-resistant *Staphylococcus aureus*

The organism known as methicillin-resistant *Staphylococcus aureus* (MRSA) is an emerging pathogen in the world of infectious diseases in pregnancy. MRSA refers to staphylococcal isolates that initially were associated with nosocomial infections but are becoming more prevalent in community settings. The skin and nares serve as sites for colonization for MRSA. The community-acquired form is a growing cause of soft tissue infections and cellulitis in both the pregnant and nonpregnant populations. The hospital-acquired form is seen in women who have been exposed to institutional organisms, such as in the setting of prolonged or frequent hospitalizations or those who have chronic medical manipulations.

The community- and hospital-acquired organisms differ from one another in three important ways. Infections caused by the community-acquired organisms are not typically associated with the usual risk factors for which hospital-acquired MRSA has become known. They may not be related to recent hospitalization or residence in a long-term care facility. They may, however, be seen in outbreak form among sports teams, in prisons or other groups. Second, they tend to be sensitive to nonbeta-lactam antibiotics that can be used orally in pregnancy. These include clindamycin and trimethoprim/sulfamethoxazole. Trimethoprim/sulfamethoxazole is preferred in patients who are able to tolerate sulfa antibiotics. Finally, the community-acquired organisms may be more likely to cause soft tissue infections such as cellulitis because of the specific

Table 16.9 Organisms associated with cellulitis and their predisposing factors

Organism	Predisposing factors
Beta-hemolytic streptococcus Group A	Most common cause of uncomplicated cellulitis
Beta-hemolytic streptococcus Group B	Infections close to anogenital region Often gastrointestinal carriage
Beta-hemolytic streptococcus Groups C or D	Interdigital spaces of lower extremities as a complication of tinea pedis
Staphylococcus aureus	Injection drug use or penetrating trauma
Pasteurella species	Cat or dog bites
Aeromonas hydrophila	Freshwater immersion
Vibrio species	Saltwater exposure
Haemophilus influenzae	Periorbital cellulitis, especially if exposed to nonimmunized children
Pseudomonas aeruginosa	Neutropenia
Helicobacter cinaedi	HIV infection
Cryptococcus neoformans	Compromised cell-mediated immunity
Streptococcus iniae or *E. rhusiopathiae*	Aquaculture or meat-packing jobs

Adapted from the IDSA treatment guidelines [102].

Box 16.8 Options for empiric therapy of cellulitis in immunocompetent pregnant women

For penicillin-tolerant patients:
- PO regimen: dicloxacillin 500 mg PO every 6 hours
- IV regimen: oxacillin 1–2 g IV every 6 hours

For penicillin-allergic patients whose prior reaction to penicillin was a rash only:
- PO regimen: cephalexin 500 mg PO every 6 hours
- IV regimen: cefazolin 1 g every 6 hours

For penicillin-allergic patients whose prior reaction to pencillin was more than just a rash:
- PO regimen: clindamycin 150–300 mg PO every 6 hours or
- IV regimen: clindamycin 600–900 mg IV every 8 hours

If MRSA is suspected:
- PO regimen: TMP/SMX 2 double-strength tablets twice daily or clindamycin 300–450 mg PO every 6–8 hours
- IV regimen: vancomycin 30 mg/kg IV every 24 hours in two equally divided doses

---

virulence genes they often harbor [104]. For severe infections or the more classic form of hospital-acquired MRSA, intravenous vancomycin is the drug of choice in pregnancy [102]. For both types of infection, incision and drainage of lesions can assist in recovery.

Individuals colonized with MRSA serve as a reservoir for transmission in hospital and the community. The nares is a common site for MRSA colonization. A number of measures to eradicate colonization with MRSA are often attempted (including topical nasal muciprocin, chlorhexidine baths and systemic antibiotics such as rifampin with doxycline) but are not supported by well-done clinical trials. At the time of this writing, most experts would support contact precautions in hospital for patients known to be colonized or infected with MRSA. The role of decolonization is likely limited to recurrent infections in one individual or to control acute institutional MRSA outbreaks and even then the efficacy will be limited.

Puerperal infections

Chorio-amnionitis

Chorio-amnionitis is a clinical syndrome of infection of the amniotic cavity during pregnancy. In its classic form, rupture of membranes has occurred and there are typical clinical signs. The criteria commonly used to diagnose chorio-amnionitis are shown in Box 16.9. Overt chorio-amnionitis can occur, however, with intact membranes. Organisms known to cause chorio-amnionitis in the setting of intact membranes include *L. monocytogenes*, *S. agalactiae* and *S. aureus*. Subclinical cases of chorio-amnionitis do occur and can be determined with amniocentesis. The following features on analysis of the amniotic fluid should raise suspicion for subclinical infection:

- >30 WBC/mm^3
- glucose concentration <15 mg/dL
- positive (≥1+) leukocyte esterase on dipstick
- bacteria on gram stain.

The presence of organisms on gram stain is the most specific of these markers. Bacterial growth on culture of the amniotic fluid remains the definitive test.

The microbiology of chorio-amnionitis is often polymicrobial. *Mycoplasma* species are commonly found. In addition, group B *Streptococcus*, gram negatives, and anaerobes are frequently grown [105]. In labor, these can be isolated by culture with collection through an intrauterine pressure catheter. Several risk factors have been shown to predispose women to the development of chorio-amnionitis. These include the presence of an intrauterine pressure catheter, internal fetal monitors, prolonged membrane rupture, multiple digital examinations, and nulliparity [106].

Chorio-amnionitis is associated with many adverse pregnancy outcomes, including increased neonatal sepsis, morbidity, and mortality [107]. It is associated with more than a threefold risk of cerebral palsy in term and near-term infants [108]. It is also known to increase a woman's risk of labor abnormalities, the need for a cesarean delivery, uterine atony, postpartum hemorrhage and postpartum endometritis [109]. Intrapartum therapy with intravenous antibiotics has been shown to decrease maternal morbidity and neonatal sepsis. Chorio-amnionitis is an indication for induction or augmentation of labor but cesarean delivery should be reserved for the usual obstetric indications and not the presence of chorio-amnionitis in itself [109–111]. Several antibiotic regimens have been shown to be effective, but a commonly used therapy in the above-noted studies for chorio-amnionitis is a dual antibiotic regimen including ampicillin and gentamicin [109,110]. Some other possible regimens are reviewed in Box 16.10.

Postpartum endometritis

Any sustained fever following delivery requires thorough evaluation. Potential causes of postpartum fever include postpartum

---

Box 16.9 Diagnosis of clinical chorio-amnionitis

Fever greater than 38°C and at least two of the following:

- Maternal leukocytosis >15,000 cells/mm^3
- Maternal tachycardia greater than 100 beats/minute
- Fetal tachycardia greater than 160 beats/minute
- Uterine tenderness
- Foul-smelling amniotic fluid

Box 16.10 Options for empiric therapy of chorio-amnionitis in immunocompetent pregnant women

For penicillin-tolerant patients:
- Ampicillin 2 g IV every 6 hours + gentamicin 1.5 mg/kg every 8 hours +/- clindamycin 900 mg every 8 hours
- Ampicillin-sulbactam 3 g IV every 6 hours
- Ticarcillin-clavulanate 3.1 g IV every 4 hours

For penicillin-allergic patients whose prior reaction to penicillin was a rash only:
- Cefuroxime 1.5 g IV every 8 hours
- Cefoxitin 2 g IV every 8 hours + gentamicin 1.5 mg/kg every 8 hours

For penicillin-allergic patients whose prior reaction to pencillin was more than just a rash:
- Clindamycin 900 mg IV every 8 hours + gentamicin 1.5 mg/kg every 8 hours
- Vancomycin + gentamicin 1.5 mg/kg every 8 hours

endometritis, mastitis, respiratory or urinary tract infection and venous thromboembolism. The incidence of postpartum endometritis is about 5% after a vaginal delivery and 10% after a cesarean [112]. Postpartum fever rarely proceeds to sepsis. However, it is mandatory that it is always regarded seriously, and fully investigated and treated because of the potentially disastrous consequences.

Classic puerperal sepsis (i.e. generalized systemic infection with *Streptococcus pyogenes* – group A streptococci (GAS) is unusual, but does still occur. The source of the organism can be either endogenous, from a carrier site in the patient, or exogenous, from procedures or attendants. GAS is found in the vagina of approximately 0.03% of women [113]. Outbreaks and isolated cases of puerperal sepsis associated with GAS still occur from time to time; hence the importance of maintaining careful aseptic technique in the delivery room.

Symptoms of GAS endometrial infection are severe. The patient is critically ill, with all the hallmarks of uncontrolled septicemia, including abdominal pain, fever, and hypotension. The lochia may or may not be malodorous, nor will it necessarily be obvious. Indeed, if a pyometra (the uterus full of inspissated purulent material) has developed, the clinician may be lulled into a false sense of security by the absence of significant discharge. This condition is an obstetric emergency, and rapid intervention with full resuscitation measures, appropriate antibiotics and serious consideration of emergency hysterectomy are necessary to avoid the high mortality of this condition [114].

The more common form of postpartum infection seen today is acute endometritis (infection of the uterus). This is usually an ascending infection from the patient's genital tract, and is characteristically a mixed infection of gram-negative and anaerobic organisms. Risk factors include prolonged labor, prolonged rupture of membranes, intrauterine fetal monitors, multiple vaginal examinations, chorio-amnionitis and cesarean section. Among women undergoing cesarean section, antibiotic prophylaxis with either a first-generation cephalosporin or ampicillin reduces the risk of postpartum endometritis and should be provided prior to making the incision.

Symptoms are similar to those seen with chorio-amnionitis. Fever and fundal tenderness are considered adequate signs to make the diagnosis of endometritis in the postpartum period. However, other sources of infection must be eliminated from the differential diagnosis. One must consider wound infection, pneumonia, pyelonephritis, and mastitis in particular. Consideration should also be given to noninfectious causes of pyrexia, including venous thromboembolism. Supporting evidence of endometritis includes abdominal pain and foul-smelling lochia.

Antimicrobial therapy must be started early. Intravenous clindamycin and once-daily gentamicin should be prescribed. This regimen has been shown to be superior to several other regimens in clinical trials with fewer treatment failures [115]. Once-daily dosing of aminoglycosides is associated with fewer treatment failures as well. Several other regimens, reviewed in Box 16.11, are reasonable, however, if women are unable to tolerate either of these drugs. Once uncomplicated endometritis has resolved with intravenous antibiotic therapy, there is no role for continued oral therapy [115].

Fevers that persist despite adequate treatment of what was clinically felt to be endometritis should prompt a careful review of the patient's history, a review of systems, her medication history and a careful physical examination. Patients should have blood cultures, urine cultures and consideration of a chest X-ray. Gentamicin levels (if this medication is being used) should be obtained. Consider whether an ultrasound to look for retained products of conception is advisable. If no explanation for the persistent fever is seen, addition of ampicillin or vancomycin to the antibiotic regimen should be considered to cover enterococci. Imaging of the pelvis by computed tomography (CT) or magnetic resonance imaging (MRI) may also be appropriate to look for septic thrombophlebitis in the ovarian or deep pelvic veins.

Tradition has entrenched the practice of giving short-course anticoagulation (until the patient is afebrile for 48 hours) in cases of unexplained persistent postpartum fever. However, the authors and editors remain skeptical about this practice as we see little evidence beyond the anecdotal to support it. If deep venous thrombosis is seen on imaging, it is our practice to treat for 3 months with anticoagulants as would be done

---

Box 16.11 Options for empiric therapy of endometritis in immunocompetent pregnant women

For penicillin-tolerant patients:
- Ampicillin-sulbactam 3 g IV every 6 hours
- Ticarcillin-clavulanate 3.1 g IV every 4 hours

For penicillin-allergic patients whose prior reaction to penicillin was a rash only:
- Cefoxitin 2 g IV every 8 hours

For penicillin-allergic patients whose prior reaction to penicillin was more than just a rash:
- Metronidazole 500 mg every 8 hours + gentamicin 5 mg/kg every 24 hours
- Clindamycin 900 mg every 8 hours + gentamicin 5 mg/kg every 24 hours

The final regimen may be preferable for all patients regardless of penicillin allergy.
Antibiotics should be stopped once the patient is afebrile for 24–48 hours. Ampicillin may be added to this regimen for refractory cases.

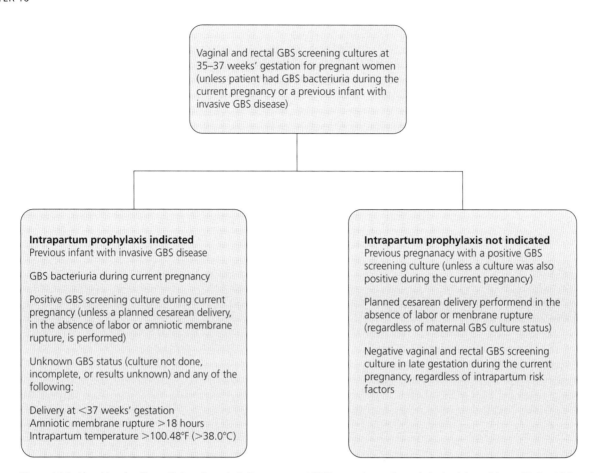

Figure 16.3 Algorithm for Group B, beta-hemolytic *Steptococcus* (GBS) screening and prophylaxis. Adapted from CDC guidelines [122].

for any other deep vein thrombosis [116]. If no thrombosis is seen it is our practice to continue to look for alternative explanations for the fever (including drug fever) while adding ampicillin or vancomycin to our antibiotic regimen for endometritis.

Group B, beta-hemolytic *Streptococcus*

Group B, beta-hemolytic *Streptococcus* (GBS) (*Streptococcus agalactiae*) is a common vaginal commensal. The prevalence varies in different reports but is generally quoted as within the range 10–30% [117]. The gastrointestinal tract is the natural reservoir for GBS. Carriage may occur in one or more of vagina, rectum and perineal skin. Furthermore, it is well established that carriage is intermittent. Thus, it is impossible to exclude carriage of the organism on a single examination. Carriage of GBS in the vagina *per se* is not usually associated with symptoms, and the presence of the organism is not an indication to treat with antibiotic therapy.

Group B *Streptococcus* is a pathogen that has had a major impact on the health and well-being of mothers and infants. It has been recognized as a leading infectious cause of infant

morbidity and mortality since the 1970s [118–121]. As a result, a massive effort to decrease the incidence of early-onset GBS disease in infants prompted the CDC to recommend a screening strategy for all pregnant women in order to provide intrapartum antibiotic prophylaxis to colonized women [122] (Figure 16.3).

Guidelines set by the CDC to identify and prevent infections from GBS using antibiotic prophylaxis have decreased the rates of GBS infection among infants [122] (Box 16.12). The two approaches of prevention are a screening-based approach, which is the preferred method, and a risk-based approach. Screening includes culturing a vaginal/rectal swab for women at 35–37 weeks gestation. Those found to have colonization are then given antibiotics before delivery. The risk-based approach includes assessing the patients for risk factors such as fever, preterm delivery, and prolonged rupture of membranes at the onset of labor and then administering antibiotics to those at risk. The screening approach has been shown to be superior to the risk-based approach in preventing neonatal sepsis [123].

Two forms of neonatal GBS infection are recognized. The early-onset form occurs within 48 hours of delivery, and is

Box 16.12 Recommended antibiotic regimens for GBS prophylaxis

• Recommended	Penicillin G, 5 million units IV initial dose, then 2.5 million units IV every 4 hours until delivery
• Alternative	Ampicillin, 2 g IV initial dose, then 1 g IV every 4 hours until delivery
• If penicillin allergic	Clindamycin and erythromycin susceptibility testing should be performed on prenatal GBS isolates from penicillin-allergic women at high risk for anaphylaxis
• Patients not at high risk for anaphylaxis	Cefazolin, 2 g IV initial dose, then 1 g IV every 8 hours until delivery
• Patients at high risk for anaphylaxis	
• GBS susceptible to clindamycin	Clindamycin 900 mg IV every 8 hours until delivery
• GBS susceptible to erythromycin	Erythromycin 500 mg IV every 6 hours until delivery
• GBS resistant to clindamycin or erythromycin or susceptibility unknown	Vancomycin 1g IV every 12 hours until delivery

Adapted from CDC guidelines 2002 [122].

characterized by rapid onset of bacteremic shock, and respiratory distress with or without meningitis. The mortality is high. This is the form of sepsis that can be largely prevented by maternal administration of antibiotics. Late-onset disease is less likely to be bacteremic, and more likely to be meningitic. The onset is more insidious and the prognosis generally better, providing diagnosis and treatment are prompt. Late-onset disease is not associated with maternal carriage or prematurity. Nosocomial infection is most likely.

Group B *Streptococcus* infection in adults is well recognized. In the postpartum woman, endometritis is the most likely manifestation, and is more common in women delivered by cesarean section. In most cases, onset of fever and fundal tenderness occurs within 48 hours of delivery. Treatment is with a penicillin, to which the organism is susceptible. Later complications such as pelvic abscess and septic shock are rare.

Obstetric anesthesia concerns related to thermoregulation and infection in pregnancy

Thermoregulatory disturbances associated with neuraxial and general anesthesia

There are five major temperature-related issues associated with labor and delivery:
• hypothermia resulting from impaired thermoregulatory control during general anesthesia
• hypothermia resulting from impaired thermoregulatory control during neuraxial anesthesia
• shivering during neuraxial anesthesia
• hyperthermia associated with prolonged epidural analgesia
• the implications of infections for anesthetic management.

Hypothermia during general anesthesia

Body temperature is normally tightly regulated. Regulation can be divided into behavioral and autonomic components. Behavioral thermoregulatory control is manifested by thermal sensation that provokes protective actions including ambient temperature modulation (i.e. air conditioning) and use of thermal insulation (i.e. putting on a sweater). The most important autonomic thermoregulatory defenses in humans are sweating, arteriovenous shunt constriction, and shivering. Each is characterized by its *threshold* (the triggering core temperature) and maximum response intensity. The sweating and vasoconstriction thresholds usually differ by only a few tenths of a degree Celsius (°C) [124], temperatures that define the *interthreshold range*.

All general anesthetics profoundly impair thermoregulatory control [125,126]. Impairment has a characteristic pattern: the sweating threshold increases only slightly, but the vasoconstriction and shivering thresholds synchronously decrease 2–3°C. Consequently, the interthreshold range increases to 3–4°C. Thermoregulatory control during general anesthesia is thus 10–20 times less precise than usual. Poor thermoregulatory control, combined with exposure to a cool operating environment, makes nearly all unwarmed surgical patients hypothermic.

Perioperative hypothermia is of considerable concern since large randomized trials have shown that reductions in core temperature of only a couple of °C markedly worsen outcomes. For example, mild hypothermia triples the risk of morbid myocardial outcomes [127], triples the risk of surgical wound infection [128], significantly increases blood loss and allogenic transfusion requirements [129], prolongs postoperative recovery [130], and lengthens the duration of hospitalization [128].

Women having general anesthesia for cesarean delivery or other obstetric procedures should thus be actively warmed to prevent hypothermia. Fortunately, inexpensive and safe warmers are available. The best combination of safety, efficacy, and ease of use probably is forced-air warming [131].

Hypothermia during neuraxial anesthesia

Epidural [132,133] and spinal [133,134] anesthesia each decrease the thresholds triggering vasoconstriction and shivering (above the level of the block) about 0.6°C (Figure 16.4). Although the magnitude is less, the pattern of impairment is thus similar to that observed with general anesthetics and opioids, suggesting that an alteration in central rather than peripheral control seems most likely. The mechanism by which peripheral administration of local anesthesia impairs centrally mediated thermoregulation remains unknown, but is proportional to the number of spinal segments blocked [135].

Since neuraxial anesthesia prevents vasoconstriction and shivering in blocked regions, it is unsurprising that epidural anesthesia decreases the maximum intensity of shivering. However, epidural anesthesia also reduces the gain

of shivering which suggests that the regulatory system is unable to compensate for lower body paralysis [136]. Sedative and analgesic medications all impair thermoregulatory control to some extent [137–140].

Interestingly, core hypothermia during regional anesthesia may not trigger a perception of cold [132,141]. The reason is that thermal perception (behavioral regulation) is largely determined by skin rather than core temperature [142]. During regional anesthesia, core hypothermia is accompanied by a real increase in skin temperature. The paradoxic result is often a perception of continued or increased warmth, accompanied by autonomic thermoregulatory responses including shivering [132,141].

Taken together, these data indicate that neuraxial anesthesia inhibits numerous aspects of thermoregulatory control. The vasoconstriction and shivering thresholds are reduced by regional anesthesia [132–135,143], and further reduced by adjuvant drugs [137,138] and advanced age [144]. Even once triggered, the gain and maximum response intensity of shivering are about half normal [145]. Finally, behavioral thermoregulation is impaired [141]. The result is that cold defenses are triggered at a lower temperature than normal during regional anesthesia, defenses are less effective once triggered, and patients frequently do not recognize that they are hypothermic. Because core temperature monitoring remains rare during regional anesthesia [146], substantial hypothermia often goes undetected in these patients [147].

Shivering during neuraxial anesthesia

Shivering-like tremor is common during neuraxial anesthesia and has at least four potential etiologies:
• normal thermoregulatory shivering in response to core hypothermia
• normal shivering in normothermic or even hyperthermic patients who are developing a fever
• direct stimulation of cold receptors in the neuraxis by injected local anesthetic
• nonthermoregulatory muscular activity that resembles thermoregulatory shivering.
Most shivering-like activity associated with neuraxial anesthesia, at least most intense muscular activity, appears to be normal shivering, the expected response to hypothermia. However, not all shivering-like tremor is thermoregulatory. It is possible to detect low-intensity shivering-like muscular activity both in surgical patients [148] and during labor [149]. The cause of this muscular activity remains unknown, but it is associated with pain and may thus result from sympathetic nervous system activation [150].

Since skin temperature contributes to control of thermoregulatory responses, shivering of any type can be treated by warming the skin surface [151]. However, the entire skin surface contributes 20% to thermoregulatory control [152,153]

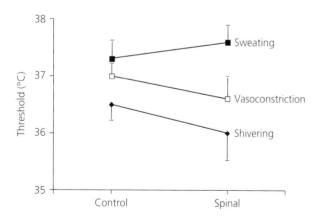

Figure 16.4 Spinal anesthesia increased the sweating threshold but reduced the thresholds for vasoconstriction and shivering. Consequently, the interthreshold range increased substantially. The vasoconstriction-to-shivering range, however, remained normal during spinal anesthesia. Results are presented as means ± SDs. From Kurz *et al.* [134].

and the lower body contributes about 10% [143], so sentient skin warming is only likely to compensate for small reductions in core temperature. As might thus be expected, skin warming is only effective in a fraction of patients. Most often, pharmacologic treatments will be required for moderate or severe shivering. Effective drugs include meperidine (25 mg IV) [154], clonidine (75 µg IV) [155], ketanserin (10 mg IV) [155], and magnesium sulfate (30 mg/kg IV) [156].

Hyperthermia during prolonged epidural anesthesia

Hyperthermia is a generic term that simply refers to elevated core body temperature (i.e. >38°C). Hyperthermia can be passive, from excessive heating or inadequate dissipation of heat to the environment. It can also result from excessive heat production, as occurs with heat stroke or malignant hyperthermia. And finally, hyperthermia can be febrile. Fever differs from the other causes of elevated body temperature in being a regulated increase mediated by endogenous pyrogens. It can be infectious, inflammatory or central in origin.

Prolonged epidural analgesia for labor and delivery is occasionally associated with hyperthermia, typically to 38.5–39.5°C. Hyperthermia develops only in a subset of women [157]. It typically develops after at least 5 hours of labor, and then increases over time [158–161]. The clinical consequence of this hyperthermia is that women given epidural analgesia for labor are more often given antibiotics than those treated conventionally, and their offspring are more commonly treated for sepsis [159,162,163]. Hyperthermia during epidural analgesia is not restricted to labor and thus must have a more general etiology.

There are several potential explanations for hyperthermia during labor analgesia. For example, it could simply be passive hyperthermia resulting from excessive heat production and inadequate heat dissipation to the environment. Similarly, a dense epidural block would inhibit sweating which might contribute to hyperthermia. However, neither mechanism seems likely. Hyperthermia during labor could also simply be a normal febrile response to infection. "Fever work-ups" and antibiotic treatments are common responses to maternal hyperthermia, and some hyperthermia surely is infectious fever [164]. Nonetheless, typical epidural-associated hyperthermia seems unlikely to result from infection and the current consensus is that infection is rarely the cause.

Inflammation is a different matter, however. There are many potential sources of noninfectious inflammation in laboring patients, to say nothing of postoperative patients who obviously have injured tissues [165]. It seems likely that inflammation provokes a regulated febrile response during labor (and in postoperative patients). Consistent with this theory, high-dose steroids (powerful anti-inflammatory drugs) nearly eliminate fever during labor [166]. In contrast, acetaminophen did not prevent hyperthermia, although the drug is usually an effective antipyretic [167]. That prolonged labor is associated with a greater risk of hyperthermia is consistent with a longer period in which to develop inflammation, especially placental inflammation which is likely to release a variety of pyrogenic cytokines. And of course, longer labor is associated with factors that promote inflammation [168].

The difficulty is that epidural analgesia surely does not augment the general inflammatory response to labor or surgery. Nor does it increase the risk of fetal malposition or need for cesarean delivery [169]. It therefore remains unclear why epidural analgesia augments the risk of hyperthermia during labor and in postoperative patients. The conventional assumption is that hyperthermia is somehow caused by the technique although no even slightly convincing mechanism has been proposed.

It is worth remembering, however, that when hyperthermia during labor is studied, pain in the "control" patients is usually treated with opioids, which themselves blunt thermoregulatory defenses [138,139] and specifically attenuate fever [170]. Fever associated with infection or tissue injury might then be suppressed by low doses of opioids that are usually given to the "control" patients while being expressed normally in patients given epidural analgesia [171]. The extent to which this mechanism contributes remains to be determined, and the theory is controversial [172]. However, no convincing alternative explanation has been advanced.

Infections and anesthetic management

Thermal perturbations *per se* have little effect on anesthetic management. In other words, anesthetics remain safe and effective in hypothermic and hyperthermic patients. Infections, though, are an issue. But to the extent that hyperthermia results from infectious fever, it needs to be considered. This is especially the case for neuraxial anesthesia which theoretically augments the risk of meningitis because spinal and epidural anesthesia requires penetration of the dura and arachnoid membranes. The extent (if any) to which neuraxial anesthesia actually increases risk of central infection remains speculative. Nonetheless, there is a consensus that patients with putative bacterial infections should first be treated with antibiotics. For the same reason, neuraxial anesthesia is avoided in patients with infectious cutaneous lesions at needle insertion sites.

References

1. Petrucco OM, Seamark RF, Holmes K, *et al*. Changes in lymphocyte function during pregnancy. Br J Obstet Gynaecol 1976;83:245–50.
2. Vaquer S, de la Hera A, Jorda J, *et al*. Diminished natural killer activity in pregnancy: modulation by interleukin 2 and interferon gamma. Scand J Immunol 1987;26(6):691–8.
3. Gehrz RC, Christianson WR, Linner KM, *et al*. A longitudinal analysis of lymphocyte proliferative responses to mitogens

and antigens during human pregnancy. Am J Obstet Gynecol 1981;140:665–70.

4. Aagard-Tillery KA. Immunology of normal pregnancy. Semin Fetal Neonat Med 2006;11:279–95.

5. Goetzl L, Zighelboim I, Badell M, et al. Maternal corticosteroids to prevent intrauterine exposure to hyperthermia and inflammation: a randomized, double-blind, placebo-controlled trial. Am J Obstet Gynecol 2006;195:1031–7.

6. Goetzl L, Rivers J, Evans T, et al. Prophylactic acetaminophen does not prevent epidural fever in nulliparous women: a double-blind placebo-controlled trial. J Perinatol 2004;24:471–5.

7. Macsween KF, Ridgway GL. The laboratory investigation of vaginal discharge. J Clin Pathol 1998;51:564–7.

8. Sobel JD. Vaginitis. N Engl J Med 1997;337:1896–902.

9. Taylor-Robinson D, McCormack WM. The genital mycoplasmas I. N Engl J Med 1980;302:1003–10.

10. Taylor-Robinson D, McCormack WM. The genital mycoplasmas II. N Engl J Med 1980;302:1063–7.

11. Amsel R, Totten PA. Non-specific vaginitis. Diagnostic criteria and microbiologic and epidemiologic associations. Am J Med 1983;74:14–22.

12. Gravett MG, Hummel D. Preterm labour associated with sub-clinical amniotic fluid infection and with bacterial vaginosis. Obstet Gynecol 1986;67:229–37.

13. Hay PE, Lamont RF. Abnormal bacterial colonisation of the genital tract and subsequent pre-term delivery and late miscarriage. BMJ 1994;308:295–8.

14. Hillier SL, Nugent RP, Eschenbach DA, et al. Association between bacterial vaginosis and preterm delivery of a low-birth-weight infant. N Engl J Med 1995;333:1737–42.

15. Royce RA, Thorp JM, Granados JL, et al. Bacterial vaginosis associated with HIV infection in pregnant women from North Carolina. J Acquir Immune Defic Syndr Hum Retrovirol 1999;20:382–6.

16. Hauth JC, Goldenberg RL, Andrews WW, et al. Reduced incidence of preterm delivery with metronidazole and erythromycin in women with bacterial vaginosis. N Engl J Med 1995;333:1732–6.

17. McDonald H, O'Loughlin J, Vigneswaran R, et al. Impact of metronidazole therapy on preterm birth in women with bacterial vaginosis flora (Gardnerella vaginalis): a randomised, placebo controlled trial. Br J Obstet Gynaecol 1997;104:1391–7.

18. Morales W, Schorr S, Albritton J. Effect of metronidazole in patients with preterm birth in preceding pregnancy and bacterial vaginosis: a placebo-controlled, double-blind study. Am J Obstet Gynecol 1994;171:345–7.

19. Carey JC, Klebanoff MA, Hauth JC, et al. Metronidazole to prevent preterm delivery in pregnant women with asymptomatic bacterial vaginosis. N Engl J Med 2000;342:534–40.

20. Krieger JN, Tam MR, Stevens CE, et al. Diagnosis of trichomoniasis: comparison of conventional wet-mount examination with cytologic studies, cultures, and monoclonal antibody staining of direct specimens. JAMA 1988;259:1223–7.

21. van der Schee C, van Belkum A, Zwijgers L, et al. Improved diagnosis of T. vaginalis infection by PCR using vaginal swabs and urine specimens compared to diagnosis by wet mount microscopy, culture, and fluorescent staining. J Clin Microbiol 1999;37:4127–30.

22. Ohlemeyer CL, Hornberger LL, Lynch DA, et al. Diagnosis of T. vaginalis in adolescent females: inpouch TV culture versus wet-mount microscopy. J Adolesc Health 1998;22:205–8.

23. Patel SR, Wiese W, Patel SC, et al. Systematic review of diagnostic tests for vaginal trichomoniasis. Infect Dis Obstet Gynecol 2000;8:248–57.

24. Grice A. Vaginal infection causing spontaneous rupture of the membranes and premature delivery. Aust NZ J Obstet Gynaecol 1974;14(1):56–8.

25. Minkoff H, Grunebaum AN, Schwarz RH, et al. Risk factors for prematurity and premature rupture of membranes: a prospective study of the vaginal flora in pregnancy. Am J Obstet Gynecol 1984;150:965–72.

26. Laga M, Manoka A, Kivuvu M, et al. Non-ulcerative sexually transmitted diseases as risk factors for HIV-1 transmission in women: results from a cohort study. AIDS 1993;7:95–102.

27. Cotch MF, Pastorek JG, Nugent RP, et al. Trichomonas vaginalis associated with low birth weight and preterm delivery. The Vaginal Infections and Prematurity Study Group. Sex Transm Dis 1997;24(6):353–60.

28. Klebanoff MA, Carey JC, Hauth JC, et al. Failure of metronidazole to prevent preterm delivery among pregnant women with asymptomatic Trichomonas vaginalis infection. N Engl J Med 2001;345(7):487–93.

29. Sobel JD. Candida vulvo-vaginitis. Clin Obstet Gynecol 1993; 36:153–66.

30. Cotch MF, Hillier SL, Gibbs RS, et al. Epidemiology and outcomes associated with moderate to heavy Candida colonization during pregnancy. Vaginal Infections and Prematurity Study Group. Am J Obstet Gynecol 1998;178(2):374–80.

31. Infertility Prevention Project; Office of Population Affairs; Local and State STD Control Programs; Centers for Disease Control and Prevention, Atlanta, GA, 2005.

32. Amstey MS, Steadman KT. Asymptomatic gonorrhea and pregnancy. J Am Vener Dis Assoc 1976;3(1):14–16.

33. Edwards LE, Barrada MI, Hamann AA, et al. Gonorrhea in pregnancy. Am J Obstet Gynecol 1978;132:637–41.

34. Centers for Disease Control and Prevention. Sexually transmitted diseases treatment guidelines 2006. MMWR 2006;55 (No. RR-11):35–54.

35. Centers for Disease Control and Prevention. Sexually transmitted disease surveillance 2005. Supplement, Chlamydia Prevalence Monitoring Project Annual Report 2005. US Department of Health and Human Services, Centers for Disease Control and Prevention, Atlanta, GA, 2006.

36. Gravett MG, Nelson HP, DeRouen T, et al. Independent associations of bacterial vaginosis and Chlamydia trachomatis infection with adverse pregnancy outcome. JAMA 1986;256: 1899–903.

37. Martin DH, Koutsky L, Eschenbach DA, et al. Prematurity and perinatal mortality in pregnancies complicated by maternal Chlamydia trachomatis infections. JAMA 1982;247:1585–8.

38. Sweet RL, Landers DV, Walker C, et al. Chlamydia trachomatis infection and pregnancy outcome. Am J Obstet Gynecol 1987; 156(4):824–33.

39. Gencay M, Koskinieme M. Chlamydia trachomatis seropositivity during pregnancy is associated with perinatal complications. Clin Infect Dis 1995;21:424–6.

40. Bell TA, Stamm WE. Delayed appearance of Chlamydia trachomatis infections acquired at birth. Pediatr Infect Dis 1987;6: 928–31.

41. Weiss SG, Newcomb RW, Beem MO. Pulmonary assessment of children after chlamydial pneumonia of infancy. J Pediatr 1986;108:659–64.

42. Davies PO, Ridgway GL. The role of polymerase chain reaction and ligase chain reaction for the detection of Chlamydia trachomatis. Int J STD AIDS 1997;8:731–8.

43. Clinical Effectiveness Group. National guidelines for the management of Chlamydia trachomatis genital tract infection. Sex Transm Infect 1999;75(suppl 1):S4–33.

44. Eschenbach DA, Nugent RP, Rao AV, et al. A randomized placebo-controlled trial of erythromycin for the treatment of Ureaplasma urealyticum to prevent premature delivery. The Vaginal Infections and Prematurity Study Group. Am J Obstet Gynecol 1991;164(3):734–42.

45. Germain M, Krohn MA, Hillier SL, et al. Genital flora in pregnancy and its association with intrauterine growth retardation. J Clin Microbiol 1994;32:2162–8.

46. Krohn MA, Hillier SL, Nugent RP, et al. The genital flora of women with intraamniotic infection. Vaginal Infection and Prematurity Study Group. J Infect Dis 1995;171:1475–80.

47. Centers for Disease Control and Prevention. Sexually transmitted disease surveillance 2005. US Department of Health and Human Services, Centers for Disease Control and Prevention, Atlanta, GA, 2006.

48. Hashisaki P, Wertzberger GG, Conrad GL, et al. Erythromycin failure in the treatment of syphilis in a pregnant woman. Sex Transm Dis 1983;10:36–8.

49. Ziaya PR, Hankins GD, Gilstrap LC 3rd, et al. Intravenous penicillin desensitization and treatment during pregnancy. JAMA 1986;256:2561–2.

50. Wendel GD Jr, Stark BJ, Jamison RB, et al. Penicillin allergy and desensitization in serious infections during pregnancy. N Engl J Med 1985;312:1229–32.

51. Lorber B. Listeriosis. Clin Infect Dis 1997;24:1–11.

52. Southwick FS, Purich DL. Intracellular Pathogenesis of Listeriosis. N Engl J Med 1996;334(12):770–6.

53. Bortolussi R, McGregor DD, Kongshavn PA, et al. Host defense mechanisms to perinatal and neonatal Listeria monocytogenes infection. Surv Synth Pathol Res 1984;3:311–32.

54. Mylonakis E, Paliou M, Hohmann EL, et al. Listeriosis during pregnancy: a case series and review of 222 cases. Medicine (Baltimore) 2002;81:260–9.

55. Ridgway GL. Bacterial Infections. In: Chamberlain G (ed) Modern antenatal care of the foetus. Blackwell Scientific Publications, Oxford, 1990:221–3.

56. Schuchat A, Zywicki SS, Dinsmoor MJ, et al. Risk factors and opportunities for prevention of early-onset neonatal sepsis: a multicenter case-control study. Pediatrics 2000;105:21–6.

57. Dubey JP. A review of toxoplasmosis in pigs. Vet Parasitol 1986;19:181–223.

58. Jones JL, Kruszon-Moran D, Wilson M, et al. Toxoplasma gondii infection in the United States: seroprevalence and risk factors. Am J Epidemiol 2001;154:357–65.

59. Cook AJC, Gilbert RE, Buffolano W, et al. Sources of toxoplasma infection in pregnant women: European multicentre case-control study. Commentary: gongenital toxoplasmosis – further thought for food. BMJ 2000;321:142–7.

60. Jenum PA, Stray-Pedersen B, Melby KK, et al. Incidence of Toxoplasma gondii infection in 35,940 pregnant women in Norway and pregnancy outcome for infected women. J Clin Microbiol 1998;36:2900–6.

61. Holliman RE. Congenital toxoplasmosis: prevention, screening and treatment. J Hosp Infect 1995;30(suppl 1):179–90.

62. Jones JL, Lopez A, Wilson M, et al. Congenital toxoplasmosis: a review. Obstet Gynecol Surv 2001;56(5):296–305.

63. Liesenfeld O, Montoya JG, Tathineni NJ, et al. Confirmatory serologic testing for acute toxoplasmosis and rate of induced abortions among women reported to have positive Toxoplasma immunoglobulin M antibody titers. Am J Obstet Gynecol 2001;184(2):140–5.

64. Hohlfeld P, MacAleese J, Capella-Pavlovski M, et al. Fetal toxoplasmosis: ultrasonographic signs. Ultrasound Obstet Gynecol 1991;1(4):241–4.

65. SYROCOT Study Group. Effectiveness of prenatal treatment for congenital toxoplasmosis: a meta-analysis of individual patients' data. Lancet 2007;369:115–22.

66. Bray RS, Anderson MJ. Falciparum malaria and pregnancy. Trans R Soc Trop Med Hyg 1979;73(4):427–31.

67. Gilles HM, Lawson JB, Sibelas M, et al. Malaria, anaemia and pregnancy. Ann Trop Med Parasitol 1969;63(2):245–63.

68. Rasheed FN, Bulmer JN, Dunn DT, et al. Suppressed peripheral and placental blood lymphoproliferative responses in first pregnancies: relevance to malaria. Am J Trop Med Hyg 1993;48(2):154–60.

69. Vleugels MPH, Eling WMC, Rolland R, et al. Cortisol and loss of malaria immunity in human pregnancy. Br J Obstet Gynaecol 1987;94:758–64.

70. Fried M, Duffy PE. Adherence of Plasmodium falciparum to chondroitin sulfate A in the human placenta. Science 1996;272(5267):1502–4.

71. Jelliffe EEP. Placental malaria and foetal growth failure. In: Avsen RN (ed) Nutrition and Infection CIBA Foundation Study Group. Churchill, London, 1967.

72. Trusell RR, Beeley L. Infestations. In: Clinics in obstetrics and gynaecology: prescribing in pregnancy. WB Saunders, London, 1981:333–40.

73. No authors listed. Malaria in pregnancy. Lancet 1983; 322(8341):84–5.

74. Wolfe MS, Cordero JF. Safety of chloroquine in chemosuppression of malaria during pregnancy. BMJ (Clin Res Ed) 1985;290:1466–7.

75. Heinonen CP, Slone D, Shapiro S. Birth defects and drugs in pregnancy. Publishing Sciences Group, Littleton, MA, 1977.

76. Looareesuwan S, White NJ, Karbwang J, et al. Quinine and severe falciparum malaria in late pregnancy. Lancet 1985;326:4–8.

77. White NJ, Warrell DA, Chanthavanich P, et al. Severe hypoglycemia and hyperinsulinemia in falciparum malaria. N Engl J Med 1983;309:61–6.

78. Phillips RE, Warrell DA, Looareesuwan S, et al. Effectiveness of SMS 201–995, a synthetic, long-acting somatostatin analogue, in treatment of quinine-induced hyperinsulinaemia. Lancet 1986; 1:713–16.

79. Treatment of malaria (guidelines for clinicians), 2007. Accessed at www.cdc.gov/malaria/ diagnosis_treatment/clinicians2.htm.

80. Nosten F, Vincenti M, Simpson J, et al. The effects of mefloquine treatment in pregnancy. Clin Infect Dis 1999;28(4):808–15.

81. Steketee RW, Wirima JJ, Slutsker WL, et al. Objectives and methodology in a study of malaria treatment and prevention in pregnancy in rural Malawi: the Mangochi Malaria Research Project. Am J Trop Med Hyg 1996;55(1 suppl):8–16.

82. Centers for Disease Control and Prevention. Health information for international travel 2005–2006. US Department of Health and Human Services, Public Health Service, Atlanta, GA, 2005.

83. Centers for Disease Control and Prevention. Reported cases of Lyme disease by year, United States, 1991–2005. Accessed at www.cdc.gov/ncidod/dvbid/lyme/ld_UpClimbLymeDis.htm.

84. Lindgren E, Jaenson TGT. Lyme borreliosis in Europe: influences of climate and climate change, epidemiology, ecology and adaptation measures. World Health Organization, Copenhagen, 2006.

85. Wormser GP, Dattwyler RJ, Shapiro ED, et al. The Clinical assessment, treatment, and prevention of Lyme disease, human granulocytic anaplasmosis, and babesiosis: clinical practice guidelines by the Infectious Diseases Society of America. Clin Infect Dis 2006;43:1089–1134.

86. MacDonald AB, Benach JL, Burgdorfer W, et al. Stillbirth following maternal Lyme disease. NY State J Med 1987;87:615–16.

87. Schlesinger PA, Duray PH, Burke BA, et al. Maternal-fetal transmission of the Lyme disease spirochete, Borrelia burgdorferi. Ann Intern Med 1985;103:67–8.

88. Shirts SR, Brown MS, Bobitt JR, et al. Listeriosis and borreliosis as causes of antepartum fever. Obstet Gynecol 1983; 62(2):256–61.

89. Weber K, Bratzke HJ, Neubert U, et al. Borrelia burgdorferi in a newborn despite oral penicillin for Lyme borreliosis during pregnancy. Pediatr Infect Dis J 1988;7:286–9.

90. Markowitz LE, Steere AC, Benach JL, et al. Lyme disease during pregnancy. JAMA 1986;255:3394–6.

91. Strobino BA, Williams CL, Abid S, et al. Lyme disease and pregnancy outcome: a prospective study of two thousand prenatal patients. Am J Obstet Gynecol 1993;169:367–74.

92. Maraspin V, Cimperman J, Lotric-Furlan S, et al. Treatment of erythema migrans in pregnancy. Clin Infect Dis 1996;22: 788–93.

93. Strobino B, Abid S, Gewitz M. Maternal Lyme disease and congenital heart disease: a case–control study in an endemic area. Am J Obstet Gynecol 1999;180:711–16.

94. Gerber MA, Zalneraitis EL. Childhood neurologic disorders and Lyme disease during pregnancy. Pediatr Neurol 1994; 11:41–3.

95. Walsh CA, Mayer EW, Baxi LV. Lyme disease in pregnancy: case report and review of the literature. Obstet Gynecol Surv 2007;62:41–50.

96. Meningococcal disease. Accessed at www.cdc.gov/ncidod/dbmd/diseaseinfo/meningococcal_g.htm.

97. Mylonakis E, Paliou M, Hohmann EL, et al. Listeriosis during pregnancy: a case series and review of 222 cases. Medicine (Baltimore) 2002;81:260–9.

98. Rotbart H. Viral meningitis and the aseptic meningitis syndrome. In: Scheld W, Whitley RJ, Durack DT (eds) Infections of the central nervous system. Raven Press, New York, 1991.

99. Mylonakis E, Hohmann EL, Calderwood SB. Central nervous system infection with Listeria monocytogenes: 33 years' experience at a general hospital and review of 776 episodes from the literature. Medicine (Baltimore) 1998;77:313–36.

100. de Gans J, van de Beek D, the European Dexamethasone in Adulthood Bacterial Meningitis Study I. Dexamethasone in adults with bacterial meningitis. N Engl J Med 2002;347:1549–56.

101. Tunkel AR, Hartman BJ, Kaplan SL, et al. Practice guidelines for the management of bacterial meningitis. Clin Infect Dis 2004;39:1267–84.

102. Stevens DL, Bisno AL, Chambers HF, et al. Practice guidelines for the diagnosis and management of skin and soft-tissue infections. Clin Infect Dis 2005;41:1373–406.

103. Hepburn MJ, Dooley DP, Skidmore PJ, et al. Comparison of short-course (5 days) and standard (10 days) treatment for uncomplicated cellulitis. Arch Intern Med 2004;164: 1669–74.

104. Dufour P, Gillet Y, Bes M, et al. Community-acquired methicillin-resistant Staphylococcus aureus infections in France: emergence of a single clone that produces Panton-Valentine leukocidin. Clin Infect Dis 2002;35:819–24.

105. Gibbs RS, Blanco JD, St Clair PJ, et al. Quantitative bacteriology of amniotic fluid from women with clinical intraamniotic infection at term. J Infect Dis 1982;145(1):1–8.

106. Newton E, Prihoda T, Gibbs R. Logistic regression analysis of risk factors for intra-amniotic infection. Obstet Gynecol 1989;73(4):571–5.

107. Lau J, Magee F, Qiu Z, et al. Chorio-amnionitis with a fetal inflammatory response is associated with higher neonatal mortality, morbidity, and resource use than chorio-amnionitis displaying a maternal inflammatory response only. Am J Obstet Gynecol 2005;193(3):708–13.

108. Wu YW, Escobar GJ, Grether JK, et al. Chorio-amnionitis and cerebral palsy in term and near-term infants. JAMA 2003;290:2677–84.

109. Gibbs RS, Dinsmoor MJ, Newton ER, et al. A randomized trial of intrapartum versus immediate postpartum treatment of women with intra-amniotic infection. Obstet Gynecol 1988;72(6): 823–8.

110. Gilstrap LC, Leveno KJ, Cox SM, et al. Intrapartum treatment of acute chorio-amnionitis: impact on neonatal sepsis. Am J Obstet Gynecol 1988;159(3):579–83.

111. Sperling RS, Ramamurthy RS, Gibbs RS. A comparison of intrapartum versus immediate postpartum treatment of intra-amniotic infection. Obstet Gynecol 1987;70(6):861–5.

112. Duff P. Pathophysiology and management of postcesarean endomyometritis. Obstet Gynecol 1986;67:269–76.

113. Mead PB, Winn WC. Vaginal-rectal colonization with group A streptococci in late pregnancy. Infect Dis Obstet Gynecol 2000;8(5–6):217–19.

114. Gergis H, Barik S, Lim K, et al. Life-threatening puerperal infection with group A streptococcus. J R Soc Med 1999;92:412–13.

115. French LM, Smaill FM. Antibiotic regimens for endometritis after delivery. Cochrane Database of Systematic Reviews, 2007;1.

116. Garcia J, AboujaoudeR, Apuzzio J, Alvarex JR. Septic pelvic thrombophlebitis; diagnosis and management. Infect Dis Obstet Gynecol 2006;2006:15614.

117. Regan JAM, Klebanoff MAMM, Nugent RPP, et al. The epidemiology of group B streptococcal colonization in pregnancy. Obstet Gynecol 1991;77(4):604–10.

118. Baker CJ, Barrett FF, Gordon RC, et al. Suppurative meningitis due to streptococci of Lancefield group B: a study of 33 infants. J Pediatr 1973;82:724–9.

119. Barton LL, Feigin RD, Lins R. Group B beta hemolytic streptococcal meningitis in infants. J Pediatr 1973;82:719–23.

120. Franciosi RA, Knostman JD, Zimmerman RA. Group B streptococcal neonatal and infant infections. J Pediatr 1973;82:707–18.

121. McCracken G. Group B streptococci: the new challenge in neonatal infections. J Pediatr 1973;82:703–6.

122. Schrag S, Gorwitz R, Fultz-Butts K, et al. Prevention of perinatal group B streptococcal disease. Revised guidelines from CDC. MMWR 2002;51(RR-11):1–22.

123. Schrag SJ, Zell ER, Lynfield R, et al. A population-based comparison of strategies to prevent early-onset group B streptococcal disease in neonates. N Engl J Med 2002;347:233–9.

124. Lopez M, Sessler DI, Walter K, Emerick T, Ozaki M. Rate and gender dependence of the sweating, vasoconstriction, and shivering thresholds in humans. Anesthesiology 1994;80: 780–8.

125. Annadata RS, Sessler DI, Tayefeh F, Kurz A, Dechert M. Desflurane slightly increases the sweating threshold, but produces marked, non-linear decreases in the vasoconstriction and shivering thresholds. Anesthesiology 1995;83:1205–11.

126. Matsukawa T, Kurz A, Sessler DI, Bjorksten AR, Merrifield B, Cheng C. Propofol linearly reduces the vasoconstriction and shivering thresholds. Anesthesiology 1995;82:1169–80.

127. Frank SM, Fleisher LA, Breslow MJ, et al. Perioperative maintenance of normothermia reduces the incidence of morbid cardiac events: a randomized clinical trial. JAMA 1997;277:1127–34.

128. Kurz A, Sessler DI, Lenhardt RA, Study of Wound Infections and Temperature Group. Perioperative normothermia to reduce the incidence of surgical-wound infection and shorten hospitalization. N Engl J Med 1996;334:1209–15.

129. Rajagopalan S, Mascha E, Na J, Sessler DI. The effects of mild perioperative hypothermia on blood loss and transfusion requirement: a meta-analysis. Anesthesiology 2008; 108:71–7.

130. Lenhardt R, Marker E, Goll V, et al. Mild intraoperative hypothermia prolongs postanesthetic recovery. Anesthesiology 1997;87:1318–23.

131. Kurz A, Kurz M, Poeschl G, Faryniak B, Redl G, Hackl W. Forced-air warming maintains intraoperative normothermia better than circulating-water mattresses. Anesth Analg 1993; 77:89–95.

132. Sessler DI, Ponte J. Shivering during epidural anesthesia. Anesthesiology 1990;72:816–21.

133. Ozaki M, Kurz A, Sessler DI, et al. Thermoregulatory thresholds during spinal and epidural anesthesia. Anesthesiology 1994;81:282–8.

134. Kurz A, Sessler DI, Schroeder M, Kurz M. Thermoregulatory response thresholds during spinal anesthesia. Anesth Analg 1993;77:721–6.

135. Leslie K, Sessler DI. Reduction in the shivering threshold is proportional to spinal block height. Anesthesiology 1996; 84:1327–31.

136. Ikeda T, Kim J-S, Sessler DI, Negishi C, Turakhia M, Jeffrey R. Isoflurane alters shivering patterns and reduces maximum shivering intensity. Anesthesiology 1998;88:866–73.

137. Kurz A, Sessler DI, Annadata R, Dechert M, Christensen R. Midazolam minimally impairs thermoregulatory control. Anesth Analg 1995;81:393–8.

138. Kurz A, Go JC, Sessler DI, Kaer K, Larson M, Bjorksten AR. Alfentanil slightly increases the sweating threshold and markedly reduces the vasoconstriction and shivering thresholds. Anesthesiology 1995;83:293–9.

139. Kurz A, Ikeda T, Sessler DI, et al. Meperidine decreases the shivering threshold twice as much as the vasoconstriction threshold. Anesthesiology 1997;86:1046–54.

140. Leslie K, Sessler DI, Bjorksten A, et al. Propofol causes a dose-dependent decrease in the thermoregulatory threshold for vasoconstriction, but has little effect on sweating. Anesthesiology 1994;81:353–60.

141. Glosten B, Sessler DI, Faure EAM, Støen R, Thisted RA, Karl L. Central temperature changes are poorly perceived during epidural anesthesia. Anesthesiology 1992;77:10–16.

142. Frank S, Raja SN, Bulcao C, Goldstein D. Relative contribution of core and cutaneous temperatures to thermal comfort, autonomic, and metabolic responses in humans. J Appl Physiol 1999;86:1588–93.

143. Emerick TH, Ozaki M, Sessler DI, Walters K, Schroeder M. Epidural anesthesia increases apparent leg temperature and decreases the shivering threshold. Anesthesiology 1994;81: 289–98.

144. Vassilieff N, Rosencher N, Sessler DI, Conseiller C. The shivering threshold during spinal anesthesia is reduced in the elderly. Anesthesiology 1995;83:1162–6.

145. Kim J-S, Ikeda T, Sessler D, Turakhia M, Jeffrey R. Epidural anesthesia reduces the gain and maximum intensity of shivering. Anesthesiology 1998;88:851–7.

146. Frank SM, Nguyen JM, Garcia C, Barnes RA. Temperature monitoring practices during regional anesthesia. Anesth Analg 1999;88:373–7.

147. Arkilic CF, Akça O, Taguchi A, Sessler DI, Kurz A. Temperature monitoring and management during neuraxial anesthesia: an observational study. Anesth Analg 2000;91:662–6.

148. Horn E-P, Sessler DI, Standl T, et al. Non-thermoregulatory shivering in patients recovering from isoflurane or desflurane anesthesia. Anesthesiology 1998;89:878–86.

149. Panzer O, Ghazanfari N, Sessler DI, et al. Shivering and shivering-like tremor during labor with and without epidural analgesia. Anesthesiology 1999;90:1609–16.

150. Horn E-P, Schroeder F, Wilhelm S, et al. Postoperative pain facilitates non-thermoregulatory tremor. Anesthesiology 1999;91:979–84.

151. Sharkey A, Lipton JM, Murphy MT, Giesecke AH. Inhibition of postanesthetic shivering with radiant heat. Anesthesiology 1987;66:249–52.

152. Cheng C, Matsukawa T, Sessler DI, et al. Increasing mean skin temperature linearly reduces the core-temperature thresholds for vasoconstriction and shivering in humans. Anesthesiology 1995;82:1160–8.

153. Lenhardt R, Greif R, Sessler DI, Laciny S, Rajek A, Bastanmehr H. Relative contribution of skin and core temperatures to vasoconstriction and shivering thresholds during isoflurane anesthesia. Anesthesiology 1999;91:422–9.

154. Brownbridge P. Shivering related to epidural blockade with bupivacaine in labour, and the influence of epidural pethidine. Anaesth Intens Care 1986;14:412–17.

155. Joris J, Banache M, Bonnet F, Sessler DI, Lamy M. Clonidine and ketanserin both are effective treatments for postanesthetic shivering. Anesthesiology 1993;79:532–9.

156. Kizilirmak S, Karakas SE, Akça O, et al. Magnesium sulphate stops postanesthetic shivering. Proc NY Acad Sci 1997; 813:799–806.

157. Goetzl L, Rivers J, Zighelboim I, Wali A, Badell M, Suresh MS. Intrapartum epidural analgesia and maternal temperature regulation. Obstet Gynecol 2007;109:687–90.

158. Fusi L, Maresh MJA, Steer PJ, Beard RW. Maternal pyrexia associated with the use of epidural analgesia in labour. Lancet 1989;1:1250–2.

159. Philip J, Alexander JM, Sharma SK, Leveno KJ, McIntire DD, Wiley J. Epidural analgesia during labor and maternal fever. Anesthesiology 1999;90:1271–5.

160. Vinson DC, Thomas R, Kiser T. Association between epidural analgesia during labor and fever. J Fam Pract 1993;36:617–22.

161. Macaulay JH, Bond K, Steer PJ. Epidural analgesia in labor and fetal hyperthermia. Obstet Gynecol 1992;80:665–9.

162. Lieberman E, Lang JM, Frigoletto F, Richardson DK, Ringer SA, Cohen A. Epidural analgesia, intrapartum fever, and neonatal sepsis evaluation. Pediatrics 1997;99:415–19.

163. Lieberman E, Cohen A, Lang J, Frigoletto F, Goetzl L. Maternal intrapartum temperature elevation as a risk factor for cesarean delivery and assisted vaginal delivery. Am J Public Health 1999;89:506–10.

164. Churgay CA, Smith MA, Blok B. Maternal fever during labor – what does it mean? J Am Board Fam Pract 1994;7:14–24.

165. Dashe JS, Rogers BB, McIntire DD, Leveno KJ. Epidural analgesia and intrapartum fever: placental findings. Obstet Gynecol 1999;93:341–4.

166. Goetzl L, Zighelboim I, Badell M, et al. Maternal corticosteroids to prevent intrauterine exposure to hyperthermia and inflammation: a randomized, double-blind, placebo-controlled trial. Am J Obstet Gynecol 2006;195:1031–7.

167. Goetzl L, Rivers J, Evans T, et al. Prophylactic acetaminophen does not prevent epidural fever in nulliparous women: a double-blind placebo-controlled trial. J Perinatol 2004;24:471–5.

168. Reilly DR, Oppenheimer LW. Fever in term labour. J Obstet Gynaecol Can 2005;27:218–23.

169. Analgesia and Cesarean Delivery Rates. ACOG Committee Opinion 339, June 2006. Obstet Gynecol 2006;107:1487–8.

170. Negishi C, Kim J-S, Lenhardt R, *et al.* Alfentanil reduces the febrile response to interleukin-2 in humans. Crit Care Med 2000;28:1295–300.

171. Negishi C, Lenhardt R, Ozaki M, *et al.* Opioids inhibit febrile responses in humans, whereas epidural analgesia does not: an explanation for hyperthermia during epidural analgesia. Anesthesiology 2001;94:218–22.

172. Gross JB, Cohen AP, Lang JM, Frigoletto FD, Lieberman ES. Differences in systemic opioid use do not explain increased fever incidence in parturients receiving epidural analgesia. Anesthesiology 2002;97:157–61.

17 Viral infections in pregnancy other than human immunodeficiency virus

Eliana Castillo[1,3] and Deborah M. Money[2,3]

[1]Department of Medicine, University of British Columbia, Vancouver, BC, Canada
[2]Department of Obstetrics and Gynecology, University of British Columbia, Vancouver, BC, Canada
[3]Women's Health Research Institute, British Columbia Women's Hospital, Vancouver, BC, Canada

Introduction

Viral infections during pregnancy are very common; it is estimated that symptomatic viral infections affect at least 5.2% of pregnancies [1]. Reported incidence rates underestimate actual rates as many infections are asymptomatic for the mother and yet can have deleterious consequences for the offspring; as an example, approximately 1% of newborns excrete cytomegalovirus (CMV) at birth. Several factors have to interact for viral infections to affect pregnancy and some of them are amenable to preventive strategies from the clinician's point of view. A key factor is the proportion of women of childbearing age susceptible to a particular virus and the exposure these women have to a population where the virus circulates. Other factors, including the virus "activity" within the population and innate characteristics of the virus such as infectivity and transmissibility, warrant awareness on the clinician's part.

Prevention is the foremost strategy to curb the occurrence of viral infections during pregnancy. Ensuring that women of reproductive age receive appropriate vaccinations in a timely manner can certainly prevent a proportion of viral infections during pregnancy, as 50–60% of pregnancies are unplanned [2,3]; preconception testing for immunity status remains an option for planned pregnancies, but this is not the most common scenario the clinician deals with. Pregnancy surveillance may allow identification of women at the highest risk for specific infections and may identify fetal infection. Screening at birth is useful if vaccination or treatment of newborns at risk is available.

Pathogenesis of viral infections during pregnancy

Viruses are obligate intracellular pathogens. They require the host cell apparatus to replicate and by doing so they compromise key cellular processes, such as nucleic acid and protein synthesis, and preservation of membrane integrity. Therefore, they invariably result in premature cell death or abnormal cell survival [4,5]. Among immunocompetent adults, the cellular damage arising from most viral infections is repairable unless infection affects not easily repairable tissues like the central nervous system. Viral infections during pregnancy pose the extra challenge of a developing fetus potentially more susceptible to permanent sequelae.

In general, viruses are composed of a nucleocapsid, consisting of viral nucleic acid, i.e. double- or single-stranded DNA or RNA, packaged in a protein coat, referred as the capsid. The viral nucleic acid often includes the enzymes required for the initial steps in viral replication, whereas the capsid allows survival in the environment and binding to host cells. For most viruses the nucleocapsid is surrounded by a lipid envelope that usually contains the immunogenic proteins that elicit antibody response.

Maternal acquisition of infectious viruses happens from inhalation of droplets or aerosols, e.g. varicella-zoster virus (VZV), ingestion of fecally contaminated food or water, e.g. hepatitis A (HAV) or polio, or exposure to contaminated body fluids or tissues (blood, saliva, urine, genital secretions, or transplanted organs), e.g. herpes simplex virus (HSV) or HIV. Viral spread to lymph nodes, skin, mucosa and viscera varies according to the virus itself, but the virus must be present in the maternal bloodstream, the birth canal or in breast milk for transmission to the fetus or neonate to happen.

The mechanisms by which viral agents may produce adverse effects on the fetus arise from direct viral injury, e.g. chromosomal damage, cellular death and/or antigen/antibody formation, or indirectly from placental dysfunction, e.g. altered

de Swiet's Medical Disorders in Obstetric Practice, 5th edition.
Edited by R. O. Powrie, M. F. Greene, W. Camann. © 2010 Blackwell Publishing.

placental circulation, placental thrombosis or placentitis, secondary to maternal fever or metabolic derangements.

The fetal or neonatal complications arising from maternal viral infections depend on several factors, including gestational age at which the fetus is exposed to the virus, as placental and fetal immunity evolves during pregnancy; type of maternal infection: primary, reactivation or reinfection, as pre-existing maternal immunity may not be 100% effective to protect the fetus, but does decrease the burden of disease; viral factors, like virulence or cellular tropism. Viral exposure during the first trimester can result in resorption of the embryo, miscarriage, teratogenesis, and/or persistent fetal infection. Viral exposure during the second half of pregnancy is more likely to result in transient fetal infection or subclinical diseases that progress after delivery. Other consequences include prematurity, intrauterine growth retardation (IUGR), neurodevelopmental delay or no apparent sequelae at all.

Modes of transmission to the fetus

Maternal viral infections during pregnancy can be transmitted to the fetus while *in utero* or at the time of delivery. Maternal viremia may result in placental infection without fetal infection, infection of both placenta and fetus, or absence of both fetal and placental infection. The mechanism for transmission of most *in utero* infections in this review is transplacental, implying maternal viremia as the starting point followed by placental infection and subsequent release of viral particles into the fetal bloodstream. However, other mechanisms for *in utero* infection, that occur very rarely, include transamniotic transmission in the setting of chronic chorio-amnionitis[6] and iatrogenic direct viral inoculation into fetal circulation during diagnostic or therapeutic procedures[7].

For the purposes of our discussion, we have classified viral infections in pregnancy according to their main impact on maternal, fetal and/or neonatal morbidity and mortality, based on the currently published data, pointing out for the reader the instances where controversy exists and further research is required (see Table 17.1).

Immune response to viral infections during pregnancy

Contrary to commonly held beliefs, pregnancy is not synonymous with general maternal immune suppression, but rather a state of complex adaptations, still poorly understood, that allow the maternal immune system to recognize and react against the foreign antigens of the fetus in a "positive way," i.e. limiting trophoblast invasion to ensure maternal corporal integrity while ensuring adequate placentation [8]. Maternal antibody production in response to vaccines is preserved in pregnancy, which presents a unique opportunity to prevent disease for the mother and her offspring, and when

challenged with various stimuli, the immune response of pregnant women is not significantly reduced when compared to nonpregnant women [9].

Epidemiologic data on increased frequency and/or severity of intracellular infections during pregnancy have led to the assumption that cell-mediated immunity is adversely affected. Effective immunity against viruses requires both arms of the immune system: innate and adaptive. Each arm has humoral (cytokines, complement and antibodies) and cellular components (granulocytes, natural killer (NK) and dendritic cells for the innate arm and T-lymphocytes, both helper and CD8+, and B-cells for the adaptive arm) (Figure 17.1). Innate immunity implies intrinsic resistance to microbes, not acquired through previous contact, like the one mediated by pattern recognition receptors (PRR) or Toll-like receptors (TLR), which recognize highly conserved sequences unique

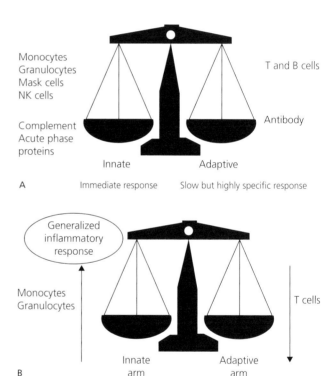

Figure 17.1 Immunology of pregnancy: overview. (A) Effective immunity against viruses requires both arms of the immune system: innate and adaptive. The two arms of the immune system, innate and adaptive, each include a cellular component (granulocytes, natural killer (NK) and dendritic cells for the innate arm, and lymphocytes (T-lymphocytes, both helper and CD8+, and B-cells) for the adaptive arm) and a humoral component (cytokines, complement and antibodies). (B) Pregnancy is associated with a generalized inflammatory response. During pregnancy, the innate immune system is activated and the adaptive immune, particularly T-cell, functions appear to be downregulated during gestation; this complex interaction is thought to be crucial for maintenance of a successful pregnancy. Adapted from Luppi [11].

Table 17.1 Consequences of viral infections during pregnancy

Viruses by predominant clinical consequences	Abortion, stillbirth	Prematurity	Symptomatic congenital infection	Developmental abnormalities/ birth defects	Neonatal disease
Fetal					
CMV	+	+	++[1]	+++	+
Rubella	+	−	+++[1]	+++	+
Parvo B−19	+−	−	+	−	−
LCV	+	−	+	++	+
Mumps	++	−	−	+	−
Materno-fetal					
Measles	+	++	−	−	+
Neonatal					
Coxsackie (mostly B1-B5 strains)	+	−	−	+[2]	++
Echovirus serotype 11	+[3]	−	−	−	++[4]
Maternal-neonatal					
Primary VZV	−+	−[5]	−	+[6]	+++[7]
HSV	−	−	+[8]	−[6]	++[9]
HPV	−	−	−	−	+[10]
Maternal					
Influenza	−	−	−	−	−
EBV[11]	−	+	−	−	−

− No documented association.
+ Documented association but true incidence unknown.
++ Well-documented association (prospective, histopathologic correlation and/or molecular data).
+++ Most clinically relevant association.
[1] Risk of congenital disease in the baby may be significant enough to warrant counseling on continuation of pregnancy.
[2] Congenital heart disease has been linked to coxsackie B3.
[3] Stillbirths reported for echovirus 27 and 11. Symptomatic congenital infections reported for echoviruses 6, 7, 9, 11, 19, 27 and 33.
[4] Neonatal sepsis-like syndrome and myocarditis associated with echovirus 11.
[5] Prospective studies have shown conflicting results regarding prematurity for offspring of gestational VZV.
[6] Congenital VZV syndrome is rare; risk is confined to maternal VZV in the first half of pregnancy (weeks 7–20).
[7] Neonatal VZV develops in 24–50% of cases of maternal chickenpox within 4 weeks of delivery.
[8] Intrauterine infection is extremely rare: 1/200,000 births.
[9] Neonatal HSV affects 1/3200 births potentially resulting in permanent sequelae or death.
[10] Incidence of JORRP in the offspring women with vaginal condyloma is 7/1000 versus 3.96/100,000 for the general pediatric population.
[11] Mononucleosis-like syndromes must be investigated, as may be secondary to CMV, LCV or EBV.
CMV, cytomegalovirus; EBV, Epstein-Barr virus; HPV, human papilloma virus; HSV, herpes simplex virus; JORRP, juvenile-onset recurrent respiratory papillomatosis; LCV, lymphocytic choriomeningitis virus; VZV, varicella-zoster virus.

to microbes such as double-stranded RNA, peptidoglycans and lipopolysacharides [10]. Adaptive immunity requires contact with the microbe; hence it is very specific but takes at least 3–4 days to reach minimally effective levels; however, it is followed by immunologic memory, which offers partial if not total protection against subsequent infections by the same organism. Activation of the adaptive immunity requires the prior activation of innate immunity and "antigen presentation" by antigen-presenting cells (APC) to T-lymphocytes. Antigens are presented by molecular histocompatibility complex (MHC) membrane proteins; MHC-I are present in all somatic cells (except neurons and red blood cells (RBC)) and MHC-II only on APC, like macrophages. Human leukocyte antigens (HLA) are the MHC in humans.

Simplistically, following infection viruses undergo rapid replication using the host cell apparatus for protein synthesis and viral replication; viral antigens then are available to be presented by HLA-I molecules to CD8+ T-cells (cytotoxic T-cells (CTL)), resulting in production of virus-specific clones of B-lymphocytes responsible for antibody production and specific T-lymphocytes.

Innate immunity against viruses (Figure 17.2) is triggered by viral destruction of cells, recognition of infected cells by NK cells (which are able to recognize cells not expressing HLA-I and otherwise evading immune surveillance) or direct interaction of complement with virions, leading to cytokine release, kinin and complement activation and recruitment of monocytes and neutrophils. Normal pregnancy is characterized by generalized upregulation of granulocytes, monocytes and complement [11]. NK cell cytotoxic function is reduced in the peripheral maternal circulation, but NK cells are the predominant leukocyte at the decidua.

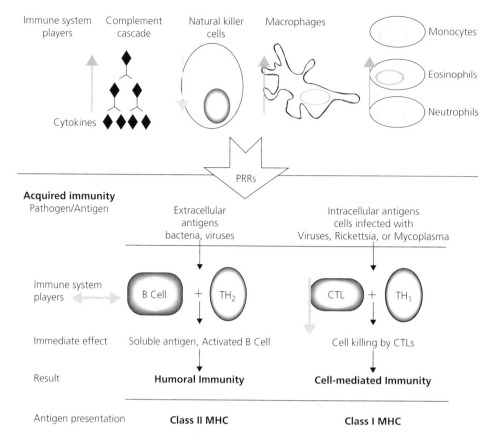

Figure 17.2 Immune response to viruses. Effective immunity against viruses requires both arms of the immune system: innate and adaptive. Innate immunity implies intrinsic resistance to microbes -not acquired through previous contact; it is mediated by pattern recognition receptors (PRRs) or toll-like receptors, which recognize highly conserved sequences unique to microbes like double stranded-RNA, peptidoglycans and lipopolysacharides. Acquired (adaptive) immunity requires contact with the microbe. Activation of the acquired immunity requires the prior activation of innate immunity and "antigen presentation" to T- lymphocytes (Th1 or Th2). Antigens are presented by MHC membrane proteins; Class I MHC are present in all somatic cells (except neurons and red blood cells) and Class II MHC only on APC, such as macrophages. HLA are the MHC in humans. Gray arrows represent the pregnancy-related changes on the immune response to viruses. Adapted from Straus JH & Strauss EG. *Viruses and Human Diseases*, 2nd edn. Elsevier, 2007.

Cell-mediated adaptive immunity changes in pregnancy as well; cytotoxic T-cell function is attenuated, and newly described immunosuppressive factors such as pregnancy-specific glycoprotein 1a (PSG1a), synthesized by the trophoblast, and prostaglandin E2 (PGE2) seem to play a role [10]. The traditionally quoted pregnancy-associated change in the pattern of cytokine production by helper T-lymphocytes toward an anti-inflammatory or "Th2" response (interleukin (IL)-4, 5 and 13) instead of a proinflammatory or "Th1" (Il-2, IFN-gamma and TNF-alpha), although well documented, is not crucial for pregnancy success [12,13], whereas IFN-gamma is crucial for adequate placentation [14] and it clearly confers protection at the materno-placental level against intracellular organisms such as malaria. [15]. B-cell function and antibody production to vaccination are normal in pregnancy. Maternal IgG transfer to fetus starts by approximately 16 weeks gestation, but is not complete until approximately 32 weeks gestation.

Diagnosis of viral infections during pregnancy

Diagnosis of viral infections during pregnancy is challenging, and relies on laboratory diagnosis for mother and fetus and/or imaging the fetus and the placenta. Maternal clinical presentation is almost never pathognomonic for a particular virus; however, if the infection is symptomatic at all, it usually fits into one of the following clinical syndromes: undifferentiated fever, fever and nonvesicular rash, fever and arthritis, fever and neurologic signs, vesicular rash, hepatitis and mononucleosis-like syndrome (Table 17.2). Laboratory diagnosis relies on viral detection, either by rapid molecular diagnostic methods or by culture, and the host immune response to the virus i.e. IgM/IgG or both, usually referred to as serology.

Table 17.2 Clinical syndromes associated with viral infections in pregnancy and diagnostic tests

Clinical syndrome	Potential viral infections	Direct viral detection	Antibodies
Undifferentiated fever	CMV, rubella[1], enteroviruses[2,6], influenza, EBV, measles[3], parvo B-19, WNV[4]	CMV, parvo B-19[5] NAAT blood Nasopharyngeal wash for influenza Throat swab for viral NAAT[6] Urine for viral culture Stool for viral culture[6]	*Single serum:* CMV, EBV IgM, IgG[7] WNV IgM Monospot *Paired serum:* Rubella IgM, IgG[8] Parvo B-19 IgM, IgG Measles IgM, IgG
Fever and nonvesicular rash	Rubella, measles, echoviruses[2], EBV, parvo B-19, CMV	Throat swab for viral NAAT[6] Stool for viral culture[6] Parvo B-19 NAAT blood	EBV IgM, IgG Monospot *Paired serum:* Rubella IgM, IgG Parvo B-19 IgM, IgG Measles IgM, IgG, CMV
Fever and arthritis	Rubella, parvo B-19, enteroviruses[2]	Throat swab for viral NAAT[6] Stool for viral culture[6] Parvo B-19 NAAT blood	Parvo B-19 IgM, IgG
Fever and neurologic signs	HSV, WNV[4], polio	WNV NAAT blood CSF for HSV, polio, WNV NAAT or viral culture Vesicle fluid/scraping for HSV	*Single serum:* WNV IgM, IgG
Vesicular rash	VZV, HSV	Vesicle fluid/scraping for VZV/HSV	VZV IgM, IgG[9]
Genital ulcers	HSV, VZV	Vesicle fluid/scraping for HSV/VZV	HSV type-specific serology
Hepatitis	CMV, EBV, hepatitis A, B, C and E	CMV NAAT blood	CMV, EBV IgM, IgG Monospot HAV IgM HBsAg[10] anti-HBc IgM[11] Anti-HCV HEV IgM, IgG[12]
Mononucleosis-like illness (recurrent fever, myalgias, sore throat +/− arthritis or rash)	CMV, LCV, EBV, HIV[13]	CMV, EBV NAAT blood	EBV IgM, IgG Monospot HIV IgG
Travel +/− any of the above	Hepatitis E, Japanese encephalitis, hemorrhagic fevers	Consultation with reference laboratory advised	

[1] Direct viral isolation of rubella not routinely done as very difficult to culture and rapid methods are not widely available.

[2] Enteroviruses – polio, coxsackie and echoviruses – to be considered particularly in the third trimester, during summer/fall season and/or in the context of aseptic meningitis.

[3] Direct viral isolation of measles not routinely done; in low-prevalence countries (USA/Canada) use paired acute and convalescent serum for anti-measles IgM and IgG: a fourfold increase in anti-measles antibody titer is indicative of infection.

[4] WNV to be considered in areas with known WNV transmission.

[5] Parvo B-19 viremia by PCR is diagnostic of acute infection and precedes development of IgM by 7–10 days.

[6] PCR for enteroviruses amplifies a highly conserved portion of the genome, allowing detection of most enteroviruses from throat swabs, blood, urine, and stool; sampling multiple sites enhances likelihood of viral detection.

[7] CMV IgG avidity test if available.

[8] Take acute phase IgG as soon as possible after rash onset (ideally within 7 days) and convalescent phase IgG 10–14 days later.

[9] Presence of IgG will rule out acute infection.

[10] Hepatitis B surface antigen is positive for 95% of patients with acute hepatitis B.

[11] Anti-hepatitis B core antibody particularly useful during "window" period when HbsAg disappears and anti-HB surface antibody appears.

[12] Available in Europe, Asia, and Canada but not in the United States.

[13] Diagnosis of HIV infection is routinely made only by serology.

CMV, cytomegalovirus; EBV, Epstein-Barr virus, HAV, hepatitis A virus; HSV, herpes simplex virus, LCV, lymphocytic choriomeningitis virus; NAAT, nucleic acid amplification test (PCR is a type of NAAT); VZV, varicella-zoster virus; WNV, West Nile virus.

Traditionally, TORCH serology has been used to aid in the diagnosis of fetal manifestations of disease like IUGR or malformations, but given its poor yield and high cost, it is not widely recommended [16,17]. TORCH testing is an acronym and refers to obtaining antibody titers for Toxoplasma, syphyllis, HBV, Rubella, CMV and HSV.

Fetal ultrasound is used to follow pregnancies with confirmed maternal viral infections or to detect findings suspicious for infection (see Table 17.3). Sequential ultrasound assessment is crucial for confirmed or suspected infections, even if initial assessment is normal, to assess fetal growth and because structural abnormalities may become apparent only with further development.

Viral infections of predominantly maternal impact

Influenza A and B

Influenza is a vaccine-preventable febrile respiratory illness, which affects 10–40% of the general population over a 6-week period every winter in temperate climates, but year round in the tropics. Pregnant patients are more susceptible to developing influenza complications, particularly pneumonia. Although influenza vaccine is widely recommended for all pregnant women throughout the flu season, vaccination rates remain low.

Virology

Influenza A and B are single-stranded RNA viruses that routinely affect humans every year (seasonal influenza). Influenza A also affects other species like swine and avian. Influenza viruses undergo frequent variations in their capsular antigens, resulting in new circulating strains every year. Small, gradual changes resulting in new strains of an existing influenza subtype are called antigenic drifts. Abrupt, major changes resulting in new influenza subtypes are called antigenic shifts; these may arise from recombination of human and animal Influenza A viruses, i.e. 2009 novel H1N1 Influenza A. These antigenic changes are responsible for the yearly influenza season and major pandemics as the population has little or no immunity against new circulating strains or subtypes.

Pathogenesis

Influenza is acquired by aspiration of small-particle aerosols (<10 µm) created by sneezing, coughing, and talking [18,19]. The incubation period varies from 18 to 72 hours.

Clinical presentation

The most common clinical course is abrupt onset of fever, malaise, headache, severe myalgias and cough. Fever typically lasts 3 days and most people recover within a week. Influenza pneumonia is more common among patients with pre-existing

Table 17.3 Common prenatal ultrasound findings of certain viral infections

Virus	CNS	Cardiac	Abdominal	Placenta	Other
CMV	Ventriculomegaly Calcifications Microcephaly Cerebellar aplasia	Cardiomegaly Septal defects Calcifications	Hepatomegaly Splenomegaly Calcifications Ascites Echogenic bowel	Placentomegaly	IUGR Hydrops Demise Oligohydramnios
Rubella	Calcifications Encephalocele Microcephaly Microphthalmia Ventriculomegaly	Septal defects Pulmonic stenosis Coarctation of aorta	Hepatomegaly Hepatic Calcifications Splenomegaly Meconium peritonitis	Calcifications	IUGR Cleft palate
VZV	Ventriculomegaly Calcifications Microphthalmia Retinal Calcifications	–	Hepatomegaly Calcifications Ascites	Small placenta Calcifications	IUGR Limb deformities Oligohydramnios
HSV	Hydranencephaly Ventriculomegaly Calcifications Microcephaly Microphthalmia	–	Hepatomegaly Splenomegaly	Calcifications	IUGR Limb hypoplasia
Parvo B-19	–	–	–	–	Hydrops Polyhydramnios Increase in MCA-Doppler velocity

CMV, cytomegalovirus; CNS, central nervous system; HSV, herpes simplex virus; IUGR, intrauterine growth retardation; VZV, varicella-zoster virus.

cardiovascular diseases or pregnancy. Epidemiologic studies during the 1918 pandemic, several epidemics until 1960 and the 2009 novel H1N1 Influenza A pandemic have consistently shown that pregnant women account for an excessive proportion of influenza-related deaths [19–22]. Pregnancy is a recognized risk factor for severe illness and hospital admission for seasonal influenza, particularly among women with asthma [23]. The risk of complications increases by threefold from weeks 16 to 36 [24], but persists through the early postpartum period (up to 2 weeks) [19]. Severity of influenza seemed even higher for 2009 novel H1N1 influenza. Late initiation of antiviral treatment (>48 hours from symptom onset) increased risk of ICU admission or death by 4-fold. [19]. Progressive increment on cardiac output, oxygen consumption, and changes in lung function may be contributing factors, making pregnant women with asthma, congenital heart disease or chronic renal disease especially susceptible. Myocarditis has been described associated with influenza in pregnancy.

Obstetric considerations

There are no consistent prospective data linking intrauterine exposure to influenza and increased rates of abortion, prematurity or congenital malformations [25]; maternal hyperthermia (which may in and of itself be associated with malformations) may well have been a confounding factor for most reported observations on birth defects [26,27].

Diagnosis

Accurate clinical diagnosis among healthy adults in the setting of an influenza outbreak is possible for 80–90% of cases, given the abrupt nature of symptoms. Recent data reinforces the notion that viral detection from the nasopharynx should be attempted in pregnancy and early postpartum period, but antiviral treatment must not be withheld pending laboratory confirmation (see below). Consultation with referral laboratory services regarding choice of diagnostic test is strongly advised. Rapid antigen detection methods, although widely available, were shown to have poor sensitivity during recent 2009 H1N1 pandemic. Availability of molecular detection methods (i.e. PCR) varies widely [19,28].

Treatment

Four antiviral agents are approved for influenza chemoprophylaxis and therapy: the adamantines (amantadine and rimantadine) and the neuraminidase inhibitors (the oral agent oseltamivir and the inhaled agent zanamivir). Increasing viral resistance to the adamantines and some concerning pregnancy animal data make this class of agents an undesirable option in pregnancy. Prompt initiation of neurominidase inhibitors

(within 48 hours of symptoms onset) was recommended for pregnant women with suspected or confirmed influenza, in light of the recently observed benefit on survival and severity of illness [29-31].

Infection control

Patients with proven or suspected influenza illness, if admitted to hospital, should be placed on droplet (mask) and contact (gloves and gowns) precautions until day 6 from symptom onset. There is no evidence that separation of infant from mother or avoidance of breastfeeding lessens the risk of the neonate developing influenza. Adjunctive measures include hand washing and contact prophylaxis.

Prevention

Vaccination is the most effective preventative measure in healthy adults, preventing 70–90% of infections in years when circulating and vaccine viruses are antigenically similar [32]. Unfortunately, vaccine administration rates during pregnancy are low, even among pregnant women with additional risk factors for increased influenza-related morbidity, i.e. asthma, congenital heart disease or chronic renal disease. Influenza vaccination is recommended for all women who will be pregnant during the influenza season (September through January) [32,33] and has been demonstrated to reduce both maternal and infant febrile respiratory illness through 6 months of age [34]. Universal vaccination for pregnant women is likely cost-effective [35]. Healthcare workers should also be vaccinated against influenza each year to help prevent the unknowing transmission of subclinical infection to patients under their care.

Epstein–Barr virus

Epstein–Barr virus (EBV) along with VZV, CMV and HSV, belongs to the human Herpesvirus family, all double-stranded DNA viruses, distributed worldwide. It causes subclinical infection in childhood and infectious mononucleosis syndrome among teenagers or adults. As with other herpes family viruses, it results in lifelong latent infection.

Primary EBV infection during pregnancy is uncommon as only 3–4% of pregnant women are susceptible [36]. Primary EBV infection, reactivation or associated complications do not happen more often in pregnancy [37,38]. Pregnant women presenting with infectious mononucleosis-like syndrome should be investigated because acute CMV infection is the most common cause of Monospot-negative mononucleosis (Monospot is a commonly used rapid test for EBV infection; see below) and, unlike EBV, CMV can have deleterious effects on the fetus and neonate.

Pathogenesis

Epstein–Barr virus is acquired by contact with infected oral secretions. Acute EBV infection results in synthesis of large amounts of IgM against antigens common to those found on the red blood cells of other mammals, called "heterophile antibodies"; this IgM is the one measured by the Monospot test. Asymptomatic reactivation of latently infected EBV cells results in shedding of EBV particles in saliva and cervical secretions.

Clinical presentation

Typical infectious mononucleosis is characterized clinically by fever, exudative sore throat in about 33% of cases and symmetric cervical adenopathy in 80–90% of patients. Splenomegaly is present about 50% of the time. Jaundice and rashes, which may be macular (nonpalpable spots <1 cm in diameter), petechial, scarlatiniform (scarlet fever-like rash, i.e. innumerable small red papules that are diffusely distributed), urticarial (hives) or erythema multiforme-like (pink-red lesions on the extremities with a pale center), are present 5% of the time. The acute phase of the illness is serologically characterized by the transient appearance of heterophile antibodies and atypical lymphocytosis (a lymphocyte count of >50% of total white blood cells or an absolute number of >4500/μL with an atypical appearance on peripheral smear). Liver function tests are elevated in approximately 90% of cases.

Obstetric considerations

Whether EBV infection during pregnancy increases the risk of abortion remains unclear. There have been no consistent anomalies associated with gestational EBV infection, and the data do not demonstrate a causal relationship [25,39]. Data from a large pregnant cohort (n=35,940) indicate that reactivation of EBV infection during pregnancy may shorten pregnancy duration and result in lower birthweight babies [40]. However, pregnant women with acute EBV infection should generally be reassured about their probable pregnancy outcome and the most important aspect of the management of this disorder in pregnancy is to firmly establish the diagnosis to ensure that the patient does not have one of the more concerning mono-like illnesses such as CMV or toxoplasmosis.

Diagnosis

The heterophile antibody test (Monospot) is positive in approximately 85% of patients who have infectious mononucleosis (and has a specificity of close to 100%), but can be falsely negative early in the illness and may remain positive for up to 18 months after acute infection. Specific anti-EBV IgM is better for the diagnosis of recent primary infection, particularly when the Monospot is initially negative. EBV DNA detection in blood by molecular methods is available in some centers and will be positive with both acute infection and reactivation.

Treatment

Treatment is generally supportive, with hydration, analgesics, acetaminophen and rest, as primary EBV infection is usually self-limiting. A meta-analysis of five randomized, controlled trials demonstrated no significant benefit of acyclovir in the treatment of infectious mononucleosis [41]. Complications including autoimmune hemolytic anemia, severe thrombocytopenia, and respiratory compromise or severe pharyngeal edema warrant the use of corticosteroids.

Viral infections of predominantly fetal impact

Human cytomegalovirus

Cytomegalovirus (CMV) is the most common infectious cause of congenital birth defects and accounts for least 15–20% of bilateral, moderate to profound sensorineural hearing loss in childhood [42,43]. CMV infections among immunocompetent hosts are subclinical, but can be devastating for immunocompromised hosts like the developing fetus, AIDS patients, and organ transplant recipients.

Epidemiology

Cytomegalovirus infections are endemic worldwide and have no seasonal variation. Age of acquisition is younger in developing countries and among those of lower socio-economic status in industrialized countries. In the US, only 58.3% of women 15–44 years have CMV antibodies [44] but specific populations have seropositivity rates close to 85%. Annual seroconversion rates range from 2% among mid/high socio-economic background to 6% for women of lower socio-economic background and up to 11% for female daycare workers [45]. Young women who care for preschool children and also become sexually active within the 2 years before delivery are at the greatest risk for delivering an infant with congenital CMV infection [46].

Virology

Cytomegalovirus is a large double-stranded DNA virus and, as all other members of the Herpesvirus family, it establishes latent infection. CMV downregulates several aspects of the immune response such as the MHC-1 pathway of antigen presentation.

Pathogenesis

The primary reservoir cell for CMV and the mechanisms by which latent CMV infection is maintained are unknown. CMV has been isolated in saliva, urine, feces, semen, vaginal secretions, breast milk, blood, donated organs and tears. Infection requires close intimate contact with persons excreting the virus in their saliva, urine or other body fluids but transmission also occurs from fomites, such as toys in the daycare setting [47].

Pathogenesis of congenital CMV infection

Congenital CMV infection refers to mother-to-child transmission of CMV *in utero* (transplacentally), has been defined as the presence of CMV on neonatal urine, blood or saliva in the first 10 days of life, and can potentially result in adverse neonatal outcomes and long-term sequelae, such as hearing loss (see below). Perinatal CMV infection refers to mother-to-child CMV transmission during birth or shortly thereafter from exposure to CMV-infected maternal blood, birth canal secretions or breastfeeding. Although far more common than congenital infection [48], perinatal infection is not usually associated with neonatal disease or long-term sequelae (except for extremely rare cases of pneumonitis among premature infants [47]).

Congenital CMV infection affects 0.7% of all livebirths in developed countries; 87.3% of these infections will be asymptomatic at birth [49] but late sequelae including hearing loss, learning difficulties and/or mental retardation will develop in at least 15% later in life [49]. Only a minority of congenital infections will manifest as fulminant cytomegalic inclusion disease (CID) with a reported mortality rate of 5%. CID is almost exclusively seen in infants of mothers who have had a primary CMV infection during pregnancy (see below for definition of primary infection). CID is characterized by hepatosplenomegaly, intrauterine growth restriction, hematologic abnormalities (including thrombocytopenia), rash (most classically purpura and petechiae described by the unfortunate term "blueberry muffin baby") and CNS abnormalities including microcephaly, cerebral atrophy, chorioretinitis, ventriculomegaly and sensorineural hearing loss [47]. Intracerebral calcifications in a periventricular distribution and microcephaly [50] appear to be predictive of a poor neurodevelopmental prognosis in this condition.

The risk of congenital CMV infection is related to the type of maternal infection, classified, according to prior immune status, as *primary* (absence of CMV antibodies prior to pregnancy) or *secondary* (presence of CMV antibodies prior to pregnancy but reactivation of latent infection or reinfection with a different CMV strain [51]). Maternal immunity decreases the risk of congenital infection at least by 69% [52]. Transmission rate is 30–40% for primary maternal CMV infections versus only 1% for secondary infections. Primary infections during the first half of pregnancy are more likely to result in CNS disease and permanent disability [53].

The pathogenesis of vertical transmission for both primary and secondary infections is not fully understood [54], and the factors preventing transmission among 60–70% of all primary maternal CMV infections are still unknown. Placental CMV infection activates the maternal immune response against the cytotrophoblast by downregulating cytotrophoblast expression of HLA-G [55,56]; this may explain the reported spontaneous abortion rates. Transport of CMV virions across the trophoblast seems to involve the fetal Fc receptor [57]. Once the fetus is infected, CMV replicates in the fetal renal tubular epithelium and virions are excreted to the amniotic fluid.

Clinical presentation

Primary CMV infection during pregnancy is asymptomatic 95% of the time. When symptomatic, its clinical manifestation does not differ from that in nonpregnant hosts. Incubation period ranges from 20 to 60 days, after which a mild mononucleosis-like syndrome ensues, with fever lasting a mean of 19 days, lymphadenopathy, high lymphocyte count and abnormal liver function test results. Rare complications include hepatitis, Guillain–Barré syndrome and myocarditis.

Other obstetric considerations

In a prospective study, when compared to control women with a 2.2% spontaneous pregnancy loss rate, women with documented primary CMV infection had a 15% rate of spontaneous pregnancy loss, a sevenfold increase [58].

Diagnosis of CMV infection in pregnancy

Despite the burden of congenital CMV infection, there is no consistent approach to the diagnosis of CMV infection during pregnancy and at present, universal screening for CMV infection in pregnancy is not recommended. There is substantial controversy regarding the appropriateness of screening in the absence of reproducible and easy-to-interpret diagnostic tests or clearly effective therapies. Identifying primary infections is difficult as in most cases there is no preconception serum available to determine if seroconversion has happened. Even if seroconversion is proven and these women are offered fetal diagnosis to decide on pregnancy continuation or treatment, CMV isolation from amniotic fluid is not sufficiently sensitive before 21–24 weeks of gestational age. In addition, secondary CMV infections still pose a risk for congenital infections and there is no appropriate testing algorithm. The appropriateness of universal screening for congenital CMV infection at birth to reduce the burden of CMV-related hearing loss is being tested in a multicenter study.

Diagnosis of primary maternal infection cannot be made on clinical grounds alone, as most infections are asymptomatic, but in general, every mononucleosis-like syndrome in pregnancy should be investigated. Several definitions of maternal CMV infection during pregnancy have been used:

- seroconversion from CMV IgG-negative status pre-pregnancy or at some point during pregnancy to CMV IgG positive
- documentation of CMV IgM only, followed by both positive CMV IgM and IgG
- fourfold or more increase on CMV IgG titer during pregnancy
- low CMV IgG avidity index (see below)
- amniotic fluid positive for CMV DNA by PCR
- presence of CMV DNA in maternal blood.

Following infection, CMV IgM appears within days and persists for as long as 16 weeks. IgG can be documented as early as 2 weeks and persists for years. However, the IgG secreted during the first months after infection is of low avidity (ability to bind antigens), ranging between 20% within 3 months of infection to 70% for remote infections. Low avidity indexes have been used to diagnose primary infections [59] and a high avidity index before 18 weeks gestation has a reported negative predictive value of 100% for congenital infection [60]. However, avidity assays are not easily reproducible, nor widely available. The level of maternal antibodies at delivery does not predict protection, but the neutralizing activity of the antibody and the avidity of the IgG may be predictive [47].

Determination of CMV DNA in maternal blood, plasma or leukocytes or one of its antigens –pp65 – is commercially available and can be used to diagnose primary CMV infections, but its role in triaging and managing CMV infection during pregnancy is not defined.

Fetal diagnosis

Cytomegalovirus detection in amniotic fluid is the gold standard for prenatal diagnosis, as the virus replicates in the fetal renal tubular epithelium and viruria is consistently found in infected newborns. Reported sensitivity has ranged between 75% and 95%, but there is a several-week delay between primary maternal infection and presence of quantifiable virus in amniotic fluid. Testing for CMV in amniotic fluid by polymerase chain reaction (PCR) is not recommended prior to the 21st week of gestation because of low sensitivity, at 45% [61], or prior to 6 weeks after maternal infection [62]. Quantitative PCR of amniotic fluid and fetal blood does not predict transmission rates or likelihood of symptomatic congenital CMV infection [63]. Fetal IgM measurement is not recommended given that many CMV-infected fetuses do not develop specific IgM until late in pregnancy and because of an estimated 1% risk of pregnancy loss associated with cordocentesis.

In utero infection is suspected by maternal seroconversion or by abnormal ultrasound markers in the fetus, including symmetric growth restriction, intracranial calcifications, ventriculomegaly or echogenic fetal bowel [64].

Treatment

Currently there are no well-studied, effective therapies for CMV during pregnancy. In 2005, one prospective interventional noncontrolled study reported on the use of CMV-specific hyper immune globulin (CMV-HIG) for confirmed and/or presumed CMV primary infection among pregnant women. CMV-HIG treatment was associated with a significantly lower risk of congenital CMV infection and disease [65]. Placental thickness was found to be a marker of CMV infection and severity, and CMV-HIG was associated with significant reductions in placental size [66]. Although this was an uncontrolled study, the magnitude of benefit reported warrants further research.

Antivirals are extensively used to treat CMV among AIDS and solid organ transplant patients, but there is a paucity of data for their use in pregnancy. Anecdotal conflicting reports on the use of ganciclovir and valganciclovir for CMV infections in pregnancy [67,68], in addition to the very narrow therapeutic range from hematologic toxicity, preclude any recommendation for their use.

Prevention and education

In the absence of effective therapies for congenital CMV infection, prevention becomes very important. A live-attenuated vaccine tested among renal transplant recipients successfully induced both humoral and cell-mediated responses and reduced severity of CMV-related illness but failed to reduce infection rates. A subunit vaccine using recombinant envelope glycoprotein B demonstrated 50% efficacy to prevent CMV infection among seronegative women [69].

Women of childbearing age should be educated about CMV and its transmission and the argument can be made to target female daycare workers in particular. Counseling about handling of potentially soiled articles such as diapers and thorough hand washing when around young children or immunocompromised hosts is feasible, and has been launched recently on the CDC website. If seroconversion is documented preconceptionally, recent evidence suggests that pregnancy should ideally be delayed for 2 years [70].

Parvovirus B-19

Parvovirus B-19 infection during pregnancy is a well-recognized cause of fetal loss, nonimmune hydrops fetalis (defined as the presence of two or more of the following abnormal fetal fluid collections: polyhydramnios, skin edema, pericardial effusion, ascites or pleural effusion) and congenital anemia; however, for the majority of children and adults, this infection is benign and self-limiting, resulting in lifelong immunity, that does not require any treatment other than symptom control. Parvovirus B-19 exhibits a characteristic tropism for precursor erythroid cell lines, inhibiting red blood cell production transiently. As a consequence, the infected fetus may be severely affected because red blood cell turnover is high and the immune response relatively immature. Pregnant women can become infected with parvovirus B-19 as these infections are commonplace in the community and occur year round, spreading primarily by respiratory secretions.

Virology

Parvovirus B-19 is a small single-stranded DNA virus, belonging to the large Parvoviridae family. Infection results in long-lasting immunity elicited by its two capsid proteins, VP2 and VP1. It cannot be cultivated in the laboratory and diagnosis relies on serology and molecular detection methods.

Epidemiology

Thirty-five to 45% of women of childbearing age are susceptible to parvovirus B-19 infection and their annual sero-conversion rate is 1.5% [71]. Higher attack and annual seroconversion rates are seen for workers in close contact with affected children, such as daycare providers and school personnel [72]. In the USA, Canada and Europe the annual incidence of acute B-19 infection in pregnancy is approximately 1–2% but may rise to >10% during epidemics; conservative estimates indicate that up to 3000 pregnancies are lost every year from B-19 infection in the US [73].

Pathogenesis

Adult patients acquire parvovirus B-19 from personal contact via aerosol or respiratory secretions and from contaminated blood products. The fetus can be infected if the mother is nonimmune at the time of exposure and she becomes viremic with parvovirus B-19, resulting in transplacental transmission. In this viral infection, transmission appears to be poorly blocked by the placenta and can occur throughout gestation.

Parvovirus B-19 binds to the P blood group antigen expressed by late erythroid cell precursors and other cells, such as synovium, cardiac endothelium, liver and lung, resulting in an acute but self-limited (4–8 days) cessation of red cell production and a corresponding decline in hemoglobin level. Among hosts with high red cell turnover, such as the fetus, this temporary failure of erythropoiesis can precipitate profound anemia and the equivalent of an aplastic crisis. By day 7 of infection, viremia peaks and IgM becomes detectable; thereafter, viral replication is contained by cell-mediated immunity driven by Th1 lymphocytes. Immune complex deposition is very common and may explain some clinical manifestations of parvovirus B-19 infection such as the polyarthritis seen in adults (see below).

Pathogenesis of mother-to-child transmission

The factors contributing to the fetal morbidity of parvovirus B-19 infection during pregnancy include the following.
• P antigen levels are highly expressed in the villous trophoblast and placental tissues during the first trimester, declining as the pregnancy progresses to undetectable levels by the third trimester [74].
• The red blood cell turnover during the hepatic stage of fetal hematopoiesis is very high during weeks 8–20 of gestation.
• The passive transfer of maternal IgG is not effective prior to week 25 of gestational age.
The maximal risk of vertical transmission is around day 7 of infection, when maternal viremia reaches its peak and IgM antibodies appear [75]. The most hazardous time for maternal infection is the early second trimester. Fetal myocardial cells express the P antigen and fetal myocarditis from parvovirus B-19 infection has been documented in the third trimester.

Clinical presentation

Parvovirus B-19 infection in pregnancy does not differ from the nonpregnant adult, but given its nonspecific symptoms and the potentially deleterious consequences to the fetus, laboratory diagnosis is recommended [76].

Following a 1-week incubation period, 80% of susceptible adults will develop a biphasic illness. The initial viremic phase is characterized by fever (rarely exceeding 39°C), malaise, myalgias and pruritus coinciding with viral shedding from the upper respiratory tract and appearance of anti-parvovirus B-19 IgM (anti-VP2). The immune complex-mediated stage (days 17–19 from initial infection) consists of rash and symmetric arthritis of the small joints of the hands, wrists, knees or ankles, seen more commonly in women. However, in many cases the symptoms are nonspecific and not recognized as parvovirus infection.

Obstetric considerations

Following exposure of a nonimmune pregnant woman, fetal infection is only a concern if the woman becomes infected. Then, the intrauterine transmission rate is 20–50% [77,78]. Despite this high rate of intrauterine transmission, many *in utero* fetal infections do not result in fetal disease [77]. Parvovirus B-19 is not teratogenic and does not result in structural anomalies in the fetus [79]. If infection results in fetal death, this usually occurs 4–6 weeks after maternal infection but has been reported at up to 12 weeks. Although fetal deaths have been reported in every trimester, the highest risk of fetal loss seems confined to the first 20 weeks of pregnancy and averages 9% [80]. Third-trimester intrauterine fetal death has been documented mostly in the absence of hydrops [81] and death has been postulated to result from fetal arrhythmias in the setting of myocarditis [82].

Nonimmune hydrops fetalis

The interval between parvovirus B-19 infection and development of nonimmune fetal hydrops ranges from 2 to 6 weeks, but up to 12 weeks in some studies [83]. Nonimmune fetal hydrops is characterized by marked fetal ascites, cardiomegaly, and pericardial effusions and, in advanced stages, generalized edema and hydropic placenta. The mechanism is severe fetal anemia, which leads to high output cardiogenic heart failure, more often during the hepatic stage (8–20 weeks gestation) of fetal hematopoiesis, when the half-life of erythrocytes is at its shortest [84]. Risk of B-19-induced hydrops fetalis is 3.9% throughout pregnancy, with a maximum of 7.1% when infection occurs between 13 and 20 weeks [85].

Diagnosis

The diagnosis of parvovirus B-19 infections during pregnancy and associated complications is a multistep process, including determination of maternal seroconversion, noninvasive fetal assessment to determine presence of fetal anemia with middle cerebral artery peak systolic velocity (MCA-PSV), and fetal blood sampling via cordocentesis for transfusion as necessary. Women infected with parvovirus B-19 (seroconverters) should be referred to a tertiary center with capability for MCA Doppler assessments or level II ultrasound capabilities for fetal assessment and surveillance, as weekly follow-up until 10–12 weeks after maternal exposure is advisable.

Pregnant women exposed to parvovirus B-19 should be tested for presence of parvovirus B-19 IgG to determine immune status. If this is negative, i.e. the woman is nonimmune and susceptible, then IgG should be repeated 2 weeks later to determine if seroconversion has occurred, i.e. she has become infected. In general, maternal recent infections (less than 1 month) are characterized by parvovirus B-19 IgM presence, high IgG titers and/or parvovirus B-19 DNA on maternal blood by PCR. At this stage, fetal complications, even if absent, can still develop [86], stressing the need for close fetal surveillance.

Fetal anemia results in a hyperdynamic pattern of blood flow in the middle cerebral artery due to the early response of brain tissue to anemia. MCA-PSV can be a very sensitive measure to identify fetal anemia secondary to parvovirus B-19 infection [87,88]. Weekly MCA-PSV measurements permit planning for cordocentesis to assess for actual fetal anemia and, if present, for fetal blood transfusions. Centers experienced in interpretation of MCA-PSV measurements and gestational age-specific comparisons should be accessed for accurate use of this tool.

Management

Opportune intrauterine transfusion (IUT) corrects fetal anemia and may reduce the mortality of B-19 infection significantly but there are no prospective data on the ideal timing to do so. Most clinicians proceed with transfusion if the fetus is anemic, even if there is already evidence of recovery of erythropoiesis by a high reticulocyte count. The neurodevelopmental prognosis of children surviving IUT for parvovirus B-19 is generally good, but some cases of delayed neurodevelopment have been associated with resolved parvovirus B-19 *in utero* infections. However, this does not seem to be related to the severity of fetal anemia and acidemia [89].

Prevention

There is no reasonable strategy to avoid B-19 exposure of pregnant women as exposure usually happens before the index case develops the rash, if symptomatic at all. For occupational exposures, the risk of occupational infection may be similar to or less than that in the community or at home. As a result, women in occupations such as school teaching do not warrant routine screening. However, if school-based outbreaks occur, selective screening may be appropriate.

Rubella

Rubella is a vaccine-preventable disease that usually causes a mild febrile rash in children and adults but it is a clearly recognized teratogenic agent. Congenital rubella syndrome (CRS), a rare occurrence in developed countries thanks to the childhood vaccination programs established 30 years ago, remains a significant cause of deafness, mental retardation and blindness in developing countries.

Virology

Rubella is a single-stranded RNA enveloped virus, with projecting glycoproteins E1, E2, and C. These glycoproteins do not undergo mutations, which makes natural and vaccine immunity attainable and long lasting.

Epidemiology

Rubella immunization dramatically decreased the incidence of infection and CRS in the United States, Canada and Western Europe. Although only a few hundred cases of rubella and less than 50 cases of CRS are reported each year in the US, up to 10% of women of reproductive age remain susceptible to rubella, in particular if they emigrated from countries where immunization has not been widely available. In developing countries 15–20% of women of reproductive age remain susceptible to rubella infection and a minimum of 100,000 cases of CRS happen every year worldwide [90].

Pathogenesis

Rubella infection is acquired by inhalation of virus particles; infection of upper respiratory tract cells is followed by lymphatic spread and subsequent viremia. The virus is detectable in blood and upper respiratory secretions 1 week before onset of symptoms. The rash develops at the same time that antibodies become detectable and viremia is cleared. Rubella-specific IgM usually persists for 8–12 weeks, but may be detected for up to a year. Immunity to rubella is lifelong, but a few cases of asymptomatic reinfection have been demonstrated [91].

Obstetric considerations

The outcomes of rubella infection during pregnancy include placental infection without fetal infection, both placental and fetal infection, resorption of the embryo, spontaneous abortion, stillbirth and congenital rubella syndrome.

Gestational age at the time of maternal rubella infection is the most important determinant of intrauterine infection risk and CRS [92–94]. Intrauterine infection (not a synonym of CRS) follows a bimodal distribution: 60–90% during the first trimester, 25% during the second trimester and 60–100% for infections acquired during the third trimester. However, the risk of CRS is confined to the first 20 weeks of pregnancy [95], as follows: 90% for maternal infections acquired prior to week 11, 33% for infections during weeks 11–12, 11% for weeks 13–14, and 24% for weeks 15–16.

Intrauterine infection arising from maternal reinfection has been the subject of much debate, but is considered very unlikely [96,97].

Clinical presentation

The clinical presentation and severity of rubella infection during pregnancy do not differ from nonpregnant adults; in general, 25% of infections are subclinical.

After an incubation period of approximately 2 weeks, adults develop fever and malaise, followed by a maculopapular rash (flat discolored areas and small raised lesions <1 cm in diameter) that starts on the face and gradually moves down to the feet. The most common complication is self-limited arthritis reported in up to 60% of women from natural infection and in 40% of women after vaccination; other complications include postinfectious encephalopathy (1:6000 cases), transient thrombocytopenia (1:3000), purpuric rash, and very rarely hemolytic anemia and Guillain–Barré syndrome [98].

Diagnosis

Acute rubella in pregnancy
Investigation of all rubella-like illnesses (fever, rash +/− arthralgias) in pregnancy is mandatory, as several other viruses have a very similar clinical presentation, including parvovirus B[19, measles, EBV, roseola, and some enteroviral infections, and yet the consequences for the fetus and the pregnancy can differ substantially among them (see Table 17.2).

In the right clinical context, acute infection is diagnosed by detection of rubella-specific IgM in one serum sample or by a fourfold increase in rubella antibody titers in paired samples (acute and convalescent) using the same assay [99]. Nevertheless, IgM may persist for up to a year after acute infection or vaccination and false-positive IgM results may arise from cross-reactivity with rheumatoid factor and other infections. IgG avidity tests (see explanation in preceding section on testing for CMV infection in pregnancy), where available, are helpful in these situations and a second rubella-specific IgM determination using a different assay is recommended as well, especially in the first 20 weeks of pregnancy [98]. Knowledge of local clinical and laboratory capabilities is critical when interpreting results, especially if pregnancy termination is being considered.

Prenatal diagnosis of fetal infection
Many cases of CRS do not have characteristic ultrasound findings. Viral detection by molecular technology (RT-PCR) in amniotic fluid is the preferred method for prenatal diagnosis of fetal infection, and has a reported sensitivity of 87–100% [100,101], when done at least 6–8 weeks after maternal infection to avoid false-negative results. Rubella virus isolation by chorionic villous sampling is used at some centers but might be misleading, as placental infection does not imply fetal infection [99].

Exposure to rubella during pregnancy
All nonimmune pregnant women exposed to close contacts of rubella or rubella-like illnesses should have rubella IgG paired serum samples (at least 2 weeks apart).

Management

There is no specific treatment for rubella infection, and postexposure prophylaxis with immunoglobulin for susceptible women is not recommended as there is no solid evidence that it prevents rubella infection. The US Centers for Disease Control and Prevention (CDC) does support its use in pregnancy only for those susceptible women who have been exposed to rubella who will not consider a termination under any circumstances. Although the immunoglobulin may ameliorate maternal symptoms to some degree, patients need to be informed that this does not imply that the fetus has been protected from infection [102].

Prevention

Rubella vaccine is a highly effective and very well-tolerated live-attenuated product. It has been usually given in combination with mumps and measles vaccines (MMR) and more recently with varicella-zoster vaccine (MMRV). Routine prenatal testing in most countries includes rubella antibody titers, and a titer >15 IU/mL is considered protective [103]. As is the case for all live-attenuated vaccines, rubella vaccine is not recommended during pregnancy [104]; women identified as seronegative should receive vaccination shortly after delivery. Inadvertent use of rubella vaccine among susceptible pregnant women against rubella has not resulted in CRS in their infants [105,106].

Mumps

Mumps is a vaccine-preventable disease that has re-emerged in the US and western Europe among young adults over the last decade. Although mumps infection usually results in a self-limited febrile illness with characteristic bilateral parotid gland swelling among children and teenagers, it does increase the risk of miscarriage if contracted during the first trimester of pregnancy and follows a more complicated course in adults.

Epidemiology

Mumps infection is prevalent worldwide and close to 90% of cases develop during childhood in developing countries. It became a rare illness in industrialized countries after the introduction of a live-attenuated vaccine 30 years ago. However, recent epidemics in the US and the UK involving thousands of adults have revealed gaps in vaccine coverage and/or systematic errors in vaccine delivery resulting in critical numbers of susceptible individuals [107].

Pathogenesis

Mumps is highly infectious. It is acquired by inhalation of infectious droplets from coughing, sneezing or talking. During the incubation period, mumps replicates in the upper respiratory tract cells; then viremia ensues, followed by localization to the central nervous system and salivary glands occurs (parotitis). Cases can transmit the infection 1 week before the onset of parotitis.

Clinical presentation

Close to 30% of infections are subclinical [108]. When symptomatic, infection in pregnant hosts does not differ from the nonpregnant. The incubation period lasts 16–18 days; then, a nonspecific prodrome of low-grade fever, anorexia, and malaise is followed by parotitis. Epididymo-orchitis is apparent in 25% of men and oophoritis in 5% of women. Adults tend to have extraglandular manifestations even in the absence of parotitis, and follow a more complicated course including CSF leukocytosis in 50% of cases, meningitis 1–15%, pancreatitis 5%, encephalitis 0.1%, transient deafness 4%, permanent deafness 1:15,000, and transient renal function abnormalities in over 60% of patients.

Obstetric considerations

In general, mumps infection during pregnancy is not an indication for termination of the pregnancy. Maternal mumps during the first trimester is associated with excessive numbers of spontaneous losses [109] (fetal demise happening within 2 weeks of maternal mumps onset). Mumps is not a recognized cause of congenital malformations [110] or prematurity [109], except for endocardial fibroelastosis (EFE), a very rare entity [111] consisting of congenital diffuse thickening of the ventricular endocardium that presents typically as heart failure in infants. Controversy exists on a potential link between juvenile diabetes mellitus and mumps, but unlike EFE, diabetes mellitus incidence has not dropped in parallel with mumps incidence [112].

Diagnosis

Diagnosis can usually be made with history of exposure and symptoms. Mumps virus can be isolated from saliva, CSF or serum. Mumps-specific IgM is detectable in serum as early as 11 days after exposure and for almost 100% of cases at the time of clinical illness. A significant rise in mumps-specific immunoglobulin titers between acute and convalescent serum samples by any standard serologic assay is diagnostic [106]. Positive IgM in saliva is the method of choice in some countries [98].

Management and prevention

The treatment of mumps and its complications is primarily supportive. Mumps vaccine is a live-attenuated product that induces detectable immunity in up to 95% of recipients. It is currently delivered with rubella and measles vaccines in the form of MMR (see Vaccination in pregnancy section). As with other live vaccines, it is not recommended in pregnancy, but inadvertent vaccination has not resulted in fetal disease. Pregnancy should be delayed for 4 weeks after administration of the MMR vaccine [104].

Viral infections that affect both maternal and fetal health

Measles

Measles is a highly contagious, vaccine-preventable disease. Measles in pregnancy can be detrimental for the mother and the fetus, stressing the need for appropriate vaccination of women of reproductive age.

Virology

Measles is an enveloped RNA virus, that remains infective (droplet form) in the air for hours under low humidity conditions (e.g. in winter) [113].

Epidemiology

Measles accounts for approximately 240,000 deaths per year among children under 5 in developing countries [90]. In North America and western Europe, outbreaks affect mostly young adults, and generally arise through travel of infected individuals from countries with lower vaccine rates [114,115].

Pathogenesis

Measles is acquired by inhalation of infectious droplets from the respiratory secretions of infected persons. Peak infectivity happens just before the rash appears when cough and sneezing are at their worst. Local replication in the upper respiratory tract leads to sequential bouts of viremia. Characteristic Koplik's spots (see below) and rash develop once specific cellular immunity appears. Protective antibodies from natural infection or immunization are life-long.

Clinical presentation during pregnancy

Clinical course in pregnancy has been observed to be more severe on the basis of primary measles pneumonia and heart failure-related mortality and morbidity [116]; this initial observation in the 1940s and 1950s was confirmed during the more recent measles resurgence in the US and Japan, when 54–60% of gestational measles cases developed respiratory complications [116–118].

In general, the incubation period of 14 days is followed by a prodromal phase lasting several days consisting of malaise, fever, conjunctivitis, cough and coryza; at the end of this phase and just before the rash starts, the characteristic Koplik's spots (bluish-gray dots on a red base) are found in the oral mucosa. The maculopapular rash (flat discolored areas and small raised lesions <1 cm in diameter) starts on the face and progresses to the extremities, involving palms and soles. The most common complication is primary measles pneumonia, followed by bacterial superinfection, sinusitis, hepatitis and encephalitis.

Obstetric considerations

It has not been established if measles causes congenital defects [119]. However, it has been associated with higher rates of spontaneous abortion and stillbirth [116,118].There is a well-documented increased risk of prematurity [109]. Mother-to-child transmission is uncommon and neonatal measles (rash up to day 10 of life) is very rare.

Diagnosis

Diagnosis can easily be made on clinical presentation, but laboratory diagnosis is recommended as measles is not common

enough in most developed countries for physicians to be familiar with its presentation. A fourfold increase in total measles antibody titers in two separate (by 2 weeks) serum samples is diagnostic in low-prevalence countries such as the UK and the US [106]. For developing nations with a high prevalence of measles, a single serum IgM measurement (preferably in the setting of negative IgG antibodies) is considered adequate. Direct viral isolation by reverse transcriptase PCR (RT-PCR) is rarely necessary and usually reserved for atypical presentations (lack of rash among immunocompromised patients) or life-threatening pneumonia [120].

Treatment

Treatment is supportive. However, given the increased rate of complications during pregnancy, mainly respiratory, a high index of suspicion is required. Admission to hospital is recommended. Although high-dose vitamin A and ribavirin have been tried outside pregnancy [121,122], these are not generally recommended in pregnancy due to their teratogenic potential.

Prevention

Measles can be prevented by a live-attenuated vaccine, which is recommended for children at the age of 18 months, in conjunction with mumps and rubella, once maternal antibodies have disappeared. Immunity induced by measles vaccine does not seem to wane with time, and reported infection in vaccine recipients likely reflects primary vaccine failures from inappropriate vaccine administration (given too early, cold-chain breakdowns, etc.).

Vaccination for nonimmune women of childbearing age should be encouraged. As with other live vaccines, measles vaccine is not recommended in pregnancy, but inadvertent vaccination has not resulted in adverse fetal outcomes (see Vaccination in pregnancy section). Susceptible pregnant women who have had close contact with a documented case of measles in the previous 6 days may benefit from passive immunization with immune globulin [104].

Viral Infections that affect both maternal and neonatal health

Varicella-zoster virus infection

Varicella-zoster virus (VZV) infection causes chickenpox, a contagious generalized vesicular rash, and herpes zoster ("shingles"), a dermatomal reactivation later in life. Chickenpox peripartum is a documented cause of severe and potentially lethal neonatal disease and chickenpox during pregnancy causes an infrequent but well-described congenital syndrome. VZV infection is vaccine preventable, and a live-attenuated vaccine is available for use in healthy children and in susceptible adults.

Virology

Varicella-zoster is a double-stranded DNA virus, a member of the Herpesviridae family, and like other members of the family, it has a short reproductive cycle, destroys the infected cells at the time of viral release, spreads from cell to cell by direct contact and establishes latency following primary infection (see Herpes simplex section).

Epidemiology

Prior to the recent inception of VZV vaccine, 90% of the population in temperate climates had suffered chickenpox by 15 years of age. Chickenpox-associated mortality during childhood is less than 2 per 100,000 cases but increases by 15-fold for adults. The true annual incidence of primary VZV infection in pregnancy is not known, but its annual rate is estimated to be 1.6–4.6 per 1000 pregnancies in North America [123]. VZV infection during the first and second trimesters may result in fetal infection in a small proportion of cases (0.45% and 2% respectively, with congenital infection essentially not reported when occurring at greater than 20 weeks of gestation [124]). The incidence of congenital varicella syndrome is unknown; the expected number of cases per year is 41 in the US, four in Canada, seven in UK and Germany [125].

The estimated incidence of herpes zoster ("shingles") in pregnancy is 1 per 10,000 pregnancies [126].

Pathogenesis

Varicella is acquired from direct contact with the vesicular fluid of the skin lesions and/or secretions from the respiratory tract. Infectivity peaks 2 days before the onset of rash (between days 15 and 19 from infection; see below under clinical presentation) but risk of contagiousness continues until the vesicles crust over, about 5 days after the onset of rash. After resolution of primary infection, the virus remains in the sensory dorsal root ganglia until reactivation happens in the form of herpes zoster (shingles). In general, immunity against VZV wanes with time which explains VZV reactivation. Reinfection is rare but may happen, particularly if the person had chickenpox in the first year of life [127].

Pathogenesis of VZV infection in the first and second trimesters of pregnancy

The risk of developing congenital varicella syndrome is confined to the first half of pregnancy, weeks 7–20 [124], yet is low at only 1–2% [119]. Congenital varicella syndrome is characterized by a combination of skin lesions (dermatomal scarring),

present in 70% of the cases, ocular and CNS abnormalities (chorioretinitis, optic atrophy, micro-ophthalmos, cortical atrophy, mental retardation) in 60% of cases and musculoskeletal abnormalities (hypoplastic lower limbs, clubbed feet) in 50% of cases. Low birthweight, gastrointestinal tract defects and zoster in infancy are observed as well.

Pathogenesis of VZV infection in the third trimester of pregnancy

Maternal VZV infection (chickenpox) within 4 weeks prior to delivery can result in transplacental infection and neonatal chickenpox, 24–50% of the time [122]. Neonatal VZV infection is defined by appearance of neonatal rash within 10 days of birth; earlier appearance of neonatal rash (days 0–4) is associated with better survival than late (days 5–10), reflecting the protective effect of maternal immunity. Neonatal chickenpox clinical presentation ranges from widespread skin rash and severe pneumonia to sparse skin lesions, without evidence of systemic disease.

Maternal rash onset between 5 days prior to 2 days after delivery is thought to be the most critical period in terms of neonatal VZV mortality and morbidity. However, severe neonatal disease has occasionally been reported with maternal rash appearing 7 days prior to delivery [128].

Clinical presentation in pregnancy

Clinical presentation in pregnancy is very similar to that in nonpregnant women. However, varicella pneumonitis, which is more likely to happen in pregnancy, results in higher rates of morbidity and mortality among pregnant patients [129,130].

Following an incubation period of 13–17 days, a prodrome of headache, fever, and malaise for 2 days is followed by the characteristic rash, which consists of maculopapules, vesicles, and scabs in varying stages of evolution as successive crops of lesions appear over a period of 2–4 days. The rash usually starts in the trunk and face and may involve the oropharynx and vagina. Adult chickenpox complications include varicella pneumonitis (1 in 400 cases), acute cerebellar ataxia, encephalitis, hepatitis and rarely thrombocytopenic purpura and myocarditis.

Risk factors for development of VZV pneumonitis in pregnancy include cigarette smoking and ≥100 skin lesions [129]. Respiratory symptoms develop 4 days after the development of the rash and include tachypnea, dyspnea, cough, hemoptysis, chest pain, and cyanosis. The classic radiographic changes include bilateral, diffuse, peribronchial nodular infiltrates but there is poor correlation between the symptoms and the auscultatory or radiographic findings.

Zoster (shingles) presentation in pregnancy is the same as that among nonpregnant immune-competent adults. Patients present with burning, stabbing or throbbing pain on a dermatomal distribution that may precede the typical dermatomal vesicular rash by days to weeks. New vesicular lesions usually stop appearing by day 7–10 and the rash resolves within 4 weeks; 10–15% of patients will develop postherpetic neuralgia that may persist for months. Lumbosacral zoster late in the third trimester may be clinically difficult to differentiate from HSV.

Diagnosis

Chickenpox and herpes zoster are diagnosed clinically in most cases but pregnancy mandates laboratory confirmation. Rapid virus identification techniques are used to confirm clinical suspicion of disease in pregnant women; maternal specimens are obtained by unroofing a vesicle, rubbing the base of the lesion with a polyester swab and sending it for PCR or direct fluorescent antibody (DFA) testing. Assessment of antibodies to VZV is very helpful in determining maternal susceptibility to VZV in the case of an exposure history [125,131].

Prenatal diagnosis of VZV infections in case of maternal infection between weeks 7 and 20 should be conducted in a systematic fashion, firstly confirming the maternal infection and then assessing the fetus by detailed ultrasound at 18–20 weeks, or at least 5 weeks following the rash in the mother to assess for *in utero* features of congenital varicella. Sequential ultrasound over the course of pregnancy is recommended to demonstrate features of *in utero* recurrent fetal infection including growth restriction, isolated limb abnormalities or CNS infection. Fetal MRI may be of assistance in further elucidating fetal anomalies, as CNS abnormalities not visualized on ultrasound, such as cerebellar hypoplasia, have been identified with MRI [132]. In addition, amniocentesis can be helpful in confirming fetal exposure with detection of VZV by PCR. However, this does not predict the severity of fetal infection [133]. Ophthalmologic exam at birth for the neonate is highly recommended.

Prevention

Women should be screened in pregnancy for VZV immunity by history and, if negative, by assessment of presence of VZV IgG. Susceptible women should be offered vaccination post partum [134]. The VZ vaccine is live-attenuated and not recommended for use in pregnancy [134].

Administration of VZ immune globulin (IG) is recommended for all susceptible pregnant women within 96 hours of exposure to chickenpox [134]. Exposure is defined as household contact, face-to-face contact with an index case for at least 5 minutes, being indoors with an index case for more than 1 hour or sharing the same hospital room with a contagious patient. Confirmation of VZV immunity prior to VZ IG administration is ideal given that 80% of adults with negative history of chickenpox are immune; however, this is not always possible in the clinical setting and VZ IG is not effective if given more than 5 days after exposure.

VZ IG only prevents 80% of cases, and if chickenpox develops despite VZ IG use, it will be delayed a mean of 3 weeks. Vaccination of susceptible women of childbearing age is recommended [134].

Management

Treatment of VZV infection or exposure during pregnancy is summarized in Table 17.4, providing maternal, fetal and neonatal considerations.

Uncomplicated maternal chickenpox in the first 20 weeks of pregnancy

In general, hospitalization is not necessary for all pregnant patients with chickenpox, but close observation and symptom control with fluids, analgesic and antipruritic agents should be provided. Treatment with acyclovir (800 mg 5 times/day for 7 days) should be considered for maternal benefit; if started within 24 hours of rash, it decreases the duration of symptoms and number of lesions by 25% [135]. However, there is no evidence of benefit on the course of fetal infection or the risk of VZV-associated embryopathy. Acyclovir is widely used in pregnancy and deemed safe for the fetus [136,137]. If admitted to the hospital, patients should be isolated from other potentially susceptible gravidas and healthcare workers; contact and air-borne precautions [138] must be followed.

Fetal surveillance with level II ultrasound at 18–20 weeks, and/or 5 weeks after onset of maternal rash, plus sequential ultrasound is indicated (see diagnosis section). Counseling regarding the risks of fetal infection, congenital varicella syndrome (CVS) and continuation of pregnancy is warranted.

Uncomplicated maternal chickenpox between 20 weeks of pregnancy to 5 days prior to delivery

The risk of CVS is extremely low in this situation, and termination of pregnancy is not indicated. Otherwise, the maternal, fetal and neonatal recommendations given above apply.

Uncomplicated maternal chickenpox 5 days before or 2 days after delivery

Infants born to women with chickenpox within this time period should be treated with VZ IG [138]. Although VZ IG may fail to prevent up to 50% of neonatal chickenpox in this setting, the severity of the infection is greatly reduced [139]. If possible, delaying delivery until 5–7 days after onset of maternal rash to allow transfer of IgG from mother to fetus is recommended. Intravenous acyclovir has been used for neonates displaying signs of infection, to prevent or ameliorate severe sequelae. Contact and air-borne isolation is indicated for both mother and infant.

Table 17.4 VZV in pregnancy: treatment and prevention

Clinical situation	Maternal intervention	Fetal surveillance	Intervention for newborn
Susceptible mother with close exposure at any point in pregnancy	• Confirm susceptible status: VZV serology • If susceptible, consider administration of VZ IG (presently only available in the US as lyophilized purified varicella immune globulin (VariZIG™) or immune globulin (IVIG)) within 96 hours of exposure	• No intervention necessary if mother not susceptible or mother does not develop clinical syndrome	• No intervention necessary if mother not susceptible or mother does not develop clinical syndrome
Uncomplicated maternal chickenpox in the first 20 weeks of pregnancy	• Symptom control for fever, pruritus and volume depletion • May consider oral acyclovir 800 mg 5 times/day for 7 days to reduce duration of rash and number of lesions • Contact (gloves, gowns) and air-borne precautions if in hospital • Discussion on risk of congenital varicella syndrome (CVS) and continuation of pregnancy is warranted	• Level II ultrasound at 18–20 weeks and/or 5 weeks after onset of maternal rash, plus • Sequential ultrasound over the course of pregnancy to detect features of *in utero* recurrent fetal infection • Consider fetal MRI for CNS abnormalities not seen on ultrasound	• Ophthalmologic exam at birth highly recommended
Uncomplicated maternal chickenpox any time between 20 weeks of gestation to 5 days prior to delivery	• Symptom control for fever, pruritus and volume depletion • May consider oral acyclovir 800 mg 5 times/day for 7 days to reduce duration of rash and number of lesions • Contact (gloves, gowns) and air-borne precautions if in hospital	• Not an indication for termination of pregnancy as risk of CVS is extremely low • Level II ultrasound at 18–20 weeks and/or 5 weeks after onset of maternal rash	• Ophthalmologic exam at birth
Uncomplicated maternal chickenpox 5 days before delivery or 2 days post partum	As above	No special monitoring required	• VZ IG at birth or as soon as maternal rash is recognized • IV acyclovir if severe illness • Contact (gloves, gowns) and air-borne precautions in the nursery
Complicated maternal chickenpox (pneumonia, CNS disease) or disseminated zoster	• Admit to hospital: respiratory support may be required • IV Acyclovir • Consider IV antibiotics for pneumonia superinfection • Contact and air-borne precautions	As above for relevant gestational age	As above for relevant gestational age
Maternal zoster in late pregnancy	• Confirm diagnosis if lumbosacral area with PCR or DFA • Consider use of acyclovir 800 mg PO 5 times/day within first 72 hours of rash appearing	No special monitoring required	Contact (gloves, gowns) and air-borne precautions in the nursery if zoster confirmed

VZV pneumonia

A high index of suspicion is required in the presence of risk factors for development of VZV pneumonia, including third trimester, smoking, co-morbidities (asthma/COPD, transplant recipients) and severe rash. Respiratory symptoms should prompt hospitalization, assessment with chest X-rays, transcutaneous oxygen saturation and treatment with intravenous acyclovir 10 mg/kg every 8 hours.

Herpes simplex viruses 1 and 2

Adult herpes simplex virus (HSV) infections are very common but remain largely unrecognized: HSV-2 is the number one cause of genital ulcer disease worldwide. Neonatal HSV infections (acquired from the maternal genital tract at or around time of delivery) are fortunately infrequent (approximately 1 in 3200 livebirths in the US [140]), but may have devastating consequences for the newborn, including death and permanent disability. A very infrequent but well-described congenital syndrome has been reported. Vaccines to prevent the burden of HSV infections are being developed but are not currently available.

Epidemiology

In general, prevalence of antibodies to HSV increases with age and demonstrates an inverse correlation with socioeconomic status. HSV-1 is usually acquired in childhood and HSV-2 later in life by means of sexual contact; however, HSV-1 accounts for 20–40% of newly diagnosed genital infections in some geographic regions [141]. Thirty percent of middle-class women attending prenatal clinics in the US have serologic evidence of HSV-2 infection [142] but only a quarter of these women are aware of their infection based on clinical history. It is estimated that 2% of pregnant women will acquire new genital HSV infection during pregnancy. However, of those newly acquired infections, 70% will not be clinically recognized [143].

Virology and pathogenesis

Herpes simplex viruses 1 and 2 are double-stranded DNA viruses, distinguished by their surface glycoprotein, that exhibit only 50% of genetic homology with one another, so infection with one type does not prevent infection with the other.

Herpes simplex virus is acquired by mucosal contact with a person excreting the virus. Following viral attachment and mucosal replication, HSV gains access to the regional dorsal root ganglia or sensory ganglia by "retrograde" transport, starting at the sensory nerve endings. From the sensory ganglia it reactivates and travels down the axon to the skin or mucosal surface, resulting in asymptomatic shedding or clinically apparent disease. Reactivation rates at 1 year following genital herpes are as high as 90% if the infection was caused by HSV-2 compared to 55% by HSV-1, yet two-thirds of all reactivations are subclinical and history and physical examination fail to identify over 50% of individuals with HSV infection [144]. Asymptomatic shedding is the most common mechanism of sexual HSV transmission [145]; anogenital HSV-2 shedding has been demonstrated 20% of the time among immunocompetent HSV-2 seropositive hosts, with a median duration of 13 hours per episode [146].

Innate immunity is very important against HSV as demonstrated by the severity of HSV infections among patients with natural killer (NK) cells and interferon-gamma deficiencies [147]. T-cell immunity is likely important to prevent visceral spread of HSV [148].

Pathogenesis of congenital and neonatal infections

In rare cases, with maternal primary infection, transplacental transmission has been described with *in utero* infection. This usually results in very severe infection with fetal demise (see section below on obstetric considerations). More commonly, neonatal infection occurs in the context of genital viral shedding at the time of delivery and is reduced by the transfer of maternal antibodies prior to birth; these two factors are determined by the type of maternal infection.

Herpes simplex virus infections are classified according to site of infection (anogenital or orolabial); state of infection (initial or recurrent); and prior immune status (primary or nonprimary (infection usually at another site)). *Primary infection* means infection by either HSV-1 or HSV-2 in a host that has not already been infected by the other virus subtype. *First episode nonprimary infection* means the host has acquired a new infection, usually HSV-2, but has antibodies against the other subtype, usually HSV-1. *Reactivation* implies active viral shedding from a latent infection by either subtype. Neonatal transmission rates for HSV infections at or near the time of labor are 50% or more for primary maternal infections, 30% for first episode nonprimary infections with either HSV-1 or HSV-2, and only 2% for reactivations [149]. Primary infections are associated with high and prolonged HSV cervical shedding($>10^6$ viral particles per 0.2 mL of inoculum for 2–3 weeks) when compared with symptomatic reactivations ($>10^2$–10^3 viral particles per 0.2 mL of inoculum for 2–5 days).

Other factors implicated in neonatal transmission have included prolonged duration of rupture of membranes (>6 hours), breach of fetal integrity of mucocutaneous barriers (i.e. use of fetal scalp electrodes) and mode of delivery – see treatment section below. Seventy percent of neonatal HSV infections occur in couples with a negative history of genital HSV infection and from asymptomatic women during both pregnancy and labor [150]. Several studies have shown that about 1% of women who are HSV-2 seropositive have their genital reactivation at delivery [149,151]; however, only about 2–4% of those exposed infants will develop neonatal herpes, presumably because of the protective effects of maternally transferred antibodies [149].

Clinical presentation

Incubation period for HSV infection averages 4–6 days. Primary HSV-1 and -2 infections may affect the oral mucosa (gingivostomatitis, pharyngitis or herpes labialis), the genital mucosa (genital herpes, usually on dermatomes S2 and S3), the central nervous system (aseptic meningitis, encephalitis, myelitis) and the eyes (conjunctivitis or keratitis).

The clinical features of primary and recurrent genital herpes do not differ between pregnant and nonpregnant women, except for the fact that recurrences appear to increase in frequency over the course of pregnancy [152,153].

Close to 70% of newly acquired HSV infections among pregnant women are asymptomatic or unrecognized [143]. Primary genital herpes, if typical, is characterized by genital vesicular lesions with an erythematous base, involving the cervix and urethra in 80% of cases, as well as the genital skin or adjacent areas. It may be accompanied by fever, headache, malaise, and myalgias. Women with HSV-2 first episode but prior HSV-1 infection report fewer systemic symptoms and faster healing than primary genital herpes. The incidence of reactivation of latent genital HSV infection and asymptomatic viral shedding on any day in pregnancy is approximately 1% (0.6–4%) [149].

Disseminated HSV should be considered in pregnant women presenting with a flu-like syndrome in the second half of pregnancy with progression to pneumonitis, hepatitis, and/or encephalitis [154]. HSV hepatitis, although rare, can present with fever, abdominal tenderness, and highly elevated transaminases with close to normal bilirubin. It is part of the differential diagnosis of acute fatty liver of pregnancy. HSV encephalitis in pregnancy (presenting with new-onset seizures) [155] and HSV endometritis (presenting with persistent puerperal fever) [156] have been described.

Obstetric considerations

Prospective studies have shown that HSV primary infections do not increase the incidence of abortion [143], premature rupture of membranes or prematurity, in contrast to case reports associating HSV infection with these events[157].

Intrauterine infection resulting in congenital HSV-related "TORCH" infection is a very uncommon but well-described occurrence. As of 2006, 30 cases of documented HSV intrauterine infections resulting from both primary and secondary infections have been reported, ranging from skin vesicles to severe CNS sequelae in the fetus/neonate; the risk of intrauterine infection following maternal infection is very small at 1:200,000 [157].

Diagnosis of symptomatic genital disease in pregnancy

Laboratory-based diagnosis of HSV infections in pregnancy is important for appropriate management [158]. Clinical diagnosis is not accurate because the manifestations of HSV can vary widely. HSV can be identified by viral culture and/or nucleic acid amplifications tests (NAAT), i.e. PCR, if sufficient virus is collected from the lesions. Scrapings of cells from the base of active lesions/ulcers or aspiration of vesicular fluid are the most useful specimens, but in order to increase the yield, swabbing multiple sites (vulva, cervix, anal canal), even in the absence of lesions, and urine viral culture are recommended. Atypical presentations or potential complications require a high index of suspicion and acquisition of clinical specimens is indicated (CSF, endometrial biopsy, etc.) [159]. Type-specific HSV serology is an important diagnostic tool for women whose cultures or PCR assays are negative; HSV-2 seropositivity does not confirm genital herpes, but it makes it very likely, particularly if there is history of lesions in the appropriate dermatomes [158]. HSV-1 seropositivity in the presence of a genital lesion warrants a viral identification test for confirmation. Nonspecific type serology is only useful if negative, to confirm susceptibility.

Diagnosis of asymptomatic infection in pregnancy

Routine antenatal type-specific HSV screening to ascertain HSV status has not been shown to decrease the burden of neonatal disease, and it is not recommended at present. However, it may have a role for pregnant women with a history of lesions suspicious for genital herpes or undiagnosed urologic or anogenital symptoms, in which viral identification tests cannot be performed or are negative. In addition, it may be useful to decrease the risk of transmission to a susceptible partner or a baby, in the case of serodiscordant couples [158].

Treatment

Treatment of primary maternal HSV infection

The maternal benefit derived from treating symptomatic primary HSV infection, including during the first trimester, likely outweighs the theoretical fetal risks. There are enough data to support the safety of acyclovir during pregnancy [136]. Acyclovir is known to cross the placenta but does not seem to accumulate in the amniotic fluid [136]. The bio-availability of oral acyclovir is very low, requiring frequent dosing to achieve therapeutic levels.

Primary infections in the third trimester when the risk of neonatal transmission is at its highest (30–50%) warrant delivery by elective cesarean section. If a first episode nonprimary rather than a primary infection is suspected, but determination of sero-status is not possible, then management as a primary infection is reasonable.

Treatment of maternal recurrent HSV infection

Treatment prior to 36 weeks for recurrent HSV infection in pregnancy is not currently recommended, unless the manifestations are clinically severe or unacceptable to the patient [158].

Beginning at 36 weeks, prophylactic use of acyclovir 400 mg three times a day or valacyclovir 500 mg twice day among women with a history of recurrent genital HSV infections (particularly patients who have had one or more genital HSV recurrences during pregnancy) has been shown to reduce the risk of clinical HSV recurrence at delivery, cesarean delivery rates for recurrent genital herpes, and risk of HSV viral shedding in randomized controlled trials [159]. Famcyclovir use in pregnancy is not recommended due to a paucity of safety or efficacy data.

Management during delivery

Cesarean section has been shown to significantly decrease the risk of neonatal HSV among women with HSV-positive genital secretions at the time of labor regardless of use of antiretrovirals and is therefore recommended for all women with active HSV genital lesions [140]. Cesarean delivery is more effective if done before the rupture of membranes, and should be done within 4–6 hours of membrane rupture. Patients with history of recurrent genital herpes should be educated about coming to the delivery room early in labor for careful examination. Routine use of viral cultures or PCR to identify asymptomatic viral shedding is not recommended at the time of this writing. Prodromal symptoms at the time of labor also warrant recommendation for an elective cesarean section as this is highly predictive of genital viral shedding [158,161,162].

Postpartum management

Maternal orolabial or anogenital HSV lesions require proper hand washing and contact precautions to avoid exposure of the infant. Breastfeeding women can use acyclovir if required for management of maternal disease and it is rated compatible with breastfeeding as per the American Academy of Pediatrics. Although acyclovir is concentrated in breast milk, the total dose received by infants of nursing mothers treated is about 1% of the effective neonatal dose [163,164]. Breastfeeding is not contraindicated unless there are active lesions on the breast.

Prevention

Herpes simplex virus vaccine trials have not been highly successful to date, and vaccines to prevent gestational and peripartum HSV infection and subsequent neonatal transmission are not currently available.

Infection control

Mothers with active genital or orolabial herpes at the time of delivery should not be isolated from their babies, as long as they can wash their hands prior to handling their children.

Human papillomavirus

Genital human papillomavirus (HPV) is the most common sexually transmitted infection in North America; 70% of sexually active women will contract the infection during their lifetime. Mother-to-child transmission of HPV is uncommon, and presence of condyloma is not an indication for cesarean delivery.

Virology

Human papillomavirus is a nonenveloped double-stranded DNA virus. Over 100 HPV types are known and approximately 40 are known to infect the genital tract. The most common types can be classified according to their oncogenic potential as low-risk types (mainly 6 and 11), being responsible for 90% of genital warts and some low-grade CIN, and high-risk types, including 16 and 18, associated with cervical, vulvar, penile, and anal cancers; 70% of cervical cancer is caused by 16 and 18.

Epidemiology

The reported prevalence of HPV infection in pregnancy has ranged from 5.5% to 65% [165]. The incidence of juvenile-onset recurrent respiratory papillomatosis (JORRP) is 3.96/100,000 in the general pediatric population [23] versus 7/1000 among children born to mothers with a history of vaginal condyloma [166]. Risk factors for JORRP include vaginal delivery, being a firstborn and maternal age younger than 20 [166].

Pathogenesis

Genital HPV is acquired through skin-to-skin contact, usually with sexual contact. HPV infects epithelium preferentially; it starts replication in the basal cell (deepest) layer of epithelium and likely gets through microtrauma or abrasion. Oncogenic HPV types disrupt normal cell architecture and function, leading to abnormal cell proliferation and accumulation of nonrepairable DNA; HPV's ability to integrate its DNA leads to its oncogenic potential as it disrupts normal cellular mechanisms that result in natural apoptosis.

Immunity to HPV is not well understood; naturally acquired antibodies against the nuclear capsid are present in 90% of infected persons but they only seem to limit but not to eradicate the infection. Decreased cell-mediated immunity (i.e. advanced HIV infection) is known to favor HPV reactivation or persistence [167].

Mother-to-child transmission

Human papillomavirus infection in children is primarily acquired by passage through an infected birth canal [168]. However, instances of cesarean section failing to prevent transmission are reported, suggesting acquisition of infection *in utero* [168] or by ascending infection in the setting of premature rupture of membranes. Breastfeeding is not a recognized route of transmission.

Clinical presentation

Although pregnancy does not seem to increase susceptibility to acquire HPV infection, increased incidence and severity of genital HPV, often with substantial growth of genital warts, are described. In general, infection with low-risk HPV types has an incubation period of 3–4 months before anogenital warts appear, usually as helophytic and hyperkeratotic papules located over the posterior introitus, but also over the labia and clitoris.

Obstetric considerations

Genital HPV infection has not been linked to any adverse fetal or neonatal outcomes except for JORRP. The reported rate of mother-to-child transmission of HPV has varied widely, but is likely to be low at 1.6% [169]. Even though HPV can be recovered in up to 30% of infants exposed to HPV at birth, only 1 in 400 children delivered vaginally in the presence of genital warts will develop JORRP, and other factors (patient immunity, timing, virus exposure, and local trauma) play a role. Almost all cases of JORRP are diagnosed by the age of 4 [170,171].

Treatment

Treatment of genital HPV during pregnancy is not routinely advocated. Because genital HPV infection may behave more aggressively during pregnancy, cryotherapy or laser treatment may be used very selectively for maternal symptom management. Usual management is observation and treatment post partum as the lesions usually decrease in size and treatment is less complicated. Treatment with podophyllin, podophyllotoxin, interferon and 5-FU are all contraindicated in pregnancy. Very little is known about imiquimod use in pregnancy and its use in pregnancy is generally not recommended.

Prevention

Two recombinant HPV vaccines (quadrivalent against types 6, 11, 16 and 18, and bivalent against types 16 and 18) are currently licensed for use at ages 11-26 years, administered as a three dose-series over the course of 6 months [172]. Although vaccination is not recommended during pregnancy, administration of quadrivalent HPV vaccine to n = 1796 women who became pregnant during licensing studies did not result on adverse pregnancy outcomes [173].

Prevention of mother-to-child HPV transmission
Cesarean delivery is not recommended to prevent HPV transmission or development of JORRP in children born to mothers with known HPV genital tract infection [166], as less than 1% of women with a history of genital warts will have children with JORRP. Yet, risk of bleeding, mechanical obstruction of birth canal and other factors need to be considered prior to deciding on mode of delivery.

Viral infections that result in increased neonatal morbidity

Enteroviruses: polio, coxsackieviruses and echoviruses

Enteroviruses include polio, coxsackie and echoviruses, among others. They account for a wide variety of illnesses, most of them subclinical or very mild, including rashes (e.g. hand-foot and mouth disease) and conjunctivitis, yet severe diseases, like poliomyelitis, aseptic meningitis, encephalitis and myocarditis, are well described. Although poliomyelitis is virtually eliminated in developed countries, other enteroviral infections are increasingly being recognized; neonates are at particular risk of severe generalized enteroviral infection acquired from the mother at the time of birth from fecal–oral contact. Poliomyelitis also has a detrimental effect on maternal heath.

Epidemiology

Enteroviruses are found worldwide. In temperate climates most infections occur in the summer and fall, but in the tropical areas they happen year round. Outbreaks of coxsackieviruses and echoviruses are now recognized to occur regularly, but the true incidence of these infections in pregnancy is unknown. Polio has been eliminated from the Americas, Europe and WHO Western Pacific regions thanks to the vaccination programs started 30 years ago[174–176] but it remains endemic in India, Pakistan and some African countries like Nigeria [177]. Sporadic cases of polio secondary to transformation of oral polio vaccine have been reported in countries where vaccination coverage and surveillance activities are low.

Pathogenesis

Enteroviral infections are acquired from ingestion of contaminated material, usually spread from person to person by the fecal–oral route. After mucosal attachment, enteroviruses replicate in the gut and/or pharynx, leading to a minor viremia by which the virus invades the reticuloendothelial system (RES; the lymph nodes, liver and spleen). Replication in the RES then leads to a major viremia which produces infection of other organs (gray matter of central nervous system and spinal cord for poliomyelitis, heart, muscle, pleura, etc. for coxsackie and echoviruses) and the clinical syndromes characteristic of each virus. Infection results in lifelong immunity specific to the infecting viral serotype.

Pathogenesis of mother-to-child transmission

Mother-to-child transmission through the birth canal from exposure to infected maternal secretions and blood seems to account for the majority of neonatal infections. Macrophage function is important to contain enteroviral replication but it is immature at the time of birth [178]. Hence timing of maternal infection is likely the most important factor to determine neonatal infection outcome, as the presence of maternally acquired antibody specific for the enteroviral serotype lessens disease manifestations [178].

Clinical presentation and obstetric considerations

Polio

Most poliovirus infections (99%) are asymptomatic. If symptomatic, poliovirus infections were severe during pregnancy, based on observations made 50 years ago when polio was endemic in the US [174–176]. Following an incubation period of 9–12 days, fever, mild headache and sore throat develop, and a small proportion of cases progress to aseptic meningitis or paralytic disease (the ratio of subclinical infection to paralytic disease ranges from 100:1 to 1000:1). Risk factors for paralytic disease include larger inoculum of virus, increasing age, pregnancy, strenuous exercise, tonsillectomy, and intramuscular injections administered while the patient is infected with poliovirus. Paralytic polio is fatal in 2–10% of cases.

Poliovirus infections during pregnancy may result in abortion, stillbirth, neonatal disease or no clinical disease at all [174–176], but neither the actual infection nor inadvertent administration of oral polio vaccine is likely to cause congenital malformations.

Coxsackieviruses and echoviruses

The clinical course and presentation of coxsackievirus and echovirus infections in pregnancy do not differ from other nonpregnant adults. In general, following a very short incubation period of 2–3 days, if symptomatic, adults develop an acute, self-limited febrile illness. Manifestations may include myocarditis, pericarditis, pleural irritation (especially an epidemic pleurodynia known as Bornholm disease, presenting with excruciating paroxysms of chest pain and associated spasms of the chest wall and abdominal muscles), rashes, hand-foot and mouth disease (a 2–3-day illness with fever and vesicles on the inner cheeks, tongue, hands feet and buttocks secondary to coxsackie A strains), herpangina (an acute febrile illness associated with small vesicular or ulcerative lesions on the posterior oropharyngeal structures), acute hemorrhagic conjunctivitis and aseptic meningitis. Maternal echovirus infection in the late second and third trimester may present with severe abdominal pain that can be mistaken for abruptio placentae. There are no specific therapies for enteroviruses and treatment is therefore supportive only.

Increased rates of abortion related to coxsackie B4 during pregnancy have been documented [179]. Congenital heart disease has been linked with coxsackie B1–B5, particularly B3 infections [112,180] using both serologic and direct viral detection methods. Third-trimester maternal infection is clearly associated with neonatal disease and these viruses appear to be particularly virulent in neonates. Manifestations of neonatal infection usually begin at day 3–7 of life and may include a maculopapular rash (in up to 40% of affected neonates), pneumonia, myocarditis, neonatal fulminant sepsis and death [181,182]. The exact incidence of neonatal disease following third-trimester maternal infection is yet to be determined. Type 1 diabetes mellitus has been proposed to be linked to maternal coxsackie B infection in pregnancy but the current data do not support such association [112]. Echoviruses are not associated with stillbirth or congenital defects [112]. In contrast, neonatal disease from maternally acquired echovirus 11 in the third trimester has resulted in neonatal sepsis-like syndrome, myocarditis and death [183].

Diagnosis

A high index of suspicion is required for nonspecific febrile maternal illnesses in the summer and fall, particularly in the third trimester, as 60–70% of women with an infected neonate reported a febrile illness during the last week of pregnancy [178]. Stool and rectal swabs are appropriate maternal specimens to be sent for "enterovirus isolation." As indicated by clinical context and season, serum, urine, throat swabs, respiratory aspirates and CSF can also be sent. Specimens can be tested for enteroviruses using cell culture (generally best if done on multiple cell lines and results can take up to 2–6 days) or RNA sequencing. Serologic testing for antibodies is impractical, not widely available, and difficult to interpret unless acute and convalescent serum is analyzed.

Prevention

Poliomyelitis is a vaccine-preventable disease and most women of reproductive age born in western Europe and the Americas have been vaccinated. As with all live vaccines, polio vaccine is not recommended during pregnancy [184], but inadvertent vaccination of thousands of pregnant women at any time during pregnancy with either live or inactivated vaccines has not resulted in increased rates of congenital anomalies, stillbirth, neonatal deaths, prematurity or neurologic abnormalities [184]. So, if a pregnant woman is at increased risk for infection and requires immediate protection against polio, polio vaccine can be administered in accordance with the recommended schedules for adults [184]. There are no preventive measures for echo or coxsackievirus infections aside from maintaining good hand hygiene.

Other viral infections in pregnancy

This section addresses rare viral diseases, relevant only if specific exposure or travel is elicited by history. They include rabies, lymphocytic choriomeningitis virus (LCV), West Nile virus (WNV) and Japanese encephalitis.

Lymphocytic choriomeningitis virus

Lymphocytic choriomeningitis virus (LCV, also known as LCM virus) is a teratogenic agent previously unrecognized as such. It belongs to the Arenavirus family with Lassa and the South American hemorrhagic fevers. LCV causes asymptomatic infection in rodents – house mice, hamsters, rabbits and laboratory rats – yet they excrete high quantities of LCV in the urine. The actual incidence of human LCV infection is unknown but 1–5% of adults in large cities of the United States have had LCV infection [185]. The specific mode of acquisition for human infection is unknown, but inhalation of aerosolized viral particles from rodent urine or secretions, followed by direct contact with rodents, and rodent bites are the likely mechanisms of transmission [186]. Unlike Lassa fever, no person-to-person transmission has been documented.

Clinical presentation and pregnancy outcomes

Ten percent of LCV cases are asymptomatic, but usually present as a biphasic febrile illness, with an initial nonspecific phase of fever, headache, nausea, myalgias, rash and lymphadenopathy lasting 3–5 days, followed by reappearance of fever with severe headache plus severe neurologic syndromes and other organ involvement (heart/liver) in some cases. The second phase usually presents with leukopenia and thrombocytopenia.

Lymphocytic choriomeningitis virus during pregnancy has resulted in intrauterine fetal infection, congenital birth defects and severe neonatal disease [187]. Although the number of intrauterine and perinatal LCV infections is likely low, the incidence of adverse pregnancy and fetal outcomes is high. Congenital birth defects mimic congenital CMV or toxoplasmosis, and include chorioretinopathy, macro- or microcephaly and hydrocephalus; overall, 63% of 26 affected pregnancies in one case series had severe neurologic sequelae. Fatal central nervous system neonatal disease following close to term maternal LCV infection has been reported as well.

Diagnosis, treatment and prevention

Lymphocytic choriomeningitis virus can readily be cultured from blood during the acute illness and from CSF late in the disease. However, LCV-specific IgM by ELISA in serum and CSF is a reliable diagnostic method, available mostly in reference laboratories. There is no specific antiviral treatment for LCV infections and there are no licensed arenavirus vaccines.

Prevention relies on avoidance of exposure. Pregnant women must avoid contact with rodents and/or rodents' excreta, as even healthy domestic mice and hamsters shed LCV.

Rabies

Rabies virus is a single-stranded RNA virus that results in fatal encephalitis if untreated. It is very common in the developing world but fortunately, rabies pre-exposure and postexposure prophylaxis is available and deemed safe for pregnant women who need it. In the developing world, most cases of human rabies are acquired from bites of rabid domestic animals (dogs), whereas in North America and developed countries where dog immunization is widespread, most human cases have been linked by molecular methods to bats, even when history of bat exposure is negative [188]. Raccoons, skunks and foxes are also major animal reservoirs in North America. The virus travels through the peripheral nerves to the CNS where it proliferates and spreads to other tissues; the incubation period is close to 90 days, followed by nonspecific symptoms, encephalitis, paralysis and death. Transplacental infection has not been reported, even in fatal cases of maternal rabies [25].

Prevention of rabies includes wound management (early thorough washing with soap and water or a virucidal agent such as povidone-iodine) and immune prophylaxis. Postexposure prophylaxis with human rabies immune globulin and human diploid cell vaccine must always be offered to pregnant women and should be administered as soon as possible after the exposure [189]. Pre-exposure prophylaxis with human diploid cell vaccine is recommended if unavoidable potential exposure to rabies happens prior to the end of pregnancy, i.e. rural, remote or nontouristic travel to an endemic area [189].

Flaviruses: Japanese encephalitis and West Nile virus

West Nile virus (WNV) and Japanese encephalitis are single-stranded RNA viruses and, like the other members of the flavivirus genus (yellow fever, dengue, dengue hemorrhagic fever, St Louis encephalitis and tick-borne encephalitis), are transmitted to humans through infected mosquito bites.

West Nile virus caused an epidemic of meningoencephalitis in New York City and the Pacific Coast between 1999 and 2002, yet 99% of human cases are asymptomatic. WNV infection in pregnancy was recognized only since this recent epidemic, and case reports confirmed mother-to-child transmission *in utero* and through breast milk [190]. Few case reports of congenital CNS defects (chorioretinitis and severe white matter loss) from maternal infections in the second trimester are available but current data are not sufficient to establish a causal relationship. Pregnant women with undifferentiated fever or acute CNS disease in an area of known active WNV transmission should have serum and CSF tested for WNV IgM [191].

Japanese encephalitis is endemic in Asia and most infections are subclinical, but symptomatic cases develop encephalitis or aseptic meningitis. JE infection during pregnancy in the first and second trimesters resulted in abortion and transplacental infection was documented in two cases [192–194].

Severe acute respiratory syndrome associated with coronavirus

Severe acute respiratory syndrome associated with coronavirus (SARS-CoV) is a recently described single0stranded RNA virus, similar to influenza, that accounted for a worldwide pneumonia outbreak involving approximately 8000 cases with a 10% mortality rate in 2003. It is transmitted from person to person by aspiration of droplets and possibly by the fecal–oral route.

Incubation period is between 4 and 7 days. Fever and other "influenza-like" symptoms are followed by cough and dyspnea within a few days without upper respiratory symptoms (i.e. rhinorrhea and sore throat). About 25% of patients progress to acute respiratory distress syndrome (ARDS). Diagnosis can be made on the basis of serologic testing (although positive antibodies may take 20 days to form and require convalescent sera for confirmation), viral culture or real-time PCR. To date, only 15 cases of SARS-CoV have been reported during pregnancy, limiting the ability to determine if the severity and mortality of SARS-CoV infection are higher among pregnant women, as suggested by some reports but not others [195–197]. Mother-to-child transmission has not been documented despite extensive testing, but miscarriage and preterm labor have been reported [164,198].

Immunization during pregnancy and breastfeeding

All women presenting for preconception counseling should have their immunization records reviewed and updated. Identification of vaccination gaps should lead to vaccination, ideally pior to conception.

Pregnancy provides a unique opportunity for vaccination, as the majority of pregnant women make contact with the healthcare system. Immunization should be provided during pregnancy or immediately after if a particular product is contraindicated during pregnancy, given that pregnancy *per se* increases the risk of acquiring and/or suffering severe outcomes from some infections. Maternal immunization may also affect fetal and neonatal well-being, as efficient placental transfer of maternal antibodies to the fetus starts at 32 weeks, conferring protection for the first 6 months of life. The objective of vaccination during pregnancy is therefore to protect the mother, the fetus, the neonate and the young infant. Postpartum vaccination is recommended to:

- protect the mother from vaccine-preventable diseases
- offer indirect protection of neonate/infant by preventing maternal infection
- confer protection in subsequent pregnancies.

Breastfeeding provides protective antibodies to the neonate/infant by means of secretory IgA. The only concern regarding maternal immunization during breastfeeding is the possible interference of IgA with the infant/neonate direct response to childhood vaccination series; however, this is only an issue for oral vaccines (like oral polio and rotavirus) which are not routinely used in the US or the UK [199].

The Advisory Committee on Immunization Practices (ACIP) has established guiding principles for vaccination recommendations during breastfeeding and pregnancy, and has defined "contraindication" and "precaution" as follows [200].

- *Contraindication*: there is a risk for serious maternal, fetal or neonatal adverse event linked to the vaccine, based on direct evidence or strong biologic plausibility and suggestive evidence that the risk of severe adverse event is elevated for at least one of those groups. A vaccine will not be administered when a contraindication is present.
- *Precaution*: there might be an increase in the risk for a serious adverse reaction linked to the vaccine or that might compromise the ability of the vaccine to produce immunity, meaning there is no supporting evidence but there is some biologic plausibility, or there is lack of data to support safety. Under usual circumstances, vaccination should be deferred. However, vaccination might be indicated because benefits outweigh the risks.

Active immunization products are classified according the type of antigen used (Table 17.5). Live or live-attenuated vaccines contain the actual pathogen and carry the biologically plausible risk of fetal damage arising from maternal viremia. Pregnancy is a contraindication to receiving the following live or live-attenuated vaccines: measles, mumps, rubella, varicella, live-attenuated influenza and vaccinia (smallpox), despite no evidence of fetal damage from vaccination during pregnancy for any of them except vaccinia [102,105,134,199,201,202]. Pregnancy is a reason to avoid vaccination with inactivated polio vaccine (IPV), yellow fever and rabies vaccines, and under normal circumstances vaccination should be deferred; however, vaccine should only be given when the benefits of vaccination outweigh the risks (in case of unavoidable travel during pregnancy to areas where exposure is likely for yellow fever or IPV) or postexposure prophylaxis after possible exposure for rabies [184,189,203,204]. Women who receive any of these vaccines are advised to avoid pregnancy for at least 1 month. However, if inadvertent vaccination during pregnancy happens or women become pregnant prior to the 1-month waiting period, termination of the pregnancy is not advised on these grounds.

Killed or inactivated vaccines against tetanus-diphtheria [205,206] and influenza are recommended in pregnancy, but unfortunately they are underutilized. Pregnant women are at increased risk of morbidity and mortality from influenza infection, and vaccination is advised for all women who

Table 17.5 Immunization: pregnancy and breastfeeding recommendations

Product (type & schedule)	Pregnancy	Post partum	Breastfeeding	Comments
Varicella • Live • 2 doses (0, 4–8 weeks)	Contraindicated	Immunize susceptible women post partum before hospital discharge or shortly thereafter whether or not they intend to breastfeed	Breastfeeding is not a contraindication or precaution to vaccination	Inadvertent use in pregnancy has not resulted in fetal or neonatal disease; not a reason for termination of pregnancy. Pregnancy to be avoided until 28 days after vaccination
Measles, mumps, rubella • Live • 1 dose	Contraindicated	Immunize susceptible women post partum before hospital discharge or shortly thereafter whether or not they intend to breastfeed	Breastfeeding is not a contraindication or precaution to vaccination	Inadvertent use in pregnancy has not resulted in fetal or neonatal disease; not a reason for termination of pregnancy. Pregnancy to be avoided until 28 days after vaccination
Vaccinia (smallpox) • Live • 1 dose	Contraindicated	Contraindicated if intention to breastfeed	Contraindicated	Has been reported to cause fetal and neonatal infection
Poliomyelitis (aka IPV or Salk vaccine) • Live attenuated • 3 doses (0, 1, 6 months)	Precaution: consider if pregnant woman needs immediate protection (high-risk situation, travel)	Immunize susceptible women post partum before hospital discharge or shortly thereafter whether or not they intend to breastfeed as per routine adult immunization schedule	Breastfeeding is not a contraindication or precaution to vaccination	No known fetal effects. Ideally defer vaccination until after 12 weeks gestation
Yellow fever • Live attenuated • 1 dose	Precaution: vaccinate during pregnancy in cases of unavoidable travel to area where exposure is likely	Precaution if intention to breastfeed due to lack of data	Breastfeeding is a precaution due to lack of data	Very limited data on pregnancy: has not resulted in fetal disease; not a reason for termination of pregnancy
Rabies • Live attenuated • 5 doses (0, 3, 7, 14 & 28 days)	Precaution: vaccinate during pregnancy only after possible exposure (postexposure prophylaxis)	Immunize women post partum at any time, whether or not they intend to breastfeed, as per routine recommendations: pre-exposure prophylaxis	Breastfeeding is not a contraindication or precaution to vaccination	Prudent to delay pre-exposure immunization unless substantial risk of exposure
Influenza • Inactivated • 1 dose annually	Recommended: for all pregnant women during the flu season, and all pregnant women as per routine recommendations based on co-morbidities or occupation (see text)	Immunize women post partum at any time, whether or not they intend to breastfeed, as per routine recommendations based on co-morbidities or occupation (see text)	Breastfeeding is not a contraindication or precaution to vaccination	
Hepatitis A • Inactivated • 2 doses (0, 6 months)	Precaution: vaccinate during pregnancy if unavoidable travel to area where exposure is likely to happen	Immunize susceptible women post partum before hospital discharge or shortly thereafter whether or not they intend to breastfeed as per routine adult immunization schedule	Breastfeeding is not a contraindication or precaution to vaccination	
Hepatitis B • Recombinant inactivated • 3 doses (0, 1, 6 months)	Precaution: recommended only for pregnant women at risk	Immunize susceptible women post partum before hospital discharge or shortly thereafter whether or not they intend to breastfeed as per routine adult immunization schedule	Breastfeeding is not a contraindication or precaution to vaccination	
Human Papilloma Virus • Recombinant • 3 doses (0, 1, 6 months)	Precaution: not recommended in pregnancy but inadvertent use has not resulted in adverse outcomes	Immunize as per adult immunization schedule	Breastfeeding is not a contraindication or precaution to vaccination	Inadvertent use in pregnancy has not resulted on fetal or neonatal disease

Table 17.5 (Continued)

Product (type & schedule)	Pregnancy	Post partum	Breastfeeding	Comments
Pneumococcus • Inactivated • 2 doses (0, 4–8 weeks)	Recommended: only for pregnant women at risk based on co-morbidities (see text)	Immunize women post partum at any time, whether or not they intend to breastfeed, as per routine recommendations (see text)	Breastfeeding is not a contraindication or precaution to vaccination	
Meningococcus Polysaccharide • Inactivated • 2 doses (0, 5 years)	Recommended: only for pregnant women at risk based on co-morbidities (see text)	Immunize women post partum at any time, whether or not they intend to breastfeed, as per routine recommendations (see text)	Breastfeeding is not a contraindication or precaution to vaccination	
Meningococcus Conjugate • Inactivated • 1 dose	Precaution: pregnancy is a precaution due to lack of data. Consider in situations where benefit outweighs risk	Breastfeeding is a precaution due to lack of data	Breastfeeding is a precaution due to lack of data	
Japanese encephalitis • Inactivated • 3 doses (0, 1, 4 weeks)	Precaution: vaccinate during pregnancy only in cases of unavoidable travel to area where exposure is likely to happen	Breastfeeding is a precaution due to lack of data	Breastfeeding is a precaution due to lack of data	
Typhoid • Some preparations live	Precaution: vaccinate during pregnancy in cases of unavoidable travel to area where exposure is likely	Breastfeeding is a precaution due to lack of data	Breastfeeding is a precaution due to lack of data	
Tetanus diphtheria • Inactivated • 3 doses (0, 1, 6 months)	Recommended: susceptible women to be vaccinated as per general guidelines for nonpregnant women.	Immunize susceptible women post partum before hospital discharge or shortly thereafter whether or not they intend to breastfeed as per routine adult immunization schedule	Breastfeeding is not a contraindication or precaution to vaccination	
Pertussis (usually given in combination with tetanus and diphtheria but also available by itself) • Inactivated • One-time dose as adult as booster to childhood pertussis immunization	Precaution: likely safe but limited pregnancy data	Recommended for all postpartum mothers prior to discharge from hospital to help protect them from acquiring pertussis and transmitting it to their infant	Breastfeeding is not a contraindication or precaution to vaccination	Tetanus diphtheria pertussis combination is only to be used if it has been more than 2 years since the last tetanus vaccine, otherwise there is an increased risk of reaction to the tetanus component

will be pregnant during the influenza season [33]. In addition, influenza vaccination is even more important for all pregnant women at increased risk of influenza-related morbidity on the basis of co-morbidities or occupation: cardiac or pulmonary disorders, diabetes mellitus and other metabolic diseases, cancer, immunodeficiency, immunosuppression, renal disease, anemia or hemoglobinopathy, conditions that compromise the management of respiratory secretions and are associated with an increased risk of aspiration, conditions treated for long periods with acetylsalicylic acid, and healthcare workers [33,207].

Hepatitis B vaccine is a recombinant vaccine recommended for pregnant women at risk for hepatitis B virus infection, including occupational risks (i.e. healthcare worker), lifestyle risks (e.g. history of intravenous drug use, sexually transmitted diseases, more than one sexual partner in the preceding 6 months), co-morbidities (i.e. hemophilia and hemodialysis)

and environmental (prison inmates, refugees, international travelers) [208,209].

Other inactivated or recombinant vaccines include hepatitis A, meningococcal (polysaccharide and conjugate), human papilloma virus (HPV) and pneumococcal (polysaccharide and conjugate). Although the safety of hepatitis A vaccination during pregnancy has not been determined, the theoretical risk to the developing fetus is expected to be very low, and vaccination during pregnancy is appropriate for women who may be at high risk for exposure, including chronic liver disease, ongoing exposure to clotting factor concentrates, occupational exposure to hepatitis A virus or unavoidable travel to countries with high endemicity of hepatitis A [210]. The meningococcal polysaccharide vaccine is safe and effective in pregnancy, and should be administered to pregnant women at increased risk of meningococcal disease, including functional or anatomic asplenia, complement, properdin or factor D deficiency [211]. Two recombinant HPV vaccines (quadrivalent against types 6, 11, 16 and 18, and bivalent against types 16 and 18) are currently licensed for use at ages 11-26 years, administered as a three dose-series ever the course of 6 months, for the prevention of cervical cancer, dysplasia and genital warts [172]. Although vaccination is not recommended during pregnancy, administration of quadrivalent HPV vaccine to n = 1796 women who became pregnant during licensing studies did not result on adverse pregnancy outcomes [173]. The safety of pneumococcal polysaccharide vaccine during the first trimester of pregnancy has not been evaluated, although no adverse consequences have been reported among newborns whose mothers were inadvertently vaccinated during pregnancy [212]; vaccination is recommended for pregnant women at high risk of pneumococcal disease: chronic lung (asthma and cigarette smoking are included) [213], cardiovascular or liver disease, diabetes mellitus, chronic alcoholism; chronic renal failure or nephrotic syndrome; functional or anatomic asplenia; cochlear implants; or cerebrospinal fluid leaks.

Recognition of epidemics of pertussis (presenting as a prolonged coughing illness in adults previously vaccinated as children against pertussis) has caused concerns related to the vulnerability of infants to this sometimes fatal condition in their first few months of life. Adults under the age of 65 are now therefore encouraged to receive the pertussis vaccine (in combination with the tetanus and diphtheria boosters) when their tetanus vaccines are next due, usually every 10 years. However, for adults (including new mothers) who are to be in contact with infants, the combined vaccine should be given if it has been less than 2 years since the tetanus vaccine was administered. (The 2-year waiting period is to decrease the risk of a reaction to the tetanus component of the combined vaccine from too frequent administration. For new mothers and family members who have had a recent tetanus shot but still need their one-time adult pertussis booster vaccination, an isolated acellular pertussis vaccine is now available.) Data about the safety of the pertussis vaccine in pregnancy are lacking, and although it is very likely to be safe in pregnancy, present recommendations are to provide this vaccine either before conception or prior to discharge from hospital after giving birth.

Breastfeeding is not a contraindication or a reason to avoid vaccination with all available vaccines, except for vaccinia (smallpox), given reported transmission of vaccinia virus from mother to child through breast milk [200].

References

1. Sever J, White LR. Intrauterine viral infections. Annu Rev Med 1968;19:471–86.
2. Finer L, Henshaw S. Disparities in rates of unintended pregnancy in the United States, 1994 and 2001. Perspect Sex Reprod Health 2006;38(2):90–6.
3. Forrest J. Epidemiology of unintended pregnancy and contraceptive use. Am J Obstet Gynecol 1994;170(5 Pt 2):1485–9.
4. Everett H, McFadden G, Everett H, McFadden G. Apoptosis: an innate immune response to virus infection. Trends Microbiol 1999;7(4):160–5.
5. Roulston A, Marcellus RC, Branton PE, Roulston A, Marcellus RC, Branton PE. Viruses and apoptosis. Annu Rev Microbiol 1999;53:577–628.
6. Chi BH, Mudenda V, Levy J, Sinkala M, Goldenberg RL, Stringer JSA. Acute and chronic chorioamnionitis and the risk of perinatal human immunodeficiency virus-1 transmission. Am J Obstet Gynecol 2006;194(1):174–81.
7. Giorlandino C, Bilancioni E, d'Alessio P, Muzii L. Risk of iatrogenic fetal infection at prenatal diagnosis. Lancet 1994;343(8902):922–3.
8. Von Rango U. Fetal tolerance in human pregnancy – a crucial balance between acceptance and limitation of trophoblast invasion. Immunol Lett 2008;115(1):21–32.
9. Thellin O, Coumans B, Zorzi W, et al. Tolerance to the foetoplacental graft. Curr Opin Immunol 2000;12:731–7.
10. Medzhitov R, Janeway C Jr. Innate immunity. N Engl J Med 2000;343(5):338–44.
11. Luppi P, Luppi P. How immune mechanisms are affected by pregnancy. Vaccine 2003;21(24):3352–7.
12. Svensson L, Arvola M, Sallstrom MA, Holmdahl R, Mattsson R, Svensson L, et al. The Th2 cytokines IL-4 and IL-10 are not crucial for the completion of allogeneic pregnancy in mice. J Reprod Immunol 2001;51(1):3–7.
13. Chaouat G. The Th1/Th2 paradigm: still important in pregnancy? Semin Immunopathol 2007;29(2):95–113.
14. Ashkar AA, di Santo JP, Croy BA. Interferon gamma contributes to initiation of uterine vascular modification, decidual integrity, and uterine natural killer cell maturation during normal murine pregnancy. J Exper Med 2000;192(2):259–70.
15. Chaisavaneeyakorn S, Moore JM, Othoro C, Otieno J, Chaiyaroj SC, Shi YP, et al. Immunity to placental malaria. IV. Placental malaria is associated with up-regulation of macrophage migration inhibitory factor in intervillous blood. J Infect Dis 2002;186(9):1371–5.
16. Khan NA, Kazzi SN. Yield and costs of screening growth-retarded infants for torch infections. Am J Perinatol 2000;17(3):131–5.
17. Abdel-Fattah SA, Bhat A, Illanes S, Bartha JL, Carrington D. TORCH test for fetal medicine indications: only CMV is necessary in the United Kingdom. Prenatal Diagn 2005;25(11):1028–31.
18. Treanor JJ. Influenza virus. In: Mandell GL, Bennett JE, Dolin R (eds) Mandell, Bennett, & Dolin: principles and practice of infectious diseases, 6th edn. Churchill Livingstone, Edinburgh, 2005.
19. Louie JK, Acosta M, Jamieson DJ, Honein MA, California Pandemic Working G. Severe 2009 H1N1 influenza in pregnant and postpartum women in California. N Engl J Med 2010;362(1):27–35.
20. Kumar A, Zarychanski R, Pinto R, Cook DJ, Marshall J, Lacroix J, et al. Critically ill patients with 2009 influenza A(H1N1) infection in Canada. JAMA 2009;302(17):1872–9.
21. ANZIC Influenza Investigators, Webb SAR, Pettila V, Seppelt I, Bellomo R, Bailey M, et al. Critical care services and 2009 H1N1 influenza in Australia and New Zealand. N Engl J Med 2009;361(20):1925–34.
22. Freeman DW, Barno A. Deaths from Asian influenza associated with pregnancy. Am J Obstet Gynecol 1959;78:1172–5.
23. Hartert TV, Neuzil KM, Shintani AK, Mitchel EF Jr, Snowden MS, Wood LB, et al. Maternal morbidity and perinatal outcomes among pregnant women with respiratory hospitalizations during influenza season. Am J Obstet Gynecol 2003;189(6):1705–12.
24. Neuzil KM, Reed GW, Mitchel EF, Simonsen L, Griffin MR, Neuzil KM, et al. Impact of influenza on acute

cardiopulmonary hospitalizations in pregnant women. Am J Epidemiol 1998;148(11):1094–102.

25. Maldonado Y. Less common viral infections. In: Remington JS, Klein J, Wilson C, Baker C (eds) Infectious diseases of the fetus and newborn infant. Elsevier Saunders, Philadelphia, 2006: 933–44.

26. Laibl VR, Sheffield JS. Influenza and pneumonia in pregnancy. Clin Perinatol 2005;32(3):727–38.

27. Edwards MJ. Review: hyperthermia and fever during pregnancy. Birth Defects Res 2006;76(7):507–16.

28 Drexler JF, Helmer A, Kirberg H, Reber U, Panning M, Muller M, et al. Poor clinical sensitivity of rapid antigen test for influenza A pandemic (H1N1) 2009 virus. Emerg Infect Dis 2009;15(10):1662–4.

29 Centers for Disease Control and Prevention. Updated interim recommendations for obstetric health care providers related to use of antiviral medications in the treatment and prevention of influenza for the 2009–2010 season. Accessed February 11, 2010, at http://www.cdc.gov/h1n1flu/pregnancy/antiviral_messages.htm.

30 CDC Health Alert Network (HAN) info service message: recommendations for early empiric antiviral treatment in persons with suspected influenza who are at increased risk of developing severe disease. Accessed February 11, 2010 at http://www.cdc.gov/H1N1flu/HAN/101909.htm.

31 Tanaka T, Nakajima K, Murashima A, Garcia-Bournissen F, Koren G, Ito S. Safety of neuraminidase inhibitors against novel influenza A (H1N1) in pregnant and breastfeeding women. CMAJ 2009;181(1–2):55–8].

32. National Advisory Committee on Influenza. Statement on influenza vaccination for the 2006–2007 season. Can Commun Dis Rep 2006;32(ACS-7):1–27. (Erratum appears in Can Commun Dis Rep 2006;32(15):175.)

33. Fiore AE, Shay DK, Broder K, Iskander JK, Uyeki TM, Mootrey G, et al. Prevention and control of influenza: recommendations of the Advisory Committee on Immunization Practices (ACIP), 2008. MMWR Recomm Rep 2008;57(RR-7):1–60.

34. Zaman K, Roy E, Arifeen SE, Rahman M, Raqib R, Wilson E, et al. Effectiveness of maternal influenza immunization in mothers and infants. N Engl J Med 2008;359(15):1555–64.

35. Roberts S, Hollier LM, Sheffield J, Laibl V, Wendel GD Jr. Cost-effectiveness of universal influenza vaccination in a pregnant population. Obstet Gynecol 2006;107(6):1323–9.

36. Icart J, Didier J, Dalens M, Chabanon G, Boucays A, Icart J, et al. Prospective study of Epstein Barr virus (EBV) infection during pregnancy. Biomedicine 1981Dec;34(3):160–3.

37. Johannsen E, Schooley R, Kaye K. Epstein-Barr virus (infectious mononucleosis). In: Mandell GL, Bennett JE, Dolin R (eds) Mandell, Bennett, & Dolin: principles and practice of infectious diseases, 6th edn. Churchill Livingstone, Edinburgh, 2005

38. Meyohas MC, Marechal V, Desire N, Bouillie J, Frottier J, Nicolas JC. Study of mother-to-child Epstein-Barr virus transmission by means of nested PCRs. J Virol 1996;70(10):6816–9.

39. Avgil M, Ornoy A. Herpes simplex virus and Epstein-Barr virus infections in pregnancy: consequences of neonatal or intrauterine infection. Reprod Toxicol 2006;21(4):436–45.

40. Eskild A, Bruu A-L, Stray-Pedersen B, Jenum P. Epstein-Barr virus infection during pregnancy and the risk of adverse pregnancy outcome. Br J Obstet Gynaecol 2005;112(12):1620–4.

41. Torre D, Tambini R. Acyclovir for treatment of infectious mononucleosis: a meta-analysis. Scand J Infect Dis 1999;31(6):543–7.

42. Grosse SD, Ross DS, Dollard SC. Congenital cytomegalovirus (CMV) infection as a cause of permanent bilateral hearing loss: a quantitative assessment. J Clin Virol 2008;41(2):57–62.

43. Nance WE, Lim BG, Dodson KM. Importance of congenital cytomegalovirus infections as a cause for pre-lingual hearing loss. J Clin Virol 2006 ;35(2):221–5.

44. Staras SAS, Dollard SC, Radford KW, Flanders WD, Pass RF, Cannon MJ. Seroprevalence of cytomegalovirus infection in the United States, 1988–1994. Clin Infect Dis 2006;43(9):1143–51.

45. Adler SP. Cytomegalovirus and child day care. Evidence for an increased infection rate among day-care workers. N Engl J Med 1989;321(19):1290–6.

46. Fowler KB, Pass RF. Risk factors for congenital cytomegalovirus infection in the offspring of young women: exposure to young children and recent onset of sexual activity. Pediatrics. 2006;118(2):e286–92.

47. Stagno S, Britt W. Cytomegalovirus infections. In: Remington JS, Klein J, Wilson C, Baker C (eds) Infectious diseases of the fetus and newborn infant. Elsevier Saunders, Philadelphia, 2006: 739–82.

48. Dworsky M, Yow M, Stagno S, Pass RF, Alford C. Cytomegalovirus infection of breast milk and transmission in infancy. Pediatrics 1983;72(3):295–9.

49. Dollard SC, Grosse SD, Ross DS. New estimates of the prevalence of neurological and sensory sequelae and mortality associated with congenital cytomegalovirus infection. Rev Med Virol 2007;17(5):355–63.

50. Noyola DE, Demmler GJ, Nelson CT, Griesser C, Williamson WD, Atkins JT, et al. Early predictors of neurodevelopmental outcome in symptomatic congenital cytomegalovirus infection. J Pediatr 2001;138(3):325–31.

51. Boppana SB, Rivera LB, Fowler KB, Mach M, Britt WJ. Intrauterine transmission of cytomegalovirus to infants of women with preconceptional immunity. N Engl J Med 2001;344(18):1366–71.

52. Fowler K, Stagno S, Pass R. Maternal immunity and prevention of congenital cytomegalovirus infection. JAMA 2003;289(8):1008–12.

53. Pass RF, Fowler KB, Boppana SB, Britt WJ, Stagno S. Congenital cytomegalovirus infection following first trimester maternal infection: symptoms at birth and outcome. J Clin Virol 2006;35(2):216–20.

54. Revello MG, Gerna G. Pathogenesis and prenatal diagnosis of human cytomegalovirus infection. J Clin Virol 2004;29(2):71–83.

55. Fisher S, Genbacev O, Maidji E, Pereira L. Human cytomegalovirus infection of placental cytotrophoblasts in vitro and in utero: implications for transmission and pathogenesis. J Virol 2000;74(15):6808–20.

56. Pizzato N, Garmy-Susini B, Le Bouteiller P, Lenfant F. Down-regulation of HLA-G1 cell surface expression in human cytomegalovirus infected cells. Am J Reprod Immunol 2003;50(4):328–33.

57. Maidji E, McDonagh S, Genbacev O, Tabata T, Pereira L. Maternal antibodies enhance or prevent cytomegalovirus infection in the placenta by neonatal Fc receptor-mediated transcytosis. Am J Pathol 2006;168:1210–26.

58. Griffiths PD, Baboonian C. A prospective study of primary cytomegalovirus infection during pregnancy: final report. Br J Obstet Gynaecol 1984;91(4):307–15.

59. Lazzarotto T, Gabrielli L, Lanari M, Guerra B, Bellucci T, Sassi M, et al. Congenital cytomegalovirus infection: recent advances in the diagnosis of maternal infection. Hum Immunol 2004;65(5):410–15.

60. Maine GT, Lazzarotto T, Landini MP. New developments in the diagnosis of maternal and congenital CMV infection. Expert Rev Mol Diagn 2001;1:19–29.

61. Donner C, Liesnard C, Brancart F, Rodesch F. Accuracy of amniotic fluid testing before 21 weeks' gestation in prenatal diagnosis of congenital cytomegalovirus infection. Prenatal Diagn 1994;14(11):1055–9.

62. Liesnard C, Donner C, Brancart F, Gosselin F, Delforge ML, Rodesch F, et al. Prenatal diagnosis of congenital cytomegalovirus infection: prospective study of 237 pregnancies at risk. Obstet Gynecol 2000;95(6 Pt 1):881–8.

63. Revello M, Lilleri D, Zavattoni M. Prenatal diagnosis of congenital human cytomegalovirus infection in amniotic fluid by nucleic acid sequence-based amplification assay. J Clin Microbiol 2003;41:1772–4.

64. Degani S. Sonographic findings in fetal viral infections: a systematic review. Obstet Gynecol Surv 2006;61:329–36.

65. Nigro G, Adler S, Torre RL. Passive immunization during pregnancy for congenital CMV infection. N Engl J Med 2005;353:1350–62.

66. La Torre R, Nigro G, Mazzocco M, Best AM, Adler SP. Placental enlargement in women with primary maternal cytomegalovirus infection is associated with fetal and neonatal disease. Clin Infect Dis 2006;43(8):994–1000.

67. Puliyanda DP, Silverman NS, Lehman D, Vo A, Bunnapradist S, Radha RK, et al. Successful use of oral ganciclovir for the treatment of intrauterine cytomegalovirus infection in a renal allograft recipient. Transplant Infect Dis 2005;7(2):71–4.

68. Nicolini U, Kustermann A, Tassis B. Prenatal diagnosis of congenital human cytomegalovirus infection. Prenat Diagn 1994;14(10):903–6.

69. Pass RF, Zhang C, Evans A, Simpson T, Andrews W, Huang M-L, et al. Vaccine prevention of maternal cytomegalovirus infection. N Engl J Med 2009;360(12): 1191–9.

70. Fowler KB, Stagno S, Pass RF. Interval between births and risk of congenital cytomegalovirus infection. Clin Infect Dis 2004;38(7):1035–7.

71. Koch WC, Harger JH, Barnstein B, Adler SP. Serologic and virologic evidence for frequent intrauterine transmission of human parvovirus B19 with a primary maternal infection during pregnancy. Pediatr Infect Dis J 1998;17(6):489–94.

72. Adler SP, Manganello AM, Koch WC, Hempfling SH, Best AM. Risk of human parvovirus B19 infections among school and hospital employees during endemic periods. J Infect Dis 1993;168(2):361–8.

73. Corcoran A, Doyle S. Advances in the biology, diagnosis and host-pathogen interactions of parvovirus B19. J Med Microbiol 2004;53(Pt 6):459–75.

74. Jordan JA, DeLoia JA. Globoside expression within the human placenta. Placenta 1999;20(1):103–8.

75. De Haan TR, Beersma MFC, Claas ECJ, Oepkes D, Kroes ACM, Walther FJ. Parvovirus B19 infection in pregnancy studied by maternal viral load and immune responses. Fetal Diagn Ther 2007;22(1):55–62.

76. Harger JH, Adler SP, Koch WC, Harger GF. Prospective evaluation of 618 pregnant women exposed to parvovirus B19: risks and symptoms. Obstet Gynecol 1998;91(3):413–20.

77. Koch WC, Adler SP, Harger J. Intrauterine parvovirus B19 infection may cause an asymptomatic or recurrent postnatal infection. Pediatr Infect Dis J 1993;12(9):747–50.

78. Rodis JF, Quinn DL, Gary GW Jr, Anderson LJ, Rosengren S, Cartter ML, et al. Management and outcomes of pregnancies complicated by human B19 parvovirus infection: a prospective study. Am J Obstet Gynecol 1990;163(4 Pt 1):1168–71.

79. Guidozzi F, Ballot D, Rothberg AD. Human B19 parvovirus infection in an obstetric population. A prospective study determining fetal outcome. J Reprod Med 1994;39(1):36–8.

80. Miller E, Fairley C, Cohen B, Seng C. Immediate and long term outcome of human parvovirus B19 infection in pregnancy. Br J Obstet Gynaecol 1998;105:174–8.

81. Tolfvenstam T, Papadogiannakis N, Norbeck O, Petersson K, Broliden K. Frequency of human parvovirus B19 infection in intrauterine fetal death. Lancet 2001;357(9267):1494–7.

82. Von Kaisenberg CS, Bender G, Scheewe J, Hirt SW, Lange M, Stieh J, et al. A case of fetal parvovirus B19 myocarditis, terminal cardiac heart failure, and perinatal heart transplantation. Fetal Diagn Ther 2001;16(6):427–32.

83. Yaegashi N, Niinuma T, Chisaka H, Uehara S, Okamura K, Shinkawa O, et al. Serologic study of human parvovirus B19 infection in pregnancy in Japan. J Infect 1999;38(1):30–5.

84. Yaegashi N, Niinuma T, Chisaka H, Watanabe T, Uehara S, Okamura K, et al. The incidence of, and factors leading to parvovirus B19-related hydrops fetalis following maternal infection: report of 10 cases and meta-analysis. J Infect 1998;37(1):28–35.

85. Enders M, Weidner A, Zoellner I, Searle K, Enders G. Fetal morbidity and mortality after acute human parvovirus B19 infection in pregnancy: prospective evaluation of 1018 cases. Prenatal Diagn 2004;24(7):513–18.

86. Beersma MFC, Claas ECJ, Sopaheluakan T, Kroes ACM. Parvovirus B19 viral loads in relation to VP1 and VP2 antibody responses in diagnostic blood samples. J Clin Virol 2005;34(1):71–5.

87. Delle Chiaie L, Buck G, Grab D, Terinde R. Prediction of fetal anemia with Doppler measurement of the middle cerebral artery peak systolic velocity in pregnancies complicated by maternal blood group alloimmunization or parvovirus B19 infection. Ultrasound Obstet Gynecol 2001;18(3):232–6.

88. Cosmi E, Mari G, delle Chiaie L, Detti L, Akiyama M, Murphy J, et al. Noninvasive diagnosis by Doppler ultrasonography of fetal anemia resulting from parvovirus infection. Am J Obstet Gynecol 2002;187(5):1290–3.

89. Nagel HTC, de Haan TR, Vandenbussche FPHA, Oepkes D, Walther FJ. Long-term outcome after fetal transfusion for hydrops associated with parvovirus B19 infection. Obstet Gynecol 2007;109(1):42–7.

90. Muller CP, Kremer JR, Best JM, Dourado I, Triki H, Reef S, et al. Reducing global disease burden of measles and rubella: report of the WHO Steering Committee on research related to measles and rubella vaccines and vaccination, 2005. Vaccine 2007;25(1):1–9.

91. Gershon AA. Rubella virus (German measles). In: Mandell GL, Bennett JE, Dolin R (eds) Mandell, Bennett, & Dolin: principles and practice of infectious diseases, 6th edn. Churchill Livingstone, Edinburgh, 2005.

92. Cradock-Watson JE, Ridehalgh MK, Anderson MJ, Pattison JR. Outcome of asymptomatic infection with rubella virus during pregnancy. J Hygiene 1981;87(2):147–54.

93. Cradock-Watson JE, Ridehalgh MK, Anderson MJ, Pattison JR, Kangro HO. Fetal infection resulting from maternal rubella after the first trimester of pregnancy. J Hygiene 1980;85(3):381–91.

94. Miller E, Cradock-Watson JE, Pollock TM. Consequences of confirmed maternal rubella at successive stages of pregnancy. Lancet 1982;2(8302):781–4.

95. Peckham C. Congenital rubella in the United Kingdom before 1970: the prevaccine era. Rev Infect Dis 1985;7(suppl 1):S11–16.

96. Morgan-Capner P, Miller E, Vurdien J, Ramsay M. Outcome of pregnancy after maternal reinfection with rubella. CDR (Lond Engl Rev) 1991;1(6):57–9.

97. De Santis M, Cavaliere AF, Straface G, Caruso A. Rubella infection in pregnancy. Reprod Toxicol 2006;21(4):390–8.

98. Banatvala J, Brown D. Rubella. Lancet 2004;363(9415): 1127–37.

99. Cooper LZ, Alford CA. Rubella. In: Remington JS, Klein J, Wilson C, Baker C (eds) Infectious diseases of the fetus and newborn infant. Elsevier Saunders, Philadelphia, 2006:893–925.

100. Tanemura M, Suzumori K, Yagami Y, et al. Diagnosis of fetal rubella infection with reverse transcription and nested polymerase chain reaction: a study of 34 cases diagnosed in fetuses. Am J Obstet Gynecol 1996;174(2):578–82.

101. Revello MG, Baldanti F, Sarasini A, Zavattoni M, Torsellini M, Gerna G, et al. Prenatal diagnosis of rubella virus infection by direct detection and semiquantitation of viral RNA in clinical samples by reverse transcription-PCR. J Clin Microbiol 1997;35(3):708–13.

102. Watson JC, Hadler SC, Dykewicz CA, *et al*. Measles, mumps, and rubella–accine use and strategies for elimination of measles, rubella, and congenital rubella syndrome and control of mumps: recommendations of the Advisory Committee on Immunization Practices (ACIP). MMWR Recomm Rep 1998;47(RR-8):1–57.

103. Robinson JL, Lee BE, Preiksaitis JK, *et al*. Prevention of congenital rubella syndrome – what makes sense in 2006? Epidemiol Rev 2006;28:81–7.

104. Watson JC, Hadler SC, Dykewicz CA, Reef S, Phillips L. Measles, mumps, and rubella – vaccine use and strategies for elimination of measles, rubella, and congenital rubella syndrome and control of mumps: recommendations of the Advisory Committee on Immunization Practices (ACIP). MMWR 1998; 47(RR-8):1–57.

105. Centers for Disease Control and Prevention. Revised ACIP recommendation for avoiding pregnancy after receiving a rubella-containing vaccine. MMWR 2001;50(49):1117.

106. Haas DM, Flowers CA, Congdon CL. Rubella, rubeola, and mumps in pregnant women: susceptibilities and strategies for testing and vaccinating. Obstet Gynecol 2005;106(2):295–300.

107. Gupta RK, Best J, MacMahon E. Mumps and the UK epidemic 2005. BMJ 2005;330(7500):1132–5.

108. Leinikki P. Mumps. In: Zuckerman AJ, Pattison JR, Griffiths PD, Schoub BD (eds) Principles and practice of clinical virology, 4th edn. Wiley, Chichester, 2004: 459–66.

109. Siegel M, Fuerst HT. Low birth weight and maternal virus diseases. A prospective study of rubella, measles, mumps, chickenpox, and hepatitis. JAMA 1966;197(9):680–4.

110. Siegel M. Congenital malformations following chickenpox, measles, mumps, and hepatitis. Results of a cohort study. JAMA 1973;226(13):1521–4.

111. Ni J, Bowles NE, Kim YH, Demmler G, Kearney D, Bricker JT, *et al*. Viral infection of the myocardium in endocardial fibroelastosis. Molecular evidence for the role of mumps virus as an etiologic agent. Circulation 1997;95(1):133–9.

112. Ornoy A, Tenenbaum A. Pregnancy outcome following infections by coxsackie, echo, measles, mumps, hepatitis, polio and encephalitis viruses. Reprod Toxicol 2006;21(4):446–57.

113. Gershon AA. Measles virus (rubeola). In: Mandell GL, Bennett JE, Dolin R (eds) Mandell, Bennett, & Dolin: principles and practice of infectious diseases, 6th edn. Churchill Livingstone, Edinburgh, 2005.

114. Rota PA, Liffick SL, Rota JS, Katz RS, Redd S, Papania M, *et al*. Molecular epidemiology of measles viruses in the United States, 1997–2001. Emerg Infect Dis 2002;8(9):902–8.

115. Tipples GA, Gray M, Garbutt M, Rota PA, Canadian Measles Surveillance Program. Genotyping of measles virus in Canada: 1979–2002. J Infect Dis 2004;189(suppl 1):S171–6.

116. Atmar RL, Englund JA, Hammill H. Complications of measles during pregnancy. Clin Infect Dis 1992;14(1):217–26.

117. Chiba ME, Saito M, Suzuki N, Honda Y, Yaegashi N. Measles infection in pregnancy. J Infect 2003;47(1):40–4.

118. Eberhart-Phillips JE, Frederick PD, Baron RC, Mascola L. Measles in pregnancy: a descriptive study of 58 cases. Obstet Gynecol 1993;82(5):797–801.

119. Gershon AA. Chickenpox, measles, and mumps. In: Remington JS, Klein J, Wilson C, Baker C (eds) Infectious diseases of the fetus and newborn infant. Elsevier Saunders, Philadelphia, 2006: 693–737.

120. Gold E. Almost extinct diseases: measles, mumps, rubella, and pertussis. Pediatr Rev 1996;17(4):120–7.

121. Huiming Y, Chaomin W, Meng M. Vitamin A for treating measles in children. Update of Cochrane Database of Systematic Reviews, 2002;1:CD001479. Cochrane Database of Systematic Reviews, 2005;4:CD001479.

122. Ni J, Wei J, Wu T. Vitamin A for non-measles pneumonia in children. Cochrane Database of Systematic Reviews, 2005;3: CD003700.

123. Enders G, Miller E. Varicella and herpes zoster in pregnancy and the newborn. In: Gershon A (ed) Varicella-zoster virus virology and clinical management. Cambridge University Press, Cambridge, 2000: 317–47.

124. Enders G, Miller E, Cradock-Watson J, Bolley I, Ridehalgh M. Consequences of varicella and herpes zoster in pregnancy: prospective study of 1739 cases. Lancet 1994;343(8912):1548–51.

125. Tan MP, Koren G. Chickenpox in pregnancy: revisited. Reprod Toxicol 2006;21(4):410–20.

126. Sterner G, Forsgren M, Enocksson E, Grandien M, Granstrom G, Sterner G, *et al*. Varicella-zoster infections in late pregnancy. Scand J Infect Dis 1990;71(suppl):30–5.

127. Hall S, Maupin T, Seward J. Second varicella infections: are they more common than previously thought? Pediatrics 2002;109:1068–73.

128. Miller E, Cradock-Watson JE, Ridehalgh MK. Outcome in newborn babies given anti-varicella-zoster immunoglobulin after perinatal maternal infection with varicella-zoster virus. Lancet 1989;2(8659):371–3.

129. Harger JH, Ernest JM, Thurnau GR, Moawad A, Momirova V, Landon MB, *et al*. Risk factors and outcome of varicella-zoster virus pneumonia in pregnant women. J Infect Dis 2002;185(4):422–7.

130. Harris RE, Rhoades ER. Varicella pneumonia complicating pregnancy. Report of a case and review of literature. Obstet Gynecol 1965;25:734–40.

131. Hollier LM, Grissom H. Human herpes viruses in pregnancy: cytomegalovirus, Epstein-Barr virus, and varicella zoster virus. Clin Perinatol 2005;32(3):671–96.

132. Verstraelen H, Vanzieleghem B, Defoort P, Vanhaesebrouck P, Temmerman M. Prenatal ultrasound and magnetic resonance imaging in fetal varicella syndrome: correlation with pathology findings. Prenatal Diagn 2003;23(9):705–9.

133. Puchhammer-Stockl E, Kunz C, Wagner G, Enders G. Detection of varicella zoster virus (VZV) DNA in fetal tissue by polymerase chain reaction. J Perinat Med 1994;22(1):65–9.

134. Marin M, Guris D, Chaves SS, Schmid S, Seward JF, Advisory Committee on Immunization Practices. Prevention of varicella: recommendations of the Advisory Committee on Immunization Practices (ACIP). MMWR Recomm Rep 2007;56(RR-4):1–40.

135. Wallace MR, Bowler WA, Murray NB, Brodine SK, Oldfield EC 3rd. Treatment of adult varicella with oral acyclovir. A randomized, placebo-controlled trial. Ann Intern Med 1992;117(5):358–63.

136. Stone KM, Reiff-Eldridge R, White AD, Cordero JF, Brown Z, Alexander ER, *et al*. Pregnancy outcomes following systemic prenatal acyclovir exposure: conclusions from the International Acyclovir Pregnancy Registry, 1984–1999. Birth Defects Res 2004;70(4):201–7.

137. Reiff-Eldridge R, Heffner CR, Ephross SA, Tennis PS, White AD, Andrews EB. Monitoring pregnancy outcomes after prenatal drug exposure through prospective pregnancy registries: a pharmaceutical company commitment. Am J Obstet Gynecol 2000;182(1 Pt 1):159–63.

138. Centers for Disease Control and Prevention. Prevention of varicella: recommendations of the Advisory Committee on Immunization Practices (ACIP). MMWR1996;45(RR-11):1–36.

139. Hanngren K, Grandien M, Granstrom G. Effect of zoster immunoglobulin for varicella prophylaxis in the newborn. Scand J Infect Dis 1985;17(4):343–7.

140. Brown ZA, Wald A, Morrow RA, Selke S, Zeh J, Corey L. Effect of serologic status and cesarean delivery on transmission rates of herpes simplex virus from mother to infant. JAMA 2003;289(2):203–9.

141. Lafferty WE, Downey L, Celum C, *et al*. Herpes simplex virus type 1 as a cause of genital herpes: impact on surveillance and prevention. J Infect Dis 2000;181(4):1454–7.

142. Nahmias AJ, Lee FK, Beckman-Nahmias S. Sero-epidemiological and -sociological patterns of herpes simplex virus infection in the world. Scand J Infect Dis 1990;69(suppl):19–36.

143. Brown ZA, Selke S, Zeh J, Kopelman J, Maslow A, Ashley RL, *et al*. The acquisition of herpes simplex virus during pregnancy. N Engl J Med 1997;337(8):509–15.

144. Enright AM, Prober CG. Neonatal herpes infection: diagnosis, treatment and prevention. Semin Neonatol 2002;7(4):283–91.

145. Mertz GJ. Asymptomatic shedding of herpes simplex virus 1 and 2: implications for prevention of transmission. J Infect Dis 2008;198(8):1098–100.

146. Mark KE, Wald A, Magaret AS, Selke S, Olin L, Huang ML, *et al*. Rapidly cleared episodes of herpes simplex virus reactivation in immunocompetent adults. J Infect Dis 2008;198(8):1141–9.

147. Bochud PY, Magaret AS, Koelle DM, *et al*. Polymorphisms in TLR2 are associated with increased viral shedding and lesional rate in patients with genital herpes simplex virus Type 2 infection. J Infect Dis 2007;196(4):505–9.

148. Koelle DM, Corey L. Recent progress in herpes simplex virus immunobiology and vaccine research. Clin Microbiol Rev 2003;16(1):96–113.

149. Brown ZA, Benedetti J, Ashley R, Burchett S, Selke S, Berry S, *et al*. Neonatal herpes simplex virus infection in relation to asymptomatic maternal infection at the time of labor. N Engl J Med 1991;324(18):1247–52.

150. Whitley R, Arvin A, Prober C, Corey L, Burchett S, Plotkin S, *et al*. Predictors of morbidity and mortality in neonates with herpes simplex virus infections. The National Institute of Allergy and Infectious Diseases Collaborative Antiviral Study Group. N Engl J Med 1991;324(7):450–4.

151. Garland SM, Lee TN, Sacks S. Do antepartum herpes simplex virus cultures predict intrapartum shedding for pregnant women with recurrent disease? Infect Dis Obstet Gynecol 1999;7(5):230–6.

152. Corey L. Herpes simplex virus. In: Mandell GL, Bennett JE, Dolin R (eds) Mandell, Bennett, & Dolin: principles and practice of infectious diseases, 6th edn. Churchill Livingstone, Edinburgh, 2005.

153. Vontver LA, Hickok DE, Brown Z, Reid L, Corey L. Recurrent genital herpes simplex virus infection in pregnancy: infant outcome and frequency of asymptomatic recurrences. Am J Obstet Gynecol 1982;143(1):75–84.

154. Frederick DM, Bland D, Gollin Y. Fatal disseminated herpes simplex virus infection in a previously healthy pregnant woman. A case report. J Reprod Med 2002;47(7):591–6.

155. Dupuis O, Audibert F, Fernandez H, Frydman R. Herpes simplex virus encephalitis in pregnancy. Obstet Gynecol 1999;94 (5 Pt 2):810–12.

156. Hollier LM, Scott LL, Murphree SS, Wendel GD Jr. Postpartum endometritis caused by herpes simplex virus. Obstet Gynecol 1997;89(5 Pt 2):836–8.

157. Arvin AM, Whitley RJ, Gutierrez KM. Herpes simplex virus infections. In: Remington JS, Klein J, Wilson C, Baker C (eds) Infectious diseases of the fetus and newborn infant. Elsevier Saunders, Philadelphia, 2006: 845–65.

158. Money D, Steben M, Society of Obstetricians and Gynecologists of Canada. Guidelines for the management of herpes simplex virus in pregnancy. J Obstet Gynaecol Can 2008;30(6):514–26.

159. Urato AC, Caughey AB. Genital herpes complicating pregnancy. Obstet Gynecol 2006;107(2 Pt 1):425–6; author reply 6.

160. Sheffield JS, Hill JB, Hollier LM, Laibl VR, Roberts SW, Sanchez PJ, *et al*. Valacyclovir prophylaxis to prevent recurrent herpes at delivery: a randomized clinical trial. Obstet Gynecol 2006;108(1):141–7. (Erratum appears in Obstet Gynecol 2006; 108(3 Pt 1):695.)

161. ACOG Practice Bulletin No. 8. Management of herpes in pregnancy. Clinical management guidelines for obstetrician-gynecologists. Int J Gynecol Obstet 2000;68(2):165–73.

162. Lam CM, Wong SF, Leung TN, Chow KM, Yu WC, Wong TY, *et al*. A case-controlled study comparing clinical course and outcomes of pregnant and non-pregnant women with severe acute respiratory syndrome. Br J Obstet Gynaecol 2004;111(8):771–4.

163. Alcorn J, McNamara PJ. Acyclovir, ganciclovir, and zidovudine transfer into rat milk. Antimicrob Agents Chemother 2002;46(6):1831–6.

164. Taddio A, Klein J, Koren G. Acyclovir excretion in human breast milk. Ann Pharmacother 1994;28(5):585–7.

165. Medeiros LR, Ethur ABdM, Hilgert JB, Zanini RR, Berwanger O, Bozzetti MC, *et al*. Vertical transmission of the human papillomavirus: a systematic quantitative review. Cadernos de Saude Publica 2005;21(4):1006–15.

166. Silverberg MJ, Thorsen P, Lindeberg H, Grant LA, Shah KV. Condyloma in pregnancy is strongly predictive of juvenile-onset recurrent respiratory papillomatosis. Obstet Gynecol 2003;101(4):645–52.

167. Strickler HD, Burk RD, Fazzari M, Anastos K, Minkoff H, Massad LS, *et al*. Natural history and possible reactivation of human papillomavirus in human immunodeficiency virus-positive women. J Natl Cancer Inst 2005;97(8):577–86.

168. Derkay CS. Recurrent respiratory papillomatosis. Laryngoscope 2001;111(1):57–69.

169. Smith EM, Ritchie JM, Yankowitz J, Swarnavel S, Wang D, Haugen TH, *et al*. Human papillomavirus prevalence and types in newborns and parents: concordance and modes of transmission. Sexual Trans Dis 2004;31(1):57–62.

170. Reeves W, Snehal S, Ruparelia M, *et al*. National registry for juvenile-onset recurrent respiratory papillomatosis. Arch Otolaryngol Head Neck Surg 2003;129:976–82.

171. Sinal SH, Woods CR. Human papillomavirus infections of the genital and respiratory tracts in young children. Semin Pediatr Infect Dis 2005;16(4):306–16.

172. Centers for Disease Control and Prevention. Recommended Adult Immunization Schedule - United States, 2010. MMWR January 15, 2010 59 (01):1-4. Last accessed February 14, 2010. www.cdc.gov/mmwr/preview/mmwrhtml/mm5901a5.htm

173. Garland SM, Ault KA, Gall SA, Paavonen J, Sings HL, Ciprero KL, *et al*. Pregnancy and infant outcomes in the clinical trials of a human papillomavirus type 6/11/16/18 vaccine: a combined analysis of five randomized controlled trials. Obstet Gynecol 2009;114(6):1179-88.

174. Siegel M, Greenberg M. Incidence of poliomyelitis in pregnancy: its relation to maternal age, parity and gestational period. N Engl J Med 1955;253(20):841–7.

175. Horn P. Pregnancy and poliomyelitis in Los Angeles county: a twenty-year report, with special emphasis on management of respirator patients. Obstet Gynecol 1955;5(4):416–22.

176. Horn P. Poliomyelitis in pregnancy: a twenty-year report from Los Angeles County, California. Obstet Gynecol 1955;6(2):121–37.

177. Centers for Disease Control and Prevention. Progress toward global eradication of poliomyelitis, 2002. MMWR 2003;52(16):366–9.

178. Modlin JF. Coxsackieviruses, echoviruses, and newer enteroviruses. In: Mandell GL, Bennett JE, Dolin R (eds) Mandell, Bennett, & Dolin: principles and practice of infectious diseases, 6th edn. Churchill Livingstone, Edinburgh, 2005.

179. Axelsson C, Bondestam K, Frisk G, Bergstrom S, Diderholm H. Coxsackie B virus infections in women with miscarriage. J Med Virol 1993;39(4):282–5.

180. Brown GC, Karunas RS. Relationship of congenital anomalies and maternal infection with selected enteroviruses. Am J Epidemiol 1972;95(3):207–17.

181. Cherry JD. Enterovirus and parechovirus infections. In: Remington JS, Klein J, Wilson C, Baker C (eds) Infectious diseases of the fetus and newborn infant. Elsevier Saunders, Philadelphia, 2006: 783–821.

182. Satosar A, Ramirez NC, Bartholomew D, Davis J, Nuovo GJ. Histologic correlates of viral and bacterial infection of the placenta associated with severe morbidity and mortality in the newborn. Hum Pathol 2004;35(5):536–45.

183. Tang JW, Bendig JWA, Ossuetta I. Vertical transmission of human echovirus 11 at the time of Bornholm disease in late pregnancy. Pediatr Infect Dis J 2005;24(1):88–9.

184. Prevots DR, Burr RK, Sutter RW, Murphy TV, Advisory Committee on Immunization Practices. Poliomyelitis prevention in the United States. Updated recommendations of the Advisory Committee on Immunization Practices (ACIP). MMWR 2000;49(RR-5):1–22; quiz CE1–7.

185. Childs J, Glass G, Ksiazek T. Human-rodent contact and infection with lymphocytic choriomeningitis and Seoul viruses in an inner-city population. Am J Trop Med Hyg 1991;44:117–21.

186. Peters CJ. Lymphocytic choriomeningitis virus, Lassa virus, and the South American hemorrhagic fevers. In: Mandell GL, Bennett JE, Dolin R (eds) Mandell, Bennett, & Dolin: principles and practice of infectious diseases, 6th edn. Churchill Livingstone, Edinburgh, 2005.

187. Barton LL, Mets MB, Beauchamp CL. Lymphocytic choriomeningitis virus: emerging fetal teratogen. Am J Obstet Gynecol 2002;187(6):1715–16.

188. Bleck TP, Ruprecht CE. Rhabdoviruses. In: Mandell GL, Bennett JE, Dolin R (eds) Mandell, Bennett, & Dolin: principles and practice of infectious diseases, 6th edn. Churchill Livingstone, Edinburgh, 2005.

189. Manning SE, Rupprecht CE, Fishbein D, Hanlon CA, Lumlertdacha B, Guerra M, et al. Human rabies prevention – United States, 2008: recommendations of the Advisory Committee on Immunization Practices. MMWR Recomm Rep 2008;57(RR-3):1–28.

190. Centers for Disease Control and Prevention. Intrauterine West Nile virus infection – New York, 2002. MMWR 2002;51(50):1135–6.

191. Centers for Disease Control and Prevention. Interim guidelines for the evaluation of infants born to mothers infected with West Nile virus during pregnancy. MMWR 2004;53(7):154–7.

192. Pogodina VV, Bochkova NG, Leshchinskaia EV, et al. Japanese encephalitis in citizens of Russia who travel abroad. Vopr Virusol 1996;41(1):8–11.

193. Mathur A, Tandon HO, Mathur KR, Sarkari NB, Singh UK, Chaturvedi UC, et al. Japanese encephalitis virus infection during pregnancy. Indian J Med Res 1985;81:9–12.

194. Chaturvedi UC, Mathur A, Chandra A, Das SK, Tandon HO, Singh UK, et al. Transplacental infection with Japanese encephalitis virus. J Infect Dis 1980;141(6):712–15.

195. Robertson CA, Lowther SA, Birch T, Tan C, Sorhage F, Stockman L, et al. SARS and pregnancy: a case report. Emerg Infect Dis 2004;10(2):345–8.

196. Stockman LJ, Lowther SA, Coy K, Saw J, Parashar UD. SARS during pregnancy, United States. Emerg Infect Dis 2004;10(9):1689–90.

197. Wong SF, Chow KM, Leung TN, Ng WF, Ng TK, Shek CC, et al. Pregnancy and perinatal outcomes of women with severe acute respiratory syndrome. Am J Obstet Gynecol 2004;191(1):292–7.

198. Shek CC, Ng PC, Fung GPG, Cheng FWT, Chan PKS, Peiris MJS, et al. Infants born to mothers with severe acute respiratory syndrome. Pediatrics 2003;112(4):e254.

199. Kroger AT, Atkinson WL, Marcuse EK, Pickering LK, Advisory Committee on Immunization Practices, Centers for Disease Control and Prevention. General recommendations on immunization: recommendations of the Advisory Committee on Immunization Practices (ACIP). MMWR 2006;55(RR-15):1–48.

200. Advisory Committee on Immunization Practices, Centers for Disease Control and Prevention. Guiding principles for development of ACIP recommendations for vaccination during pregnancy and breastfeeding. MMWR 2008 30;57(21):580.

201. Centers for Disease Control and Prevention. Recommended adult immunization schedule – United States, 2002–2003. MMWR 2002;51(40):904–8. (Erratum appears in MMWR 2003;52(15):345.)

202. Rotz LD, Dotson DA, Damon IK, Becher JA, Advisory Committee on Immunization Practices. Vaccinia (smallpox) vaccine: recommendations of the Advisory Committee on Immunization Practices (ACIP), 2001. MMWR Recomm Rep 2001;50(RR-10):1–25; quiz CE1–7.

203. Cetron MS, Marfin AA, Julian KG, Gubler DJ, Sharp DJ, Barwick RS, et al. Yellow fever vaccine. Recommendations of the Advisory Committee on Immunization Practices (ACIP), 2002. MMWR Recomm Rep 2002;51(RR-17):1–11; quiz CE1-4.

204. Advisory Committee on Immunization Practices. Human rabies prevention – United States, 1999. MMWR Recomm Rep 1999;48(RR-1):1–21. (Erratum appears in MMWR 1999;48(1):16.)

205. Gall SA. Vaccines for pertussis and influenza: recommendations for use in pregnancy. Clin Obstet Gynecol 2008;51(3):486–97.

206. Murphy TV, Slade BA, Broder KR, Kretsinger K, Tiwari T, Joyce PM, et al. Prevention of pertussis, tetanus, and diphtheria among pregnant and postpartum women and their infants. Recommendations of the Advisory Committee on Immunization Practices (ACIP). MMWR Recomm Rep 2008;57(RR-4):1–51. (Erratum appears in MMWR 2008;57(26):723.)

207. National Advisory Committee on Immunization (NACI). Statement on influenza vaccination for the 2007–2008 season. Can Commun Dis Rep 2007;33(11):23–4.

208. Mast EE, Weinbaum CM, Fiore AE, Alter MJ, Bell BP, Finelli L, et al. A comprehensive immunization strategy to eliminate transmission of hepatitis B virus infection in the United States: recommendations of the Advisory Committee on Immunization Practices (ACIP). Part II: immunization of adults. MMWR Recomm Rep 2006;55(RR-16):1–33; quiz CE1-4. (Erratum appears in MMWR 2007;56(42):1114.)

209. Kroger AT, Atkinson WL, Marcuse EK, Pickering LK, Advisory Committee on Immunization Practices, Centers for Disease Control and Prevention. General recommendations on immunization: recommendations of the Advisory Committee on Immunization Practices (ACIP). MMWR Recomm Rep. 2006;55(RR-15):1–48. (Erratum appears in MMWR 2006;55(48):1303.)

210. Advisory Committee on Immunization Practices, Fiore AE, Wasley A, Bell BP. Prevention of hepatitis A through active or passive immunization: recommendations of the Advisory Committee on Immunization Practices (ACIP). MMWR Recomm Rep 2006;55(RR-7):1–23.

211. Bilukha OO, Rosenstein N, National Center for Infectious Diseases. Prevention and control of meningococcal disease. Recommendations of the Advisory Committee on Immunization Practices (ACIP). MMWR Recomm Rep 2005;54(RR-7):1–21.

212. Canadian Immunization Guide 2006, 7th edition. Public Health Agency of Canada under the authority of Public Works and Government Services Canada, 2007. HP40-3/006E.

213. Advisory Committee on Immunization P. Recommended adult immunization schedule: United States, 2010. Ann Intern Med 2010;152(1):36–9.

Human immunodeficiency virus infection in pregnancy

Ruth E. Tuomala[1], Judith S. Currier[2], Susan Cu-Uvin[3]
with Roshan Fernando[4]

[1]Department of Obstetrics, Gynecology, and Reproductive Biology, Harvard Medical School and Brigham and Women's Hospital, Boston, MA, USA
[2]Division of Infectious Diseases, Center for Clinical AIDS Research and Education, David Geffen School of Medicine at UCLA, Los Angeles, CA, USA
[3]Departments of Medicine and Obstetrics and Gynecology, Brown University and The Immunology Center, The Miriam Hospital, Providence, RI, USA
[4]Department of Anaesthesia, Royal Free Hospital, London, UK

Introduction

Medical management for human immunodeficiency virus (HIV-1) infected pregnant women encompasses both prevention of mother-to-child transmission (MTCT) of HIV-1 and contemporary standards for evaluation and treatment of HIV-infected adults. This chapter will present an overview of HIV disease including its diagnosis and treatment in adults, discuss counseling for HIV-infected women of reproductive age, and outline specifics of the obstetric, medical, anesthetic, and postpartum management of HIV-infected pregnant women.

Epidemiology of human immunodeficiency virus infection in women

Over half of the 39.5 million people living with HIV in 2006 were women. In sub-Saharan Africa, 60% of the 25 million HIV-infected adults are women. The number of HIV-infected females continues to rise, with the greatest increases in Eastern Europe, Asia, and Latin America. In North America an estimated 350,000 women are living with HIV, an increase of 50,000 from 2004 to 2006 [1]. The primary mode of transmission among women is heterosexual transmission.

In the United States, HIV disproportionately affects women of color. In 2004, HIV was the leading cause of death among African American women aged 25–34 and the third and fourth leading cause among ages 35–44 and 45–54 years respectively. The incidence of AIDS for African American women (49.9/100,000) is 24 times and four times higher than for white women (2.1/100,000) and Hispanic women (12.2/100,000), respectively [2]. Lack of perception of risk and relationship dynamics, including inability to negotiate condom use and fear of violence, contribute to growing rates of HIV infection among young women.

Screening for human immunodeficiency virus infection in pregnancy

Human immunodeficiency virus testing of all pregnant women is recommended [3]. Recommendations are for testing to be performed unless declined ("opt out"), without separate written informed consent unless required by specific law. Testing should be done early in pregnancy, and repeated in the third trimester if early testing was not done or was initially negative in "at-risk" women. Risk factors include high-prevalence geographic areas or healthcare facilities, and personal factors, including injection drug use, exchanging sex for money or drugs, sex partners of HIV-infected persons or drug users, and a new or more than one sex partner during this pregnancy. Rapid HIV testing at the time of labor is recommended if HIV infection status has not previously been documented during the index pregnancy.

de Swiet's Medical Disorders in Obstetric Practice, 5th edition.
Edited by R. O. Powrie, M. F. Greene, W. Camann. © 2010 Blackwell Publishing.

Diagnostic tests for human immunodeficiency virus infection

The diagnosis of HIV infection is made by detecting either antibodies to HIV or HIV viral ribonucleic acid (RNA) in blood by polymerase chain reaction (PCR) testing (HIV RNA-PCR). The standard antibody assay is the enzyme-linked immunoassay (EIA, also known as ELISA) performed on serum. In addition, there are several different rapid EIA tests that utilize blood, and the Oraquick test can be performed on oral fluid samples. An initial positive EIA test must be confirmed with a second, more specific test: a Western blot, immunoflorescence assay or HIV RNA-PCR [3,4]. The Western blot detects antibodies to specific HIV antigens; positivity requires the presence of antibodies to two of the following: p 24, gp 41, and gp 120/160. Testing is indeterminate if the EIA is positive and the Western blot shows antibody to only a single HIV antigen. Negative confirmatory testing should be repeated in the third trimester in "at-risk" women, and indeterminate testing should prompt both repeat testing and referral to a specialist.

Causes of indeterminate results include partial seroconversion, advanced acquired immune deficiency syndrome (AIDS) with decreased antibody titers, blood transfusions, organ transplantation, autoimmune disease and experimental HIV vaccines. Risk factors must be assessed when evaluating an indeterminate test. HIV infection is unlikely in low-risk patients with repeat indeterminate testing in 3 months. Patients in the process of seroconversion will usually have a positive Western blot within 1 month.

Gestational age must be considered in making decisions about treatment in the case of indeterminate testing [5]. Waiting 1 and 3 months to repeat testing is reasonable in early pregnancy. Viral testing can be used and if negative, treatment can be deferred pending follow-up antibody testing. Close to delivery, indeterminate tests should prompt antiretroviral treatment, as should any positive antibody testing at the time of labor and delivery.

Pathogenesis of human immunodeficiency virus infection

Principles of therapy are based on the pathogenesis of HIV infection. The clinical features and pathogenesis of primary infection have been recently reviewed [6,7]. Primary HIV infection is followed by a dramatic increase in plasma viremia, sometimes accompanied by a distinct clinical syndrome consisting of fever, adenopathy, malaise, myalgia, pharyngitis, rash and in some cases aseptic meningitis. Cells with CD4+ receptors become infected and viral replication begins within them. Infected cells release virions by surface budding or lysis, leading to infection of additional cells.

HIV-directed sequences become incorporated into host DNA during replication and remain so until cell death. A reservoir of long-lived, infected resting T-cells is established early on and persists for many years, even in the presence of treatment. This reservoir can harbor drug-resistant virus when patients are exposed to suboptimal treatment regimens.

The number of CD4+ T-lymphocytes declines acutely, stabilizes, and then rebounds as the immune system, CD8+ T-lymphocytes in particular, works to control viral replication. After a new equilibrium is reached in which the rate of production of new CD4+ T-cells equals the rate of destruction, a person may remain asymptomatic for a number of years. Viral replication continues, and over time the plasma viral load increases and the number of CD4 + T-lymphocytes declines. Monitoring the CD4+ cell count helps to establish the stage of HIV disease. Mild symptoms such as weight loss, lymphadenopathy, and a variety of skin problems (mucocutaneous ulcers and/or rash with the initial seroconversion and oral hairy leukoplakia, thrush, persistent vaginal candidiasis with early symptomatic disease) often occur early in the course of symptomatic HIV disease. Most AIDS-related opportunistic infections do not occur until the CD4+ cell count falls below 200 cells/mm^3. This typically develops 10 or more years after infection [8]. The risk of disease progression increases with time and is thought to ultimately be very high without treatment.

Although mild symptoms can occur early in the course of HIV disease, patients can remain completely asymptomatic for a long period of time. The absence of symptoms should not preclude HIV testing.

Human immunodeficiency virus mutates readily and several viral variants emerge over time in an individual, some of which are capable of immune control. Chronic immune system activation is thought to contribute to CD4+ cell loss and reduced efficacy of B-cell responses to bacterial pathogens.

More severe symptoms and development of AIDS-defining illnesses occur when a significant number of CD4+ T-lymphocytes has been destroyed and production cannot match destruction (Table 18.1). PCP pneumonia caused by *Pneumocystis jiroveci* remains the most common initial opportunistic infection (OI), although with PCP prophylaxis the incidence has decreased. Other OI occurring early in the course of AIDS include cryptococcal meningitis, cerebral toxoplasmosis, recurrent bacterial infections, including bacteremia and pneumococcal pneumonia, and severe herpes simplex infection. Later complications include disseminated cytomegalovirus (CMV) and *Mycobacterium avium complex* (MAC) infection.

Several cohort studies have contributed to understanding the natural history and outcomes of women with HIV infection [9–11]. Kaposi's sarcoma is more common in men, and esophageal candidiasis and bacterial infections may be more common in women, but otherwise HIV-related complications are similar in men and women [12,13]. There is no indication

Table 18.1 Time course of HIV infection without treatment

Stage	Acute infection	Early disease	Mid-range disease	Advanced HIV/AIDS
Time since exposure	Weeks	Months to years	Years	Years
CD4+ T-cells	Usually >500 but can drop acutely	350–500	200–350	<200
HIV RNA	Usually >25,000 Often >500,000	Varies	Varies	Varies
Clinical symptoms	Fever, rash, pharyngitis, lymphadenopathy	Often no symptoms Night sweats Zoster	Weight loss Lymphadenopathy Oral thrush Night sweats Diarrhea	All of the previous symptoms and AIDS-defining opportunistic infections

Table 18.2 Current recommendations for initiation of antiretroviral therapy for nonpregnant patients [20]

Clinical category	CD4+ cell count (cells/mm^3)	Plasma HIV-RNA (copies/mm^3)	Recommendations
Symptomatic, history of AIDS-defining illness	Any value	Any value	Treat
Asymptomatic, AIDS	<200	Any value	Treat
Asymptomatic	>200 but <350	Any value	Treat
HIV-associated nephropathy	Any value	Any value	Treat
Co-infection with hepatitis B needing HBV treatment	Any value	Any value	Treat with fully suppressive antiviral drugs active against both HIV and HBV
None of above conditions	>350	Any value	No clear benefit to treatment (currently recommended by some experts)

that women have a different course once OI have occurred or that they respond differently to commonly used therapies. Women have lower HIV-1 RNA levels than do men, especially early in disease [14]. Early studies suggested that HIV-infected women had a more rapid rate of disease progression and shortened survival after diagnosis compared to men [15]. Other studies have not found gender differences in survival or attribute survival differences to stage of disease when diagnosed, or differential utilization of healthcare resources including antiretroviral therapy (ART) [16,17].

Antiretroviral therapy prolongs life and extends disease-free survival in HIV infection [18,19]. Efficacy is judged by clinical criteria, improvement in CD4+ cell count, and suppression or decrease in viral load. Current recommendations for ART initiation balance efficacy, long-term ART toxicity and development of drug resistance (Table 18.2). Combinations of at least three separate highly active antiretroviral agents (HAART) are associated with the greatest efficacy and least development of resistance. The major classes of agents include nucleoside and nucleotide analog reverse transcriptase inhibitors (NRTI),

non-nucleoside reverse transcriptase inhibitors (NNRTI), and protease inhibitors (PI), although drugs with other modes of actions have entered into the armamentarium. Combination regimens for initial ART typically consist of two separate NRTI and either an NNRTI or a PI. US Public Health Service guidelines for treatment of HIV-infected adults are published, posted online, and continually updated [20].

Preconception counseling

With the advent of HAART, HIV-infected women are living longer and healthier lives. Attitudes towards having children are more positive. All HIV-infected women of reproductive age should receive preconception counseling, starting early during HIV care. Preconception counseling should include information about MTCT, the importance of maximizing health and minimizing viral load surrounding pregnancy, utilization of ART, and potential short- and long-term implications of HIV treatments during pregnancy for women and their infants.

Preconception counseling also offers the opportunity to advise on safe sex practices and discuss methods to prevent unintended pregnancies. HIV testing of sex partners should be encouraged. For discordant couples, options such as intravaginal or intrauterine insemination and other assisted reproductive technologies to achieve pregnancy should be discussed. Counseling and referrals for cessation of smoking and illicit drug use are also appropriate.

A substantial number of women are identified as HIV infected during prenatal testing. These women need to receive the same information about MTCT, ART, their own health, and long-term follow-up as provided during preconception counseling.

Without ART, the MTCT rate centers around 25%. Transmission occurs antepartum, intrapartum, and postnatally through breastfeeding. Two-thirds to three-quarters occurs during or close to the intrapartum period [21]. In resource-limited settings, breastfeeding accounts for approximately 40% of peripartum/postnatal HIV transmission [22].

Maternal factors associated with MTCT include advanced HIV disease, high plasma viral load, low CD4+ cell count, poor maternal nutrition, and maternal illicit drug use, smoking, and sexually transmitted diseases [23–26]. Obstetric factors include prolonged rupture of membranes, chorio-amnionitis, and route of delivery [25,27,28]. Fetal factors include low birthweight, prematurity, and genetic susceptibility [25,29]. Viral phenotype and genotype may also affect transmission rates [30]. The two most important factors affecting MTCT are maternal viral load and ART use during pregnancy.

Viral load near term correlates with risk of MTCT among both untreated women and women treated with ART during pregnancy. Women with HIV RNA levels <1000 copies have very low rates of MTCT [24,26]. However, HIV transmission has been documented even with low or undetectable maternal viral levels [31]. Although plasma and genital tract HIV levels correlate well, discordance between these two compartments [32,33] may explain some cases of MTCT despite low peripheral blood virus concentrations.

Since 1994, recommendations for ART for HIV-infected pregnant women have evolved in parallel with evolving standards for other adults. Combinations of three or more antiretroviral (ARV) agents maximally decrease MTCT compared with no ARV or zidovudine (ZDV, AZT) alone, and viral load and ART independently affect MTCT risk [34]. Current guidelines recommend antepartum, intrapartum, and postnatal infant ARV for fetal and neonatal protection regardless of viral load [35]. Finally, breastfeeding is not recommended in resource-rich countries to prevent postnatal HIV transmission.

Women should be told of the most common side effects of ARV, and informed of safety concerns, described in detail later in this chapter. They should be informed of the need for short- and long-term monitoring of both women and infants for potential effects of exposure to ARV during pregnancy.

Pregnancy does not accelerate immunologic decline or affect disease progression and survival among HIV-infected women [36,37]. There are reports of postpartum increases in HIV-1 RNA regardless of continuation of ART after delivery [38,39]. Decreased adherence or changes in ART postpartum may explain some of this increase.

Antepartum management

Basic care for HIV infected pregnant women consists of:
• evaluation and therapy for maternal HIV disease
• ART for fetal protection and as appropriate for maternal health
• monitoring for ART toxicities
• PERIPARTUM management, including selection of route of delivery
• neonatal ART
• arrangements for long-term healthcare for both mother and infant.

Comprehensive care entails a team approach with co-ordinated efforts by multiple service providers (Box 18.1). Community-based

Box 18.1 Referrals for HIV-infected pregnant women

• Maternal-fetal medicine specialist with expertise in perinatal HIV
• HIV specialist (internist or ID physician)
• Case manager/care co-ordinator
• Psychiatric/social services
• Drug treatment program
• Pediatrics

obstetric care should be supplemented by consultation with specialists in maternal-fetal medicine or infectious diseases; alternatively care may be transferred to referral centers with expertise in HIV/AIDS. Management issues include:
• HIV education and counseling
• HIV testing of sexual partners and family members
• psychologic assessment and ongoing counseling
• drug abuse management
• supportive services
• adherence strategies for healthcare visits and ART.

If a woman is receiving HIV care prior to pregnancy, results of recent laboratory evaluations and the currently prescribed ART should be confirmed. If a woman has not been receiving medical care or was recently diagnosed, the obstetric provider must initiate evaluations for HIV disease staging, and frequently co-existing conditions including OI, sexually transmitted diseases, illicit drug use, alcohol use, and both smoking and respiratory tract complications. Initial laboratory assessment of HIV-infected pregnant women is outlined in Box 18.2.

Antiretrovirals: choice of agents and initiation of therapy

Comprehensive guidelines for the use of ARV during pregnancy have been published and are posted online and continually updated [35]. All women should receive combination regimens of at least three ARV agents during pregnancy for fetal protection, regardless of the necessity of ART for maternal health. The exact ARV regimen should be individualized based on stage of maternal HIV disease, prior history of ART, and genotypic resistance to ARV. Regimens recommended for women who have not previously received ART are those recommended as initial therapy for HIV-infected adults. If possible, zidovudine should be included.

If a woman is on stable ART that has achieved good virologic control and immunologic effect, this should not be stopped during pregnancy. Discontinuation of ART can lead to viral rebound with the possibility of *in utero* fetal infection and emergence of resistant virus. No major teratogenic effects of commonly used ARV agents have been demonstrated [40]. The exception to this is the drug efavirenz (Sustiva), classified by the FDA as category D. Efavirenz is associated with neural

Box 18.2 Initial laboratory assessment of HIV-infected pregnant women

Staging/antiretroviral management

- CD4 + cell count
- Viral load (HIV RNA-PCR)
- HIV genotype

Co-existing conditions

- Hepatitis B surface antigen (if positive, hepatitis B DNA-PCR)
- Hepatitis C antibody (if positive, hepatitis C RNA-PCR)
- Serologic test for syphilis
- Toxoplasmosis IgG
- Cytomegalovirus IgG
- *Gonorrhea, Chlamydia* lower genital tract assessments
- Pap smear

Baseline laboratory tests for ARV toxicity monitoring

- CBC – platelet count
- Liver function tests
- BUN, creatinine
- Electrolytes
- Amylase
- G6PD

including financial assistance, drug abuse services, and management of psychiatric issues. Hospitalization for directly observed therapy (DOT) and treatment of side effects may also be an effective strategy to maximize adherence.

The pharmacokinetics during pregnancy of many of the ARV agents currently in use have been elucidated [35]. A summary of results of pharmacokinetics studies is presented in Table 18.3. In general, the pharmacokinetics of NRTI

Table 18.3 Pharmacokinetic properties of antiretroviral agents during pregnancy

Drug	Cord blood/maternal drug level ratio	Maternal pharmacokinetic changes	Dosage change in agent necessary during Pregnancy
NRTI			
Zidovudine (ZDV, AZT)	0.85	No change	No
Lamivudine (3TC)	1.0	No change	No
Stavudine (d4t)	0.76–1.3	No change	No
Didanosine (ddI)	0.5	No change	No
Abacavir	0.85	No change	No
Tenofovir	yes	No change	No
NNRTI			
Nevirapine	1.0	No change	No
Efavirenz	Yes		
Protease inhibitors			
Indinavir	Minimal	Antepartum <postpartum; low levels compared to nonpregnant	Yes*
Ritonavir	Minimal	Antepartum <postpartum; low levels compared to nonpregnant	Used only as low dose for "boosting"
Nelfinavir	Minimal	Antepartum <postpartum; low levels compare to nonpregnant	Yes*
Saquinavir	Minimal	Low levels compared to nonpregnant	Yes*
Kaletra (lopinavir/ritonavir)		Antepartum <postpartum; low levels c ompared to nonpregnant	Some experts increase from 2 to 3 tablets twice daily in third trimester; some administer 2 tablets twice daily and monitor response and drug levels. Studies of new formulations underway

*Dose adjustment may involve co-administration with low-dose ritonavir and/or increase in dosing of primary agent.

tube defects in primates and four reported cases of significant CNS defects in infants exposed *in utero* to efavirenz during the first trimester, including three neural tube defects and one Dandy–Walker syndrome [41]. Other agents should be substituted for efavirenz during preconception counseling or as early as possible once pregnancy has been documented.

The timing of initiation of ART during pregnancy is determined by indication for use. If maternal viral load is low, immunologic suppression minimal, and the indication is fetal protection, ARV can be started after the first trimester. If indicated for maternal health, ART should be started as soon as possible.

Effectiveness and safety of ART are influenced by adherence to drug regimens as prescribed [42,43]. Inconsistent use with time periods of subtherapeutic drug levels promotes the development of genotypic resistance and virologic failure. In the case of hyperemesis gravidarum, all ARV should be stopped, or not instituted, until the medications can be taken as prescribed. If initiation of ART is associated with nausea and vomiting, antiemetics should be utilized. A variety of strategies to otherwise promote adherence have been suggested, and NNRTI agents are not affected by pregnancy, and dose alterations are not necessary. There are substantial differences during pregnancy in the pharmacokinetic profiles of the PI that have been studied, with lower drug levels observed, often requiring dose modifications. Negligible levels of PI in cord blood have also been noted. The PI are metabolized in the liver by the cytochrome P450 system; pharmacokinetic changes are likely due to alterations in hepatic metabolism during pregnancy as well as placental protein synthesis and drug metabolism.

Some of the PI and the NNRTI efavirenz can induce or inhibit the hepatic metabolism of other medications, thereby altering drug levels or enhancing toxicities (Table 18.4). Of particular note, the concomitant use of ergotamines and PI or efavirenz has been associated with exaggerated vasoconstrictive responses. If a woman on PI develops uterine atony and bleeding, methergine should be used only if absolutely necessary.

HIV viral load and CD4+ cell counts are checked within 2–4 weeks after initiating or changing ART. Once an effective regimen has been established, CD4+ cell counts are checked every 3 months and HIV viral loads are checked every 2 months and between 34 and 36 weeks of gestation in order to assist in determination of mode of delivery. The goal is to achieve a nondetectable viral load prior to delivery.

Laboratory monitoring for common hematologic, renal, hepatic, and metabolic side effects of ARV should occur periodically antepartum (see Table 18.5) and whenever suggestive signs or symptoms occur. Many experts recommend third-trimester monitoring for fetal growth and well-being, if women are receiving an ARV that has not been commonly used during pregnancy.

Table 18.4 Drug–drug interactions, antiretrovirals and commonly used drugs

Antiretroviral	Other drug	Effect	Action to take
Nevirapine Lopinavir/ritonavir Saquinavir/ritonavir	Methadone	↓ methadone levels; can precipitate withdrawal	↑ methadone dose
Protease inhibitors Efavirenz	Ergot alkaloids (methergine)	Vasospasm, ischemia	Avoid if possible (use other uterotonic agents)
Protease inhibitors Efavirenz	Midazolam, other benzodiazepines	Prolonged sedation	Avoid if possible (give lorazepam)
Ritonavir Lopinavir/ritonavir Saquinavir/ritonavir	Meperidine	Prolonged sedation	Avoid if possible (give oxycodone)
Ritonavir Lopinavir/ritonavir Saquinavir/ritonavir	Bupropion, clozapine	↑ drug levels	Avoid if possible (give other agents, lower doses)

Table 18.5 Laboratory evaluations/testing during pregnancy

Assessment	Frequency
CD4+cell count Quantitative HIV viral load	Every trimester, one month after initiating or changing ARV and as needed for evaluating or adjusting therapy
HIV genotype	When viral load increased while on ARV or when virus detected when previously suppressed while on ARV
PPD Chest X-ray Complete blood count Liver function tests Electrolytes Amylase	Early in pregnancy; for suggestive symptoms Each trimester and for signs or symptoms of possible toxicity
50 g glucose loading test	Early in pregnancy, repeat in third trimester
Ultrasound	Per obstetric standard; every 4–6 weeks for assessment of fetal growth and amniotic fluid volume
Nonstress test/ biophysical profile	Weekly as indicated for assessment of fetal well-being according to ARV regimen

PPD, purified protein derivative.

Safety data for individual agents and for ARV combinations during pregnancy come largely from case reports, small phase I/II trials, and observational databases. The commonly used ARV regimens are not associated with patterns of toxicities or side effects concerning enough to limit their use [40,44,45].

Most ARV can cause gastrointestinal side effects, particularly during initial use. Rates are not higher during pregnancy, if initiation is after the first trimester. Anemia is a known side effect of NRTI, in particular ZDV. Anemia occurs more frequently in HIV-infected pregnant women receiving any ARV than in those not on medications. Long-term use of PI-containing ART is associated with hyperglycemia, including new-onset diabetes mellitus [46] in adults. Most studies to date have not associated PI use with increased risk for gestational diabetes [44,47]. The potential for glucose intolerance remains of concern among women with long-duration PI use and patients may benefit from an early diabetic screen in addition to the usual screen between 24 and 28 weeks gestation [45].

Deaths from hepatic failure have been reported in pregnant women commenced on combination ART containing nevirapine during pregnancy [48,49]. Severe nevirapine hepatotoxicity in adults has been observed to occur soon after onset of use, more commonly in women, often in association with a rash, and almost exclusively among those with CD4+ cell counts >250/mm³ [50]. Its true rate of occurrence is unknown, as is whether or not it is more common during pregnancy. Chronic nevirapine should not be initiated if CD4+ count is >250/mm³. If therapy with nevirapine is initiated during pregnancy, liver function should be monitored frequently for the first 18 weeks. Most cases of hepatotoxicity resolve upon discontinuing the medication. Nevirapine-containing regimens that have been used since before pregnancy do not need to be discontinued.

Maternal deaths in the third trimester from lactic acidosis and hepatic steatosis in association with use of ddI (dida-nosine) and d4t (stavudine) throughout pregnancy have been reported [51]. Symptoms are nonspecific, including nausea, vomiting, and malaise; symptoms and laboratory findings can mimic those of pregnancy-related disorders such as the HELLP syndrome and fatty liver of pregnancy. Discontinuation of the ARV and supportive therapy most often results in recovery. The combination of d4T and ddI should not be used during pregnancy. The possibility of metabolic syndrome with hepatic dysfunction should be investigated in pregnant women receiving NRTI agents who present with suggestive symptoms.

In general, ARV use is not associated with adverse obstetric outcomes. Some reports have shown improvement in obstet-ric outcomes in women receiving ARV compared to untreated women [44,45]. There are conflicting data as to whether the use of combination ART containing PI is associated with pre-term delivery. European cohort studies and one from a single-center US cohort have found 2–4-fold increased odds for preterm delivery in association with combination ART con-taining PI [52–54]. However, similar studies from the US and Brazil and a meta-analysis of studies from resource-rich countries have shown no such association [55–57].

The few studies that have assessed maternal outcomes after pregnancy-specific ARV use for fetal protection have not shown any short-term deleterious effects [37,58]. There is theoretical concern that short-term exposure to ART for one or more pregnancies could result in the emergence of antiret-roviral resistance, limiting options for maternal health in the future, but long-term outcome data are lacking.

The advantage of ARV use during pregnancy for fetal protection outweighs any neonatal and infant toxicities observed to date. Immediate toxicities are limited to tran-sient anemia associated with neonatal ZDV [59]. Concerns have been raised about two potential long-term effects.

In rodents, the occurrence of squamous tumors of the skin, lung, liver, and genital tract at mid-life has been noted in offspring with *in utero* exposure to ZDV [60]. Analyses of observational cohorts show no increase in tumors or childhood cancers through age 6 in ARV-exposed infants [61,62].

Reports from France have suggested an association between *in utero* exposure to NRTI drugs and mitochondrial disease in infants [63,64]. Mitochondrial disease is a rare, progressive, multisystem disorder due to mutations of mitochondrial DNA. Symptoms range in severity from laboratory abnormalities to severe disease, including death. In clinically apparent disease, neurologic involvement, including seizures, hypotonia, enceph-alopathy and developmental delay, is typical and myopathy, pancreatitis, and cardiac toxicity can also occur. An increased rate of febrile seizures in NRTI-exposed infants has also been suggested [65]. Analyses of data from other cohorts have failed to document an association between *in utero* NRTI exposure and mitochondrial disease [66].

The potential for delayed effects of *in utero* ARV exposure requires close communication between obstetric and pediatric providers. Documentation of such exposure should be part of the permanent pediatric medical record and all appropriate monitoring for long-term toxicities should be assured.

Other management concerns

During pregnancy, HIV management also includes providing therapy for all HIV-related and co-existing conditions as well as providing appropriate obstetric care.

Women with evidence of advanced immune suppression should receive prophylaxis for prevention of OI as recom-mended for HIV-infected adults [67,68]. This includes proph-ylaxis for primary prevention of infections, such as PCP, disseminated MAC, and encephalitis (and less commonly chorioretinitis or pneumonitis) caused by *Toxoplasma gondii* as well as secondary prophylaxis, or chronic therapy, to pre-vent OI recurrences. New clinical symptoms or signs should be investigated with appropriate diagnostic procedures, and appropriate therapy given upon diagnosis.

Most OI prophylaxis or treatment is the same for preg-nant women as for other nonpregnant adults. The following should be noted.
• *PCP*: trimethoprim/sulfamethoxazole is the preferred prophy-laxis. Pregnancy-related respiratory changes may affect absorp-tion and distribution of aerosolized pentamidine.
• *MAC*: azithromycin is preferred for prophylaxis and treatment of disseminated MAC infection during pregnancy. Clarithromycin is a teratogen and abortifacient in animal models.
• *Fungal opportunistic infections* (e.g. candidiasis, histoplas-mosis, cryptococcosis, coccidioides, aspergillosis): amphoter-icin is preferred for prophylaxis or treatment during the first trimester. The azoles, fluconazole and itraconazole, are animal teratogens; safety of high dose or continuous therapy in pregnancy is unknown.
• *Cytomegalovirus*: all CMV treatment drugs are animal embryotoxins or teratogens. During pregnancy, ganciclovir is preferred. Treatment of pre-existing CMV infection solely for fetal protection is not indicated.
• *Toxoplasmosis*: *in utero* transmission of toxoplasmosis to the fetus has occurred in HIV-infected women who are antibody positive pre-pregnancy. Prophylaxis is generally accomplished with trimethoprim/sulfamethoxazole in anti-body-positive women and with avoidance of exposure in antibody-negative women.
• *Tuberculosis* (TB): isoniazid (INH), rifampin, pyrazinamide (PZA), ethambutol are preferred treatments due to wider experience in human pregnancy. INH hepatotoxicity may

be increased during pregnancy; monitor liver function tests monthly.

• *Respiratory infections*: administer influenza vaccine every year and pneumococcal vaccine every 5 years as indicated. Do not use clarithromycin or quinolones for treatment if alternatives are available.

The management of other conditions seen with increased prevalence in association with HIV infection is the same as for non-HIV-infected adults, with some notable exceptions.

• *Syphilis of undetermined or advanced stage*: evaluate and consider treatment for neurosyphilis.

• *Hepatitis C co-infection*: perinatal transmission of both agents is increased [69,70]. However, there is no evidence for decreased rates of perinatal hepatitis C transmission with elective cesarean section [71] and treatment of hepatitis C in pregnancy is not routinely recommended.

• *Hepatitis B co-infection* [20,35]: hepatotoxicity of ARV may be enhanced. If ARV includes agents with activity against hepatitis B (lamivudine, tenofovir, and emtricitabine), hepatitis B disease may flare upon discontinuation of ARV postpartum. Co-manage with hepatitis specialist.

Women who are HIV infected should be offered appropriate antenatal genetics testing including amniocentesis and chorionic villus sampling as indicated. Although of theoretical concern, in utero transmission of HIV infection during these procedures has not been documented. It is, however, advisable when possible to control HIV viral load prior to performing these procedures.

Management of labor and delivery

All women should receive intravenous ZDV during labor unless contraindicated due to allergy. This is given intravenously, as one loading dose of 2 g/kg over an hour, followed by 1 g/kg/h throughout labor. Other ARV are continued orally during labor. Discontinue ART given solely for fetal protection after delivery. The infant should receive 6 weeks of ZDV.

Duration of ruptured membranes increases the risk for MTCT in women not receiving ART; the effect in women on ART with viral load suppression is not known. Consider oxytocin augmentation to shorten the length of labor in women with ruptured membranes. Perform artificial rupture of membranes and invasive monitoring only when obstetrically indicated.

Elective cesarean delivery before labor onset or ruptured membranes decreases MTCT by 55–80% compared to other modes of delivery in women receiving either no ART or ZDV monotherapy [28,72]. In women receiving ART, with undetectable viral load, it is unlikely that elective cesarean section confers substantial additional fetal protection. Similarly, after labor onset or ruptured membranes, cesarean delivery for fetal protection is not indicated. See Box 18.3 for recommendations for cesarean delivery to decrease MTCT [35,73].

Box 18.3 Recommendations for cesarean delivery to decrease MTCT

• Elective cesarean section prior to labor onset and ruptured membranes if:
  • HIV-1 RNA >1000 copies/mL
  • unknown HIV-1 RNA level
• Perform at 38 weeks gestation
• Administer intravenous ZDV starting 3 hour prior to procedure
• Use perioperative antibiotic prophylaxis

For HIV-infected women who have not received ART prior to labor, alternative recommendations for ARV for fetal protection to maximize efficacy are as follows:

• intrapartum intravenous ZDV followed by 6 weeks of ZDV for the baby

• some experts would administer single-dose mother/infant nevirapine in addition to the intrapartum 6-week newborn ZDV regimen [35].

Rates of nevirapine resistance ranging from 20–69% of women and 33–87% of infants after exposure to single-dose nevirapine [74,75] have been reported, likely due to the long half-life of nevirapine. If single-dose nevirapine is given alone or in combination with intrapartum ZDV, the additional administration of ZDV plus 3TC to the mother for 7 days post partum is recommended to prevent development of resistance.

Anesthetic concerns

Most HIV-infected parturients are otherwise healthy, with a low viral load and a CD4+ cell count > 200 cells/mm^3. Some women will undergo an elective cesarean delivery to reduce MTCT. Those undergoing labor may request epidural analgesia; some may need emergency cesarean delivery. Most women will require input from an obstetric anesthesiologist.

Labor analgesia

Labor analgesia can be instituted with a standard epidural or combined spinal epidural (CSE) technique using a low-dose mixture of local aesthetic and opioid (e.g. 0.1% bupivacaine with 2 μg/mL fentanyl).

Cesarean delivery

There is no evidence that general anesthesia (GA) or regional anesthesia (RA) alters immunity or has other adverse effects [76,77].

For an elective or emergency cesarean delivery under RA, single-shot spinal, CSE or epidural techniques can be used. An epidural catheter inserted for labor analgesia can be topped up for emergency cesarean delivery or to provide anesthesia for operative vaginal delivery.

Regional anesthesia

The human immunodeficiency virus is a neurotropic virus; the central nervous system (CNS) is infected early in the course of disease with isolation of virions and antibodies in the CSF at the time of initial diagnosis. RA does not cause CNS HIV infection.

Regional anesthesia does not increase neurologic or infectious problems in the HIV-infected patient [76]. Therefore when indicated and no routine contraindications exist (e.g. coagulopathy), RA can be utilized.

Hypotension is a common side effect of spinal anesthesia that is treated with fluids and vasopressors. The use of phenylephrine has also been associated with improved fetal umbilical cord blood gases [78] when used to maintain baseline systolic blood pressure during spinal anesthesia has [79]. Such regimens can also be used in HIV-infected parturients [80].

Postdural puncture headache (PDPH) after spinal anesthesia or accidental dural puncture with an epidural needle is one of the most common complications of RA. The use of an epidural blood patch (EBP), injection of the patient's own blood into the epidural space, is an effective treatment for PDPH. There have been no serious complications related to EBP in the HIV-infected patient [81]. Conversely, not treating a PDPH appropriately and promptly may lead to neurologic sequelae [82].

Drug interactions

There is the potential for significant interactions between HAART and anesthetic drugs. PI reduce the metabolism of multiple anesthetics and analgesics, such as midazolam and fentanyl, and cardiac drugs such as amiodarone and quinidine [83]. Nevirapine and efavirenz are inducers of CYP450; increased doses of anesthetic drugs may be needed with these drugs [84]. In practice, with careful titration of anesthetic drugs, problems are uncommon [85].

Other anesthetic considerations

For patients with advanced HIV disease the following should be noted.

• *Respiratory*: OI such as PCP and TB may cause respiratory distress and hypoxemia, aggravated by a decreased functional residual capacity seen during pregnancy. RA may be preferable in these patients. A high motor block with intercostal muscle weakness may increase respiratory problems.

• *Cardiovascular*: long-standing ART can cause hyperglycemia, hyperlipidemia, lipodystrophy and accelerated coronary arteriosclerosis [86]. Pulmonary hypertension has also been reported [87]. Preoperative evaluation of cardiac function needs to include consideration of more extensive testing, e.g. echocardiography and stress testing, in patients who have been on long-term ART.

• *Central nervous system*: HIV infection, intracranial masses or OI may lead to cerebral edema and increased intracranial pressure (ICP). RA is contraindicated in the presence of raised ICP due to an increased risk of brainstem coning.

• *Hematologic*: bone marrow suppression and coagulation abnormalities, including thrombocytopenia, may result from HIV infection, ARV drugs or bone marrow infiltration by OI or neoplastic disease. RA may be contraindicated due to an increased risk of spinal hematoma.

• *Co-infection with hepatitis*: the concurrent presence of hepatitis B or C infection, causing liver abnormalities, may alter anesthetic management.

• *Occupational exposure*: universal precautions should always be used when handling body fluids, tissue, blood and blood products regardless of patients' HIV status.

Postpartum management

Women with HIV may be at increased risk for postpartum complications. Some studies have suggested that complications due to infection, including fever, endometritis, wound infection, urinary tract infection and sepsis, are increased, in particular among those who undergo cesarean section [88–92] and among those with more advanced HIV infection [88,93]. In addition, two reports have suggested an increase in blood loss requiring transfusion or resulting in anemia. These complications must be anticipated and treated accordingly.

In resource-rich countries, where risks for infant morbidity and mortality from infectious and diarrheal illnesses are small, avoidance of all breastfeeding among HIV-infected women is recommended.

Women are at particular risk for self-discontinuing ART and dropping out of healthcare post partum [94,95]. Postpartum depression and relapse in drug use are both common. Women may ignore their healthcare in deference to that of the infant. Specific contact with HIV providers should be facilitated during the immediate postpartum period. Prior to hospital discharge, all necessary medications or prescriptions should be given and visits for healthcare, including drug treatment, scheduled. Case management and social services should be arranged.

Contraceptive services should be provided. Although the use of male and female condoms can prevent HIV/STD transmission, they may not be highly effective in preventing pregnancies. Combination hormonal contraceptives are highly effective in preventing pregnancies. Significant drug

Table 18.6 Antiretroviral therapy and its interactions with oral contraceptives

ART increases hormonal levels	ART decreases hormonal levels
Efavirenz (EE ↑ 37%)	Nevirapine (EE ↑ 20%)
Indinavir (EE ↑ 24%, NE ↑ 26%)	Ritonavir (EE ↑ 40%)
Atazanavir (EE ↑ 48%, NE ↑ 110%)	Nelfinavir (EE ↑ 47%, NE ↑ 18%)
	Lopinavir/ritonavir (EE ↑ 42%)
Etravirine (EE ↑ 22%)	Darunavir (EE ↓ 44%, NE ↓ 14%)
	Tipranavir (EE ↓ 50%)

ART, antiretroviral therapy; EE, ethinylestradiol; NE, norethindrone.

interactions with ARV agents can complicate their use among HIV-infected women (Table 18.6). In addition, oral hormonal contraception decreases amprenavir levels and these drugs should not be co-administered. Alternative methods or back-up contraception can be used simultaneously with oral contraceptives in women receiving ART. Transdermal or intravaginal hormonal contraceptives may be other options, but their pharmacokinetics in the setting of ART have not yet been determined. Medroxyprogesterone levels appear to be unaffected by ART [96].

Intrauterine devices are safe and effective contraception for selected HIV-infected women. Studies from Kenya show equal safety of the copper T IUD among HIV-infected and uninfected women [97]. Increased HIV genital tract shedding has not been found with IUD use [98]. The levonorgestrel-releasing IUD has an added advantage of decreased menstrual bleeding compared to the copper T IUD [99].

Spermicides have *in vitro* activity against HIV but non-oxynol-9 (N-9) has been associated with increased vaginal irritation, inflammation, and decreased lactobacilli. These changes may theoretically increase HIV shedding in the genital tract. In a randomized, placebo-controlled clinical trial among sex workers, N-9 increased vaginal lesions and possibly increased HIV acquisition [100].

Transitioning care post partum

Women receiving ART solely for fetal protection may elect to discontinue ARV post partum. Regular monitoring of CD4+ cell counts and viral load every 4–6 months should be maintained among women who stop treatment. A recent randomized clinical trial involving nonpregnant subjects demonstrated the potential risks (increased rates of OI and death) of discontinuing ART among patients with established HIV infection, even for those with CD4 counts above 350 cells/mm^3 [101]. In contrast, short-term follow-up of pregnant women who have discontinued ART post partum has not demonstrated a detrimental effect [58,102]. Other chronic conditions (such as active hepatitis B or HIV nephropathy) may also influence the decision to continue ART post partum. All plans for continuing medical care with an HIV specialist should be developed prior to delivery and instituted post partum.

Conclusion

Human immunodeficiency virus infection should be viewed as are other chronic medical conditions during pregnancy. Up-to-date knowledge of maternal, obstetric, anesthetic and fetal concerns and appropriate attention to current standards of adult management will result in optimum outcomes for both women and their neonates.

References

1. www.unaids.org/pub/EpiReport/2006.
2. Centers for Disease Control and Prevention. HIV/AIDS Surveillance Report, 2005. Vol. 17. US Department of Health and Human Services, Centers for Disease Control and Prevention, Atlanta, GA, 2006:1–46.
3. Panel on Antiretroviral Guidelines for Adults and Adolescents. Guidelines for the Use of Antiretroviral Agents in HIV-1-Infected Adults and Adolescents. Department of Health and Human Services. December 1, 2009; 1-161. Available at http://www.aidsinfo.nih.gov/ContentFiles/AdultandAdolescentGL.pdf. Accessed February, 2010.
4. Centers for Disease Control and Prevention. Rapid HIV-1 antibody testing during labor and delivery for women of unknown HIV status: a practical guide and model protocol. Centers for Disease Control and Prevention, Atlanta, GA, 2004:1–44. www.cdc.gov/hiv/topics/testing/resources/guidelines/pdf/Labor&DeliveryRapidTesting.pdf.
5. Doran TI, Parra E. False-positive and indeterminate human immunodeficiency virus test results in pregnant women. Arch Fam Med 2000; 9:924–9.
6. Picker LJ. Immunopathogenesis of acute AIDS virus infection. Curr Opin Immunol 2006;18:399–405.
7. Wilkinson J, Cunningham AL. Mucosal transmission of HIV-1: first stop dendritic cells. Curr Drug Targets 2006;7:1563–9.
8. Munoz A, Wang MC, Bass S, et al. Acquired immunodeficiency syndrome (AIDS)-free time after human immunodeficiency virus type 1 (HIV-1) seroconversion in homosexual men. Am J Epidemiol 1989;130:530–9.
9. Anastos K, Barron Y, Cohen MH, et al. The prognostic importance of changes in CD4+cell count and HIV-1 RNA level in women after initiating highly active antiretroviral therapy. Ann Intern Med 2004;140:256–64.
10. Anastos K, Barron Y, Miotti P, et al. Risk of progression to AIDS and death in women infected with HIV-1 initiating highly active antiretroviral treatment at different stages of disease. Arch Intern Med 2002;162:1973–80.
11. Levine AM. Evaluation and management of HIV-infected women. Ann Intern Med 2002;136:228–42.
12. Clark RA, Brandon W, Dumestre J, Pindar C. Clinical manifestations of infection with the human immunodeficiency virus in women in Louisiana. Clin Infect Dis 1993;17:165–72.
13. Clark RA, Squires KE. Gender-specific considerations in the antiretroviral management of HIV-infected women. Expert Rev Anti Infect Ther 2005;3:213–27.
14. Sterling TR, Lyles CM, Vlahov D, Astemborski J, Margolick JB, Quinn TC. Initial plasma HIV-1 RNA levels and progression to AIDS in women and man. N Engl J Med 2001;344:720–5.
15. Montgomery JP, Gillespie BW, Gentry AC, Mokotoff ED, Crane LR, James SA. Does access to health care impact survival time after diagnosis of AIDS? AIDS Patient Care STDS 2002:16:223–31.

16. Hader SL, Smith DK, Moore JS, Holmberg SD. HIV infection in women in the United States: status at the Millennium. JAMA 2001;285:1186–92.

17. Poundstone KE, Chaisson RE, Moore RD. Differences in HIV disease progression by injection drug use and by sex in the era of highly active antiretroviral therapy. AIDS 2001;15:1115–23.

18. Vittinghoff E, Scheer S, O'Malley P, et al. Combination antiretroviral therapy and recent declines in AIDS incidence and mortality. J Infect Dis 1999;179:717–20.

19. Egger M, May M, Chene G, et al. Prognosis of HIV-1-infected patients starting highly active antiretroviral therapy: a collaborative analysis of prospective studies. Lancet 2002;360:119–29.

20. Panel on Antiretroviral Guidelines for Adults and Adolescents. Guidelines for the use of antiretroviral agents in HIV-infected adults and adolescents. US Department of Health and Human Services, Washington, DC, 2006: 1–113. http://aidsinfo.nih.gov/ContentFiles/ AdultandAdolescentGL.pdf.

21. Mofenson LM. Interaction between timing of perinatal human immunodeficiency virus infection and the design of preventive and therapeutic interventions. Acta Paediatr 1997;421(suppl):1–9.

22. Coutsoudis A, Dabis F, Fawzi W, et al. Late postnatal transmission of HIV-1 in breast-fed children: an individual patient data meta-analysis. J Infect Dis 2004;189:2154–66.

23. Fawzi WW, Msamanga GI, Spiegelman D, et al. Randomised trial of effects of vitamin supplements on pregnancy outcomes and T cell counts in HIV-1-infected women in Tanzania. Lancet 1998;351:1477–82.

24. Garcia PM, Kalish LA, Pitt J, et al. Maternal levels of plasma human immunodeficiency virus type 1 RNA and the risk of perinatal transmission. N Engl J Med 1999;341:394–402.

25. Landesman SH, Kalish LA, Burns DN, et al. Obstetrical factors and the transmission of human immunodeficiency virus type 1 from mother to child. N Engl J Med 1996;334:1617–23.

26. Mofenson LM, Lambert JS, Stiehm ER, et al. Risk factors for perinatal transmission of human immunodeficiency virus type 1 in women treated with zidovudine. N Engl J Med 1999;341:385–93.

27. Minkoff H, Mofenson LM. The role of obstetric interventions in the prevention of pediatric human immunodeficiency virus infection. Am J Obstet Gynecol 1994;171:1167–75.

28. International Perinatal HIV Group. The mode of delivery and the risk of vertical transmission of human immunodeficiency virus type 1 – a meta-analysis of 15 prospective cohort studies. N Engl J Med 1999;340:977–87.

29. Minkoff HL. HIV disease in pregnancy. Obstet Gynecol Clin North Am 1997;24:xi–xvii.

30. Reinhardt PP, Reinhardt B, Lathey JL, Spector SA. Human cord blood mononuclear cells are preferentially infected by non-syncytium-inducing, macrophage-tropic human immunodeficiency virus type 1 isolates. J Clin Microbiol 1995;33:292–7.

31. Ioannidis JPA, Abrams EJ, Ammann A, et al. Perinatal transmission of human immunodeficiency virus type 1 by pregnant women with RNA virus loads <1000 copies/mL. J Infect Dis 2001;183:539–45.

32. De Pasquale MP, Leigh Brown AJ, Uvin SC, et al. Differences in HIV-1 pol sequences from female genital tract and blood during antiretroviral therapy. J Acquir Immune Defic Syndr 2003;34:37–44.

33. Rasheed S, Li Z, Xu D, Kovacs A. Presence of cell-free human immunodeficiency virus in cervicovaginal secretions is independent of viral load in the blood of human immunodeficiency virus-infected women. Am J Obstet Gynecol 1996;175:122–9.

34. Cooper ER, Charurat M, Mofenson L, et al. Combination antiretroviral strategies for the treatment of pregnant HIV-1-infected women and prevention of perinatal HIV-1 transmission. J Acquir Immune Defic Syndr 2002;29:484–94.

35. Perinatal HIV Guidelines Working Group. Public Health Service Task Force Recommendations for Use of Antiretroviral Drugs in Pregnant HIV-Infected Women for Maternal Health and Interventions to Reduce Perinatal HIV Transmission in the United States. April 29, 2009; pp 1-90. Available at http://aidsinfo.nih.gov/ContentFiles/PerinatalGL_.pdf. Accessed February, 2010.

36. French R, Brocklehurst P. The effect of pregnancy on survival in women infected with HIV: a systematic review of the literature and meta-analysis. Br J Obstet Gynaecol 1998;105:827–35.

37. Minkoff H, Hershow R, Watts DH, et al. The relationship of pregnancy to human immunodeficiency virus disease progression. Am J Obstet Gynecol 2003;189:552–9.

38. Cao Y, Krogstad P, Korber BT, et al. Maternal HIV-1 viral load and vertical transmission of infection: the Ariel Project for the prevention of HIV transmission from mother to infant. Nat Med 1997;3:549–52.

39. Watts DH, Lambert J, Stiehm ER, et al. Progression of HIV disease among women following delivery. J Acquir Immune Defic Syndr 2003;33(5):585–93.

40. www.apregistry.com.

41. De Santis M, Carducci B, de Santis L, Cavaliere AF, Straface G. Periconceptional exposure to efavirenz and neural tube defects. Arch Intern Med 2002;162:355.

42. Paterson DL, Swindells S, Mohr J, et al. Adherence to protease inhibitor therapy and outcomes in patients with HIV infection. Ann Intern Med 2000;133:21–30.

43. Le Moing V, Chene G, Carrieri MP, et al. Clinical, biologic, and behavioral predictors of early immunologic and virologic response in HIV-infected patients initiating protease inhibitors. J Acquir Immune Defic Syndr 2001;27:372–6.

44. Tuomala RE, Watts DH, Li D, et al. Improved obstetric outcomes and few maternal toxicities are associated with antiretroviral therapy, including highly active antiretroviral therapy during pregnancy. J Acquir Immune Defic Syndr 2005;38:449–73.

45. Watts DH, Balasubramanian R, Maupin RT Jr, et al. Maternal toxicity and pregnancy complications in human immunodeficiency virus-infected women receiving antiretroviral therapy: PACTG 316. Am J Obstet Gynecol 2004;190:506–16.

46. Dube MP, Sattler FR. Metabolic complications of antiretroviral therapies. AIDS Clin Care 1998;10:41–4.

47. Hitti J, Andersen J, McComsey G, et al. Protease inhibitor-based antiretroviral therapy and glucose tolerance in pregnancy: AIDS Clinical Trials Group A5084. Am J Obstet Gynecol 2007;196:331.e1–7.

48. Lyons F, Hopkins S, Kelleher B, et al. Maternal hepatotoxicity with nevirapine as part of combination antiretroviral therapy in pregnancy. HIV Med 2006;7:255–60.

49. Hitti J, Frenkel LM, Steck AM, et al. Maternal toxicity with continuous nevirapine in pregnancy: results from PACTG 1022. J Acquir Immune Defic Syndr 2004;36:772–6.

50. Stern JO, Robinson PA, Love J, et al. A comprehensive hepatic safety analysis of nevirapine in different populations of HIV infected patients. J Acquir Immune Defic Syndr 2003;34:S21–33.

51. www.fda.gov/medWatch/SAFETY/2001/pregwarnfinalBMS.pdf.

52. European Collaborative Study and the Swiss Mother + Child HIV Cohort Study. Combination antiretroviral therapy and duration of pregnancy. AIDS 2000;14:2913–20.

53. Thorne C, Patel D, Newell ML. Increased risk of adverse pregnancy outcomes in HIV-infected women treated with highly active antiretroviral therapy in Europe. AIDS 2004;18:2337–9.

54. Cotter AM, Garcia AG, Duthely ML, Luke B, O'Sullivan MJ. Is antiretroviral therapy during pregnancy associated with an increased risk of preterm delivery, low birth weight, or stillbirth? J Infect Dis 2006;193:1195–201.

55. Tuomala RE, Shapiro D, Mofenson LM, et al. Antiretroviral therapy during pregnancy and the risk of an adverse outcome. N Engl J Med 2002;346:1863–70.

56. Szyld EG, Warley EM, Freimanis L, et al. Maternal antiretroviral drugs during pregnancy and infant low birth weight and preterm birth. AIDS 2006;20:2345–53.

57. Kourtis AP, Schmid CH, Jamieson DJ, Lau J. Use of antiretroviral therapy in pregnant HIV-infected women and the risk of premature delivery: a meta-analysis. AIDS 2007;21:607–15.

58. Bardeguez A, Shapiro D, Mofenson LM, et al. Effect of cessation of zidovudine prophylaxis to reduce vertical transmission on maternal HIV disease progression and survival. J Acquir Immune Defic Syndr Hum Retrovirol 2003;32:170–81.

59. Connor EM, Sperling RS, Gelber R, et al. Reduction of maternal-infant transmission of human immunodeficiency virus type 1 with zidovudine treatment. N Engl J Med 1994;331:1173–80.

60. Olivero OA, Anderson LM, Diwan BA, et al. Transplacental effects of 3¢-azido-2¢, 3¢-dideoxythymidinet (AZT): tumorigenicity in mice and genotoxicity in mice and monkeys. J Natl Cancer Inst 1997;89:1602–8.

61. Culnane M, Fowler MG, Lee SS, et al. Lack of long-term effects of in utero exposure to zidovudine among uninfected children born to HIV-infected women. JAMA 1999;281:151–7.

62. Hanson IC, Antonelli TA, Sperling RS, et al. Lack of tumors in infants with perinatal HIV-1 exposure and fetal/neonatal exposure to zidovudine. J Acquir Immune Defic Syndr Hum Retrovirol 1999;20:463–7.

63. Blanche S, Tardieu M, Rustin P, et al. Persistent mitochondrial dysfunction and perinatal exposure to antiretroviral nucleoside analogues. Lancet 1999;354:1084–9.

64. Barret B, Tardieu M, Rustin P, et al. Persistent mitochondrial dysfunction in HIV-1-exposed but uninfected infants: clinical screening in a large prospective cohort. AIDS 2003;17:1769–85.

65. Landreau-Mascaro A, Barret B, Mayaux MJ, et al. Risk of early febrile seizure with perinatal exposure to nucleoside analogues. Lancet 2002;359:583–4.

66. Perinatal Safety Review Working Group. Nucleoside exposure in the children of HIV-infected women receiving antiretroviral drugs: absence of clear evidence for mitochondrial disease in children who died before 5 years of age in five United States cohorts. J Acquir Immune Defic Syndr Hum Retrovirol 2000;25:261–8.

67. Centers for Disease Control and Prevention. Treating opportunistic infections among HIV-infected adults and adolescents. MMWR 2004;3(RR-15):1–112.

68. US Public Health Service/Infectious Disease Society of America. Guidelines for the prevention of opportunistic infections in persons infected with human immunodeficiency virus. 2002. http://aidsinfo.nih.gov.

69. Polis CB, Shah SN, Johnson KE, Gupta A. Impact of maternal HIV coinfection on the vertical transmission of hepatitis C virus: a meta-analysis. Clin Infect Dis 2007;44:1123–31.

70. Hershow RC, Riester KA, Lew J, et al. Increased vertical transmission of human immunodeficiency virus from hepatitis C virus-coinfected mothers. J Infect Dis 1997;176:414–20.

71. McIntyre PG, Tosh K, McGuire W. Caesarean section versus vaginal delivery for preventing mother to infant hepatitis C virus transmission. Cochrane Database of Systematic Reviews, 2006;4:CD005546.

72. European Mode of Delivery Collaboration. Elective cesarean-section versus vaginal delivery in prevention of vertical HIV-1 transmission: a randomised clinical trial. Lancet 1999;353:1035–9.

73. ACOG Committee on Obstetric Practice. ACOG Committee Opinion. Scheduled Cesarean Delivery and the Prevention of Vertical Transmission of HIV Infection. Int J Gynecol Obstet 2001;73:279-81.

74. Cunningham CK, Chaix ML, Rekacewica C, et al. Development of resistance mutations in women on standard antiretroviral therapy who received intrapartum nevirapine to prevent perinatal HIV-1 transmission: a substudy of pediatric AIDS clinical trials group protocol 316. J Infect Dis 2002;186:181–8.

75. Eshleman SH, Mracna M, Guay LA, et al. Selection and fading of resistance mutations in women and infants receiving nevirapine to prevent HIV-1 vertical transmission (HIVNET 012). AIDS 2001;15:1951–7.

76. Gershon RY, Manning-Williams D. Anesthesia and the HIV infected parturient: a retrospective study. Int J Obstet Anesth 1997;6:76–81.

77. Hughes SC, Dailey PA, Landers D, Dattel BJ, Crombleholme WR, Johnson JL. Parturients infected with human immunodeficiency virus and regional anesthesia. Clinical and immunologic response. Anesthesiology1995;82:32–7.

78. Lee A, Ngan Kee WD, Gin T. A quantitative, systematic review of randomized controlled trials of ephedrine versus phenylephrine for the management of hypotension during spinal anesthesia for cesarean delivery. Anesth Analg 2002;94:920–6.

79. Ngan Kee WD, Khaw KS, Ng FF. Comparison of phenylephrine infusion regimens for maintaining maternal blood pressure during spinal anaesthesia for Caesarean section. Br J Anaesth 2004;92:469–74.

80. Avidan MS, Groves P, Blott M, et al. Low complication rate associated with cesarean section under spinal anesthesia for HIV-1-infected women on antiretroviral therapy. Anesthesiology 2002;97:320–4.

81. Tom DJ, Gulevich SJ, Shapiro HM, Heaton RK, Grant I. Epidural blood patch in the HIV-positive patient. Review of clinical experience. San Diego HIV Neurobehavioral Research Center. Anesthesiology 1992;76:943–7.

82. Loo CC, Dahlgren G, Irestedt L. Neurological complications in obstetric regional anaesthesia. Int J Obstet Anesth 2000;9:99–124.

83. Olkkola KT, Palkama VJ, Neuvonen PJ. Ritonavir's role in reducing fentanyl clearance and prolonging its half-life. Anesthesiology 1999;91:681–5.

84. Sahai J. Risks and synergies from drug interactions. AIDS 1996;10(suppl 1):S21-5.

85. Hughes SC. HIV and anesthesia. Anesthesiol Clin North Am 2004;22:379–404.

86. Prendergast BD. HIV and cardiovascular medicine. Heart 2003;89:793–800.

87. Bonnin M, Mercier FJ, Sitbon O, et al. Severe pulmonary hypertension during pregnancy: mode of delivery and anesthetic management of 15 consecutive cases. Anesthesiology 2005;102:1133–7.

88. Read JS, Tuomala R, Kpamegan E, et al. Mode of delivery and postpartum morbidity among HIV-infected women: the Women and Infants Transmission Study. J Acquir Immune Defic Syndr 2001;26:236–45.

89. Marcollet A, Goffinet F, Firtion G, et al. Differences in postpartum morbidity in women who are infected with the human immunodeficiency virus after elective cesarean delivery, emergency cesarean delivery, or vaginal delivery. Am J Obstet Gynecol 2002;186:784–9.

90. Maiques-Montesinos V, Cervera-Sanchez J, Bellver-Pradas J, *et al.* Post-cesarean section morbidity in HIV-positive women. Acta Obstet Gynecol Scand 1999;78:789–92.

91. Grubert TA, Reindell D, Kastner R, *et al.* Complications after caesarean section in HIV-1-infected women not taking antiretroviral treatment. Lancet 1999;354:1612–13.

92. Rodriguez EJ, Spann C, Jamieson D, Lindsay M. Postoperative morbidity associated with cesarean delivery among human immunodeficiency virus-seropositive women. Am J Obstet Gynecol 2001;184:1108–11.

93. Semprini AE, Castagna C, Ravizza M, *et al.* The incidence of complications after caesarean section in 156 HIV-positive women. AIDS 1995;9:913–17.

94. Ickovics JR, Wilson TE, Royce RA, *et al.* Prenatal and postnatal zidovudine adherence among pregnant women with HIV. J Acquir Immune Defic Syndr 2002;30:311–15.

95. Bardeguez A, Lindsey J, Shannon M, *et al.* Adherence to antiretroviral therapy in US women during and after pregnancy. 13th Conference on Retroviruses and Opportunistic Infections, 2006 (abstract #706).

96. Cohn SE, Watts DH, Lertora J, Park JG, Yu S. An open-label, non-randomized study of the effect of depo-medroxyprogesterone acetate on the pharmacokinetics (PK) of selected protease inhibitors and non-nucleoside reverse transcriptase inhibitors therapies among HIV-infected women. 12th Conference on Retroviruses and Opportunistic Infections, Boston, Massachusetts, 2005.

97. Morrison CS, Sekadde-Kigondu C, Sinei SK, Weiner DH, Kwok C, Kokonya D. Is the intrauterine device appropriate contraception for HIV-1-infected women? Br J Obstet Gynaecol 2001;108:784–90.

98. Richardson BA, Morrison CS, Sekadde-Kigondu C, *et al.* Effect of intrauterine device use on cervical shedding of HIV-1 DNA. AIDS 1999;13:2091–7.

99. Sivin I, Stern J. Health during prolonged use of levonorgestrel 20 micrograms/d and the copper TCu 380Ag intrauterine contraceptive devices: a multicenter study. International Committee for Contraception Research (ICCR). Fertil Steril 1994;61:70–7.

100. Hiller SL, Moench T, Shattock R, Black R, Reichelderfer P, Veronese F. In vitro and in vivo: the story of nonoxynol-9. J Acquir Immun Defic Syndr 2005;39:1–8.

101. El-Sadr WM, Lundgren JD, Neaton JD, *et al.* CD4+ count-guided interruption of antiretroviral treatment. N Engl J Med 2006;355:2283–96.

102. Watts DH, Mofenson L, Lu M, *et al.* Treatment interruption after pregnancy and disease progression: a report from the women and infants transmission study. 14th Conference on Retroviruses and Opportunistic Infections, 2007 (abstract #751).

19 Substance misuse in pregnancy

Ilana B. Crome[1], *Khaled M. K. Ismail*[2] *with David Birnbach*[3]

[1]Academic Psychiatry Unit, Keele University Medical School, St George's Hospital, Stafford, UK

[2]Keele University Medical School and The Maternity Center, University Hospital of North Staffordshire, Stoke-on-Trent, UK

[3]Department of Anesthesia, University of Miami and Jackson Memorial Hospital, Miami, FL, USA

Introduction

There are three main reasons why an understanding of substance misuse in pregnancy is important. The first is to appreciate that substance use, misuse, harmful use and dependence are associated with considerable mortality and physical and psychologic morbidity in the mother. The second reason is to understand the likely impact on the fetus, neonate and infant through childhood to adolescence, and even into adult life. The third main reason is to develop effective services, which detect problems early and deliver appropriate interventions.

Definitions

The terms 'substance" and "drug" are used interchangeably. The term "drug" may be used to cover licit substances (tobacco and alcohol) and illicit substances such as central nervous system depressants (opiates and opioids, e.g. heroin and "street" methadone), stimulants (cocaine, crack, amphetamines and ecstasy), volatile substances and cannabis. It includes prescription drugs (such as benzodiazepines) taken in a manner that was not indicated or intended by a medical practitioner, and failing to use over-the-counter preparations such as codeine-based products (e.g. cough medicines, decongestants) in accordance with instructions. A combination of prescribed medications is known as "polypharmacy." Combinations of substances may result in "polydrug" "misuse," "harmful use" or "dependence" (or addiction). All may be associated with physical or psychologic co-morbidity [1].

It should be noted that just one dose of a drug can sometimes be fatal and, therefore, any substance "use" must be considered in detail. A working definition of "substance misuse" is the use of substances that is socially, medically or legally unacceptable or that has the potential for harm.

In order to reach a diagnosis, the two similar (though not identical) systems that have emerged are the *International classification of diseases* (ICD-10) [2] and the American Psychiatric Association's *Diagnostic and statistical manual* (DSM-IV) [3]. A diagnosis of harmful use can be made if there is a pattern of psychoactive substance use that is causing physical or mental damage to health. A diagnosis of dependence syndrome (or addiction) can be made if three of the criteria outlined in Box 19.1 are present. Table 19.1 summarizes the symptoms of intoxication for commonly misused substances.

Prevalence of substance use in young women

There is great variability in prevalence rates in different countries and regions of countries, and in different ethnic groups [4]. This may be explained in part by differences in definitions,

> **Box 19.1** Criteria for diagnosis of dependence syndrome (addiction)
>
> - A strong desire or sense of compulsion to take the substance.
> - Difficulties in controlling substance use.
> - A withdrawal state when substance use ceases, which is relieved by the use of the substance (for details on each substance, please see Table 19.1).
> - Evidence of tolerance, i.e. more of the substance is required to give the same effect.
> - Neglect of activities and interests in order to obtain substances or recover from use.
> - Persisting in substance use, despite evidence of overtly harmful consequences.

de Swiet's Medical Disorders in Obstetric Practice, 5th edition. Edited by R. O. Powrie, M. F. Greene, W. Camann. © 2010 Blackwell Publishing.

Table 19.1 Symptoms of intoxication and withdrawal [224]

Substance	Intoxication	Withdrawal	Substance	Intoxication	Withdrawal
Alcohol	Disinhibition Argumentativeness Aggression Interference with personal functioning Labile mood Impaired judgment and attention Unsteady gait and difficulty in standing Slurred speech Nystagmus Decreased level of consciousness Flushed face Conjunctival injection	Tremor (tongue, eyelids, hands) Agitation, insomnia, malaise Convulsions Visual, auditory, tactile illusions or hallucinations		Depersonalization and derealization Increased appetite Dry mouth Conjunctival injection Tachycardia	
			Nicotine	Insomnia Bizarre dreams Fluctuating mood Derealization Interference with personal functioning Nausea Sweating	Craving Malaise or weakness Anxiety, irritability, moodiness Insomnia Increased appetite Increased cough and mouth ulceration Difficulty concentrating Tachycardia and cardiac arrhythmias
Opiates	Apathy Sedation, drowsiness, slurred speech Disinhibition Psychomotor retardation Impaired attention and judgment Pupillary constriction Decreased level of consciousness Interference with personal functioning	Craving Sneezing, yawning, runny eyes Muscle aches, abdominal pains Nausea, vomiting, diarrhea Goose flesh, recurrent chills Pupillary dilation Restless sleep	Stimulants	Euphoria and increased energy Hypervigilance Repetitive stereotyped behaviors Grandiose beliefs and actions Paranoid ideation Abusiveness, aggression and argumentativeness Auditory, tactile and visual hallucinations Sweats, chills, muscular weakness Nausea or vomiting, weight loss Pupillary dilation, convulsions Tachycardia, arrhythmias, chest pain, hypertension Agitation	Lethargy Psychomotor retardation or agitation Craving Increased appetite Insomnia or hypersomnia Bizarre and unpleasant dreams
Cannabis	Euphoria and disinhibition Anxiety and agitation Suspiciousness and paranoid ideation Impaired reaction time, judgment and attention Hallucinations with preserved orientation	Anxiety Irritability Tremor Sweating Muscle aches			

in patterns and modes of use, in screening, assessment and diagnostic tools, the time window during which use is being measured (e.g. lifetime, previous year or previous month usage), measurement techniques, and study settings, as well as by wider environmental influences such as availability, price, social acceptability, seizure and arrest policies.

Alcohol

In general, abstention rates are consistently higher among women than men. The UK has a relatively low abstention rate (14%, compared with 38% in the USA) [5]. However, drinking among young women is increasing and consumption in many young women is in excess of the sensible drinking benchmarks. Among women aged 16–24 years heavy drinking (above a weekly benchmark of 14 units – see Box 19.2) has more than doubled, from 15% in 1988–89 to 33% in 2002–3 [6] (one unit = 8 g or 10 mL of alcohol). Among young women in the UK aged 16–24, 40% exceeded

three units on at least one day in the previous week [6,7]. This is important information because the safe threshold of drinking in pregnancy is not established and, therefore, comprehensive assessment is essential and extremely careful consideration of appropriate advice is required.

Box 19.2 Units of alcohol

- 1 unit of alcohol is 10 mL or 8 g of alcohol.
- More than 2–3 units of alcohol per day is considered a health concern for nonpregnant women.
- 1 half pint (284 mL) of beer with 3.5–4% alcohol has 1 unit of alcohol.
- 175 mL of wine with 12% alcohol has 2 units of alcohol.
- 25 mL of spirits with 40% alcohol has 1 unit of alcohol.

Illicit substance misuse

Illicit substance misuse is a substantial problem. A million people in the UK aged 16–59 used class A drugs in the past year and this increased between 1998 and 2005–6 [8]. One and a half million young people in the UK aged 16–24 have used an illicit drug over the previous year. Men more commonly report use. Class A drug use by young women and men remains stable (for details of the classes of substances laid out in the Misuse of Drugs Act 1971, see Table 19.2). However, young women are 1.5–3 times more likely to use substances than older women. International studies demonstrate that about one-quarter to one-fifth of women in younger age groups have used illicit drugs in the past year.

Nicotine use in young women

There was a fall in the overall prevalence of cigarette smoking between 1998–99 and 2004–5, from 28% to 25% of people aged 16 and over. In 2004–5, 26% of men and 23%

of women were cigarette smokers, compared with the early 1970s when around 50% of men and 40% of women smoked. Male smokers smoked more cigarettes a day on average than female smokers. In each year since 1998–99, men smoked on average 15 cigarettes a day compared with 13 for women.

In recent years, girls have been more likely to smoke than boys. In 2004, 7% of boys aged 11–15 in England were regular smokers (that is, they usually smoked at least one cigarette a week), compared with 10% of girls. Since the early 1990s the prevalence of cigarette smoking has been higher among 20–24 year olds than in any other age group in Britain. The proportion of respondents smoking on average 20 or more cigarettes a day fell from 14% of men in 1990 to 9% in 2004–5 and from 9% of women to 6% [9].

Substance use during pregnancy

Alcohol

Alcohol exposure varies from 0.2% to 14.8% depending upon stage of pregnancy, definition of exposure, diagnostic classification and method of assessment. A recent Swedish study reported risky use of alcohol during the first 6 weeks of pregnancy at 15% [10], where risky drinking was defined as drinking more than 70 g/week (see Box 19.2) during any 2 or more weeks and/or two or more episodes of more than 60 g/episode. A Norwegian study demonstrated similar findings: binge drinking was reported in 25% during the first 6 weeks of pregnancy [11]. The behavioral risk factor surveillance system survey in the USA reported that approximately 10% of pregnant women aged 18–44 used alcohol and approximately 2% engaged in binge drinking (five or more drinks on one occasion) or frequent use of alcohol (seven or more drinks per week). It also showed that more than half of the women in this age group who did not use birth control (and therefore might become pregnant) reported alcohol use and 12.4% reported binge drinking [12]. Other findings in the USA, which reveal that 4.1% of pregnant women aged 15–44 report binge drinking in the past month, are broadly consistent [13,14]. This compares to a rate of binge drinking during the past month of 23.2% among nonpregnant women. Moreover, an Australian national survey revealed that 47% of pregnant and/or breastfeeding women were using alcohol up to 6 months post partum [15].

Illicit substance misuse

In the UK, since 6.1% of women aged 16–24 have used a class A drug and 20.6% have used any illicit drug in the past year, there is clear evidence that substance use in this population is an issue of real and potentially serious clinical concern [8].

There is some consistency from several US and Australian studies that report on substance use in pregnancy. The American National Pregnancy Health Survey found that 5.5% of pregnant women were using any illicit drug (cannabis, cocaine,

Table 19.2 Summary of the classes of the Misuse of Drugs Act 1971

Class	Main drugs in each class	Maximum penalties for possession	Maximum penalties for possession with intent to supply
A	Heroin, cocaine (and crack cocaine); ecstasy, LSD, methadone, methylamphetamine[2], morphine, opium, dipipanone and mepiridine (pethidine) Class B drugs when designed for injection become class A	Six months or a fine of £5000 or both (in a magistrates' court) Seven years or an unlimited fine or both (in a jury trial)	Six months or a fine of £5000 or both (in a magistrates' court) Life or an unlimited fine or both (in a jury trial)
B	Amphetamines, barbiturates, codeine and dihydrocodeine, cannabis[1] (herbal and resin)	Three months or a fine of £2500 or both (in a magistrates' court) Five years or an unlimited fine or both (in a jury trial)	Six months or a fine or of £5000 or both (in a magistrates' court) Fourteen years or an unlimited fine or both (in a jury trial)
C	Benzodiazepines, buprenorphine, anabolic steroids, gamma hydroxybutyrate (GHB)	Three months or a fine of £1000 or both (in a magistrates' court) Two years or an unlimited fine or both (in a jury trial)	Three months or a fine of £2500 or both (in a magistrates' court) Fourteen years or an unlimited fine or both (in a jury trial)

[1] Cultivation of the cannabis plant carries a maximum penalty of 6 months or a fine of £5000 or both in a magistrates' court, or in a trial by jury, 14 years or an unlimited fine or both.
[2] From 18 January 2007.

amphetamines, opiates, inhalants, hallucinogens, nonmedical use of psychotherapeutics) [16]. A study using birth certificate reports of substance misuse showed 5.2% of pregnant women to be using illicit drugs [17]. The Australian National Drug Strategy Household Survey reported any illicit drug use in 6% of those women who stated that they were pregnant and/or breastfeeding in the last 12 months [18].

Opiates/opioids

Opiates/opioids/narcotics are taken orally (often from misuse of prescription medications), intravenously or intranasally. Intravenous heroin is a short-acting drug with a half-life of minutes. Withdrawal may begin in as little as 6–8 hours after the last dose is taken. The reported prevalence of opiate use during pregnancy ranges from 1.6% to 8.5% [19,20]. The Maternal Lifestyle Study in the USA [21] reported a prevalence of 2.3% detected through meconium analysis, though there was considerable variation (1.6–7.2%) in the reported prevalence.

Cocaine

Cocaine can be snorted, injected intravenously or subcutaneously or smoked and inhaled as crack cocaine. It is a short-acting drug with peak levels in 15–60 minutes. It readily crosses the placenta. The reported prevalence varies from 0.3% [22] to 9.5% [21]. Cocaine exposure in the UK was reported as less than 1.1% among pregnant women [23–25]. Based on maternal self-report and meconium analysis, one American study reported 9.5% exposure to cocaine [21] while another reported 1.1% of pregnant women to be using this substance [16].

Cannabis

Marijuana is generally inhaled through smoking. Cannabis use among pregnant women varies greatly, from 1.8% [22] to 15% [23]. Between 8.5% and 14.5% of pregnant women in urban UK samples are smoking cannabis at 12 weeks gestation [24,25]. In a perinatal sample from Glasgow, meconium analysis showed that 15% of mothers had used cannabis in the second or third trimester [23] compared with 7.2% in a multi-center American study [21]. The Australian study reported that 5% of those women who stated that they were pregnant and/or breastfeeding in the last 12 months had used cannabis [18]. Since cannabis was used by 16.6% of women aged 16–24 years and 5.9% of those aged 16–59 years during the last year in the UK, the potential impact on the fetus must be considered [8].

Amphetamine

Methamphetamine use is increasing throughout the world. It is used clinically to treat attention deficit hyperactivity disorder. It comes in different forms that may be smoked, swallowed,

snorted or injected and may be known as meth, speed or crank. It can be manufactured from common cough and cold remedies. The effects are similar to cocaine but often accompanied by hallucinations. The half-life is much longer than that of cocaine, ranging from 10 to 20 hours. While data about the use of these agents in pregnancy are still evolving, there appear to be an increasing number of infants in Western countries who were exposed to these agents *in utero*.

Cigarette smoking

Similar methodologic issues to those described above pertain to smoking estimates. However, in industrialized countries, between 20% and 30% of pregnant women report smoking [26]. Between 11% and 48% of pregnant smokers quit at some stage during pregnancy [27–30]. In the UK, an estimated 27% of pregnant women continue to smoke throughout pregnancy [31]. Up to a quarter of women who smoke before pregnancy are likely to stop before their first antenatal visit without professional help. A further 10% are likely to stop following their first antenatal visit. However, the majority of those who do not quit prior to becoming pregnant continue to smoke [32].

Mortality

The mortality associated with alcohol and drugs is 9–16 times higher than in the general population and substance misuse is a very strong predictor of completed suicide [33–38]. The Confidential Enquiry into Maternal Deaths in the UK from 2002–4 found that, when all deaths up to 1 year from delivery were taken into account, 8% were caused by substance misuse [39] (Figure 19.1). Injecting drug users have a mortality rate 12–22 times greater than that of their peers [35] and age-standardized alcohol-related death rates for women aged 25–44 have tripled over the last 30 years [40].

Morbidity

The interactions of substance misuse with health are multiple and complex. The effects may be very rapid or insidious, by a direct pharmacologic or physiologic action or indirectly due to associated behaviors. Substance misuse, which may involve a range of substances, must be seen in the context of social and medical difficulties. These may include poor diet and nutrition and/or chaotic lifestyle, e.g. homelessness, social isolation, social deprivation, and medical and psychiatric complications [41–43].

Practitioners working with substance misusers need to be aware of the relationship of a history of substance misuse to presenting physical or psychologic problems such as coma, confusion, delirium, memory problems, fever, agitation, convulsions, tremor, paranoia or hallucinations. Substance misusers may

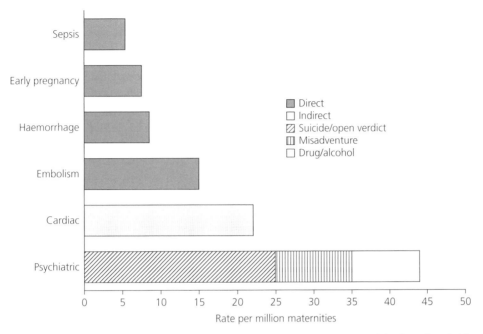

Figure 19.1 Maternal mortality rate per million maternities from leading causes of death as identified by ONS linkage study for England and Wales; 2000–02.

have vascular, infectious, carcinogenic or traumatic conditions directly related to their misuse. This may connect previous difficulties to a current acute presentation for which life-saving measures could be required. For these reasons, it is obligatory to establish whether recent substance use (including the types, quantities, route and the time course of use) may have a bearing on overt and covert physical and psychologic symptomatology. Even where the incidence of serious adverse effects is low, it is the unpredictability of these events that makes the health consequences significant.

Alcohol, drugs and nicotine affect all organs of the body, but a detailed account of these physiologic effects is beyond the scope of this chapter [1]. The acute effects of intoxication, as well as the impact of chronic use and including the development of withdrawal and dependence, can lead to an array of physical and psychologic problems and social consequences. Dependence on some substances can develop very rapidly, within weeks or months. Intoxication, addiction and perhaps even an underlying tendency to seek out risk may all work together to further increase high-risk behaviors such as injecting drug use, needle sharing, unsafe sex and the repeated use of substances to the point of intoxication (e.g. binge drinking). The psychologic symptoms or psychiatric syndromes may be either cause or effect. These include behaviors such as impulsivity, aggression and disinhibition and disorders including anxiety, depression, psychotic illness, post-traumatic stress disorder, personality disorder and eating disorders. Self-harm may result, with eventual suicide. These difficulties can lead to homelessness, unemployment, poverty and criminality, as well as disengagement from families, communities and services.

Patients with co-morbid conditions have a poorer prognosis and place a heavy burden on services because of higher rates of relapse and rehospitalization, serious infections such as hepatitis and HIV, prostitution, violence, arrest and even imprisonment.

It should be borne in mind that co-morbid conditions might constitute up to 75% of some clinical populations [36]. In the National Treatment Outcome Study [37], as in other studies, females were more likely to report a co-morbid psychiatric condition, especially depression or borderline personality disorder, whilst males were more likely to suffer from antisocial personality disorder. Compared with controls, pregnant women with affective disorder or schizophrenia still smoke very heavily [44].

The impact of ethnic and cultural factors must be considered when undertaking an assessment of pregnant women, as their substance-using behavior may be a marker of other attitudes and behaviors that could influence their perceptions of pregnancy and health. In the UK, ethnic minorities use alcohol less than whites, but those of mixed ethnicity use drugs more frequently [45–48].

Effect of substance misuse on pregnancy and the neonate (Table 19.3)

Substance misusers are poor candidates for pregnancy. They are frequently underweight, anemic and socially disadvantaged. They are often poor attendees to antenatal clinics and young users tend to present to maternity services late in their

Table 19.3 Fetal and neonatal effects of substance misuse (modified) [71,147,225,226]

Substance	Fetal and neonatal effects
Alcohol	Abortion, microcephaly, growth restriction (IUGR), orofacial clefts, neonatal unit admissions, low APGAR scores, cognitive dysfunction and behavioral abnormalities
Cigarette smoking	IUGR, preterm birth, placental abruption and (possibly) oral clefts and digital anomalies
Cannabis	Shorter gestation and low birthweight
Cocaine	*In utero* hyperactivity, symmetric IUGR, placental abruption, cerebral infarctions, neonatal necrotizing enterocolitis
Opiates	IUGR, reduced breathing movements, preterm delivery, preterm rupture of membranes, intrauterine withdrawal
Metamphetamine	Growth restriction

Box 19.3 Some facts about alcohol use in pregnancy

- Up to 15% of women may be using alcohol.
- About 5% may be using illicit drugs.
- The proportion of women using substances is less at term compared with in the early stages of pregnancy.
- Substance use rises sharply in the first six months postpartum.
- Detection of substance use in obstetric units is low.
- Effective screening and intervention strategies should be implemented.

pregnancies. Substance misuse also increases the risk for other conditions, for example sexually transmitted diseases, hepatitis B, hepatitis C, HIV and domestic violence. These associated problems can, in themselves, present a significant risk to the pregnant mother and her unborn child. Moreover, intravenous drug users are at increased risk for cellulitis, phlebitis, thrombosis, endocarditis, septicemia, septic osteomyelitis and, importantly, difficult intravenous access. Substances may affect the growth and maturation of the fetus [49,50].

Alcohol misuse

Antenatal alcohol use is the leading preventable cause of birth defects, growth restriction and neurodevelopmental disorders [51] yet half of all pregnant women report drinking before pregnancy; one-fifth of these drink at moderate or high levels and one-fifth report that they continue drinking throughout the pregnancy [52,53]. There is evidence that those reporting moderate alcohol intake (≥ 5 drinks per week) are at increased risk of first-trimester spontaneous abortion and stillbirth [54,55]. A recent review has established that alcohol in pregnancy is an important factor independently associated with an increased incidence of a broader range of congenital anomalies than was previously recognized [Box 19.3] [56].

Estimates vary as to the incidence of children affected by prenatal alcohol exposure. A reasonable conclusion based on a review of US data would be that around 1 in 1000 infants is born with the full fetal alcohol syndrome (defined below) and that 1 in 100 is born with some features of the effects of alcohol (fetal alcohol spectrum disorder). These abnormalities may include facial dysmorphic features, cognitive abnormalities, central nervous system abnormalities, birth defects or growth restriction [57–61].

Stratton *et al.* have developed diagnostic criteria for fetal alcohol syndrome [59].

- Confirmed maternal alcohol exposure.
- Evidence of a characteristic pattern of facial anomalies that includes features such as short palpebral fissures and abnormalities in the premaxillary zone (e.g. flat upper lip, flattened philtrum, flat midface).
- Evidence of growth retardation, as in one of the following: (a) low birthweight for gestational age, (b) decelerating weight over time not due to nutrition, (c) disproportional low weight to height ratio.
- Evidence of CNS neurodevelopmental abnormalities, as in at least one of the following – decreased cranial size at birth, structural brain abnormalities (e.g. microcephaly, partial or complete agenesis of the corpus callosum, cerebellar hypoplasia), neurologic hard or soft signs (as age appropriate), such as impaired fine motor skills, neurosensory hearing loss, poor tandem gait or poor eye–hand co-ordination.

Central nervous system effects include hyperactivity and attention deficits and poor impulse control, as well as language and motor development delays [62]. Affected children continue to manifest developmental disabilities, psychiatric disorders and cognitive delay as they mature. In terms of dysmorphic features, those who were more severely damaged also showed the more prevalent and marked psychiatric symptoms. Milder difficulties, such as poor attention span, distractibility and poorer performance on IQ and neurobehavioral tests, were noted in mothers drinking more than 250 g of alcohol per week. In a follow-up study, Streissguth *et al.* identified dose–response effects of alcohol prenatally on neurobehavioral attention, speed of information processing and learning function at 14 years [63].

There is no conclusive evidence of adverse effects on either growth or IQ at levels of consumption below 120 g (15 units) per week. However, Day & Richardson note a linear relationship between growth and alcohol use below one drink a day [64]. Interestingly, children who live in privileged environments can make up these deficits as they develop. However, although one study reported that binge drinking does appear to increase behavioral characteristics that might predispose to later dysfunction [65], it should be noted that a meta-analysis of prenatal alcohol exposure and infant mental development has urged caution in interpreting this relationship because of the small, inconclusive literature and heterogeneity in analytic techniques and measurements [66].

There is also recent evidence that maternal alcohol misuse, particularly during early pregnancy, is associated with adult alcohol disorders in the offspring [67,68]. Furthermore, some very intriguing work by Zhang and colleagues describes the adverse impact of alcohol on immune competence and the increased vulnerability of alcohol-exposed offspring to the immunosuppressive effects of stress. These researchers postulate that fetal programming of hypothalamic-pituitary-adrenal axis activity may underlie some of the long-term behavioral, cognitive and immune deficits that are observed following prenatal alcohol exposure [69]. Nonetheless, despite lack of certainty regarding the immediate, short- and long-term effects of alcohol on the fetus and later development, it is recommended that women should be careful about alcohol consumption in pregnancy and limit this to no more than one standard drink per day [70].

Illicit substance misuse

Using record linkage methodology, Burns *et al.* have confirmed that births in drug misusers (opioids, stimulants or cannabis) occurred in women who were younger, had a higher number of previous pregnancies, were indigenous, smoked heavily and were not privately insured [71]. These women also presented later to antenatal services and were more likely to arrive at hospital without having had any antenatal care. Neonates were more likely to be premature and admitted to the neonatal intensive care unit and special care nursery. This is in keeping with the findings of the National Confidential Enquiry into Maternal Deaths in the UK [39] and other studies [72].

Opiates/opioids

A classic opiate abstinence withdrawal syndrome occurs in at least 50% of babies born to mothers using opiates. No clear teratogenic effect has been identified, although consistent findings include low birthweight, prematurity and reduced intrauterine growth [73]. Heroin is a short-acting opiate and many of the problems associated with its use result from withdrawal effects. Withdrawal causes contraction of smooth muscle; this can lead to spasm of the placental blood vessels, reduced placental blood flow and, consequently, reduced birthweight in babies. However, methadone, the opioid substitute, has a longer lasting effect, thus eliminating fluctuations in blood levels and leading to less severe withdrawals.

Cocaine

Maternal cocaine use is associated with restricted intrauterine brain growth [73,74] and placental abruption [75]. These complications probably occur secondary to its powerful vasoconstrictor effect. Cocaine use during pregnancy does not cause withdrawal symptoms in the newborn baby. However, Scher and colleagues [49,50] have reported electroencephalographic effects at birth and 1 year. There is some evidence [76] that prenatal cocaine use is associated with specific cognitive impairment at 4 years of age. However, cocaine effects on cognitive function can be related to associated environmental risk, social status and exposure to multiple and cumulative risks, which compromise outcomes and may overshadow any prenatal effect from cocaine [77].

Amphetamines and ecstasy

"Ecstasy" is associated with congenital cardiovascular and musculoskeletal abnormalities [78]. However, there is no evidence that use of either amphetamines or ecstasy directly affects pregnancy outcomes, although, again, there may be indirect effects due to associated problems. Amphetamines and ecstasy do not cause withdrawal symptoms in the newborn baby. Prenatal exposure should be seen as a possible marker for multiple medical and social risk factors, such as social isolation, maternal psychopathology, violence and child abuse.

Methamphetamine is an increasing problem. A study by Smith *et al.* has exposed a three times greater likelihood of being small for gestational age than in an unexposed group, after adjustment for co-variates [79].

Cannabis

Cannabis is frequently used together with tobacco and the latter could be the main contributor to the associated side effects. Cannabis exposure has been linked to shorter gestation and low birthweight and later effects on the central nervous system, cognitive development and behavior [49,80,81]. A mild withdrawal syndrome has been reported and disturbed sleep with potentiation of the effects of alcohol on the fetus has been described [82,83]. Moreover, a recent report suggests that prenatal exposure is a significant predictor of marijuana use at age 14 [84].

Benzodiazepines

Benzodiazepine use has been associated with poorer outcomes (especially low birthweight, premature birth, cleft lip and cleft palate). Benzodiazepine misuse during pregnancy also causes withdrawal symptoms in the newborn baby, which can be particularly severe if there is "poly" drug misuse [85]. However, once again, its use is frequently associated with medical and social problems, making it difficult to know whether these adverse effects are a direct result of the substance or of the related difficulties.

Solvents

Limited attention has been paid to these easily obtainable substances, which may be associated not only with behavioral problems, CNS stimulation and disinihibition in the mother, but also with fetal growth restriction, preterm delivery and perinatal mortality [86].

Cigarette smoking and nicotine

Smoking is a common occurrence in drug and alcohol users, making it difficult to be certain that the effects ascribed to drugs are not wholly or partly due to cigarettes. The amount of daily smoking prior to pregnancy also seems to be associated with spontaneous abortion [87]. Cigarette smoking during pregnancy results in low birthweight and intrauterine growth restriction associated with developmental delay. It has even been suggested that the reduction in birthweight secondary to tobacco is greater than that due to heroin [85]. A recurring theme is the association between maternal smoking during pregnancy and sudden infant death syndrome [73] and the correlation of passive smoking with respiratory difficulties in infants [88]. The use of snuff or nicotine substitutes has also been investigated, but there is no significant impact on birthweight, though there is a slight increase in congenital malformation [89,90]. Duration of smoking, exposure to environmental smoke (such as smoking in partners and family), self-efficacy and educational status have been demonstrated to influence the mother's reduction in nicotine use during and after pregnancy [91]. It is notable that the background socio-economic status factors also require attention [89]. See also Chapter 1.

The impact of parental substance misuse on children

Long-term developmental neurocognitive, physical and psychosocial effects resulting from *in utero* exposure to opioids and other drugs are poorly understood. Moreover, it is increasingly common that substance misusers take a combination of different drugs at different times during their pregnancy and, because of the complex psychosocial context in which they use substances, such research can face serious methodologic problems. However, generally, parental substance misuse poses significant risks for children. Child and adolescent mental health services report that a parent's long-standing drug and/or alcohol misuse is a substantial risk factor for poor mental health in children [92]. Children may also be at high risk of maltreatment, emotional or physical neglect or abuse, family conflict,

and inappropriate parental behavior [93–95]. Children may be exposed to, and involved in, drug-related activities and associated crimes [96]. They are more likely to display behavioral problems [97], experience social isolation and stigma [98], misuse substances themselves when older [99], and develop problem drug use [100].

Parents with chronic drug addiction spend considerable time and attention on accessing and using drugs, which reduces their emotional and actual availability for their children. Conflicting pressures may be especially acute in economically deprived, lone-parent households and where there is little support from relatives or neighbors [101]. In the long term, children of substance-misusing parents may have severe social difficulties, including strong reactions to change, isolation, difficulty in learning to have fun and estrangement from family and peers [95]. Despite this, substance misusers should not automatically be stereotyped as poor parents.

Effect of pregnancy on substance misuse

Pregnancy may motivate individuals to spontaneously modify their behaviors or to be susceptible to advice for the health of the baby [102]. Indeed, about two-thirds of American women who drank prior to conceiving, as well as up to 40% of those who smoked, stopped spontaneously during pregnancy [103]. In the USA, the 1995 behavioral risk factor survey showed that 51% of women of childbearing age drank prior to pregnancy, but only 16% drank during pregnancy [103]. A telephone survey of pregnant women found that 65.6% were drinking before pregnancy compared with 5.2% during pregnancy [104]. Hispanic ethnicity and younger age were significantly associated with spontaneous alcohol abstinence. The Australian national data [18] showed that women who were pregnant either abstained from alcohol (38%) or drank less (59%). It is encouraging to note that only 3% continued to drink the same amount of alcohol after becoming pregnant.

Among those who smoked prior to pregnancy 39% quit after becoming pregnant, a rate eight times that reported among smokers in the general population [105]. Among low-income, predominantly unmarried American women, spontaneous cessation of smoking and alcohol was reported by 28% and 80% of the women respectively. Factors associated with decreased likelihood of spontaneous smoking cessation in pregnancy such as less education [27,106], less concern about the effects of smoking on the fetus [107], worse mood or emotional well-being [108], having partners who smoke [109,110], and greater severity of addiction [27] could also be relevant to other substances.

Research has also shown that up to 60% of those who stop smoking when pregnant will return to smoking within the first 6 months post partum and 80–90% will have experienced a relapse by 12 months post partum [105,111]. There is some indication that this might be applicable to drugs and

- Late booking
- Irregular attendance due to social problems, homelessness or chaotic lifestyles
- Attendance at different hospitals
- Concealment of drug problems because women may perceive services to be judgmental or due to the concern that they may lose their children
- Reluctance to provide samples
- Concerns of obstetricians and midwives regarding screening possibly due to:
  - lack of training in this field
  - lack of time
  - worries about interfering with their relationship with antenatal women
  - difficulties in accessing treatment services for women with addictions

alcohol. A longitudinal study of pregnant substance users found that the use of cigarettes, alcohol and marijuana was lowest during pregnancy, increased sharply at 6 months post partum and remained level at 12 months post partum [112]. Although the evidence demonstrates that the proportion of women using substances is less at term compared with in the early stages of pregnancy, which might indicate that use of substances diminishes as pregnancy advances, this has not been studied in a longitudinal design over the long term.

Overarching principles of treatment

The main objectives of a pregnant drug users (PDU) service are a safe pregnancy with a healthy baby and mother – the welfare of both the unborn child and the mother is a paramount consideration. In order to achieve this, promotion of engagement with substance misuse treatment and antenatal care within a co-ordinated framework is a key concern (Box 19.4). This should involve different phases of reproductive healthcare: preconception, pregnancy, childbirth and postnatal (including parenting) [113]. In this chapter we will focus on management during pregnancy and childbirth.

Screening and detection

In order to develop the optimal treatment plan, the substance problem must be recognized by professionals and acknowledged by the patient. It is well documented that a substantial number of women treated in obstetric settings have unrecognized and untreated psychiatric disorders, as well as substance use [114].

All pregnant women should be screened for substance misuse. Questions should be asked in a nonjudgmental manner, beginning with inquiries about legal substances, followed by illegal ones beginning with marijuana. Patients who admit to substance misuse should be asked to quantify their use and about route of administration. As terminology varies by region and changes with time, practitioners should be comfortable asking patients to explain terms with which they are unfamiliar [224, 227].

Routine antenatal assessment is unlikely to detect all women with a past or present history of alcohol and/or illicit drug misuse (Figures 19.2 and 19.3). Various studies have underlined the poor detection rate of fetal alcohol syndrome (FAS) in general practice and by obstetricians and pediatricians [115]. In one study, less than half of the general practitioners studied were competent in the recognition of FAS [116]; 73% of obstetric case notes made no record of maternal alcohol consumption (despite the mothers being known to be in a high-risk group) and routine pediatric care did not identify cases from high-risk mothers that had been detected by a trained researcher [117].

Self-report as a measure of substance misuse is unreliable and could potentially lead to underestimation of the problem. Screening questionnaires have been shown to identify correctly more than two-thirds of current prenatal drinkers, only 20% of whom were identified and documented in obstetric records [118]. An intensive screening interview in Sweden has been able to detect five times more antenatal women as drinking excessively compared with regular antenatal screening [10]. In the case of illicit drugs, biologic markers are more reliable [119] but test accuracy is dependent upon the tissue tested and the type of substance misused. Urine analysis can lead to false-negative results if the duration between the last drug use and providing of urine sample is prolonged. Hair analysis has a high sensitivity for opiates and cocaine but low for cannabis; it is also associated with a 13% false-positive rate for cocaine and opiates, which may be due to passive exposure [120]. Table 19.4 lists the duration of a positive urine drug screen after use for some commonly misused substances.

The CAGE, AUDIT and TWEAK questionnaires have been identified as optimal for identifying problem alcohol use in antenatal settings [121]. The AUDIT-C (a brief version of the AUDIT) [122] and the T-ACE (a modified version of the CAGE questionnaire) [118] have also proved useful in pregnancy and are reviewed in Box 19.5 and Box 19.6. The use of biomarkers, though helpful in the detection of alcohol use in pregnancy, requires more development [123].

Management of substance misuse in pregnancy

The most important issue is to be able to determine whether patients are engaging in harmful use or are dependent on one or more substances. This differentiation is critical in

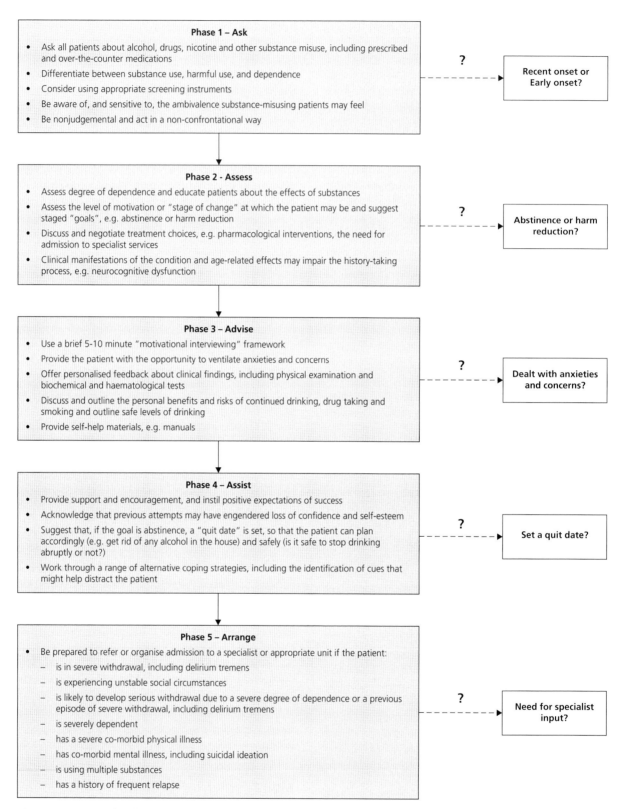

Phase 1 – Ask
- Ask all patients about alcohol, drugs, nicotine and other substance misuse, including prescribed and over-the-counter medications
- Differentiate between substance use, harmful use, and dependence
- Consider using appropriate screening instruments
- Be aware of, and sensitive to, the ambivalence substance-misusing patients may feel
- Be nonjudgemental and act in a non-confrontational way

? → Recent onset or Early onset?

Phase 2 - Assess
- Assess degree of dependence and educate patients about the effects of substances
- Assess the level of motivation or "stage of change" at which the patient may be and suggest staged "goals", e.g. abstinence or harm reduction
- Discuss and negotiate treatment choices, e.g. pharmacological interventions, the need for admission to specialist services
- Clinical manifestations of the condition and age-related effects may impair the history-taking process, e.g. neurocognitive dysfunction

? → Abstinence or harm reduction?

Phase 3 – Advise
- Use a brief 5-10 minute "motivational interviewing" framework
- Provide the patient with the opportunity to ventilate anxieties and concerns
- Offer personalised feedback about clinical findings, including physical examination and biochemical and haematological tests
- Discuss and outline the personal benefits and risks of continued drinking, drug taking and smoking and outline safe levels of drinking
- Provide self-help materials, e.g. manuals

? → Dealt with anxieties and concerns?

Phase 4 – Assist
- Provide support and encouragement, and instil positive expectations of success
- Acknowledge that previous attempts may have engendered loss of confidence and self-esteem
- Suggest that, if the goal is abstinence, a "quit date" is set, so that the patient can plan accordingly (e.g. get rid of any alcohol in the house) and safely (is it safe to stop drinking abruptly or not?)
- Work through a range of alternative coping strategies, including the identification of cues that might help distract the patient

? → Set a quit date?

Phase 5 – Arrange
- Be prepared to refer or organise admission to a specialist or appropriate unit if the patient:
  - is in severe withdrawal, including delirium tremens
  - is experiencing unstable social circumstances
  - is likely to develop serious withdrawal due to a severe degree of dependence or a previous episode of severe withdrawal, including delirium tremens
  - is severely dependent
  - has a severe co-morbid physical illness
  - has co-morbid mental illness, including suicidal ideation
  - is using multiple substances
  - has a history of frequent relapse

? → Need for specialist input?

Figure 19.2 Suggested outline for schedule of issues to be covered in assessment. Adapted from Raw *et al.* [227].

Table 19.4 Duration of positive urine drug screens after use

Drug	Duration
Amphetamines	48 hours
Alcohol	12 hours
Barbiturates	10–30 days
Diazapam (Valium)	4–5 days
Cocaine	24–72 hours
Heroin	24 hours
Marijuana	3–30 days
Methaqualone	4–24 days
Phencyclidine	3–10 days
Methadone	3 days

Box 19.5 AUDIT-C (Alcohol Use Disorders Identification Test © WHO 1990)

Q1: How often did you have a drink containing alcohol in the past year?

Answer	Points
Never	0
Monthly or less	1
Two to four times a month	2
Two to three times a week	3
Four or more times a week	4

Q2: How many drinks did you have on a typical day when you were drinking in the past year?

Answer	Points
None, I do not drink	0
1 or 2	0
3 or 4	1
5 or 6	2
7 to 9	3
10 or more	4

Q3: How often did you have six or more drinks on one occasion in the past year?

Answer	Points
Never	0
Less than monthly	1
Monthly	2
Weekly	3
Daily or almost daily	4

The AUDIT-C is scored on a scale of 0–12 (scores of 0 reflect no alcohol use). In men, a score of 4 or more is considered positive; in women, a score of 3 or more is considered positive. Generally, the higher the AUDIT-C score, the more likely it is that the patient's drinking is affecting his/her health and safety.

Box 19.6 TACE screen for alcohol problems

T **Tolerance:** How many drinks does it take to make you feel high?

A Have people **annoyed** you by criticizing your drinking?

C Have you ever felt you ought to **cut down** on your drinking?

E **Eye-opener:** Have you ever had a drink first thing in the morning to steady your nerves or get rid of a hangover?

The TACE, which is based on the CAGE, is valuable for identifying a range of use, including lifetime use and prenatal use, based on the DSM–IIIR criteria. A score of 2 or more is considered positive. Affirmative answers to questions A, C, or E = 1 point each. Reporting tolerance to more than two drinks (the T question) = 2 points.

terms of decisions around the selection of appropriate treatment interventions (in terms of type and intensity) and suitability of settings. It is also important when designing and assessing research because a range of terms may be used that do not equate to each other, so that the findings are not comparable.

Whatever the available options, they need to be discussed and agreed with the patient, the patient's partner (if feasible), and the multidisciplinary team. Regular individual monitoring and attendance are a priority. Liaison with other services is essential. Group work has the benefit of providing a social network and group cohesion, and may more efficiently support both health education (about effects of substance misuse on mother and baby, diet and nutrition, health visitors, sexual health), and support with core problems (e.g. housing, benefits). However, some mothers prefer individual treatment.

Available options

Over the last 10 years there has been a steady accumulation of research on the treatment of substance misusers. It is beyond the scope of this chapter to review this in detail, but readers are referred to several recent comprehensive reviews [124–132]. However, these studies demonstrate that, in very general terms, effective treatments are available for people who have problems with alcohol, drugs and nicotine. Treatment can be effective, but it does have limitations. Not all people who have problems will seek treatment. Nor is everyone who uses substances in need of treatment. Treatment is not always available or accessible. Treatment may not be a "cure" but may reduce substance misuse and associated problems. There is the recognition that conditions may be chronic and thus the model of care that is adopted should be tailored so that the goals and aspirations are manageable and attainable.

There is also the recognition that treatment in the 21st century is usually dictated by clinical trials.

The groups of patients studied are often unrepresentative; those who are pregnant and/or co-morbid are usually excluded. Results are then extrapolated to unstudied groups. Combined treatments (of the essence in pregnancy) are rarely studied, and practice guidelines are usually not centered on special groups such as young people or pregnant substance misusers. Thus, there does need to be a degree of caution when translating general guidance to the treatment of pregnant substance misusers.

Specific interventions of proven value in pregnant substance misusers

This section will outline a selection of interventions (both psychologic and pharmacologic) that have been evaluated in pregnancy. Perinatal substance misuse intervention in obstetric clinics has been shown to reduce adverse neonatal outcomes. Babies of those who received the intervention did as well as the control infants on rates of assisted ventilation, low birthweight and preterm delivery [132]. Most pregnant women seek prenatal care during their first trimester; this is an opportune time to help them to make the changes necessary for a healthy pregnancy. All these interventions are best provided in the context of harm reduction programs, which may lead to abstinence, that have services specific for female clients including social services, parenting classes and on-site child care.

Psychosocial interventions

There are a variety of psychosocial interventions potentially available for pregnant substance misusers, including motivational enhancement therapy (MET – evokes from clients their own motivation for change, consolidates a personal decision and plan for change, and requires an empathic, nonjudgmental style), cognitive behavioral therapy (CBT – client learns to recognize and avoid situations in which they are most likely to misuse substances, and to cope with other problems and behaviors which may also lead to misuse) and contingency treatment (client receives explicit incentives for improvement).

Alcohol

Brief interventions (usually lasting about an hour in total) have been recommended as the first step in approaching people with mild-to-moderate alcohol problems. Because pregnant women generally are motivated to change their behaviors and only infrequently have severe alcohol problems [133], they may be especially receptive to brief interventions. In addition, studies show that people who change their drinking behavior do so within 6 months of receiving the brief intervention [134]. A trial for early alcohol treatment in women of childbearing age demonstrated a significant treatment effect when two 15-minute physician-delivered counseling sessions were provided. Both 7-day alcohol use and binge drinking were reduced at 48 months [118,133,135–137].

In a recent study, 304 pregnant women were assigned either to receive a single session of a brief intervention or to be in a control group. Women received the intervention together with their partners. Results indicated that the women with the highest levels of drinking had the greatest reductions in drinking when they received the brief intervention. The effects of the brief intervention were much greater when a partner participated [138].

An innovative approach in the prenatal setting, the Protecting the Next Pregnancy Project, involves intervening with women who have been identified as drinking during their last pregnancy. The goal of this approach is to reduce alcohol use during the women's future pregnancies. Following the intervention, these women not only drank significantly less than those in a control group during their later pregnancies, they also had fewer low-birthweight babies and fewer premature deliveries [133,139]. Moreover, children born to women in the brief intervention group had better neurobehavioral performance at 13 months when compared with control group children [133].

Similarly, initial results of a clinical trial of an RCT using a motivational intervention in women exposed to alcohol at risk of pregnancy are promising, though follow-up was only for 1 month [140].

Substance misuse
Opiates/opioids
As described below, methadone treatment as part of a comprehensive package of care for pregnant heroin users has been shown to improve birth outcomes and maternal psychosocial function [141,142].

Cocaine
A study on pregnant indigent women using crack pointed to improved treatment retention when specialized interventions are provided [143].

Nicotine
A recent update on treating nicotine use and dependence in pregnant and parenting smokers has relevance for all substance misuse treatment in pregnancy. As can be seen from Figure 19.2, the "five As": Ask, Advise, Assess, Assist and

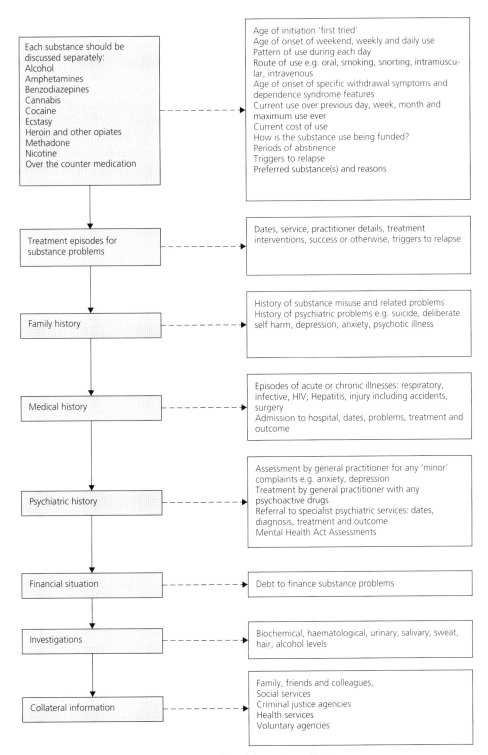

Figure 19.3 A framework for assessment. Adapted from Crome [224].

Arrange, are key components of a treatment plan [227]. Support should also be given to those patients who have managed to quit spontaneously. A meta-analysis of 64 trials involving 20,931 women has shown that a smoking cessation program in pregnancy reduces the proportion of women who continue to smoke, as well as low birthweight and preterm birth [26]. However, the studies could not detect reductions in perinatal mortality or very low birthweight. Smoking interventions resulted in a 20% reduction in preterm birth and low birthweight and an absolute difference in the proportion continuing to smoke in late pregnancy of 6% [132]. Higgins *et al.* have described a voucher-based incentive scheme that promoted abstinence for 24 weeks post partum [144]. Other issues to be considered include barriers to implementation of effective interventions in medical settings and the impact of partner substance misuse [145].

Pregnant women should be advised of the harms associated with substances, including that of secondhand smoke. Further assessment with regard to motivation to stop and goals of treatment (i.e. reduction or abstinence) is necessary. Following assessment, in which a judgment about degree of dependence and polysubstance misuse or dependence is made, decisions in partnership with the patient and partner should revolve around intensity of treatment, including pharmacotherapy and community or inpatient treatment for, for example, detoxification. See also Chapter 1.

Pharmacologic treatment options

There is a growing variety of pharmacologic treatments available [146]. Pharmacologic treatments may be used for stabilization, detoxification, reduction, maintenance and relapse prevention, in addition to treatment for psychiatric disorder or physical problems [147]. Most of these treatments can be administered in the community with close supervision, but patients may need to be admitted to hospital or to a rehabilitation unit. These decisions are clinically complex and depend upon a range of factors, including degree of dependence, polysubstance misuse, social stability, support network, and stage of pregnancy. The treatment must be individualized to the patient's needs. The benefits must, where possible, be weighed against the potential risks, which the patient must understand and, of course, there can be no medical or social contraindication to the therapy.

It cannot be emphasized enough that pharmacologic treatments must always be delivered in the context of the psychosocial situation and in combination with psychologic support, which may be individual, group or family interventions. It should also be stressed that substance misuse may co-occur with a psychiatric condition that may require pharmacotherapy in its own right [148].

Alcohol
Detoxification

There are no research data available specifically for pregnancy. It is not known whether detoxification is preferable at any particular trimester, though the impact of heavy alcohol use on the fetus is detrimental at all stages of pregnancy. While alcohol withdrawal does not appear to be worse in pregnancy, good practice involves inpatient admission for detoxification so that the mother can be carefully monitored, since severe withdrawal is potentially fatal. Treatment with benzodiazepines is appropriate for short-term treatment for alcohol withdrawal in pregnancy but should not be prolonged beyond the acute period unless the medication

is needed to treat a co-morbid psychiatric condition and the benefits are believed to outweigh the risks. Withdrawal usually begins within 12–24 hours of the last drink and can last for 5 days. If the mother is poorly nourished, vitamin B6 (thiamine) replacement should be considered to avert Wernicke–Korsakoff's syndrome. Glucose, potassium, magnesium and phosphate should be monitored and replaced if deficient. Benzodiazepine therapy is best given in response to symptoms titrated to an objective scale such as the Clinical Institute Withdrawal Assessment of Alcohol Scale (CIWA-Ar; Box 19.7). Patients with a CIWR-Ar score of greater than 8 (maximum score of 67) measured every 15–60 minutes should be given diazepam 5 mg IV [149]. If an alcohol-dependent mother delivers in withdrawal, the fetus may suffer from withdrawal symptoms. After detoxification in an acute care hospital, patients should be transferred to treatment programs for ongoing management.

Maintaining abstinence

Since there is no information about the safety or effectiveness of acamprosate, disulfiram and naltrexone in pregnancy, it is advisable not to prescribe these medications at this time.

Illicit substance misuse
Methadone
Detoxification

For those mothers who may not wish to take methadone throughout pregnancy, partly to avoid neonatal withdrawal, it is recommended that detoxification be undertaken in the second trimester. There are many protocols for establishing methadone maintenance prior to tapering but one such approach is to begin methadone at a dose of 20 mg per day. In the first 24–48 hours after introduction of methadone, additional doses of 5 mg may be given if the patient has symptoms for narcotic withdrawal. The total 24-hour dose of methadone required to prevent symptoms of narcotic withdrawal is then administered as a once-daily dose. The dose of methadone is then decreased at a rate of 1 mg per day or 2–5 mg weekly or every 2 weeks, depending on whatever is manageable for the patient [150]. This can be carried out as an outpatient if done gradually or more rapidly as an inpatient. Detoxification in the first trimester may be associated with increased risk of spontaneous abortion and in the third trimester there may be increased risk of premature labor and fetal death. Thus, if possible, detoxification should be avoided in the first trimester and carried out very cautiously in the third [151]. The risks must be explained to the patient, but in a manner that does not unduly alarm her.

Substitution and maintenance

Methadone is the mainstay of the management of opioid abuse in pregnancy. It has been used safely for many years, although it lacks a license for this usage in the UK. Methadone

Box 19.7 Clinical Institute Withdrawal Assessment of Alcohol Scale, Revised (CIWA-Ar)

NAUSEA AND VOMITING: Ask "Do you feel sick to your stomach? Have you vomited?"

Observation

0   No nausea and no vomiting
1   Mild nausea with no vomiting
2
3
4   Intermittent nausea with dry heaves
5
6
7   Constant nausea, frequent dry heaves and vomiting

TACTILE DISTURBANCES: Ask "Have you any itching, pins and needles sensations, any burning, any numbness, or do you feel bugs crawling on or under your skin?"

Observation

0   None
1   Very mild itching, pins and needles, burning or numbness
2   Mild itching, pins and needles, burning or numbness
3   Moderate itching, pins and needles, burning or numbness
4   Moderately severe hallucinations
5   Severe hallucinations
6   Extremely severe hallucinations
7   Continuous hallucinations

TREMOR: Arms extended and fingers spread apart

Observation

0   No tremor
1   Not visible, but can be felt fingertip to fingertip
2
3
4   Moderate, with patient's arms extended
5
6
7   Severe, even with arms not extended

AUDITORY DISTURBANCES: Ask "Are you more aware of sounds around you? Are they harsh? Do they frighten you? Are you hearing anything that is disturbing to you? Are you hearing things you know are not there?"

Observation

0   Not present
1   Very mild harshness or ability to frighten
2   Mild harshness or ability to frighten
3   Moderate harshness or ability to frighten
4   Moderately severe hallucinations
5   Severe hallucinations
6   Extremely severe hallucinations
7   Continuous hallucinations

PAROXYSMAL SWEATS

Observation

0   No sweat visible
1   Barely perceptible sweating, palms moist
2
3
4   Beads of sweat obvious on forehead

(Continued on p. 492)

Box 19.7 (Continued)

5
6
7   Drenching sweats

VISUAL DISTURBANCES: Ask "Does the light appear to be too bright? Is its color different? Does it hurt your eyes? Are you seeing anything that is disturbing to you? Are you seeing things you know are not there?"
Observation
0   Not present
1   Very mild sensitivity
2   Mild sensitivity
3   Moderate sensitivity
4   Moderately severe hallucinations
5   Severe hallucinations
6   Extremely severe hallucinations
7   Continuous hallucinations

ANXIETY: Ask "Do you feel nervous?"
Observation
0   No anxiety, at ease
1   Mildly anxious
2
3
4   Moderately anxious or guarded, so anxiety is inferred
5
6
7   Equivalent to acute panic states as seen in severe delirium or
      acute schizophrenic reactions

HEADACHE, FULLNESS IN HEAD: Ask "Does your head feel different? Does it feel like there is a band around your head?"
Do not rate for dizziness or lightheadedness. Otherwise, rate severity.
0   Not present
1   Very mild
2   Mild
3   Moderate
4   Moderately severe
5   Severe
6   Very severe
7   Extremely severe

AGITATION
Observation
0   Normal activity
1   Somewhat more than normal activity
2
3
4   Moderately fidgety and restless
5
6
7   Paces back and forth during most of the interview, or constantly thrashes about

ORIENTATION AND CLOUDING OF SENSORIUM: Ask "What day is this? Where are you? Who am I?"
0   Oriented and can do serial additions
1   Cannot do serial additions or is uncertain about date
2   Disoriented for date by no more than 2 calendar days

3   Disoriented for date by more than 2 calendar days

4   Disoriented for place/or person

Total CIWA-Ar Score: _____

Maximum possible score: 67

This assessment for monitoring withdrawal symptoms requires approximately 5 minutes to administer. The maximum score is 67 (see instrument). Patients scoring less than 10 do not usually need additional medication for withdrawal.

Reproduced with permission from Sullivan JT, Sykora K, Schneiderman J, Naranjo CA, Sellers EM. Assessment of alcohol withdrawal: the revised Clinical Institute Withdrawal Assessment for Alcohol Scale (CIWA-Ar). Br J Addiction 1989; 84: 1353–7.

maintenance treatment decreases illicit opioid use, maternal mortality and morbidity, criminality, drug-seeking behavior and prostitution, sexually transmitted diseases and incidence of obstetric complications. It decreases the incidence of preterm delivery and the need for neonatal intensive care and ensures improved compliance with obstetric care [152]. Methadone can be taken orally, is difficult to inject, and has low street value. Its long half-life means it can be taken once daily, though it may be helpful in some cases to split the daily dose. Methadone reduces withdrawal in the fetus and little is secreted in the breast milk, so that it is safe to breast-feed. There are disadvantages associated with methadone: it is a potentially addictive opiate, it is associated with neonatal withdrawal and it can cause neonatal thrombocytopenia, albeit very rarely [147].

Methadone dose does not always correlate with neonatal abstinence syndrome. The daily dose may vary between 50 and 150 mg, but more may be required in the third trimester due to physiologic changes [153]. Methadone dosage needs to be taken into account when pain relief is assessed during labor. Neonatal withdrawal may not emerge until 48 hours after delivery. The American Academy of Pediatrics considers methadone to be compatible with breastfeeding.

The relationship between maternal methadone dose and both maternal opiate supplementation and neonatal withdrawal syndrome has been studied by a number of authors. Berghella *et al.* and McCarthy *et al.* found that higher doses of methadone were associated with less heroin supplementation, but at the cost of neonatal withdrawal [154,155]. Conversely, Dashe *et al.* indicated that heroin supplementation was less in women receiving lower doses of methadone (20 mg or under) and that the rate and severity of neonatal withdrawal increased with increasing doses [156,157]. These conflicting findings may be explained by differences in the populations studied, differing cut-off thresholds or by the fact that the neonate may be exposed to low maternal serum levels, despite high methadone doses. Maternal methadone doses in the studies by Berghella *et al.* and McCarthy and colleagues were uniformly high, reflecting the recent trend towards the use of higher doses in nonpregnant subjects.

It appears that higher maternal doses may be necessary to minimize heroin supplementation, but that doses over 40 mg/day at delivery are associated with a high incidence of neonatal withdrawal syndrome.

Mothers who continue to use heroin with methadone have a higher neonatal mortality than those who only use heroin [158–160]. Current practice suggests that it is important to try to stabilize the mother on an effective maintenance dose, as this has significant implications, especially for those with erratic maternal opiate levels, repeated withdrawal or risk of hepatitis or HIV infection. In cases where stabilization is difficult and heroin supplementation is problematic, measurement of maternal methadone trough levels can be helpful [161]. Splitting the daily dose and increased levels of psychosocial support are alternatives to simply increasing the dose of methadone. In managing the dose of methadone, it is necessary to balance the risks of maternal heroin supplementation against the risk of neonatal withdrawal syndrome. At all times, optimal stability is the objective [162]. There is more to treatment than methadone.

Data to date suggest that methadone-exposed infants function normally at 1–2 year cognitive evaluation [163]. A small study compared 51 pregnant women and nonpregnant women enrolled in a methadone program. Although in both groups the majority continued to use illicit drugs, the nonpregnant group had more psychiatric disorders [164].

Buprenorphine

Buprenorphine (a centrally acting partial mu agonist and a kappa and delta opioid receptor antagonist) has become available relatively recently and a number of small-scale studies have been undertaken [165–169]. At this stage it is not clear whether there is any advantage over methadone. The most recent study reported that buprenorphine is not inferior to methadone on neonatal abstinence syndrome (NAS) and neonatal and maternal safety in the second trimester of pregnancy.

Fischer *et al.* have compared methadone and buprenorphine in 18 patients [165]. They found that retention was greater with buprenorphine, but that less illicit drug use occurred with methadone. Forty-three percent in both groups did not require NAS treatment, but there was earlier onset of NAS in the methadone group than in the buprenorphine group.

A prospective observational study by Lejeune *et al.* of 260 infants born to opiate-dependent mothers (39% of whom were on methadone and 61% on high-dose buprenorphine) is of interest. This study was carried out in 35 centers within a multidisciplinary treatment framework. It concluded that the perinatal medical and social prognoses for mothers and infants were similar for methadone and buprenorphine substitution when provided in the context of specialized prenatal care. Subsequent data have largely confirmed this study [170–175].

However, despite considerable progress in engaging and retaining pregnant substance users in treatment, illicit use and its subsequent complications should not be downplayed [176] and therefore, the use of contingency management as an adjunct has been described [177]. In the United States, buprenorphine has the advantage that it can be dispensed by prescription, rather than at federally certified methadone clinics [178].

Currently, "good practice" must encompass prescribing within a comprehensive care plan. Furthermore, an increasing number of pregnant teenagers are using substances and, potentially, accessing services. Consideration needs to be given, therefore, to a further set of complex issues, such as identification and diagnosis, treatment and follow-up, which may involve multiple health and social service professionals. This group is often the most vulnerable and disadvantaged.

Cocaine

There is no evidence to suggest that substitution is effective and safe.

Amphetamines and ecstasy

Use of dexamphetamine substitution is not yet established as an effective therapy for amphetamine users [146]. A recent study has reported that, although dexamphetamine treatment in pregnancy ensures that patients receive adequate antenatal care, it should be used "with caution and used as a last line treatment." This cannot be emphasized sufficiently [179].

Cannabis

There is no pharmacotherapy for cannabis dependence and psychosocial support should be provided.

Nicotine

Clinical trials in nonpregnant smokers indicate that nicotine gum, patches, inhaler and nasal spray are similar in efficacy and that they double quit rates compared with placebo [180]. A recent study has shown that cigarette smoking during pregnancy is of far greater risk than nicotine alone [181]. This is

important as it puts the concern that nicotine is toxic to the developing fetus in perspective and therefore, despite the fact that "three trials of nicotine replacement were borderline" [26], women should be encouraged to stop smoking and to use intermittent forms of nicotine replacement therapy (NRT), for example gum, spray and inhaler rather than patches, which is the formulation in NRT trials in pregnancy to date. The UK National Institute for Health and Clinical Excellence (NICE) approves the use of NRT in pregnancy, as long as the patient seeks a medical recommendation [182].

The dose should be at the level that is judged to be effective, but this should be the lowest dose necessary, so as to avoid harm to the fetus. The formulation should be chosen that best suits the patient, e.g. if she has vomiting and nausea due to pregnancy then this should be taken into account. Patches may be as effective for 16–24 hours. Pharmacotherapy should be initiated as early as possible during the pregnancy, once it is clear that psychosocial treatments are not effective. Cessation in the first 16 weeks diminishes the adverse effects. On the basis of Benowitz & Dempsey's review, nicotine replacement should be used in combination with behavioral therapy [181].

Since evidence is inconclusive, Coleman *et al.* outline a protocol to determine whether or not standard doses of NRT are safe and effective for pregnant smokers and their babies [183]. Smokers will be randomized to NRT or placebo and will receive behavioral support. Pregnant women may require higher doses and there is concern about increased risk of fetal damage. Thus, although NRT is likely to be safer than smoking, this study will produce direct evidence and investigate effectiveness. There are no trials of bupropion in pregnancy and it is best avoided at present, as advised by NICE.

Postnatal interventions

Given the fact that many new mothers appear to revert to substance misuse after delivery, it has become more and more clear that continuation of the interventions or re-establishment of treatment is as vital a component of the "treatment episode" as that delivered during the pregnancy. A short-term intensive intervention by trained counselors for postpartum women with a drug problem can increase the number of women attending drug and alcohol services [150,158,159,165,166,184]. The value of partners should not be overlooked [185].

Special groups

Since substance misuse has increased in teenagers over the last decade, this group is of great immediate and future concern [186]. Many studies described above have noted the vulnerability of young and disadvantaged women who are at increased risk of substance use, imprisonment as a result of activities associated with substance use, and even death and the possibility of leaving bereaved children. There is, as yet, little information on the extent and impact of substance problems in ethnic minority groups.

Child protection

This is clearly a very complicated and emotionally driven area for understandable and justifiable reasons [187]. The rights of the parents and needs of the child have to be carefully balanced. It is of paramount importance that a thorough assessment is undertaken, including the ability of the parents (and perhaps the extended family) to provide shelter, food, safety and emotional security. The nature and extent of the substance misuse, the impact on the child, the social circumstances and wider support network need to be taken into consideration. In the final analysis, services would prefer to work together to retain the integrity of the family if feasible, by engaging the family in treatment and support. The situation may be monitored regularly under the Child Protection Register. Nevertheless, on the occasions when the child is considered to be at immediate risk, it is in the best interests of the infant or child that other suitable arrangements are made. This could result in the child being removed permanently, which might follow an Emergency Protection Order and court case. In some countries it is routine for children of addicts to be placed on a Child Protection Register. Fear that this might happen is a strong force in pregnant women and mothers not seeking treatment early on, so it is necessary to encourage an atmosphere that appeals to their needs.

Model service development

In the UK it appears that women are accessing drug services in proportion to the problem in the community; this is not the case for alcohol misusers [188,131]. However, barriers to user engagement and practitioner involvement remain. Patients may opt not to participate [189] although a high proportion of pregnant women express a desire to stop smoking and appreciate the benefits. In the UK, only 5% of pregnant smokers make use of free behavioral support for smoking cessation [190]. Some of the methods that seem acceptable include behavioral support and self-help materials on an individual basis, preferably from a counselor [191,192]. As ethnicity, occupational status, age, partner attitude and confidence all had an impact on which interventions and methods (e.g. telephone, internet) were acceptable, a focus on these factors may enhance uptake for smokers and other substance misusers [193]. Of note, though, was the evidence that, at most, two-thirds of practitioners had

"told pregnant smokers" to stop and only 5% of pregnant smokers had received help. This further underlines the need to train practitioners in substance misuse intervention, so that this skill can be integrated readily into the overall care plan [194–196].

It is well documented that substance misusers do better if supported by a wide range of comprehensive services and there is no reason to suppose that pregnant women are exceptional [197]. Routine screening in obstetric offices may prove to be vital in preventing drinking and smoking during pregnancy – the leading causes of preventable birth defects. Not only should health practitioners undertake screening, but counseling needs to be provided [198]. Educational programs for providers are necessary and should be orientated to increasing confidence in the provision of effective treatment strategies [199–201].

Health providers may embrace multiple roles in addition to that of clinician, for example advocate, mediator, broker, and educator [202]. There is also the suggestion that the value of less intensive or briefer psychologic treatment should be tested in women who have lower levels of psychopathology [203].

However, while there is no evidence about which models of care are more effective, there is some guidance about the components of care. Ideally, this should consist of a multidisciplinary team, including an obstetrician/gynecologist, midwife, neonatologist/pediatrician, pharmacist, general practitioner, substance misuse and/or liaison psychiatrist, substance misuse worker, and social worker. The skills of these professionals must be accessible, even if a comprehensive service is not available.

Care and discharge plans should be developed, to include all key service providers such as maternity, substance misuse, primary care and health visitor, social worker and family and community support workers. Where appropriate, child protection safeguards should be put in place at the time of diagnosis, at 32 weeks gestation and 5 days after the birth of the baby but prior to discharge. It should also be noted that unrecognized psychiatric illness with or without substance misuse is well documented, so if a patient has a substance problem, assessment of mental illness should be undertaken [204]. It is important to try to identify those patients who are likely to leave treatment early, e.g. due to craving and withdrawal, not being prescribed methadone, reporting more treatment episodes or having more psychosocial problems, but fewer drug and medical problems [205]. A recent study in Aberdeen suggests that women like a one-stop shop (a multidisciplinary clinic) where staff are nonjudgmental and consistent, provide reliable information and come from a variety of agencies [206]. Home visits during pregnancy and after the birth have been demonstrated to increase engagement, but whether this improves the health of the baby and mother has yet to be determined [207]. Social circumstances should be taken into account when planning treatment and services [208].

One model of integrated care: the North Staffordshire PDU service

This service is provided by two units: the Edward Myers Centre (EMC), a specialist substance misuse unit based at Harplands Hospital (the local psychiatric hospital), and a specialized antenatal clinic (ANC) based at the maternity unit of the University Hospital of North Staffordshire NHS Trust. These units are in close proximity on the hospital site so that pregnant women can be seen in both units within an hour. The multidisciplinary team which manages this service includes a consultant addiction psychiatrist, an associate specialist in substance misuse, a family therapist, designated staff nurses on the EMC, a consultant obstetrician, and a named midwife based at the maternity unit. The service has close links to the University Hospital of North Staffordshire NHS Trust Neonatology Unit. The objective of the service is to target the social, physical, psychologic and pharmacologic needs of the mother, fetus, neonate and family.

Women treated at the PDU service are reviewed weekly in the EMC. The center offers a range of physical, psychosocial and pharmacologic interventions on an inpatient or outpatient basis. Pharmacologic treatments for smoking cessation and alcohol dependence are also provided by the center. Women are reviewed in the ANC at the booking visit when they are offered routine antenatal screening, at 20 weeks gestation with the results of the fetal anomaly scan, and then every 2 weeks starting from 24 weeks gestation, with serial ultrasound scans to monitor fetal growth and liquor (amniotic fluid) volume and more detailed assessment with biophysical profiles, cardiotocograms and uterine artery Doppler where the scan identifies a problem. Review by both units is organized to take place on the same day to decrease the risk of defaulting antenatal appointments. Substitution therapy prescriptions for patients at high risk for defaulting are given after the antenatal appointment has been completed. Another feature is that patients continue to be seen in the EMC for 6 months postnatally.

Cost-effectiveness

There is relatively little work in this key area. Petrou *et al.* investigated the long-term economic implications of smoking during pregnancy, i.e. hospital inpatient service utilization and costs through the first 5 years of the infant's life [209]. Infants born to mothers who smoked were hospitalized for a significantly greater number of days than infants born to mothers who did not smoke. The study generated mean cost differences of between £138 and £462 over the first 5 years of life, when infants born to women who reported smoking during pregnancy were compared to infants born to women who reported either never smoking or smoking in the past. This indicates an annual economic burden for smoking during pregnancy of £46.7 million. Another piece of work demonstrated that specialized treatment settings are more cost-effective than standard residential treatment, and this research needs to be extended and replicated [210].

Policy recommendations

Alcohol

As outlined above, binge drinking is relatively common among women and may lead to unplanned pregnancies, which in turn may be at more risk from the adverse effects of alcohol. Though there is no evidence of harm from low levels of consumption, this does not mean that it is safe to drink during pregnancy. Therefore, the safest approach must be to avoid any alcohol intake [41]. Since 1981 the US Surgeon General's Office has given consistent advice that women who are pregnant (or considering a pregnancy) should not drink alcoholic beverages and alcohol-containing products carrying a health warning. However, the Royal College of Obstetricians and Gynaecologists notes that while "there is an increasing body of evidence suggesting harm to the fetus from alcohol consumption during pregnancy, it remains the case that there is no evidence of harm from low levels of alcohol consumption defined as no more than 1 or 2 units of alcohol once or twice a week" [211]. Absence of evidence does not equate to evidence of absence. The Department of Health's sensible drinking guidance stresses the need to avoid episodic intoxication during periods when pregnancy could occur, because it appears that women do change their behavior to some degree, especially after a pregnancy is confirmed [212,213].

Illicit substance misuse

The continued use of illicit substances during pregnancy calls for policy initiatives to enable primary care providers to identify, treat and refer pregnant users, but also for an integrated public health program [214]. In the United Kingdom a series of policy initiatives has evolved, including *Hidden harm* (2003), *Hidden harm: three years on* (2007), *Every child matters* (2003), the National Service Framework for Children, Young People and Maternity Services, the updated Drugs Strategy, *Every child matters: change for children, young people and drugs*, the updated *Working together to safeguard children* (2006) and the updated and revised *Models of care for drug treatment* (2005) [114,215–221]. These policies, taken as a whole, acknowledge and prioritize the needs of children, whether from the perspective of service development and provision, assessment and treatment interventions, planning and commissioning, or standards. The main themes involve strong leadership to bridge child and adult health and social care services, collaborative working by integrated and multidisciplinary and multiagency teams, training and practical resources such as checklists, protocols, briefings and conferences.

Nicotine

Pregnant smokers have been targeted as a "hard to reach" group in the National Stop Smoking Services roll-out [222]. Techniques to engage women have included appointed champions, dedicated services and sharing good practice. This is high on the government's agenda, in an effort to reduce the 4000 deaths annually attributed to miscarriage, stillbirth and prematurity.

There is an urgent need for well-designed longitudinal studies to assess the impact of substance misuse on the mother, fetus and developing child, as well as the effectiveness of interventions. Randomized controlled trials which combine psychologic and pharmacologic treatments may help to determine whether, why and how women appear to abstain during pregnancy but may later reinstate their substance misuse. This will have implications for substance misuse interventions in general and for the development of prevention measures and models of service that enhance detection and treatment as early as possible in particular [223].

Obstetric anesthesia concerns in relation to substance misuse

Illicit substance abuse is a major health concern. During recent years, drug abuse has risen to epidemic proportions, especially in our inner cities. Drug use, either acute or chronic, comes with consequences and changes affecting the pulmonary, cardiovascular, nervous, renal and hepatic systems. Anesthesiologists come into contact with and treat these patients in emergency and everyday situations, so they need to know about these drugs of abuse, its effects and risks. Due to the diverse clinical presentations that may arise from substance or polysubstance abuse, the anesthetic management should be tailored to each individual and universal precautions should always be followed when providing care.

Anesthesiologists need to be aware of the use of illicit drugs because of the long-term negative consequences it may have on health and how it impacts on anesthetic care. Medical adverse effects range from pulmonary and cardiovascular effects to irreversible brain damage (that could manifest or worsen while under anesthesia, when these substances interact with the anesthetics provided). Illicit drugs may encourage reckless driving and thus increase the potential for motor vehicle accidents and suicide attempts, often requiring anesthesia for emergency and trauma situations. Injected drugs and high-risk sexual

---

Box 19.8 Future research directions

- Prevalence
- Prevalence of children affected by substance misuse
- Methods of improving disclosure of substance use
- Taking account of the views of children
- Resilience
- Partner involvement
- Siblings and grandparents
- Safety and efficacy of pharmacotherapies
- Use of biomarker feedback as incentives to quit, e.g. smoking
- Service needs assessment
- Service provision evaluation
- Special groups: teenage pregnancy, ethnic minorities, bereaved children, children whose parents are in prison
- Mental health needs of pregnant women
- Professional training from undergraduate, postgraduate through to continued professional development level
- Improvement of compliance with best practice guidelines

Adapted from Scottish Executive [225].

---

behaviors are key risk factors for the transmission of blood-borne diseases such as HIV, AIDS, and hepatitis C.

Anesthetizing pregnant women who use illicit drugs is particularly complex and difficult, especially when the effects of drug abuse mimic disease such as pre-eclampsia. Drug users have more health problems and more pregnancy complications but measuring the impact of drug exposure on the fetus has proven to be difficult.

Cocaine abuse has become a serious health concern throughout the world. The drug was first introduced as a local anesthetic due to its topical anesthetic properties, commercially available in a hydrochloride form as powder, granules or crystals. But the hydrochloride form, converted back to its alkalinized form by the addition of baking soda or ammonia plus water followed by heating, is the alkalinized form widely smoked and known as "crack" or "free base." This "crack" form of cocaine is highly addictive and smoked in a base pipe, injected, snorted or orally ingested. Its low molecular weight and high lipid solubility allow easy diffusion across lipid membranes. It has a biologic half-life of 0.5–1.5 hours as it is metabolized by plasma and liver cholinesterases to water-soluble metabolites which are excreted in the urine. Only 1–5% of the ingested drug is cleared unmetabolized in the urine, allowing its detection only 3–6 hours after its use. On the other hand, two of its metabolites (ecgonine methyl ester and benzoylecgonine) account for 75–90% of its metabolism and can be detected in urine for 15–60 minutes after intake of cocaine.

Cocaine interferes with presynaptic uptake of sympathomimetic neurotransmitters (e.g. norepinephrine, serotonin, and dopamine). Blood flow to arteries in areas like the heart and brain may be compromised as these vessels vasoconstrict temporarily, severely compromising oxygenation and supply; this may lead to irreversible brain damage, stroke and myocardial infarction or depression. At higher doses, cocaine can depress ventricular function and slow electrical conduction of the heart. Other adverse effects, many of which have implications, include infection or perforation of the nasal septum, anxiety, restlessness, irritability, confusion, papillary dilation, seizures, tachycardia, peripheral blood vessel constriction, hypertension, angina or myocardial infarction, ventricular arrhythmias and death. Pulmonary complications associated with cocaine range from simple asthma to pulmonary hemorrhage.

Serious complications are associated with both regional and general anesthesia when administered to cocaine abusers. Although it is controversial whether a platelet count is required for an otherwise healthy cocaine abuser, cocaine-induced thrombocytopenia can occur. Many theories for this have been proposed, including that this is the result of platelet activation due to arterial vasospasm or part of an autoimmune response. When regional anesthesia is provided, the hemodynamic consequences of cocaine use should be taken into consideration: profound hypertension may occur (a result of the peripheral vasoconstriction) as well as hypotension, and cardiac arrhythmias or myocardial dysfunction are common. Ephedrine-resistant hypotension may be encountered; however, it appears that low doses of phenylephrine, titrated to effect, usually restore blood pressure. Patients under regional anesthesia may also show combative behavior and altered pain perception, perhaps due to changes in mu and kappa opioid receptor densities and abnormal endorphin levels.

Cocaine-abusing patients under general anesthesia may also exhibit hypertension and cardiac arrhythmias, with their subsequent complications. The pathogenesis of cocaine-related myocardial ischemia is due to increased myocardium oxygen demand, the result of the vasoconstriction of the coronary arteries, and/or enhanced platelet aggregation, leading to thrombus formation. Severe hypertension may also occur as a result of direct laryngoscopy in cocaine-intoxicated patients undergoing general anesthesia. To reduce this complication, it is recommended that blood pressure be controlled with medications, prior to induction. However, beta-blockers, such as propranolol, are contraindicated in these patients because of the potential for unopposed alpha-adrenergic stimulation. Although some may consider that

the short elimination half-life of esmolol is advantageous, its beta-blockade may also enhance cocaine-induced coronary vasoconstriction. Intravenous hydralazine has also been used for the treatment of hypertension in these patients because of its beneficial vasodilation and decrease in systemic vascular resistance. However, a suboptimal aspect of this medication would be the occurrence of reflex tachycardia, in a patient already tachycardic. Labetalol has been another medication recommended, but its use is also controversial. Its nonselective beta- and alpha-adrenergic blockade which acts fast and restores blood pressure without changes in heart rate seems useful in cocaine toxicity cardiovascular changes. However, unopposed alpha-stimulation may occur. Other drugs which may be used include nitroglycerin, nitroprusside, and calcium channel blockers. Cocaine-related chest pain has been treated with phentolamine (alpha-adrenergic blocker), nitroglycerin, verapamil, benzodiazepines and aspirin.

The potent volatile anesthetics may also produce cardiac arrhythmias and increase the systemic vascular resistance in patients acutely intoxicated with cocaine. Halothane is an example of a volatile agent best avoided, because of its sensitizing effects on the myocardium to catecholamines. Ketamine should be used with caution or avoided since it may stimulate the central nervous system and increase cathecholamine levels, potentiating cardiac affects, or alternatively, cause myocardial depression in the abscense of catecholamines. Etomidate administration should also be used with caution because of possible myoclonus, seizures and hyper-reflexia. Induction with propofol and thiopental has proven to be safe in cocaine-abusing patients. It is controversial whether or not succinylcholine produces prolonged blockade because of depletion of cholinesterase by cocaine metabolism or a competition between cocaine and succinylcholine for plasma cholinesterases. Dexmedetomidine, a highly selective alpha-2-adrenoreceptor agonist recently introduced into anesthesia practice for its sedative and analgesic properties, has demonstrated in rats that it delays the onset of cocaine-induced seizure activity and consequently increases the cumulative doses of cocaine necessary to produce seizures.

Lack of prenatal care, history of premature labor and cigarette smoking are associated risk factors which may raise suspicion of cocaine use in pregnancy. Careful and nonjudgmental history taking, physical examination and toxicology screening are necessary to confirm the diagnosis. Pregnancy enhances the cardiovascular toxicity of cocaine and its complications worsen due to the increased oxygen demand and limited or decreased supply, due to the increases in heart rate, blood pressure and left ventricular contractility. Decreased uteroplacental blood flow may lead to uteroplacental insufficiency, acidosis, hypoxia and fetal distress. Acute effects from cocaine intake in parturients include "fetal distress," placental abruption, preterm delivery, fetal tachycardia, hypertension and intrauterine fetal death.

Key points

• Cocaine abuse remains a major public health problem, and all pregnant women should be questioned about illicit drug use.

• Drug abuse should be considered in the differential diagnosis for pregnant patients with severe hypertension and placental abruption.

• Cocaine abuse represents a relative contraindication to the use of pure beta-blockade, because beta-adrenergic receptor blockade may cause unopposed alpha-stimulation and thus an exacerbation of hypertension.

• A pregnant woman who is known or suspected to be an opioid addict should not receive an opioid antagonist or agonist-antagonist.

Conclusion

There is a rapidly growing range of effective interventions for substance misuse. Many of these can be offered to women presenting at obstetric services during pregnancy, which is an opportune moment for detection and treatment, if generalists have the skills to manage less severe problems and referral to specialists is possible. It is important to be able to determine when a patient requires specialist referral for the health and safety of the patient, their baby and the family and for the integrity of provision by professionals involved in their care. Knowledge of the epidemiology of substance use and associated problems demonstrates that a sizeable minority of pregnant women are using substances, to the detriment of themselves and their babies. The data on the relationship with disadvantage and deprivation have not escaped our notice and point to the importance of harnessing support where needs are great. This information can provide the basis for expert assessment and judgment regarding appropriate service development and the need for specialist services [114,216,217]. Finally, in the UK, up to 1.3 million children are affected by alcohol problems in the family and approximately 300,000 live in households where one or both parents have serious drug problems [41,115,215]. Pregnancy may be a turning point.

Acknowledgments

The expert administrative assistance of Corrina Knight was much appreciated. We would like to thank Dr Rosana McAuley and Dr Norman Smalldridge for comments made on a draft of this chapter.

The authors would like to thank Dr C Henshaw for seeking our expert opinion and for including some of our suggested changes to her chapter entitled Henshaw C, Cox J, Barton J. *Modern Management of Perinatal Psychiatric Disorders*. The Royal College Psychiatrists Publications, London, 2009.

References

1. Crome IB, Ghodse AH. Drug misuse in medical patients. In: Lloyd G, Guthrie E (eds) Handbook of liaison psychiatry. Cambridge University Press, Cambridge, 2009.
2. World Health Organization. International classification of diseases 10 (ICD-10). World Health Organization, Geneva, 1992.
3. American Psychiatric Association. Diagnostic and statistical manual IV. American Psychiatric Association, Washington, DC, 1994.
4. Crome IB, Kumar M. Epidemiology of drug and alcohol use in young women. Semin Fetal Neonatal Med 2007;12:98–105.
5. World Health Organization. Global status report: alcohol policy. World Health Organization, Geneva, 2004.
6. Office for National Statistics. General household survey 2003. Office for National Statistics, London, 2003.
7. Office for National Statistics, Department of Health. Statistics on alcohol: England 2004. Office for National Statistics/Department of Health, London 2004.
8. Roe S, Man L. Drug misuse declared: findings from the 2005/6 British Crime Survey – England and Wales. Home Office, London, 2006.
9. Office for National Statistics. Smoking habits in Great Britain. www.statistics.gov.uk/cci/nugget.asp?id5313.
10. Magnusson A, Goransson M, Helig M. Unexpectedly high prevalence of alcohol use among pregnant Swedish women: failed detection by antenatal care and simple tools that improve detection. J Stud Alcohol 2005;66:157–64.
11. Alvik A, Heyerdahl S, Haldorsen T, Lindemon R. Alcohol use before and during pregnancy: a population based study. Acta Obstet Gynecol Scand 2006;85:1292–8.
12. Centers for Disease Control and Prevention (CDC). Behavioral risk factor surveillance system. www.cdc.gov/brfss.
13. Substance Abuse and Mental Health Services Administration (SAMHSA). Results from the 2003 National Survey on Drug Use and Health: national findings. SAMHSA, Rockville, MD, 2004.
14. Caetano R, Ramisetty-Mikler S, Floyd LR, McGrath C. The epidemiology of drinking among women of child-bearing age. Alcohol Clin Exp Res 2006;30:1023–30.
15. Turner C, Russell A, Brown W. Prevalence of illicit drug use in young Australian women: patterns of use and associated risk factors. Addiction 2003;98:1419–26.
16. National Institute on Drug Abuse. National Pregnancy Health Survey. NIH, Rockville, MD, 1996.
17. Slutsker L, Smith R, Higginson G, Fleming D. Recognizing illicit drug use by pregnant women: reports from Oregon birth attendants. Am J Public Health 1993;83:61–4.
18. Australian Institute of Health and Welfare. Statistics on drug use in Australia. Australian Institute of Health and Welfare, Canberra, 2004.
19. Pichini S, Puig C, Zuccaro P, *et al*. Assessment of exposure to opiates and cocaine during pregnancy in a Mediterranean city: preliminary results of the "Meconium Project". Forensic Sci Int 2005;153:59–65.
20. Bauer CR, Shankaran S, Bada HS, *et al*. The Maternal Lifestyle Study: drug exposure during pregnancy and short-term maternal outcomes. Am J Obstet Gynecol 2002;186:487–95.
21. Lester B, El Sohly M, Wright LL, *et al*. The Maternal Lifestyle Study: drug use by meconium toxicology and maternal self-report. Pediatrics 2001;107:309–17.
22. Buchi KF, Zone S, Langheinrich K, Varner MW. Changing prevalence of prenatal substance abuse in Utah. Obstet Gynecol 2003; 102:27–30.

23. Williamson S, Jacobson L, Skeoch C, Azzim G, Anderson R. Prevalence of maternal drug misuse by meconium analysis. Arch Dis Child 2003;88:A17–21.

24. Sherwood R, Keating J, Kawadia V, Greenough A, Peters T. Substance misuse in early pregnancy and relationship to fetal outcome. Neonatology 1999;158:488–92.

25. Farkas AG, Colbert DL, Erskine KJ. Anonymous testing for drug abuse in an antenatal population. J Obstet Gynaecol 1995;102: 563–5.

26. Lumley J, Oliver SS, Chamberlain C, Oakley L. Interventions for promoting smoking cessation during pregnancy (Cochrane review). Cochrane Library, 2004;4.

27. Cnattingius S, Lindmark G, Mierik O. Who continues to smoke while pregnant? J Epidemiol Community Health 1992;46:218–21.

28. Cnattingius S, Thorsland M. Smoking behaviour among pregnant women prior to antenatal care registration. Soc Sci Med 1990;31:1271–8.

29. Morales AW, Marks MN, Kumar R. Smoking in pregnancy: a study of psychosocial and reproductive risk factors. J Psychosom Obstet Gynaecol 1997;18:247–54.

30. Isohanni M, Oja H, Moilanen I, Koiranen M, Rantakallio P. Smoking or quitting during pregnancy: association with background and future social factors. Scand J Soc Med 1995;23: 32–8.

31. Owen LA, Penn GL. Smoking and pregnancy: a survey of knowledge, attitudes and behaviour, 1992–1999. Health Education Authority, London, 1999.

32. Haslam C, Draper ES, Goyder E. The pregnant smoker: a preliminary investigation of the social and psychological influences. J Public Health Med 1997;19:187–92.

33. National Confidential Inquiry into Suicide and Homicide by People with Mental Illness. Safety first. Department of Health, London, 2001.

34. National Confidential Inquiry into Suicide and Homicide by People with Mental Illness. Avoidable deaths. Centre for Suicide Prevention, Manchester, 2006.

35. Wilcox HC, Conner KR, Caine ED. Association of alcohol and drug use disorders and completed suicide: an empirical review of cohort studies. Drug Alcohol Depend 2004;76S:S11–19.

36. Weaver T, Madden P, Charles V, et al., Comorbidity of Substance Misuse and Mental Illness Collaborative Study Team. Comorbidity of substance misuse and mental illness in community mental health and substance misuse services. Br J Psychiatry 2003;183:304–13.

37. Marsden J, Gossop M, Stewart D, Rolfe A, Farrell M. Psychiatric symptoms among clients seeking treatment for drug dependence. Br J Psychiatry 2000;176:285–9.

38. National Confidential Inquiry into Suicide and Homicide by People with Mental Illness. Safer services. Department of Health, London, 1999.

39. Lewis G (ed) Why mothers die 2000–2002: Confidential Enquiry into Maternal and Child Health – The Sixth Report. CEMACH, London, 2004.

40. Prime Minister's Strategy Unit. Alcohol Harm Reduction Strategy for England. Cabinet Office, London, 2004.

41. Velez ML, Montoya ID, Jansson LM, et al. Exposure to violence among substance dependent pregnant women and their children. J Subst Abuse Treat 2006;30:31–8.

42. Little M, Shah R, Vermeulen MJ, et al. Adverse perinatal outcomes associated with homelessness and substance use in pregnancy. CMAJ 2005;173:615–18.

43. Okah FA, Cai J, Hoff GL. Term-gestation low birth weight and health-compromising behaviors during pregnancy. Obstet Gynecol 2005;105:543–50.

44. Henriksson KM, McNeil TF, Larmark G. Letter: Smoking in pregnancy and its correlates among women with a history of schizophrenia or affective disorder. Schizophr Res 2006;81: 121–3.

45. Erens B, Primatesta P, Prior G. Health survey of England: the health of minority groups 1999. Stationery Office, London, 2001.

46. Office for National Statistics. How do you define ethnicity? www.statistics.gov.uk/about/ethnic_group_statistics/how_define/default.asp.

47. Kershaw C, Chivite-Matthews N, Thomas G, Aust R. The 2001 British Crime Survey. Office for National Statistics, London, 2001.

48. Fuller E (ed) Smoking, drinking and drug use among young people in England in 2004. Health and Social Care Information Centre, Leeds, 2004.

49. Scher MS, Richardson GA, Robles N, et al. Effects of prenatal substance exposure: altered maturation of visual evoked potentials. Pediatr Neurol 1998;18:236–43.

50. Scher MS, Richardson GA, Day NL. Effects of prenatal cocaine/ crack and other drug exposure on electroencephalographic sleep studies at birth and one year. J Am Acad Pediatr 2000;105: 39–48.

51. O'Leary CM. Fetal alcohol syndrome: diagnosis, epidemiology and developmental outcomes. J Paediatr Child Health 2004;40: 2–7.

52. Floyd RL, Decoufle P, Hungerford DW. Alcohol use prior to pregnancy recognition. Am J Prev Med 1999;17:101–7.

53. Morse BA, Hutchins E. Reducing complications from alcohol use through screening. J Am Med Womens Assoc 2000;55: 225–7.

54. Kesmodel U, Wisborg K, Olsen SF, Henriksen TB, Secher NJ. Moderate alcohol intake during pregnancy and the risk of stillbirth and death in the first year of life. Am J Epidemiol 2002; 155:305–12.

55. Kesmodel U, Wisborg K, Olsen SF, Henriksen TB, Secher NJ. Moderate alcohol intake in pregnancy and the risk of spontaneous abortion. Alcohol Alcohol 2002;37:87–92.

56. Baumann P, Schild C, Hume RF, Sokol RJ. Alcohol abuse – a persistent preventable risk for congenital abnormalities. Int J Gynecol Obstet 2006;95:66–72.

57. Abel EL, Sokol R. A revised conservative estimate of the incidence of fetal alcohol syndrome and its economic impact. Alcohol Clin Exp Res 1991;15: 514–24.

58. May PA, Gossage JP. Estimating the prevalence of fetal alcohol syndrome: a summary. Alcohol Res Health 2001;25:159–67.

59. Stratton K, Howe C, Battaglia FC (eds). Fetal alcohol syndrome: diagnosis, epidemiology, prevention and treatment. National Academy Press, Washington, DC, 1996.

60. Jones K, Smith D. Recognition of the fetal alcohol syndrome in early infancy. Lancet 1973; ii: 999–1001.

61. Lemoine P, Harousseau H, Borteyru JP, Menuet JC. Children of alcoholic parents – observed anomalies: discussion of 127 cases. Ther Drug Monit 2003;25:132–6.

62. Young NK. Effects of alcohol and other drugs on children. J Psychoactive Drugs 1997;29:23–42.

63. Streissguth AP, Sampson PD, Olson HC, et al. Maternal drinking during pregnancy: attention and short-term memory in 14-year-old offspring – a longitudinal prospective study. Alcohol Clin Exp Res 1994;18:202–18.

64. Day NL, Richardson GA. An analysis of the effects of prenatal alcohol exposure on growth: a teratologic model. Am J Med Genet C Semin Med Genet 2004;127:28–34.

65. Nulman I, Rovet J, Kennedy D, Wasson C, Gladstone J, Fried S, Koren G. Binge alcohol consumption by non-alcohol-dependent women during pregnancy affects child behaviour, but not general intellectual functioning: a prospective controlled study. Arch Womens Ment Health 2004;7:173–81.

66. Testa M, Quigley BM, Das Eiden R. The effects of prenatal alcohol exposure on infant mental development: a meta-analytical review. Alcohol Alcohol 2003;38:295–304.

67. Alati R, Al Mamun A, Williams GM, O'Callaghan M, Najman JM, Bor W. In utero alcohol exposure and prediction of alcohol disorders in early adulthood. Arch Gen Psychiatry 2006;63: 1009–16.

68. Barr HM, Bookstein FL, O'Malley KD, Connor PD, Huggins JE, Streissguth AP. Binge drinking during pregnancy as a predictor of psychiatric disorders on the Structured Clinical Interview for DSM-IV in young adult offspring. Am J Psychiatry 2006;163: 1061–5.

69. Zhang X, Sliwowska JH, Weinberg J. Prenatal alcohol exposure and fetal programming: effects on neuroendocrine and immune function. Exp Biol Med 2005;230:376–88.

70. Royal College of Obstetricians and Gynaecologists. Alcohol consumption in pregnancy (guideline no. 9). Royal College of Obstetricians and Gynaecologists, London, 1999.

71. Burns L, Mattick RP, Cooke M. The use of record linkage to examine illicit drug use in pregnancy. Addiction 2006;101: 873–82.

72. Fajemirokun-Odudeyi O, Sinha C, Tutty S, et al. Pregnancy outcome in women who use opiates. Eur J Obstet Gynaecol Reprod Biol 2006;126:170–5.

73. Bauer CR. Perinatal effects of prenatal drug exposure. Clin Perinatol 1999;26:87–106.

74. Bateman DA, Chiriboga CA. Dose response effect of cocaine on newborn head circumference. Pediatrics 2000;106:33–9.

75. Hladsky K, Yankowitz J, Hansen WF. Placental abruption. Obstet Gynecol Surv 2002;57:299–305.

76. Singer LT, Minnes S, Short E, et al. Cognitive outcomes of preschool children with prenatal cocaine exposure. JAMA 2004; 291: 2448–56.

77. Tronick E, Beeghly M. Prenatal cocaine exposure, child development and the compromising effects of cumulative risk. Clin Perinatol 1999;26:151–71.

78. McElhatton PR, Bateman DN, Evans C, Pughe KR, Thomas SH. Congenital anomalies after prenatal ecstasy exposure. Lancet 1999;354:1441–2.

79. Smith LM, LaGasse LL, Derauf C, et al. The infant development, environment and lifestyle study: effects of prenatal methamphetamine exposure, polydrug exposure and poverty on intrauterine growth. Pediatrics 2006;118:1149–56.

80. Fergusson DM, Horwood, LJ, Northstone K, ALSPAC Study Team. Maternal use of cannabis and pregnancy outcome. Br J Obstet Gynecol 2002;109:21–7.

81. Martin BR, Hall W. The health effects of cannabis: key issues of policy reference (United Nations Bulletin on Drugs and Crime Bulletin on Narcotics). www.unodc.org/unodc/en/bulletin/bulletin_1997-01-01_1_page005.html.

82. Fried PA. Marijuana use during pregnancy: consequences for the offspring. Semin Perinatol 1991;15:280–7.

83. Dahl RE, Scher MS, Williamson DE, Robles N, Day N. A longitudinal study of prenatal marijuana use: effects on sleep and arousal at age 3 years. Arch Pediatr Adolesc Med 1995;149: 145–50.

84. Day NL, Goldschmidt L, Thomas CA. Prenatal marijuana exposure contributes to the prediction of marijuana use at age 14. Addiction 2006;101:1313–22.

85. Scottish Executive. Getting our priorities right: policy and practice guidelines for working with children and families affected by problem drug use. Scottish Executive, Edinburgh, 2003.

86. Kuczkowski KM. Letter: Solvents in pregnancy: an emerging problem in obstetrics and obstetric anaesthesia. Anaesthesia 2003;58:1036–7.

87. Nielsen A, Hannibal CG, Lindekilde BE, et al. Maternal smoking predicts the risk of spontaneous abortion. Acta Obstet Gynecol 2006;85:1057–65.

88. Spencer N. Maternal education, lone parenthood, material hardship, maternal smoking and longstanding respiratory problems in childhood: testing a hierarchical conceptual framework. J Epidemiol Community Health 2005;59:842–6.

89. Steyn K, de Wet T, Saloojee Y, Nel H, Yach D. The influence of maternal cigarette smoking, snuff use and passive smoking on pregnancy outcomes: the Birth to Ten study. Paediatr Perinat Epidemiol 2006;20:90–9.

90. Morales-Suárez-Varela MM, Bille C, Christiansen K, Olsen J. Smoking habits, nicotine use and congenital malformations. Obstet Gynecol 2006;107:51–7.

91. Woodby LL, Windsor RA, Snyder SW, Kohler CL, DiClemente CC. Predictors of smoking cessation during pregnancy. Addiction 1999;94:283–92.

92. Mountenay J. Children of drug using parents (Highlight No. 163). National Children's Bureau, London, 1998.

93. Famularo R, Kinscherff R, Fenton T. Parental substance abuse and the nature of child maltreatment. Child Abuse Negl 1992; 16:475–83.

94. Wasserman DR, Leventhal JM. Maltreatment of children born to cocaine dependent mothers. Am J Dis Child 1993;147:1324–28.

95. Barlow J. HIV and children – a training manual. Children in Scotland, Edinburgh, 1996.

96. Hogan DM. Annotation: the psychological development and welfare of children of opiate and cocaine users: review and research needs. J Child Psychol Psychiatry 1998;39:609–20.

97. Wilens TE, Biederman J, Kiely K, Bredin E, Spencer TJ. Pilot study of behavioural and emotional disturbances in the high risk children of parents with opioid dependence. J Am Acad Child Adolesc Psychiatry 1995;34:779–85.

98. Kumpfer KL, DeMarsh J. Family environmental and genetic influences on children's future chemical dependence. In: Griswold-Ezekoye S (ed) Childhood and chemical abuse: prevention and intervention. Haworth Press, New York, 1986;49–91.

99. McIntosh J, Gannon M, McKeganey N, MacDonald F. Exposure to drugs among pre-teenage schoolchildren. Addiction 2003;98:1615–23.

100. Hoffman JP, Su SS. Parental substance use disorder, mediating variables and adolescent drug use: a non-recursive model. Addiction 1998;93:1351–64.

101. Rosenbaum M. Difficulties in taking care of business: women addicts as mothers. Am J Drug Alcohol Abuse 1979;6:431–6

102. McBride CM, Emmons KM, Lipkus MT. Understanding the potential of teachable moments: the case of smoking cessation. Health Educ Res Theory Pract 2003;18:156–70.

103. Durham J, Owen P, Bender B, et al. Alcohol consumption among pregnant and childbearing-aged women: United States, 1991 and 1995. MMWR 1997;46:3–10.

104. Pirie P, Lando H, Curry S, McBride C, Grothaus L. Tobacco, alcohol and caffeine use and cessation in early pregnancy. Am J Prev Med 2000;18:54–61.

105. Fingerhurt LA, Klienman JC, Kendrik JS. Smoking before, during and after pregnancy. Am J Public Health 1990;80:541–4.

106. Mathews T. Smoking during pregnancy in the 1990s. Natl Vital Stat Rep 2001;49:1–14.

107. Edwards N, Sims-Jones N. Smoking and smoking relapse during pregnancy and postpartum: results of a qualitative study. Birth 1998;25:94–100.

108. Anda R, Williamson D, Escobedo L, Mast E, Giovino G, Remington P. Depression and the dynamics of smoking: a national perspective. JAMA 1990;264:1541–5.

109. McBride C, Curry S, Grothaus L, Nelson J, Lando H, Pirie P. Partner smoking status and pregnant smokers' perceptions of support for and likelihood of smoking cessation. Health Psychol 1998;17:63–9.

110. Appleton P, Pharoah P. Partner smoking behaviour change is associated with women's smoking reduction and cessation during pregnancy. Br J Health Psychol 1998;3:361–74.

111. Floyd RL, Rimer BK, Giovino GA, Mullen PD, Sullivan SE. A review of smoking in pregnancy: effects on pregnancy outcomes and cessation efforts. Annu Rev Public Health 1993; 14: 379–411.

112. Morrison D, Spencer M, Gillmore M. Beliefs about substance use among pregnant and parenting adolescents. J Res Adoles 1998;8:69–95.

113. Effective Interventions Unit. Integrated care pathways guide 8: drug misuse in pregnancy and reproductive health. Scottish Executive, Edinburgh, 2005.

114. Advisory Council on the Misuse of Drugs (ACMD). Hidden harm. Home Office, London, 2003.

115. Vik T, Jacobsen G, Vatten L, Bakketeig LS. Pre- and post-natal growth in children of women who smoked in pregnancy. Early Hum Dev 1996;45:245–55.

116. Nanson JL, Bolaria R, Snyder RE, Morse BA, Weiner L. Physician awareness of fetal alcohol syndrome: a survey of pediatricians and general practitioners. CMAJ 1995;152:1071–6.

117. Stoler JM, Holmes LB. Under-recognition of prenatal alcohol effects in infants of known alcohol abusing women. J Pediatr 1999;134:430–6.

118. Chang G, Wilkins-Haug L, Berman S, et al. Alcohol use and pregnancy: improving identification. Obstet Gynecol 1998;91:892–8.

119. Markovic N, Ness R, Cefilli D. Substance use measures among women in early pregnancy. Am J Obstet Gynecol 2000;183: 627–32.

120. Ostrea J, Knapp DK, Tannenbaum L, et al. Estimates of illicit drug use during pregnancy by maternal interview, hair analysis and meconium analysis. J Pediatr 2001;138:344–8.

121. Bradley KA, Boyd-Wickizer J, Powell SH, Burman ML. Alcohol screening questionnaires in women: a critical review. JAMA 1998;280:166–71.

122. Dawson DA, Grant BF, Stinson FS, Zhou Y. Effectiveness of the derived Alcohol Use Disorders Identification Test (AUDIT-C) in screening for alcohol use disorders and risk drinking in the US general population. Alcohol Clin Exp Res 2005;29:844–54.

123. Bearer CF. Markers to detect drinking during pregnancy. Alcohol Res Health 2001;25:210–18.

124. Curran V, Drummond C. Psychological treatments of substance misuse and dependence. www.foresight.gov.uk/previous_projects/brain_science_addiction_and_drugs/reports_and_publications/sciencereviews/Psychological 520Treatments.pdf.

125. Wanigaratne S, Davis P, Pryce K, Brotchie J. The effectiveness of psychological therapies on drug misusing clients (research briefing 11). National Treatment Agency, London, 2005.

126. UKATT Research Team. Effectiveness of treatment for alcohol problems: findings of the randomised UK alcohol treatment trial (UKATT). BMJ 2005;331:541–5.

127. Project MATCH Research Group. Matching alcoholism treatments to client heterogeneity: treatment main effects and matching effects on drinking during treatment. J Stud Alcohol 1998; 59:631–9.

128. Gossop M, Marsden J, Stewart D, Kidd T. The National Treatment Outcome Research Study (NTORS): 4–5 year follow-up results. Addiction 2003;98:291–303.

129. West R, McNeill A, Raw M. Smoking cessation guidelines for health professionals: an update. Thorax 2000;55:987–99.

130. Raistrick D, Heather N, Godfrey C. Review of the effectiveness of treatment for alcohol problems. National Treatment Agency, London, 2006.

131. National Institute for Health and Clinical Excellence (NICE). Methadone and buprenorphine for the management of opioid dependence (NICE Technology Appraisal Guidance 114). National Institute for Health and Clinical Excellence, London, 2007.

132. Armstrong MA, Osejo VG, Carpenter DM, Pantoja PM, Escobar GJ. Perinatal substance abuse intervention in obstetric clinics decreases adverse neonatal outcomes. J Perinatol 2003; 23:3–9.

133. Hankin J, McCaul ME, Heussner J. Pregnant, alcohol abusing women. Alcohol Clin Exp Res 2000;24:1276–86.

134. Wutzke SE, Conigrave KM, Saunders JB, Hall WD. The long-term effectiveness of brief interventions for unsafe alcohol consumption: a 10-year follow-up. Addiction 2002;97:665–75.

135. Manwell LB, Fleming MF, Mundt MP, Stauffacher EA, Lawton K. Treatment of problem alcohol use in women of childbearing age: results of a brief intervention trial. Alcohol Clin Exp Res 2000;24:1517–24.

136. Peterson PL, Lowe JB. Preventing fetal alcohol exposure: a cognitive behavioural approach. Int J Addict 1992;27:613–26

137. Handmaker NS, Miller WR, Manicke M. Findings of a pilot study of motivational interviewing with pregnant drinkers. J Stud Alcohol 1999;60:285–7.

138. Chang G, McNamara TK, Orav EJ, et al. Brief interventions for prenatal alcohol use: a randomised trial. Obstet Gynecol 2005; 105:991–8.

139. Hankin JR, Sokol RJ. Identification and care of problems associated with alcohol ingestion in pregnancy. Semin Perinatol 1995;19:286–92.

140. Ingersoll KS, Ceperich SD, Nettleman MD, et al. Reducing alcohol-exposed pregnancy risk in college women: initial outcomes of a clinical trial of a motivational intervention. J Subst Abuse Treat 2005;29: 173–80.

141. Batey RG, Weissel K. A 40 month follow-up of pregnant drug using women treated at Westmead Hospital. Drug Alcohol Rev 1993;12:265–70.

142. Lejeune C, Simmat-Durand L, Gourarier L, Aubisson S. Prospective multicentre observational study of 260 infants born to 259 opiate-dependent mothers on methadone or high-dose buprenorphine substitution. Drug Alcohol Depend 2006;82: 250–7.

143. Weisdorf T, Parran TV Jr, Graham A, Snyder C. Comparison of pregnancy-specific interventions to a traditional treatment program for cocaine addicted pregnant women. J Subst Abuse Treat 1999;16:39–45.

144. Higgins ST, Heil SH, Solomon LJ, et al. A pilot study on voucher based incentives to promote abstinence from cigarette smoking during pregnancy. Nicotine Tob Res 2004;6: 1015–20.

145. Stanton WR, Lowe JB, Moffat J, del Mar CB. Randomised trial of a smoking cessation intervention directed at men whose partners are pregnant. Prev Med 2004;38:6–7.

146. Lingford-Hughes AR, Welch S, Nutt DJ. Evidence-based guidelines for the pharmacological management of substance misuse, addiction and comorbidity: recommendations from the British

Association for Psychopharmacology. J Psychopharmacol 2004; 18:293–335.

147. Rayburn WF, Bogenschutz MP. Pharmacotherapy for pregnant women with addictions. Am J Obstet Gynecol 2004;191: 1885–97.

148. Chandler G, McCaul M. Co-occurring psychiatric disorders in women with addictions. Obstet Gynecol Clin North Am 2003; 30:469–81.

149. Saitz R, Mayo-Smith MF, Roberts MS, et al. Individualized treatment for alcohol withdrawal. A randomized double-blind controlled trial. JAMA 1994;272(7):519–23.

150. Kendall SR, Doberczak TM, Jantunen M, Stein J. The methadone maintained pregnancy. Clin Perinatol 1999;26:173–83.

151. Luty J, Niikolaou V, Bearn J. Is opiate detoxification unsafe in pregnancy? J Subst Abuse Treat 2003;24:363–7.

152. Burns L, Mattick RP, Lim K, Wallace C. Methadone in pregnancy: treatment retention and neonatal outcomes. Addiction 2006;102:264–270.

153. Jarvis MA, Wu-Pong S, Kniseley JS, Schnoll SH. Alterations in methadone metabolism during late pregnancy. J Addict Dis 1999;18:51–61.

154. Berghella C, Lim PJ, Hill MK, Cherpes J, Chennat J, Kaltenbach K. Maternal methadone dose and neonatal withdrawal. Am J Obstet Gynecol 2003;189:312–17.

155. McCarthy JJ, Leamon MH, Parr MS, Anania B. High-dose methadone maintenance in pregnancy: maternal and neonatal outcomes. Am J Obstet Gynecol 2005;193:606–10.

156. Dashe JS, Sheffield JS, Wendel GD Jr. Letter: Improving the management of opioid-dependent pregnancies. Am J Obstet Gynecol 2004;190:1806.

157. Dashe JS, Sheffield JS, Olscher DA, et al. Relationship between maternal methadone dosage and neonatal withdrawal. Obstet Gynecol 2002;100:1244–9.

158. Hulse GK, Milne E, English DR, Holman CD. The relationship between maternal use of heroin and methadone and infant birth weight. Addiction 1997;92:1571–9.

159. Hulse GK, Milne E, English DR, Holman CD. Assessing the relationship between maternal opiate use and neonatal mortality. Addiction 1998;93:1033–42.

160. Hulse GK, O'Neill G. Methadone and the pregnant drug user: a matter for careful clinical consideration. Aust NZ J Obstet Gynaecol 2001;41:329–32.

161. Drozdick J III, Berghella V, Hill M, Kaltenbach K. Methadone trough levels in pregnancy. Am J Obstet Gynecol 2002;187: 1184–5.

162. Dashe JS, Jackson GL, Olscher DA. Opioid detoxification in pregnancy. Obstet Gynecol 1998;92:854–8

163. Kaltenbach KA, Finnegan LP. Prenatal narcotic exposure: perinatal and developmental effects. Neurotoxicology 1989;10: 597–604.

164. Crandall C, Crosby RD, Carlson GA. Does pregnancy affect outcome of methadone maintenance treatment? J Subst Abuse Treat 2004;26:295–303.

165. Fischer G, Ortner R, Rohrmeister K, et al. Methadone versus buprenorphine in pregnant addicts: a double-blind, double-dummy comparison study. Addiction 2006;101:275–81.

166. Fischer G, Johnson RE, Eder H, et al. Treatment of opioid-dependent pregnant women with buprenorphine. Addiction 2000;95:239–44.

167. Lacroix I, Berrebi A, Chaumerliac C, Lapeyre-Mestre M, Montastruc JL, Damase-Michel C. Buprenorphine in pregnant opioid-dependent women: first results of a prospective study. Addiction 2004;99:209–14.

168. Jones HE, Johnson RE, Jasinski DR, et al. Buprenorphine versus methadone in the treatment of pregnant opioid-dependent

169. Johnson K, Gerada C, Greenough A. Substance misuse during pregnancy. Br J Psychiatry 2003;187–9.

170. Hytinantti T, Kahila H, Renlund M, et al. Neonatal outcome of 58 infants exposed to maternal buprenorphine in utero. Acta Paediatr 2008; 97(8):1040–4.

171. Minozzi S, Amato L, Vecchi S, Davoli M. Maintenance agonist treatments for opiate dependent pregnant women. Cochrane Database of Sysematic Reviews, 2008;2:CD006318.

172. Kakko J, Heilig M, Sarman I. Buprenorphine and methadone treatment of opiate dependence during pregnancy: comparison of fetal growth and neonatal outcomes in two consecutive case series. Drug Alcohol Depend 2008;96(1–2):69–78.

173. Farid WO, Dunlop SA, Tait RJ, Hulse GK. The effects of maternally administered methadone, buprenorphine and naltrexone on offspring: review of human and animal data. Curr Neuropharmacol 2008;6(2):125–50.

174. Bakstad B, Sarfi M, Welle-Strand GK, Ravndal E. Opioid maintenance treatment during pregnancy: occurrence and severity of neonatal abstinence syndrome. A national prospective study. Eur Addict Res 2009;15(3):128–34.

175. Kacinko SL, Jones HE, Johnson RE, et al. Urinary excretion of buprenorphine, norbuprenorphine, buprenorphine-glucuronide, and norbuprenorphine-glucuronide in pregnant women receiving buprenorphine maintenance treatment. Clin Chem 2009;55(6):1177–87.

176. Kashiwagi M, Arlettaz R, Lauper U, Zimmerman R, Hebisch G. Methadone maintenance program in a Swiss perinatal center: (I): Management and outcome of 89 pregnancies. Acta Obstet Gynecol Scand 2005;84:140–4.

177. Jones HE, Haug N, Silverman K, Stitzer M, Dvikis D. The effectiveness of incentives in enhancing treatment attendance and drug abstinence in methadone-maintained pregnant women. Drug Alcohol Depend 2001;61:297–306.

178. Nocon JJ. Letter: Buprenorphine in pregnancy: the advantages. Addiction 2006;101:608–9.

179. White R, Thompson M, Windsor D, et al. Dexamphetamine substitute-prescribing in pregnancy: a 10-year retrospective audit. J Subst Use 2006;11:205–16.

180. Fiore MC, Bailey WC, Cohen SJ, et al. Treating tobacco use and dependence (clinical practice guideline). Department of Health and Human Services, Rockville, MD, 2000.

181. Benowitz NL, Dempsey DA. Pharmacotherapy for smoking cessation during pregnancy. Nicotine Tob Res 2004; 6(suppl 2): S189–202.

182. National Institute for Clinical Excellence. Guidance on the use of nicotine replacement therapy (NRT) and bupropion for smoking cessation. National Institute for Clinical Excellence, London, 2002.

183. Coleman T, Thornton J, Britton J, et al. Protocol for the Smoking, Nicotine and Pregnancy (SNAP) trial: double blind, placebo-randomised, controlled trial of nicotine replacement therapy in pregnancy. BMC Health Serv Res 2007;7:2.

184. Dakof GA, Quille TJ, Tejeda MJ, et al. Enrolling and retaining mothers of substance-exposed infants in drug abuse treatment. J Consult Clin Psychol 2003;71:764–72.

185. Tuten M, Jones HE. A partner's drug-using status impacts women's drug treatment outcome. Drug Alcohol Depend 2003; 70:327–30.

186. Crome I, Ghodse H, Gilvarry E, McArdle P (eds) Young people and substance misuse. Gaskell, London, 2004.

187. Ghodse H. Drugs and addictive behaviour. Cambridge University Press, Cambridge, 2002.

patients: effects on the neonatal abstinence syndrome. Drug Alcohol Depend 2005;79:1–10.

188. Best D, Abdulrahim D. Women in drug treatment services (NTA research briefing no. 6). National Treatment Agency, London, 2005.

189. Hotham ED, Gilbert AL, Atkinson ER. A randomised-controlled pilot study using nicotine patches with pregnant women. Addict Behav 2006;31:641–8.

190. Taylor TR, Hajek P. Smoking cessation services for pregnant women: survey of English health authorities. Health Development Agency, London, 2001.

191. Ussher M, West R, Hibbs N. A survey of pregnant smokers' interest in different types of smoking cessation support. Patient Educ Couns 2004;54:67–72.

192. Ussher M, Etter J-F, West R. Perceived barriers to and benefits of attending a stop smoking service during pregnancy. Patient Educ Couns 2006;61:467–72.

193. Rigotti, NA, Park ER, Regan S, et al. Efficacy of telephone counselling for pregnant smokers. Obstet Gynecol 2006;108: 83–92.

194. Amarin ZO. Obstetricians, gynaecologists and the anti-smoking campaign: a national survey. Eur J Obstet Gynaecol Reprod Biol 2005;119:156–60.

195. Jordan TR, Dake JA, Price JH. Best practices for smoking cessation in pregnancy: do obstetricians/gynaecologists use them in practice? J Womens Health 2006;15:400–11.

196. Hajek P, West R, Lee A, et al. Randomised controlled trial of midwife-delivered brief smoking cessation intervention in pregnancy. Addiction 2001;96: 485–94.

197. McLellan AT, Hagan TA, Levine M, et al. Does clinical case management improve outpatient addiction treatment? Drug Alcohol Depend 1999;55:91–103.

198. Moran S, Thorndike AN, Armstrong K, Rigotti NA. Physicians' missed opportunities to address tobacco use during prenatal care. Nicotine Tob Res 2003;5:363–8.

199. Bonollo DP, Zapka JG, Stoddard AM, et al. Treating nicotine dependence during pregnancy and postpartum: understanding clinician knowledge and performance. Patient Educ Couns 2002;48:265–74.

200. Melvin CL, Gaffney CA. Treating nicotine use and dependence of pregnant and parenting smokers. Nicotine Tob Res 2004; 6(suppl 2):S107–24.

201. Handmaker NS, Hester RK, Delaney HD. Videotaped training in alcohol counselling for obstetric care practitioners: a randomised controlled trial. Obstet Gynecol 1999;93:213–18.

202. Sun A-P. Principles for practice with substance abusing pregnant women: a framework based on the five social work intervention roles. Social Work 2004;49:383–94.

203. Ingersoll KS, Knisely JS, Dawson KS, Schnoll SH. Psychopathology and treatment outcome of drug dependent women in a perinatal program. Addict Behav 2004;29: 731–41.

204. Kelly RH, Zatzick DF, Anders T. The detection and treatment of psychiatric disorders and substance use among pregnant women cared for in obstetrics. Am J Psychiatry 2001;158: 213–19.

205. Kissin WB, Svikis DS, Moylan P, Haug NA, Stitzer ML. Identifying pregnant women at risk for early attrition from substance abuse treatment. J Subst Abuse Treat 2004;27: 31–8.

206. Hall JL, van Teijlingen ER. A qualitative study of an integrated maternity, drugs and social care service for drug using women. BMC Pregnancy Childbirth 2006;6:1–11.

207. Doggett C, Burrett S, Osborn DA. Home visits during pregnancy and after birth for women with an alcohol or drug problem (Cochrane review). Cochrane Library, 2005;4.

208. Penn G, Owen L. Factors associated with continued smoking during pregnancy: analysis of sociodemographic pregnancy and smoking related factors. Drug Alcohol Rev 2002;21:17–25.

209. Petrou S, Hockley C, Mehta Z, Goldacre M. The association between smoking during pregnancy and hospital inpatient costs in childhood. Soc Sci Med 2005;60:1071–85.

210. French MT, McCollister KE, Cacciola J, Durrell J, Stephen RL. Benefit of cost analysis of addiction treatment in Arkansas: specialty and standard residential programs for pregnant and parenting women. Substance Abuse 2002;23:31–51.

211. Fraser RB. Alcohol consumption and the outcomes of pregnancy (RCOG statement no. 5). Royal College of Obstetricians and Gynaecologists, London, 2006.

212. Department of Health. Alcohol and health. www.dh.gov.uk / Policy And Guidance / Health And Social CareTopics/Alcohol Misuse/ Alcohol Misuse General Information / Alcohol Misuse General Article /fs/en?CONTENT_ID 5 4062199 & chk5 J782BY.

213. Tough S, Tofflemire K, Clarke M, Newburn-Cook C. Do women change their drinking behaviors while trying to conceive? An opportunity for preconception counselling. Clin Med Res 2006;4:97–105.

214. Ebrahim SH, Gfroerer J. Pregnancy-related substance use in the United States during 1996–1998. Obstet Gynecol 2003;101: 374–9.

215. Advisory Council on the Misuse of Drugs (ACMD). Hidden harm – three years on: realities, challenges and opportunities. www.drugs.gov.uk/Hidden_Harm_3_Years_On_Fina1.pdf.

216. HM Government. Every child matters. Stationery Office, London, 2003.

217. Department of Health, Department for Education and Skills. National service framework for children, young people and maternity services. Department of Health, London, 2004.

218. Home Office. Updated drug strategy 2002. Home Office, London, 2002.

219. HM Government. Every child matters: change for children. Stationery Office, London, 2004.

220. HM Government. Working together to safeguard children. Stationery Office, London, 2006.

221. National Treatment Agency. Models of care for treatment of adult drug users: update 2006. National Treatment Agency, London, 2006.

222. Pound E, Coleman T, Adams C, Bauld L. Targeting smokers in priority groups: the influence of government targets and policy statements. Addiction 2005;100(suppl 2):28–35.

223. Scottish Executive. Looking beyond risk. Scottish Executive, Edinburgh, 2006.

224. Crome IB. The process of assessment. In: Crome I, Ghodse H, Gilvarry E, McArdle P (eds) Young people and substance misuse. Gaskell, London, 2004:129–39.

225. Wyszinski DF, Duffy DL, Beatty TH. Maternal cigarette smoking and oral clefts: a meta-analysis. Cleft Palate Craniofac J 1997;34:206–10.

226. Munger RG, Romitti PA, Daack-Hirsch S, Burns TL, Murray JC, Hanson J. Maternal alcohol use and risk of orofacial birth defects. Int J Pediatr Otorhinolaryngol 1997;40:217–18.

227. Raw M, McNeill A, West R. Smoking cessation guidelines for health professionals: a guide to effective smoking cessation interventions for the health care system. Thorax 1998;53 (suppl 5).

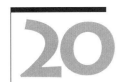

Skin diseases in pregnancy

Mark Davis[1], Brian Brost[2] with Nollag O'Rourke[3]

[1]Department of Dermatology, Mayo Clinic, Rochester, MN, USA
[2]Department of Obstetrics and Gynecology, Mayo Clinic, Rochester, MN, USA
[3]Department of Anesthesia, Perioperative and Pain Medicine, Brigham and Women's Hospital, Harvard Medical School, Boston, MA, USA

Drug therapy during pregnancy

Pregnancy is a period of profound temporary hormonal change, which may affect the skin in numerous ways. Many are so common that they are not considered abnormal and are classified as "physiological skin changes." Other dermatoses occur less frequently and are specifically associated with the gravid state. Finally, pregnancy may modify pre-existing dermatologic conditions. This chapter offers a summary of all these phenomena and is indebted to several helpful review articles previously published on this topic[1–3]. Table 20.1 defines many commonly used dermatologic descriptive terms to aid the reader and other additional terms are defined in the text.

Physiologic skin changes in pregnancy

There are a number of common skin changes in pregnancy that are thought to be related to hormonal changes.

Pigmentation

Hyperpigmentation is very common during pregnancy and occurs in up to 90% of women [4]. It is one of the most commonly recognized signs of pregnancy and may be generalized or restricted to areas of normal hyperpigmentation such as nipples, areolae, inner thighs, perineum, vulva and perianal region. The linea alba, a tendinous median line on the anterior abdominal wall, frequently hyperpigments to become the linea nigra and may extend from the symphysis pubis to the xiphisternum. Pigmentation increases in the first trimester, particularly in dark-haired, dark-complexioned women,

and fades post partum, although it seldom returns to the pre-pregnancy level. Freckles and melanocytic nevi tend to darken and may increase in number. Recent scars may also hyperpigment.

Melasma

Irregular, sharply demarcated patches of facial pigmentation known as melasma (see Plate 20.1) develop in approximately 70% of women during the second half of pregnancy [4,5]. Melasma also occurs in up to 30% of women taking oral contraceptives [6] and in essentially healthy women between early adulthood and the menopause [7]. The most common pattern is centrofacial, involving the forehead, cheeks, upper lip, nose and chin. The malar pattern is limited to cheeks and nose, and the mandibular type involves the ramus of the mandible [8]. Histologically, there are two patterns of pigmentation: the epidermal type, which occurs in 72% of cases, in which the melanin is deposited mainly in the basal melanocytes, and the dermal type, which affects 13% of patients, where the melanin is mainly in the superficial and deep dermis [8]. Examination under Wood's light shows enhancement of color contrast if melanin is primarily in the epidermis, and not if the melanin is located only in the dermis. Nearly 90% of women with chloasma due to oral contraception have a past history of melasma of pregnancy [6].

Pathogenesis

Eestrogen and progesterone are known to be strong melanogenic stimulants [9] and these hormones may be responsible for the hyperpigmentation of pregnancy. Serum and urinary melanocyte-stimulating hormone (MSH) levels have been reported as elevated during pregnancy with a rapid decrease post partum [10]. Other work has, however, demonstrated no difference in beta-MSH levels in the third trimester and after parturition [11]. Levels of beta-MSH were higher than the mean level obtained from nonpregnant controls but were

de Swiet's Medical Disorders in Obstetric Practice, 5th edition.
Edited by R. O. Powrie, M. F. Greene, W. Camann. © 2010 Blackwell Publishing.

Table 20.1 Common dermatologic definitions

Term	Description
Bulla	Raised well-delineated fluid-filled blisters >1.0 cm in diameter
Ecchymosis (plural ecchymoses)	Nonblanching, purpuric macules or patches of greater than 3 mm caused by extravasated blood in the skin
Excoriations	Superficial skin abrasions due to scratching of the skin
Erythema nodosum	An eruption of painful, tender, erythematous, subcutaneous, firm nodules most commonly found on the extensor surfaces of the lower legs
Erythema multiforme	An acute, symmetric eruption of multiple lesion types (papules, macules, and vesicles), the most characteristic of which is the "target" lesion (see below)
Erythema chronicum migrans	The classic skin lesion of primary Lyme disease, which occurs at the site of the bite by an infected tick
Hyperkeratosis	Increased keratinization (cornification) of the epidermis, appearing clinically as thickening of the skin
Macule	A circumscribed flat area (<1 cm) of discoloration. There should be no elevation or depression of the lesion's surface relative to surrounding skin
Maculopapular	A term used to denote an eruption that has both macular (flat and <1 cm) and papular (raised and <1 cm) features
Nodule	A palpable, solid lesion, <1 cm in diameter, that extends deeper than a papule and may be above, level with or below the skin surface
Onycholysis	Separation of the nail plate from the nail bed usually beginning at the free borders of the nail plate
Papule	A well-circumscribed, elevated, solid lesion, usually <1 cm. Often dome shaped
Patch	A circumscribed flat area of discoloration, >1 cm. It should be neither elevated or depressed relative to the surrounding skin (a large macule)
Petechiae	Small, nonblanching, red macules pinpoint to pinhead in size), caused by rupture of small blood vessels leading to hemorrhage
Plaque	A well-circumscribed, elevated, superficial, solid lesion, >1 cm in diameter. Often flat-topped or "plateau-like"
Purpura	Hemorrhage into skin or mucous membranes which varies in size and ranges in color related to duration. Types of purpura include ecchymosis and petechiae. Lesions are typically nonblanching and purple in color and may be palpable or nonpalpable
Pustule	A small (<1 cm in diameter), circumscribed superficial elevation of the skin that is filled with purulent material
Target lesion	Resembling, an archer's bull's eye, a target lesion has a central erythematous papule, macule or vesicle, a surrounding area of pale edema and a peripheral area of erythema
Telangiectasias	Small, superficial blood vessels
Urticaria	Also known as hives. An eruption of transient pruritic, elevated papules and plaques, typically with erythematous lesions known as wheals that have sharply defined borders and pale centers. Each lesion resolves within 24 hours
Vesicle	A small, superficial, circumscribed elevation of the skin, <1 cm, which contains serous fluid

Adpated from materials developed for the Dermatology Lexicon Project at www.dermatologylexicon.org and the Dermatology Glossary at http://missinglink.ucsf.edu/lm/DermatologyGlossary/index.html

within the normal range and therefore thought unlikely to be responsible for the pigmentary changes.

The patterns of pigmentation may relate to differences in end-organ sensitivity or distribution of melanocytes. Sun exposure may also exacerbate the development of melasma.

Treatment

Treatment is unsatisfactory and consists of minimizing exposure to sunlight by sun avoidance, or covering the skin with clothing when out in the sun, and avoidance of oral contraceptives. Sunscreens should be used and cosmetic camouflage with nonallergic products is helpful. Postpartum use of depigmenting agents may be effective and Kligman & Willis [12] report success in 14 out of 16 patients using twice-daily application of 5% hydroquinone, 0.1% tretinoin and 0.1% dexamethasone in ethanol and propylene glycol for 5–7 weeks. Sanchez *et al.* [8] recommend the use of 2% hydroquinone and 0.05% tretinoin on the epidermal type of persistent melasma and believe that the dermal types respond poorly if at all to this therapy. Depigmenting agents should always be used with caution as dermatitis, further hyperpigmentation or even hypopigmentation may ensue. Melasma usually fades within 1 year of delivery [13], although in one study 30% of cases persisted after 10 years [10].

Pruritus gravidarum

This term refers to intense pruritus that occurs as a manifestation of pregnancy, without any associated rash or clinical jaundice and usually in early pregnancy. Pruritus from all causes occurs in 17% of pregnant women [14] and may be due to conditions unrelated to pregnancy (such as dry skin, scabies, pediculosis (lice), urticaria, atopic eczema, drug eruptions, candidiasis, trichomonal vaginitis or neurodermatitis) or conditions that only occur in pregnancy (cholestasis of pregnancy, pruritic urticarial papules and plaques of pregnancy, pruritic folliculitis of pregnancy, prurigo of pregnancy and pemphigoid gestationis, also known as herpes gestationis). All of these listed conditions (with the notable exception of cholestasis of pregnancy) are associated with a typical rash that should be looked for by a careful complete skin examination.

Early scabies may be the most subtle of these rashes and should be looked for by examining the space between the fingers, the flexing surfaces of the wrists and armpits, the areolae of the breasts, along the belt line, and on the lower buttocks. The face usually does not become involved in adults. Examination in this areas may reveal only small, barely noticeable bumps that may be slightly shiny and dark in color rather than red. Initially the itching may not exactly correlate to the location of these bumps.

If no rash is found, the main differential diagnosis of persistent itch in pregnancy is obstetric cholestasis and this condition should be tested for on several occasions by obtaining a serum bile salts and liver function tests in any pregnant patient with persistent itch (see Chapter 9 where obstetric cholestasis is discussed in detail). In the absence of rash and in the presence of repeatedly normal serum liver enzymes and bile salts, patients with new-onset persistent itch in pregnancy can be presumed to have pruritus gravidarum.

Treatment

Mild forms of pruritus gravidarum may be treated with bland topical antipruritic creams such as calamine or moisturizers. Antihistamines may be a useful adjunct. However, in some patients the pruritus may be so severe that preterm delivery is necessary. Pruritus gravidarum (just like obstetric cholestasis) can recur in up to 50% of subsequent pregnancies or with oral contraceptive use. Unlike obstetric cholestasis, the condition is not associated with an increased fetal risk. It usually resolves rapidly in the postpartum period.

Vascular changes

Edema

Clinically apparent edema of the face and hands occurs in approximately 50% of pregnant women, whilst edema of the legs not associated with pre-eclampsia develops in about 80% [4]. It is usually nonpitting in nature and worse in the morning. It is probably due to several factors: increased fluid retention (approximately 2.5 L during pregnancy), increased vascular permeability, increased blood flow [15] and decreased colloid osmotic pressure of plasma. It warrants no treatment except for reassurance. In extreme cases of lower limb edema, compression stockings may be necessary.

Spider nevi

Vascular spiders (also known as spider nevi) are superficial vascular structures that consist of a central pulsating arteriole with radiating thin-walled vessels. Compression of the center causes the lesion to fade but when compression is released, the spider leg-like vessels quickly refill from the center of the lesion. Clinically they are indistinguishable from the spider nevi of chronic liver disease. Spider nevi develop between the second and fifth months of pregnancy and are present in about 57% of white women and 10% of black women by the third trimester [16]. This difference is probably due to difficulty in visualizing them on dark skin. In comparison, spider nevi are said to occur in 15% of normal nonpregnant white women. They occur in the areas drained by the superior vena cava on the upper trunk and face, increase in size and number throughout pregnancy and fade post partum. The majority (75%) have disappeared by the 7th week after delivery [16]; the remainder persist and recurrence may occur at the same sites in subsequent pregnancies. Treatment for persistent lesions is with cold point cautery or pulsed dye laser.

Palmar erythema

Palmar erythema develops during pregnancy in 70% of white women and 35% of black women [16]. Its onset is in the first trimester and it fades within 1 week of delivery. There are two clinical patterns: (i) diffuse mottling of the whole palm; and (ii) erythema confined to the thenar and hypothenar eminences. The former is the more common. It frequently occurs in patients who also have spider nevi and both are thought to be due to high estrogen levels. The increases in blood volume and blood flow are other possible factors.

Varices

Varices may affect as many as 40% of pregnant women and may involve the saphenous system or small superficial vessels in the legs, as well as the hemorrhoidal and vulvar networks. Venous congestion of the labial tissue can also lead to significant edema and pain. Factors contributing to venous congestion include increased venous pressure in femoral and pelvic vessels due to compression from the gravid uterus, increase in the blood volume, increased collagen fragility and a hereditary tendency to varicose veins. Varices tend to regress post partum, although not always completely.

Treatment is elevation of the legs and elastic support stockings. Several maxi-type pads can be placed in the undergarments to provide symptomatic relief of significant labial edema. Vulvar support garments have also been developed for this indication. Thrombosis may occur in leg varices or in hemorrhoids. Varices are a risk factor for thromboembolism which is discussed in Chapter 4.

Hemangiomata

Hemangiomata are red to purple papules on the skin that are vascular in origin. The term includes such diverse lesions as port wine stain (vascular birthmarks), Campbell de Morgan spots (nonblanching red or violet spots that appear with age, usually on the chest or trunk, and are typically less than 6 mm in diameter) and strawberry nevi (red firm dome-shaped hemangiomas present at birth or soon after that typically occur on the head or neck and grow rapidly but then regress and involute without scarring). Capillary hemangiomata develop on the head and neck in 5% of pregnant women, appearing at the end of the first trimester and enlarging until term [13]. Pre-existing hemangiomata of any type may also increase in size during pregnancy. High estrogen levels are probably an etiologic factor. Surgical removal is the treatment for lesions which persist post partum.

The "pregnancy tumor" or telangiectatic epulis is a specific pregnancy lesion composed of fibrous and vascular tissue. It is clinically and histologically similar to pyogenic granuloma (a misnamed noninfectious and nongranulomatous vascular lesion of skin and mucosa typically seen in children and young adults that appears as a solitary glistening papule or nodule prone to bleeding or ulceration). Telangiectatic epulis is sited on the oral mucosa or gingiva and arises from interdental papillae on the buccal or lingual surfaces of the gingiva. It is usually associated with extensive gingivitis and may bleed or ulcerate. It often grows rapidly and may represent a vascular and fibrous response to injury It usually develops at between 2 and 5 months gestation and affects 2% of pregnant women. Treatment is not usually necessary because these lesions typically regress after delivery. For cases with persistent bleeding in pregnancy cautery or excision may be performed.

Purpura

This may occur on the legs during the second half of pregnancy due to increased capillary permeability and fragility [13]. Vasculitis and thrombocytopenia must be excluded with a complete blood count and consideration of the need for biopsy if a systemic vascultis is suspected.

Connective tissue and collagen

Striae gravidarum (gravidarum distensae)

Striae gravidarum, commonly known as stretch marks, develop during the second half of pregnancy in most women. They occur on the abdomen, breasts and thighs. Initially they are pink or violaceous linear wrinkles, which develop perpendicular to skin tension lines. They become white and atrophic with time, although never disappear completely. They are identical to the striae associated with puberty, obesity, Cushing's disease and steroid therapy.

The etiology of striae is multifactorial: stretching is a localizing factor and striae do tend to occur more with overweight mothers or those carrying heavier babies or with multiple pregnancy but their occurrence does not correlate directly with the degree of skin distension or weight gain [17,18]. There is also a familial tendency [19]. Rupture of collagen and elastic fibers [20] and increased adrenocortical activity have been considered important [17]. It has also been suggested that estrogen and relaxin increase the collagen and sulfate-free mucopolysaccharides and that subsequent stretching leads to easier separation of collagen [19]. Histologically, striae consist of areas of broken and curled elastic fibers in the upper dermis with parallel bands of collagen and elastic fibers in the center [21]. Fibrillin microfibrils in the elastic fiber network appear to be reduced and reorganized in skin affected by striae [22]. There is no specific treatment for striae and it is controversial as to whether emollient massage is effective in their prevention [17]. Topical tretinoin cream 0.025% does not appear to have any beneficial effect and should not be used in pregnancy because of the teratogenic effects of vitamin A compounds [23].

Skin tags or molluscum fibrosum gravidarum

Soft, fleshy, pendunculated, skin-colored or slightly pigmented papillomata (papules or plaques with fine multiple surface projections) may develop on the face, neck, upper anterior chest, axillae and under the breasts during the second half of pregnancy. They are about 1–5 mm in diameter and clinically and histologically identical to skin tags [24]. They are probably due to hormonal factors and regress post partum. Persisting lesions may be removed by electrodesiccation.

Glandular activity

Sweat and apocrine glands

Eccrine sweating (the watery sweating that can be produced by glands throughout the skin) is increased during pregnancy [25] and may be associated with milia (also known as milk spots, these are benign keratin-filled cysts under the epidermis that typically occur in the area around the nose and eyes due to occlusion of the eccrine sweat ducts) and intertrigo (inflammation of skin in the body folds, especially the inner thighs, genitalia, armpits, under the breasts and belly, behind the ears and between digits). Palmar eccrine sweating is, however, diminished [26]. Apocrine (the oily sweating that occurs only in areas such as the axilla, periareolar and pubic area) activity is also reduced with subsequent improvement of conditions such as Fox–Fordyce disease (a noninfectious inflammation behind chronically blocked sweat gland ducts which most commonly presents as a pruritic papular eruption) and hidradenitis suppurativa (a bacterial infection occurring behind chronically blocked sweat glands with the formation of pus-draining sinuses) [3], which may, however, rebound post partum.

Sebaceous glands

Sebaceous activity (sebum- or oil-producing glands usually associated with hair follicles anywhere but also occurring on the lips, areola, and genitals) increases during the third trimester, and acne occasionally develops during pregnancy. Sebaceous glands associated with lactiferous ducts on the areolae hypertrophy as early as 6 weeks gestation and appear as Montgomery's tubercles (tiny bumps scattered around the areola). They are one of the signs of early pregnancy.

Hair changes

Telogen effluvium

Normally about 85% of scalp hairs are in the anagen (growing) phase and 15% are in the telogen (resting or non-growing) phase. A hair usually grows in anagen phase for 4 years and then rests in telogen phase for 4 months. At the end of the telogen phase, a hair is dead, fully keratinized and falls out. The scalp end of the hair lost at the end of the telogen phase has a characteristic shape of a club or bulb while hair lost in the anagen phase has a tapered or pointed end. Typically adults lose about 100 hairs a day, with most hairs having the club-shaped end indicating the end of the hair life cycle.

During pregnancy the proportion of hairs in anagen (the growing phase) increases [27] to 95% of hair follicles, creating the thickening of scalp hair in pregnancy reported by many women. Post partum, the conversion from anagen (growing) hairs to telogen (resting) hairs is accelerated and the proportion of growing hairs drops within a few months

to 75%. This creates a phenomenon of postpartum hair loss known as "telogen effluvium" that typically follows delivery by 4–20 weeks [3]. The hair loss is generally diffuse, although may be more marked in the frontoparietal hairline in women with a tendency to male-pattern baldness. Baldness seldom, if ever, occurs, and spontaneous recovery usually takes place within 6 months of delivery [28], although it may take as long as 15 months [3]. Recovery is usually complete unless the telogen effluvium is severe, repeated in several pregnancies or associated with male-pattern alopecia. With successive pregnancies hair loss tends to be less marked.

The diagnosis of telogen effluvium is made by finding large numbers of "club hairs" when hair is pulled gently or falls from the patient's scalp. Histologically, the follicles in telogen are normal. Increased adrenocorticosteroids and ovarian androgens probably account for the increase in anagen hairs, and estrogens prolong the anagen phase [5]. Telogen effluvium is probably caused by several factors including changes in endocrine balance, the stress of delivery, difficult labor and blood loss. No specific treatment is required apart from reassurance.

Some women develop male-pattern or diffuse hair loss in late pregnancy. This is usually due to inhibition of anagen in some follicles and not to increased loss. The postpartum regrowth of hair in women with male-pattern hair loss in pregnancy is unlikely to be complete.

There is no significant change in the anagen/telogen ratio of body hair [29].

Hirsutism

Hypertrichosis (increased hair growth not localized to androgen-dependent areas of the skin), most marked on face, arms and legs, is quite common in pregnancy but marked hirsutism (male-pattern hair growth) is rare. It resolves post partum but frequently recurs in subsequent pregnancies.

Hirsutism may be accompanied by acne, deepening of the voice and clitoral enlargement and is probably due to increased adrenocorticosteroid and ovarian androgen secretion. Other causes of hirsutism, namely androgen-secreting ovarian tumors (luteomas and theca lutein cysts) and polycystic ovaries, should be excluded. Androgenization of a female fetus is unlikely in these circumstances. Treatment of the mother's hirsutism (which will persist after the pregnancy) is with reassurance and cosmetic removal (depilatory creams, electrolysis or ruby laser).

Nails

Nail changes, consisting of transverse grooving, brittleness, distal onycholysis (separation of the distal nail plate from the underlying nail bed starting at the distal free margin and progressing proximally) and subungual keratosis (excessive proliferation of the nail bed) may occur from the 6th week of pregnancy. The pathogenesis of these changes is not known. There is no effective treatment.

Breasts and nipples

Sore nipples with cracks and fissures commonly develop in the first few days of breastfeeding. The soreness may limit sucking, and stasis, mastitis or breast abscess may follow. Nipple eczema may also develop and involve the breast. Secondary infection must be excluded. Fissures and eczema are avoided by gentle washing to remove saliva and milk and by use of emollients after each feeding session. Removal of excess emollients prior to the next breastfeeding session is important. To help heal fissures, the breasts should be left exposed if possible for 5–10 minutes after breastfeeding to allow air drying; alternatively, a hair drier on the cool, low setting can be used when in a hurry. Any secondary infection should be treated with antibiotics. Severely affected patients are often atopic.

Dermatoses specific to pregnancy

A number of dermatoses are specific to pregnancy, to the puerperium or occur as a result of trophoblastic tumors. Severe pruritus is the leading symptom in all these dermatoses of pregnancy, and can considerably impair maternal quality of life. Intrahepatic cholestasis of pregnancy is the only condition that is also associated with significant fetal risks. Unequivocal diagnostic tests are only available for pemphigoid gestationis (indirect immunofluorescence) and intrahepatic cholestasis of pregnancy (serum bile acids with liver function tests). In the largest case series to date of pregnancy dermatoses, the following classification system was proposed with associated distribution of relative frequencies [4]:

- pemphigoid gestationis (herpes gestationis) 4.2%
- polymorphic eruption of pregnancy 21.6%
- prurigo of pregnancy 0.8%
- pruritic folliculitis of pregnancy 0.2%
- intrahepatic cholestasis of pregnancy 3%
- eczema in prengnacy 49.7%
- miscellaneous dermatoses 20.6%.

Pemphigoid gestationis

Pemphigoid gestationis (PG) (see Plates 20.2 and 20.3) (also known as herpes gestationis) is an intensely pruritic bullous eruption that occurs in one in 60,000 pregnancies [30] or in association with the trophoblastic tumors choriocarcinoma [31] and hydatidiform mole [32]. Fortunately, it is a rare cause of significant pruritius during pregnancy. Because of the connotations of the term herpes to patients and other medical providers (and the fact that it is not caused by the herpes virus), it is best to use the term pemphigoid

gestationis (rather than herpes gestationis) in conversation with the patient and in the medical record.

The eruption initially consists of pruritic erythematous urticarial papules and plaques often with target lesions and ring-like (annular) patterns. Vesicles develop after a delay varying between a few days and a month and enlarge to become tense bullae. In 90% of patients the lesions begin in the periumbilical region and spread to involve thighs, breasts, palms and soles (see Plate 20.2). The face and oral mucosa are only rarely involved. PG may begin during the first or any subsequent pregnancy and typically arises during the second and third trimesters but has been reported as early as 9 weeks gestation or as late as 1 week post partum [33]. In subsequent pregnancies recurrence usually occurs with an earlier onset and more severe disease. When PG develops during the mid-trimester, there is usually a period of relative remission in the last few weeks of pregnancy followed by an abrupt postpartum flare [15]. The bullous lesions tend to resolve within a month of delivery, but the urticated plaques may persist for over a year [33].

The etiology of PG is unknown, but recent work highlights the immunopathologic findings in this disease. Paternal histocompatibility antigens (human leukocyte antigens (HLA)) were considered important following a study in which 50% of the consorts were HLA-DR2 compared to 25% of the controls [34]. However, this was not confirmed in another study in which the frequency of paternal HLA was normal [35]. A paternal factor is likely, as in some patients with pregnancies by several consorts the onset of PG has coincided with a change in partner, and in one case a patient had PG in her first and second pregnancies and then had an unaffected pregnancy by a new consort [35–37].

Maternal HLA studies have revealed a significantly increased frequency of DR3 with DR4 [34]. DR3 and DR4 are associated with other diseases with an immune pathogenesis such as Graves' disease, rheumatoid arthritis and insulin-dependent diabetes mellitus, which suggests that their presence confers an increase in immune susceptibility in the patients with PG. One study has confirmed the association between PG and other autoimmune diseases, particularly Graves' disease [38]. The antigenic trigger is probably paternally derived as PG occurs not only in pregnancy but also in association with hydatidiform mole and choriocarcinoma, and in these trophoblastic tumors, the chromosomes are all paternally derived. There is also evidence that DR compatibility between mother and fetus favors a spared pregnancy [39]. Once initiated, PG is undoubtedly hormonally modulated.

Exacerbations may occur with ovulation or premenstrually, suggesting that estrogen may also be a contributing factor. It tends to be in a phase of relative remission in late pregnancy and flares post partum when the most significant hormonal change is a fall in progesterone. Progesterone has been shown to have immunosuppressive effects similar to glucocorticoids and may exert an inhibiting effect on PG [40]. Exacerbations may also be induced by taking the contraceptive pill [41]. Holmes *et al.* [39] prescribed oral contraceptives to eight patients and four experienced exacerbations; three were given combined estrogen and progesterone, but the patient who flared most severely was given estrogen alone. Two patients were given progesterone alone and their PG was unaffected. There is experimental evidence that at certain concentrations estrogen may have immuno-enhancing properties [42] and this may account for its effect in PG. Holmes *et al.* [39] also demonstrated that breastfeeding was associated with a shorter and less severe postpartum illness, suggesting that prolactin may have an immunosuppressant effect on the disease.

Fetal prognosis

It has been stated that PG is associated with an increased fetal and maternal risk [43], although other workers have disagreed and found that fetal prognosis was unaffected [44]. In a study of 50 infants from affected pregnancies, there was a significant increase in babies of low birthweight and small-for-dates babies which did not correlate with the severity or duration of PG [43,45]. There were no stillbirths or maternal deaths and none of the four neonatal deaths was ascribed to PG. One infant developed a bullous eruption resembling PG, which resolved within a week. A more recent study [38] has once again indicated a tendency for premature delivery to be associated with PG. Serial ultrasound screening for growth starting at 24–28 weeks gestation may be warranted in women with PG, as small-for-dates infants have an increased morbidity. Regular antenatal testing with nonstress tests or biophysical profiles should be reserved for the fetus with intrauterine growth restriction or those who are falling off their growth curve. It is recommended that when possible, patients with PG be delivered in maternity units with access to special care facilities since prematurity and low birthweight may be an issue.

Pathology

Histologically, the early urticated lesions of PG show epidermal and papillary dermal edema with occasional foci of eosinophilic spongiosis (intercellular edema of the epidermis) [46]. The bullae are subepidermal and contain numerous eosinophils. Ultrastructurally, the "split" occurs within the lamina lucida (a component of the basement membrane zone between the epidermis and dermis of the skin) [46,47].

Direct immunofluorescence demonstrates C3 at the basement membrane zone in all patients with active PG [40]. Indirect immunofluorescence usually shows a C3 binding factor [47]. This PG factor is an IgG of the IgG1 or IgG3 subclass [48] and although it is only positive in 25% of cases by conventional techniques, it can be demonstrated more reliably by immunoelectron microscopy [49].

Differential diagnosis

The main differential diagnoses are from the much more common polymorphic eruption of pregnancy (PEP), and from bullous pemphigoid. Table 20.2 compares the characteristics of the two conditions.

Polymorphic eruption of pregnancy (also known as pruritic urticarial plaques and papules of pregnancy (PUPPP); see below) usually affects primigravidae, and the eruption starts in prominent striae. Urticarial plaques, wheals and vesicles may occur in both disorders but only become frankly bullous in PG [40]. Histologically, there are no features of early lesions to distinguish between the two but on direct immunofluorescence, PEP (PUPPP) is consistently negative [33,40].

Pemphigoid gestationis and bullous pemphigoid share several features. Both are characterized by pruritic, urticarial and bullous eruptions. Histologic and immunofluorescent findings are also closely similar. However, the lesions of PG occur predominantly on the lower abdomen and thighs, whilst the distribution in bullous pemphigoid is more variable. The clinical activity of PG is affected by estrogen and progesterone, but there is no evidence that these have any effect on bullous pemphigoid. Finally, unlike the previously mentioned association of PG with certain HLA types, there does not appear to be any assoiation between bullous pemphigoid and HLA type. Nevertheless, considerable similarities between PG and bullous pemphigoid led to the suggestion that "pemphigoid" gestationis is a more appropriate term than "herpes" gestationis [33,40]. Two cases have been reporting as evolving from PG into bullous pemphigoid, again demonstrating the close links between these two dermatoses [50].

Treatment

Mild cases of PG respond to treatment with antihistamines and topical fluorinated corticosteroids. Systemic steroids are indicated in more severe disease with bullae. Most cases respond to 40 mg daily of prednisolone and this can usually be reduced fairly rapidly to a daily maintenance dose of 10 mg. Use of systemic steroids in pregnancy is reviewed in Chapter 47. It should be increased again in anticipation of the postpartum flare, which occurs frequently and can persist for months. While systemic steroids remain the mainstay of treatment of PG, treatment failures do occur. Plasmapheresis should be considered for severe cases unresponsive to steroids[51]. Dapsone (an antibacterial agent used to treat bullous pemphigoid) is usually avoided for this indication during pregnancy as it can cause hemolytic disease of the newborn [52], although it has been given safely

Table 20.2 Comparison of pemphigoid gestationis and polymorphic eruption of pregnancy [33]

	Pemphigoid gestationis	Polymorphic eruption of pregnancy
Incidence per 100,000 pregnancies	2	420
Onset	Second trimester or earlier	Last few weeks of pregnancy
Postpartum exacerbations	75% Can persist for 12–60 weeks	15% Generally clears with delivery but can persist for 3–4 weeks
Recurrence with subsequent pregnancies	Yes	Not usually
Location of lesions	Begins and remains most prominent around the umbilicus in 87%	Begins within abdominal striae. Umbilicus affected in only 12%
Morphology		
Urticarial lesions	+	+
Vesicles	+	+
Bullae	+	−
Prominent striae	3%	81%
Fetal risk	Possible increased risk of prematurity and small for gestational age babies	None
Treatment	Systemic steroids	Topical steroids, antihistamines, colloidal baths. Systemic steroids rarely needed
Positive direct immunofluorescence	100%	0%
HLA-DR3	84%	46%
Associated autoimmune phenomena	+	−

to treat leprosy during pregnancy [53]. A single case has been reported of complete remission of severe PG during treatment with ritodrine commenced for premature labor [54]. The use of the luteinizing hormone-releasing hormone (LHRH) analog goserelin led to a complete temporary remission in a longstanding case of PG [55].

Maternal prognosis

Once a patient has had an affected pregnancy, PG will usually recur in subsequent pregnancies [15], with an earlier onset and more severe disease. Thus, many would caution against further pregnancy. However, occasional "skipped" pregnancies can occur and some mothers are prepared to risk another pregnancy. HLA-DR3 typing may be a useful prognostic indicator as the absence of DR3 is associated with milder disease.

Polymorphic eruption of pregnancy

This is more commonly known as pruritic urticarial plaques and papules of pregnancy in the US (see Plate 20.4).

This pruritic urticarial eruption develops in and around abdominal striae in approximately one in 240 pregnancies.

It has previously been named pruritic urticarial papules and plaques of pregnancies (given the unfortunate acronym "PUPPP") [56,57], toxemic rash of pregnancy [58] or late-onset prurigo of pregnancy [59,60]. It has been suggested that these are all synonyms for the same eruption and the adoption of the uniform term PEP has been proposed [61].

Three clinical subtypes of PEP have been described [62]: type I, mainly urticarial papules and plaques; type II, non-urticarial erythema; type III, papules or vesicles and combinations of the two forms. Seventy-six percent of affected women are primigravidae, and recurrence with subsequent pregnancies is rare [61]. PEP is significantly associated with increased abdominal skin distension and multiple pregnancies [63,64]. If a second episode does occur, it is generally much less severe than the first, which is in direct contrast to PG. Severe cases of PEP can closely mimic the early stages of PG and thus direct immunofluorescence can be a useful diagnostic test [65].

A prospective study of 44 cases of PEP showed low cortisol levels compared to controls, suggesting a hormonal influence [66]. Furthermore, a male/female ratio of 2/1 was found in the offspring of affected women [66]. This may be relevant in the light of a preliminary study of male DNA detection in the skin of women with PEP [67]. The results of this study indicate that fetal cells can migrate to maternal skin during pregnancy (a phenomenon known as microchimerism). Such migration of fetal DNA may be an important factor in the pathogenesis of PEP and was not seen in the skin of pregnant women without skin disease [67].

Polymorphic eruption generally begins in the last 5 weeks of pregnancy and rarely persists for more than a few weeks. It usually begins in prominent abdominal striae and may remain confined to the abdomen with relative sparing of the umbilicus. Sometimes it becomes widespread, involving buttocks, shoulders and limbs. The lesions consist of urticarial papules, plaques and polycyclic wheals (see Plate 20.4). Vesicles occur in approximately 45% and target lesions in 19%, but the vesicles rarely enlarge beyond 2 mm [61] and thus bullous lesions as in PG are hardly ever seen. The condition is more common in multiple gestations.

The differential diagnosis includes pemphigoid gestationis, idiopathic urticaria and drug eruption. If bullae are prominent and the skin eruption occurs remote from term, a skin biopsy may be necessary. Histology of the urticarial papules in PEP shows epidermal and upper dermal edema with a perivascular infiltrate of lymphocytes, histiocytes and eosinophils. With the vesicular lesions, vesicular spongiosis occurs. Immunofluorescence, however, is consistently negative in distinction from pemphigoid gestationis [61].

Polymorphic eruption of pregnancy is generally not associated with significant adverse maternal or fetal outcomes other than the itching. Treatment is with antihistamines, colloidal oatmeal baths, lubrication and mild topical steroids. Systemic corticosteroids have been effective in extensive disease but are not generally necessary or recommended for mild to moderate cases [68]. In very severe cases elective delivery may be the only way to relieve pruritus [69].

Prurigo of pregnancy

Prurigo is a general term used to describe itchy eruptions of the skin. Prurigo of pregnancy is a pruritic papular eruption unique to pregnancy that affects one in 300 pregnancies [60] and begins earlier in pregnancy than PEP. It is also referred to as prurigo gestationis of Besnier and "early-onset prurigo of pregnancy." The onset is usually between 25 and 30 weeks gestation and although the pruritus settles at delivery, the papules tend to persist for several months. The lesions consist of groups of excoriated papules on the extensor surface of limbs and abdomen, although they may become widespread.

Histology of the lesions demonstrates parakeratosis (persistence of the nuclei of keratinocytes in the outermost layer of the epidermis), acanthosis (an abnormal thickening of the stratum spinosum or "prickle cell layer" of the epidermis) and perivascular lymphocytic infiltrate. Immunofluorescence is negative.

The cause is unknown, but many patients appear to be atopic. It has been suggested that prurigo of pregnancy may be the result of pruritus gravidarum developing in atopic individuals [33].

The rash may recur in subsequent pregnancies and there is no increased risk to mother or fetus. Treatment is symptomatic with antihistamines and topical corticosteroids.

Pruritic folliculitis of pregnancy

Pruritic folliculitis of pregnancy is a pruritic folliculitis (inflammation of hair follicles) that begins between the 4th month of gestation and term and usually resolves by 2 weeks post partum [70]. The eruption is acneiform with widespread follicular erythematous papules.

As the clinical appearance resembles the monomorphic type of acne seen in some patients taking systemic corticosteroids, it is possible that pruritic folliculitis may be a form of hormonally induced acne rather than a specific dermatosis of pregnancy. Histopathology demonstrates acute folliculitis with focal spongiosis (intercellular fluid in the epidermis) and exocytosis (the process by which a cell directs the contents of secretory vesicles out of the cell membrane) of polymorphonuclear and mononuclear cells. In the dermis, there is edema and a perivascular infiltrate. Direct immunofluorescence is negative. The maternal and fetal prognosis is normal. Treatment is with topical 10% benzoyl peroxide and 1% hydrocortisone. Serum androgens do not appear to be elevated in this condition [71,72].

A prospective study of 14 cases showed a male/female ratio of 2/1 in the offspring of affected women and a significant reduction in birthweight compared to controls [71]. Serial ultrasound screening from 24–28 weeks gestation is important, as small-for-dates infants have increased morbidity. Regular antenatal testing should be reserved for fetuses with intrauterine growth restriction or who are falling off their growth curve.

Intrahepatic cholestasis of pregnancy

Intrahepatic cholestasis of pregnancy (ICP) is discussed in detail in Chapter 10 but will be briefly summarized here. Patients present with sudden onset of generalized pruritus with exclusively secondary skin changes (caused by scratching) and elevated total serum bile acid levels. The hallmark is a sudden onset of generalized pruritus starting during the second or third trimester, followed by secondary skin lesions, such as excoriations and excoriated papules caused by scratching, localized on the extensor surfaces of the limbs and also on the abdomen and back. The incidence has been estimated to be between 1:146–1293 pregnancies in the US. The condition usually resolves post partum.

The etiology of this condition is unclear: it is occasionally familial, tends to recur in subsequent pregnancies, and patients may have a family history of cholelithiasis and a higher risk of gallstones. The condition is associated with a risk of premature delivery, meconium-stained amniotic fluid, and intrauterine death (predominantly after 37 weeks gestation). Fetal risk may be higher in patients with higher bile acid levels.

Diagnosis is based on the clinical picture of pruritus without primary skin lesions, and laboratory markers of cholestasis: elevated bile acid levels are the most reliable markers with increases of 10–100-fold. Alkaline phosphatase may be raised but is also raised in healthy pregnant women; therefore this marker is less useful. Cholestasis and jaundice in ICP may be associated with vitamin K deficiency and coagulopathy.

Treatments include oral antihistamines for mild itching while ursodeoxycholic acid may be used for more severe itching. Weekly maternal injections of vitamin K may be prudent to decrease the risk of intracranial hemorrhage in the newborn.

Fetal risks include an increased risk of stillbirth. Patients should receive increased antenatal surveillance at the time of diagnosis although antepartum testing can be unreliable and a negative antepartum test is not necessarily reassuring. In the past, some authorities recommended delivery by 38 weeks gestation; given the less predictive nature of antenatal surveillance, providers should consider amniocentesis at 36 weeks gestation with delivery if the amniotic sample is suggestive of fetal lung maturity. The impact of early delivery on perinatal complications is unclear.

Papular dermatitis of pregnancy

This was described as a distinct entity by Spangler *et al.* [73] as a widespread papular dermatitis associated with a significant fetal mortality of 30% [74]. The authors found characteristic biochemical changes with elevated urinary chorionic gonadotropin levels in the last trimester and reduced plasma cortisol and urinary estriol. Spangler *et al.* [73] felt that the clinical feature that distinguished those with papular dermatitis of pregnancy from those with prurigo of pregnancy was that the lesions were widespread rather than grouped on the extensor surfaces of limbs. Holmes & Black, however, suggested that these cases of Spangler *et al.* do not justify a separate classification and may simply represent more florid examples of prurigo of pregnancy or PEP [61]. It is important to point out that similar biochemical studies have not been performed in other specific dermatoses of pregnancy. Spangler *et al.* [73,74] claimed that administration of systemic steroids or diethylstilbestrol dramatically improved the fetal mortality to approximately 12%. However, in the following year in a letter to the editor, this statement was withdrawn [75].

The fetal mortality of 30% that was reported [73] has not been confirmed subsequently. Vaughan Jones *et al.* [66], in their prospective study of 200 women with pregnancy dermatoses, showed an overall fetal mortality of less than 5%. Furthermore, no cases of papular dermatitis were identified

in this study. Thus, papular dermatitis is no longer considered to be a separate pregnancy dermatosis, but probably forms part of the spectrum of PEP or prurigo of pregnancy.

Autoimmune progesterone dermatitis of pregnancy

A single case of autoimmune progesterone dermatitis of pregnancy was described by Bierman [76]. It consisted of a nonpruritic acneiform eruption with papules, pustules and comedones on the fingers, arms, legs and buttocks. The eruption recurred in a subsequent pregnancy and both pregnancies terminated in spontaneous abortion. The striking histopathologic features were of intense accumulation of eosinophils in hair follicles, epidermis, dermis and subcutis. Intradermal testing with aqueous progesterone produced a delayed hypersensitivity reaction, and administration of an oral contraceptive containing norethindrone and mestranol resulted in a severe flare of the eruption. No premenstrual flares occurred. The dermatitis, which resolved rapidly on treatment with conjugated estrogens, probably represents hypersensitivity to endogenous progesterone. No similar cases have since been reported.

The more common autoimmune progesterone dermatitis not associated with pregnancy is clinically distinct and consists of a polymorphic rash with urticaria, papulopustular vesicular or erythema multiforme-like lesions that recur on the trunk and extremities in the premenstrual period [77]. It is associated with previous use of progesterone-containing oral medication, which appears to sensitize the body to endogenous progesterone [77]. There is usually a positive intradermal skin test to progesterone and treatments include conjugated estrogens or oophorectomy [78]. Tamoxifen 30 mg has also caused complete remission but with consequent amenorrhea [79]. The anabolic androgen danazol (200 mg twice daily given just before the onset of a period) has also proved effective in two cases [80].

The effect of pregnancy on other dermatoses

The effect of pregnancy on other skin disorders is generally unpredictable, although individual patients may react consistently.

Eczema

Atopic dermatitis (also known as eczema) is present in 10–20% of the population. Most patients develop the condition in early childhood. It is strongly associated with allergies, allergic rhinitis and asthma. Environmental irritants such as soap, cleansers, lotions and perfumes can worsen the condition. In adults lesions are typically dry, red to brownish gray and may be scaly or appear thickened. Commonly affected sites include the elbows, knees, hands, feet, wrists, ankles, face, neck and upper chest.

Atopic dermatitis is frequently exacerbated during pregnancy. Hand and nipple eczema are both common in the puerperium. A prospective study of 200 women with pregnancy dermatoses showed eczema to be the most common skin complaint during pregnancy [66]. In some cases it presented *de novo* during pregnancy. In addition, if pruritus gravidarum develops, there may be further exacerbation with development of prurigo. Atopic dermatitis is not associated with an increase in adverse fetal outcomes.

Treatment of atopic dermatitis includes avoidance of triggers such as heat, perspiration, stress and low humidity, limiting exposure to irritants with the use of gloves for dishwashing and cleaning, use of topical emollients with high oil content such as petroleum jelly, and mild to moderately potent topical corticosteroids. Topical calcineurin inhibitors such as tacrolimus and pimecrolimus are also used but their safety in pregnancy is not established.

Acne vulgaris

Acne vulgaris is a disease of the pilosebaceous follicles and is the most common skin disorder in the United States with up to half of women of reproductive age affected. The effect of pregnancy on acne vulgaris is variable. Some patients improve whilst others develop acne for the first time. In these patients acne is often limited to the chin and may be associated with hirsutism. Withdrawal of acne medication at any time may cause a flare of the condition and this includes the withholding of medication during gestation.

Treatments for acne vulgaris outside of pregnancy include topical retinoids, benzoyl peroxide, azelaic acid, salicylic acid by themselves or in combination, systemic oral antibiotics such as the tetracyclines, erythromycin, clindamycin or trimethoprim sulfamethoxazole (TMP/SMX) in combination with a topical agent, oral contraceptive therapy and oral isotretinoin. Topical retinoids (theoretically) and isotretinoin (definitively) are teratogens and should not be used to treat acne in pregnancy. Tetracyclines can cause staining of bone and teeth in the infant and although conception on these agents is likely not of major concern, stopping these agents before or early in pregnancy is recommended. Topical agents other than retinoids are readily justifiable in pregnancy. The use of erythromycin may be warranted for severe cases but TMP/SMX is not generally used for this indication during pregnancy.

Psoriasis and impetigo herpetiformis

Psoriasis (Plate 20.5) is a chronic skin disorder affecting 0.6–4.8% of the population. It often presents between ages 20 and 30. It is characterized by erythematous plaques with sharply defined margins covered by a thick silvery scale.

The most common form of psoriasis (plaque psoriasis) typically affects the scalp, elbows, knees, back, ears and nails. Psoriasis may remain unchanged, clear or worsen and may also only manifest itself during pregnancy.

Treatment for psoriasis outside pregnancy includes topical agents (salicylic acid, steroids, vitamin D derivatives, tar and dithranol and the vitamin A derivative tazorotene), ultraviolet B phototherapy, PUVA (psoralen, a light-sensitizing medication, and ultraviolet light A together), biologic agents (such as infliximab and adalimumab), cyclosporine, methotrexate, soriatane (an oral vitamin A derivative) and other immunosuppressive agents. Use of these agents in pregnancy is briefly reviewed below in the section on medications in pregnancy.

Impetigo herpetiformis is a rare form of pustular psoriasis, which may be triggered by pregnancy, infections or sudden withdrawal of glucocorticoids. It can develop at any stage of gestation. The eruption consists of urticated erythema, which begins in the flexures, especially in the inguinal region. Superficial sterile pustules form at the margins of the lesions and the eruption may become widespread with involvement of mucosal surfaces. Fever, malaise, neutrophilia, hypocalcemia and tetany are associated. Abnormal liver enzymes can also be seen with this condition.

The histopathology is similar to that of pustular psoriasis with intraepidermal and subcorneal spongiform pustules of Kogoi and a perivascular infiltrate [81].

Pregnancy-related impetigo herpetiformis usually remits at delivery but may recur with each subsequent pregnancy and with oral contraceptive therapy [82]. The main obstetric problem is placental insufficiency, which can lead to stillbirth, neonatal death and fetal abnormalities which persist despite adequate maternal treatment [83]. Management requires intensive medical care with fluid and electrolyte replacement and correction of hypocalcemia. Antibiotics are indicated for secondary infection, and systemic corticosteroids may be helpful (see Chapter 47 on the use of steroids in pregnancy). Fetal well-being should be carefully monitored with daily maternal assessment of fetal movements and serial antenatal testing. An elective cesarean section may be necessary to improve fetal morbidity Low-dose methotrexate can be substituted post partum to prevent rebound pustulation, but is contraindicated during pregnancy and lactation. Gonadotropins are also reported to be helpful [84,85].

Leprosy

Leprosy is a deforming disease caused by *Mycobacterium leprae* and although it is seen throughout the world, it is now most common in Brazil, India, Madagascar, Mozambique, Myanmar and Nepal. It typically manifests as hypopigmented or erythematous papules, nodules and macules. Sensory and/or motor loss occurs in the area of the lesions and later in the distal extremities. Treatment is usually with dapsone, rifampin and clofazimine and the course of treatment is typically

6 months to 2 years. The course of leprosy can be complicated by immunologic reactions of two types: a delayed type hypersensitivity reaction (also known as a type 1 reaction) characterized by edema, erythema and even ulceration of existing lesions accompanied by neuritis, and erythema nodosum leprosum (also known as a type 2 reaction) characterized by a systemic inflammatory syndrome with fever, multiple erythematous tender nodules, neuritis and joint, eye, bone, and kidney involvement.

In general, patients with leprosy (Hansen's disease) do well in pregnancy. Treatment with dapsone, rifampin and clofazimine is generally offered in pregnancy although dapsone may cause hemolytic disease of the newborn both with *in utero* exposure and through breast milk [53,54]. Both type 1 and type 2 reactions and relapse are more common in pregnancy. Active lepromatous leprosy may also have an increased incidence of obstetric complications including low-birthweight infants. There is also an increased incidence of twins in lepromatous patients [53].

Pregnancy and collagen disease

Collagen vascular dieasese with skin manifestations such as systemic lupus erythematosus (SLE), discoid lupus, dermatomyositis, polyarteritis nodosa and systemic sclerosis are discussed in Chapter 8.

Pregnancy and inflammatory skin disease

Urticaria (hives)

Urticaria may develop in late pregnancy, and dermographism is also common. The specific dermatoses of pregnancy such as PG and prurigo of pregnancy may have an urticarial component and are part of the differential diagnosis. While food, medication or environmental triggers should be sought, for many cases no etiology is found. Treatment is with antihistamines.

Erythema multiforme

Erythema multiforme (EM) is an acute hypersensitivity reactiovn with a characterisitic symmetric eruption of multiple lesion types (papules, macules, and vesicles), the most characteristic of which is the "target" lesion (see Table 20.1). EM can be triggered by infection (especially herpes simplex) or medications. It typically is preceded by a nonspecific viral-like prodrome and lasts 2–4 weeks. EM may also be caused by pregnancy and has been reported to recur in successive pregnancies in some women. The differential diagnosis includes PG and the two conditions can be differentiated histologically and on immunofluorescence [15]. Treatment involves treatment of or discontinuance of the underlying cause. Steroids should not be given routinely but may be considered in the most severe cases.

Erythema nodosum

Erythema nodosum and sarcoidosis are discussed in Chapter 1.

Pregnancy and benign and malignant skin tumors

Neurofibromatosis

Neurofibromatosis (also known as von Recklinghausen's disease) is a genetic neurocutaneous disorder that occurs in 1 in 3000 individuals. Patients with neurofibromatosis type 1 (the most common type) have multiple café au lait spots (flat hyperpigmented lesions the color of coffee with milk) and associated cutaneous neurofibromas.

Pregnancy usually has an adverse effect on neurofibromatosis. Women with neurofibromatosis were reported to have a higher than expected rate of first-trimester spontaneous abortions, stillbirths and intrauterine growth restriction so that close monitoring of pregnancy was deemed essential [86,87]. However, the largest and most recent series did not find an increased risk of obstetric complications aside from an increased rate of cesarean delivery at 36%. However, 60% of patients did report growth of new neurofibroma and 52% reported the growth of pre-existing ones during pregnancy. Many patients have associated hypertension that can further complicate the pregnancy [88] (see Chapter 6). Other complications include neuropathies associated with tumor growth and occasional sudden hemorrhage into neurofibromata. Major blood vessels can also rupture and should be considered as part of the differential diagnosis of acute medical complaints in these patients [89]. Antental genetic screening (or preimplantation genetic diagnosis) for neurofibromatosis is available to parents.

Melanoma

Malignant melanoma accounts for nearly 50% of all metastases to the placenta and approximately 90% involving the fetus, both of which are nevertheless exceedingly rare (see below). Although this was not always thought to be the case, good evidence now exists that survival rates for melanoma do not appear to be affected by pregnancy and nor does a subsequent pregnancy increase the risk of recurrence [90]. Treatment of melanoma in pregnancy is as for melanoma in the nonpregnant state and termination of pregnancy appears to offer no appreciable maternal benefit [91]. Transplacental transmission of melanoma to the fetus is extremely rare, and maternal melanoma usually has no adverse effects on the fetus [91]. However, the placenta should be sent to a pathologist after delivery for evaluation for evidence of metastasis. Women who have had malignant melanoma excised should be advised to delay future pregnancy by at least 2 years after diagnosis, as 83% of patients with primary melanoma who later present with metastatic disease do so within 2 years [92].

General recommendations about dermatologic medication use during pregnancy

Prescribing for common skin disorders in pregnancy

The general principles guiding prescribing in pregnancy are reviewed in Chapter 30 and apply as much to the treatment of skin disorders in pregnancy as they do to any other disease group. Ideally, pregnancy safety issues related to medication should be considered with every prescription given to a woman during her reproductive years. Decisions regarding what medications to use during a pregnancy require a good understanding of the disease being treated, the efficacy of the various options available and a review of the usually very limited pregnancy safety data. This usually requires direct conversation between a dermatologist and the obstetrician. Complicating matters further is the importance of the patient's own perspective on what is and what is not tolerable in terms of disease control and fetal risk during the 40 weeks of gestation.

While potential guidelines for some dermatologic drug prescribing in pregnancy or lactation are available [93], new drug formulations are constantly being developed. There remains little published experience with many of these medications in human pregnancy. Decisions to use any medication in pregnancy need always to be made on the basis of careful consideration of the potential benefits, therapeutic alternatives and the potential risks, be they known or unknown.

Topical agents

Topical corticosteroids present a distinct problem in terms of pregnancy safety rating as there are many formulations and the absorption will vary significantly with the formulation, the area being treated and the lesion being treated. Meaningful pregnancy safety data are rarely available for individual formulations and clinical decisions about use of topical steroids in pregnancy must be extrapolated from the overwhelmingly favorable data about the use of systemic steroids in pregnancy (reviewed in Chapter 47). Table 20.3 provides a list of common topical steroids and classifies them according to strength. Although all of these agents are likely safe for use in pregnancy, many clinicians will gravitate towards agents containing hydrocortisone, triamcinolone, betamethasone, mometasone, and fluticasone because of the extensive experience with these agents in the treatment of asthma.

Topical antibiotics (used for acne vulgaris and rosacea) are not significantly absorbed and may be used in pregnancy.

Topical tretinoin (used for acne), while minimally absorbed, is not generally used in pregnancy because of the marked teratogenic effects of systemic vitamin A derivatives.

Topical dithranol and tar (used for treatment of psoriasis) have minimal systemic absorption and appear to be safe.

Topical calcipotriene (used for psoriasis) is a vitamin D3 derivative with systemic absorption of approximately 6% of the applied dose through psoriatic lesions. High doses of calcipotriene administered systemically to pregnant animals are associated with skeletal abnormalities but a dose consistent with the systemic absorption anticipated from topical use is not. While human data on the use of this agent in pregnancy are limited, its use when topical steroids are not enough to contol significant psoriasis seems justifiable.

Topical tacrolimus (used for atopic dermatitis) is an unknown in pregnancy and should only be used when alternatives have failed.

Psoralen (a light-sensitizing medication) and ultraviolet light A (UVA), known together as PUVA, are used to treat moderately severe psoriasis. There is no evidence to suggest that psoralen (administered topically or orally) and UVA (PUVA) are teratogenic when used to treat psoriasis. However, because PUVA is mutagenic, it is considered advisable to avoid PUVA as first-line treatment during pregnancy [94] even though no adverse effects in pregnancies conceived during PUVA treatment have been identified [95]. Its use to control severe psorisiasis in pregnancy is therefore justifiable when other options are limited.

Systemic agents

Most of the commonly used antihistamines appear to be safe during pregnancy after the first trimester. Diphenhydramine has the best safety record and is the most effective antihistamine although the drowsiness associated with its use makes it difficult for some patients to tolerate.

The use of antibiotics such as penicillins, cephalosporins and the macrolides is justifiable when warranted. Less is known about the effects of chronic use of metronidazole and trimethoprim but their short-term use is safe and their long-term use is justifiable when other options have failed.

The use of systemic corticosteroids in pregnancy is discussed in Chapter 47. These agents should not be withheld when indicated in pregnancy despite a very small possibility of being associated with adverse outcomes.

The use of various biologic agents (such as infliximab and adalimumab) and immunosuppressive agents (such as cyclosporine) in pregnancy is discussed in detail elsewhere in this text. Despite much reassuring data about their use in pregnancy for severe medical illness, their use for dermatologic conditions in pregnancy needs to be carefully considered with recognition that most skin conditions are not life threatening. Some comments about the more commonly prescribed of these agents follow below.

Choroquine appears to be very well tolerated in pregnancy.

Although cyclosporine was once felt to be contraindicated for the treatment of dermatologic illness in pregnancy, experience from transplant patients indicates that there is no conclusive evidence of any teratogenic effect [96]. A paper in 2000 reported the first British case of the successful use of cyclosporine to control pustular psoriasis in pregnancy from 25 weeks gestation [97]. The experience with the biologic agents (tumor necrosis factor antagonists such as infliximab) in pregnancy for the treatment of inflammatory bowel disease and rheumatologic conditions had been encouraging, with initial reports reporting no evidence of teratogenicity. A recent report of a possible association between these agents and congenital anomalies in the exposed infants has made their role in pregnancy less clear at the time of this writing [98].

Thalidomide, now being advocated for the treatment of erythema nodosum leprosum, should never be used in pregnancy because of the well-known risk of limb reduction defects. Hydroxyurea and griseofulvin should also not be used because of potential toxicity.

Skin disorders and neuraxial anesthesia

Most skin disorders are completely compatible with neuraxial anesthesia. However, lesions in the area of planned insertion of the epidural or spinal catheter can be a cause for concern.

Table 20.3 Topical corticosteroids available in the US and their relative potency

Group	Brand name	%	Generic name	Tube size (g unless noted)
I Superpotent	Condran tape		Flurandrenolide	Small roll, large roll, patches
	Cormax cream	0.05	Clobetasol propionate	15, 30, 45
	Cormax ointment	0.05		15, 30, 45
	Cormax scalp solution	0.05		25 mL, 50 mL
	Ultravate cream	0.05	Halobetasol propionate	15, 50
	Ultravate ointment	0.05		15, 50
	Diprolene lotion	0.05	Augmented betamethasone dipropionate	30 mL, 60 mL
	Diprolene ointment	0.05		15, 50
	Diprolene gel	0.05		15, 50
	Olux foam	0.05	Clobetasol propionate	50 gm, 100 gm can
	Psorcon ointment	0.05	Diflorasone diacetate	15, 30, 60
	Temovate-E cream	0.05	Clobetasol propionate	15, 30, 45, 60
	Temovate ointment	0.05	Clobetasol propionate	15, 30, 45, 60
	Temovate gel	0.05	Clobetasol propionate	15, 30, 60
II. Potent	Cyclocort ointment	0.1	Amcinonide	15, 30, 60
	Diprolene AF cream	0.05	Augmented betamethasone dipropionate	15, 50
	Diprosone ointment	0.05	Betamethasone dipropionate	15, 45
	Diprosone aerosol	0.1	Betamethasone dipropionate	85 gm can
	Elocon ointment	0.1	Momethasone furoate	
	Halog cream	0.1	Halcinonide	15, 30, 60
	Halog ointment	0.1		15, 30, 60
	Halog solution	0.1		20, 60 mL
	Halog-E cream	0.1		30, 60
	Lidex cream	0.05	Fluocinonide	15, 30, 60, 120
	Lidex-E	0.05	Fluocinonide	15, 30, 60
	Lidex gel	0.05		15, 30, 60
	Lidex ointment	0.05		30, 60
	Lidex solution	0.05		20, 60 mL
	Psorcon-E cream	0.05	Diflorasone diacetate	15, 30, 60
	Psorcon-E ointment	0.05		15, 30, 60
	Topicort cream	0.25	Desoximethasone	15, 60
	Topicort gel	0.05		15, 60
	Topicort ointment	0.25		15, 60
III. Upper mid-strength	Alphatrex cream	0.05	Betamethasone dipropionate	45
	Alphatrex ointment	0.05		45
	Aristocort A cream	0.5	Triamcinolone acetonide	15
	Betatrex ointment	0.1	Betamethasone valerate	45
	Cutivate ointment	0.005	Fluticasone propionate	15, 30, 60
	Cyclocort lotion	0.1	Amcinonide	20, 60 mL

Table 20.3 (Continued)

Group	Brand name	%	Generic name	Tube size (g unless noted)
	Cyclocort cream	0.1	Amcinonide	15, 30, 60
	Diprosone cream	0.05	Betamethasone dipropionate	15, 45
	Diprosone lotion	0.05	Betamethasone dipropionate	20, 60 mL
	Elocon ointment	0.1	Momethasone furoate	15, 45
	Kenalog cream	0.5	Triamcinolone acetonide	20
IV. Mid-strength	Aristocort A ointment	0.1	Triamcinolone acetonide	15, 60
	Cordran ointment	0.05	Flurandrenolide	15, 30, 60
	Cyclocort cream	0.1	Amcinonide	15, 30, 60
	Dermatop-E ointment	0.1	Prednicarbate	15, 60
	Elocon cream	0.1	Momethasone furoate	15, 45
	Elocon lotion	0.1		30, 60 mL
	Kenalog ointment	0.1	Triamcinolone acetonide	15, 60
	Luxig foam	0.12	Betamethasone valerate	50 gm, 100 gm can
	Synalar ointment	0.025	Fluocinolone acetonide	15, 60
	Westcort ointment	0.2	Hydrocortisone	15, 45, 60
V. Lower mid-strength	Aristocort cream	0.1	Triamcinolone acetonide	15
	Betatrex cream	0.1	Betamethasone valerate	45
	Cloderm cream	0.1	Clocortolone pivalate	15, 45
	Cordran SP cream	0.05	Flurandrenolide	15, 30, 60
	Cordran lotion	0.5		15, 60 mL
	Cordran ointment	0.025		15, 30, 60
	Cutivate cream	0.05	Fluticasone propionate	15, 30, 60
	Dermatop-E cream	0.1	Prednicarbate	15, 60
	DesOwen ointment	0.05	Desonide	15, 60
	Kenalog cream	0.1	Triamcinolone acetonide	15, 60, 80
	Kenalog lotion	0.1		60 mL
	Locoid lipocream	0.1	Hydrocortisone butyrate	15, 45
	Locoid cream	0.1	Hydrocortisone butyrate	15, 45
	Locoid ointment	0.1		15, 45
	Locoid solution			20, 60 cc
	Synalar cream	0.025	Fluocinolone acetonide	15, 60
	Synemol cream	0.025	Fluocinolone acetonide	60
	Tridesilon ointment	0.05	Desonide	15, 60
	Westcort cream	0.2	Hydrocortisone valerate	15, 45, 60
VI. Mild	Aclovate cream	0.05	Prednicarbate	15, 45, 60
	Aclovate ointment	0.05	Prednicarbate	15, 45, 60
	Aristocort A cream	0.025	Triamcinolone acetonide	15, 60
	Capex shampoo	0.01	Fluocinolone acetonide	120 mL
	Dermasmooth	0.01	Fluocinolone acetonide	4 oz
	Cordran SP cream	0.025	Flurandrenolide	30, 60
	DesOwen cream	0.05	Desonide	15, 60, 90
	DesOwen lotion	0.05		2, 4 oz
	Kenalog lotion	0.025	Triamcinalone acetonide	60 mL
	Synalar solution	0.01		20, 60 mL
VII. Least potent	Epifoam	1.0	Hydrocortisone acetate	10 gm can
	Hytone cream	2.5	Hydrocortisone	1, 2 oz
	Hytone lotion	2.5		2 oz
	Hytone ointment	2.5		1 oz
	Lacticare HC lotion	1.0	Hydrocortisone	4 oz
		2.5		2 oz
	Pramosone	1.0	Hydrocortisone acetate 1 pramoxine	2, 4, 8 oz lotion
				1, 2 oz cream
				1 oz ointment
		2.5		2, 4, oz lotion
				1, 2 oz cream
				1 oz ointment
		1.0	Hydrocortisone	Many brands

Tropical steroids in this table are classified by potency: group I is the most potent and group VII the least potent.
Reproduced with permission from Habif T. Clinical dermatology, 4th edn. Mosby, St Louis, 2004.

Dermatitis in the region of insertion may be associated with secondary bacterial infection or colonization of the disrupted skin. Even untreated infection elsewhere on the skin or in the body may promote either local or hematogenous contamination of the neuraxial site. Tattoos may lead to concern that pigment could be introduced into the spinal or epidural space.

Lesions in close proximity to the site of needle insertion may be viewed as a relative contraindication to neuraxial techniques, although individual judgment may be utilized depending on the extent and type of lesion and exact proximity to the needle insertion site.

There are a number of steps that are recommended in order to avoid contamination during epidural catheter insertion [99]. These apply in all cases but are particularly important when possible infected or contaminated skin lesions are in the vicinity of the insertion site. These include:

• adequate drying time of skin "prep"
• number of attempts should be minimized
• catheter should be covered by a clear adhesive dressing at the time of insertion
• examine all catheters daily (including intravenous lines) and remove them if there is any indication of infection at the puncture site
• maintain a high index of suspicion of an epidural abscess when catheters are placed at the time of localized infection or skin eruptions, especially if patient factors which predispose to immunosuppression are also present.

Epidural anesthesia has and can be used in the presence of distant abscess or infected wounds without complications but deep or superficial epidural infection is more likely in patients in intensive care with prolonged catheters, receiving immunosuppressive therapy or low-dose anticoagulation, or with diabetes or cancer [100,101]. It is important to take into consideration these patient factors when considering the use of neuraxial techniuques in patients with skin disorders, especially if the lesions are excoriated and therefore possibly infected.

Tattoos have become popular fashion accessories worldwide. More than 50% of all tattoos are being done on women. In recent years body tattooing in unconventional sites including the lumbar region has gained increasing popularity. Fortunately, all epidural and spinal anesthesia is administered with styletted (rather than hollow) needles, and the stylet is not removed until the needle has passed through the superficial (and pigment-containing) layers of skin. Therefore, most anesthesiologists do not find that a lower back tattoo precludes the use of regional anesthesia [102,103]. Some anesthesiologists feel otherwise and counsel patients against the use of regional anesthesia. However, there is no published evidence to support any danger of a regional anesthetic in the presence of a tattoo. Thankfully, even if the anesthesiologist is uncomfortable with passing an epidural or spinal needle through tattooed skin,

an area of nontattooed skin can generally be found that will allow regional anesthesia. If there is concern about a patient's suitability for neuraxial anestheisa, it is always worth seeking anesthesia consultation in advance of the delivery date.

Polymorphic eruption of pregnancy (PEP, also known as pruritic urticarial papules and plaques of pregnancy (PUPPP)) is worth some separate additional consideration here. As previously outlined, these lesions are typically found over the lower abdomen and proximal extremities [104,105]. Most anesthesiologists will find that epidural analgesia is appropriate as long as the lesions do not directly involve the injection site or if the back does not seem to be involved with widespread superinfection. Individual clinical judgment is necessary, and patients with PEP who are considering epidural analgesia should avail themselves of an anesthetic consultation early in labor.

A recent report describes the occurrence of an epidural abscess 1 week post partum in a 33 year old who had severe PEP and had received an epidural anesthetic during labor [106]. She had a diffuse papular rash with several excoriated areas and had received prednisolone therapy. Notably her back was free of lesions. The patient underwent emergency decompressive laminectomy and wound cultures revealed methicillin-sensitive *Staphylococcus aureus*. The infection could have resulted from direct seeding whereby, despite the strict aseptic technique described, some contamination with skin flora may have been introduced with the epidural needle. The epidural abscess could also have resulted from hematogenous spread as she had a diffusely pruritic rash with several excoriated areas. It is therefore reasonable to hypothesize that the scratching could have resulted in colonization of lesions and transient bacteremia. Microtrauma to the epidural vessels during epidural placement or removal during a bacteremic period could then have resulted in seeding of the epidural space. In either case, her immunosuppression from her steroids and her extensive excoriations from scratching likely contributed to her complication. However, despite this case, most experts would not consider regional anesthesia to be contraindicated in the majority of patients with PEP.

References

1. Catanzarite V, Quirk SG. Papular dermatoses of pregnancy. Clin Obstet Gynecol 1990; 33: 754–8.
2. Hayashi RH. Bullous dermatoses and prurigo of pregnancy. Clin Obstet Gynecol 1990; 33: 746–53.
3. Winton GB. Skin diseases aggravated by pregnancy. J Am Acad Dermatol 1989; 20: 1–13.
4. Fitzpatrick TB, Eisen AZ, Wolff K. Dermatology in general medicine. McGraw-Hill, New York, 1987: 2082.
5. Wade TR, Wade SL, Jones HE. Skin changes and diseases associated with pregnancy. Obstet Gynecol 1978; 52: 233–42.
6. Resnick S. Melasma induced by oral contraceptive drugs. JAMA 1967; 199: 601–5.

7. Newcomer VD, Lindberg MC, Sternberg TH. A melanosis of the face ("chloasma"). Arch Dermatol 1961; 83: 284–97.

8. Sanchez NP, Pathak MA, et al. Melasma: a clinical, light microscopic, ultrastructural and immunofluorescence study. J Am Acad Dermatol 1981; 4: 698–710.

9. Snell R. The pigmentary changes occurring in breast skin during pregnancy and following oestrogen treatment. J Invest Dermatol 1964; 43: 181–6.

10. Schizume K, Lerner AB. Determination of melanocyte stimulating hormone in urine and blood. J Clin Endocrinol Metab 1954; 14: 1491.

11. Thody AJ, Plummer NA, et al. Plasma SS-melanocyte stimulating hormone levels in pregnancy. J Obstet Gynaecol Br Commonwealth 1974; 81: 875–7.

12. Kligman AM, Willis I. A new formula for depigmenting human skin. Arch Dermatol 1975; 111: 540–7.

13. Hellreich PD. The skin changes of pregnancy. Cutis 1974; 13: 82–6.

14. Aldercreutz H, Tenhunen R. Some aspects of the interaction between natural and synthetic female sex hormones and the liver. Am J Med 1970; 49: 630–8.

15. Iffy L, Kaminetzky HA. Skin diseases in pregnancy. In: Iffy L, Kaminerzky H (eds) Principles and practice of obstetrics and perinatology. John Wiley, Chichester, 1981: 1361–79.

16. Bean WB, Cogswell R, et al. Vascular changes in the skin in pregnancy. Surg Gynaecol Obstet 1949; 88: 739–52.

17. Davey CMH. Factors associated with the occurrence of striae gravidarum. J Obstet Gynaecol Br Commonwealth 1972; 79: 113.

18. Thomas RG, Liston WA. Clinical associations of striae gravidarum. J Obstet Gynaecol 2004; 24: 270–1.

19. Liu DTY. Striae gravidarum. Lancet 1974; i: 625.

20. Shuster S. The cause of striae distense. Acta Dermatovenereol (Stockh) 1979; 59(suppl): 161–9.

21. Pinkus H, Keech MK, Mehregan AH. Histopathology of striae distensae with special reference to striae and wound healing in the Marfan syndrome. J Invest Dermatol 1966; 46: 293–9.

22. Watson REB, Parry EJ, et al. Fibrillin microfibrils are reduced in skin exhibiting striae distensae. Br J Dermatol 1998; 138: 931–7.

23. Pribanich S, Simpson FG, Held B, Yarbrough CL, White SN. Low-dose tretinoin does not improve striae distensae: a double blind, placebo-controlled study. Cutis 1994; 54: 121–4.

24. Cummings K, Derbes VJ. Dermatoses associated with pregnancy. Cutis 1967; 3: 120–6.

25. Demis DB, Dobson RL, McGuire J. Clinical dermatology. Harper and Row, New York, 1972.

26. MacKinnon PCB, McKinnon IL. Palmar sweating in pregnancy. J Obstet Gynaecol Br Empire 1955; 62: 298–9.

27. Lyndfield YL. Effect of pregnancy on the human hair cycle. J Invest Dermatol 1960; 35: 323–7.

28. Schiff BL, Pawtucket RI, Kern AB. Study of postpartum alopecia. Arch Dermatol 1963; 87: 609–11.

29. Trotter M. The activity of hair follicles with reference to pregnancy. Surg Gynaecol Obstet 1935; 60: 1092–5.

39. Kolodny RC. Herpes gestationis. A new assessment of incidence, diagnosis and foetal prognosis. Am J Obstet Gynecol 1969; 104: 39–45.

31. Tillman WG. Herpes gestationis with hydatidiform mole and chorion epithelioma. BMJ 1950; i: 1471.

32. Dupont C. Herpes gestationis with hydatidiform mole. Trans St Johns Dermatol Soc 1974; 60: 103.

33. Holmes RC, Black MM. The specific dermatoses of pregnancy. J Am Acad Dermatol 1983; 8: 405–12.

34. Shornick JK, Stastny P, Gilliam JN. High frequency of histocompatibility antigens HLA-DR3 and DR4 in herpes gestationis. J Clin Invest 1981; 68: 553–5.

35. Holmes RC, Black MM, James DCO. Paternal responsibility for herpes gestationis. In: MacDonald DM (ed) Immunodermatology. Butterworths, London, 1984: 251–3.

36. Villegas M. Goff HW, Kraus EW, Usatine RP. Blisters during pregnancy – just with the second husband. J Fam Pract 2006; 55: 953–6.

37. Parodi A, Rebora A. Pemphigoid gestationis postpartum after changing husband. Int J Dermatol 2005;44:1057–8.

38. Jenkins RE, Hern S, Black MM. Clinical features and management of 87 patients with pemphigoid gestationis. Clin Exp Dermatol 1999; 24: 255–9.

39. Holmes RC, Black MM, et al. Clues to the aetiology and pathogenesis of herpes gestationis. Br J Dermatol 1983; 109: 131–9.

40. Holmes RC, Black MM, et al. A comparative study of toxic erythema of pregnancy and herpes gestationis. Br J Dermatol 1982; 106: 499–510.

41. Lynch FN, Albrecht RJ. Hormonal factors in herpes gestationis. Arch Dermatol 1966; 3: 465–6.

42. Kenny JF, Pangburn PC, Trail G. Effect of oestradiol on immune competence: in vivo and in vitro studies. Infect Comm 1976; 13: 448.

43. Lawley TJ, Stingl G, Katz ST. Foetal and maternal risk factors in herpes gestationis. Arch Dermatol 1978; 114: 552–5.

44. Shornick JK, Bangert JL, et al. Herpes gestationis. Clinical and histologic features of twenty eight cases. J Am Acad Dermatol 1983; 8: 214.

45. Shornick JK, Black MM. Fetal risk in herpes gestationis. J Am Acad Dermatol 1992; 26: 63–8.

46. Borrego L, Peterson EA, et al. Polymorphic eruption of pregnancy and herpes gestationis: comparison of granulated cell proteins in tissue and serum. Clin Exp Dermatol 1999; 24: 213–25.

47. Provost TT, Tomasi TB. Evidence of complement activiation via the alternative pathway in skin diseases I. Herpes gestationis, systemic lupus erythematosus and bullous pemphigoid. J Clin Invest 1973; 52: 1779–87.

48. Kelly SE, Cerio R, Bhogal BS, Black MM. The distribution of IgG subclasses in pemphigoid gestationis: PG factor is an IgG1 autoantibody. J Invest Dermatol 1989; 92: 695–8.

49. Jureka W, Holmes RC, et al. An immunoelectron microscopy study of the relationship between herpes gestationis and polymorphic eruption of pregnancy. Br J Dermatol 1983; 108: 147–51.

50. Jenkins RE, Vaughan Jones SA, Black MM. Conversion of pemphigoid gestationis to bullous pemphigoid – two refractory cases highlighting this association. Br J Dermatol 1996; 135: 595–8.

51. Van Der Wiel A, Hart H, et al. Plasma exchange in herpes gestationis. BMJ 1980; 281: 1041.

52. Hocking DR. Neonatal haemolytic disease due to dapsone. Med J Aust 1968; 1: 1130.

53. Lockwood DNJ, Sinha HH. Pregnancy and leprosy. A comprehensive literature review. Int J Lepr 1999; 167: 6–12.

54. MacDonald KJS, Raffle EJ. Ritodrine therapy associated with remission of pemphigoid gestationis. Br J Dermatol 1984; 111: 630.

55. Garvey MP, Handfield-Jones SE, Black MM. Pemphigoid gestationis response to chemical oophorectomy with goserelin. Clin Exp Dermatol 1992; 17: 443–5.

56. Andersen B, Felding C. Pruritic urticarial papules and plaques of pregnancy. J Obstet Gynaecol 1992; 12: 1–3.

57. Lawley TJ, Hertz KC, *et al.* Pruritic urticarial papules and plaques of pregnancy. JAMA 1979; 241: 1696–9.

58. Boume G. Toxaemic rash of pregnancy. J R Soc Med 1962; 55: 462–4.

59. Cooper AJ, Fryer JA. Prurigo of late pregnancy. Austral J Dermatol 1980; 21: 79–84.

60. Nurse DS. Prurigo of pregnancy. Austral J Dermatol 1968; 9: 258–67.

61. Holmes RC, Black MM. The specific dermatoses of pregnancy. A reappraisal with special emphasis on a proposed simplified classification. Clin Exp Dermatol 1982; 7: 65–73.

62. Aronson IK, Bond S, *et al.* Pruritic urticarial papules and plaques of pregnancy: clinical and immunopathologic observations in 57 patients. J Am Acad Dermatol 1998; 39: 933–9.

63. Bunker CB, Erskine K, *et al.* Severe polymorphic eruption of pregnancy occurring in twin pregnancies. Clin Exp Dermatol 1990; 15: 228–31.

64. Cohen LM, Capeless EL, *et al.* Pruritic urticarial papules and plaques of pregnancy and its relationship to metemalfetal weight gain and twin pregnancy. Arch Dermatol 1989; 125: 1534–6.

65. Vaughan Jones SA, Dunnill MGS, Black MM. Pruritic urticarial papules and plaques of pregnancy (polymorphic eruption of pregnancy): two unusual cases. Br J Dermatol 1996; 135: 102–5.

66. Vaughan Jones SA, Hern S, *et al.* A prospective study of 200 women with dermatoses of pregnancy correlating the clinical findings with hormonal and immunopathological profiles. Br J Dermatol 1999; 141: 71–81.

67. Aractingi S, Berkane N, *et al.* Fetal DNA in skin of polymorphic eruptions of pregnancy. Lancet 1998; 352: 1898–901.

68. Yancey KB, Hall RB, Lawley T. Pruritic urticarial papules and plaques of pregnancy. J Am Acad Dermatol 1984; 10: 473–80.

69. Beltrani VP, Beltrani VS. Pruritic urticarial papules and plaques of pregnancy: a severe case requiring early delivery from relief of symptoms. J Am Acad Dermatol 1992; 26: 266–7.

70. Zoberman E, Farmer ER. Pruritic folliculitis of pregnancy. Arch Dermatol 1981; 117: 20–2.

71. Vaughan Jones SA, Hern S, Black MM. Pruritic folliculitis and serum androgen levels. Clin Exp Dermatol 1999; 24: 392–5.

72. Wilkinson SM, Buckler H, Wilkinson N, *et al.* Androgen levels in pruritic folliculitis of pregnancy. Clin Exp Dermatol 1995; 20: 234–6.

73. Spangler AS, Reddy W, *et al.* Papular dermatitis of pregnancy. JAMA 1962; 181: 577–81.

74. Spangler AS, Emerson K. Estrogen levels and estrogen therapy in papular dermatitis of pregnancy. Am J Obstet Gynaecol 1971; 110: 534–7.

75. Spangler AS, Emerson K. Diethylstilbestrol in the management of papular dermatitis of pregnancy. A reply to the editor. Am J Obstet Gynecol 1972; 113: 571.

76. Bierman SM. Autoimmune dermatitis of pregnancy. Arch Dermatol 1973; 107: 896–901.

77. Hart RH. Autoimmune progesterone dermatitis. Arch Dermatol 1977; 113: 427–30.

78. Rodenas JM, Herranz MT, Tercedor J. Autoimmune progesterone dermatitis: treatment with oophorectomy. Br J Dermatol 1998; 139: 508–11.

79. Stephens CJM, Wojnarowska FT, Wilkinson JD. Autoimmune progesterone dermatitis responding to tamoxifen. Br J Dermatol 1989; 121: 135–7.

80. Shahar E, Bergman R, Pollack S. Autoimmune progesterone dermatitis: effective prophylactic treatment with Danazol. Int J Dermatol 1997; 36: 708–11.

81. Lever WF. Histopathology of the skin. JB Lippincott, Philadelphia, 1985: 145.

82. Oumeish OY, Farraj SE, Bataineh AS. Some aspects of impetigo herpetiformis. Arch Dermatol 1982; 118: 103–5.

83. Lotem M, Katzenelson V, *et al.* Impetigo herpetiformis: a variant of pustular psoriasis or a separate entity? J Am Acad Dermatol 1989; 20: 338–41.

84. Rasmussen KA, Ehrenskjold MI. Impetigo herpetiformis. A case in a pregnant woman treated with antex. Acta Obstet Gynaecol Scand 1965; 44: 563.

85. Beveridge GW, Harkness RA, Livingstone JRB. Impetigo herpetiformis in two successive pregnancies. Br J Dermatol 1966; 78: 106–12.

86. Segal D, Holcberg G, *et al.* Neurofibromatosis in pregnancy. Eur J Obstet Gynaecol Reprod Biol 1999; 84(1): 59–61.

87. Weissman A, Jakobi P, *et al.* Neurofibromatosis and pregnancy. An update. J Reprod Med 1993; 38(11): 890–6.

88. Dugoff L, Sujansky E. Neurofibromatosis type 1 in pregnancy. Am J Med Genet 1996; 6(1): 7–10.

89. Brady DB, Bolan JC. Neurofibromatosis and spontaneous hemothorax in pregnancy: two case reports. Obstet Gynecol 1984; 63(3 suppl): 35S-38S.

90. Driscoll MS, Grant-Kels JM. Nevi and melanoma in the pregnant woman. Clin Dermatol 2009; 27(1): 116–21.

91. Colburn DS, Nathanson L, Belilos E. Pregnancy and malignant melanoma. Semin Oncol 1989; 16: 377–87.

92. Mackie RM, Bufalino R, *et al.* Lack of effect of pregnancy on outcome of melanoma. Lancet 1991; i: 653–5.

93. Stockton DL, Paller AS. Drug administration to the pregnant or lactating woman: a reference guide for dermatologists. J Am Acad Dermatol 1990; 23: 87–103.

94. Stern RS, Lange R. Outcomes of pregnancies among women and partners of men with a history of exposure to methoxsalen photochemotherapy (PUVA) for the treatment of psoriasis. Arch Dermatol 1991; 127: 347–400.

95. Gunnarskog JG, Kallen AJB, *et al.* Psoralen photochemotherapy (PUVA) and pregnancy. Arch Dermatol 1993; 129: 320–3.

96. Wright S, Glover M, Baker H. Psoriasis, cyclosporin and pregnancy. Arch Dermatol 1991; 127: 426.

97. Finch TM, Tan CY. Pustular psoriasis exacerbated by pregnancy and controlled by cyclosporin A. Br J Dermatol 2000; 142: 582–4.

98. Carter JD, Ladhani A, Ricca LR, Valeriano J, Vasey FB. A safety assessment of tumor necrosis factor antagonists during pregnancy: a review of the Food and Drug Administration database. J Rheumatol 2009;36(3):635–41.

99. O'Rourke N, Khan K, Hepner DL. Contraindications to epidural anesthesia. In: Wong C (ed) Spinal and epidural anesthesia. McGraw Hill, New York, 2007.

100. Brookman CA, Rutledge ML. Epidural abscess: case report and literature review. Reg Anesth Pain Med 2000; 25: 428.

101. Wang LP, Hauerberg J, Schmidt JF. Incidence of spinal epidural abscess after epidural analgesia: a national 1-year survey. Anesthesiology 1991; 91: 1928–36.

102. Society for Obstetric Anesthesia and Perinatology. Newsletter, summer 2001. www.soap.org.

103. Bryant A, Chen KT, Camann WR, Norwitz ER. Coping with the complications of tattooing and body piercing. Contemp OB/GYN 2005; 50(1): 40–7.

104. Bucculo LS, Viera AJ. Pruritic urticarial papules and plaques of pregnancy presenting in the postpartum period. A case report. J Reprod Med 2005; 50: 61–3.

105. Hugh WA, Huang MP, Miller MD. Pruritic urticarial papules and plaques of pregnancy with unusual and extensive palmo-plantar involvement. Obstet Gynecol 2005; 105: 1261–4.

106. Cummings KC, Dolak JA. Case report: epidural abscess in a parturient with pruritic urticarial papules and plaques of pregnancy (PUPPPs). Can J Anaesth 2006; 53: 1010–14.

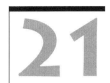

21 Psychiatric disorders in pregnancy

Teri Pearlstein[1] and Jami Star[2]

[1]Department of Psychiatry and Human Behavior, Warren Alpert Medical School of Brown University and Women's Behavioral Health Program, Women & Infants' Hospital of Rhode Island, Providence, RI, USA

[2]Department of Obstetrics and Gynecology, University of Massachusetts Medical School, University of Massachusetts Memorial Medical Center, Worcester, MA, USA

Introduction

This chapter will present a selected review of studies about the course and treatment of psychiatric disorders through pregnancy. The research on the influence of untreated psychiatric disorders and symptoms on birth outcome will be described. The potential adverse effects on the fetus and neonate from psychotropic medications will be reviewed. Management of the pregnant woman with a psychiatric disorder should consider the consequences of fetal exposure to untreated maternal psychiatric illness, fetal exposure to psychotropic medications, and available alternative treatments [1]. Unfortunately, there are no risk-free decisions for pregnant women with a psychiatric disorder. However, the evidence predominantly supports present practice that ongoing treatment of psychiatric disorders in pregnancy is preferable to withholding treatment during gestation. Postpartum blues and postpartum depression (PPD) are in the section on depression. Postpartum psychosis is discussed in the section on bipolar disorder.

Major depressive disorder

The World Health Organization (WHO) ranks depression as a leading contributor to the global burden of disease in men and women of reproductive age as measured by disability-adjusted life-years (DALYs – the sum of years of potential life lost due to premature mortality and the years of productive life lost due to disability). It tends to be a relapsing diagnosis with up to 40% of patients having a recurrence within 2 years after their first episode of depression and 75% of patients having a recurrence within 5 years of their second episode of depression.

Diagnosis and epidemiology

The definition of major depressive disorder (MDD) is reviewed in Box 21.1 [2]. The prevalence of depression in women during the reproductive years is 10–15%, approximately twice the prevalence rate in men [3]. Depression is under-recognized and undertreated in obstetric clinics [4]. Short two-item or three-item screening questionnaires for depression can be used to identify patients who may warrant further assessment for a depressive disorder [5,6]. The self-report Edinburgh Postnatal Depression Scale (EPDS) [7] (Box 21.2), which was developed to identify PPD, is also commonly used to screen for depression during pregnancy. A seven-item clinician-rated scale has recently been developed specifically to screen for depression in pregnant women [8]. The diagnosis of depression in pregnant women can be complicated due to symptoms of normal pregnancy (e.g. sleep changes, appetite change, and fatigue) overlapping with some of the diagnostic symptoms of MDD [8].

> **Box 21.1** Diagnostic criteria for major depressive disorder (MDD)
>
> Requires a period of at least 2 weeks of low mood, or loss of interest or pleasure, associated with at least five of the following:
> 1. change in appetite or weight
> 2. insomnia or hypersomnia
> 3. psychomotor symptoms such as restlessness or retardation (slowed speech, thought or movements)
> 4. decreased energy or fatigue
> 5. sense of worthlessness or guilt, hopelessness or helplessness
> 6. difficulty concentrating or making decisions
> 7. recurrent thoughts of death, dying or suicide.

de Swiet's Medical Disorders in Obstetric Practice, 5th edition.
Edited by R. O. Powrie, M. F. Greene, W. Camann. © 2010 Blackwell Publishing.

In a systematic review of studies in which depression was evaluated by structured clinical interview, the point prevalence of depression (MDD and less severe depression) was 11% in the first trimester with a drop to 8.5% in the second and third trimesters [9]. The point prevalence of MDD ranged from 1% to 5.6% through pregnancy [9]. Pregnancy does not appear to be a time of increased risk of depression compared to other times during women's reproductive years [10–12]. An increased risk of depression during pregnancy occurs in women who are adolescent, unmarried, financially disadvantaged, African American, Hispanic, have a lack of social support, have had recent negative life events, and have had a previous MDD [13]. Recent studies have reported an association of prenatal depression with nicotine dependence [14], high interpersonal conflict and low social support [15], intimate partner violence (IPV) [16], and high obstetric risk [17]. Women who have had a previous reproductive loss may experience depression, anxiety and unresolved grief

---

Box 21.2 Edinburgh Postnatal Depression Scale (EPDS)

This scale can be used to screen for postnatal depression in new mothers at 4–6 weeks post partum. Response categories are scored 0, 1, 2, and 3 according to increased severity of the symptoms. Items marked with an asterisk are reverse scored (i.e. 3, 2, 1, and 0). The total score is calculated by adding together the scores for each of the 10 items. The maximum possible score is 30 and a score of 10 or greater is considered to be suggestive of postnatal depression and warrants further evaluation. Regardless of the total score, examiners should always look at the patient answer to item 10 and directly address the answer if the patient admits to periodic suicidal thoughts.

Edinburgh Postnatal Depression Scale (EPDS)

Adapted from Cox JL, Holden JM, Sagovsky R. Detection of postnatal depression: development of the 10-item. Edinburgh Postnatal Depression Scale. British Journal of Psychiatry 1987;150: 782–786.

As you have recently had a baby, we would like to know how you are feeling. Please circle the answer which comes closest to how you have felt IN THE PAST 7 DAYS, not just how you feel today.

1. I have been able to laugh and see the funny side of things.
   (1) As much as I always could
   (2) Not quite so much now
   (3) Definitely not so much now
   (4) Not at all
2. I have looked forward with enjoyment to things.
   (1) As much as I ever did
   (2) Rather less than I used to
   (3) Definitely less than I used to
   (4) Hardly at all
3. *I have blamed myself unnecessarily when things went wrong.
   (1) Yes, most of the time
   (2) Yes, some of the time
   (3) Not very often
   (4) No, never
4. I have been anxious or worried for no good reason.
   (1) No, not at all
   (2) Hardly ever
   (3) Yes, sometimes
   (4) Yes, very often
5. *I have felt scared or panicky for no very good reason.
   (1) Yes, quite a lot
   (2) Yes, sometimes
   (3) No, not much
   (4) No, not at all
6. *Things have been getting on top of me.
   (1) Yes, most of the time I haven't been able to cope at all
   (2) Yes, sometimes I haven't been coping as well as usual
   (3) No, most of the time I have coped quite well
   (4) No, I have been coping as well as ever
7. *I have been so unhappy that I have had difficulty sleeping.
   (1) Yes, most of the time
   (2) Yes, sometimes
   (3) Not very often
   (4) No, not at all
8. *I have felt sad or miserable.
   (1) Yes, most of the time
   (2) Yes, quite often
   (3) Not very often
   (4) No, not at all
9. *I have been so unhappy that I have been crying.
   (1) Yes, most of the time
   (2) Yes, quite often
   (3) Only occasionally
   (4) No, never
10. *The thought of harming myself has occurred to me.
    (1) Yes, quite often
    (2) Sometimes
    (3) Hardly ever
    (4) Never

in a subsequent pregnancy [18,19]. The American College of Obstetricians and Gynecologists (ACOG) recommends screening pregnant women for psychosocial risk factors such as barriers to care, unstable housing, economic burdens, lack of social support, unintended or unwanted pregnancy, communication barriers, poor nutrition, tobacco use, substance use, psychiatric symptoms, safety issues, IPV, and stress [20].

Recurrence with antidepressant discontinuation

Women who are euthymic (i.e. have a neutral mood) on an antidepressant medication may choose to discontinue it prior to conceiving, or once they have conceived, in an effort to minimize exposure of the fetus to the antidepressant. In a prospective observational study of women with prior depression who were euthymic on an antidepressant at conception, 68% of 44 women who discontinued their antidepressant had a depression relapse compared to 26% of 82 women who maintained their antidepressant through pregnancy [21]. In addition, 60% of women who relapsed following discontinuation of their medication restarted an antidepressant during pregnancy. Depressive symptoms may increase even in women who maintain antidepressant medication through pregnancy [21,22]. It is clear that the recurrence of depression is likely when women discontinue antidepressants before or during pregnancy.

Untreated depression, anxiety, and stress and pregnancy outcome

Untreated depression can adversely affect maternal and fetal health due to potential harmful prenatal health behaviors such as poor nutrition, poor prenatal medical care, smoking, alcohol, other substance misuse, and suicidal risk [23]. The obstetric and neonatal complications reported with untreated prenatal stress, anxiety and depression have been reviewed elsewhere [24–28]. These complications include miscarriage, pre-eclampsia, preterm delivery (PTD), low birthweight (LBW), small-for-gestational-age infants, low Apgar scores, elevated infant cortisol levels at birth and neonatal complications. A recent study reported that the risk of PTD increased with increasing severity of depression scores [29]. However, other recent studies have reported that untreated prenatal depressive symptoms were not associated with younger gestational age at birth [30] or LBW [31].

Untreated depression, anxiety, and stress and child development

Prenatal anxiety and depression have been associated with increased infant salivary cortisol levels [32], frontal electroencephalogram (EEG) asymmetry [33], and increased sleep problems in children at 18 and 30 months [34]. A recent large prospective cohort study reported that prenatal depression in mothers who did not report postpartum depressive symptoms was associated with developmental delay in 18-month-old offspring [35]. Prenatal stress, anxiety and depression have also been associated with impaired attachment, altered infant temperament, language and cognitive impairment, impulsivity, behavioral dyscontrol, attention deficit disorder, depression and other psychiatric disorders [36–38]. Theories about the influence of maternal stress and depression during pregnancy on neonatal variables and subsequent childhood development include elevated corticotropin-releasing hormone and cortisol [39–41], decreased heart rate variability [42], reduced uterine artery blood flow, alterations in immune function and increased catecholamines [27,28,43–45]. Of particular concern is the risk for antenatal depression continuing into the postpartum period, and PPD has well-established negative effects on maternal-infant attachment and child development.

Suicidality during pregnancy

A study reported that 17–28% of 383 pregnant women presenting to a neuropsychiatric clinic endorsed suicidal ideation by self-report or clinician ratings, higher than the 5–7% prevalence in community samples [46]. Suicidal ideation was associated with unplanned pregnancy, current MDD, and comorbid anxiety disorder. In spite of the elevated prevalence of suicidal ideation during pregnancy, completed suicide rate appears to be low during pregnancy. The rate of suicide during pregnancy described in the 2003–2005 UK Confidential Enquiry into Maternal and Child Health (CEMACH) report was 0.85 per 100,000 maternities when counting suicides that occurred only during pregnancy or the first 6 weeks post partum and 1.8 per 100,000 maternities if the time frame is extended to include the first postpartum year [47,48]. Despite this low prevalence, suicide remains one of the leading causes of maternal mortality in the developed world and when pregnant women do complete suicide, it is by more violent and lethal means than when not pregnant [49]. Low rates of suicide attempts in spite of elevated suicidal ideation during pregnancy may be due to neuroendocrine factors, the impending responsibility of motherhood or misclassification of cause of death in public reporting. [46]

Serious adverse neonatal outcomes may follow a suicide attempt during pregnancy. A study compared women who had attempted suicide (mostly by drug overdose) during their pregnancy to women who had not attempted suicide [50]. Suicide attempts were correlated with psychiatric illness, substance abuse, younger age, being single, less education, multiparity, being African American, and poor prenatal care. The women who delivered at the hospitalization for attempted suicide had an increased risk of neonatal and infant death. Later consequences included cesarean delivery, PTD, LBW, and infant respiratory distress syndrome. The authors emphasized the importance of screening pregnant women for untreated psychiatric and substance use disorders and risk factors for suicide [50].

Postpartum blues

Postpartum blues occur in up to 85% of women, peak at day 5, and usually resolve by day 10 [51]. Common symptoms include mood swings, irritability, tearfulness, confusion and fatigue; elation and mild hypomanic symptoms may also occur [51]. Postpartum blues are usually brief and do not necessitate treatment beyond reassurance and support; however, a proportion of women with postpartum blues will develop PPD [52].

Postpartum depression

The prevalence of depression (mild to severe) ranges from 7% to 13% through the first 6 postpartum months, while the point prevalence (the proportion of postpartum women who have depression on any particular day) of MDD ranges from 1% to 6% through the same 6 months [9]. Although the strict definition of PPD is onset of MDD within the first month post partum [2], depressive symptoms may have started during pregnancy, or may start beyond the first month [53]. The EPDS (see Box 21.2) is a validated and extensively utilized 10-item self-report screening measure, with a score of 12 or higher indicating probable PPD [7]. A recent study suggested that the three anxiety subscale items of the EPDS may be a sufficient screen for PPD [54]. Another self-report screening scale, the Postpartum Depression Screening Scale [55], includes additional clinically relevant questions but has higher false-positive rates [56]. Postpartum women with depression should also be screened for manic and hypomanic symptoms (listed below in section on bipolar disorder in pregnancy) [57], suicidal thoughts [49], and thoughts of harm toward the infant [58].

Postpartum obstetrician or primary care physician visits, and well-baby pediatrician visits, afford opportunities to screen for PPD and initiate or refer for treatment when indicated. Variation in clinician beliefs, lack of knowledge about resources, perceived barriers to care, and time constraints conspire to decrease the likelihood of screening for PPD [59–61]. Even when PPD is identified, compliance with treatment recommendations is variable. The screening and treatment of PPD are of public health significance due to the well-established negative effects of persistent maternal depression on child cognitive, motor and behavioral development [62–64].

Treatment of depression

Treatment of depression outside pregnancy

Depression can be treated with psychotherapy, antidepressant medication or both.

Psychotherapy for depression typically entails 12–16 weekly visits using either interpersonal therapy or cognitive behavioral therapy and is particularly well suited to the highly motivated patient with mild depression who can comply with regular therapeutic visits. Although many modalities of psychotherapy exist for depression, the two most common are cognitive behavior therapy (CBT) and interpersonal therapy (IPT). CBT is a time-limited, instructive psychotherapy that focuses on how changing the way a person thinks about their situation can improve how they feel or act. Interpersonal therapy is a time-limited psychotherapy that focuses on the interpersonal context and on building interpersonal skills. Response rates to psychotherapy for mild depression are similar to those seen with antidepressant medication with approximately 50% of patients going into remission.

Medical treatment typically involves use of an antidepressant medication for 6–9 months. Recurrent depression is often treated with prolonged use of antidepressant to prevent relapse. The presently available antidepressants fit into one of the four following categories based on their assumed mechanism of action:
- tricyclic antidepressant (TCA, such as amitriptyline or nortriptyline)
- serotonin reuptake inhibitors (SSRI, such as fluoxetine, paroxetine and sertraline)
- inhibitors of the reuptake of both serotonin and norepinephrine (SNRI, such as venlafaxine)
- far less commonly, the monoamine oxidase inhibitors (MAOI, such as phenelzine and tranylcypromine).

Specific agents in each of these classes are listed in Table 21.1. The response rate to any of these classes of medications is typically around 50–60% in a primary care setting with most of the responders having improved by 6–7 weeks after initiation of treatment. There are no data to clearly show that one of these agents is more effective than another and treatment decisions outside pregnancy are usually based on side effect profile, previous response to medication, price and reproductive plans. Unlike TCA and MAOI, intentional overdoses of SSRI and SNRI have the advantage that they are unlikely to lead to a successful suicide.

Nonpharmacologic treatments of MDD during pregnancy

Pregnant women with depression often prefer psychosocial treatments to antidepressant medications [65]. The systematic evaluation of psychotherapy in pregnant women has been minimal. Interpersonal psychotherapy (IPT) is an established treatment for PPD [66], and depressed pregnant women similarly can benefit from the exploration of role transitions and interpersonal issues. A randomized controlled study (RCT) reported that IPT administered in a group format was superior to a parenting education program in improving mood in pregnant women with depression [67]. A recent study reported positive results with CBT started during pregnancy

Table 21.1 Antidepressant medications with some pregnancy-specific recommendations

Class of agent	Specific agents (with US marketed name)	Comments
Tricyclics and tetracyclics	Amitriptyline (Elavil) Amoxapine (Asendin) Clomipramine (Anafranil) Desipramine (Norpramin) Doxepin (Adapin, Sinequan) Imipramine (Tofranil) Maprotiline (Ludiomil) Nortriptyline (Pamelor) Protriptyline (Vivactil) Trimipramine (Surmontil)	Among the tricyclic antidepressants, nortriptyline likely has the most data for pregnancy at the time of this writing and may be the preferred agent for use in pregnancy and breastfeeding from this class. Initiation of these agents is usually done in a stepwise fashion with initial doses of nortriptyline starting at 25 mg at night and gradually increased to 50–200 mg per day over 4–6 weeks based on tolerance and response. Serum levels should be monitored. Main side effects include dry mouth, blurred vision, constipation, urinary retention, and tachycardia. These agents also carry the potential for fatal arrhythmias if taken as an overdose.
Selective serotonin reuptake inhibitors	Citalopram (Celexa) Escitalopram (Lexapro) Fluoxetine (Prozac) Fluvoxamine (Luvox) Paroxetine (Paxil) Paroxetine CR (Paxil CR) Sertraline (Zoloft)	At the time of writing, fluoxetine has the most published data for pregnancy but is used less currently due to concerns about PPHN. Sertraline is likely the preferred agent for both pregnancy and breastfeeding from this class. Also at the time of writing, paroxetine has accumulated the most concerning pregnancy data among agents in this class and should likely be avoided when possible in pregnant women but may be used in breastfeeding mothers. Present data do not, however, preclude the use of paroxetine in pregnant women who enter a pregnancy on this agent and for whom this medication has been of unique benefit or medication changes are felt to represent a significant risk to the mother's well-being. Sertraline is usually initiated at a dose of 50 mg daily and this dose may be adequate for many patients. However, it can be titrated up to a dose of 200 mg daily based on tolerance and response. The main side effects include headache, jitteriness, restlessness, nausea, diarrhea, insomnia and decreased libido. Jitteriness, restlessness and headache usually resolve after the first week of treatment and patients should be informed of these potential side effects and encouraged to "wait them out."
Serotonin-norepinephrine reuptake inhibitors	Venlafaxine (Effexor) Venlafaxine XR (Effexor XR) Desvenlafaxine (Pristiq) Duloxetine (Cymbalta)	Published pregnancy data on these agents are limited and at the time of writing, recommendations as to the "safest" of this class of agents for use in pregnancy cannot be made. Use of an SSRI or TCA would generally be preferable when initiating treatment in pregnancy or women considering pregnancy. Continuing the use of this class of agents in pregnancy should be done on the basis of a careful consideration of both their unknown (but likely small) risks and the risk of medication changes on the mother's well-being. These agents have similar side effects to SSRI although at higher doses they can cause sweating and dizziness. Venlafaxine can cause hypertension at doses >300 mg per day.
Dopamine-norepinephrine reuptake inhibitors	Bupropion (Wellbutrin) Bupropion SR (Wellbutrin SR) Bupropion XL (Wellbutrin XL)	Published pregnancy safety data on this agent are limited and at the time of writing, recommendations as to the "safety" of this agent for use in pregnancy cannot be made. Use of an SSRI or TCA would generally be preferable when initiating treatment in pregnancy or women considering pregnancy. Continuing these agents in pregnancy should be done on the basis of a careful consideration of both its unknown (but likely small) risks and the risk of medication changes to the mother's well-being.
Serotonin modulators	Nefazodone (Serzone) Trazodone (Desyrel)	Published pregnancy safety data on this agent are limited and at the time of writing, recommendations as to the "safety" of this agent for use in pregnancy cannot be made. Use of an SSRI or TCA would generally be preferable when initiating treatment in pregnancy or women considering pregnancy. Continuing these agents in pregnancy should be done on the basis of a careful consideration of both its unknown (but likely small) risks and the risk of medication changes to the mother's well-being.

Table 21.1 (Continued)

Class of agent	Specific agents (with US marketed name)	Comments
Noradrenergic and specific serotonergic antidepressant	Mirtazapine (Remeron)	Published pregnancy safety data on this agent are limited and at the time of writing, recommendations as to the "safety" of this agent for use in pregnancy cannot be made. Use of an SSRI or TCA would generally be preferable when initiating treatment in pregnancy or women considering pregnancy. Continuing these agents in pregnancy should be done on the basis of a careful consideration of both its unknown (but likely small) risks and the risk of medication changes to the mother's well-being.
Monamine oxidase inhibitors	Phenelzine (Nardil) Selegiline (Ensam) Tranylcypromine (Parnate)	Published pregnancy safety data on this agent are limited and at the time of writing, recommendations as to the "safety" of this agent for use in pregnancy cannot be made. Use of an SSRI or TCA would generally be preferable when initiating treatment in pregnancy or women considering pregnancy. Continuing these agents in pregnancy should be done on the basis of a careful consideration of both its unknown (but likely small) risks and the risk of medication changes to the mother's well-being.

When initiating medical treatment of depression in women who are pregnant or considering a pregnancy, the tricyclic antidepressant nortriptyline or the SSRI sertraline are probably the preferred agents for pregnancy at the time of writing. Psychotherapy, when feasible, is an excellent alternative for patients with mild to moderate depression who are able to commit to the necessary 12–16 weekly appointments

If a patient is considering a pregnancy or is already pregnant on an agent other than sertraline or nortriptyline the options include:
1. continuing their present agent (none of the above listed agents are absolutely contraindicated in pregnancy)
2. switching to sertraline or nortriptyline (done by gradually tapering the dose their present agent over 2–6 weeks while gradually introducing and tapering up the dose of the new agent gradually increasing their new agent)
3. tapering and discontinuing treatment over 0–4 weeks.

Factors to guide the decision between these three options include:
1. severity of depression being treated (including whether there have been suicide attempts or hospitalizations. "Lifestyle" use of these agents to cope with irritability or minor stress is not indicated in pregnancy)
2. duration of present treatment (typically depression is treated for 9 months)
3. number of prior episodes of depression (≥3 recurrences generally warrants maintenance medication)
4. response to previous medications (patients are likely not to respond to medication that has not worked for them in the past but clinicians should also make a distinction between ineffectiveness or intolerance and premature discontinuance of an antidepressant because of patient ambivalence about treatment or impatience with the initial jitteriness or headaches often seen in the first week of treatment with SSRI)
5. potential dangers of medication adjustments on maternal (and thereby also fetal) well-being.

for depressed women that continued into the postpartum months. In this study, CBT administered by community-based primary health workers improved maternal mood up to 1 year compared to enhanced routine care [68]. Although effective, and from a safety standpoint ideal for pregnancy, use of psychotherapy is hampered by both limited access to trained psychotherapists and the logistic difficulties that many women face in committing to 12–16 weekly sessions of therapy when it is available.

Randomized controlled trials have reported efficacy with acupuncture [69,70], massage [71], and bright light therapy [72] for prenatal depression. Moderate exercise has been reported to improve maternal well-being without adverse effects on birth outcomes although exercise has not been specifically studied in depressed pregnant women [73]. RCT with omega-3 supplementation have yielded positive [74] and negative results [75,76] for depression during pregnancy. The use of these modalities for treatment of anything more than mild depression would generally be discouraged.

Women with severe depression not responsive to pharmacotherapy or nonpharmacologic treatments may need electroconvulsive therapy (ECT). Although ECT has been used safely in pregnancy, there are specific maternal and fetal precautions [77]. Of concern are recent case reports of fetal cerebral infarcts, fetal cardiac arrhythmias and premature birth with ECT during pregnancy [77–79].

Antidepressant treatment of MDD during pregnancy

Treatment of MDD during pregnancy should follow the general guidelines for the treatment of MDD in the nongravid woman. The ACOG has recommended that preferred medications in pregnancy are those with the best safety data, fewer metabolites, higher protein binding to decrease placental passage, and fewer interactions with other medications [1]. Desipramine and nortriptyline are the TCA recommended in pregnancy because they are less anticholinergic and less likely to precipitate orthostatic hypotension [80]. However, SSRI and SNRI have generally replaced TCA as first-line treatments for depression. Up to one-quarter of pregnant women in North America and Europe take a SSRI at some point during their pregnancy [81–85]. SSRI and their metabolites have been detected in both umbilical cord blood [86] and amniotic fluid [87]. Fetal drug exposure may be determined by fetal genotypes for drug metabolism and transporter proteins located in the placenta in addition to the concentration of medication found in the mother's serum, umbilical cord blood and amniotic fluid [88,89].

Antidepressants and miscarriage

One meta-analysis of studies reported that exposure to antidepressant medication was associated with a 1.45 relative risk of miscarriage compared to nonexposure; however, the miscarriage rate of 12.4% with exposure was within range of normal population rates [90]. Another meta-analysis of studies reported a significant odds ratio of 1.7 for miscarriage with SSRI use [91]. Two studies conducted subsequent to these meta-analyses also reported increased miscarriage rates with bupropion [92], mirtazapine and other antidepressants [93]. Many of the studies included in both of these meta-analyses did not control for confounding variables such as age, smoking and underlying depression.

Antidepressants and birth outcome

Recent studies have reported an increased risk of PTD with *in utero* exposure to TCA and SSRI [94,95] as well as SNRI [96]. A retrospective review conducted in a Canadian population cohort reported that maternal use of SSRI increased the risk of LBW, PTD, fetal death and neonatal seizures compared to nonexposed infants [97]. LBW, younger gestational age at birth, and lower Apgar scores have been reported with third-trimester exposure of fluoxetine compared to first- or second-trimester exposure [98] and with SSRI exposure compared to TCA exposure or no exposure [99]. LBW has been associated with higher doses of fluoxetine compared to lower doses or use of other SSRI [100]. However, other studies have failed to find birthweight differences between SSRI-exposed and nonexposed infants [101,102] or between early and late SSRI-exposed infants [103,104]. Another study reported that birthweight, gestational age, premature birth and 5-minute Apgar scores did not differ between neonates exposed to various antidepressants and nonexposed neonates, although 1-minute Apgar scores were lower in exposed neonates [105]. Many of the studies examining birth outcomes with antidepressant exposure have not controlled for untreated prenatal maternal depression, concomitant medications, maternal age or other sociodemographic variables, smoking, alcohol or drug use. These potential confounding factors could underlie the mixed results from studies evaluating the effect of SSRI exposure on pregnancy outcomes.

Two studies have controlled for untreated prenatal depression. One study reported that compared to birth outcomes of untreated women with depression and healthy controls, prenatal SSRI use was associated with an increased risk of PTD and lower gestational age at birth, but not with LBW or lower Apgar scores [30]. Another study examining more than 119,000 births compared birth outcomes of infants of depressed mothers treated with SSRI, depressed mothers not treated with SSRI, and nonexposed control mothers, while controlling for maternal depression severity [83]. Although not a RCT, this large study used linked population health data and propensity score matching. Compared to infants of depressed mothers not treated with SSRI, infants of depressed mothers treated with SSRI were more likely to have LBW, younger gestational age, and a higher proportion born earlier than 37 weeks. Longer prenatal SSRI exposure increased these risks [106]. Both maternal depression and SSRI use were significantly associated with increased risk of birthweight below the 10th percentile when maternal illness severity was controlled for in the analyses. These results suggest (but do not prove – a large randomized control trial would be necessary for this) that exposure to SSRI adds to the negative birth outcomes due to the effect of exposure to underlying depression alone (LBW and younger gestational age) [83].

Antidepressants and congenital malformations

Studies examining the prevalence of congenital malformations with first-trimester exposure to antidepressants have yielded mixed results. Two meta-analyses reported that newer antidepressants were not associated with an increased risk of major or minor malformations above the 1–3% population baseline risk [91,107]. Studies have reported a lack of increased congenital malformation rates with fluoxetine exposure [98,100,108–110] and with exposure to sertraline, paroxetine, fluvoxamine or citalopram [95,100,101,110–113]. No increased risk of congenital malformations has been reported with trazodone and nefazodone [114], bupropion [92,115], mirtazapine [93], venlafaxine [116], and TCA [117].

Two large case–control studies reported an association of sertraline with omphalocele and of paroxetine with right ventricular outflow tract obstruction defects [118], and an association of omphalocele, craniosynostosis, and anencephaly with several SSRI [119]. These results suggested a very small increase in absolute risk and a lack of specific malformations linked to specific antidepressants. A study conducted in Denmark reported an adjusted relative risk of 1.34 for congenital malformations (cardiovascular, gastrointestinal, muscle and bone) in infants born to mothers who took SSRI early in pregnancy compared to nonexposed infants [120]. A recent prospective study reported increased cardiovascular abnormalities in infants exposed to fluoxetine compared to paroxetine or no exposure [113]. The risk of congenital malformations was recently reported to not be associated with the duration of antidepressant use during the first trimester [121]. Most of the studies of congenital malformations have not controlled for underlying maternal psychiatric disease. A recent study that did control for maternal illness variables reported that the risk of cardiovascular malformations is increased with first-trimester combined SSRI and benzodiazepine use [122].

In 2005, a retrospective analysis of GlaxoSmithKline data reported an adjusted odds ratio of 2.08 for cardiovascular malformations (mostly ventricular septal defects) and an adjusted odds ratio of 2.2 for overall major congenital malformations with paroxetine use compared to other antidepressants. The FDA issued a public health advisory about paroxetine use in pregnancy in December 2005 and paroxetine's FDA pregnancy category was changed from "C" to "D." Subsequently, the elevated risk of cardiac malformations with first-trimester use of paroxetine was confirmed by a meta-analysis [123] and a retrospective cohort study from Sweden [124]. A large study of a healthcare organization database reported a slight increase in the prevalence of several congenital malformations with paroxetine compared to exposure with other antidepressants [125]. However, a recently published study of prospective cohorts reported that first-trimester paroxetine use was not associated with an increased risk of cardiovascular defects [126]. In addition, a recent meta-analysis [127] reported a lack of increased cardiovascular abnormalities with first-trimester paroxetine use. The ACOG has advised that paroxetine not be used during pregnancy and that the use of SSRI should be individualized [128].

In summary, the relationship between congenital malformations and antidepressants, including paroxetine, is unclear. If first-trimester antidepressant exposure does increase the risk of congenital malformations, the magnitude of the increase is not large and the use of these agents to treat major depression in pregnancy is justifiable when potential risks of treatment are weighed against the potential risks of untreated depression.

Antidepressants and poor neonatal adaptation

Exposure to antidepressants at the end of the third trimester may lead to a poor neonatal adaptation (PNA), also described as neonatal behavioral syndrome, neonatal toxicity or neonatal abstinence syndrome. PNA includes poor muscle tone, jitteriness, respiratory distress, weak or absent cry, hypoglycemia, poor temperature regulation, low Apgar score and seizures [95,129–131]. The symptoms are usually mild and transient, but supportive care in special care nurseries may be necessary [103,105,111,132,133]. PNA has been reported to occur in up to 30% of exposed neonates [134]. A comprehensive review reported that third-trimester SSRI exposure carried an overall risk ratio of 3.0 compared to first-trimester exposure or no exposure [132]. Even with control for severity level of maternal prenatal depression, the risk for respiratory distress at birth was greater with exposure to SSRI during pregnancy compared to nonexposure [83] and with longer gestational exposure to SSRI [106].

An increased risk of PNA with third-trimester use of paroxetine and fluoxetine has been reported in seminal studies [132,135]. Subsequent cases of neonatal symptoms have been reported with third-trimester use of paroxetine [136], citalopram [111,137], venlafaxine [96,133,138,139], mirtazapine [96,140], and duloxetine [141]. A recent study reported a prolonged neonatal QTc interval with SSRI use prior to delivery [142]. Neonatal jitteriness, irritability, respiratory difficulties, poor suck reflex, urinary retention, functional bowel obstruction, and, rarely, seizures have also been described with third-trimester TCA use [95,143]. In 2005, the FDA issued an advisory about the potential for neonatal symptoms with late third-trimester use in the prescribing information of antidepressants.

The signs and symptoms of the PNA have not been systematically defined, but they have similarities with some of the signs and symptoms of adult serotonin toxicity, SSRI discontinuation syndrome and cholinergic overdrive [129–132,144,145]. Future studies of PNA need to include use of a validated neonatal behavioral symptom scale, assessments of infants by evaluators blind to maternal SSRI use, control for maternal psychiatric and other variables, and follow-up to evaluate long-term sequelae [146].

Antidepressants and persistent pulmonary hypertension of the newborn

A case–control study reported an association between SSRI use after week 20 of pregnancy and an increased risk of persistent pulmonary hypertension of the newborn (PPHN) after controlling for maternal Body Mass Index, diabetes, smoking and nonsteroidal anti-inflammatory drug (NSAID) use [84]. The absolute risk was small (7/1000), and compares to the risk of PPHN in unexposed newborns (1/700). Although all f cases of PPHN observed in this study were relatively mild and self-limited, PPHN can be fatal in 10–20% of newborns. The FDA issued an alert about the increased risk of PPHN with SSRI use in the second half of pregnancy in July 2006. A subsequent study from Sweden confirmed a smaller increased risk of PPHN with SSRI late in pregnancy [147]. However, two recent studies failed to find an association between SSRI use in pregnancy and PPHN [148, 149]. It has been suggested that SSRI may promote pulmonary artery constriction after birth by direct effects on pulmonary smooth muscle cells or by inhibiting the vasodilator nitric oxide [84]. *In utero* fluoxetine exposure induced pulmonary hypertension in rats by an increase in pulmonary artery smooth muscle proliferation [150]. PPHN may fall at the severe end of the spectrum of respiratory problems that can occur after third-trimester SSRI use [84,147].

Long-term effects of antidepressants during pregnancy

Few long-term studies exist that have followed the cognitive, neurologic and behavioral development of children exposed to antidepressant medications or untreated disease during pregnancy. A review of studies about the long-term development of children with prenatal and postpartum SSRI exposure reported that most studies (involving 306 children) have demonstrated no impairment with exposure, while two studies (involving 81 children) have suggested mild adverse effects of motor control and development [151]. Normal neurodevelopment at 1 year was reported in a prospective study of infants with fetal exposure to citalopram compared to nonexposed infants [152]. Normal neurodevelopment, language development and IQ were also reported in prospective cohorts of children up to age 5 exposed to TCA or fluoxetine, compared to no exposure [153,154]. Two more recent studies reported that in a cohort of 4-year-old children, concurrent maternal depression, but not exposure to SSRI during pregnancy, was associated with externalizing (aggression and increased activity) behaviors [155] and internalizing (withdrawal, depression, emotional reactivity, anxiety) behaviors [156]. Since both untreated illness and medication exposure pose risks to the fetus, there is a critical need for future systematic studies of long-term developmental effects of exposure to both untreated illness and antidepressant medication during each trimester.

Treatment dilemmas for pregnant women with depression

A pregnant woman with depression faces significant treatment dilemmas given the growing evidence that fetal risk exposure occurs with depression, stress, and anxiety as well as psychotropic medications (see Box 21.5). The decision about how to treat psychiatric illness in pregnancy involves the woman, her partner, her clinician, and an ongoing discussion about research results of medication versus untreated disease exposure. However, patients, their partners and clinicians must rely on results from observational, cohort and administrative database studies in the absence of definitive studies [157]. Moreover, the results of these studies are difficult to interpret due to the confounding effects of medication, underlying illness and unhealthy behaviors due to illness Also, there is minimal evidence-based research suggesting efficacy of psychotherapies or alternative treatments for MDD during pregnancy. Treatment options are governed by the current severity of symptoms, psychiatric history and response to treatment, clinician presentation of treatment choices with their risks and benefits, patient perception of the risks and benefits of treatment choices, cultural expectations, and plans for breastfeeding. A recent study of pregnant women with depression identified cost, lack of transportation, distrust of mental health clinicians, and lack of knowledge of available resources as barriers to pursuing psychiatric care [158].

A woman who is euthymic on her antidepressant may wish to taper her medication prior to a planned conception, or following conception, in an effort to decrease the exposure of the fetus to medication. However, the risk for relapse of MDD is significant and there are clear risks of exposure to untreated depression. If a pregnant woman decides to start, restart or continue medication, monotherapy and the minimum effective dosage of an antidepressant without known teratogenicity should be used. At the time of writing, the SSRI sertraline and the TCA nortriptyline would appear to be the "safest" medication choices for treatment of depression when initiating therapy in pregnancy or changing antidepressant medication in preparation for (or early on during) a pregnancy. However, the literature suggests that some risk likely exists with any antidepressant use during pregnancy. The risk of miscarriage is increased slightly with first-trimester exposure compared to nonexposure. Antidepressants are not considered major teratogens and, overall, they are not linked to significantly increased rates of specific congenital malformations [1]. However, a controversy exists as to whether first-trimester exposure to paroxetine increases the risk of cardiovascular malformations. Exposure to SSRI in the second half of pregnancy does appear to increase the risk of PPHN.

Neonatal symptoms due to antidepressant toxicity or withdrawal are generally mild and transient, but deserve systematic study. The tapering of antidepressant medication approximately 2 weeks prior to delivery in an attempt to decrease possible PNA is currently controversial and it is not our present practice to do so [159]. Although PNA symptoms might be decreased, the timing of delivery cannot be predicted, a taper could predispose a woman to MDD prior to delivery as well as post partum, and a decrease in PNA following a taper has not been confirmed [132,160].

The long-term effects of exposure to antidepressants during pregnancy, as well as to untreated psychiatric symptoms, are largely unstudied to date. Thus, pregnant women with depression must choose the risks of exposure to untreated disease or to medication without clear data about the long-term effects of both on the development of their infant and child. Table 21.1 lists the presently available antidepressant medications and offers some practical advice about their use in pregnancy. Although these data are up to date at the time of writing, the reader should be aware that the literature on the use of antidepressants in pregnancy is rapidly evolving.

Treatment of postpartum depression

The treatment of PPD is assumed to be similar to the treatment of MDD at nonpuerperal periods. However, a new infant brings about significant role change with new demands, sleep loss and fatigue, each of which can exacerbate depressive symptoms. In addition, women who are breastfeeding need to consider potential exposure of the infant to psychotropic medications through breast milk. Breastfeeding mothers with PPD may prefer psychotherapy to medications [161–163]. Systematic reviews report that psychotherapies have at least moderate efficacy for PPD [164,165], an example of which is IPT which addresses role change, social support, the marital relationship, and life stressors [66].

Women with PPD may choose antidepressant medication or may need to add it to psychotherapy if improvement does not occur. Two placebo-controlled RCT demonstrated superiority of paroxetine [166] and fluoxetine [167]. Two active comparator RCT reported that sertraline and nortriptyline were equally effective [168] and that both paroxetine and combined paroxetine/CBT were effective in women with PPD and co-morbid anxiety disorders [169]. Antidepressant studies in PPD to date have not uniformly included breastfeeding women and have not systematically assessed adverse effects in breastfeeding infants. Other treatments studied in PPD have included estrogen, exercise, and light therapy [170]. Two recent RCT failed to demonstrate superiority of fish oil over placebo in PPD [75,76].

Breastfeeding

The breastfeeding woman with PPD must take into account the known negative effects of not treating her depression on child development and the potential risks of exposure of her infant to antidepressant medication through breast milk. In addition to potential short-term adverse effects, the long-term effects of antidepressant exposure through breast milk on child cognitive, motor, neurologic and behavioral development are unknown [149]. Reviews of antidepressants and breastfeeding suggest that sertraline, paroxetine and nortriptyline usually yield undetectable infant serum levels and an absence of adverse effects in infants, while adverse effects have been reported with fluoxetine, citalopram and doxepin [171–173]. Lactation risk categories currently exist [174], and the FDA has suggested a future reclassification [175]. Breast milk analysis and measurement of infant antidepressant serum levels are not routinely obtained in clinical care [1], and adverse effects in the infant may not correlate with milk-to-plasma ratios [176]. Administration of an antidepressant should include a low initial dose followed by gradual titration of the dose while monitoring the infant for adverse effects such as irritability, sedation, poor weight gain or a change in feeding patterns [172,177]. If adverse effects in the infant are noted, the pediatrician should be consulted, and the options include decreasing the dose, changing to partial or full bottlefeeding or changing the medication. If a postpartum woman is already doing well on an antidepressant that may be associated with potential adverse effects or high infant serum levels, carefully monitoring the infant rather than switching the antidepressant may be indicated [172,177].

Bipolar disorder

Background

Bipolar disorder is the occurrence of one or more manic episodes, with or without depressive episodes [2]. Mania is characterized by a period of persistently elevated, expansive or irritable mood lasting at least 1 week that is associated with at least three of the following:

- inflated self-esteem or grandiosity
- decreased need for sleep
- pressured or rapid speech
- flight of ideas or racing thoughts
- distractibility
- increase in goal-directed activity such as starting multiple projects
- excessive engagement in activities with potentially painful consequences such as spending sprees, hypersexuality, risk taking, reckless driving, and substance use [2].

The prevalence of bipolar disorder is 0.4–1.6% in both genders. Women experience more depressive episodes, mixed episodes (combined manic and depressive symptoms), and rapid cycling compared to men [178,179].

Bipolar disorder runs a relapsing and remitting course with episodes of depression usually predominating but an episode of mania being necessary for the diagnosis. It is ranked by the WHO as the sixth leading cause of DALY worldwide in persons of reproductive age. Addiction is common among patients with bipolar disorder, likely as some form of self-treatment to manage the commonly associated anxiety. Between 25% and 50% of patients with this diagnosis will attempt suicide at some time in their lives and 15% of patients with bipolar disorder will die from suicide.

The usual first-line therapeutic medications for management of acute mania outside pregnancy are lithium, carbamazepine or valproate. The usual first-line therapeutic medications for acute depression in patients with bipolar disorder outside pregnancy are lithium or quetiapine. Antidepressants should be used cautiously for bipolar-related depression due to the risk of inducing mania if not used simultaneously with a mood stabilizer. Other atypical antipsychotics such as olanzapine or risperidone can also be used for any of these indications outside pregnancy. ECT is effective for treating both severe depression and mania when there is a lack of response to medications.

Pregnancy

Pregnancy appears to be neither protective nor a time of increased risk for bipolar episodes. Recent studies confirm that the risk for relapse is increased if a mood stabilizer is discontinued during pregnancy [180,181] and a rapid rate of medication discontinuation further increases the risk of relapse [181]. Manic relapse in the pregnant woman can lead to poor health behaviors, poor compliance with prenatal care, substance abuse, risk-taking behavior, and suicide. There are few studies of the effect of untreated bipolar disorder on fetal outcome. One study reported that women with a previous bipolar episode were at increased risk of LBW, PTD, and small-for-gestational-age infants [182]. Women with bipolar disorder have a greater than 50% risk for having a postpartum bipolar episode [183], so mood stabilizer prophylaxis needs to be discussed even with bipolar women who have remained euthymic through pregnancy without psychotropic medication. The postpartum episode is depressive in a substantial proportion of bipolar women, and bipolar women who receive an antidepressant need to be closely monitored for hypomanic and manic symptoms because of the possibility that antidepressant therapy might precipitate a "mood switch" to mania. [184].

Postpartum psychosis

Postpartum psychosis occurs in 0.2% of postpartum women with rapid onset in the first 4 weeks after delivery and is more common in women with bipolar affective disorder [185]. Postpartum psychosis includes confused thinking, delusions, paranoia, mood swings, disorganized behavior, impaired functioning, and impaired judgment [186]. Women with postpartum psychosis usually require an inpatient psychiatric hospitalization. Risk factors include recent discontinuation of mood stabilizers, previous postpartum psychosis, previous hospitalization for a manic or psychotic episode, primiparity, obstetric complications, sleep deprivation, environmental stressors, and a family history of postpartum psychosis or bipolar disorder [186–190]. Women who have had postpartum psychosis are likely to have a longitudinal course consistent with bipolar disorder [186].

Neonaticide and infanticide

The rate of homicide of infants up to 1 year of age (infanticide) is 8 per 100,000 in the United States [191], but while postpartum psychosis is associated with an increased risk of infant homicide, the prevalence of infanticide in women with this condition is unknown. Infanticide may occur with a postpartum mother who has psychotic symptoms such as delusions or command hallucinations, has sleep deprivation, and has the increased responsibilities of the care of a newborn [192]. However, infanticide may also occur with mothers without psychosis, such as with those with severe PPD, due to neglect and abuse, or as revenge against the infant's father [192,193]. A significant proportion of mothers who kill their children also kill themselves [191]. Neonaticide is defined as killing a newborn within 24 hours of birth. It is associated with denial of pregnancy, lack of prenatal care, depersonalization, dissociation, and amnesia about the delivery [191,194]. Sporadic thoughts of intentionally harming an infant or of accidental harm occurring to an infant are common [58], and

most women with these thoughts respond to reassurance that such thoughts are common, frightening and rarely acted upon. A postpartum woman with persistent thoughts of harming her infant that do not resolve needs psychiatric evaluation.

Antenatal and postpartum issues with bipolar disorder

Bipolar disorder that is untreated or undertreated during pregnancy can lead to life-threatening consequences to the mother and fetus. The risks of acute mood symptoms and decompensated behavior must be weighed against the risks of the medications used for mood stabilization in pregnancy. Psychosocial treatment should be considered [195]. Factors to be considered include the severity of mania, depression, psychosis and suicidality, illness history and previous response to treatment, patient preferences, and plans for breastfeeding [183,195]. Active collaboration between the patient, her family, the psychiatrist, the obstetrician, and the pediatrician is necessary in order to optimize stability for women with bipolar disorder during pregnancy and the postpartum period [195]. Postpartum psychosis is treated as a manic or psychotic episode would be treated when a woman is nonpuerperal, i.e. with mood stabilizers, antipsychotics, and ECT if necessary.

Mood stabilizers and pregnancy

Table 21.2 reviews the typical dosing of mood stabilizers and recommends features to monitor for pregnant patients who are on these medications. The discussion below reviews the data about the use of these medications in pregnancy.

Lithium

Lithium is the first-line medication for the acute and maintenance treatment of bipolar disorder. First-trimester lithium exposure (up to day 56 after conception or day 42 after the last menstrual period, when the embryologic development of the heart is completed) has been associated with an increased risk of cardiac anomalies, specifically Ebstein's anomaly (apical displacement of the septal and posterior tricuspid valve leaflets, leading to atrialization of the right ventricle – see Chapter 5). The 0.05–0.1% (1 in 1000) risk of Ebstein's anomaly with lithium exposure is 10–20 times higher than the risk in the general population (1 in 20,000) [196]. However, the absolute risk is small and must be weighed against the risks of untreated or undertreated bipolar disorder. Increased dosage and more frequent dosing of lithium may be necessary as pregnancy progresses to maintain stable serum levels. A level II ultrasound and fetal echocardiogram at 18–20 weeks are suggested in women who have had first-trimester exposure to lithium [179]. Such testing offers the woman the option of termination of pregnancy and if this is not her desire, allows the patient and her medical team

Table 21.2 Medications used to treat bipolar affective disorder

Medication	Dosing	Patient monitoring in pregnancy
Lithium	Typical dose 900–1200 mg per day for maintenance and 1200–2400 mg per day for acute episodes with goal of maintaining lithium concentration of 0.6–1.0 mEq/L. Toxicity occurs at levels >1.2 mEq/L. Anticipate need to increase lithium dosing with increasing blood volume and glomerular filtration rate (GFR) in pregnancy. Both GFR and blood volume drop rapidly post partum so lithium dosing usually needs reduction to pre-pregnancy doses shortly after birth. Monitor levels every 2–4 weeks initially then up to weekly in the third trimester. Consider checking levels with any nausea/vomiting/diarrhea significant enough to cause dehydration at any point in the pregnancy.	Obtain baseline thyroid function tests and repeat every 3 months in pregnancy. Watch for excessive polydypsia and polyuria which may suggest nephrogenic diabetes insipidus. Watch for forgetfulness, sleepiness and tremor which may suggest toxicity. Obtain level II fetal ultrasound at 18–20 weeks gestation to look for Ebstein's anomaly.
Carbamazepine	Typically starting at 200 mg PO twice a day of extended-release formulations (or 100 mg four times a day of standard formulation) and increased by 200 mg/day increments as needed to be effective. Maximum dose is 1600 mg per day total. Therapeutic blood levels typically run from 4 to 12 µg/mL. Dosing may need to be increased in pregnancy based on either blood levels or therapeutic effect. Check levels at least every 3 months in pregnancy and more frequently if symptoms increase or there are signs of potential toxicity. U Upward adjustments in dosing made during pregnancy may need to be reduced post partum.	Level II fetal ultrasound recommended to look for craniofacial and neurologic anomalies at 18–20 weeks gestation. Patient on carbamazepine should also take 4 mg daily of folic acid throughout gestation starting prior to pregnancy. Addition of vitamin K 10 mg PO daily from 36 weeks gestation may decrease risk of vitamin K deficiency-related bleeding in mother and newborn. Watch patient for signs of toxicity which include double or blurred vision, dizziness, lethargy and headache. Monitor serum sodium, liver function tests and complete blood count every 6 months while on therapy. Deemed compatible with breastfeeding by the American Academy of Pediatrics.
Valproic acid	Dosing typically initiated at 750 mg total per day divided between 1–4 times a day depending on formulation used. Dose is increased 5–10 mg/kg/day every week until therapeutic effect and/or levels are achieved. Maximum dose is 60/mg/kg per day. Clinical response typically seen with levels 85–125 µg/mL. Toxicity may be seen above these levels.	Level II fetal ultrasound recommended looking for craniofacial and neurologic anomalies at 18–20 weeks gestation. Patient on valproic acid should also take 4 mg daily of folic acid throughout gestation starting prior to pregnancy. Addition of vitamin K 10 mg PO daily likely not necessary for this medication. Watch patient for signs of toxicity which include double or blurred vision, dizziness, lethargy and headache. Monitor liver function tests and complete blood count every 6 months while on therapy. Watch for tremor as a sign of toxicity. Although deemed compatible with breastfeeding by the American Academy of Pediatrics, increasing data about the neurologic sequelae of valproic use in pregnancy have led to increasing concerns about its use in breastfeeding mothers until further data become available.
Lamotrigine	Typically initiated at 25 mg daily for 2 weeks and gradually increased to 200 mg daily over 6 weeks. Response is monitored clinically as a reliable therapeutic range for this agent has not been established.	Level II fetal ultrasound at 18–20 weeks gestation. recommended to look for craniofacial and neurologic anomalies. Watch patient for signs of toxicity which include dizziness and somnolence. Agent can cause Stevens Johnson syndrome in first 8 weeks of therapy or if suddenly stopped and then resumed at regular dose rather than being started at low dose and gradually increased. Likely compatible with breastfeeding but data are limited.

to prepare to care for an infant with congenital disease. Lithium toxicity due to the rapid decrease in vascular volume at delivery can be avoided by holding lithium prior to and at delivery. However, to prevent a postpartum bipolar episode, immediately following delivery, lithium should be restarted and serum levels monitored [197]. Neonatal effects in infants exposed to lithium include floppy infant syndrome, hypotonicity and cyanosis. Third-trimester lithium use can lead to rare complications such as neonatal diabetes insipidus, hypothyroidism, low muscle tone, hepatic abnormalities, respiratory difficulties, lethargy and polyhydramnios [179,197]. There have been no reported negative long-term consequences on child neurobehavioral development after gestational lithium exposure but few studies exist.

Carbamazepine

First-trimester exposure to carbamazepine is associated with an elevated risk of neural tube defects (0.5–1%), as well as increased risks of craniofacial abnormalities, growth restriction, LBW, decreased head circumference and fingernail hypoplasia [179]. A serum alpha-fetoprotein level at 14–16 weeks and a level II ultrasound at 18–20 weeks can screen for neural tube defects and other major malformations [198,199]. Supplemental folic acid (4 mg/day) is recommended following a baseline B12 level, ideally before conception occurs, since most neural tube defects occur in the first month after conception [198]. However, it has not been clearly demonstrated that folic acid supplementation reduces the risk of neural tube defects in pregnant women taking anticonvulsants [198]. Vitamin K 10–20 mg/day is recommended in the last month of pregnancy to avoid a bleeding diathesis since carbamazepine can reduce vitamin K levels [179,195]. Reports of neonatal toxicity with third-trimester carbamazepine use have been few, and there are no reports of negative long-term neurobehavioral development in children exposed to carbamazepine in pregnancy.

Valproate

Although a common treatment of bipolar disorder in non-pregnant patients, valproate should be used with caution in pregnancy as it is associated with a greater incidence of major congenital abnormalities than other antiepileptics, particularly at doses above 1000 mg/day [200–202]. Neural tube defects occur in 1–2% of neonates after first-trimester exposure [178,179]. A fetal valproate syndrome has been described which includes craniofacial abnormalities, cardiovascular abnormalities, and growth restriction [179,203]. Neonatal symptoms include decelerations in heart rate, hypoglycemia, jitteriness, liver toxicity, difficulty feeding and abnormal muscle tone [178,179]. A serum alpha-fetoprotein level (at 14–16 weeks) and a level II ultrasound (ideally at 18–20 weeks) can screen for neural tube defects and other major malformations [198,199].

Valproate should be administered in divided doses and serum valproate levels should be monitored [204]. Supplemental folic acid (4 mg/day) is recommended following a baseline B12 level. Vitamin K supplementation is likely not necessary for patients on valproate. Neurobehavioral outcome studies have suggested lower IQ scores, developmental delays, and increased use of special educational interventions in children exposed to valproate throughout pregnancy and the use of this agent in pregnancy is most justifiable in patients who cannot tolerate or have failed trials of alternative agents [198,205,206].

Lamotrigine and other newer antiepileptic medications

Lamotrigine is an antiepileptic that is increasingly used in the treatment of bipolar disorder and its use during pregnancy and the postpartum period is increasing. Some studies suggested that the 2–3% risk of teratogenicity reported with monotherapy was similar to the risk rate in the general population [201,202,207]. Recent data from some of the ongoing international prospective pregnancy registries have suggested an increased risk of oral clefts with lamotrigine exposure [205,208] as well as no increased risk [209]. Malformations are more likely to occur at higher lamotrigine doses [201]. Serum concentrations may fall due to altered pharmacokinetics during pregnancy, and serum monitoring has been suggested although the effective therapeutic range is not well established [204]. Neonatal symptoms with lamotrigine use prior to delivery have not been reported. As in adults, in infants there can be a risk of hepatotoxicity and skin rash [178,179]. Minimal safety data are available about gabapentin, oxcarbazepine, levetiracetam, zonisamide and pregabalin use during pregnancy.

Using combinations of mood stabilizers in pregnancy

Topiramate use as part of polytherapy may be associated with oral clefts and hypospadias [210]. Teratogenic risks increase with the use of multiple antiepileptics compared to antiepileptic monotherapy [199,202]. However, in more severe or refractory cases of bipolar disorder, multiple medications may be required to maintain mood stability. To avoid using two antiepileptic mood stabilizers, antipsychotic medications may be useful for mood stabilization and reduction of psychotic symptoms, if present.

Mood stabilizers and breastfeeding

Mood stabilizers have been used with breastfeeding. Even though it was recently reported that lithium could be used during breastfeeding with careful infant serum level monitoring [211], lithium has been deemed incompatible with breastfeeding by the American Academy of Pediatrics due to reports of hypotonia, hypothermia, cyanosis, T wave inversion and lethargy in infants [179,186,203,212]. Breast milk levels readily reach 50% of maternal serum levels and milk and infant serum levels are approximately equal. Carbamazepine and valproate are both deemed compatible with breastfeeding by the American Academy of Pediatrics although there is increasing concern about the use of valproic acid because of the association of pregnancy exposure with long-term adverse intellectual effects in the child. There are minimal published data about the safety of the newer antiepileptic drugs with breastfeeding [213]. Preliminary data have suggested that lamotrigine, oxcarbazepine, topiramate, gabapentin and levetiracetam are not associated with adverse effects [186,212,213] although serum levels of lamotrigine may be high after breastfeeding in some infants [214].

Summary

In summary, lithium appears to be safer during pregnancy than carbamazepine and valproate in terms of teratogenicity, while carbamazepines (and possibly valproate) are preferable to lithium with breastfeeding. Lamotrigine use in pregnancy and with breastfeeding is increasing and future data from the international registries should either identify or alleviate concerns about specific adverse effects from exposure during pregnancy and breastfeeding.

Schizophrenia

Epidemiology and diagnosis

The prevalence of schizophrenia in the adult population is 0.5–1.5% [2] and the peak age of onset for women is 25–35 years of age [215]. Schizophrenia is defined as having two or more of the following symptoms for at least 1 month: delusions, hallucinations, disorganized speech, grossly disorganized behavior and negative symptoms such as flat affect. These symptoms are generally associated with significant impairment of social and occupational functioning [2]; 10% of patients will have a single episode of schizophrenia and recover. However, the majority will suffer either a chronic or intermittent course. Schizophrenia is also associated with a 20% reduction in life expectancy and a twofold increased risk of death at any age compared with age- and sex-matched controls without schizophrenia. Homelessness, medication side effects and access to healthcare contribute to this mortality gap as does a high incidence of alcohol and tobacco use. Five to 10% of patients with schizophrenia end their life in suicide.

Previously, patients with psychosis were routinely treated with "traditional" or first-generation antipsychotics (FGA) or neuroleptics, such as phenothiazines (chlorpromazine, fluphenazine) and butyrophenones (haloperidol). The main disadvantage of these medications is the associated risk of dyskinesias and pseudoparkinsonism. One of the other common side effects of the FGA is hyperprolactinemia which leads to infertility in many women with schizophrenia. In recent years, "atypical" or second-generation antipsychotics (also known as SGA but for the purposes of this chapter and context, we will use the nonstandard abbreviation SGAp to avoid confusion with SGA as an abbreviation for small for gestational age), such as olanzapine, risperidone, quetiapine, aripiprazole and ziprasidone, have become first-line treatments for psychotic disorders. These agents have the advantage of a lower risk of extrapyramidal side effects but the additional disadvantages of a much higher cost and metabolic side effects such as glucose intolerance and weight gain. The SGAp have minimal effect on prolactin levels and the increasing use of SGAp is presumed to be increasing rates of unplanned pregnancy in women with chronic psychosis [216,217].

Box 21.3 reviews and classifies the presently available FGA and SGAp.

Box 21.3 Antipsychotic medications and their US trade names

First-generation antipsychotics
- Chlorpromazine (Thorazine)
- Chlorprothixene (Taractan)
- Flupenthixol (Derpixol/Fluanxol)
- Fluphenazine (Prolixin)
- Haloperidol (Haldol)
- Levomepromazine (Nozinan)
- Penfluridol (Semap/Micefal)
- Perphenazine (Trilafon)
- Pimozide (Orap)
- Prochlorperazine (Compazine)
- Promethazine (Phenergan)
- Thiethylperazine (Torecan)
- Thioridazine (Mellaril)
- Thiothixene (Navane)
- Trifluoperazine (Stelazine)
- Zuclopenthixol (Cloxipixol/Acuphase)

Second-generation Antipsychotics
- Amisulpride (Solian)
- Clozapine (Clozaril)
- Olanzapine (Zyprexa)
- Quetiapine (Seroquel)
- Risperidone (Risperdal)
- Sertindole (Serdolect)
- Ziprasidone (Geodon)

Third-generation antipsychotics
- Ariprazole (Abilify)

At the time of writing, the jury is still out on whether FGA or SGAp should be considered the standard first-line treatment of schizophrenia. While avoidance of extrapyramidal side effects is desirable, there is increasing concern that the SGAp increase cardiovascular risk without offering substantial improvements in efficacy over the FGA.

Acutely agitated nonpregnant patients may be given intramuscular olanzapine, ziprasidone, ariprazole or haloperidol or dissolving oral tablets of risperidone or olanzapine. Stabilization and maintenance therapy are achieved with any of the FGA or SGAp, with practice in the US presently favoring SGAp agents. Long-acting depot forms are usually preferred for maintenance therapy and although both haloperidol and fluphenazine are available in a long-acting injectable form, risperidone is the only SGAp available for depot treatment in the US. Discontinuation of antipsychotic therapy is associated with relapse, with 80% of patients experiencing relapse of psychotic symptoms within a year of stopping medications (contrasted with a 30% recurrence rate in patients with good compliance with their antipsychotic medications).

Pregnancy

Patients with schizophrenia are at greatest risk of relapse within the first 3 months after discontinuing their antipsychotic medication. Tapering medications over less than 2 weeks increases the risk of relapse 5–6 times compared with tapering medications over 2 months or more [218]. Therefore, a woman who conceives while stable on antipsychotic medication is at high risk of relapse if she abruptly discontinues the medication. Untreated psychosis can lead to poor prenatal care, poor nutrition, poor prenatal health behaviors, relationship disruptions, increased use of alcohol, drugs and smoking, and increased risks of suicide or injury to others. A psychotic decompensation usually leads to inpatient psychiatric hospitalization. Some population-based studies have reported an association of schizophrenia with cardiovascular congenital malformations, placental abruption, LBW, fetal distress and hypoxia, increased admissions to the neonatal intensive care [219–221], and increased risk of sudden infant death syndrome independent of the treatment used [222]. The postpartum period is a time of risk of relapse of schizophrenia, possibly due to the rapid decrease in estrogen's antidopaminergic activity [223].

Antipsychotics and pregnancy

For all the reasons listed above, most experts strongly support the ongoing active treatment and prevention of psychotic symptoms in pregnancy. However, studies have reported mixed results in terms of an increased risk of congenital malformations with FGA [224–228]. A meta-analysis of first-trimester phenothiazine exposure reported a small increase in relative risk of congenital anomalies (2.4%) relative to the 2.0% risk in the general population, particularly with phenothiazines with aliphatic side chains (those in which carbon atoms are linked in open chains rather than rings, e.g. chlorpromazine) [117]. However, a recent systematic review suggested that chlorpromazine was the "safest" FGA to use in pregnancy and identified it as the only antipsychotic with (favorable) follow-up data on school-aged children exposed *in utero* [228].

Although there is no long-term follow-up of infants exposed to haloperidol in pregnancy, most data suggest that this is a reasonable agent to use in pregnancy and it is in fact favored over chlorpromazine in pregnancy by many experts because of its potentially better efficacy and side effect profile. Case reports of limb defects with haloperidol exposure have led some to recommend level II ultrasounds at 18–20 weeks in patients taking haloperidol during the first trimester [229].

Less is known about the safety of the other FGA in pregnancy but none of them have been shown to be a human teratogen. Use of FGA other than haloperidol and chlorpromazine in pregnancy should probably be limited to patients for whom the risk of relapse related to medication adjustment is prohibitive and those patients who have previously failed or not tolerated these agents. The use of FGA at the end of the third trimester has been associated with neonatal dyskinesias, hypertonia tremor, motor restlessness, difficulty with oral feeding, and cholestatic jaundice [224,225,228]. While some experts recommend decreasing medication doses close to term to try and prevent such neonatal effects, most would agree that the risks of relapse make such an approach undesirable. Studies are few, but no adverse long-term effects on behavioral and cognitive functioning in children with *in utero* FGA exposure have been identified to date [224,225].

As stated previously, the SGAp are used more frequently in the US than FGA due to their easier tolerability and decreased risk for tardive dyskinesia. A prospective cohort study of first-trimester pregnancy exposures to SGAp did not reveal an increased risk of major malformations compared to a nonexposed comparison group [215]. A review reported a lack of congenital abnormalities with olanzapine, risperidone and clozapine [224] but other reports have reported slightly higher malformation rates with SGAp [223,228,230–232]. However, safety data about SGAp are limited and remain too sparse at this time to recommend a preferred SGAp for use in pregnancy. Many of the SGAp are associated with glucose intolerance and weight gain and this should be discussed with patients, in the context of pregnancy [228]. Screening for diabetes with a fasting glucose prior to pregnancy and in the early third trimester seems therefore advisable in patients on SGAp. SGAp have been reported to be associated with LBW [89,215], but a recent systematic review [228] and a prospective study [230] reported that SGAp were associated with increased birthweight and large-for-gestational-age infants compared to FGA or no exposure. SGAp use overall may be associated with an increased risk of neonatal complications (neonatal intensive care admissions and low birthweight) but the data are too sparse to tell if any particular SGAp is more hazardous than another [89,228]. It has been suggested that infants with third-trimester exposure to clozapine should have a complete blood count obtained at birth to rule out agranulocytosis, a known side effect of this medication in adults [223,232]. There is a need for studies of the long-term effects of SGAp use during pregnancy on long-term child development.

In summary, women with schizophrenia, their families, and their clinicians must weigh the risks of psychosis versus the potential risks of psychotropic medication during pregnancy and the postpartum period. At the time of writing, the evidence would suggest that the risks of antipsychotic medication in pregnancy (a potential slight increased risk of congenital malformations and a moderate increase in neonatal complications) are small and the benefits of ongoing treatment for most patients considerable [227,228].

Most patients with schizophrenia will present to the obstetrician already pregnant and on an antipsychotic agent. In this situation, we would recommend continuing the presently effective medication. None of the presently available data on FGA or SGAp suggest that the risk of any of these agents is great enough to warrant either discontinuing an effective agent or carrying out an abrupt medication adjustment. For patients with untreated schizophrenia who are pregnant or desiring a pregnancy, treatment with chlorpromazine or haloperidol seems preferable on the basis of the presently available data. If a patient is already well controlled on another agent and desiring a planned pregnancy, consideration should be given to switching her to either chlorpromazine or haloperidol gradually and under the supervision of an experienced psychiatrist.

Legal and ethical concerns can arise regarding the validity of informed consent for treatment of patients with severe mental illness during pregnancy. However, most patients with schizophrenia will be able to make treatment decisions (and their ability to do so will be helped with their treatment). When there is doubt about competency, guidance can be provided by the consulting psychiatrist. Factors for clinicians to consider with the patient when counseling her about antipsychotic use in pregnancy include the severity of the woman's illness, her previous response to treatment, the developmental stage of the fetus or infant, plans for breastfeeding, the woman's perceptions and preferences, and any confounding psychosocial issues [234,237]. It is important also to involve partners and/or family members in these decisions whenever possible as their understanding of the rationale for treatment may have significant effects on the patient's compliance. It is well worth spending time helping schizophrenic mothers and their partners and families understand the advantages of accepting a possible modest increase in risk of adverse pregnancy outcome over the risks of unstable mental health during a pregnancy.

Other treatment issues during and following a pregnancy

The management of the pregnant woman with psychosis is challenging and usually requires a team approach. Psychotic women often have limited supports, are financially disadvantaged, and their pregnancies are often unplanned [233]. Psychosocial interventions that have demonstrated benefit in patients with schizophrenia include individual therapy, family therapy, social skills training, vocational rehabilitation and multidisciplinary case management [234,235]. Helping patients to identify potential alternative child caregivers if they are needed at a later time can be of benefit. Addressing additional risks such as alcohol, nicotine and street drug use and unprotected sexual activity will help improve both maternal well-being and pregnancy outcome.

Nonpharmacologic treatment strategies should be administered during pregnancy to increase prenatal functioning, improve healthy behaviors, potentially limit the need for medication during pregnancy, and improve pregnancy outcomes [224]. Special instruction in parenting skills may be particularly helpful for the postpartum woman with chronic psychosis.

Antipsychotic therapy and breastfeeding

Data about the safety of FGA and SGAp with breastfeeding [213] are scarce but sporadic adverse effects in breastfeeding infants have been reported with olanzapine and clozapine [236]. Breastfeeding infants should be monitored for the same potential adverse events as adults taking antipsychotics [213]. It is often difficult for a pregnant woman experiencing psychotic symptoms to make an informed decision about whether to start, continue or discontinue psychotropic medication.

Panic disorder and generalized anxiety disorder

Panic disorder is characterized by recurrent unexpected panic attacks with at least 1 month's duration of concern about future panic attacks, worry about the consequences of the panic attacks (e.g. having a heart attack), and a change in behavior due to the panic attacks [2]. Panic attacks involve intense symptoms such as palpitations, chest pain, sensation of shortness of breath, feeling of choking, trembling, sweating, lightheadedness, and fear of losing control or going crazy [2]. Agoraphobia (avoidance of places where help may not be available, or escape not possible, in the event of a panic attack) often accompanies panic disorder [2].

While panic attacks an be experienced occasionally by almost anyone, the prevalence rates of true panic disorder during pregnancy and the postpartum period are similar to the 1–2% prevalence rates in the general population [238,239]. A recent large population survey reported that nicotine dependence during pregnancy was associated with an increased risk of panic disorder [14]. Case–control studies of more than 20,000 birth records in Hungary have reported that untreated panic disorder during pregnancy was associated with isolated cleft lip with or without cleft palate, other congenital abnormalities, PTD, and anemia [240,241].

The course of panic disorder through pregnancy is variable, with some women finding no change in rates of panic attacks while others report fewer or more panic attacks [242–244]. Although a few studies report new-onset or an increase in panic symptoms postpartum or following weaning, the results of studies are mixed [238,245]. Medical conditions that should be ruled out as part of the work-up of new-onset pregnancy or postpartum panic attacks or generalized anxiety include anemia, thyroid dysfunction, pre-eclampsia and pheochromocytoma [238].

Treatment of panic disorder outside pregnancy is successfully achieved by psychotherapy, antidepressant therapy (SSRI or TCA) and often a combination of both these modalities. It is a chronic illness that often requires indefinite treatment although psychotherapy can provide skills that persist after therapy has ceased. Benzodiazepines (typically alprazolam, lorazepam or clonazepam, with the long half-life of clonazepam making rebound anxiety between dosing less likely) may be used in patients who do not benefit from or cannot tolerate an adequate trial of antidepressants. Abuse of and addiction to benzodiazepines is a potential problem, however, and their chronic use is best undertaken with the supervision of a psychiatrist.

Generalized anxiety disorder (GAD) is characterized by chronic excessive anxiety and worry and at least 6 months of restlessness, fatigue, difficulty concentrating, irritability, muscle tension or sleep disturbance [2]. It often occurs in association with other psychiatric diagnoses such as depression, panic disorder or phobias. It can be difficult to differentiate GAD from the normal worries of a pregnant or postpartum woman [238]. The few studies that have examined the prevalence of GAD during pregnancy and the postpartum period have suggested prevalence rates of 4.4–8.5% compared to 5% in the general population [238].

Treatment of GAD outside pregnancy is successfully achieved with psychotherapy (particularly CBT, see above), antidepressants (TCA or SSRI) or a combination of the two therapies. Buspirone is also an effective alternative. While benzodiazepines also have a role in the treatment of GAD, the same cautions apply for their use for this condition as were stated above for panic disorder. One-third of patients with GAD will have long-term recovery with treatment and the rest will require either intermittent or chronic maintenance treatment.

Treatment of panic disorder and GAD in pregnancy

Both panic disorder and GAD have a chronic course; discontinuation of medication often leads to a relapse of symptoms, and maintenance psychotropic medication is common. The reproductive safety of antidepressant and anxiolytic medications needs to be discussed with the pregnant women with panic disorder or GAD and decisions made jointly by the patient and her physician as to the best course for management during a pregnancy. If the woman wishes to attempt to discontinue (or switch) medication, the medication should be tapered (and the new agent introduced) slowly to decrease the likelihood of relapse. CBT or other nonpharmacologic treatments for anxiety disorders could be alternative or adjunctive options for the pregnant and breastfeeding woman with panic disorder or GAD. Ideally, these adjustments should be made prior to conception.

The use of antidepressants in pregnancy is discussed in detail in the preceding section on depression in pregnancy and as stated previously, sertraline and nortriptyline are the preferred agents for use in pregnancy at this time. When possible, transitioning patients to these medications prior to pregnancy is desirable but most clinicians would not make such an adjustment if the patient presents in pregnancy already on one of the other agents.

Little is known about the safety of buspirone in pregnancy but the limited data that exist suggest the agent is not a major teratogen. However, many clinicians find that this medication has only limited efficacy for management of anxiety disorders and decisions to continue this agent in pregnancy should likely occur in the context of documented benefit that was not achieved with an antidepressant agent.

Benzodiazepines are effective treatment for panic disorder, and are also commonly used for other anxiety disorders, insomnia, and depression with co-morbid anxiety. One study reported on birth outcomes in Sweden after *in utero* exposure to either benzodiazepines or hypnotic benzodiazepine receptor agonists such as zolpidem, zaleplon and zopiclone [246]. Both drug classes were associated with pyloric stenosis and alimentary tract atresia, but not orofacial clefts. First-trimester exposure was associated with LBW and PTD, and third-trimester exposure was associated with an increased risk of respiratory problems and low Apgar scores [246]. A previous study had suggested possible association between *in utero* lorazepam exposure and anal atresia [247]. A review of studies published from 1966 to 2000 on the effect of *in utero* exposure to diazepam, chlordiazepoxide, clonazepam, lorazepam and alprazolam suggested an increased risk of oral clefts with first-trimester diazepam exposure [248]. One meta-analysis reported that the increased risk of oral cleft with *in utero* exposure to benzodiazepines was only 0.01%, i.e. an increase from 6 in 10,000 to 7 in 10,000 [117]. Another meta-analysis reported an elevated odds ratio for oral cleft with first-trimester benzodiazepine use of 1.19 from cohort studies and 1.79 from case–control studies [249]. A large case–control study of infants with congenital abnormalities did not identify an association between first-trimester exposure to benzodiazepines and congenital malformations [250] with the exception of possible increased cardiovascular malformations with chlordiazepoxide [251]. A recent study reported that the risk of cardiovascular malformations was increased with first-trimester combined SSRI and benzodiazepine use [122]. Thus, the association of benzodiazepines and hypnotic benzodiazepine receptor agonists with alimentary tract atresia, pyloric stenosis, orofacial clefts and other congenital malformations is unclear. If possible, benzodiazepine use should be avoided during the first-trimester organogenesis period. If anxiolytics are used, shorter half-life benzodiazepines, monotherapy, the lowest possible dose, and divided doses should be considered [248].

Neonatal benzodiazepine withdrawal and floppy infant syndrome are both potential neonatal complications with third-trimester use of benzodiazepines. Neonatal symptoms after third-trimester exposure include irritability, restlessness, hyper-reflexia, hypertonia, abnormal sleep patterns, diarrhea, vomiting, apnea, tremors or jerking of the extremities, and suckling difficulties may persist for weeks [248,252]. Floppy infant syndrome is characterized by hypothermia, lethargy, feeding difficulties, and poor respiratory effort [248,252]. The combined use of clonazepam and paroxetine during the third trimester produced more problematic neonatal symptoms than paroxetine alone [253]. Neonatal symptoms need to be monitored if maternal use of benzodiazepines has occurred close to delivery and slow tapering of benzodiazepines prior to delivery should be attempted if clinically tolerated [252]. Few studies have been conducted on the long-term effects of *in utero* benzodiazepine exposure on child development, but both developmental delays and normal neurobehavioral development have been reported [252].

Overall, the use of benzodiazepines in pregnancy should generally be viewed as a short-term option used to control disease while antidepressant therapy and/or psychotherapy is introduced. Their chronic use is best justified in patients who have failed or not responded to adequate trials of antidepressants and/or psychotherapy and should be done under the supervision of a psychiatrist.

Treatment of anxiety disorders and breastfeeding

Use of antidepressant agents and breastfeeding has been discussed in the section on depression above. Sertraline, paroxetine and nortriptyline are presently considered the preferred antidepressants for breastfeeding mothers. Data to guide recommendations for the use of buspirone are scarce but the medication is unlikely to have significant adverse effects in this setting. However, its limited efficacy should lead clinicians to question whether the breastfeeding mother might benefit more from a medication with more extensive breastfeeding data. Sedation and poor feeding have been reported in breastfeeding infants exposed to benzodiazepines [1] and their use is rated by the American Academy of Pediatrics as "of concern" in breastfeeding mothers. When necessary, they are best used as short-term solutions while awaiting the effects of either an antidepressant or psychotherapy. If

chronic benzodiazepines are given to a breastfeeding mother (and there are many circumstances where this may be justifiable), close observation of the infant for evidence of excessive sleepiness or poor feeding should occur and the lowest effective dose of a benzodiazepine with no active metabolites (e.g. lorazepam or clonazepam) should be used.

Obsessive compulsive disorder

Obsessive compulsive disorder (OCD) is characterized by recurrent and persistent intrusive thoughts and images (obsessions) or excessive repetitive behaviors that the person feels driven to perform (compulsions) [2]. The 1-year prevalence of OCD in the general population is 1.5–2.1% [2]. Psychotherapy and/or antidepressant therapy (particularly the TCA clomipramine or one of the SSRI) are helpful to most patients but this disorder can be particularly difficult to treat.

The prevalence of OCD has been reported to be 0.2–1.2% during pregnancy and 2.7–3.9% during the postpartum period [238]. Several studies report a variable course of OCD during pregnancy [254,255]. Up to one-third of women with OCD retrospectively date the onset of the disorder to pregnancy or the postpartum period [255,256]. Recent studies conducted in Turkey reported an OCD prevalence rate of 3.5% during the third trimester of pregnancy [257] and a 4% incidence of new-onset OCD at 6 weeks post partum [258]. An elevated rate of obstetric complications was reported in a small study of women with OCD [259]. Women with OCD during pregnancy report more contamination obsessions and washing or cleaning rituals, while women with postpartum OCD report more unwanted intrusive obsessional thoughts of harming the infant along with phobic avoidance of fear cues [255]. Concerns about harming the infant accidentally or intentionally also occur in PPD and in new parents not seeking care [58,238]. Once a clinician has ruled out a postpartum psychosis or infanticidal ideation, women with postpartum OCD or obsessional thought about harming the infant should be reassured that the likelihood of acting on thoughts of harm is extremely low.

Pregnancy and postpartum treatment issues

Serotonergic antidepressants (SSRI and clomipramine) are the first-line pharmacologic treatments for OCD, and the safety of these medications with pregnancy and lactation should be discussed with a woman with OCD who is either pregnant or considering a pregnancy. These data are reviewed in the section on depression above. Exposure and response prevention therapy (exposure to the anxiety-producing situations while blocking the rituals) and CBT are effective nonpharmacologic options for OCD. These therapies could be alternative or adjunctive options for the pregnant and breastfeeding woman with OCD.

Post-traumatic stress disorder

Post-traumatic stress disorder (PTSD) occurs after a traumatic event and involves the persistent re-experiencing of the trauma (e.g. recollections, dreams), avoidance of stimuli associated with the trauma, and increased arousal. To meet criteria for this disorder, symptoms should be present for more than 1 month and should have caused impairment both socially and at work [2]. Treatment is typically multifaceted. Nonpharmacologic treatments for PTSD include CBT, exposure therapy, stress inoculation training and eye movement desensitization [276]. Antidepressant medications are the first-line pharmacotherapy for PTSD [276]. Mood stabilizers and antipsychotic medication may be tried in patients unresponsive to standard treatment. Anxiolytics are not helpful and should be avoided.

PTSD in pregnancy

Point prevalence rates of PTSD in pregnant women range from 2.3% to 8.1% [238,260–262], similar to the range of point prevalence rates in nongravid women [238]. PTSD during pregnancy has been associated with higher rates of poor prenatal care, high-risk health behaviors, ectopic pregnancies, miscarriages, hyperemesis, preterm contractions, PTD and LBW [263–267].

A pronounced fear of the upcoming delivery during the late third trimester, or a "pretraumatic stress" syndrome, occurs in some women [268]. This syndrome has been associated with anxiety and depressive symptoms during pregnancy, lack of support, dissatisfaction with partners [268,269], and childhood sexual or physical abuse [270]. Psychoeducation about pain and the delivery process and cognitive techniques can decrease anxiety about delivery and requests for cesarean birth [271]. Fear of childbirth is not necessarily associated with postpartum PTSD or depression [272].

A systematic review reported the development of PTSD in 1.5–6% and of post-traumatic stress symptoms in 24–34% of women following childbirth [273]. Risk factors included obstetric procedures, feelings of loss of control, lack of partner support, trait anxiety, and negative aspects of staff–patient contact [273]. Current interpersonal violence (IPV) [274] and prior trauma and sexual abuse have also been associated with antepartum PTSD [238,261]. Postpartum PTSD has been associated with low mood, avoidance of the baby, impaired mother–infant relationship, impaired relationship with the partner, sexual dysfunction, and avoidance of future childbearing [238,275].

Screening for risk factors and providing extra education and support during the birth process may help prevent the occurrence of PTSD or post-traumatic stress symptoms [277]. A screening measure (Box 21.4) specific to perinatal trauma may identify women who need specific referral [278].

Box 21.4 Modified Perinatal Post-traumatic Stress Disorder Questionnaire (Modified PPQ) [278]

(1) Did you have bad dreams of giving birth or of your baby's hospital stay?

(2) Did you have upsetting memories of giving birth or of your baby's hospital stay?

(3) Did you have any sudden feelings as though your baby's birth was happening again?

(4) Did you try to avoid thinking about childbirth or your baby's hospital stay?

(5) Did you avoid doing things that might bring up feelings you had about childbirth or your baby's hospital stay (e.g. not watching a TV show about babies)?

(6) Were you unable to remember parts of your baby's hospital stay?

(7) Did you lose interest in doing things you usually do (e.g. did you lose interest in your work or family)?

(8) Did you feel alone and removed from other people (e.g. did you feel like no one understood you)?

(9) Did it become more difficult for you to feel tenderness or love with others?

(10) Did you have unusual difficulty falling asleep or staying asleep?

(11) Were you more irritable or angry with others than usual?

(12) Did you have greater difficulties concentrating than before you gave birth?

(13) Did you feel more jumpy (e.g. did you feel more sensitive to noise or more easily startled)?

(14) Did you feel more guilt about the childbirth than you felt you should have felt?

Note: The answer to each question is scored as follows:
(0) if the answer is "not at all";
(1) for "once or twice";
(2) for "sometimes";
(3) for "often, but for less than 1 month";
(4) for "often, for more than a month."
Mothers with a total score of 19 or higher are at high risk for PTSD and should be considered for a referral to a behavioral health specialist for early intervention.

PTSD in pregnancy treatment issues

The detection and treatment of PTSD are important due to the negative consequences of PTSD for the mother and infant [274,276]. As described earlier in the section on depression in pregnancy, the known safety data of antidepressants during pregnancy and lactation should be discussed with women with PTSD who are either pregnant or considering a pregnancy. Similar principles apply as were discussed in the section above dealing with panic and anxiety disorders in pregnancy. Again, nonpharmacologic treatments could be alternative or adjunctive options for the pregnant and breastfeeding woman with PTSD but many women will need to stay on an antidepressant to control their symptoms adequately.

Eating disorders

Eating disorders and pregnancy

The diagnosis, epidemiology and treatment of anorexia nervosa, bulimia nervosa and binge-eating disorder have been reviewed elsewhere in detail [279–282]. The lifetime prevalence for women is 0.9% for anorexia and 3.5% for bulimia. Treatment for both disorders requires an interdisciplinary team of a medical provider, mental health provider and a dietitian. Psychotherapy and antidepressants (particularly SSRI such as fluoxetine) are used for both conditions but are more effective for bulimia. The literature describing outcome for patients with eating disorders is biased toward the description of patients with more severe disease who present to tertiary care centers. Overall, 32–70% of patients have recovered at 20-year follow-up.

Anorexia nervosa and bulimia nervosa in pregnancy

The course of anorexia nervosa and bulimia nervosa through pregnancy has had mixed reports. Several, but not all, studies have suggested improvement in anorexic and bulimic symptoms through pregnancy, perhaps secondary to concern about fetal and infant health [283–285]. Elevated rates of MDD during pregnancy have been observed with both previous and active eating disorders [286]. Women with bulimia nervosa have an increased risk for pregnancy-related nausea and vomiting but do not necessarily have an increased risk for hyperemesis gravidarum [287].

Eating disorders and birth outcome

Active eating disorders have been associated with an increased rate of delivery by cesarean section [288,289]. Several studies have reported negative pregnancy outcomes in women with active or prior eating disorders. A recent study reported that anorexia or bulimia nervosa was associated with fetal growth restriction, PTD, anemia, genitourinary tract infections and labor induction [290]. Another study reported that pregnant women with past or current eating disorders were at greater risk compared to control women for delivering small-for-gestational-age infants, LBW and smaller head circumference [291]. A study reported that

eating disorders identified prior to pregnancy were associated with LBW, PTD and small-for-gestational-age infants [292]. A study in which previous eating disorder diagnosis was ascertained by a "yes/no" question reported that anorexia nervosa was significantly associated with LBW and that bulimia nervosa was significantly associated with increased rates of miscarriage compared with the general population [293]. Another study reported that active bulimia during pregnancy was associated with miscarriage and PTD [294]. However, a prospective cohort study reported that in women with normal weight at the time of conception, a history of anorexia nervosa was not associated with negative birth outcomes [295]. Negative birth outcomes may be due to weight-controlling behaviors and decreased nutrition to the fetus. Negative effects on the fetus may also result from some of the potential medical complications of eating disorders.

Medical complications of anorexia nervosa include bradycardia, hypotension, cardiac conduction abnormalities, arrhythmias, electrolyte and hematologic abnormalities, dehydration, endocrinologic abnormalities and gastrointestinal complications due to food restriction or refeeding [280,296]. Medical complications of bulimia nervosa include electrolyte abnormalities and gastrointestinal complications from purging, and cardiac abnormalities from ipecac use [281,297]. Binge-eating disorder has been associated with higher birth-weight infants and large-for-gestational-age infants, but women with this disorder had higher pre-pregnancy weight and increased weight gain during pregnancy [289].

Treatment of eating disorders in pregnancy and postpartum

Antenatal care should include an assessment of current eating habits as well as previous or current eating disorders. Particularly when poor weight gain or hyperemesis is present, specific inquiries should be made about food restriction, weight preoccupation, binge eating and purging. Women with eating disorders may exhibit shame, denial and secrecy about an eating disorder, and emphasis about the importance of maternal nutrition for fetal well-being may help a woman with an eating disorder to disclose her symptoms to a concerned clinician. Women with known eating disorders need to be monitored after giving birth due to the elevated risks of an exacerbation of the eating disorder and the development of PPD [284,288,294,298,299]. The postpartum period may be a time of altered infant feeding and maternal–infant attachment for mothers with eating disorders [299].

It is clear that current and previous eating disorders can lead to negative birth outcomes. The treatment of the pregnant and postpartum woman with an eating disorder should involve the co-ordinated efforts of a multidisciplinary team including the obstetrician, the primary care clinician, a mental health clinician and dietitian [300,301]. Individual and/or family psychotherapy are the first-line treatments for anorexia nervosa in pregnancy, and CBT is the first-line psychotherapy treatment option for bulimia nervosa [282,302]. Eating disorders in pregnancy that do not respond to psychotherapy and that are interfering with maternal health and nutritional intake may need adjunctive pharmacotherapy. As stated above, medications are not generally effective for anorexia nervosa [303], but emerging data suggest that olanzapine may increase food intake and decrease anxiety associated with eating [304,305]. However, the risk of metabolic syndrome and relative lack of safety data with olanzapine use in pregnancy and breastfeeding have to be considered.

Antidepressant medications are known to be effective in reducing symptoms of bulimia nervosa, at least in the short term [306,307], and their use may be indicated in women with severe binge-eating and purging symptoms during pregnancy. The safety profile of antidepressants with pregnancy and breastfeeding must be considered and is discussed earlier in this chapter.

Conclusion

The screening and identification of psychiatric disorders at prenatal visits need improvement. Multidisciplinary management involving the obstetrician, mental health clinician, and pediatrician is often necessary to optimize care [1]. Even when pregnant women acknowledge the need for treatment of psychiatric disorders, there are many barriers to accessing effective treatment. In addition, the pregnant woman with a psychiatric disorder faces difficult treatment decisions. Untreated stress, anxiety, depression and psychosis, as well as psychotropic medications, each involve exposure to the fetus with potential short-term and long-term adverse effects (summarized in Box 21.5). Women, their partners, and their clinicians should discuss current knowledge about the safety and efficacy of treatment options, the woman's previous psychiatric history and treatment response, and her own preferences, expectations and concerns. Clinicians and patients can monitor websites that update and review published information frequently such as www.otispregnancy.org, www.motherisk. org, www.womensmentalhealth.org, www.mededppd.org, and www.postpartum.net. Although certain medications at the present time have more favorable pregnancy data than others (e.g. sertraline for depression), often maintaining the pregnant woman on the antidepressant or other psychotropic medication that is currently working, and monitoring the fetus, is the optimal treatment course.

Psychiatric illness is perhaps the most common serious nonobstetric condition to complicate pregnancy and there remains a pressing need for systematic longitudinal studies examining the effects of psychotropic medication exposure as well as exposure to untreated psychiatric disease on child cognitive, motor, neurologic and behavioral development. Future

Box 21.5 Risks of untreated psychiatric illness and psychotropic medications during pregnancy

Untreated stress, anxiety and depression

- Obstetric complications, e.g. low birthweight, preterm delivery
- Elevated cortisol levels, developmental delay, sleep problems, cognitive impairment, impulsivity, attention deficit disorder, and other psychiatric disorders in childhood

Antidepressants (SSRI)

- Small increase in miscarriages
- Possible small increase in nonspecific congenital malformations
- Possible small increase of cardiac congenital malformations with paroxetine
- Possible lower birthweight, premature delivery
- Persistent pulmonary hypertension of the newborn (PPHN) with exposure after week 20
- Transient poor neonatal adaptation (e.g. jitteriness, respiratory distress, poor muscle tone)

Benzodiazepines

- Possible small increased risk of oral cleft and other congenital malformations
- "Floppy infant syndrome": neonatal hypotonicity, cyanosis, feeding difficulties
- Neonatal benzodiazepine withdrawal
- Possible developmental delay in children

Lithium

- Increased risk of Ebstein's cardiac malformation
- "Floppy infant syndrome": neonatal hypotonicity, cyanosis, feeding difficulties
- Rare: hypothyroidism, diabetes insipidus, polyhydramnios

Carbamazepine

- Spina bifida, craniofacial abnormalities, growth restriction

Valproate

- Spina bifida, craniofacial abnormalities, cardiovascular abnormalities, growth restriction
- Transient neonatal effects
- Possible lower intelligence in children

Lamotrigine

- Possible increased risk of oral cleft

Antipsychotics

- Possible small increased risk of congenital malformations
- Transient neonatal effects

studies are needed to confirm the efficacy of antidepressants and psychotherapies in pregnancy-related and postpartum depression. Systematic studies of nonpharmacologic and alternative treatments are also needed.

References

1. American College of Obstetricians and Gynecologists. ACOG practice bulletin: clinical management guidelines for obstetrician-gynecologists number 92. Use of psychiatric medications during pregnancy and lactation. Obstet Gynecol 2008;111:1001–20.
2. American Psychiatric Association. Diagnostic and Statistical manual of mental disorders, 4th edn. American Psychiatric Press Washington, DC, 2000.
3. Weissman MM, Bland RC, Canino GJ, et al. Cross-national epidemiology of major depression and bipolar disorder. JAMA 1996;276:293–9.
4. Marcus SM, Flynn HA, Blow FC, Barry KL. Depressive symptoms among pregnant women screened in obstetrics settings. J Womens Health 2003;12:373–80.
5. Bennett IM, Coco A, Coyne JC, et al. Efficiency of a two-item pre-screen to reduce the burden of depression screening in pregnancy and postpartum: an IMPLICIT network study. J Am Board Fam Med 2008;21:317–25.
6. Mitchell AJ, Coyne JC. Do ultra-short screening instruments accurately detect depression in primary care? A pooled analysis and meta-analysis of 22 studies. Br J Gen Pract 2007;57:144–51.
7. Cox JL, Holden JM, Sagovsky R. Detection of postnatal depression. Development of the 10-item Edinburgh Postnatal Depression Scale. Br J Psychiatry 1987;150:782–6.
8. Altshuler LL, Cohen LS, Vitonis AF, et al. The Pregnancy Depression Scale (PDS): a screening tool for depression in pregnancy. Arch Womens Ment Health 2008;11:277–85.
9. Gavin NI, Gaynes BN, Lohr KN, Meltzer-Brody S, Gartlehner G, Swinson T. Perinatal depression: a systematic review of prevalence and incidence. Obstet Gynecol 2005;106:1071–83.
10. Mota N, Cox BJ, Enns MW, Calhoun L, Sareen J. The relationship between mental disorders, quality of life, and pregnancy: findings from a nationally representative sample. J Affect Disord 2008;109:300–4.
11. Vesga-Lopez O, Blanco C, Keyes K, Olfson M, Grant BF, Hasin DS. Psychiatric disorders in pregnant and postpartum women in the United States. Arch Gen Psychiatry 2008;65:805–15.
12. Dietz PM, Williams SB, Callaghan WM, Bachman DJ, Whitlock EP, Hornbrook MC. Clinically identified maternal depression before, during, and after pregnancies ending in live births. Am J Psychiatry 2007;164:1515–20.
13. Halbreich U. Prevalence of mood symptoms and depressions during pregnancy: implications for clinical practice and research. CNS Spectr 2004;9:177–84.
14. Goodwin RD, Keyes K, Simuro N. Mental disorders and nicotine dependence among pregnant women in the United States. Obstet Gynecol 2007;109:875–83.
15. Westdahl C, Milan S, Magriples U, Kershaw TS, Rising SS, Ickovics JR. Social support and social conflict as predictors of prenatal depression. Obstet Gynecol 2007;110:134–40.
16. Martin SL, Li Y, Casanueva C, Harris-Britt A, Kupper LL, Cloutier S. Intimate partner violence and women's depression before and during pregnancy. Violence Against Women 2006;12:221–39.
17. Brandon AR, Trivedi MH, Hynan LS, et al. Prenatal depression in women hospitalized for obstetric risk. J Clin Psychiatry 2008;69:635–43.
18. O'Leary J. Grief and its impact on prenatal attachment in the subsequent pregnancy. Arch Womens Ment Health 2004;7:7–18.
19. Geller PA, Kerns D, Klier CM. Anxiety following miscarriage and the subsequent pregnancy: a review of the literature and future directions. J Psychosom Res 2004;56:35–45.
20. American College of Obstetricians and Gynecologists Committee on Health Care for Underserved Women. ACOG committee opinion no. 343: psychosocial risk factors: perinatal screening and intervention. Obstet Gynecol 2006;108:469–77.
21. Cohen LS, Altshuler LL, Harlow BL, et al. Relapse of major depression during pregnancy in women who maintain or discontinue antidepressant treatment. JAMA 2006;295:499–507.
22. Marcus SM, Flynn HA, Blow F, Barry K. A screening study of antidepressant treatment rates and mood symptoms in pregnancy. Arch Womens Ment Health 2005;8:25–7.
23. Zuckerman B, Amaro H, Bauchner H, Cabral H. Depressive symptoms during pregnancy: relationship to poor health behaviors. Am J Obstet Gynecol 1989;160:1107–11.
24. Hobel CJ, Goldstein A, Barrett ES. Psychosocial stress and pregnancy outcome. Clin Obstet Gynecol 2008;51:333–48.
25. Alder J, Fink N, Bitzer J, Hosli I, Holzgreve W. Depression and anxiety during pregnancy: a risk factor for obstetric, fetal and neonatal outcome? A critical review of the literature. J Matern Fetal Neonatal Med 2007;20:189–209.
26. Beydoun H, Saftlas AF. Physical and mental health outcomes of prenatal maternal stress in human and animal studies: a review of recent evidence. Paediatr Perinat Epidemiol 2008;22:438–66.
27. Bonari L, Pinto N, Ahn E, Einarson A, Steiner M, Koren G. Perinatal risks of untreated depression during pregnancy. Can J Psychiatry 2004;49:726–35.
28. Halbreich U. The association between pregnancy processes, preterm delivery, low birth weight, and postpartum depressions – the need for interdisciplinary integration. Am J Obstet Gynecol 2005;193:1312–22.
29. Li D, Liu L, Odouli R. Presence of depressive symptoms during early pregnancy and the risk of preterm delivery: a prospective cohort study. Hum Reprod 2009;24:146–53.
30. Suri R, Altshuler L, Hellemann G, Burt VK, Aquino A, Mintz J. Effects of antenatal depression and antidepressant treatment on gestational age at birth and risk of preterm birth. Am J Psychiatry 2007;164:1206–13.
31. Evans J, Heron J, Patel RR, Wiles N. Depressive symptoms during pregnancy and low birth weight at term: longitudinal study. Br J Psychiatry 2007;191:84–5.
32. Brennan PA, Pargas R, Walker EF, Green P, Newport DJ, Stowe Z. Maternal depression and infant cortisol: influences of timing, comorbidity and treatment. J Child Psychol Psychiatry 2008;49:1099–107.
33. Field T, Diego M. Maternal depression effects on infant frontal EEG asymmetry. Int J Neurosci 2008;118:1081–108.
34. O'Connor TG, Caprariello P, Blackmore ER, Gregory AM, Glover V, Fleming P. Prenatal mood disturbance predicts sleep problems in infancy and toddlerhood. Early Hum Dev 2007;83:451–8.
35. Deave T, Heron J, Evans J, Emond A. The impact of maternal depression in pregnancy on early child development. Br J Obstet Gynaecol 2008;115:1043–51.
36. Van den Bergh BR, Mulder EJ, Mennes M, Glover V. Antenatal maternal anxiety and stress and the neurobehavioural development of the fetus and child: links and possible mechanisms. A review. Neurosci Biobehav Rev 2005;29:237–58.
37. Hollins K. Consequences of antenatal mental health problems for child health and development. Curr Opin Obstet Gynecol 2007;19:568–72.

38. Pawlby S, Hay DF, Sharp D, Waters CS, O'Keane V. Antenatal depression predicts depression in adolescent offspring: prospective longitudinal community-based study. J Affect Disord 2009:113:236–43.

39. Rich-Edwards JW, Mohllajee AP, Kleinman K, et al. Elevated mid-pregnancy corticotropin-releasing hormone is associated with prenatal, but not postpartum, maternal depression. J Clin Endocrinol Metab 2008;93:1946–51.

40. Field T, Diego M. Cortisol: the culprit prenatal stress variable. Int J Neurosci 2008;118:1181–205.

41. Weinstock M. The long-term behavioural consequences of prenatal stress. Neurosci Biobehav Rev 2008;32:1073–86.

42. Shea AK, Kamath MV, Fleming A, Streiner DL, Redmond K, Steiner M. The effect of depression on heart rate variability during pregnancy. A naturalistic study. Clin Auton Res 2008;18:203–12.

43. Diego MA, Field T, Hernandez-Reif M, Schanberg S, Kuhn C, Gonzalez-Quintero VH. Prenatal depression restricts fetal growth. Early Hum Dev 2009;85:65–70.

44. Wadhwa PD. Psychoneuroendocrine processes in human pregnancy influence fetal development and health. Psychoneuroendocrinology 2005;30:724–43.

45. Talge NM, Neal C, Glover V. Antenatal maternal stress and long-term effects on child neurodevelopment: how and why? J Child Psychol Psychiatry 2007;48:245–61.

46. Newport DJ, Levey LC, Pennell PB, Ragan K, Stowe ZN. Suicidal ideation in pregnancy: assessment and clinical implications. Arch Womens Ment Health 2007;10:181–7.

47. Marzuk PM, Tardiff K, Leon AC, et al. Lower risk of suicide during pregnancy. Am J Psychiatry 1997;154:122–3.

48. Appleby L. Suicide during pregnancy and in the first postnatal year. BMJ 1991;302:137–40.

49. Lindahl V, Pearson JL, Colpe L. Prevalence of suicidality during pregnancy and the postpartum. Arch Womens Ment Health 2005;8:77–87.

50. Gandhi SG, Gilbert WM, McElvy SS, et al. Maternal and neonatal outcomes after attempted suicide. Obstet Gynecol 2006;107:984–90.

51. Henshaw C. Mood disturbance in the early puerperium: a review. Arch Womens Ment Health 2003;6:S33–42.

52. Reck C, Stehle E, Reinig K, Mundt C. Maternity blues as a predictor of DSM-IV depression and anxiety disorders in the first three months postpartum. J Affect Disord 2009; 113:77–87.

53. Stowe ZN, Hostetter AL, Newport DJ. The onset of postpartum depression: implications for clinical screening in obstetrical and primary care. Am J Obstet Gynecol 2005;192:522–6.

54. Kabir K, Sheeder J, Kelly LS. Identifying postpartum depression: are 3 questions as good as 10? Pediatrics 2008;122:e696–702.

55. Beck CT, Gable RK. Further validation of the Postpartum Depression Screening Scale. Nurs Res 2001;50:155–64.

56. Hanusa BH, Scholle SH, Haskett RF, Spadaro K, Wisner KL. Screening for depression in the postpartum period: a comparison of three instruments. J Womens Health 2008;17:585–96.

57. Sharma V, Khan M, Corpse C, Sharma P. Missed bipolarity and psychiatric comorbidity in women with postpartum depression. Bipolar Disord 2008;10:742–7.

58. Fairbrother N, Woody SR. New mothers' thoughts of harm related to the newborn. Arch Womens Ment Health 2008;11:221–9.

59. Lieferman JA, Dauber SE, Heisler K, Paulson JF. Primary care physicians' beliefs and practices toward maternal depression. J Womens Health 2008;17:1143–50.

60. Gjerdingen DK, Yawn BP. Postpartum depression screening: importance, methods, barriers, and recommendations for practice. J Am Board Fam Med 2007;20:280–8.

61. Chaudron LH, Szilagyi PG, Campbell AT, Mounts KO, Mcinerny TK. Legal and ethical considerations: risks and benefits of postpartum depression screening at well-child visits. Pediatrics 2007;119:123–8.

62. Lyons-Ruth K, Wolfe R, Lyubchik A. Depression and the parenting of young children: making the case for early preventive mental health services. Harv Rev Psychiatry 2000;8:148–53.

63. Grace SL, Evindar A, Stewart DE. The effect of postpartum depression on child cognitive development and behavior: a review and critical analysis of the literature. Arch Womens Ment Health 2003;6:263–74.

64. Weissman MM, Wickramaratne P, Nomura Y, Warner V, Pilowsky D, Verdeli H. Offspring of depressed parents: 20 years later. Am J Psychiatry 2006;163:1001–8.

65. O'Mahen HA, Flynn HA. Preferences and perceived barriers to treatment for depression during the perinatal period. J Womens Health 2008;17:1301–9.

66. O'Hara MW, Stuart S, Gorman LL, Wenzel A. Efficacy of interpersonal psychotherapy for postpartum depression. Arch Gen Psychiatry 2000;57:1039–45.

67. Spinelli MG, Endicott J. Controlled clinical trial of interpersonal psychotherapy versus parenting education program for depressed pregnant women. Am J Psychiatry 2003;160:555–62.

68. Rahman A, Malik A, Sikander S, Roberts C, Creed F. Cognitive behaviour therapy-based intervention by community health workers for mothers with depression and their infants in rural Pakistan: a cluster-randomised controlled trial. Lancet 2008;372:902–9.

69. Manber R, Schnyer RN, Allen JJ, Rush AJ, Blasey CM. Acupuncture: a promising treatment for depression during pregnancy. J Affect Disord 2004;83:89–95.

70. Bosco Guerreiro da Silva J. Acupuncture for mild to moderate emotional complaints in pregnancy – a prospective, quasi-randomised, controlled study. Acupunct Med 2007;25:65–71.

71. Field T, Diego MA, Hernandez-Reif M, Schanberg S, Kuhn C. Massage therapy effects on depressed pregnant women. J Psychosom Obstet Gynaecol 2004;25:115–22.

72. Epperson CN, Terman M, Terman JS, et al. Randomized clinical trial of bright light therapy for antepartum depression: preliminary findings. J Clin Psychiatry 2004;65:421–5.

73. Morris SN, Johnson NR. Exercise during pregnancy: a critical appraisal of the literature. J Reprod Med 2005;50:181–8.

74. Su KP, Huang SY, Chiu TH, et al. Omega-3 fatty acids for major depressive disorder during pregnancy: results from a randomized, double-blind, placebo-controlled trial. J Clin Psychiatry 2008;69:644–51.

75. Rees A-M, Austin M-P, Parker GB. Omega-3 fatty acids as a treatment for perinatal depression: randomized double-blind placebo-controlled trial. Aust NZ J Psychiatry 2008;42:199–205.

76. Freeman MP, Davis M, Sinha P, Wisner KL, Hibbeln JR, Gelenberg AJ. Omega-3 fatty acids and supportive psychotherapy for perinatal depression: a randomized placebo-controlled study. J Affect Disord 2008;110:142–8.

77. Pinette MG, Santarpio C, Wax JR, Blackstone J. Electroconvulsive therapy in pregnancy. Obstet Gynecol 2007;110:465–6.

78. Bozkurt A, Karlidere T, Isintas M, Ozmenler NK, Ozsahin A, Yanarates O. Acute and maintenance electroconvulsive therapy for treatment of psychotic depression in a pregnant patient. J ECT 2007;23:185–7.

79. Kasar M, Saatcioglu O, Kutlar T. Electroconvulsive therapy use in pregnancy. J ECT 2007;23:183–4.

80. Eberhard-Gran M, Eskild A, Opjordsmoen S. Treating mood disorders during pregnancy: safety considerations. Drug Saf 2005;28:695–706.

81. Cooper WO, Willy ME, Pont SJ, Ray WA. Increasing use of antidepressants in pregnancy. Am J Obstet Gynecol 2007;196:544, e1–5.

82. Ramos E, Oraichi D, Rey E, Blais L, Berard A. Prevalence and predictors of antidepressant use in a cohort of pregnant women. Br J Obstet Gynaecol 2007;114:1055–64.

83. Oberlander TF, Warburton W, Misri S, Aghajanian J, Hertzman C. Neonatal outcomes after prenatal exposure to selective serotonin reuptake inhibitor antidepressants and maternal depression using population-based linked health data. Arch Gen Psychiatry 2006;63:898–906.

84. Chambers CD, Hernandez-Diaz S, van Marter LJ, et al. Selective serotonin-reuptake inhibitors and risk of persistent pulmonary hypertension of the newborn. N Engl J Med 2006;354:579–87.

85. Bakker MK, Kolling P, van den Berg PB, de Walle HE, de Jong van den Berg LT. Increase in use of selective serotonin reuptake inhibitors in pregnancy during the last decade, a population-based cohort study from the Netherlands. Br J Clin Pharmacol 2008;65:600–6.

86. Hendrick V, Stowe ZN, Altshuler LL, Hwang S, Lee E, Haynes D. Placental passage of antidepressant medications. Am J Psychiatry 2003;160:993–6.

87. Loughhead AM, Fisher AD, Newport DJ, et al. Antidepressants in amniotic fluid: another route of fetal exposure. Am J Psychiatry 2006;163:145–7.

88. DeVane CL, Stowe ZN, Donovan JL, et al. Therapeutic drug monitoring of psychoactive drugs during pregnancy in the genomic era: challenges and opportunities. J Psychopharmacol 2006;20:54–9.

89. Newport DJ, Calamaras MR, DeVane CL, et al. Atypical antipsychotic administration during late pregnancy: placental passage and obstetrical outcomes. Am J Psychiatry 2007;164:1214–20.

90. Hemels ME, Einarson A, Koren G, Lanctot KL, Einarson TR. Antidepressant use during pregnancy and the rates of spontaneous abortions: a meta-analysis. Ann Pharmacother 2005;39:803–9.

91. Rahimi R, Nikfar S, Abdollahi M. Pregnancy outcomes following exposure to serotonin reuptake inhibitors: a meta-analysis of clinical trials. Reprod Toxicol 2006;22:571–5.

92. Chun-Fai-Chan B, Koren G, Fayez I, et al. Pregnancy outcome of women exposed to bupropion during pregnancy: a prospective comparative study. Am J Obstet Gynecol 2005;192:932–6.

93. Djulus J, Koren G, Einarson TR, et al. Exposure to mirtazapine during pregnancy: a prospective, comparative study of birth outcomes. J Clin Psychiatry 2006;67:1280–4.

94. Maschi S, Clavenna A, Campi R, Schiavetti B, Bernat M, Bonati M. Neonatal outcome following pregnancy exposure to antidepressants: a prospective controlled cohort study. Br J Obstet Gynaecol 2008;115:283–9.

95. Davis RL, Rubanowice D, McPhillips H, et al. Risks of congenital malformations and perinatal events among infants exposed to antidepressant medications during pregnancy. Pharmacoepidemiol Drug Saf 2007;16:1086–94.

96. Lennestal R, Kallen B. Delivery outcome in relation to maternal use of some recently introduced antidepressants. J Clin Psychopharmacol 2007;27:607–13.

97. Wen SW, Yang Q, Garner P, et al. Selective serotonin reuptake inhibitors and adverse pregnancy outcomes. Am J Obstet Gynecol 2006;194:961–6.

98. Chambers CD, Johnson KA, Dick LM, Felix RJ, Jones KL. Birth outcomes in pregnant women taking fluoxetine. N Engl J Med 1996;335:1010–15.

99. Simon GE, Cunningham ML, Davis RL. Outcomes of prenatal antidepressant exposure. Am J Psychiatry 2002;159:2055–61.

100. Hendrick V, Smith LM, Suri R, Hwang S, Haynes D, Altshuler L. Birth outcomes after prenatal exposure to antidepressant medication. Am J Obstet Gynecol 2003;188:812–15.

101. Kulin NA, Pastuszak A, Sage SR, et al. Pregnancy outcome following maternal use of the new selective serotonin reuptake inhibitors: a prospective controlled multicenter study. JAMA 1998;279:609–10.

102. Suri R, Altshuler L, Hendrick V, Rasgon N, Lee E, Mintz J. The impact of depression and fluoxetine treatment on obstetrical outcome. Arch Womens Ment Health 2004;7:193–200.

103. Malm H, Klaukka T, Neuvonen PJ. Risks associated with selective serotonin reuptake inhibitors in pregnancy. Obstet Gynecol 2005;106:1289–96.

104. Cohen LS, Heller VL, Bailey JW, Grush L, Ablon JS, Bouffard SM. Birth outcomes following prenatal exposure to fluoxetine. Biol Psychiatry 2000;48:996–1000.

105. Pearson KH, Nonacs RM, Viguera AC, et al. Birth outcomes following prenatal exposure to antidepressants. J Clin Psychiatry 2007;68:1284–9.

106. Oberlander TF, Warburton W, Misri S, Aghajanian J, Hertzman C. Effects of timing and duration of gestational exposure to serotonin reuptake inhibitor antidepressants: population-based study. Br J Psychiatry 2008;192:338–43.

107. Einarson TR, Einarson A. Newer antidepressants in pregnancy and rates of major malformations: a meta-analysis of prospective comparative studies. Pharmacoepidemiol Drug Saf 2005;14:823–7.

108. Pastuszak A, Schick-Boschetto B, Zuber C, et al. Pregnancy outcome following first-trimester exposure to fluoxetine (Prozac). JAMA 1993;269:2246–8.

109. Goldstein DJ, Corbin LA, Sundell KL. Effects of first-trimester fluoxetine exposure on the newborn. Obstet Gynecol 1997;89:713–18.

110. McElhatton PR, Garbis HM, Elefant E, et al. The outcome of pregnancy in 689 women exposed to therapeutic doses of antidepressants. A collaborative study of the European Network of Teratology Information Services (ENTIS). Reprod Toxicol 1996;10:285–94.

111. Sivojelezova A, Shuhaiber S, Sarkissian L, Einarson A, Koren G. Citalopram use in pregnancy: prospective comparative evaluation of pregnancy and fetal outcome. Am J Obstet Gynecol 2005;193:2004–9.

112. Ericson A, Kallen B, Wiholm BE. Delivery outcome after the use of antidepressants in early pregnancy. Eur J Clin Pharmacol 1999;55:503–8.

113. Diav-Citrin O, Schechtman S, Weinbaum D, et al. Paroxetine and fluoxetine in pregnancy: a prospective, multicentre, controlled, observational study. Br J Clin Pharmacol 2008;66:695–705.

114. Einarson A, Bonari L, Voyer-Lavigne S, et al. A multicentre prospective controlled study to determine the safety of trazodone and nefazodone use during pregnancy. Can J Psychiatry 2003;48:106–10.

115. Cole JA, Modell JG, Haight BR, Cosmatos IS, Stoler JM, Walker AM. Bupropion in pregnancy and the prevalence of congenital malformations. Pharmacoepidemiol Drug Saf 2007;16:474–84.

116. Einarson A, Fatoye B, Sarkar M, et al. Pregnancy outcome following gestational exposure to venlafaxine: a multicenter prospective controlled study. Am J Psychiatry 2001;158:1728–30.

117. Altshuler LL, Cohen L, Szuba MP, Burt VK, Gitlin M, Mintz J. Pharmacologic management of psychiatric illness during pregnancy: dilemmas and guidelines. Am J Psychiatry 1996;153:592–606.

118. Louik C, Lin AE, Werler MM, Hernandez-Diaz S, Mitchell AA. First-trimester use of selective serotonin-reuptake inhibitors and the risk of birth defects. N Engl J Med 2007;356:2675–83.

119. Alwan S, Reefhuis J, Rasmussen SA, Olney RS, Friedman JM, Study NBDP. Use of selective serotonin-reuptake inhibitors in pregnancy and the risk of birth defects. N Engl J Med 2007;356:2684–92.

120. Wogelius P, Norgaard M, Gislum M, et al. Maternal use of selective serotonin reuptake inhibitors and risk of congenital malformations. Epidemiology 2006;17:701–4.

121. Ramos E, St-Andre M, Rey E, Oraichi D, Berard A. Duration of antidepressant use during pregnancy and risk of major congenital malformations. Br J Psychiatry 2008;192:344–50.

122. Oberlander TF, Warburton W, Misri S, Riggs W, Aghajanian J, Hertzman C. Major congenital malformations following prenatal exposure to serotonin reuptake inhibitors and benzodiazepines using population-based health data. Birth Defects Res B Dev Reprod Toxicol 2008;83:68–76.

123. Bar-Oz B, Einarson T, Einarson A, et al. Paroxetine and congenital malformations: meta-analysis and consideration of potential confounding factors. Clin Ther 2007;29:918–26.

124. Kallen BA, Otterblad Olausson P. Maternal use of selective serotonin re-uptake inhibitors in early pregnancy and infant congenital malformations. Birth Defects Res A Clin Mol Teratol 2007;79:301–8.

125. Cole JA, Ephross SA, Cosmatos IS, Walker AM. Paroxetine in the first trimester and the prevalence of congenital malformations. Pharmacoepidemiol Drug Saf 2007;16:1075–85.

126. Einarson A, Pistelli A, DeSantis M, et al. Evaluation of the risk of congenital cardiovascular defects associated with use of paroxetine during pregnancy. Am J Psychiatry 2008;165:749–52.

127. O'Brien L, Einarson TR, Sarkar M, Einarson A, Koren G. Does paroxetine cause cardiac malformations? J Obstet Gynaecol Can 2008;30:696–701.

128. ACOG Committee on Obstetric Practice. Committee opinion no. 354: treatment with selective serotonin reuptake inhibitors during pregnancy. Obstet Gynecol 2006;108:1601–3.

129. Koren G, Matsui D, Einarson A, Knoppert D, Steiner M. Is maternal use of selective serotonin reuptake inhibitors in the third trimester of pregnancy harmful to neonates? CMAJ 2005;172:1457–9.

130. Nordeng H, Spigset O. Treatment with selective serotonin reuptake inhibitors in the third trimester of pregnancy: effects on the infant. Drug Saf 2005;28:565–81.

131. Boucher N, Bairam A, Beaulac-Baillargeon L. A new look at the neonate's clinical presentation after in utero exposure to antidepressants in late pregnancy. J Clin Psychopharmacol 2008;28:334–9.

132. Moses-Kolko EL, Bogen D, Perel J, et al. Neonatal signs after late in utero exposure to serotonin reuptake inhibitors: literature review and implications for clinical applications. JAMA 2005;293:2372–83.

133. Ferreira E, Carceller AM, Agogue C, et al. Effects of selective serotonin reuptake inhibitors and venlafaxine during pregnancy in term and preterm neonates. Pediatrics 2007;119:52–9.

134. Levinson-Castiel R, Merlob P, Linder N, Sirota L, Klinger G. Neonatal abstinence syndrome after in utero exposure to selective serotonin reuptake inhibitors in term infants. Arch Pediatr Adolesc Med 2006;160:173–6.

135. Sanz EJ, de-las-Cuevas C, Kiuru A, Bate A, Edwards R. Selective serotonin reuptake inhibitors in pregnant women and neonatal withdrawal syndrome: a database analysis. Lancet 2005;365:482–7.

136. Knoppert DC, Nimkar R, Principi T, Yuen D. Paroxetine toxicity in a newborn after in utero exposure: clinical symptoms correlate with serum levels. Ther Drug Monit 2006;28:5–7.

137. Franssen EJ, Meijs V, Ettaher F, Valerio PG, Keessen M, Lameijer W. Citalopram serum and milk levels in mother and infant during lactation. Ther Drug Monit 2006;28:2–4.

138. Pakalapati RK, Bolisetty S, Austin M-P, Oei J. Neonatal seizures from in utero venlafaxine exposure. J Paediatr Child Health 2006;42:737–8.

139. Koren G, Moretti M, Kapur B. Can venlafaxine in breast milk attenuate the norepinephrine and serotonin reuptake neonatal withdrawal syndrome. J Obstet Gynaecol Can 2006;28:299–302.

140. Sokolover N, Merlob P, Klinger G. Neonatal recurrent prolonged hypothermia associated with maternal mirtazapine treatment during pregnancy. Can J Clin Pharmacol 2008;15:e188–90.

141. Eyal R, Yaeger D. Poor neonatal adaptation after in utero exposure to duloxetine. Am J Psychiatry 2008;165:651.

142. Dubnov-Raz G, Juurlink DN, Fogelman R, et al. Antenatal use of selective serotonin-reuptake inhibitors and QT interval prolongation in newborns. Pediatrics 2008;122:e710–15.

143. Loughhead AM, Stowe ZN, Newport DJ, Ritchie JC, DeVane CL, Owens MJ. Placental passage of tricyclic antidepressants. Biol Psychiatry 2006;59:287–90.

144. ter Horst PG, Jansman FG, van Lingen RA, Smit JP, de Jong-van den Berg LT, Brouwers JR. Pharmacological aspects of neonatal antidepressant withdrawal. Obstet Gynecol Surv 2008;63:267–79.

145. Haddad PM, Pal BR, Clarke P, Wieck A, Sridhiran S. Neonatal symptoms following maternal paroxetine treatment: serotonin toxicity or paroxetine discontinuation syndrome? J Psychopharmacol 2005;19:554–7.

146. Austin MP. To treat or not to treat: maternal depression, SSRI use in pregnancy and adverse neonatal effects. Psychol Med 2006;36:1663–70.

147. Kallen B, Olausson PO. Maternal use of selective serotonin re-uptake inhibitors and persistent pulmonary hypertension of the newborn. Pharmacoepidemiol Drug Saf 2008;17:801–6.

148. Andrade SE, McPhillips H, Loren D, et al. Antidepressant medication use and risk of persistent pulmonary hypertension of the newborn. Pharmacoepidemiol Drug Saf. 2009;18:246–52.

149. Wichman CL, Moore KM, Lang TR, St Sauver JL, Heise RH Jr, Watson WJ. Congenital heart disease associated with selective serotonin reuptake inhibitor use during pregnancy. Mayo Clin Proc 2009;84:23–7.

150. Fornaro E, Li D, Pan J, Belik J. Prenatal exposure to fluoxetine induces fetal pulmonary hypertension in the rat. Am J Respir Crit Care Med 2007;176:1035–40.

151. Gentile S. SSRIs in pregnancy and lactation: emphasis on neurodevelopmental outcome. CNS Drugs 2005;19:623–33.

152. Heikkinen T, Ekblad U, Kero P, Ekblad S, Laine K. Citalopram in pregnancy and lactation. Clin Pharmacol Ther 2002;72:184–91.

153. Nulman I, Rovet J, Stewart DE, et al. Neurodevelopment of children exposed in utero to antidepressant drugs. N Engl J Med 1997;336:258–62.

154. Nulman I, Rovet J, Stewart DE, et al. Child development following exposure to tricyclic antidepressants or fluoxetine throughout fetal life: a prospective, controlled study. Am J Psychiatry 2002;159:1889–95.

155. Oberlander TF, Reebye P, Misri S, Papsdorf M, Kim J, Grunau RE. Externalizing and attentional behaviors in children of depressed mothers treated with a selective serotonin reuptake inhibitor antidepressant during pregnancy. Arch Pediatr Adolesc Med 2007;161:22–9.

156. Misri S, Reebye P, Kendrick K, et al. Internalizing behaviors in 4-year-old children exposed in utero to psychotropic medications. Am J Psychiatry 2006;163:1026–32.

157. Yonkers KA. The treatment of women suffering from depression who are either pregnant or breast feeding. Am J Psychiatry 2007;164:1457–9.

158. Kopelman RC, Moel J, Mertens C, Stuart S, Arndt S, O'Hara MW. Barriers to care for antenatal depression. Psychiatr Serv 2008;59:429–32.

159. Miller LJ, Bishop JR, Fischer JH, Geller SE, Macmillan C. Balancing risks: dosing strategies for antidepressants near the end of pregnancy. J Clin Psychiatry 2008;69:323–4.

160. Gentile S. Serotonin reuptake inhibitor-induced perinatal complications. Paediatr Drugs 2007;9:97–106.

161. Pearlstein TB, Zlotnick C, Battle CL, et al. Patient choice of treatment for postpartum depression: a pilot study. Arch Womens Ment Health 2006;9:303–8.

162. Battle CL, Zlotnick C, Pearlstein T, et al. Depression and breastfeeding: which postpartum patients take antidepressant medications? Depress Anxiety 2008;25:888–91.

163. Chabrol H, Teissedre F, Armitage J, Danel M, Walburg V. Acceptability of psychotherapy and antidepressants for postnatal depression among newly delivered mothers. J Reprod Infant Psychol 2004;22:5–12.

164. Dennis CL, Hodnett E. Psychosocial and psychological interventions for treating postpartum depression. Cochrane Database of Systematic Reviews, 2007;Oct 17;(4):CD006116.

165. Cuijpers P, Brannmark JG, van Straten A. Psychological treatment of postpartum depression: a meta-analysis. J Clin Psychol 2008;64:103–18.

166. Yonkers KA, Lin H, Howell HB, Heath AC, Cohen LS. Pharmacologic treatment of postpartum women with new-onset major depressive disorder: a randomized controlled trial with paroxetine. J Clin Psychiatry 2008;69:659–65.

167. Appleby L, Warner R, Whitton A, Faragher B. A controlled study of fluoxetine and cognitive-behavioural counselling in the treatment of postnatal depression. BMJ 1997;314:932–6.

168. Wisner KL, Hanusa BH, Perel JM, et al. Postpartum depression: a randomized trial of sertraline versus nortriptyline. J Clin Psychopharmacol 2006;26:353–60.

169. Misri S, Reebye P, Corral M, Milis L. The use of paroxetine and cognitive-behavioral therapy in postpartum depression and anxiety: a randomized controlled trial. J Clin Psychiatry 2004;65:1236–41.

170. Pearlstein T. Perinatal depression: treatment options and dilemmas. J Psychiatry Neurosci 2008;33:302–18.

171. Weissman AM, Levy BT, Hartz AJ, et al. Pooled analysis of antidepressant levels in lactating mothers, breast milk, and nursing infants. Am J Psychiatry 2004;161:1066–78.

172. Hallberg P, Sjoblom V. The use of selective serotonin reuptake inhibitors during pregnancy and breast-feeding: a review and clinical aspects. J Clin Psychopharmacol 2005;25:59–73.

173. Gentile S. Use of contemporary antidepressants during breastfeeding: a proposal for a specific safety index. Drug Saf 2007;30:107–21.

174. Hale TW. Medications and mother's milk: a manual of lactational pharmacology. Hale Publising, Amarillo, TX, 2008.

175. Pregnancy and Lactation Labeling on www.fda.gov

176. Gentile S, Rossi A, Bellantuono C. SSRIs during breastfeeding: spotlight on milk-to-plasma ratio. Arch Womens Ment Health 2007;10:39–51.

177. Abreu AC, Stuart S. Pharmacologic and hormonal treatments for postpartum depression. Psychiatr Ann 2005;35:568–76.

178. McElroy SL. Bipolar disorders: special diagnostic and treatment considerations in women. CNS Spectr 2004;9:5–18.

179. Yonkers KA, Wisner KL, Stowe Z, et al. Management of bipolar disorder during pregnancy and the postpartum period. Am J Psychiatry 2004;161:608–20.

180. Newport DJ, Stowe ZN, Viguera AC, et al. Lamotrigine in bipolar disorder: efficacy during pregnancy. Bipolar Disord 2008;10:432–6.

181. Viguera AC, Whitfield T, Baldessarini RJ, et al. Risk of recurrence in women with bipolar disorder during pregnancy: prospective study of mood stabilizer discontinuation. Am J Psychiatry 2007;164:1817–24.

182. MacCabe JH, Martinsson L, Lichtenstein P, et al. Adverse pregnancy outcomes in mothers with affective psychosis. Bipolar Disord 2007;9:305–9.

183. Cohen LS. Treatment of bipolar disorder during pregnancy. J Clin Psychiatry 2007;68:4–9.

184. Payne JL. Antidepressant use in the postpartum period: practical considerations. Am J Psychiatry 2007;164:1329–32.

185. Heron J, Robertson Blackmore E, McGuinness M, Craddock N, Jones I. No 'latent period' in the onset of bipolar affective puerperal psychosis. Arch Womens Ment Health 2007;10:79–81.

186. Sit D, Rothschild AJ, Wisner KL. A review of postpartum psychosis. J Womens Health 2006;15:352–68.

187. Harlow BL, Vitonis AF, Sparen P, Cnattingius S, Joffe H, Hultman CM. Incidence of hospitalization for postpartum psychotic and bipolar episodes in women with and without prior prepregnancy or prenatal psychiatric hospitalizations. Arch Gen Psychiatry 2007;64:42–8.

188. Blackmore ER, Jones I, Doshi M, et al. Obstetric variables associated with bipolar affective puerperal psychosis. Br J Psychiatry 2006;188:32–6.

189. Sharma V. Pharmacotherapy of postpartum psychosis. Expert Opin Pharmacother 2003;4:1651–8.

190. Jones I, Craddock N. Familiality of the puerperal trigger in bipolar disorder: results of a family study. Am J Psychiatry 2001;158:913–17.

191. Friedman SH, Horwitz SM, Resnick PJ. Child murder by mothers: a critical analysis of the current state of knowledge and a research agenda. Am J Psychiatry 2005;162:1578–87.

192. Spinelli MG. Maternal infanticide associated with mental illness: prevention and the promise of saved lives. Am J Psychiatry 2004;161:1548–57.

193. Krischer MK, Stone MH, Sevecke K, Steinmeyer EM. Motives for maternal filicide: results from a study with female forensic patients. Int J Law Psychiatry 2007;30:191–200.

194. Spinelli MG. A systematic investigation of 16 cases of neonaticide. Am J Psychiatry 2001;158:811–13.

195. Ward S, Wisner KL. Collaborative management of women with bipolar disorder during pregnancy and postpartum: pharmacologic considerations. J Midwifery Womens Health 2007;52:3–13.

196. Cohen LS, Friedman JM, Jefferson JW, Johnson EM, Weiner ML. A reevaluation of risk of in utero exposure to lithium. JAMA 1994;271:146–50.

197. Newport DJ, Viguera AC, Beach AJ, Ritchie JC, Cohen LS, Stowe ZN. Lithium placental passage and obstetrical outcome: implications for clinical management during late pregnancy. Am J Psychiatry 2005;162:2162–70.

198. Cramer JA, Gordon J, Schachter S, Devinsky O. Women with epilepsy: hormonal issues from menarche through menopause. Epilepsy Behav 2007;11:160–78.

199. Vajda FJ. Treatment options for pregnant women with epilepsy. Expert Opin Pharmacother 2008;9:1859–68.

200. Eadie MJ. Antiepileptic drugs as human teratogens. Expert Opin Drug Saf 2008;7:195–209.

201. Perucca E. Birth defects after prenatal exposure to antiepileptic drugs. Lancet Neurol 2005;4:781–6.

202. Morrow J, Russell A, Guthrie E, *et al.* Malformation risks of antiepileptic drugs in pregnancy: a prospective study from the UK Epilepsy and Pregnancy Register. J Neurol Neurosurg Psychiatry 2006;77:193–8.

203. Iqbal MM, Gundlapalli SP, Ryan WG, Ryals T, Passman TE. Effects of antimanic mood-stabilizing drugs on fetuses, neonates, and nursing infants. South Med J 2001;94:304–22.

204. Tomson T, Battino D. Pharmacokinetics and therapeutic drug monitoring of newer antiepileptic drugs during pregnancy and the puerperium. Clin Pharmacokinet 2007;46:209–19.

205. Viguera AC, Koukopoulos A, Muzina DJ, Baldessarini RJ. Teratogenicity and anticonvulsants: lessons from neurology to psychiatry. J Clin Psychiatry 2007;68:29–33.

206. Adab N, Kini U, Vinten J, *et al.* The longer term outcome of children born to mothers with epilepsy. J Neurol Neurosurg Psychiatry 2004;75:1575–83.

207. Cunnington M, Tennis P. Lamotrigine and the risk of malformations in pregnancy. Neurology 2005;64:955–60.

208. Holmes LB, Baldwin EJ, Smith CR, *et al.* Increased frequency of isolated cleft palate in infants exposed to lamotrigine during pregnancy. Neurology 2008;70:2152–8.

209. Dolk H, Jentink J, Loane M, Morris JB, de Jong van den Berg LT. Does lamotrigine use in pregnancy increase orofacial cleft risk relative to other malformations? Neurology 2008;71:714–22.

210. Hunt S, Russell A, Smithson WH, *et al.* Topiramate in pregnancy: preliminary experience from the UK Epilepsy and Pregnancy Register. Neurology 2008;71:272–6.

211. Viguera AC, Newport DJ, Ritchie J, *et al.* Lithium in breast milk and nursing infants: clinical implications. Am J Psychiatry 2007;164:342–5.

212. Gentile S. Prophylactic treatment of bipolar disorder in pregnancy and breastfeeding: focus on emerging mood stabilizers. Bipolar Disord 2006;8:207–20.

213. Stowe ZN. The use of mood stabilizers during breastfeeding. J Clin Psychiatry 2007;68:22–8.

214. Newport DJ, Pennell PB, Calamaras MR, *et al.* Lamotrigine in breast milk and nursing infants: determination of exposure. Pediatrics 2008;122:e223–31.

215. McKenna K, Koren G, Tetelbaum M, *et al.* Pregnancy outcome of women using atypical antipsychotic drugs: a prospective comparative study. J Clin Psychiatry 2005;66:444–9.

216. Howard LM. Fertility and pregnancy in women with psychotic disorders. Eur J Obstet Gynecol Reprod Biol 2005;119:3–10.

217. Gregoire A, Pearson S. Risk of pregnancy when changing to atypical antipsychotics. Br J Psychiatry 2002;180:83–4.

218. Gilbert PL, Harris J, McAdams LA, Jeste DV. Neuroleptic withdrawal in schizophrenic patients. A review of the literature. Arch Gen Psychiatry 1995;52:173–88.

219. Ellman LM, Huttunen M, Lonnqvist J, Cannon TD. The effects of genetic liability for schizophrenia and maternal smoking during pregnancy on obstetric complications. Schizophr Res 2007;93:229–36.

220. Jablensky AV, Morgan V, Zubrick SR, Bower C, Yellachich LA. Pregnancy, delivery, and neonatal complications in a population cohort of women with schizophrenia and major affective disorders. Am J Psychiatry 2005;162:79–91.

221. Nilsson E, Lichtenstein P, Cnattingius S, Murray RM, Hultman CM. Women with schizophrenia: pregnancy outcome and infant death among their offspring. Schizophr Res 2002;58:221–9.

222. Bennedsen BE, Mortensen PB, Olesen AV, Henriksen TB. Congenital malformations, stillbirths, and infant deaths among children of women with schizophrenia. Arch Gen Psychiatry 2001;58:674–9.

223. Yaeger D, Smith HG, Altshuler LL. Atypical antipsychotics in the treatment of schizophrenia during pregnancy and the postpartum. Am J Psychiatry 2006;163:2064–70.

224. Trixler M, Gati A, Fekete S, Tenyi T. Use of antipsychotics in the management of schizophrenia during pregnancy. Drugs 2005;65:1193–206.

225. Pinkofsky HB. Effects of antipsychotics on the unborn child: what is known and how should this influence prescribing? Paediatr Drugs 2000;2:83–90.

226. McElhatton PR. The use of phenothiazines during pregnancy and lactation. Reprod Toxicol 1992;6:475–90.

227. Reis M, Kallen B. Maternal use of antipsychotics in early pregnancy and delivery outcome. J Clin Psychopharmacol 2008;28:279–88.

228. Gentile S. Antipsychotic therapy during early and late pregnancy. A systematic review. Schizophr Bull 2008;Sep 11 [Epub ahead of print].

229. Diav-Citrin O, Shechtman S, Ornoy S, *et al.* Safety of haloperidol and penfluridol in pregnancy: a multicenter, prospective, controlled study. J Clin Psychiatry 2005;66:317–22.

230. Newham JJ, Thomas SH, MacRitchie K, McElhatton PR, McAllister-Williams RH. Birth weight of infants after maternal exposure to typical and atypical antipsychotics: prospective comparison study. Br J Psychiatry 2008;192:333–7.

231. Howard L, Webb R, Abel K. Safety of antipsychotic drugs for pregnant and breastfeeding women with non-affective psychosis. BMJ 2004;329:933–4.

232. Ernst CL, Goldberg JF. The reproductive safety profile of mood stabilizers, atypical antipsychotics, and broad-spectrum psychotropics. J Clin Psychiatry 2002;63:42–55.

233. McCauley-Elsom K, Kulkarni J. Managing psychosis in pregnancy. Aust NZ J Psychiatry 2007;41:289–92.

234. Wisner KL, Sit DK, Moses-Kolko EL. Antipsychotic treatment during pregnancy: a model for decision making. Adv Schizophr Clin Psychiatry 2007;3:48–55.

235. Lenroot R, Bustillo JR, Lauriello J, Keith SJ. Integrated treatment of schizophrenia. Psychiatr Serv 2003;54:1499–507.

236. Gentile S. Infant safety with antipsychotic therapy in breast-feeding: a systematic review. J Clin Psychiatry 2008; 69:666–73.

237. Seeman MV. Relational ethics: when mothers suffer from psychosis. Arch Womens Ment Health 2004;7:201–10.

238. Ross LE, McLean LM. Anxiety disorders during pregnancy and the postpartum period: a systematic review. J Clin Psychiatry 2006;67:1285–98.

239. Navarro P, Garcia-Esteve L, Ascaso C, Aguado J, Gelabert E, Martin-Santos R. Non-psychotic psychiatric disorders after childbirth: prevalence and comorbidity in a community sample. J Affect Disord 2008;109:171–6.

240. Banhidy F, Acs N, Puho E, Czeizel AE. Association between maternal panic disorders and pregnancy complications and delivery outcomes. Eur J Obstet Gynecol Reprod Biol 2006; 124:47–52.

241. Acs N, Banhidy F, Horvath-Puho E, Czeizel AE. Maternal panic disorder and congenital abnormalities: a population-based case-control study. Birth Defects Res A Clin Mol Teratol 2006;76:253–61.

242. Bandelow B, Sojka F, Broocks A, Hajak G, Bleich S, Ruther E. Panic disorder during pregnancy and postpartum period. Eur J Psychiatry 2006;21:495–500.

243. Dannon PN, Iancu I, Lowengrub K, Grunhaus L, Kotler M. Recurrence of panic disorder during pregnancy: a 7-year naturalistic follow-up study. Clin Neuropharmacol 2006; 29:132–7.

244. Hertzberg T, Wahlbeck K. The impact of pregnancy and puerperium on panic disorder: a review. J Psychosom Obstet Gynaecol 1999;20:59–64.

245. Guler O, Koken GN, Emul M, et al. Course of panic disorder during the early postpartum period: a prospective analysis. Compr Psychiatry 2008;49:30–4.

246. Wikner BN, Stiller CO, Bergman U, Asker C, Kallen B. Use of benzodiazepines and benzodiazepine receptor agonists during pregnancy: neonatal outcome and congenital malformations. Pharmacoepidemiol Drug Saf 2007;16:1203–10.

247. Bonnot O, Vollset SE, Godet PF, d'Amato T, Robert E. Maternal exposure to lorazepam and anal atresia in newborns: results from a hypothesis-generating study of benzodiazepines and malformations. J Clin Psychopharmacol 2001;21:456–8.

248. Iqbal MM, Sobhan T, Ryals T. Effects of commonly used benzodiazepines on the fetus, the neonate, and the nursing infant. Psychiatr Serv 2002;53:39–49.

249. Dolovich LR, Addis A, Vaillancourt JM, Power JD, Koren G, Einarson TR. Benzodiazepine use in pregnancy and major malformations or oral cleft: meta-analysis of cohort and case-control studies. BMJ 1998;317:839–43.

250. Eros E, Czeizel AE, Rockenbauer M, Sorensen HT, Olsen J. A population-based case-control teratologic study of nitrazepam, medazepam, tofisopam, alprazolam and clonazepam treatment during pregnancy. Eur J Obstet Gynecol Reprod Biol 2002;101:147–54.

251. Czeizel AE, Rockenbauer M, Sorensen HT, Olsen J. A population-based case-control study of oral chlordiazepoxide use during pregnancy and risk of congenital abnormalities. Neurotoxicol Teratol 2004;26:593–8.

252. Levey L, Ragan K, Hower-Hartley A, Newport DJ, Stowe ZN. Psychiatric disorders in pregnancy. Neurol Clin 2004;22:863–93.

253. Oberlander TF, Misri S, Fitzgerald CE, Kostaras X, Rurak D, Riggs W. Pharmacologic factors associated with transient neonatal symptoms following prenatal psychotropic medication exposure. J Clin Psychiatry 2004;65:230–7.

254. Williams KE, Koran LM. Obsessive-compulsive disorder in pregnancy, the puerperium, and the premenstruum. J Clin Psychiatry 1997;58:330–4.

255. Abramowitz JS, Schwartz SA, Moore KM, Luenzmann KR. Obsessive-compulsive symptoms in pregnancy and the puerperium: a review of the literature. J Anxiety Disord 2003;17:461–78.

256. Pigott TA. Anxiety disorders in women. Psychiatr Clin North Am 2003;26:621–72.

257. Uguz F, Gezginc K, Zeytinci IE, et al. Obsessive-compulsive disorder in pregnant women during the third trimester of pregnancy. Compr Psychiatry 2007;48:441–5.

258. Uguz F, Akman C, Kaya N, Cilli AS. Postpartum-onset obsessive-compulsive disorder: incidence, clinical features, and related factors. J Clin Psychiatry 2007;68:132–8.

259. Maina G, Albert U, Bogetto F, Vaschetto P, Ravizza L. Recent life events and obsessive-compulsive disorder (OCD): the role of pregnancy/delivery. Psychiatry Res 1999;89:49–58.

260. Ayers S, Pickering AD. Do women get posttraumatic stress disorder as a result of childbirth? A prospective study of incidence. Birth 2001;28:111–18.

261. Loveland Cook CA, Flick LH, Homan SM, Campbell C, McSweeney M, Gallagher ME. Posttraumatic stress disorder in pregnancy: prevalence, risk factors, and treatment. Obstet Gynecol 2004;103:710–17.

262. Smith MV, Poschman K, Cavaleri MA, Howell HB, Yonkers KA. Symptoms of posttraumatic stress disorder in a community sample of low-income pregnant women. Am J Psychiatry 2006;163:881–4.

263. Seng JS, Low LK, Ben-Ami D, Liberzon I. Cortisol level and perinatal outcome in pregnant women with posttraumatic stress disorder: a pilot study. J Midwifery Womens Health 2005;50:392–8.

264. Seng JS, Oakley DJ, Sampselle CM, Killion C, Graham-Bermann S, Liberzon I. Posttraumatic stress disorder and pregnancy complications. Obstet Gynecol 2001;97:17–22.

265. Rogal SS, Poschman K, Belanger K, et al. Effects of posttraumatic stress disorder on pregnancy outcomes. J Affect Disord 2007;102:137–43.

266. Morland L, Goebert D, Onoye J, et al. Posttraumatic stress disorder and pregnancy health: preliminary update and implications. Psychosomatics 2007;48:304–8.

267. Rosen D, Seng JS, Tolman RM, Mallinger G. Intimate partner violence, depression, and posttraumatic stress disorder as additional predictors of low birth weight infants among low-income mothers. J Interpers Violence 2007;22:1305–14.

268. Soderquist J, Wijma K, Wijma B. Traumatic stress in late pregnancy. J Anxiety Disord 2004;18:127–42.

269. Saisto T, Halmesmaki E. Fear of childbirth: a neglected dilemma. Acta Obstet Gynecol Scand 2003;82:201–8.

270. Heimstad R, Dahloe R, Laache I, Skogvoll E, Schei B. Fear of childbirth and history of abuse: implications for pregnancy and delivery. Acta Obstet Gynecol Scand 2006;85:435–40.

271. Saisto T, Salmela-Aro K, Nurmi J-E, Kononen T, Halmesmaki E. A randomized controlled trial of intervention in fear of childbirth. Obstet Gynecol 2001;98:820–6.

272. Fairbrother N, Woody SR. Fear of childbirth and obstetrical events as predictors of postnatal symptoms of depression and post-traumatic stress disorder. J Psychosom Obstet Gynaecol 2007;28:239–42.

273. Olde E, van der Hart O, Kleber R, van Son M. Posttraumatic stress following childbirth: a review. Clin Psychol Rev 2006;26:1–16.

274. Kendall-Tackett KA. Violence against women and the perinatal period: the impact of lifetime violence and abuse on pregnancy, postpartum, and breastfeeding. Trauma Violence Abuse 2007;8:344–53.

275. Ayers S, Eagle A, Waring H. The effects of childbirth-related post-traumatic stress disorder on women and their relationships: a qualitative study. Psychol Health Med 2006;11:389–98.

276. Seedat S, Stein DJ, Carey PD. Post-traumatic stress disorder in women: epidemiological and treatment issues. CNS Drugs 2005;19:411–27.

277. Ayers S. Delivery as a traumatic event: prevalence, risk factors, and treatment for postnatal posttraumatic stress disorder. Clin Obstet Gynecol 2004;47:552–67.

278. Callahan JL, Borja SE. Psychological outcomes and measurement of maternal posttraumatic stress disorder during the perinatal period. J Perinat Neonatal Nurs 2008;22:49–59.

279. Mehler PS. Clinical practice. Bulimia nervosa. N Engl J Med 2003;349:875–81.

280. Yager J, Andersen AE. Clinical practice. Anorexia nervosa. N Engl J Med 2005;353:1481–8.

281. Rome ES. Eating disorders. Obstet Gynecol Clin North Am 2003;30:353–77.

282. American Psychiatric Association. Treatment of patients with eating disorders, 3rd edn. Am J Psychiatry 2006;163 (7 suppl):4–54.

283. Bulik CM, von Holle A, Hamer R, et al. Patterns of remission, continuation and incidence of broadly defined eating disorders during early pregnancy in the Norwegian Mother and Child Cohort Study (MoBa). Psychol Med 2007;37:1109–18.

284. Blais MA, Becker AE, Burwell RA, et al. Pregnancy: outcome and impact on symptomatology in a cohort of eating-disordered women. Int J Eat Disord 2000;27:140–9.

285. Crow SJ, Agras WS, Crosby R, Halmi K, Mitchell JE. Eating disorder symptoms in pregnancy: a prospective study. Int J Eat Disord 2008;41:277–9.

286. Mazzeo SE, Slof-Op't Landt MC, Jones I, et al. Associations among postpartum depression, eating disorders, and perfectionism in a population-based sample of adult women. Int J Eat Disord 2006;39:202–11.

287. Torgersen L, von Holle A, Reichborn-Kjennerud T, et al. Nausea and vomiting of pregnancy in women with bulimia nervosa and eating disorders not otherwise specified. Int J Eat Disord 2008;41:722–7.

288. Franko DL, Blais MA, Becker AE, et al. Pregnancy complications and neonatal outcomes in women with eating disorders. Am J Psychiatry 2001;158:1461–6.

289. Bulik CM, von Holle A, Siega-Riz AM, et al. Birth outcomes in women with eating disorders in the Norwegian Mother and Child cohort study (MoBa). Int J Eat Disord 2009;42:9–18.

290. Bansil P, Kuklina EV, Whiteman MK, et al. Eating disorders among delivery hospitalizations: prevalence and outcomes. J Womens Health 2008;17:1523–8.

291. Kouba S, Hallstrom T, Lindholm C, Hirschberg AL. Pregnancy and neonatal outcomes in women with eating disorders. Obstet Gynecol 2005;105:255–60.

292. Sollid CP, Wisborg K, Hjort J, Secher NJ. Eating disorder that was diagnosed before pregnancy and pregnancy outcome. Am J Obstet Gynecol 2004;190:206–10.

293. Micali N, Simonoff E, Treasure J. Risk of major adverse perinatal outcomes in women with eating disorders. Br J Psychiatry 2007;190:255–9.

294. Morgan JF, Lacey JH, Chung E. Risk of postnatal depression, miscarriage, and preterm birth in bulimia nervosa: retrospective controlled study. Psychosom Med 2006;68:487–92.

295. Ekeus C, Lindberg L, Lindblad F, Hjern A. Birth outcomes and pregnancy complications in women with a history of anorexia nervosa. Br J Obstet Gynaecol 2006;113:925–9.

296. Mehler PS, Krantz M. Anorexia nervosa medical issues. J Womens Health 2003;12:331–40.

297. Mehler PS, Crews C, Weiner K. Bulimia: medical complications. J Womens Health 2004;13:668–75.

298. Morgan JF, Lacey JH, Sedgwick PM. Impact of pregnancy on bulimia nervosa. Br J Psychiatry 1999;174:135–40.

299. Astrachan-Fletcher E, Veldhuis C, Lively N, Fowler C, Marcks B. The reciprocal effects of eating disorders and the postpartum period: a review of the literature and recommendations for clinical care. J Womens Health 2008;17:227–39.

300. Wolfe BE. Reproductive health in women with eating disorders. J Obstet Gynecol Neonatal Nurs 2005;34:255–63.

301. Franko DL, Spurrell EB. Detection and management of eating disorders during pregnancy. Obstet Gynecol 2000;95:942–6.

302. Wilson GT, Grilo CM, Vitousek KM. Psychological treatment of eating disorders. Am Psychol 2007;62:199–216.

303. Bulik CM, Berkman ND, Brownley KA, Sedway JA, Lohr KN. Anorexia nervosa treatment: a systematic review of randomized controlled trials. Int J Eat Disord 2007;40:310–20.

304. Bissada H, Tasca GA, Barber AM, Bradwejn J. Olanzapine in the treatment of low body weight and obsessive thinking in women with anorexia nervosa: a randomized, double-blind, placebo-controlled trial. Am J Psychiatry 2008;165:1281–8.

305. Mehler-Wex C, Romanos M, Kirchheiner J, Schulze UM. Atypical antipsychotics in severe anorexia nervosa in children and adolescents – review and case reports. Eur Eat Disord Rev 2008;16:100–8.

306. Mitchell JE, Agras S, Wonderlich S. Treatment of bulimia nervosa: where are we and where are we going? Int J Eat Disord 2007;40:95–101.

307. Shapiro JR, Berkman ND, Brownley KA, Sedway JA, Lohr KN, Bulik CM. Bulimia nervosa treatment: a systematic review of randomized controlled trials. Int J Eat Disord 2007;40:321–36.

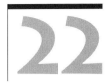

22 Cancer in pregnancy

Sunanda Sadanandan[1]*, Timothy Hurley*[2]*, Carolyn Muller*[3]*,
Claire Verschraegen*[4]*, Marianne Berwick*[5]*, Charles L. Wiggins*[6]
and Kimberly K. Leslie[7]

Departments of Obstetrics and Gynecology[1,2,3,7] and Internal Medicine[4,5,6] and the Cancer Research and Treatment Center[4,5,6,7] of the University of New Mexico Health Sciences Center, Albuquerque, NM, USA

Introduction

Cancer complicates approximately one in 1000 pregnancies. Assisted by new technologies, older women are successfully achieving pregnancies at a higher rate than in the past. As a result, the incidence of cancer complicating pregnancy may increase in the future. The purpose of this chapter is to review the known literature on the diagnosis and management of some of the most common malignancies encountered during pregnancy. Cervical cancer is the most frequent tumor type, followed by breast cancer and melanoma. Other malignancies seen more rarely are ovarian cancer, leukemia, and lymphoma, which will also be discussed. The management of pregnant women with cancer presents a major challenge to the caregiving team: the risks and benefits of treatment must be weighed for both the mother and the fetus. In addition, patients who are pregnant not infrequently present at a later stage compared to nonpregnant women, fueling a debate as to whether pregnancy itself accelerates the progression of some types of tumors. Regardless of whether pregnancy increases the risk for cancer progression or not, it is likely that clinicians will encounter a disproportionate number of women with more advanced disease in pregnancy necessitating aggressive management to achieve a cure. This chapter provides an overview and some guidelines to assist physicians treating patients with pregnancy-associated malignancies.

Cervical neoplasia complicating pregnancy

Cervical cancer is the most common malignancy diagnosed in pregnancy. This may be related to the fact that it is the one

de Swiet's Medical Disorders in Obstetric Practice, 5th edition.
Edited by R. O. Powrie, M. F. Greene, W. Camann. © 2010 Blackwell Publishing.

type of cancer for which screening is routinely performed on the first prenatal visit. The incidence of cervical cancer is 0.45–1 per 1000 livebirths in the United States, with carcinoma *in situ* occurring in 1 in 750 pregnancies [1]. In the United States from 2001 to 2005 the median age of diagnosis for cervical cancer was 48 years of age. Approximately 0.1% were diagnosed under age 20, 15.2% between 20 and 34, 25.9% between 35 and 44, 23.4% between 45 and 54, 15.5% between 55 and 64, 10.4% between 65 and 74, 6.8% between 75 and 84, and 2.5% at 85 years and above [2].

Screening and preinvasive cervical disease

Cervical dysplasia and cancer are strongly associated with infection from the human papilloma virus (HPV). HPV is the most commonly diagnosed sexually transmitted disease in the United States. It is a double-stranded DNA virus that causes condyloma acuminata (low-risk types) and cancer of the vagina, vulva, and anus as well as cervical dysplasia and cancer (oncogenic types). Oncogenic HPV types 16 and 18 account for nearly 70% of invasive cervical cancers in the US and are more frequently isolated in cervical cancer tissue than either intermediate (31,33,35,39,45,51,52,58) or low-risk types (6,11,42,43,44), with type 16 accounting for approximately 50% of cases [3]. However, not all infections with HPV types 16 or 18 progress to cervical cancer. In general, HPV infections in pregnancy that cause cervical dysplasia do not seem to be more aggressive despite the presumed immunosuppressed state [4–6]. However, the low-risk HPV types that account for the condylomatous changes can rapidly proliferate in pregnancy, presumably due to hormonal influences.

Screening in pregnancy is recommended at the first prenatal visit and again at 6 weeks post partum. Most experts advocate using liquid-based cytology because of a lower false-negative rate; this technique also allows for reflex HPV typing if an abnormality is found. During pregnancy Pap smears should be interpreted and evaluated as in the nonpregnant state following the 2006 Bethesda guidelines [7]. For the diagnosis of atypical squamous cells of unknown significance (ASCUS), it is appropriate to request HPV reflex testing and refer the patient for colposcopy only if the lesion is positive for a high- or intermediate-risk HPV type. If dysplasia is diagnosed, reflex HPV typing should be performed, but colposcopy is indicated regardless of the HPV type.

Colposcopy should be performed by an experienced practitioner who is familiar with the cervical changes associated with pregnancy, including the proliferation of the glandular epithelium. Endocervical curettage (ECC) is contraindicated during pregnancy. All squamous intraepithelial lesions, including both low and high grades (LSIL and HSIL, respectively) and any patient with HIV and an ASCUS Pap should undergo colposcopy [7]. Due to the increased risk of bleeding, biopsies should only be performed if an area is suspicious for invasive disease. Cervical conization should be performed only if invasive disease cannot be ruled out by biopsy and should be done by an expert with complete understanding of the potential impact to the pregnancy. Most of the time, conservative management is all that is required, with follow-up throughout gestation if needed, because cervical dysplasia rarely progresses to invasive cancer during the relatively short period of gestation [6]. The timing of the repeat Pap or colposcopy evaluation depends on the initial diagnosis and the point in gestation [6]. It is customary to repeat the Pap and colposcopy every 8–12 weeks [1], particularly for high-grade lesions in women at high risk for developing cervical cancer. In women at low risk for invasive cervical cancer, such as pregnant adolescent and young women, it is reasonable to defer colposcopy until after birth [7]. Postpartum colposcopy should be performed at 6 weeks for all cases of dysplasia followed during pregnancy. Regression of high- and low-grade lesions is not uncommon after delivery. Low-grade lesions are more likely to regress, just as in the nonpregnant state, and rates of regression for LSIL are reported to be 36–70% [8–10]. High-grade lesions and carcinoma *in situ* regress at rates of 48–70%, with the overall progression of premalignant lesions to cancer reported as being only 0.4% [6,10,11].

Treatment of cervical cancer

Treatment of cervical cancer during pregnancy is complicated by the need to preserve fertility and the ongoing pregnancy, and therapeutic options will be partly determined by the gestational age at presentation. As reviewed above, cervical conization should be reserved for definitive diagnosis of invasive malignant disease. The pregnant cervix is significantly more vascular than in the nonpregnant state. Therefore, if conization is required, caution must be exercised because of the increased risk of hemorrhage. If invasive disease is suspected early in gestation, between 16 and 20 weeks, a cone biopsy should be performed, and consideration should be given to the placement of a cerclage to maintain cervical competence [6]. At later gestational ages, a cone biopsy can also be performed when invasive cancer is suspected; however, it should not be performed

within 4 weeks of anticipated delivery. This is due to the fact that cervical healing may not be complete by the time of labor, and the risk of hemorrhage could be significantly increased [6]. Instead of a complete cone biopsy, some providers perform a "wedge biopsy" or "coin-shaped resection" which may provide enough information without causing excessive bleeding or other deleterious effects on the pregnancy. Complications of cone biopsies of the cervix during pregnancy include preterm premature rupture membranes (PPROM) and preterm labor. A retrospective study showed a 1.9- and 2.7-fold increase in PPROM with loop electrocautery excision procedures (LEEP) or laser conization, respectively [12]. However, no difference was noted in preterm delivery rates, and the increased risk of PPROM was proportional to the amount of tissue that was removed [12]. Other data have supported an increased risk of preterm delivery with cone ablations of 10 mm depth or greater [13].

The management of pregnant patients diagnosed with invasive disease depends upon the stage, the gestational age, and whether the pregnancy is highly desired. Cervical cancer staging is described in Box 22.1. Each case should be individualized, and a multidisciplinary approach including input from obstetricians, gynecologists, oncologists, and neonatologists is required. For cancers diagnosed in the third trimester, there is substantial evidence that early-stage cancers are unlikely to spread significantly during pregnancy, and delay of definitive treatment until after pregnancy does not adversely affect outcome. For more advanced cases, it is often acceptable to delay therapy but to deliver early so that definitive treatment can be undertaken. However, the work-up of more advanced-stage cancers may require special imaging and are more difficult to manage with an ongoing pregnancy to consider. Fortunately, many pregnant women diagnosed with cervical cancer have early-stage cancer (IA1, IA2 microinvasive) or stages IB1 and IB2 (visible lesion confined to the cervix). If the stage has been diagnosed as very early microinvasive without lymphovascular invasion, a vaginal delivery is acceptable with therapeutic conization in the postpartum period. If the stage is IA1 (+lymphovascular invasion), IA2, IB1 or IB2, a cesarean radical hysterectomy should be considered with appropriate adjuvant therapy individualized to the patient following delivery. Vaginal delivery is contraindicated with any visible invasive cervical lesions (IB) [14–17].

In the first and second trimesters, the diagnosis of cervical cancer is more challenging. Accurate dating is important and may dictate the management. Prior to 20 weeks, management will first depend upon how strongly the patient wishes to maintain this pregnancy. If the pregnancy is not highly desired, then termination followed by the appropriate surgery may be offered. As viability approaches, particularly between 22 and 24 weeks of gestation, termination may be more difficult to accomplish depending on state and ethical concerns. Regardless of gestational age, if the pregnancy is desired, treatment for early-stage disease can generally be delayed to allow for fetal lung maturity. Advanced-stage cancers diagnosed early in the pregnancy are

Box 22.1 Cervical cancer staging

Stage 0: The tumor is carcinoma *in situ*. If your cancer is in this stage, it is very superficial (only affecting the surface), is found only in the layer of cells lining the cervix, and has not invaded deeper tissues of the cervix.

Stage I: If your cancer is this stage, it has invaded the cervix, but it has not spread anywhere else.

Stage IA: This is the earliest form of stage I. There is a very small amount of cancer, and it can be seen only under a microscope.

- **Stage IA1:** The area of invasion is less than 3 mm (about 1/8 inch) deep and less than 7 mm (about 1/4-inch) wide.
- **Stage IA2:** The area of invasion is between 3 mm and 5 mm (about 1/5 inch) deep and less than 7 mm (about 1/4 inch) wide.

Stage IB: In this stage, the cancer usually can be seen without a microscope. But this stage also includes cancers that have spread deeper than 5 mm (about 1/5 inch) into connective tissue of the cervix or are wider than 7 mm and can only be seen using a microscope.

- **Stage IB1:** The cancer is visible but no larger than 4 cm (about 1 3/5 inches).
- **Stage IB2:** The cancer is visible and larger than 4 cm.
- **Stage II:** In this stage, the cancer has spread beyond the cervix to nearby areas, but it is still inside the pelvic area.
- **Stage IIA:** The cancer has spread beyond the cervix to the upper part of the vagina. It is not in the lower third of the vagina.
- **Stage IIB:** The cancer has spread to the tissue next to the cervix, called the parametrial tissue.

Stage III: The cancer has spread to the lower part of the vagina or the pelvic wall. The cancer may be blocking the ureters (tubes that carry urine from the kidneys to the bladder).

> **Stage IIIA:** The cancer has spread to the lower third of the vagina but not to the pelvic wall.

> **Stage IIIB:** The cancer extends to the pelvic wall and/or blocks urine flow to the bladder.

Note: In the alternative staging system by the American Joint Committee on Cancer, stage IIIB is defined by the fact that the cancer has spread to lymph nodes in the pelvis.

Stage IV: This is the most advanced stage of cervical cancer. The cancer has spread to nearby organs or other parts of the body.

> **Stage IVA:** The cancer has spread to the bladder or rectum, which are organs close to the cervix.

> **Stage IVB:** The cancer has spread to distant organs beyond the pelvic area, such as the lungs.

more difficult to manage, especially for desired pregnancies. For advanced disease, it is not as clear what risks may be incurred by waiting for definitive therapy. However, evidence suggests no difference in prognosis with delay in many cases [18]. For cases involving advanced cervical cancers diagnosed early in pregnancy, extensive counseling as to management options is warranted and documentation of informed consent is required.

Breast cancer in pregnancy

Breast cancer is considered to be associated with pregnancy if the diagnosis is made during a pregnancy or within 1 year of delivery [19]. Approximately one in 3000–10,000 women will be diagnosed with a malignant breast tumor that is associated with a pregnancy [20–23]. For premenopausal women, it is striking that one in three to four breast cancers is associated with pregnancy according to the precise definition [24,25]. In addition, given the potentially prolonged occult growth period of breast tumors, it is likely that many more cancers are present during and influenced by a preceding pregnancy, perhaps years before the diagnosis is actually made.

The breast undergoes remarkable epithelial cell hypertrophy during pregnancy. Breast hypertrophy is related to hormonal changes during pregnancy with a rise in estradiol, estrone, estriol, progesterone, cortisol, insulin, and prolactin. The normal physiologic breast changes of pregnancy may mask a developing malignant mass and result in a significant delay in diagnosis [26] and this may partially explain why pregnancy is a risk factor for more advanced presentation of breast cancer.

Largent *et al.* described a study of 254 women diagnosed with invasive breast cancer under the age of 35 [27]. Compared with nulliparous women, those with three or more births were more likely to be diagnosed with a nonlocalized tumor, a poor prognostic finding. In addition, they found that women with two or more full-term pregnancies were more likely to die from their disease compared to women with one or no term pregnancy. These data appear to indicate that among younger women, tumors associated with pregnancy are more aggressive and more difficult to treat. A delay in diagnosis also contributes to the poor prognosis.

For women who carry either *BRCA1* or *BRCA2* mutations, the lifetime risk for breast cancer approaches 80%.

Recent reports have addressed the effect of pregnancy on life-time risk for breast cancer in this population. Interestingly, the effect of parity appears to be different depending upon whether the patient carries a mutation in *BRCA1* or *BRCA2*, with *BRCA1* carriers enjoying a modest protective effect from pregnancy, while *BRCA2* carriers appear to have an increased risk due to pregnancy [28].

Screening, diagnosis, and staging of breast cancer in pregnancy

The diagnosis of breast cancer can be challenging during pregnancy. Mammography, the most important diagnostic test used in the work-up of a breast mass, is less reliable due to the density of the pregnant breast. In pregnancy, mammography is acceptable from the standpoint of radiation exposure to the fetus; however, the test is likely to be nondiagnostic due to the density of the pregnant breast and cannot be relied upon to rule out malignancy. In a small study of eight pregnant women with breast cancer who underwent mammograms, six of the eight studies were negative [29]. Ultrasonography can be used to distinguish fluid-filled cysts from solid masses. If cystic, aspiration of the fluid should be carried out, and the fluid should be sent for cytologic evaluation if it is bloody. Fine needle aspiration of a solid mass is less accurate in pregnancy due to the normal hyperplastic epithelial changes and must be interpreted by an experienced pathologist. Not infrequently, fine needle aspirations of breast masses during pregnancy are nondiagnostic and may be falsely labeled as malignant [30].

In general, if a solid mass is found, surgical excision is the standard practice and can usually be carried out under local anesthesia (although general anesthesia is certainly not contraindicated in pregnancy) [31]. Excisional biopsies may be complicated by infection, hematomas, and milk fistulas. Therefore, prophylactic antibiotics should be given, and patients should consider ceasing lactation if the biopsy is performed in the postpartum period. Byrd and colleagues reported that of 134 biopsies performed during pregnancy or lactation, 29 proved to be cancer [32].

Once the diagnosis of malignancy is established, the patient should be staged. Breast cancer staging is based upon the criteria in Boxes 22.2 and 22.3. Magnetic resonance imaging (MRI) and computed tomography (CT) scans are not contraindicated in pregnancy and should be performed if indicated.

For clinical stage I and II disease, bone scans are not indicated unless the patient has symptoms or serum chemistries suggestive of bone involvement; however, for clinical stage III disease, a modified bone scan using maternal hydration, as reported by Baker, will reduce the fetal radiation exposure to a very acceptable 76 millirems (mrem) resulting from the isotope ^{99m}Tc [33]. Unless the patient has central nervous system symptoms, a brain scan is rarely performed.

Box 22.2 Breast cancer T, N and M categories

Primary tumor (T)

TX: Primary tumor cannot be assessed.
T0: No evidence of primary tumor.
Tis: Carcinoma *in situ* (DCIS, LCIS or Paget disease of the nipple with no associated tumor mass)
T1: Tumor is 2 cm (3/4 of an inch) or less across
T2: Tumor is more than 2 cm but not more than 5 cm (2 inches) across
T3: Tumor is more than 5 cm across
T4: Tumor of any size growing into the chest wall or skin. This includes inflammatory breast cancer

Nearby lymph nodes (N) (based on looking at them under a microscope)

NX: Nearby lymph nodes cannot be assessed (for example, removed previously)
N0: Cancer has not spread to nearby lymph nodes
N1: Cancer has spread to 1–3 axillary (underarm) lymph node(s), and/or tiny amounts of cancer are found in internal mammary lymph nodes (those near the breast bone) on sentinel lymph node biopsy
N2: Cancer has spread to 4–9 axillary lymph nodes under the arm, or cancer has enlarged the internal mammary lymph nodes.
N3: One of the following applies:
- cancer has spread to 10 or more axillary lymph nodes
- cancer has spread to the lymph nodes under the clavicle
- cancer has spread to the lymph nodes above the clavicle
- cancer involves axillary lymph nodes and has enlarged the internal mammary lymph nodes.
- cancer involves 4 or more axillary lymph nodes, and tiny amounts of cancer are found in internal mammary lymph nodes on sentinel lymph node biopsy

Metastasis

MX: Presence of distant spread (metastasis) cannot be assessed
M0: No distant spread
M1: Spread to distant organs is present

Treatment of breast cancer in pregnancy

The usual recommendation is to treat pregnant patients with breast cancer surgically with a modified radical mastectomy. An acceptable alternative for many nonpregnant patients is a lumpectomy followed by radiation. Most clinicians believe

Box 22.3 Breast cancer stage grouping

Once the T, N, and M categories have been determined, this information is combined in a process called *stage grouping*. Cancers with similar stages tend to have a similar outlook and thus are often treated in a similar way. Stage is expressed in Roman numerals from stage I (the least advanced stage) to stage IV (the most advanced stage). Noninvasive cancer is listed as stage 0.

Stage 0: Tis, N0, M0: This is *ductal carcinoma in situ (DCIS)*, the earliest form of breast cancer. In DCIS, cancer cells are still within a duct and have not invaded deeper into the surrounding fatty breast tissue. *Lobular carcinoma in situ (LCIS)* is sometimes classified as stage 0 breast cancer, but most oncologists believe it is not a true breast cancer. In LCIS, abnormal cells grow within the lobules or milk-producing glands, but they do not penetrate through the wall of these lobules. Paget disease of the nipple (without an underlying tumor mass) is also stage 0. In all cases the cancer has not spread to lymph nodes or distant sites.

Stage I: T1, N0, M0: The tumor is 2 cm (about 3/4 of an inch) or less across and has not spread to lymph nodes or distant sites.

Stage IIA: T0, N1, M0/T1, N1, M0/T2, N0, M0: One of the following applies.
- The tumor is 2 cm or less across (or is not found) and has spread to 1–3 axillary lymph nodes.
- The tumor is 2 cm or less across (or is not found) and tiny amounts of cancer are found in internal mammary lymph nodes on sentinel lymph node biopsy.
- The tumor is 2 cm or less across (or is not found), has spread to 1–3 axillary lymph nodes, and tiny amounts of cancer are found in internal mammary lymph nodes on sentinel lymph node biopsy.
- The tumor is larger than 2 cm across and less than 5 cm but hasn't spread to the lymph nodes.

In all cases, the cancer hasn't spread to distant sites.

Stage IIB: T2, N1, M0/T3, N0, M0: One of the following applies.
- The tumor is larger than 2 cm and less than 5 cm across. It has spread to 1–3 axillary lymph nodes and/or tiny amounts of cancer are found in internal mammary lymph nodes on sentinel lymph node biopsy.
- The tumor is larger than 5 cm across but does not grow into the chest wall or skin and has not spread to lymph nodes.
- The cancer hasn't spread to distant sites.

Stage IIIA: T0–2, N2, M0/T3, N1–2, M0: One of the following applies.
- The tumor is not more than 5 cm across (or cannot be found). It has spread to 4–9 axillary lymph nodes, or it has enlarged the internal mammary lymph nodes.
- The tumor is larger than 5 cm across but does not grow into the chest wall or skin. It has spread to 1–9 axillary nodes, or to internal mammary nodes.

In all cases, the cancer hasn't spread to distant sites.

Stage IIIB: T4, N0–2, M0: The tumor has grown into the chest wall or skin, and one of the following applies.
- It has not spread to the lymph nodes.
- It has spread to 1–3 axillary lymph nodes and/or tiny amounts of cancer are found in internal mammary lymph nodes on sentinel lymph node biopsy.
- It has spread to 4–9 axillary lymph nodes, or it has enlarged the internal mammary lymph nodes.

The cancer hasn't spread to distant sites.

Inflammatory breast cancer is classified as stage IIIB unless it has spread to distant lymph nodes or organs, in which case it would be stage IV.

Stage IIIC: T0–4, N3, M0: The tumor is any size (or can't be found), and one of the following applies.
- Cancer has spread to 10 or more axillary lymph nodes.
- Cancer has spread to the lymph nodes under the clavicle (collar bone).
- Cancer has spread to the lymph nodes above the clavicle.
- Cancer involves axillary lymph nodes and has enlarged the internal mammary lymph nodes.
- Cancer involves 4 or more axillary lymph nodes, and tiny amounts of cancer are found in internal mammary lymph nodes on sentinel lymph node biopsy.

The cancer hasn't spread to distant sites.

Stage IV: T0–4, N0–3, M1: The cancer can be any size and may or may not have spread to nearby lymph nodes. It has spread to distant organs (the most common sites are the bone, liver, brain or lung), or to lymph nodes far from the breast.

that this alternative is contraindicated during pregnancy because the dose of radiation exceeds recommended limits for the fetus. However, at least one review refutes this assertion; hence this is controversial [34]. For surgery, general anesthesia is indicated. Antacids should be given to raise the gastric pH. This is required because of the increased risk of aspiration with pregnancy. Prolonged preoxygenation prior to endotracheal intubation should be undertaken, and intraoperative fetal monitoring should be considered during the procedure so that anesthesia can be adjusted to avoid fetal hypoxia. The patient should also undergo fetal and uterine monitoring in the early postoperative period to identify a nonreassuring fetal heart rate pattern and/or preterm labor. Postoperative tocolysis should be instituted if necessary.

For stage II or greater disease, chemotherapy is the standard of care. Regardless of stage or node status, for tumors with high-risk factors, including lack of hormone receptors and high cellular ploidy, adjuvant and/or neo-adjuvant chemotherapy has been reported to improve clinical outcome and should not be withheld during pregnancy. Chemotherapy with a combination of cyclophosphamide, adriamycin, and 5-fluorouracil (CAF) versus cyclophosphamide alone is commonly employed. However, other regimens, including those with paclitaxel, have been reported [35–37]. Most clinicians avoid the folate inhibitor methotrexate during pregnancy because of the high malformation rate of 17–25% associated with this agent [38]. The most common anomaly associated with methotrexate is microcephaly, which is more common with exposure early in pregnancy.

Malignant melanoma in pregnancy

Malignant melanoma originates from melanocytes, which are cells of neural crest origin that produce the pigment melanin [39,40]. Incidence rates for malignant melanoma have increased in the United States and other countries in recent decades and are highest among fair-skinned populations. Exposure to solar ultraviolet radiation is considered to be the primary risk factor for the disease; however, hormonal effects are also postulated to play a role [41].

Effect of pregnancy on melanoma

Malignant melanoma is one of the most common tumors reported in pregnancy [42,43]. Although the real incidence of malignant melanoma during pregnancy is unknown, it is estimated that melanoma accounts for about 8% of all malignant tumors diagnosed during gestation [43–45]. Smith & Randall published an incidence of 2.8 per 1000 deliveries in a report from 1969 [46]. Other studies have reported an incidence of 2.8–5 per 100,000 pregnancies [47]. Additionally, Lens *et al.* estimated that melanoma during pregnancy accounted for 967 cases per 100,000 women diagnosed with melanoma during reproductive years [48].

A number of case reports indicate that melanoma is more aggressive during pregnancy [49–53]; melanoma rates are higher in general in young women compared to men during the reproductive years [49] and pregnancy results in cutaneous hyperpigmentation (also seen with the use of exogenous hormones), suggesting that hormonal factors play a role in melanocyte proliferation [54]. In addition, preclinical models of melanoma strongly suggest that pregnancy has an effect on melanoma cell proliferation and angiogenesis, possibly in response to placental growth factors [55]. However, most epidemiologic studies have shown no association between prior pregnancy and an increased risk of developing melanoma, so the link between hormones and melanoma remains controversial.

Stage and prognosis of malignant melanoma in pregnancy

The maternal outcome depends upon well-established prognostic factors for melanoma. Melanoma staging is based upon the criteria in Box 22.4. The prognosis of melanoma is strongly associated with Breslow thickness, which is measured as the depth of the lesion from the granular cell layer of the epidermis to the deepest identifiable tumor cells. The location of the lesion is also associated with prognosis. Those that occur on the head, neck, and trunk are associated with lower survival [56].

Interestingly, melanoma is the most common tumor type that metastasizes to the placenta and/or the fetus. More than 28 cases of metastatic melanoma to the fetal compartment have been reported [57, 58]. It is important to notify the pathologist of the need to do a complete evaluation of the placenta after birth for any patient delivered with melanoma to rule out occult metastasis. In the setting of frank fetal metastasis, the outcome can be fatal for the neonate.

Treatment of melanoma during pregnancy

Most studies have indicated no overall difference in survival between pregnant and nonpregnant women with melanoma. When detected at an early stage, melanoma is highly curable with surgery alone. However, patients with lymph node involvement or thicker primary tumors with ulceration – stages IIB/IIC/III – require adjuvant therapy after surgery. Unfortunately cytotoxic chemotherapy has limited benefit; however, immunotherapy with adjuvant interferon-alpha-2b significantly reduces recurrences and results in a survival benefit for some patients [59–62]. Interferon therapy is considered to be generally contraindicated during pregnancy but because of its importance in the treatment of melanoma, it is important to understand the basis for the advice not to use it. Some studies do indicate an increased risk for early fetal loss and later growth restriction [63]; other investigators report no difference in pregnancy outcome in women treated with interferon during pregnancy [64–67]. Therefore,

Box 22.4 TNM staging for melanoma (American Cancer Society, 2007)

T categories

The T category is based on an exam of the skin biopsy. Measuring the size and thickness of a melanoma under a microscope is believed to be the best way to determine a patient's prognosis.

TX: Primary tumor cannot be assessed
T0: No evidence of primary tumor
Tis: Melanoma *in situ* (Clark level I – it remains in the epidermis)
T1a: The melanoma is less than or equal to 1.0 mm thick (1.0 mm = 1/25 or 0.04 inches), without ulceration and Clark level II or III
T1b: The melanoma is less than or equal to 1.0 mm thick, Clark level IV or IV, or with ulceration
T2a: The melanoma is between 1.01 and 2.0 mm thick without ulceration
T2b: The melanoma is between 1.01 and 2.0 mm thick with ulceration
T3a: The melanoma is between 2.01 and 4.0 mm thick without ulceration
T3b: The melanoma is between 2.01 and 4.0 mm thick with ulceration
T4a: The melanoma is thicker than 4.0 mm without ulceration
T4b: The melanoma is thicker than 4.0 mm with ulceration

N categories

The possible values for N depend on whether or not a sentinel lymph node biopsy was done.
   The *clinical staging* of the lymph nodes is listed below; it is done without the sentinel node biopsy.

NX: Regional lymph nodes cannot be assessed
N0: No spread to nearby lymph nodes
N1: Spread to 1 nearby lymph node
N2: Spread to 2 or 3 nearby lymph nodes, or spread of melanoma in the skin toward a nearby lymph node area (without reaching the lymph nodes)
N3: Spread to 4 or more lymph nodes, or spread to lymph nodes that are clumped together, or spread of melanoma in the skin toward a lymph node area and into the lymph node(s)

Following a lymph node biopsy, the *pathologic stage* can be determined. The involvement of any lymph nodes can be subdivided as follows.
- Any Na (N1a, N2a, etc.) means that the melanoma in the lymph node is only seen under the microscope.
- Any Nb (N1b, N2b, etc.) means that the melanoma in the lymph node is visible to the naked eye.
- N2c means the melanoma has spread to very small areas of nearby skin (satellite tumors) or has spread to skin lymphatic channels around the tumor (without reaching the lymph nodes).

M categories

The M values are:

MX: Presence of distant metastasis cannot be assessed
M0: No distant metastasis
M1a: Distant metastases to skin or subcutaneous (below the skin) tissue or distant lymph nodes
M1b: Metastases to lung
M1c: Metastases to other organs or distant spread to any site along with an elevated blood LDH level

given the activity of this agent against melanoma and the need to optimize treatment during pregnancy on behalf of the mother, it is wise to consider using interferon if the need is encountered during the second and early third trimesters of pregnancy. Delaying adjuvant interferon treatment until after pregnancy is appropriate for pregnancies in the late third trimester on a case-by-case basis.

Malignant ovarian masses in pregnancy

While benign ovarian cysts are common during pregnancy, malignancies are rare.

Functional, simple ovarian cysts consistent with corpus lutea are required for progesterone production and pregnancy maintenance in the early first trimester. After the first trimester, ovarian masses are less common. A review of the literature from 1954 to 1998 reveals that 1 in 79–2334 pregnancies are associated with persistent ovarian masses, with an average incidence of 1 in 800 pregnancies [68–89]. Of these masses, 5% of the cases were malignant, with an overall incidence of 1:16,000 pregnancies [90]. In order of prevalence, the types of malignancies diagnosed during pregnancy are germ cell tumors (45%), epithelial tumors (37.5%), sex cord-stromal tumors (10%), and other pathologies (7.5%).

Diagnosis of ovarian cancer during pregnancy

Masses can be found on initial pelvic exam, on pelvic ultrasound or at the time of cesarean section. Patients are often asymptomatic but this can vary depending upon the type and size of the mass. Symptomatic women may present with abdominal pain, torsion or even obstructed labor [90–92]. The best modality for imaging in pregnancy is ultrasound. Unilateral, simple masses less than 5 cm in diameter noted in the first trimester are usually benign functional cysts and resolve by 14 weeks gestation. However, masses that are larger than 5 cm, are bilateral or have solid or septated areas, particularly those with papillary projections, require further work-up. In one study that evaluated 125 pregnant women after 12 weeks gestation, 131 masses larger than 4 cm were studied. Most of the lesions were expected to be benign based upon ultrasound evaluation, and this was confirmed at final pathologic diagnosis. However, of the 14 patients (10.7%) in whom the ultrasound was suggestive of malignancy, only one actually had cancer, indicating a high false-positive rate for ultrasound [88,90].

Magnetic resonance imaging is another imaging modality that is useful when evaluating an adnexal mass during pregnancy and should be considered for any lesions suspected of being malignant by ultrasound. An important aspect to remember is that there are several non-neoplastic ovarian lesions associated with pregnancy that may be confused with a true ovarian neoplasm [93]. They include pregnancy luteoma, hyper-reactio luteinalis, large luteal follicles, intra-follicular granulosa cell proliferations, hilus cell hyperplasia, and ectopic decidual lesions. These conditions usually resolve spontaneously after pregnancy [90].

Management of ovarian malignancies during pregnancy

Germ cell tumors comprise the most abundant ovarian malignancies diagnosed during pregnancy. Histologic subtypes include dysgerminomas, endodermal sinus tumors, immature malignant teratomas, choriocarcinomas, embryonal carcinomas, polyembryomas, and mixed germ cell tumors. The most common of these is the dysgerminoma. These solid tumors are generally unilateral but 10–15% are bilateral [94,95].

Histologically, dysgerminomas demonstrate dispersed sheets or cords separated by scant fibrous stroma [94]. These tumors contain syncytiotrophoblastic giant cells that produce lactate dehydrogenase (LDH) which can be used as a marker for treatment response. LDH is more reliable as a tumor marker than CA-125, which may be elevated simply because of the pregnancy.

Fortunately, most dysgerminomas present at an early stage. The treatment for suspected ovarian malignant tumors is surgery. In early pregnancy and if surgery is not urgent, i.e. there is no torsion, it is reasonable to wait until 16–18 weeks gestation before proceeding. The rationale for this strategy is that surgery during the first trimester increases the risk for spontaneous abortion. The recommended surgical approach is a midline incision, avoiding uterine manipulation. Most patients will require a unilateral salpingo-oophorectomy with preservation of the contralateral ovary unless affected. Appropriate staging should be performed including pelvic washings, omental and peritoneal biopsies and sampling of suspicious pelvic and peri-aortic lymph nodes. Adjunctive chemotherapy may not be needed in pregnancy, given the low recurrence rate of early-stage disease after surgery.

Endodermal sinus tumors are the second most common germ cell malignancies diagnosed during pregnancy [94,96]. They are composed of tubules lined with cuboidal cells and produce alpha-fetoprotein (AFP). AFP is usually elevated in early pregnancy but the levels observed with this tumor are much higher than in normal pregnancy. Endodermal germ cell tumors often grow rapidly and may present with acute symptoms such as torsion and hemorrhage into the tumor [97–99]. Survival depends upon aggressive management which includes surgery combined with chemotherapy. Compared to surgery alone with a 5-year survival rate of only 13% [99], the addition of chemotherapy confers an 80% survival for early-stage disease. The multidrug regimen recommended for endodermal sinus tumors is bleomycin, etoposide, and cisplatin (BEP). Several studies have reported reassuring pregnancy outcomes with BEP when used after the first trimester [100–105]. Thus, the decision to start chemotherapy must be balanced with the gestational age of the fetus, the patient's desire for the pregnancy and whether the tumor markers AFP and LDH are persistently elevated.

Epithelial ovarian cancer, the most common ovarian malignancy in older women, is rare in pregnancy. Ovarian masses of epithelial origin can be benign, borderline (low malignant potential) or invasive. The different pathologic types of invasive tumors are as follows: serous (75%), mucinous (10%), endometrioid (10%), and the remainder made up of clear cell, transitional cell, Brenner, epidermal-stromal, undifferentiated, carcinosarcoma, and mesodermal mixed tumors. Most borderline ovarian tumors are either serous or mucinous. Pathologically, invasive tumors appear cystic and have complex growth patterns with papillary structures [94].

Mucinous tumors are made up of large, multicystic structures. These tumors also contain solid compartments and may be associated with pseudomyxoma peritonei. Endometrioid cancers contain both solid and cystic components and exhibit a glandular pattern very similar to endometrial cancer. Another important point is the frequency of bilateral tumors. Approximately 65% of invasive serous, 40% of endometrioid, and 5% of mucinous tumors are bilateral [94,106]. Clinical symptoms of malignant ovarian epithelial tumors include abdominal distension, intra-abdominal pressure, dyspepsia, and urinary frequency; however, the diagnosis may be delayed because these symptoms are also quite common in normal pregnancies. CA-125 is a commonly used marker for ovarian epithelial cancer but, as mentioned above, this may not be reliable during pregnancy. In particular, CA-125 levels are increased in pregnancy up to the 10th week, so caution should be used when interpreting these levels in the first trimester [107].

Treatment of epithelial ovarian cancer varies by stage and gestational age. If the patient has stage IA epithelial ovarian cancer, unilateral oophorectomy with close observation may be considered (see Box 22.5 for ovarian cancer staging).

Box 22.5 Ovarian cancer staging

Stage I: The cancer is still contained within the ovary (or ovaries).

Stage IA (T1a, N0, M0): Cancer has developed in one ovary, and the tumor is confined to the inside of the ovary. There is no cancer on the outer surface of the ovary. Laboratory examination of washings from the abdomen and pelvis did not find any cancer cells.

Stage IB (T1b, N0, M0): Cancer has developed within both ovaries without any tumor on their outer surfaces. Laboratory examination of washings from the abdomen and pelvis did not find any cancer cells.

Stage IC (T1c, N0, M0) The cancer is present in one or both ovaries and one or more of the following are present:

- cancer on the outer surface of at least one of the ovaries
- in the case of cystic tumors (fluid-filled tumors), the capsule (outer wall of the tumor) has ruptured (burst)
- laboratory examination found cancer cells in fluid or washings from the abdomen.

Stage II: The cancer is in one or both ovaries and has involved other organs (such as the uterus, fallopian tubes, bladder, the sigmoid colon, or the rectum) within the pelvis.

Stage IIA (T2a, N0, M0): The cancer has spread to or has actually invaded (grown into) the uterus or the fallopian tubes, or both. Laboratory examination of washings from the abdomen did not find any cancer cells.

Stage IIB (T2b, N0, M0): The cancer has spread to other nearby pelvic organs such as the bladder, the sigmoid colon, or the rectum. Laboratory examination of fluid from the abdomen did not find any cancer cells.

Stage IIC (T2c, N0, M0): The cancer has spread to pelvic organs as in stages IIA or IIB and laboratory examination of the washings from the abdomen found evidence of cancer cells.

Stage III: The cancer involves one or both ovaries, and one or both of the following are present: (1) cancer has spread beyond the pelvis to the lining of the abdomen; (2) cancer has spread to lymph nodes.

Stage IIIA (T3a, N0, M0): During the staging operation, the surgeon can see cancer involving the ovary or ovaries, but no cancer is grossly visible (can be seen without using a microscope) in the abdomen and the cancer has not spread to lymph nodes. However, when biopsies are checked under a microscope, tiny deposits of cancer are found in the lining of the upper abdomen.

Stage IIIB (T3b, N0, M0): There is cancer in one or both ovaries, and deposits of cancer large enough for the surgeon to see, but smaller than 2 cm (about 3/4 inch) across, are present in the abdomen. Cancer has not spread to the lymph nodes.

Stage IIIC: The cancer is in one or both ovaries, and one or both of the following are present:

- cancer has spread to lymph nodes (any T, N1, M0)
- deposits of cancer larger than 2 cm (about 3/4 inch) across are seen in the abdomen (T3c, N0, M0).

Stage IV: (any T, any N, M1): This is the most advanced stage of ovarian cancer. In this stage the cancer has spread to the inside of the liver, the lungs or other organs located outside the peritoneal cavity. (The peritoneal cavity or abdominal cavity is the area enclosed by the peritoneum, a membrane that lines the inner abdomen and covers most of its organs.) Finding ovarian cancer cells in the fluid around the lungs (called pleural fluid) is also evidence of stage IV disease.

Recurrent ovarian cancer: This means that the disease has come back (recurred) after completion of treatment.

This management is similar to how early-stage disease is handled in the nonpregnant state. However, for more advanced-stage disease, the treatment in the nonpregnant state is a total hysterectomy, bilateral salpingo-oophorectomy, omentectomy, and tumor debulking followed by chemotherapy. Obviously, an ongoing pregnancy requires an alternative strategy, and there are few case reports of treatment of invasive ovarian epithelial cancer during pregnancy upon which to base recommendations. One option is to perform an oophorectomy followed by adjuvant single-agent chemotherapy with carboplatin during pregnancy. After delivery, the patient should undergo a hysterectomy and tumor debulking followed by additional, multiagent chemotherapy [90]. Borderline epithelial tumors are confined to the ovary in 70–75% cases. In the nonpregnant state, the treatment is primarily surgical staging consisting of total abdominal hysterectomy, bilateral salpingo-oophorectomy, and omentectomy, although in young women desiring fertility, surgery may be limited with the goal of preserving fertility [90]. Adjuvant chemotherapy is usually not recommended unless disease is found outside the ovary, and most epithelial tumors of low malignant potential have a very good prognosis. Recurrent cases are treated with surgery first followed by chemotherapy if needed based upon the extent of the disease.

Sex cord-stromal tumors are rarely found in pregnancy. The cell types include granulosa, theca, Sertoli, Leydig and fibroblasts. These tumors are typically composed of one or more cell types which may include fibromas, thecomas, granulosa (granulosa-theca) cell tumors, Sertoli–Leydig cell tumors, and gynandroblastoma. Fibromas and thecomas are benign, but granulosa cell tumors are malignant and are the most frequent type [90]. Granulosa cell tumors can be cystic or solid. Histologically, they have small cuboidal to polygonal cells which spread in cords, strands or sheets [90,94]. These tumors produce estrogen. They are bilateral in 2–8% of cases and 78–91% are stage I at diagnosis. In addition to estrogen, inhibin is produced by granulosa cell tumors and may be used as a diagnostic or treatment marker. However, inhibin is not specific for granulosa cell tumors and may also be elevated in mucinous epithelial malignancies.

Sertoli–Leydig cell tumors are usually solid and lobulated [90]. The well-differentiated tumors are hollow or solid tubules made up of Sertoli or Leydig cells with fibrous stroma [90,94]. Loss of structure occurs in undifferentiated tumors. Sertoli–Leydig tumors are rarely bilateral (less than 5%) [94,108–112]. The clinical presentation is similar to other ovarian malignancies, with abdominal pain and possible torsion as considerations. In the nonpregnant state, many patients may have infertility and may exhibit disruption of normal menstrual cycles due to the estrogen and androgen produced by such tumors. Fortunately, most patients with sex cord-stromal tumors present at an early stage, and conservative therapy is recommended for

young patients with stage I tumors [94,95,113]. For more advanced stages, the recommended chemotherapy for patients with granulosa and Sertoli–Leydig tumors is BEP, which can be given during the later trimesters of pregnancy without undue concern.

Carcinosarcomas or malignant mixed mesodermal tumors usually occur in older patients and are rarely diagnosed in pregnancy. Pathologically, these tumors contain malignant epithelial and mesenchymal components. The tumors are aggressive, and metastases are more common than with other ovarian cancer types [114,115]. Accordingly, conservative surgical approaches should not be considered; tumor debulking is important and a determinant of prognosis. Surgery should be followed by aggressive chemotherapy. If at all possible, pregnancy should not affect treatment. Even so, the prognosis of carcinosarcoma remains poor.

Hematologic malignancies in pregnancy

Twenty-five percent of all cancers diagnosed during pregnancy are hematologic. In women aged 15–24, the most frequent malignancy is Hodgkin's lymphoma. The incidence of Hodgkin's lymphoma in pregnancy is 1:1000 to 1:1600. Unlike Hodgkin's lymphoma which peaks in the reproductive years, non-Hodgkin's lymphoma occurs at a mean age of 42 years. Although the exact prevalence of non-Hodgkin's lymphoma during pregnancy is unknown, the estimated incidence is thought to be 0.8:100,000 [116]. In comparison to the lymphoma, the incidence of leukemia in pregnancy is 1:75,000 to 1:100,000 [117–119]. In this section, the diagnosis and management of Hodgkin's lymphoma, non-Hodgkin's lymphoma, and leukemia will be addressed.

Hodgkin's lymphoma in pregnancy

Hodgkin's lymphoma accounts for 51% of all hematologic malignancies and is the fourth most common cancer in pregnancy [117–119]. The average age at diagnosis is 25.5 years. This neoplasm begins in the lymph nodes and spreads throughout the lymphatic system. Accordingly, the principal clinical sign is lymphadenopathy, usually of the cervical (neck), submaxillary or axillary nodes. The etiology is unknown and is probably multifactorial, involving both environmental and genetic factors. The diagnosis is based upon the presence of clonal malignant Hodgkin cells or multinucleated Reed Sternberg cells within a mixture of reactive, inflammatory and stromal cells. Reed Sternberg cells are of the B-cell lineage [120].

Hodgkin's lymphoma can be subclassified based on histopathologic characteristics, as defined by the World Health Organization (WHO), with nodular sclerosis occurring most

Box 22.6 Ann Arbor staging system

The staging system most often used to describe the spread of non-Hodgkin's lymphoma in adults is called the Ann Arbor staging system. The stages are described by Roman numerals I through IV (1–4). Lymphomas that affect organs outside the lymph system (extranodal organs) have E added to their stage (for example, stage IIE), while those affecting the spleen have S added.

Stage I: If either of the following is present it means the disease is stage I.
- The lymphoma is in a lymph node or nodes in only 1 region, such as the neck, groin, underarm, and so on.
- The cancer is found only in 1 area of a single organ outside the lymph system (IE).

Stage II: If either of the following is present it means the disease is stage II.
- The lymphoma is in 2 or more groups of lymph nodes on the same side of (above or below) the diaphragm (the muscle that aids breathing and separates the chest and abdomen). For example, this might include nodes in the underarm and neck area but not the combination of underarm and groin nodes.
- The lymphoma extends locally from a single group of lymph node(s) into a nearby organ (IIE). It may also affect other groups of lymph nodes on the same side of the diaphragm.

Stage III: If either of the following is present it means the disease is stage III.
- The lymphoma is found in lymph node areas on both sides of (above and below) the diaphragm.
- The cancer may also have extended into an area or organ next to the lymph nodes (IIIE), into the spleen (IIIS) or both (IIIE,S).

Stage IV: If either of the following is present it means the disease is stage IV.
- The lymphoma has spread outside the lymph system into an organ that is not right next to an involved node.
- The lymphoma has spread to the bone marrow, liver, brain or spinal cord, or the pleura (thin lining of the lungs).

Along with the Roman numeral, each stage is also assigned an A or B. The letter A is added if the person doesn't have any symptoms of lymphoma. The letter B is added (stage IIIB, for example) if any of the following symptoms are present:
- unexplained weight loss (more than 10% of weight)
- soaking night sweats
- unexplained fever >100°.

Although the type and stage of the lymphoma provide useful information about a person's prognosis, for some types of lymphomas (especially fast-growing ones) the stage is not too helpful on its own. Other factors are looked at to help overcome this.

frequently in pregnancy. However, the two most important prognostic factors are the stage of the disease (modified Ann Arbor system) and the patient's age (see Box 22.6 for Ann Arbor staging). Patients with Ann Arbor stage I and II, characterized by the absence of bulky disease (tumor <10 cm) and without symptoms, are considered to have an early-stage neoplasm with a good prognosis [121]. The expected long-term survival rate for patients less than 60 years of age and who have early-stage disease is 90%.

Pregnancy does not appear to affect the stage of the disease, response to therapy, or overall survival compared to age- and stage-equivalent nonpregnant patients [122,123]. Additionally, termination of pregnancy does not improve maternal outcome. Seventy percent of pregnant patients present with stage I or II disease with 8-year survival rates of 83% [122, 124]. In the past, staging was accomplished by clinical and pathologic diagnosis, with pathologic staging

determined by laparotomy. However, with recent advances employing new-generation CT and MRI, laparotomy is uncommon.

When lymphoma is suspected, the initial evaluation should include a complete history and a thorough examination of all node-bearing areas. A complete differential blood cell count, erythrocyte sedimentation rate, liver and renal function tests, lactate dehydrogenase, and alkaline phosphatase should be determined. Additionally, radiographic studies should be performed, including a chest radiograph, as well as a MRI evaluation of the chest, abdomen, and pelvis. Although usually negative, a bone marrow biopsy is recommended [125]. Most imaging studies are safe in pregnancy but lymphangiograms, occasionally recommended for the work-up of Hodgkin's lymphoma, are usually avoided secondary to fetal radiation exposure. Fortunately, this procedure is rarely used in current practice.

With respect to maternal or fetal outcome, it is unknown if Hodgkin's lymphoma adversely affects pregnancy. A report of patients choosing to delay treatment until after delivery did not show a significant difference in birthweight, mean gestational age or mode of delivery compared to healthy women [123,126]. In a study of 26 pregnant patients with advanced-stage Hodgkin's lymphoma treated during pregnancy using combined chemotherapy (doxorubicin, bleomycin, vinblastine, and dacarbazine; mechlorethamine, vincristine, prednisone and procarbazine; or epirubicin, bleomycin, vinblastine, and dacarbazine), there was no evidence of long-term complications such as congenital anomalies, hematologic malignancies or neurodevelopmental abnormalities in the newborns [126]. However, other reports suggest that intensive chemotherapy started in the first trimester increases the risk for fetal anomalies, fetal demise, growth restriction, premature deliveries, and neonatal pancytopenia.

The treatment of Hodgkin's lymphoma has shifted over the years. In the past, the treatment for early-stage disease was external beam radiation therapy, with the mantle field (axillary, cervical, mediastinal, and pulmonary hilar lymph nodes) used for supradiaphragmatic disease. Later a combined approach was instituted by using multiagent chemotherapy with low-dose field radiotherapy. This combination regimen produced an overall survival of 93% in one study [127]. Even during pregnancy, it is recommended that patients with early-stage disease begin multiagent chemotherapy (preferably doxorubicin, bleomyocin, vinblastine, and dacarbazine with or without involved-field radiotherapy) after the first trimester.

While radiotherapy during the second and third trimesters may sound concerning for the pregnancy, interestingly, in a study performed by Woo et al. with women that required involved-field radiotherapy, none of the infants demonstrated adverse effects from the treatment. In this study, 11 women with stage IA and IIA nodular sclerosing Hodgkin's lymphoma were treated at various gestational ages with mantle radiation (4000 centi-gray units (cGy) – 1 cGy is equivalent to 1 rad). Precautions were taken with proper shielding, resulting in the highest calculated fetal dose equal to 13.6 cGy [128]. The risks of ionizing radiation to the fetus are very much dependent on gestational age and dose, with concerns of congenital malformations and miscarriage highest in the first trimester with doses over 18–20 cGy. The threshold dose that may increase the risk for mental retardation at 8–15 weeks of gestation is reported to be 18 cGy, and the effect is greatest within the first trimester. Therefore, it may be reasonable to wait until the second or third trimesters to start treatment. Chemotherapy in the first trimester also poses a risk; therefore, delaying treatment with either chemotherapy or radiation must be balanced with the stage of the disease and the patient's desire to avoid harm to the fetus. If the diagnosis is made in the first trimester, termination of

pregnancy to allow intensive therapy is also an option that should be discussed.

When Hodgkin's disease is diagnosed in the third trimester, consideration of early delivery before treatment is appropriate. Particularly after 32 weeks, administration of corticosteroids to accelerate fetal lung maturity followed by delivery is an option when intensive chemotherapy and radiation are indicated. If early delivery is not desired, or if the diagnosis is made prior to 32 weeks, treatment should be instituted. If possible, delivery should be planned at least 2 weeks after the last dose of chemotherapy to decrease the risk of neonatal myelosuppression [125]. There is no evidence that mode of delivery (vaginal versus cesarean section) is important. After delivery, the placenta should be examined for metastases, which are rare but would prompt closer evaluation and follow-up of the newborn if found [125]. Importantly, cord blood banking should be offered to the patient as a source of HLA-compatible stem cells for the future [125]. Patients who decide to maintain their fertility after delivery should be advised not to get pregnant for at least 2 years, because relapses may be more common in the postpartum period.

Non-Hodgkin's lymphoma in pregnancy

Non-Hodgkin's lymphoma constitutes a heterogeneous group of lymphoid malignancies that originate in lymphoreticular tissues. Non-Hodgkin's lymphoma is differentiatied from Hodgkin's lymphoma by the absence of Reed Sternberg cells. These tumors can be of T- or B-cell origin and are variable in presentation, stage at diagnosis and prognosis [125]. Some lymphomas of the non-Hodgkin's type follow an indolent course, while others are very aggressive. These neoplasms are derived from monoclonal populations of B-cells approximately 88% of the time [129]. However, in pregnancy and in patients under the age of 35, a disproportionate number of T-cell and intermediate phenotypes are found [130,131]. The mean age at diagnosis is 42 years compared to Hodgkin's lymphoma, which typically occurs earlier during the reproductive years. Although the exact prevalence is unknown, the incidence in pregnancy is estimated to be approximately 0.8 cases per 100,000 women [116]. In a review of the literature, Hurley and co-workers found only 103 reported cases of non-Hodgkin's lymphoma complicating pregnancy [125].

The cause of non-Hodgkin's lymphoma has not been fully elucidated, although there are a number of risk factors. Epstein–Barr virus, human T-cell lymphotropic virus, hepatitis C, and HIV have all been associated with the later development of non-Hodgkin's lymphoma [116,132]. Additionally, autoimmune conditions including Sjögren's disease, lupus erythematosus, and rheumatoid arthritis have been associated with non-Hodgkin's lymphoma, and immunosuppression from any cause is a well-established risk factor [116,132,133]. Pregnancy itself is considered an immunosuppressed state, and non-Hodgkin's lymphoma tends to present at a more advanced stage in pregnant women. However, it is not clear whether the later stage presentation during pregnancy is due to immune changes or to a delay in diagnosis [134,135].

The clinical presentation is variable. Most patients present with lymphadenopthy (66%), but only 20% of patients with B-cell tumors have night sweats, weight loss or fever. Involvement of the bone marrow is more frequent with the indolent lymphomas (39%) than with more aggressive types [125,136]. Patients with T-cell lymphomas present more often with constitutional symptoms and extranodal disease and have a worse prognosis than patients with B-cell lymphomas [137]. However, Burkitt's lymphoma (a B-cell non-Hodgkin's lymphoma) is an exception, and this disease often progress rapidly.

The treatment approach to non-Hodgkin's lymphoma is similar to Hodgkin's lymphoma and is based upon the Ann Arbor staging system (see Box 22.6). Even in the pregnant patient, it is important to perform CT scans of the chest, abdomen and pelvis for staging. The MRI can provide additional information about extranodal involvement and may be helpful in detecting bone marrow involvement; MRIs are considered safe during pregnancy. Both gallium and thallium scanning, although prognostic, are not usually obtained in pregnancy, however, their use might be justifiable if the information obtained was felt to justify the likely minimal but definitely unknown risk [125].

In addition to the Ann Arbor staging system, the WHO classification provides important information. It incorporates morphologic, genetic, immunophenotypic, and clinical features of non-Hodgkin's lymphomas. Although the stage (more advanced) and the most common histoimmunologic types (more T-cell and intermediate phenotypes) of non-Hodgkin's lymphoma may be different in pregnancy, their clinical behavior, when appropriately treated, is the same as in the nonpregnant state. Treatment choices are based on stage, classification, and the International Prognostic Index [125]. Standard therapy for non-Hodgkin's lymphoma includes cyclophosphamide, doxorubicin, vincristine, and prednisone resulting in a 3-year overall survival of 53–62%. Similar long-term survival rates are seen with pregnant patients [138]. Generally, women diagnosed in the third trimester and those with early-stage disease have a better prognosis [125]. Unfortunately, many pregnant women present with aggressive, advanced-stage disease so it is important that treatment not be delayed. Those patients diagnosed in the first trimester should weigh their options of worsening disease and potential risk of chemotherapy to the fetus. Those women unwilling to accept the potential risk to the fetus should be offered a termination. In the second and third trimesters, exposure to multiagent chemotherapy has been reported to be associated with fetal growth restriction and myeleosuppression; however, other studies indicate that the risk of these complications may be lower than previously reported [126,139].

Maternal to fetal transmission of non-Hodgkin's lymphoma is a potential risk during pregnancy [125,140]. Pathologic examination of the placenta should be routinely performed with maternal hematologic malignancies and, as with Hodgkin's lymphoma, cord blood should be collected for a potential source of HLA-compatible progenitor cells which may be used for bone marrow transplantation if necessary. If possible, delivery should be timed to minimize fetal lung immaturity as well as the risk of neonatal myelosuppression, which may occur in the first few weeks after administration of chemotherapy.

Leukemia and pregnancy

Leukemias comprise a heterogeneous group of malignancies that arise from genetically altered lymphoid or myeloid progenitor cells in the bone marrow. The incidence in pregnancy is estimated to be 1:75,000 to 1:100,000 [117–119]. First described by Virchow in 1845, clonal leukemic blasts invade the bloodstream and infiltrate into the liver, spleen and other tissues [141,142]. Leukemias are classified based on morphologic characteristics as being myeloid or lymphoid in origin. The types include acute myeloid leukemia (AML), chronic myeloid leukemia (CML), acute lymphoid leukemia (ALL), and chronic lymphoid leukemia (CLL). Recent advances in technology (immunophenotyping and molecular genetics) have produced a more complex but prognostically more accurate classification of leukemia [143]. Forty-three percent of leukemias are classified as acute and 41% as chronic. In the pregnant population, 90% are acute [144,145]. In addition, 68% are myeloid (61% AML and 7% CML) and 31% are lymphoid (28% AML and 3% CLL) [146].

The cause of leukemia is unknown but numerous associations including environmental, socio-economic, infectious, and genetic factors are postulated to play a role. There does appear to be a higher incidence of certain leukemias among monozygotic twins and patients with aneuploidy including Down's, Patau's and Klinefelter's syndromes. Other conditions such as Bloom's syndrome and X-linked agammaglobulinemia also are associated with a higher incidence of leukemia [147–150]. In addition, environmental factors such as radiation, exposure to alkylating agents, and viral infections have been implicated in the pathogenesis.

The clinical signs and symptoms of acute leukemia are nonspecific (fatigue, weakness, dyspnea, and lack of energy), and many of these symptoms are common in normal pregnancy.

In the presence of acute leukemia, bone marrow infiltration by the leukemic clonal cells occurs, resulting in a suppression of normal hematopoiesis [125]. This results in pancytopenia, causing episodes of epistaxis, bruising, and recurrent infections [125]. On exam, these patients may present with pallor, petechiae or ecchymoses. Lymphadenopathy and hepatosplenomegaly are uncommon. Usually, the chest radiograph is negative, but occasionally may demonstrate an enlarged mediastinum. This is particularly true in patients with T-cell leukemia.

The diagnosis of acute leukemia is usually made by a peripheral blood smear demonstrating a normocytic, normochromic anemia with mild thrombocytopenia. The white blood cell count can be variable but blasts are almost always present [148]. A lumbar puncture is recommend to evaluate disease in the central nervous system, and a bone marrow aspiration and biopsy are necessary for diagnosis and for morphologic, immunophenotypic and cytogenetic classification [148]. Age is a very important prognostic factor, with younger patients having a better prognosis [125]. The patient's response to the induction chemotherapy and the time until the bone marrow normalizes are the most powerful indicators of the ultimate outcome [148]. Today, with treatment, most children with ALL respond, and clinicians anticipate a cure rate of 80%. Even for adults, outcomes have improved. A complete remission can be expected in 70–85% of patients, with 25–50% of patients experiencing long-term disease-free periods [148]. The primary goals of chemotherapy for acute leukemia are to reduce the leukemic blasts in the bone marrow to a level less than 5% to normalize hematopoiesis [125]. Goals of therapy are to achieve a granulocyte count $>1000/\mu L$ and platelets $>100,000/\mu L$). The next goal is to prevent the emergence of resistant clones by using multiagent chemotherapy, which is usually divided into three phases: induction, consolidation, and maintenance [148,151].

Blast cytogenetic abnormalities are common and help to predict patient outcome in leukemia. The Philadelphia chromosome, translocation t (9; 22), occurs more frequently in adult ALL (25%) compared to children (3%) and is associated with a poor prognosis. For chronic leukemia, the common cytogenetic anomaly is the reciprocal translocation t (9:22) (q34; q11) and its bcr-abl fusion gene product which is found in 95% of cases.

The most common chemotherapeutic regimen for ALL is vincristine, anthracycline, steroids, and L-asparaginase. For AML patients less than 60 years of age, the regimen for induction is anthracycline (daunorubicin or idarubicin) and cytarabine. Those patients who do not go into remission are candidates for allogenic hematopoietic stem cell transplantation. It is important to consider that while patients are being treated with chemotherapeutic drugs, they may also require other medications such as allopurinol to reduce the risk of urate nephropathy. Antibiotics are generally recommended for *Pneumocystis jiroveci* prophylaxis as well as fluconazole to reduce the risk of yeast infections.

The treatment of chronic leukemia is more individualized. CLL staging is based upon criteria in Box 22.7. If the median survival is determined to be greater than 10 years, immediate treatment may not be required [152]. For patients with CLL who require treatment, fludarabine is recommended [125]. For CML in the chronic phase and for those who are not candidates for bone marrow transplantation, imatinib or interferon-alpha have been shown to improve survival [153].

The management of chronic leukemia in pregnancy is controversial [125]. In general, maternal and fetal outcomes are good regardless of whether or not therapy is instituted, with rates of maternal survival over 90%. Treatment, when instituted, is used to control splenomegaly, leukocytosis, and constitutional symptoms. Interferon-alpha does not appear to cross the placenta readily and has been used in 10 cases of CML in pregnancy from one report, with only one case of transient thrombocytopenia in a newborn as a side effect [65,66].

On the other hand, unlike chronic leukemia, there is a consensus that acute leukemia is adversely affected when treatment is delayed due to pregnancy [125]. Therefore, the induction of chemotherapy is the primary objective in management, regardless of gestational age. When deciding on a multidrug regimen, the pregnancy should be taken into account. Pregnancy is a hypercoagulable state, with a risk of thromboembolism six times higher than the nonpregnant state. L-Asparginase, which is part of the multidrug regimen for ALL, significantly decreases antithrombin III and has been associated with an increased risk for thromboembolism particularly in the upper limbs in association with central lines but also with cerebral venous thrombosis [154–157]. Therefore, the use of L-asparaginase is controversial in pregnancy although the benefits may outweigh the risks. In addition, long-term, high-dose steroid administration increases the risk for insulin resistance and gestational diabetes, a complication which is undesirable but readily treatable when identified.

Despite the risks of these medications, delaying treatment for acute leukemia during pregnancy is not recommended, and patients are faced with a difficult decision if the diagnosis is made in the first or second trimester [144,146,158]. Early delivery after steroids in the third trimester to minimize fetal exposure to chemotherapy is a consideration. The specific risks of chemotherapy to the fetus are reviewed by drug category in Tables 22.1–22.8 [159].

Box 22.7 Staging for chornic lymphocytic leukemia

There are two different systems for staging CLL:
- Rai system – used more often in the United States
- Binet system – used more widely in Europe.

There are also other factors that have been found to affect prognosis, which are discussed below.

Rai staging system

The Rai system divides CLL into five stages.
- **Rai stage 0:** Lymphocytosis is present (the blood lymphocyte count is too high, usually defined as over 10,000 lymphocytes/mm^3 of blood. Some doctors will diagnose CLL if the count is over 5000/mm^3 and the cells all have the same chemical pattern on special testing). The lymph nodes, spleen, and liver are not enlarged and the red blood cell and platelet counts are near normal.
- **Rai stage I:** Lymphocytosis plus enlarged lymph nodes. The spleen and liver are not enlarged and the red blood cell and platelet counts are near normal.
- **Rai stage II:** Lymphocytosis plus an enlarged spleen (and possibly an enlarged liver), with or without enlarged lymph nodes. The red blood cell and platelet counts are near normal.
- **Rai stage III:** Lymphocytosis plus anemia (too few red blood cells), with or without enlarged lymph nodes, spleen, or liver. Platelet counts are near normal.
- **Rai stage IV:** Lymphocytosis plus thrombocytopenia (too few blood platelets), with or without anemia, enlarged lymph nodes, spleen, or liver.

The Rai stages can be separated into low-, intermediate- and high-risk groups, which are often used to assess outlook and treatment options. Stage 0 is considered low risk, stages I and II are considered intermediate risk, and stages III and IV are considered high risk.

Binet staging system

In the Binet staging system, CLL is classified by the number of affected lymphoid tissue groups (neck lymph nodes, groin lymph nodes, underarm lymph nodes, spleen, and liver) and the presence of anemia (too few red blood cells) or thrombocytopenia (too few blood platelets).
- **Binet stage A**: Fewer than three areas of lymphoid tissue are enlarged, with no anemia or thrombocytopenia.
- **Binet stage B**: Three or more areas of lymphoid tissue are enlarged, with no anemia or thrombocytopenia.
- **Binet stage C**: Anemia and/or thrombocytopenia are present.

Both the Rai and Binet staging systems are useful and have been in use for many years.

Table 22.1 Alkylating agents used for chemotherapy and a summary of pregnancy safety data [159]

Drug	Mechanism of action	Tissue distribution	Indications	Maternal side effects	US FDA pregnancy safety category	Fetal effects	Breastfeeding
Cyclophosphamide (Cytoxin, CTX, CPM, Neosar)	Cyclophosphamide is activated by the liver cytochrome P450 microsomal system to cytotoxic metabolites phosphoramide mustard and acrolein. The metabolites form cross-links with DNA resulting in inhibition of DNA synthesis. This agent is active in all stages of the cell cycle	Cyclophosphamide is distributed throughout the body including the brain, CSF, milk, saliva and, presumably, the amniotic fluid. The drug is given either orally or intravenously	Breast cancer, non-Hodgkin's lymphoma, chronic lymphocytic leukemia, ovarian cancer, bone and soft tissue sarcoma, rhabdomyosarcoma, neuroblastoma and Wilms' tumor	Myelosuppression is dose limiting	D	Normal as well as malformed fetuses have been reported from first-trimester exposures. A total of seven isolated reports of defects have appeared in the literature and have been reviewed. The defects reported include oculofacial malformations, missing digits and nail abnormalities, coronary artery defects, umbilical hernia, hemangioma, imperforate anus, rectovaginal fistula, cleft palate, microcephaly, growth restriction, and developmental delays. Second- and third-trimester exposures are not associated with malformations, but are linked to growth restriction, microcephaly and, possibly, neonatal pancytopenia. As with alkylating agents in general, the use of cyclophosphamide is also associated with subsequent menstrual difficulties and premature ovarian failure, although a recent study suggests that successful post-therapy pregnancies are not uncommon	Breastfeeding is contraindicated and may be associated with neonatal neutropenia, immune suppression, and risk for the development of cancer

Drug	Pharmacology	Distribution/Administration	Indications	Toxicity	Category	Pregnancy	Risk
Thiotepa (triethylenethiophosphoramide, TSPA, Thioplex)	Thiotepa is an ethylenamine analog chemically related to nitrogen mustard that alkylates the N-7 position of guanine. This damages DNA and inhibits DNA, RNA, and protein synthesis. The drug is active in all phases of the cell cycle.	Thiotepa is widely distributed throughout the body including, presumably, the amniotic fluid. Intravenous infusion is required	Breast cancer, ovarian cancer, superficial transitional cell cancer of the bladder, and Hodgkin's and non-Hodgkin's lymphoma	Myelosuppression is dose limiting	D	Little is known, but thiotepa has been used during the second and third trimesters without apparent harm in one pregnancy	The risks are unknown
Chlorambucil (Leukeran)	Chlorambucil is an analog of nitrogen mustard that cross-links with DNA and inhibits DNA synthesis and function. It is active in all phases of the cell cycle.	given orally; distribution is not adequately studied.	Chronic lymphocytic leukemia, low-grade non-Hodgkin's lymphoma.	Myelosuppression is dose-limiting and nadirs at 25–30 days after therapy.	D	Normal pregnancies as well as pregnancies complicated by fetal malformations have been reported after chlorambucil use in pregnancy. Potential effects on the fetus include unilateral agenesis of one kidney and ureter in male fetuses following first trimester exposure as well as cardiac defects.	No information is available.
Melphalan (Alkeran, phenylalanine mustard, L-PAM)	Melphalan is an analog of nitrogen mustard. It forms interstrand and intrastrand cross-links with DNA resulting in inhibition of DNA synthesis and function. The drug is active in all phases of the cell cycle.	melphalan is widely distributed throughout the body including, presumably, the amniotic fluid. It can be given orally or intravenously.	multiple myeloma, breast cancer, ovarian cancer.	myelosuppression.	D	No reports linking melphalan with congenital defects have appeared, although it is possible that this drug has similar effects to other alkylating agents in pregnancy (see cyclophosphamide).	No information is available.

(Continued on p. 570)

Drug	Mechanism of action	Tissue distribution	Indications	Maternal side effects	US FDA pregnancy safety category	Fetal effects	Breastfeeding
Busulfan (Myleran, Busulfex)	This is a methanesulfonate-like bifunctional alkylating agent that interacts with thiol groups and causes nucleic acid and protein cross-links. Busulfan is active in all phases of the cell cycle	The drug distributes rapidly in all tissues and crosses into the amniotic fluid and the blood–brain barrier. It is given orally or intravenously	Chronic myelogenous leukemia	Myelosuppression is dose limiting and, rarely, a severe and life-threatening form of pulmonary fibrosis results which may occur 1–10 years after therapy	D	Six of 22 fetuses exposed in the first trimester demonstrated malformations including liver and spleen abnormalities, pyloric stenosis, cleft palate, microphthalmia, cytomegaly, hypoplasia of the ovaries and the thyroid, growth restriction, hydronephrosis and absent kidney and ureter	Should be avoided
Cisplatin (cisdiamine-dechloroplatinum, CDDP, Platinol)	Cisplatin covalently binds to DNA preferentially at the N-7 position of guanine and adenine causing cross-links. It also binds to nuclear and cytoplasmic proteins and causes cytotoxic effects	Cisplatin is widely distributed in all tissues with highest concentrations in the liver and kidneys. The drug is given intravenously or directly into the peritoneal cavity (not absorbed orally)	Ovarian cancer, bladder cancer, head and neck cancer, cancer of the esophagus, small cell and nonsmall cell lung cancer, non-Hodgkin's lymphoma, and choriocarcinoma	Nephrotoxicity and neurotoxicity are dose limiting. Myelosuppression is also a factor	D	Limited use has been reported in pregnancy without known complications that were clearly attributable to cisplatin alone	The advice is conflicting. Some references suggest that breastfeeding is possible "with caution" (Perinatology Network and American Academy of Pediatrics); however, other references state that breastfeeding should be avoided based upon a report of excretion into breast milk

570

Drug	Mechanism	Pharmacokinetics	Indications	Toxicity	Category	Use in pregnancy	Breastfeeding
Carboplatin (Paraplatin, CBDCA)	Carboplatin forms DNA cross-links preferentially by binding to the N-7 position of guanine and adenine. It is cell cycle nonspecific	Carboplatin is widely distributed throughout all body tissues, including, presumably, the amniotic fluid. It is given intravenously and is not absorbed orally	Ovarian cancer, germ cell tumors, head and neck cancer, small cell and nonsmall cell lung cancer, bladder cancer, relapsed and refractory acute leukemia, endometrial cancer	Myelosuppression is significant and dose limiting; nephrotoxicity and neurotoxicity are less than with cisplatin	D	Information is not available for carboplatin specifically; refer to the information on cisplatin above	The risks are unknown
Dacarbazine (DIC, DTIC-Dome, imidazole carboxamide)	Dacarbazine is a nonclassic alkylating agent that prevents the biosynthesis of purines. It methylates nucleic acids and inhibits DNA, RNA, and protein synthesis	This agent is distributed throughout the body and fluid spaces. It is loosely bound to plasma proteins. Dacarbazine is given intravenously	Indicated for the treatment of melanoma, Hodgkin's disease, soft tissue sarcomas, and neuroblastoma	Myelosuppression is dose limiting	C	Little information on dacarbazine in pregnancy is available; however, it has been reported in the treatment of metastatic melanoma in pregnancy during the second and third trimesters in combination with other medications (carmustine, tamoxifen, cisplatin) with no apparent ill effects. In this case, the baby was delivered prematurely at 30 weeks, but was otherwise healthy	No data are available

Table 22.2 Antibiotic agents used for chemotherapy and a summary of pregnancy safety data [159]

Drug	Mechanism of action	Tissue distribution	Indications	Maternal side effects	Pregnancy category	Fetal effects	Breastfeeding
Dactinomycin-D (actinomycin-D, Act-D, Cosmegen)	Dactinomycin-D is a product of *Streptomyces* that is composed of a tricyclic phenoxazone chromophore linked to two cyclic polypeptides. This agent binds to guanine-cytidine base pairs and inhibits DNA synthesis and function. It also causes the accumulation of intracellular oxygen-free radicals that further damage DNA	This drug must be given intravenously and is not absorbed orally. It concentrates in nucleated blood cells and is highly protein bound	Wilms' tumor, rhabdomyosarcoma, germ cell tumors, gestational trophoblastic disease, Ewing's sarcoma	Myelosuppression is dose limiting	C	Reports of the use of dactinomycin-D in the second and third trimesters have appeared. These pregnancies have resulted in apparently normal neonates	Dactinomycin-D is excreted in breast milk; hence, breastfeeding is not recommended
Bleomycin (Blenoxane)	Bleomycin is a small peptide antibiotic that binds iron to create activated oxygen-free radicals causing breaks in DNA	Bleomycin is given IV or directly into the pleural space (not absorbed orally). Found in the intra- and extracellular fluid where less than 10% is bound to proteins	Hodgkin's disease and non-Hodgkin's lymphoma, germ cell tumors, head and neck cancer, and squamous cell carcinomas of the skin, cervix, and vulva	Pneumonitis is dose limiting	D	While chromosomal aberrations in human bone marrow cells have been reported, no congenital defects have been linked to the use of bleomycin in pregnancy. Second- and third-trimester exposures in combination with other agents have resulted in the delivery of normal babies	The risks are unknown

Table 22.3 Antimetabolite agents used for chemotherapy and a summary of pregnancy safety data [159]

Drug	Mechanism of action	Tissue distribution	Indications	Maternal side effects	Pregnancy category	Fetal effects	Breastfeeding
Methotrexate (MTX, Amethopterin)	Folic acid analog, specific for the S-phase of the cell cycle. The drug enters the cell through the folate transport system and inhibits the enzyme dihydrofolate reductase, thus depleting the level of reduced folates necessary for cell function. Methotrexate also inhibits *de novo* thymidylate and purine synthesis	Methotrexate is widely distributed throughout the body including fluid spaces such as the amniotic fluid. The drug is given by the IV, IM or oral routes	Breast cancer, head and neck cancer, osteogenic sarcoma, acute lymphocytic leukemia, non-Hodgkin's lymphoma, meningeal leukemia and carcinomatous meningitis, bladder and colorectal cancers, gestational trophoblastic disease	Myelosuppression is dose limiting. Also, acute renal failure due to intratubular precipitation of methotrexate or its metabolites can occur	D	Congential anomalies associated with first-trimester exposure have been described, and methotrexate is clearly associated with teratogenicity. Malformations include severe cephalic and skull abnormalities with the absence of sutures, absence of the frontal bone, hypertelorism, a depressed or widened nasal bridge, hypoplasia of the mandible, heart defects such as dextroposition, and other conditions including the absence of digits. The attack rate appears to be relatively high with three of the 10 exposed fetuses demonstrating malformations. In addition, late effects of methotrexate on brain development are possible and should be studied further	Breastfeeding is contraindicated due to a low level of excretion in breast milk that may result in immune suppression, neutropenia and poor growth, and may be related to subsequent carcinogenesis
5-Fluorouracil (5FU, Efudex)	5-Fluorouracil is a pyrimidine analog specific for the S-phase of the cell cycle. Metabolic forms are incorporated into DNA and RNA to disrupt cell function	Given IV, it is widely distributed in tissues and fluid spaces, including, presumably, the amniotic fluid	Colorectal and breast cancers, GI malignancies, head and neck cancer, skin cancer, hepatoma, and ovarian cancer	Myelosuppression and mucositis and/or diarrhea may each be dose limiting. Hand-foot syndrome, manifested by tingling, skin and nail changes, pain and/or numbness, may also be	D	Normal as well as malformed fetuses have resulted from pregnancies treated with 5-fluorouracil. In one report, first-trimester exposure was associated with multiple anomalies including radial dysplasia, absent digits, hypoplasias of thoracic and abdominal organs such as the lungs, aorta, esophagus, duodenum, and ureters, among other defects	The risk is unknown

Table 22.4 Nucleoside analogs used for chemotherapy and a summary of pregnancy safety data [159]

Drug	Mechanism of action	Tissue distribution	Indications	Maternal side effects	Pregnancy category	Fetal effects	Breastfeeding
Cytarabine (cytosine arabinoside, Ara-C, Cytosar-U)	Cytarabine is a deoxycytidine analog synthesized by the sponge *Cryptotethya crypta*. Its activity is specific for the S-phase of the cell cycle where the drug incorporates as a metabolite, ara-CTP, into DNA. This results in the termination of DNA chain synthesis	IV administration results in wide tissue distribution throughout the body including fluid spaces such as the amniotic cavity. The drug is inactive orally	Acute myelogenous leukemia, acute lymphocytic leukemia, chronic myelogenous leukemia, and leptomeningeal carcinomatosis	Myelosuppression is dose limiting	D	First-trimester exposures have been associated with anomalies such as micro-otis and auditory canal atresia, lobster claw hand and other digit anomalies, as well as lower limb defects. As well as the potential for the usual growth restriction in fetuses exposed later in pregnancy, reports of fetal death *in utero* associated with cytarabine or combinations including cytarabine have appeared in the literature	No data are available
Gemcitabine (Gemzar)	Fluorine-substituted deoxycytidine analog that inhibits the cell cycle at the S-phase. Drug exposure results in the incorporation of a metabolic triphosphate nucleotide product, dFdCTP, into DNA that causes chain termination and stops DNA synthesis and function	Gemcitabine is administered IV and the drug is not extensively distributed in the body; however, it does cross the blood–brain barrier and may cross the placenta	Cancer of the pancreas, bladder cancer, nonsmall cell lung cancer, soft tissue sarcoma	Myelosuppression is dose limiting	D	No information on humans is available at this time; however, gemcitabine is teratogenic in mice and rabbits	No information is available

Table 22.5 Topoisomerase I inhibitors used for chemotherapy and a summary of pregnancy safety data [159]

Drug	Mechanism of action	Tissue distribution	Indications	Maternal side effects	Pregnancy category	Fetal effects	Breastfeeding
Topotecan (Hycamtin)	Topotecan is an alkaloid derivative from the *Camptotheca acuminata* tree that inhibits topoisomerase I function. Topotecan binds to and stabilizes the topoisomerase I-DNA complex and prevents the release of DNA after it has been cleaved by topoisomerase I. The complex collides with the advancing replication fork and stops DNA synthesis	This agent is widely distributed in body tissues and is given IV	Ovarian cancer, small cell lung cancer, acute myelogenous leukemia	Myelosuppression is dose limiting with the neutropenic nadir occurring at 7–10 days	D	No information from humans is available at this time; however, topotecan is teratogenic in animals in dosages that approximate recommended human regimens	Breastfeeding should be avoided according to the manufacturer; however, it is not known if topotecan is secreted in breast milk
Irinotecan (Camptosar, CPT-II)	Irinotecan is a synthetic derivative of camptothecin, an alkaloid derivative of the *Camptotheca acuminata* tree. The active metabolite of irinotecan, SN-38, stabilizes the topoisomerase I-DNA complex and prevents normal DNA synthesis and function. The drug is cell cycle nonspecific	This agent is widely distributed throughout the body and is administered IV	Colorectal cancer and nonsmall cell lung cancer	Myelosuppression is dose limiting	D	No studies reporting its use in pregnancy have appeared	Breastfeeding should be avoided according to the manufacturer

Table 22.6 Topoisomerase II inhibitors used for chemotherapy and a summary of pregnancy safety data [159]

Drug	Mechanism of action	Tissue distribution	Indications	Maternal side effects	Pregnancy category	Fetal effects	Breastfeeding
Etoposide (VePesid, VP-16)	A plant alkaloid extracted from the *Podophyllum peltatum* mandrake plant that inhibits toposiomerase II by stabilizing the topoisomerase II-DNA complex and preventing DNA unwinding. Etoposide is active during the S- and G2-phases of the cell cycle	Etoposide is rapidly distributed into all body fluids and tissues when administered either IV or PO. Decreased albumin, as may occur during pregnancy, may result in elevated free drug levels and toxicity	Germ cell tumors, small cell lung cancer, nonsmall cell lung cancer, non-Hodgkin's lymphoma, and gastric cancer	Myelosuppression is dose limiting, and etoposide may prolong the prothombin time and the INR	D	Use of etoposide in pregnancy has not resulted in fetal malformations; however, intrauterine growth restriction and pancytopenia in neonates have been reported [33,34]	The risk is unknown, but breastfeeding after a recent dose may lead to bone marrow suppression in the baby
Doxorubicin (Adriamycin, Adria, Hydroxydaunorubicin, DOX, Rubex)	Doxorubicin is an anthracycline antibiotic isolated from *Streptomyces* that intercalates into DNA resulting in inhibition of DNA synthesis. The drug also inhibits transcription by inhibiting DNA-dependent RNA polymerase and the function of topoisomerase II	This agent is widely distributed when given IV; about 75% of the drug and metabolites are bound to plasma proteins	Breast cancer, Hodgkin's and non-Hodgkin's lymphoma, soft tissue sarcoma, ovarian cancer, nonsmall cell and small cell lung cancer, bladder cancer, thyroid cancer, hepatoma, gastric cancer, Wilms' tumor, neuroblastoma, and acute lymphoblastic leukemia	Myelosuppression is dose limiting; however, cardiotoxicity, both acute and chronic, is well described. The acute form presents with arrhythmias and conduction abnormalities and is not dose related; however, chronic cardiotoxicity is dose related and results in dilated cardiomyopathy	D	First-trimester exposures, sometimes in combination with other drugs or radiation, have resulted in normal and abnormal neonates. Imperforate anus and rectovaginal fistula have been described as well as microcephaly. The effects of doxorubicin on the hearts of exposed fetuses and neonates are under evaluation [36] but no definitive information is available	Breastfeeding should be avoided because doxorubicin is excreted in breast milk
Daunorubicin (Daunomycin, DNR, Cerubidine, Rubidomycin)	Daunomycin intercalates into DNA and causes damage by forming a complex between DNA and topoisomerase II	Daunorubicin is widely distributed throughout the major organ systems and is highly lipid soluble. It is given IV	Acute myelogenous leukemia and acute lymphoblastic leukemia	Myelosuppression is dose limiting, and cardiotoxicity is usually transient, but can persist in a chronic form that leads to dilated cardiomyopathy	D	Specific reports on daunorubicin in pregnancy are lacking; however, see comments on doxorubicin above	Breastfeeding should be avoided

Table 22.7 Vinca alkaloids used for chemotherapy and a summary of pregnancy safety data [159]

Drug	Mechanism of action	Tissue distribution	Indications	Maternal side effects	Pregnancy category	Fetal effects	Breastfeeding
Vincristine (Oncovin, VCR)	Vincristine is a vinca alkaloid, antimicrotubule agent derived from the periwinkle plant *Catharanthus roseus*. Vincristine inhibits tubulin polymerization and disrupts mitosis; hence this drug is principally active during the M-phase of the cell cycle	This agent is rapidly distributed throughout the body but with relatively poor penetration of the blood–brain barrier. Vincristine is given IV, not orally	Acute lymphoblastic leukemia, Hodgkin's and non-Hodgkin's lymphoma, multiple myeloma, rhabdomyosarcoma, neuroblastoma, Ewing's sarcoma, Wilms' tumor, chronic leukemias, thyroid cancer, brain tumors, and choriocarcinoma	Neurotoxicity is dose limiting. The clinical manifestations include peripheral neuropathy, autonomic nervous system dysfunction, cranial nerve palsies, seizures, cortical blindness, and coma	D	Various sporadic reports of vincristine use in pregnancy and associated fetal anomalies have appeared. These include the presence of an atrial septal defect, renal hypoplasia, and pancytopenia	The risks are unknown
Vinblastine (Velban)	Vinblastine is a plant alkaloid from the periwinkle plant (*Catharanthus roseus*). It inhibits tubulin polymerization and disrupts microtubules during the M-phase of the cell cycle	Vinblastine is widely distributed to most body tissues, but with poor penetration of the blood–brain barrier. It is given IV	Hodgkin's and non-Hodgkin's lymphoma, testicular and breast cancers, Kaposi's sarcoma, and renal cell carcinoma	Myelosuppression is dose limiting, and neurotoxicity is less than with vincristine	D	Exposure during the first trimester has been associated with normal outcomes, and no malformations are known to be uniquely associated with vinblastine; however, digit abnormalities have been reported with multiple drug use including vinblastine	No data are available
Vinorelbine (Navelbine)	Vinorelbine is a semi-synthetic form of vinblastine with similar actions	This agent is widely distributed throughout the body and 80% protein bound. It is given IV	Nonsmall cell lung cancer, breast cancer, ovarian cancer, and Hodgkin's lymphoma	Myelosuppression is dose limiting	D	No information is available in humans; however, vinorelbine is teratogenic in animals	Breastfeeding should be avoided according to the manufacturer; however, it is not known if the drug is excreted in milk

Table 22.8 Taxanes used for chemotherapy and a summary of pregnancy safety data [159]

Drug	Mechanism of action	Tissue distribution	Indications	Maternal side effects	Pregnancy category	Fetal effects	Breastfeeding
Paclitaxel (Taxol)	Paclitaxel is isolated from *Taxus brevifolia*, the Pacific yew tree. The drug acts by binding to microtubules and enhancing polymerization. Mitosis is inhibited in the M-phase of the cell cycle	This agent is widely distributed throughout the body, including fluid spaces; however it has poor blood–brain barrier penetration. It is given IV	Ovarian cancer, breast cancer, nonsmall cell and small cell lung cancers, head and neck cancer, esophageal cancer, prostate cancer, bladder cancer, and AIDS-related Kaposi's sarcoma	Myelosuppression is dose limiting and neurotoxicity is a consideration. Rare cases of fatal anaphylaxis have been reported	D	No information is available in humans; however, in rabbits paclitaxel caused fetal death and resorption but not fetal malformations	Paclitaxel is highly lipophilic, and minimal kinetic information is available. It is not known if paclitaxel enters milk, but due to its potential toxicity, breastfeeding should be avoided

References

1. Brown D, Berran P, Kaplan KJ, Winter WE 3rd, Zahn CM. Special situations: abnormal cervical cytology during pregnancy. Clin Obstet Gynecol 2005;48(1):178–85.

2. National Cancer Institute. SEER Cancer Statistics Review 1975–2005. National Cancer Institute, Rockville, MD, 2007.

3. Bosch FX, Manos MM, Munoz N, Sherman M, Jansen AM, Peto J, et al. Prevalence of human papillomavirus in cervical cancer: a worldwide perspective. International biological study on cervical cancer (IBSCC) Study Group. J Natl Cancer Inst 1995;87(11):796–802.

4. Creasman WT. Cancer and pregnancy. Ann NY Acad Sci 2001;943:281–6.

5. Connor JP. Noninvasive cervical cancer complicating pregnancy. Obstet Gynecol Clin North Am 1998;25(2):331–42.

6. Muller CY, Smith HO. Cervical neoplasia complicating pregnancy. Obstet Gynecol Clin North Am 2005;32(4):533–46.

7. Wright TC Jr, Massad LS, Dunton CJ, Spitzer M, Wilkinson EJ, Solomon D. 2006 consensus guidelines for the management of women with abnormal cervical cancer screening tests. Am J Obstet Gynecol 2007;197(4):346–55.

8. Kaplan KJ, Dainty LA, Dolinsky B, Rose GS, Carlson J, McHale M, et al. Prognosis and recurrence risk for patients with cervical squamous intraepithelial lesions diagnosed during pregnancy. Cancer 2004;102(4):228–32.

9. Paraskevaidis E, Koliopoulos G, Kalantaridou S, Pappa L, Navrozoglou I, Zikopoulos K, et al. Management and evolution of cervical intraepithelial neoplasia during pregnancy and post-partum. Eur J Obstet Gynecol Reprod Biol 2002;104(1):67–9.

10. Siddiqui G, Kurzel RB, Lampley EC, Kang HS, Blankstein J Cervical dysplasia in pregnancy: progression versus regression post-partum. Int J Fertil Womens Med 2001;46(5):278–80.

11. Yost NP, Santoso JT, McIntire DD, Iliya FA. Postpartum regression rates of antepartum cervical intraepithelial neoplasia II and III lesions. Obstet Gynecol 1999;93(3):359–62.

12. Sadler L, Saftlas A, Wang W, Exeter M, Whittaker J, McCowan L. Treatment for cervical intraepithelial neoplasia and risk of preterm delivery. JAMA 2004;291(17):2100–6.

13. Raio L, Ghezzi F, Di Naro E, Gomez R, Luscher KP. Duration of pregnancy after carbon dioxide laser conization of the cervix: influence of cone height. Obstet Gynecol 1997;90(6):978–82.

14. Nguyen C, Montz FJ, Bristow RE. Management of stage I cervical cancer in pregnancy. Obstet Gynecol Surv 2000; 55(10):633–43.

15. Goldman NA, Goldberg GL. Late recurrence of squamous cell cervical cancer in an episiotomy site after vaginal delivery. Obstet Gynecol 2003;101(5 Pt 2):1127–9.

16. Sood AK, Sorosky JI, Mayr N, Anderson B, Buller RE, Niebyl J Cervical cancer diagnosed shortly after pregnancy: prognostic variables and delivery routes. Obstet Gynecol 2000;95 (6 Pt 1):832–8.

17. Abramovici A, Shaklai M, Pinkhas J. Myeloschisis in a six weeks embryo of a leukemic woman treated by busulfan. Teratology 1978;18(2):241–6.

18. Sood AK, Sorosky JI, Mayr N, Krogman S, Anderson B, Buller RE, et al. Radiotherapeutic management of cervical carcinoma that complicates pregnancy. Cancer 1997;80(6):1073–8.

19. Petrek JA. Breast cancer and pregnancy. J Natl Cancer Inst Monogr 1994;16:113–21.

20. White TT. Carcinoma of the breast and pregnancy; analysis of 920 cases collected from the literature and 22 new cases. Ann Surg 1954;139(1):9–18.

21. White TT. Prognosis of breast cancer for pregnant and nursing women: analysis of 1,413 cases. Surg Gynecol Obstet 1955; 100(6):661–6.

22. Peete CH Jr, Huneycutt HC Jr, Cherny WB. Cancer of the breast in pregnancy. N C Med J 1966;27(11):514–20.

23. Anderson JM. Mammary cancers and pregnancy. BMJ 1979;1(6171):1124–7.

24. Wallack MK, Wolf JA Jr, Bedwinek J, Denes AE, Glasgow G, Kumar B, et al. Gestational carcinoma of the female breast. Curr Probl Cancer 1983;7(9):1–58.

25. Gemignani ML, Petrek JA. Pregnancy-associated breast cancer: diagnosis and treatment. Breast J 2000;6(1):68–73.

26. Petrek JA, Dukoff R, Rogatko A. Prognosis of pregnancy-associated breast cancer. Cancer 1991;67(4):869–72.

27. Largent JA, Ziogas A, Anton-Culver H. Effect of reproductive factors on stage, grade and hormone receptor status in early-onset breast cancer. Breast Cancer Res 2005;7(4):R541–54.

28. Cullinane CA, Lubinski J, Neuhausen SL, Ghadirian P, Lynch HT, Isaacs C, et al. Effect of pregnancy as a risk factor for breast cancer in BRCA1/BRCA2 mutation carriers. Int J Cancer 2005;117(6):988–91.

29. Max MH, Klamer TW. Pregnancy and breast cancer. South Med J 1983;76(9):1088–90.

30. Finley JL, Silverman JF, Lannin DR. Fine-needle aspiration cytology of breast masses in pregnant and lactating women. Diagn Cytopathol 1989;5(3):255–9.

31. Fiorica JV. Special problems. Breast cancer and pregnancy. Obstet Gynecol Clin North Am 1994;21(4):721–32.

32. Byrd BF Jr, Bayer DS, Robertson JC, Stephenson SE Jr. Treatment of breast tumors associated with pregnancy and lactation. Ann Surg 1962;155:940–7.

33. Baker J, Ali A, Groch MW, Fordham E, Economou SG. Bone scanning in pregnant patients with breast carcinoma. Clin Nucl Med 1987;12(7):519–24.

34. Kal HB, Struikmans H. Radiotherapy during pregnancy: fact and fiction. Lancet Oncol 2005;6(5):328–33.

35. Ring AE, Smith IE, Jones A, Shannon C, Galani E, Ellis PA. Chemotherapy for breast cancer during pregnancy: an 18-year experience from five London teaching hospitals. J Clin Oncol 2005;23(18):4192–7.

36. Mathelin C, Annane K, Liegeois P, Bergerat JP, Dufour P. Chemotherapy for breast cancer during pregnancy. Eur J Obstet Gynecol Reprod Biol 2005;123(2):260–2.

37. Gadducci A, Cosio S, Fanucchi A, Nardini V, Roncella M, Conte PF, et al. Chemotherapy with epirubicin and paclitaxel for breast cancer during pregnancy: case report and review of the literature. Anticancer Res 2003;23(6D):5225–9.

38. Doll DC, Ringenberg QS, Yarbro JW. Management of cancer during pregnancy. Arch Intern Med 1988;148(9):2058–64.

39. Urist MM, Heslin MJ, Miller DM. Malignant melanoma. In: Lenhard Jr RE, Osteen RT, Gansler T (eds) Clinical oncology. American Cancer Society/Blackwell Science, Malden, MA, 2001:553–61.

40. Morton DL, Essner R, Kirkwood JM. Malignant melanoma. In: Bast Jr RC, Kaufe DW, Pollock RE (eds) Cancer medicine. American Cancer Society/BC Decker, Hamilton, Ontario, Canada, 2000:1849–69.

41. Leslie KK, Espey E. Oral contraceptives and skin cancer: is there a link? Am J Clin Dermatol 2005;6(6):349–55.

42. Weisz B, Schiff E, Lishner M. Cancer in pregnancy: maternal and fetal implications. Hum Reprod Update 2001;7(4):384–93.

43. Potter JF, Schoeneman M. Metastasis of maternal cancer to the placenta and fetus. Cancer 1970;25(2):380–8.

44. Silipo V, de Simone P, Mariani G, Buccini P, Ferrari A, Catricala C. Malignant melanoma and pregnancy. Melanoma Res 2006;16(6):497–500.

45. Slingluff CL Jr, Seigler HF. Malignant melanoma and pregnancy. Ann Plast Surg 1992;28(1):95–9.

46. Smith RS, Randall P. Melanoma during pregnancy. Obstet Gynecol 1969;34(6):825–9.

47. Dillman RO, Vandermolen LA, Barth NM, Bransford KJ. Malignant melanoma and pregnancy ten questions. West J Med 1996;164(2):156–61.

48. Lens MB, Rosdahl I, Ahlbom A, Farahmand BY, Synnerstad I, Boeryd B, et al. Effect of pregnancy on survival in women with cutaneous malignant melanoma. J Clin Oncol 2004;22(21):4369–75.

49. Wiggins CL, Berwick M, Bishop JA. Malignant melanoma in pregnancy. Obstet Gynecol Clin North Am 2005;32(4):559–68.

50. Pack GT, Scharnagel IM. The prognosis for malignant melanoma in the pregnant woman. Cancer 1951;4(2):324–34.

51. Byrd BF Jr, McGanity WJ. The effect of pregnancy on the clinical course of malignant melanoma. South Med J 1954;47(3):196–200.

52. Riberti C, Marola G, Bertani A. Malignant melanoma: the adverse effect of pregnancy. Br J Plast Surg 1981;34(3):338–9.

53. Sato T, Ishiko A, Saito M, Tanaka M, Ishimoto H, Amagai M. Rapid growth of malignant melanoma in pregnancy. J Dtsch Dermatol Ges 2008;6(2):126–9.

54. Sadoff L, Winkley J, Tyson S. Is malignant melanoma an endocrine-dependent tumor? The possible adverse effect of estrogen. Oncology 1973;27(3):244–57.

55. Marcellini M, de Luca N, Riccioni T, Ciucci A, Orecchia A, Lacal PM, et al. Increased melanoma growth and metastasis spreading in mice overexpressing placenta growth factor. Am J Pathol 2006;169(2):643–54.

56. Stadelmann WK, Rapaport DP, Soong S-J. Prognostic, clinical, and pathologic features. In: Balck CM, Houghton AN, Sober AJ (eds) Cutaneous melanoma. Quality Medical Publishing, St Louis, MO, 1998:11–35.

57. Altman JF, Lowe L, Redman B, Esper P, Schwartz JL, Johnson TM, et al. Placental metastasis of maternal melanoma. J Am Acad Dermatol 2003;49(6):1150–4.

58. Alexander A, Samlowski WE, Grossman D, Bruggers CS, Harris RM, Zone JJ, et al. Metastatic melanoma in pregnancy: risk of transplacental metastases in the infant. J Clin Oncol 2003;21(11):2179–86.

59. Hauschild A, Gogas H, Tarhini A, Middleton MR, Testori A, Dreno B, et al. Practical guidelines for the management of interferon-alpha-2b side effects in patients receiving adjuvant treatment for melanoma: expert opinion. Cancer 2008;112(5):982–94.

60. Kirkwood JM, Ibrahim JG, Sondak VK, Richards J, Flaherty LE, Ernstoff MS, et al. High- and low-dose interferon alfa-2b in high-risk melanoma: first analysis of intergroup trial E1690/S9111/C9190. J Clin Oncol 2000;18(12):2444–58.

61. Kirkwood JM, Ibrahim JG, Sosman JA, Sondak VK, Agarwala SS, Ernstoff MS, et al. High-dose interferon alfa-2b significantly prolongs relapse-free and overall survival compared with the GM2-KLH/QS-21 vaccine in patients with resected stage IIB-III melanoma: results of intergroup trial E1694/S9512/C509801. J Clin Oncol 2001;19(9):2370–80.

62. Kirkwood JM, Strawderman MH, Ernstoff MS, Smith TJ, Borden EC, Blum RH. Interferon alfa-2b adjuvant therapy of high-risk resected cutaneous melanoma: the Eastern Cooperative Oncology Group Trial EST 1684. J Clin Oncol 1996;14(1):7–17.

63. Boskovic R, Wide R, Wolpin J, Bauer DJ, Koren G. The reproductive effects of beta interferon therapy in pregnancy: a longitudinal cohort. Neurology 2005;65(6):807–11.

64. Hiratsuka M, Minakami H, Koshizuka S, Sato I. Administration of interferon-alpha during pregnancy: effects on fetus. J Perinat Med 2000;28(5):372–6.

65. Mubarak AA, Kakil IR, Awidi A, Al-Homsi U, Fawzi Z, Kelta M, et al. Normal outcome of pregnancy in chronic myeloid leukemia treated with interferon-alpha in 1st trimester: report of 3 cases and review of the literature. Am J Hematol 2002;69(2):115–18.

66. Mesquita MM, Pestana A, Mota A. Successful pregnancy occurring with interferon-alpha therapy in chronic myeloid leukemia. Acta Obstet Gynecol Scand 2005;84(3):300–1.

67. Sandberg-Wollheim M, Frank D, Goodwin TM, Giesser B, Lopez-Bresnahan M, Stam-Moraga M, et al. Pregnancy outcomes during treatment with interferon beta-1a in patients with multiple sclerosis. Neurology 2005;65(6):802–6.

68. Grimes WH Jr, Bartholomew RA, Colvin ED, Fish JS, Lester WM. Ovarian cyst complicating pregnancy. Am J Obstet Gynecol 1954;68(2):594–605.

69. Struyk AP, Treffers PE. Ovarian tumors in pregnancy. Acta Obstet Gynecol Scand 1984;63(5):421–4.

70. Booth RT. Ovarian tumors in pregnancy. Obstet Gynecol 1963;21:189–93.

71. White KC. Ovarian tumors in pregnancy. A private hospital ten year survey. Am J Obstet Gynecol 1973;116(4):544–50.

72. Buttery BW, Beischer NA, Fortune DW, Macafee CA. Ovarian tumours in pregnancy. Med J Aust 1973;1(7):345–9.

73. Hess LW, Peaceman A, O'Brien WF, Winkel CA, Cruikshank DP, Morrison JC. Adnexal mass occurring with intrauterine pregnancy: report of fifty-four patients requiring laparotomy for definitive management. Am J Obstet Gynecol 1988;158(5):1029–34.

74. Thornton JG, Wells M. Ovarian cysts in pregnancy: does ultrasound make traditional management inappropriate? Obstet Gynecol 1987;69(5):717–21.

75. Tawa K. Ovarian tumors in pregnancy. Am J Obstet Gynecol 1964;90:511–16.

76. Hill LM, Johnson CE, Lee RA. Ovarian surgery in pregnancy. Am J Obstet Gynecol 1975;122(5):565–9.

77. Hasan A, Amr S, Issa A, Bata M. Ovarian tumors complicating pregnancy. Int J Gynaecol Obstet 1983;21(4):279–82.

78. Ballard CA. Ovarian tumors associated with pregnancy termination patients. Am J Obstet Gynecol 1984;149(4):384–7.

79. Hopkins MP, Duchon MA. Adnexal surgery in pregnancy. J Reprod Med 1986;31(11):1035–7.

80. Nelson MJ, Cavalieri R, Graham D, Sanders RC. Cysts in pregnancy discovered by sonography. J Clin Ultrasound 1986;14(7):509–12.

81. Ashkenazy M, Kessler I, Czernobilsky B, Nahshoni A, Lancet M. Ovarian tumors in pregnancy. Int J Gynaecol Obstet 1988;27(1):79–83.

82. Tchabo JG, Stay EJ, Limaye NS. Ovarian tumors in pregnancy. A community hospital's five year experience. Int Surg 1987;72(4):227–9.

83. Koonings PP, Platt LD, Wallace R. Incidental adnexal neoplasms at cesarean section. Obstet Gynecol 1988;72(5):767–9.

84. Sunoo CS, Terada KY, Kamemoto LE, Hale RW. Adnexal masses in pregnancy: occurrence by ethnic group. Obstet Gynecol 1990;75(1):38–40.

85. el-Yahia AR, Rahman J, Rahman MS, al-Suleiman SA. Ovarian tumours in pregnancy. Aust NZ J Obstet Gynaecol 1991;31(4):327–30.

86. Platek DN, Henderson CE, Goldberg GL. The management of a persistent adnexal mass in pregnancy. Am J Obstet Gynecol 1995;173(4):1236–40.

87. Ueda M, Ueki M. Ovarian tumors associated with pregnancy. Int J Gynaecol Obstet 1996;55(1):59–65.

88. Bromley B, Benacerraf B. Adnexal masses during pregnancy: accuracy of sonographic diagnosis and outcome. J Ultrasound Med 1997;16(7):447–52; quiz 53–4.

89. Whitecar MP, Turner S, Higby MK. Adnexal masses in pregnancy: a review of 130 cases undergoing surgical management. Am J Obstet Gynecol 1999;181(1):19–24.

90. Sayar H, Lhomme C, Verschraegen CF. Malignant adnexal masses in pregnancy. Obstet Gynecol Clin North Am 2005;32(4):569–93.

91. Jubb ED. Primary ovarian carcinoma in pregnancy. Am J Obstet Gynecol 1963;85:345–54.

92. Creasman WT, Rutledge F, Smith JP. Carcinoma of the ovary associated with pregnancy. Obstet Gynecol 1971;38(1):111–16.

93. Clement PB. Tumor-like lesions of the ovary associated with pregnancy. Int J Gynecol Pathol 1993;12(2):108–15.

94. Kumar V, Fausto N, Abbas A. Pathologic basis of disease, 7th edn. WB Saunders/Elsevier, St Louis, MO, 2005.

95. DiSaia PJ, Creasman WT. Clinical gynecologic oncology, 6th edn. Mosby, St Louis, MO, 2002.

96. Fujita M, Inoue M, Tanizawa O, Minagawa J, Yamada T, Tani T. Retrospective review of 41 patients with endodermal sinus tumor of the ovary. Int J Gynecol Cancer 1993;3(5):329–35.

97. Schwartz RP, Chatwani AJ, Strimel W, Putong PB. Endodermal sinus tumor in pregnancy: report of a case and review of the literature. Gynecol Oncol 1983;15(3):434–9.

98. Kurman RJ, Norris HJ. Endodermal sinus tumor of the ovary: a clinical and pathologic analysis of 71 cases. Cancer 1976;38(6):2404–19.

99. Tewari K, Cappuccini F, Disaia PJ, Berman ML, Manetta A, Kohler MF. Malignant germ cell tumors of the ovary. Obstet Gynecol 2000;95(1):128–33.

100. Talerman A, Haije WG, Baggerman L. Serum alphafetoprotein (AFP) in diagnosis and management of endodermal sinus (yolk sac) tumor and mixed germ cell tumor of the ovary. Cancer 1978;41(1):272–8.

101. Malone JM, Gershenson DM, Creasy RK, Kavanagh JJ, Silva EG, Stringer CA. Endodermal sinus tumor of the ovary associated with pregnancy. Obstet Gynecol 1986;68(3 suppl):86S–9S.

102. Kim DS, Park MI. Maternal and fetal survival following surgery and chemotherapy of endodermal sinus tumor of the ovary during pregnancy: a case report. Obstet Gynecol 1989;73(3 Pt 2):503–7.

103. Metz SA, Day TG, Pursell SH. Adjuvant chemotherapy in a pregnant patient with endodermal sinus tumor of the ovary. Gynecol Oncol 1989;32(3):371–4.

104. Malhotra N, Sood M. Endodermal sinus tumor in pregnancy. Gynecol Oncol 2000;78(2):265–6.

105. Han JY, Nava-Ocampo AA, Kim TJ, Shim JU, Park CT. Pregnancy outcome after prenatal exposure to bleomycin, etoposide and cisplatin for malignant ovarian germ cell tumors: report of 2 cases. Reprod Toxicol 2005;19(4):557–61.

106. Seidman JD, Kurman RJ. Pathology of ovarian carcinoma. Hematol Oncol Clin North Am 2003;17(4):909–25, vii.

107. Kobayashi F, Sagawa N, Nakamura K, Nonogaki M, Ban C, Fujii S, et al. Mechanism and clinical significance of elevated CA 125 levels in the sera of pregnant women. Am J Obstet Gynecol 1989;160(3):563–6.

108. Fox H, Agrawal K, Langley FA. A clinicopathologic study of 92 cases of granulosa cell tumor of the ovary with special reference to the factors influencing prognosis. Cancer 1975;35(1):231–41.

109. Pankratz E, Boyes DA, White GW, Galliford BW, Fairey RN, Benedet JL. Granulosa cell tumors. A clinical review of 61 cases. Obstet Gynecol 1978;52(6):718–23.

110. Stenwig JT, Hazekamp JT, Beecham JB. Granulosa cell tumors of the ovary. A clinicopathological study of 118 cases with long-term follow-up. Gynecol Oncol 1979;7(2):136–52.

111. Evans AT 3rd, Gaffey TA, Malkasian GD Jr, Annegers JF. Clinicopathologic review of 118 granulosa and 82 theca cell tumors. Obstet Gynecol 1980;55(2):231–8.

112. Ohel G, Kaneti H, Schenker JG. Granulosa cell tumors in Israel: a study of 172 cases. Gynecol Oncol 1983;15(2):278–86.

113. Schumer ST, Cannistra SA. Granulosa cell tumor of the ovary. J Clin Oncol 2003;21(6):1180–9.

114. Barwick KW, LiVolsi VA. Malignant mixed mesodermal tumors of the ovary: a clinicopathologic assessment of 12 cases. Am J Surg Pathol 1980;4(1):37–42.

115. Brown E, Stewart M, Rye T, Al-Nafussi A, Williams AR, Bradburn M, et al. Carcinosarcoma of the ovary: 19 years of prospective data from a single center. Cancer 2004;100(10):2148–53.

116. Kuzel TM, Benson AB. Non-Hodgkin's lymphoma. In: Gleicher N (ed) Principles and practice of medical therapy in pregnancy. Appleton and Lange, East Norwalk, CT, 1992:1078–81.

117. Smith LH, Danielsen B, Allen ME, Cress R. Cancer associated with obstetric delivery: results of linkage with the California cancer registry. Am J Obstet Gynecol 2003;189(4):1128–35.

118. Dildy GA 3rd, Moise KJ Jr, Carpenter RJ Jr, Klima T. Maternal malignancy metastatic to the products of conception: a review. Obstet Gynecol Surv 1989;44(7):535–40.

119. Pavlidis NA. Coexistence of pregnancy and malignancy. Oncologist 2002;7(4):279–87.

120. Jox A, Zander T, Kornacker M, Kanzler H, Kuppers R, Diehl V, et al. Detection of identical Hodgkin–Reed Sternberg cell specific immunoglobulin gene rearrangements in a patient with Hodgkin's disease of mixed cellularity subtype at primary diagnosis and in relapse two and a half years later. Ann Oncol 1998;9(3):283–7.

121. Connors JM. Hodgkin's lymphoma, 3rd edn. Elsevier, Philadelphia, 2004.

122. Ward FT, Weiss RB. Lymphoma and pregnancy. Semin Oncol 1989;16(5):397–409.

123. Lishner M, Zemlickis D, Degendorfer P. Maternal and fetal outcome following Hodgkin's disease in pregnancy. In: Koren G, Lishner M, Farine D (eds) Cancer in pregnancy: maternal and fetal risk. Cambridge University Press, Cambridge, 1996:107–15.

124. Peleg D, Ben-Ami M. Lymphoma and leukemia complicating pregnancy. Obstet Gynecol Clin North Am 1998;25(2):365–83.

125. Hurley TJ, McKinnell JV, Irani MS. Hematologic malignancies in pregnancy. Obstet Gynecol Clin North Am 2005;32(4):595–614.

126. Aviles A, Neri N. Hematological malignancies and pregnancy: a final report of 84 children who received chemotherapy in utero. Clin Lymphoma 2001;2(3):173–7.

127. Vassilakopoulos TP, Angelopoulou MK, Siakantaris MP, Kontopidou FN, Dimopoulou MN, Kokoris SI, et al. Combination chemotherapy plus low-dose involved-field radiotherapy for early clinical stage Hodgkin's lymphoma. Int J Radiat Oncol Biol Phys 2004;59(3):765–81.

128. Woo SY, Fuller LM, Cundiff JH, Bondy ML, Hagemeister FB, McLaughlin P, et al. Radiotherapy during pregnancy for clinical stages IA-IIA Hodgkin's disease. Int J Radiat Oncol Biol Phys 1992;23(2):407–12.

129. Economopoulos T, Papageorgiou S, Dimopoulos MA, Pavlidis N, Tsatalas C, Symeonidis A, et al. Non-Hodgkin's lymphomas in Greece according to the WHO classification of lymphoid neoplasms. A retrospective analysis of 810 cases. Acta Haematol 2005;113(2):97–103.

130. Carbone A, Franceschi S, Gloghini A, Russo A, Gaidano G, Monfardini S. Pathological and immunophenotypic features of adult non-Hodgkin's lymphomas by age group. Hum Pathol 1997;28(5):580–7.

131. Ioachim HL. Non-Hodgkin's lymphoma in pregnancy. Three cases and review of the literature. Arch Pathol Lab Med 1985;109(9):803–9.

132. Weinshel EL, Peterson BA. Hodgkin's disease. CA Cancer J Clin 1993;43(6):327–46.

133. Hoover RN. Lymphoma risks in populations with altered immunity – a search for mechanism. Cancer Res 1992;52 (19 suppl):5477s–8s.

134. Giovannini M, Saccucci P, Cannone D, Damiani G, Pomini P. Can pregnancy aggravate the course of non-Hodgkin's lymphoma? Eur J Gynaecol Oncol 1989;10(4):287–9.

135. Selvais PL, Mazy G, Gosseye S, Ferrant A, van Lierde M. Breast infiltration by acute lymphoblastic leukemia during pregnancy. Am J Obstet Gynecol 1993;169(6):1619–20.

136. Conlan MG, Bast M, Armitage JO, Weisenburger DD. Bone marrow involvement by non-Hodgkin's lymphoma: the clinical significance of morphologic discordance between the lymph node and bone marrow. Nebraska Lymphoma Study Group. J Clin Oncol 1990;8(7):1163–72.

137. Escalon MP, Liu NS, Yang Y, Hess M, Walker PL, Smith TL, et al. Prognostic factors and treatment of patients with T-cell non-Hodgkin lymphoma: the M. D. Anderson Cancer Center experience. Cancer 2005;103(10):2091–8.

138. Aviles A, Diaz-Maqueo JC, Torras V, Garcia EL, Guzman R. Non-Hodgkin's lymphomas and pregnancy: presentation of 16 cases. Gynecol Oncol 1990;37(3):335–7.

139. Cardonick E, Iacobucci A. Use of chemotherapy during human pregnancy. Lancet Oncol 2004;5(5):283–91.

140. Walker JW, Reinisch JF, Monforte HL. Maternal pulmonary adenocarcinoma metastatic to the fetus: first recorded case report and literature review. Pediatr Pathol Mol Med 2002;21(1):57–69.

141. Yahia C, Hyman GA, Phillips LL. Acute leukemia and pregnancy. Obstet Gynecol Surv 1958;13(1):1–21.

142. Armitage J, Longo D. Malignancies of lymphoid cells. In: Braunwald E, Hausser S, Fancis A (eds) Harrison's principles of internal medicine. McGraw-Hill, New York, 2001:715–27.

143. Kantanjiano HM, Faderl S. Acute lymphoid leukemia in adults. In: Meloni D, Morrissey D, O'Keefe K (eds) Abeloff: clinical oncology. Elsevier, Philadelphia, 2004:2793–8.

144. Reynoso EE, Shepherd FA, Messner HA, Farquharson HA, Garvey MB, Baker MA. Acute leukemia during pregnancy: the Toronto Leukemia Study Group experience with long-term follow-up of children exposed in utero to chemotherapeutic agents. J Clin Oncol 1987;5(7):1098–106.

145. Applegaum FF. Acute myeloid leukemia in adults. In: Meloni D, Morrissey D, O'Keefe K (eds) Abeloff: clinical oncology. Elsevier, Philadelphia, 2004:2825–42.

146. Caligiuri MA, Mayer RJ. Pregnancy and leukemia. Semin Oncol 1989;16(5):388–96.

147. McDunn SH, Winter JN. Acute leukemia. In: Gleicher N (ed) Principles and practice of medical therapy in pregnancy. Appleton and Lange, New York, 1992:1064–8.

148. Hoelzer D, Gokbuget N. Acute lymphocytic Philadelphia: leukemia in adults. In: Hoffman R, Benz EJ, Shattil SJ (eds) Hematology: basic principles and practice. Elsevier, Philadelphia, 2005:1177.

149. Shaw MP, Eden OB, Grace E, Ellis PM. Acute lymphoblastic leukemia and Klinefelter's syndrome. Pediatr Hematol Oncol 1992;9(1):81–5.

150. Janik-Moszant A, Bubala H, Stojewska M, Sonta-Jakimczyk D. Acute lymphoblastic leukemia in children with Fanconi anemia. Wiad Lek 1998;51(suppl 4):285–8.

151. Todeschini G, Tecchio C, Meneghini V, Pizzolo G, Veneri D, Zanotti R, et al. Estimated 6-year event-free survival of 55% in 60 consecutive adult acute lymphoblastic leukemia patients treated with an intensive phase II protocol based on high induction dose of daunorubicin. Leukemia 1998;12(2):144–9.

152. Baustian GH, Fenni FF, Clark OA. Chronic lymphocytic leukemia: treatment. In: Clark OA (ed) wwwfirstconsultcom Elsevier, Oxford, 2005:1 (Part 4).

153. Kabonjo M, O'Handon KM, Clark OA. Chronic myelogenous leukemia: summary. In: Clark OA (ed) wwwfirstconsultcom Elsevier, Oxford, 2005:1 (Part 4).

154. Elliott MA, Wolf RC, Hook CC, Pruthi RK, Heit JA, Letendre LL, *et al.* Thromboembolism in adults with acute lymphoblastic leukemia during induction with L-asparaginase-containing multi-agent regimens: incidence, risk factors, and possible role of antithrombin. Leuk Lymphoma 2004;45(8):1545–9.

155. Beinart G, Damon L. Thrombosis associated with L-asparaginase therapy and low fibrinogen levels in adult acute lymphoblastic leukemia. Am J Hematol 2004;77(4):331–5.

156. Mauz-Korholz C, Junker R, Gobel U, Nowak-Gottl U. Prothrombotic risk factors in children with acute lymphoblastic leukemia treated with delayed E. coli asparaginase (COALL-92 and 97 protocols). Thromb Haemost 2000;83(6):840–3.

157. Jaime-Perez JC, Gomez-Almaguer D. The complex nature of the prothrombotic state in acute lymphoblastic leukemia of childhood. Haematologica 2003;88(7):ELT25.

158. Greenlund LJ, Letendre L, Tefferi A. Acute leukemia during pregnancy: a single institutional experience with 17 cases. Leuk Lymphoma 2001;41(5–6):571–7.

159. Leslie KK, Koil C, Rayburn WF. Chemotherapeutic drugs in pregnancy. Obstet Gynecol Clin North Am 2005;32(4):627–40.

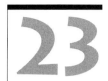

23 Critical care in pregnancy

Uma Munnur[1], *Dilip R. Karnad*[2], *Edward R. Yeomans*[3]
and Kalpalatha K. Guntupalli[4]

[1]Department of Anesthesiology, Baylor College of Medicine, Houston, TX, USA
[2]Seth G S Medical College and Medical Intensive Care Unit, KEM Hospital, Mumbai,
India, and Baylor College of Medicine, Houston, TX, USA
[3]Department of Obstetrics and Gynecology, University of Texas Medical School at
Houston and Texas Tech University Health Sciences Center, Lubbock, TX, USA
[4]Pulmonary, Critical Care and Sleep Medicine, Baylor College of Medicine, Houston,
TX, USA

Introduction

Critical care refers to the intensive monitoring and aggressive and often invasive treatment of severely ill patients with potentially fatal but reversible conditions, usually in the intensive care unit (ICU). The critically ill obstetric patient presents several challenges. Common illnesses may present differently in pregnant women due to altered anatomy and physiology [1,2]. The impact of less severe disorders may be more devastating due to decreased physiologic reserve during pregnancy [3,4]. Thresholds for instituting therapy may differ in pregnant women because of the threat to fetal well-being [5]. Finally, some diagnostic modalities and drugs which are commonly used in the ICU may have undesirable effects on the fetus [6].

Epidemiology of critical illness in pregnancy

Acute disorders requiring ICU admission complicate 1–9/1000 pregnancies [7]. ICU admission rates range from 100 to 1700 per 100,000 deliveries in individual series [8,9]. Admission rates are generally higher in ICU with a large referral base [9–11] and in hospitals with dedicated obstetric ICU [12,13]. While intercurrent medical disorders account for some of these critical illnesses, a large proportion of women have obstetric disorders like pre-eclampsia, which can usually be detected before they reach a critical stage. In most economically developed countries, a combination of meticulous antenatal care, excellent obstetric anesthesia, skilled intrapartum management and high-quality neonatal intensive care has decreased maternal mortality rates to <20 per 100,000 deliveries [8,14,15]. The absence of one or more of these critical components of care contributes to the extremely high maternal and perinatal morbidity and mortality in underdeveloped countries [10,16].

Organization of the intensive care unit

Care of critically ill obstetric patients involves a multidisciplinary team consisting of an obstetrician or maternal-fetal medicine specialist familiar with obstetric physiology and its derangements, an intensive care physician trained in the detection and treatment of failing organs, an anesthesiologist for pain control, airway management and for anesthesia during emergency surgical delivery, and a neonatologist to manage a preterm neonate who may have suffered intrauterine insult due to severe maternal illness. Nurses with experience in a labor and delivery unit and additional training in advanced life support techniques are essential [17]. The nurse-to-patient ratio must be at least 1:1; two nurses (ideally one with an extensive labor and delivery background and the other with an extensive intensive care background) will be required to provide optimum care during delivery [17]. Ideally a senior member of both the obstetric and intensive care teams should interface in person at least daily to discuss these cases directly to ensure that both team members have a good understanding of the other's concerns.

Proximity to the labor suite or obstetric operating room is an issue that needs attention. In a majority of hospitals, obstetric patients are managed in the general ICU [8]. Equipment to monitor uterine activity and fetal well-being is usually transported to the ICU when needed. In the 1990s there was great enthusiasm for having a dedicated ICU for

de Swiet's Medical Disorders in Obstetric Practice, 5th edition.
Edited by R. O. Powrie, M. F. Greene, W. Camann. © 2010 Blackwell
Publishing.

obstetric patients [13]. It is now believed that such units may only be justified in hospitals that receive >100 admissions/year requiring obstetric intensive care; smaller numbers may not allow staff to maintain their critical care skills [17]. Moreover, to be economically viable, at least 1% of obstetric hospital admissions would have to be admitted to the ICU [9,13]. Even with admission rates above 100/year, individual familiarity with the management of many critical care cases will still be lacking and the best practice for obstetric critical care units may need to involve formal arrangements to allow co-management of obstetric patients in the obstetric intensive care by intensivists and obstetricians in collaboration with a bedside team of both an obstetric and a critical care nurse.

Indications for intensive care unit admission

The Society of Critical Care Medicine guidelines assign highest priority for ICU admission to unstable patients who need intensive monitoring or treatment that cannot be provided outside the ICU [18]. These would include women with hypotension, coagulopathy, renal failure, hepatic encephalopathy, coma, seizures or respiratory failure. The next priority is assigned to patients who require intensive monitoring and may potentially need immediate intervention [18]. Women

with severe pre-eclampsia, HELLP syndrome, jaundice, severe community-acquired infections and pre-existing medical disorders fall in this category [19]. Conditions commonly leading to organ dysfunction and ICU admission in pregnancy are listed in Table 23.1. Previous studies have shown that maternal age >35 years, high parity, multiple pregnancy, ethnic minority status, and transfer from another hospital for delivery are associated with increased need for ICU admission [8,15,20,21].

Transfers within hospital from one unit to the critical care unit are potentially dangerous times when errors may be made. Clear hand-over communications between physicians and nurses are essential. Transport of patients should be carried out by experienced medical personnel who have ready access to the following equipment while en route: an adequately full oxygen tank and appropriate oxygen delivery device, a bag and mask should the patient stop breathing, continuous cardiac monitoring, a manual suction device, manual blood pressure cuff and stethoscope, good intravenous access, and any medications that might reasonably needed during the time frame involved in the transfer. This list is summarized in Box 23.1.

Obstetric versus medical disorders

Primary obstetric disorders account for 50–80% of ICU admissions during pregnancy and the puerperium in all parts of the

Table 23.1 Important conditions that may cause severe organ dysfunction or failure during pregnancy or postpartum period

Obstetric disorders	Increased susceptibility during pregnancy	Pre-existing conditions that may worsen during pregnancy
Obstetric hemorrhage	Renal	Cardiovascular
Adherent, retained placenta	Acute renal failure	Valvular disease
Pregnancy-induced hypertension	Infections	Coarctation of aorta
HELLP syndrome	Urinary tract infection	Systemic hypertension
Acute fatty liver of pregnancy	Listeriosis	Congenital cyanotic heart disease
Chorioamnionitis	Viral hepatitis E	Ischemic heart disease
Septic abortion	*Plasmodium falciparum* malaria	Pulmonary hypertension
Puerperal sepsis	Varicella pneumonia	Respiratory
Amniotic fluid embolism	Hematologic	Cystic fibrosis
Intrauterine fetal demise	Disseminated intravascular	Lung transplant
Ruptured ectopic pregnancy	coagulation	Renal
Pelvic septic thrombophlebitis	Postpartum HUS/TTP	Chronic renal insufficiency
Peripartum cardiomyopathy	Venous thrombosis	Endocrine
Tocolytic-induced pulmonary edema	Endocrine	Prolactinoma
Uterine inversion	Gestational diabetes	Diabetes mellitus
	Sheehan's syndrome	Liver
	Neurologic	Cirrhosis
	Intracranial hemorrhage	Hematologic
	Respiratory	Sickle cell disease
	Pulmonary thromboembolism	Rheumatologic
	Air embolism	Scleroderma
	Aspiration	Polymyositis
		Neurologic
		Epilepsy
		Intracranial tumors

Adapted from Soubra & Guntupalli [15].
HELLP, hemolysis, elevated liver enzymes, low platelets; HUS, hemolytic uremic syndrome; TTP, thrombotic thrombocytopenic purpura.

Box 23.1 Checklist in preparation for transfer of patient to an intensive care setting

- Full oxygen tank
- Device to provide oxygen and a double check to ensure it is working (nasal prongs/mask/"100% nonrebreather"/transport ventilator)
- Bag-mask to ventilate patient should breathing cease in transport
- Oxygen saturation monitor with good waveform and alarms on
- EKG monitor with alarms on and adequate paper to print
- Transport defibrillator with batteries checked
- Adequate volume in any active intravenous drips for a transfer that includes unanticipated delays en route
- Syringes, intravenous fluid, and medications that may be needed in transit (e.g. fluid bolus for sepsis patient, an antihypertensive for a pre-eclamptic patient, a benzodiazepine for a patient with recurrent seizures)
- Critical care team has expressed their readiness to receive patient and have received or will receive detailed hand-over including list of medications and results of recent testing

Final "pause" before mobilizing:
- Patient vitals are stable (if patient recently unstable, consider having physician accompany transfer)
- Patient able to protect airway or airway that has been placed is secure

world [8,15]. Over 80% of these are due to pre-eclampsia and its complications, obstetric hemorrhage and pelvic sepsis. On the other hand, nonobstetric or medical disorders in pregnancy show large geographic variations. In developed countries, asthma [16,20], pneumonia [12,16], drug abuse [16,22], complicated urinary infections [12,16], pre-existing autoimmune disorders, chronic pulmonary disease [23], endocrine disorders [12], trauma [24,25] and pulmonary thromboembolism [3,26] are common. Medical disorders commonly seen in developing countries include severe malaria, vital hepatitis, cerebral venous sinus thrombosis, tetanus, tuberculosis, rheumatic valvular heart disease, anemia and attempted suicide (poisoning or burns) [8,10,27].

Intensive care units in developed countries are increasingly seeing a unique subgroup of pregnant women. Advances in healthcare have resulted in survival to child-bearing age of women with disorders such as surgically corrected complex congenital heart disease, organ transplant and chronic disorders like cystic fibrosis. Pregnant women with these conditions develop increased morbidity and sometimes require intensive medical care [28,29].

Antepartum versus postpartum intensive care unit admissions

Postpartum women comprise approximately 60–80% of obstetric ICU admissions [8,10,15]. Almost 80% of postpartum admissions occur during the first 24 hours after delivery, usually for obstetric disorders like postpartum hemorrhage and its consequences, aspiration and eclampsia [8]. Late postpartum admissions are usually for puerperal sepsis, cerebral venous thrombosis, acute renal failure and worsening thrombocytopenia in women with the HELLP syndrome [10,30]. Antepartum admissions are more frequently due to co-existing medical disorders. Some of these disorders may precede the pregnancy (e.g. valvular heart disease, asthma, epilepsy) while others may develop acutely during pregnancy (e.g. peripartum cardiomyopathy, viral hepatitis, severe community-acquired pneumonia, acute pyelonephritis) [15,16]. Respiratory failure is the most common problem seen in antepartum ICU admissions [10–12.22].

Initial assessment of a critically ill patient

As in a nonpregnant critically ill patient, the initial assessment of a parturient is focused on airway, breathing, and circulation.

Airway

Airway evaluation and management remain the first priority. Supplemental oxygen may be required in some patients. Tracheal intubation is needed in the setting of persistent hypoxemia, airway obstruction, impaired laryngeal reflexes or altered mental status [31,32]. Pregnant women are at high risk for aspiration of gastric contents and are often more difficult to intubate than nonpregnant patients. Therefore, endotracheal intubation should be performed sooner rather than later, to protect the airway, and should be attempted by the most experienced individual available (who should be notified early of the potential need for intubation) [32–34]. Box 23.2 provides a checklist to ensure the right equipment is available in the room when intubation is attempted in areas where such care is not routine. If the airway exam indicates that tracheal intubation is likely to be difficult [32], awake intubation should be performed with good topical anesthesia [31,33]. Rapid-sequence induction with cricoid pressure and orotracheal intubation is recommended in the obtunded or unconscious parturient without a potentially difficult airway

Box 23.2 Checklist in preparation for endotracheal intubation

For maternal monitoring
- Continuous EKG monitoring of mother
- Blood pressure monitor on patient's arm
- Pulse oximeter

For resuscitation
- High-flow oxygen source
- Securely fitting mask with manual inflation bag
- Two large-bore (18 G or greater) intravenous catheters in place
- Plan in place for next step if attempt at endotracheal intubation fails (e.g. laryngeal mask airway)

For person doing intubation
(who should be the most experienced person available and have an assistant working with them)
- Oropharyngeal suction equipment
- Laryngoscope with light working
- Stylet
- Gloves, mask, goggles and gown for person doing intubation
- Medications for sedation and (if necessary) paralysis of patient (e.g. IV thiopental 3–5 mg/kg for sedation, etomidate 0.3 mg/kg over 60 seconds for muscle relaxation and succinyl choline 1–1.5 mg/kg up to 150 mg for paralysis)

For verification of correct tube placement
- Ideally a method of verifying that CO_2 is being exhaled from endotracheal tube but chest X-ray and bilateral auscultation may be used as additional assessment tools

[31,33]. A set of instruments for difficult airway management must always be available in the ICU and the labor and delivery room [32,34].

Breathing

Adequacy of respiration must be established rapidly. Supplemental oxygen and bag-mask ventilation may be required initially. Noninvasive positive pressure ventilation is an option for some patients (see Chapter 1). If respiratory effort is inadequate, tracheal intubation is performed and mechanical ventilation initiated.

Circulation

Hypotension and shock should be treated promptly in order to maintain uteroplacental perfusion. After 20 weeks of pregnancy, pressure of the gravid uterus on the inferior vena cava and abdominal aorta in the supine position can decrease cardiac output by up to 30% [2,4,35]. The parturient should therefore be positioned on either the left or right side. Two large-bore intravenous cannulae (14 G or 16 G) should be placed to administer fluids and a Foley catheter should be placed to monitor urine output [36]. Central venous access may be needed for volume resuscitation, bolus drug administration and infusion of vasopressors. Femoral vein

catheterization should be avoided due to the risk of thromboembolism and sepsis [37]. The jugular route is preferred over the subclavian in patients with coagulopathy as the subclavian site cannot be compressed in the event of excessive bleeding or accidental arterial puncture [37]. Hypotension is treated by aggressive volume resuscitation [3,6,36]. If hemorrhage is life-threatening, blood group O Rh-negative packed red blood cells are transfused until type-specific or cross-matched blood is available [38]. It is preferable to place an arterial line at the earliest opportunity to measure the blood pressure continuously. Severe maternal hypotension may require treatment with vasopressors [39]. In pulseless, severely hypotensive patients, intravenous epinephrine (0.5–1 mg) may be given [40].

Comprehensive maternal and fetal evaluation

After stabilization of the airway, breathing and circulation, a thorough evaluation with a detailed history and physical examination is performed. Routine ICU monitoring includes electrocardiogram (EKG), pulse oximetery and noninvasive blood pressure monitoring. Besides blood grouping and cross-matching, blood should be sent for analysis of arterial pH and blood gases, hemoglobin concentration, electrolytes, glucose, renal and liver function. Platelet count, prothrombin time (PT), partial thromboplastin time (PTT) and serum fibrinogen and fibrin degradation product levels are ordered (DIC screen). Thromboelastography (TEG) is an alternative test that measures viscoelastic properties of clot formation and lysis and can diagnose thrombocytopenia, platelet dysfunction and coagulation factor abnormalities [41]. The Kleihauer-Betke test is done in Rh-negative mothers with trauma to look for fetomaternal transfusion. Ultrasonography is performed to evaluate fetal and uteroplacental status and for any abdominal disease.

Methods of assessing and ensuring fetal well-being are reviewed in Chapter 49. There is no standard practice for how fetal monitoring should be carried out in the setting of critical care for patients. The plan should be individualized based on the condition of the mother, the gestational age of the pregnancy, and the preferences of the patient or her healthcare proxy which will determine the purpose of fetal monitoring. Generally, the primary concern and intervention strategy should be to optimize maternal health as this will generally be the safest and most effective route to improving fetal status. At gestational ages prior to *ex utero* viability, continuous fetal monitoring is difficult to perform and interpret and would not be used as the basis for emergency delivery. Evidence of apparently nonreassuring fetal assessment might be used only to help optimize maternal physiology (e.g. blood pressure and volume status) for maximal fetal and maternal benefit. Once a gestational age has been reached that is compatible with *ex utero* survival, frequent or even continuous assessment of fetal well-being may be appropriate to inform a decision for delivery for fetal benefit as well as to optimize maternal physiology. Decisions about moving toward delivery should be based upon both fetal assessment and an assessment of the risk of delivery to the mother. Decisions regarding delivery under these circumstances can be among the most difficult in maternal-fetal medicine and should be made in consultation with a multidisciplinary team ideally including intensivists, anesthesiologists, any specialists appropriate for the maternal condition (e.g. cardiology, neurology, etc.), neonatologists and maternal-fetal medicine. If preterm delivery is anticipated and there is no medical contraindication, betametasone (two intramuscular doses of 12 mg, 24 hours apart) may be given to enhance fetal lung maturity [42].

Organ dysfunction and failure

Approximately 65% of obstetric ICU admissions have failure of at least one organ system and 33% have multiple organ failure [8,15]. Organ failure may result from worsening of pre-existing medical diseases like valvular heart disease or onset of a new illness like pneumonia. Many obstetric conditions also may precipitate acute severe organ dysfunction (Table 23.2) [8]. The pattern of initial organ failure in most diseases is predictable. However, it must be realized that function of most organs is interdependent and prolonged failure of one or more organs may secondarily result in a domino effect, culminating in severe multiple organ system failure [43,44]. The Sequential Organ Failure Assessment (SOFA) system is commonly used to define organ failure (Table 23.3)

Table 23.2 Pattern of severe organ system dysfunction in obstetric disorders. Although the organs primarily affected in each obstetric disorder are indicated here, prolonged shock and severe DIC may ultimately result in secondary dysfunction of almost all organ systems

Obstetric disorder	Cardiovascular	Respiratory	Renal	Hepatic	Central nervous system	Hematologic	Endocrine/metabolic
Pre-eclampsia/eclampsia	++[a]	±	+++	+	+++	+++	−
Postpartum hemorrhage	+++	±	+++[b]	−	+	+++	+[c,d]
Intrauterine fetal demise	−	±	−	−	−	++	−
Puerperal sepsis	++	++	++	+	−	++	−
Chorioamnionitis	+	+	+	−	−	+	−
HELLP syndrome	−	−	±	++	+	+++	−
Acute fatty liver of pregnancy	±	−	++	+++	+++	+++	++[e]
Abruptio placentae	+	−	++[b]	−	−	+++	−
Amniotic fluid embolism	+++	+++	±	−	++	+++	−
Adherent placenta	+	−	−	−	−	−	−
Uterine rupture	+++	−	−	−	−	−	−
Tocolytic-induced pulmonary edema	−	+++	−	−	−	−	−
Ruptured ectopic pregnancy	+++	−	±	−	−	−	−

+++very common; ++common; +sometimes encountered; ±rarely encountered; −not seen.
[a]Hypertensive crisis; [b]acute cortical necrosis is common; [c]acute ischemic pituitary necrosis (Sheehan's syndrome); [d]hypocalcemia due to massive blood transfusion; [e]hypoglycemia, hepatic encephalopathy, and rarely diabetes insipidus.

Table 23.3 Sequential Organ Failure Assessment (SOFA) criteria for diagnosis of organ dysfunction or failure. Each of the six organ systems is assigned scores ranging from 0 (normal function) to 4 (severe failure). Scores 1 and 2 indicate organ dysfunction and 3 and 4 indicate organ failure. The scores of all six systems could be added to give a composite score which has prognostic significance

Organ system	Score			
	1	2	3	4
Cardiovascular				
Hypotension, inotropes or vasopressors administered for at least 1 hour	MAP <70 mmHg	Dopamine ≤5 µg/kg/min or dobutamine (any dose)	Dopamine >5 µg/kg/min or epinephrine or norepinephrine ≤0.1 µg/kg/min	Dopamine >15 µg/kg/min or epinephrine or norepinephrine >0.1 µg/kg/min
Respiratory				
PaO_2/FiO_2	<400	<300	<200 (with respiratory support)	<100 (with respiratory support)
Renal				
Serum creatinine				
mg/dL	1.2–1.9	2.0–3.4	3.5–4.9	>5.0
µmol/L	110–170	171–299	300–440	>440
urine output (mL/day)			200–499	<200
Liver				
Serum bilirubin				
mg/dL	1.2–1.9	2.0–5.9	6.0–11.9	>12.0
µmol/L	20–32	33–101	102–204	>204
Central nervous system				
Glasgow Coma Score	13–14	10–12	6–9	<6
Coagulation				
Platelet count $\times 10^3/mm^3$	100–149	50–99	20–49	<20

as it permits quantification of individual organ dysfunction as well as a combined assessment [45].

The frequency of failure of individual organs shows considerable geographic variation. In an American ICU, Afessa *et al.* observed that the most common organ system to fail was the respiratory system (32%) followed by hematologic (28%), cardiovascular (28%), renal (9%), liver (8%), and neurologic failure (1.5%) [22]. In Indian ICU patients, neurologic failure is the most common (63%) followed by hematologic (56%), renal (49%), respiratory (46%), cardiovascular (38%) and hepatic failure (36%) [16]. An Argentinean study found that respiratory failure was the most common (37%) followed by cardiovascular (28%), hematologic (13%) and renal failure (12%) [11].

Cardiovascular dysfunction

Shock

Shock is the most common manifestation of cardiovascular dysfunction in obstetric ICU patients (Box 23.3). Shock presents as tachycardia, tachypnea, hypotension, oliguria, altered mental status and lactic acidosis [42,44,46]. Orthostatic hypotension can be the only manifestation of early hemorrhagic shock; the diagnosis may be missed in the supine patient. Signs of external or internal hemorrhage may be present. Rales on auscultation are found in left ventricular failure or acute respiratory distress syndrome (ARDS), a third heart sound in peripartum cardiomyopathy and pulmonary thromboembolism, and cardiac murmurs in valvular heart disease.

Box 23.3 Causes of shock in obstetric patients

Hypovolemic shock	Hyperemesis gravidarum, ruptured ectopic pregnancy, concealed placental abruption, placenta previa, postpartum hemorrhage, uterine rupture, trauma
Septic shock	Chorioamnionitis following intrauterine fetal demise, puerperal sepsis, septic abortion, community-acquired pneumonia, pyelonephritis
Cardiogenic shock	Valvular heart disease, peripartum cardiomyopathy, acute myocardial infarction, myocarditis
Miscellaneous	Pulmonary thromboembolism, amniotic fluid embolism*, uterine inversion†, Sheehan's syndrome, dissecting aneurysm of the aorta

*Amniotic fluid embolism initially produces circulatory obstruction (obstructive shock) and cardiac dysfunction, and later vasodilation and increased capillary permeability (distributive shock).

†Uterine inversion produces a combination of hemorrhagic and neurogenic shock.

Patients with shock require invasive monitoring of arterial and central venous pressures [44,47]. A central venous catheter (CVC) should be placed in most patients with shock. It can be used to infuse intravenous fluids, blood products and medications, draw blood, and monitor both the central venous pressure (CVP – with a goal of keeping it between 8 and 12 mmHg) and the central venous oxyhemoglobin saturation (ScvO$_2$ – with a goal of keeping this >70%) which is adequate for many cases of shock. Pulmonary artery catheterization (PAC) may be useful in some patients to monitor pulmonary artery wedge pressure (PAWP – a measure of the left ventricular filling pressure), pulmonary arterial pressure and cardiac output [35,48]. However, the role of PAC is controversial as its use was associated with increased mortality in a retrospective analysis. Recent prospective studies show that it does not increase mortality when used by experienced intensive care practitioners at tertiary care centers, but have failed to show any benefit [35,43,48]. The use of PAC by less experienced teams is less likely to be "neutral" in its effects and may even be harmful. While PAC continues to have a potential role in expert hands, echocardiography may be preferred in many patients, especially if they are coagulopathic or require only a single hemodynamic evaluation in order to classify their disease [35].

In the second half of pregnancy, right or left lateral positioning of the pregnant woman will avoid aortocaval compression by the gravid uterus [2–4]. Cardiac filling should be optimized with rapid intravenous infusion of crystalloids such as normal saline or lactated Ringer's solution [43,44,46,47]. Approximately 3 liters of crystalloids are required to replenish 1 liter of lost blood [36]. Colloids like polymerized gelatin, hetastarch or albumin remain in the circulation longer than crystalloids [36]. However, in a large randomized study, fluid replacement with normal saline was as effective as human albumin, and considerably cheaper, and preferred by the authors [49]. Low CVP or PAWP indicates decreased cardiac preload requiring fluid replacement [43]. However, a normal CVP or PAWP does not rule out hypovolemia [43] and should be treated by repeated fluid challenges with 200–500 mL of crystalloids infused over 10–15 minutes until the CVP or PAWP increases by ≥3 mmHg and stays persistently elevated [46].

If the mean arterial pressure (MAP) remains below 65 mmHg after fluid replacement, vasopressor therapy is started with infusion of dopamine (2–30 µg/kg/min) or norepinephrine (0.5–20 µg/min) through the central line [43,46]. Vasopressin (0.01–0.04 units/min) infusion may work if hypotension does not respond to norepinephrine or dopamine [43,46]. In cardiogenic shock, inotropic agents like dobutamine (intravenous infusion at 2–30 µg/kg/min) can be started when the MAP exceeds 65 mmHg [43,46]. Many patients with septic shock have relative adrenal insufficiency and may also benefit from systemic glucocorticoids (see below) [46].

Once hypotension is corrected, adequacy of tissue oxygenation can be assessed by the ScvO$_2$, especially in sepsis [43]. It is monitored continuously using a special central venous catheter with an oxygen sensor at its tip, or intermittently, by blood gas analysis of venous blood drawn from a regular central venous catheter. ScvO$_2$ values of <70% indicate tissue hypoperfusion and oxygen delivery must be further enhanced by augmenting cardiac output with dobutamine or by increasing oxygen-carrying capacity by blood transfusion [43]. Normally, hemoglobin level of <7.0 g/dL is considered as the appropriate threshold for packed red blood cell transfusion in ICU patients [43]. However, in patients with ScvO$_2$ <70% transfusion may be considered if the hematocrit is <30% [43]. Administration of corticosteroids (hydrocortisone 100 mg IV every 8 hours for 5–7 days) to patients with severe septic shock and persistent hypotension despite fluid resuscitation may also be of benefit. Recombinant activated protein C is a very costly therapy that is recommended in septic shock for patients with an APACHE II score ≥25. APACHE stands for "acute physiology and chronic health evaluation" and is a widely used ICU scoring system. Scores range from 0 to 71 and are based on multiple parameters. Higher scores imply disease that is more severe and a greater risk of mortality. Use of recombinant activated protein C in higher risk patients is associated with a 15% reduction in relative risk of 26-day all-cause mortality but does not appear to benefit patients with less severe disease [48]. Experience with this agent in pregnant women is limited. Major hemorrhage is a side effect in 3.5% of patients [48].

The cause of shock should also be aggressively managed. Septic shock is treated with antibiotics and control of the source of sepsis. Multiple possible antibiotic regimens exist depending on the probable source of the sepsis, but in pregnant or postpartum patients with no clear source, one such possible regimen is meropenem and vancomycin. Antibiotic therapy should be adjusted once the etiology is determined and generally continued for a minimum of 10 days. Blunt curettage of the infected uterus or aspiration or surgical drainage of pelvic abscesses may be required. Severe mitral stenosis may require emergency balloon or surgical mitral valvotomy [48]. In postpartum hemorrhage, correction of coagulopathy and thrombocytopenia is vital [44]. Useful temporizing measures include uterotonic drugs, bimanual uterine compression and sterile packing or balloon tamponade of the uterine cavity [36,44]. Subsequent treatment should be guided by the obstetrician's best assessment of the reason for the hemorrhage. If the best assessment is that the bleeding is due to uterine atony, then failure of the measures above may require uterine artery embolization by interventional radiologists or surgical ligation of the internal iliac arteries or compressive uterine compression sutures like the B-Lynch suture [36,44]. Although hysterectomy is the last resort for persistent hemorrhage due to atony, the obstetrician should proceed to hysterectomy promptly if the most likely cause is placenta accreta, increta or percreta [36,44].

Hypertensive crisis

Arterial pressure >160/110 mmHg in pre-eclampsia can result in pulmonary edema, seizures and intracerebral hemorrhage and requires rapid blood pressure control [50]. Oral short-acting nifedepine (5 or 10 mg) is safe and effective, but is not approved for this indication in the United States [50]. An excellent alternative is intravenous labetalol, 20 mg initially followed by a 40 mg dose and two 80 mg doses at 10-minute intervals until blood pressure is controlled or a cumulative dose of 220 mg is reached [50–52]. Intravenous hydralazine, 5–10 mg every 20 minutes (maximum of 40 mg) until blood pressure is controlled, is also effective [50–52]. Reduction of pressure to normal levels (<140/90 mmHg) should be avoided as it may compromise placental perfusion [51]. Hypertension refractory to these drugs is an indication for intravenous nitroglycerine (10–100 μg/min) or sodium nitroprusside (2–8 μg/min). Prolonged use of nitroglycerine produces methemoglobinemia [3,51]. Cyanide toxicity in the mother and fetus may occur with sodium nitroprusside, particularly with higher rates of infusion or maternal renal dysfunction, and use of higher doses or prolonged use of any dose should be avoided [3,51].

Dissecting aneurysm of the aorta is a rare complication of hypertension in pregnancy, presenting as interscapular or retrosternal pain and discrepancy of pulse volume in the upper and lower extremities due to occlusion of one or more branches of the aorta. Intravenous beta-blockers like esmolol or metoprolol are the drugs of choice in this condition.

Cardiopulmonary resuscitation in pregnancy

The 2005 American Heart Association guidelines for cardiopulmonary resuscitation recommend some modification of the standard procedures in pregnant women [40]. The patient should be positioned 15–30° back from the left lateral position by placing a rolled blanket or other object under the right hip and lumbar area. Alternatively, one rescuer should kneel on the patient's left side and pull the gravid uterus laterally to relieve aortocaval pressure. Cricoid pressure is applied during bag and mask ventilation and endotracheal intubation. Chest compressions are performed with hands placed slightly higher on the sternum. Endotracheal tube diameter should be 0.5–1 mm smaller than that used for nonpregnant women. Emergency drugs should not be administered via intravenous access placed in the lower extremity as they may not reach the heart. Fetal and uterine monitors must be disconnected before defibrillation. If magnesium sulfate has been administered for pre-eclampsia/eclampsia prior to the cardiac arrest, empiric intravenous calcium gluconate (1 g (10 mL of a 100 mg/mL solution) diluted in 150 mL of D5W and administered over 10 minutes) may help reverse magnesium toxicity, if present. The decision regarding emergency hysterotomy and delivery must be made early during resuscitation. Hysterotomy is not indicated before 20 weeks of gestation. Between 20 and 23 weeks, hysterotomy likely increases the success of resuscitation for the mother by relieving aortocaval compression and enhancing efficacy of chest compressions. It likely will not help survival of the fetus at this gestational age. At 24 weeks' gestation or greater, hysterotomy increases chances of both maternal and fetal survival. The benefit is maximal if hysterotomy is performed within 5 minutes of the onset of cardiac arrest. It should therefore be started if maternal cardiac activity is not established by the fourth minute [6,34,40]. In ICU caring for pregnant women, an obstetrician skilled in emergency hysterotomy and a neonatologist or pediatrician to look after the neonate must therefore be part of the resuscitation team.

Respiratory failure

Respiratory failure is the leading reason for admission of obstetric patients to the ICU. Respiratory failure is classified into two categories: type 1 and type 2.

Type I respiratory failure refers to hypoxemia due to impaired alveolar gas exchange and carbon dioxide washout due to compensatory hyperventilation [3,5,22]. Severe hypocapnia can cause uterine artery vasoconstriction and uteroplacental insufficiency, and worsen fetal hypoxia [5,53]. Common causes of respiratory failure (Box 23.4) include lung infections, cardiogenic pulmonary edema, volume overload associated with beta-adrenergic tocolytic therapy or pre-eclampsia-related pulmonary edema and ARDS [53,54]. ARDS is characterized by damage to the alveolar-capillary membrane due to direct toxic injury or indirect damage by proinflammatory cytokines, free oxygen radicals, complement, prostaglandins, leukotrienes and enzymes released from leukocytes and macrophages [53]. The resultant exudation of intravascular fluid into the pulmonary interstitium and alveoli produces noncardiogenic pulmonary edema with ventilation perfusion mismatch and severe derangement of gas exchange [53,55]. Damage to surfactant-producing pneumocytes results in alveolar collapse and intrapulmonary shunting of blood [53,55]. Diagnosis of ARDS is made by the following criteria: (1) acute onset, (2) bilateral shadows on chest radiograph, (3) severe hypoxemia defined as a ratio of arterial pO_2 (PaO_2)/fraction of inspired oxygen (FiO_2) ≤200 and (4) absence of clinical evidence of left atrial hypertension or pulmonary arterial wedge pressure <18 mmHg [53,55]. PaO_2/FiO_2 between 200 and 300 in the presence of the other three criteria is termed acute lung injury (ALI), a less severe form of ARDS [53,55].

Although many cases of respiratory failure related to tocolytics, pre-eclampsia or infection may meet criteria for ALI or ARDS, most of these cases will run a distinctly shorter course, improving within a day or two of treatment or removal of the underlying cause. The aim of management of type I respiratory failure is to maintain the arterial pO_2 >60 mm Hg or SpO_2 >90%. Oxygen administered by

Box 23.4 Causes of acute respiratory failure in obstetric patients

Infections	
Respiratory	Severe bacterial
Systemic	pneumonia*, varicella
Pelvic	pneumonia*
	Pyelonephritis[†], *falciparum*
	malaria[†]
	Puerperal sepsis[†], septic
	abortion[†], chorioamnionitis[†]
Obstetric disorders	Amniotic fluid embolism*, tocolytic-induced pulmonary edema*, eclampsia[†], obstetric hemorrhage[†]
Chronic pulmonary conditions	Asthma, cystic fibrosis, primary pulmonary hypertension
Cardiogenic pulmonary edema	Valvular heart disease, peripartum cardiomyopathy, severe hypertension, myocarditis in autoimmune disorders
Miscellaneous	Aspiration of gastric contents*, massive blood transfusions*, polytrauma[†], acute pancreatitis[†]

*Cause acute respiratory distress syndrome (ARDS) due to direct lung injury.

[†]Cause ARDS due to a systemic inflammatory response syndrome (SIRS).

nasal prongs can provide FiO_2 of 24–32% [56]. Masks, with or without a Venturi device, deliver up to 60% oxygen [56]. Nonrebreathing masks with a reservoir bag provide higher oxygen concentrations [56]. Patients with respiratory distress and PaO_2 <60 mmHg despite oxygen supplementation require tracheal intubation and mechanical ventilation [56].

Mechanical ventilation in ARDS is typically initiated using high FiO_2 along with application of positive end expiratory pressure (PEEP – usually starting at 5 cmH_2O) to open collapsed alveoli, and low tidal volumes (6 mL/kg of ideal bodyweight) to limit the inspiratory plateau pressure to <30 cmH_2O [48,53,55]. Use of higher tidal volumes causes pulmonary volutrauma (overdistension injury) but the low tidal volumes used in the management of ARDS can cause maternal hypercapnia which may not be ideal for the fetus but may be warranted to maintain maternal and thereby fetal health (see Chapter 1). Prolonged ventilation with FiO_2 >60% can worsen the course of ARDS due to oxygen toxicity [53]. High PEEP decreases venous return

and may cause barotrauma manifesting as pneumothorax, pneumomediastinum or subcutaneous emphysema [53]. Therefore, the lowest combination of FiO_2 and PEEP that can achieve a PaO_2 of >60 mmHg and SpO_2 of >90% is used.

Ventilated patients with ARDS require sedation and neuromuscular paralysis [53]. If hypoxemia persists, an attempt is made to forcibly open nonfunctioning collapsed alveoli by lung recruitment maneuvers where the airway pressure is maintained at 40 cm for 40 seconds [55]. Other modes of ventilation such as inverse inspiratory/expiratory ratio ventilation, airway pressure release ventilation and high-frequency oscillatory ventilation have been tried for persistent hypoxia [53,55]. In nonpregnant patients, prone positioning improves oxygenation in 70–80% [53,55]. However, this may not be advisable during the later part of gestation.

Type II respiratory failure is characterized by hypoventilation and hypercapnia and is usually caused by respiratory depression in patients with status epilepticus, cerebral edema, cerebral hemorrhage, cerebral venous sinus thrombosis, and following drugs such as magnesium sulfate, chlorpromazine, opioids, barbiturates and benzodiazepines [5]. These patients require tracheal intubation and mechanical ventilation until the underlying abnormality recovers [5].

Renal failure

Oliguria (urine output <0.5 mL/kg/h), azotemia and metabolic acidosis are the hallmarks of acute renal failure [57]. Prerenal azotemia occurs when hypovolemia results in renal hypoperfusion and decreased glomerular filtration [57]. Prolonged hypoperfusion due to shock or renal microvascular obstruction (pre-eclampsia, disseminated intravascular coagulation, malaria) may cause ischemic acute tubular necrosis (Box 23.5) [8]. Toxic acute tubular necrosis can be caused by drugs and toxins. Prerenal azotemia can be distinguished from acute tubular necrosis by low urinary sodium (<20 mmol/L), urine/plasma creatinine ratio >40 and fractional excretion of sodium <1% [57] (see Chapter 7). Severe albuminuria suggests glomerular disease and occurs in severe pre-eclampsia, systemic lupus erythematosus and glomerulonephritis [57]. Postpartum hemolytic uremic syndrome is suspected if there is no evident cause for renal failure and schistocytes (fragmented red blood cells) are found in the peripheral blood smear [3].

While poor urine output with a transient slight rise in creatinine is commonly seen in pre-eclamptic patients, most of these will improve rapidly with delivery and as long as they appear to be euvolemic, do not generally need large fluid resuscitation which may precipitate pulmonary edema. Persistent and severe acute renal failure in most obstetric patients is associated with hypovolemia with low CVP and hyperuricemia. Timely hydration, often using invasive hemodynamic monitoring, can prevent progression to ischemic acute tubular necrosis [58].

Box 23.5 Causes of acute renal failure in obstetric patients

Obstetric disorders	Pre-eclampsia, eclampsia, placental abruption, acute fatty liver of pregnancy, postpartum hemorrhage, HELLP syndrome, postpartum HUS
Infections	Pyelonephritis, *falciparum* malaria, puerperal sepsis, septic abortion, chorioamnionitis
Shock	Prolonged shock due to any cause
Toxins	Methanol, ethylene glycol, illegal abortifacients, acetaminophen overdose
Drugs	Aminoglycoside antibiotics, radiologic contrast, NSAID
Miscellaneous	Hemoglobinuria (mismatched transfusion, malaria), myoglobinuria (status epilepticus, eclampsia), DIC, systemic lupus erythematosus

After hydration, some experts will administer 40–100 mg of furosemide as a single intravenous dose or a continuous infusion of 5–20 mg/h, sometimes in conjunction with albumin to achieve greater diuresis [59]. However, randomized studies have shown that while furosemide causes a diuresis, it has only a questionable effect on the subsequent need for dialysis and does not alter mortality. Renal dose dopamine (2–5 μg/kg/min) is no longer used as it is ineffective, causes arrhythmias, and decreases uteroplacental perfusion in animals [57]. Diet is modified to prevent fluid overload and hyperkalemia, and to limit azotemia [57]. Fluid intake is restricted to urine output plus 600 mL per 24 hours. Dietary potassium is avoided. High-quality protein (0.6 g/kg bodyweight) rich in essential amino acids is prescribed. Inadequate caloric intake promotes catabolism which worsens azotemia by increasing nitrogen breakdown, as does excessive protein intake. Metabolic acidosis is treated if arterial pH drops <7.2 [57]. Many drugs need dose reduction in renal failure; blood levels of antibiotics must be monitored.

Approximately 30% of patients with acute renal failure will require dialysis [10,16]. Indications for dialysis are severe azotemia (serum creatinine >9 mg/dL or blood urea nitrogen >100 mg/dL), refractory acidosis, serum potassium >6 mMol/L, fluid overload, acute pulmonary edema, uremia (drowsiness, seizures) or severe catabolic state [57]. Conventional intermittent dialysis is useful when acute renal failure occurs as a single organ disease. In critically ill patients, with multiple organ failure, slow continuous arteriovenous or venovenous dialysis using high-flux biocompatible dialyzers is preferred as it causes fewer hemodynamic fluctuations and less activation of inflammatory mediators [57].

Seven to 20% of obstetric renal failure is due to acute cortical necrosis, a form of severe ischemic renal damage rarely seen in nonpregnant individuals [57,60]. It is common with shock and DIC due to a combination of hypotension and microvascular occlusion, and is characterized by anuria (urine output <100 mL/day) rather than oliguria [60]. While most patients with acute tubular necrosis have complete recovery of renal function in 4–12 weeks [58], women with acute cortical necrosis have residual renal dysfunction and some remain dialysis dependent [3,57,60].

Acute hepatic dysfunction

Common causes of acute hepatic dysfunction in pregnancy are listed in Table 23.4. Elevated aminotransferases are common in pre-eclampsia, but progression to hepatic failure is rare [61]. Potentially fatal liver diseases in pregnancy are acute fatty liver of pregnancy (AFLP), HELLP (hemolysis, elevated liver enzymes, low platelets) syndrome and acute viral hepatitis [62]. Acute fulminant viral hepatitis A and E is common in pregnant women in tropical countries [10,16,63]. In India, incidence of hepatitis E infection is higher in pregnant women and 33–50% of hepatitis E infections in pregnancy lead to fulminant hepatic failure versus 3% in nonpregnant women [63,64]. It is difficult to differentiate between viral hepatitis and acute fatty liver of pregnancy [61]. Proteinuria, thrombocytopenia and hyperuricemia are common in acute fatty liver of pregnancy but rare in viral hepatitis [61,62]. Women with the HELLP syndrome have lower platelet counts, higher serum LDH levels and lower bilirubin than with fatty liver of pregnancy [61,62]. Unlike the HELLP syndrome, fatty liver of pregnancy is associated with severely prolonged PT and hypoglycemia [62].

Cerebral edema is an important cause of coma in fulminant hepatic failure [65,66]. It is treated by elevation of the head of the bed and administration of intravenous mannitol.

Table 23.4 Causes of acute hepatic failure in obstetric patients

Liver dysfunction	Disorders
Severe	Pre-eclampsia
	Sepsis with multiple organ failure
	Acute fatty liver of pregnancy
	Hemolysis, elevated liver enzymes, low platelets (HELLP) syndrome
	Acute fulminant hepatitis
	Shock (ischemic hepatitis)
	Acetaminophen overdose

Short periods of mechanical hyperventilation are useful to control transient surges in intracranial pressure. Maintenance of fluid balance requires central venous pressure monitoring. Hypotension may occur due to systemic vasodilation and responds to hydration and vasopressors. Renal failure co-exists in 40% of patients. Lactic acidosis, hyperammonemia, hyponatremia and hypoglycemia are common [61,62,65,66].

Intestinal ammonia production is controlled by restriction of dietary protein and administration of oral neomycin (avoided in renal failure and usually before delivery despite poor maternal absorption), ampicillin or metronidazole to eliminate ammonia-producing bacteria [65,66]. Lactulose (30 mL 3–4 hourly, until diarrhea occurs) maintains an acidic intestinal pH and reduces ammonia absorption. Parenteral alimentation is usually necessary to meet protein and energy needs [65,66]. Stress ulcer prophylaxis helps prevent gastric hemorrhage. Coagulopathy, characterized by a prolonged PT, is common and bleeding is managed with vitamin K, blood transfusion and fresh-frozen plasma [65,66]. Liver hematomas are common in patients with the HELLP syndrome with a platelet count <20,000/μL [30,62]. Subcapsular hematomas may rupture, causing hemorrhagic shock and death, and require prompt surgical exploration [30,62].

Corticosteroids produce transient increase in platelets in the HELLP syndrome but their effect on long-term outcomes is less clear [30,62]. In acute fatty liver of pregnancy and HELLP syndrome liver function improves rapidly after delivery [3,62]. However, delivery does not improve maternal survival in viral hepatitis [61]. In a recent study, there was a threefold increase in maternal mortality with acute liver failure. However, on multivariate analysis, liver failure itself did not increase mortality unless caused by acute viral hepatitis or accompanied by failure of other organs [10].

Central nervous system dysfunction

Central nervous system (CNS) dysfunction may manifest as seizures or coma (Box 23.6) [27]. Seizures in late pregnancy are commonly due to eclampsia [67,68]; other causes include epilepsy, intracerebral hemorrhage, severe hypertension, cerebral cortical venous thrombosis and cerebral malaria [10,16,27,69]. Comatose patients have a depressed cough reflex and endotracheal intubation is essential to prevent aspiration. Raised intracranial pressure due to cerebral edema, intracranial hemorrhage or space-occupying lesions may cause transtentorial herniation with brainstem compression [3,27]. It is treated by elevation of the head end of the bed to 20° and administration of intravenous mannitol (100 mL of 20% mannitol over 5 minutes, repeated 4–8 hourly) [27,65,66]. If intracranial pressure is being monitored invasively (commonly done for closed head injuries, stroke and intracerebral hemorrhage with coma), short periods of mechanical hyperventilation are useful when transient surges

Box 23.6 Causes of central nervous system dysfunction in obstetric patients

Vascular	Cerebral infarction, intracerebral hemorrhage, cerebral venous sinus thrombosis, subarachnoid hemorrhage, hypertensive encephalopathy
Infections	Bacterial meningitis, septic encephalopathy, cerebral malaria
Intracranial space-occupying lesions	Gliomas, meningiomas, acoustic neuromas, pituitary tumors
Metabolic disorders	Hypoglycemia, hepatic encephalopathy, hyponatremia, acute intermittent porphyria
Drugs and toxins	Magnesium sulfate, sedative overdose, ethanol, illicit drug abuse, poisoning
Miscellaneous	Epilepsy, eclampsia, thrombotic thrombocytopenic purpura, postpartum pituitary necrosis (Sheehan's syndrome)

in intracranial pressure occur. Cerebral perfusion pressure (difference between mean arterial and intracranial pressure) must be maintained at ≥50 mmHg [27]. Infusion of 5% dextrose is avoided as it is hypo-osmolar and may worsen cerebral edema.

While a single seizure may not affect fetal well-being, status epilepticus is associated with high fetal and maternal mortality [70]. Seizures during labor may produce prolonged fetal bradycardia, accidental rupture of membranes and, rarely, placental abruption [27]. Intravenous lorazepam (2–4 mg boluses administered every 5 minutes) is the preferred treatment of seizures in pregnancy [71]. Diazepam is an effective alternative. Intravenous phenytoin (18 mg/kg at a rate not exceeding 50 mg/min) is given to prevent recurrence of seizures [71]. Magnesium sulfate is clearly superior to phenytoin for the treatment of seizures due to eclampsia [27,51,68]. However, patients convulsing despite magnesium sulfate should receive phenytoin [3,27]. If seizures persist after intravenous phenytoin, phenobarbital (20 mg/kg at a rate of 50–75 mg/min intravenously) or midazolam (0.2 mg/kg bolus followed by infusion at 0.1–0.2 mg/kg/h) may be given [27,70]. Respiratory depression is common with these drugs and mechanical ventilation is invariably required [27,70]. Benzodiazepines may also cause neonatal hypothermia and hypotonia.

Supportive treatment of status epilepticus includes an intravenous injection of 50% dextrose (50 mL) and thiamine (100 mg) if alcoholism is suspected [27]. Prolonged seizures cause severe metabolic acidosis, rhabdomyolysis, myoglobinuria and hyperthermia [70]. Renal failure due to myoglobinuria may be prevented by forced alkaline diuresis [57].

Coagulation failure

Subclinical disturbances of hemostasis are common in pre-eclampsia. Significant thrombocytopenia occurs in up to 18% of patients with severe pre-eclampsia, 15% develop the HELLP syndrome and 11% develop DIC [71]. Severe DIC may occur in patients with eclampsia, placental abruption, amniotic fluid embolism and intrauterine fetal death if the dead fetus is retained for 5 weeks [71–73]. In an Indian ICU pregnant women accounted for 41% of all cases of DIC [73] and DIC was present in 19% of obstetric patients in the ICU [16].

Disseminated intravascular coagulation manifests primarily as postpartum hemorrhage [71–73]. Other hemorrhagic manifestations include bleeding from venepuncture sites, hematuria, bleeding gums, upper gastrointestinal hemorrhage, and rarely intracranial hemorrhage [73]. Elevation of fibrin spilt products to >40 µg/mL along with thrombocytopenia (platelet count <100,000/mm^3) and abnormal coagulation tests are characteristic of DIC [72,73]. Patients with DIC commonly develop uterine atony which further aggravates postpartum hemorrhage; rarely hemorrhage within the myometrium is also seen [72].

Treatment of DIC consists of replacement of lost blood with packed cells and correction of clotting factor and platelet deficiency by blood component therapy [71–73]. The aim is to maintain the platelet count at 50,000/µL and the serum fibrinogen level at 100 mg/dL [73]. One unit of single-donor platelets will increase the platelet count by 5000–10,000 µL and one unit of fresh-frozen plasma will raise the fibrinogen level by 5–10 mg/dL [44,73]. Cryoprecipitate (1 unit/10 kg bodyweight) may be given if fresh-frozen plasma does not correct the coagulopathy [44,72,73]. It is also preferred in renal failure since a smaller volume of cryoprecipitate is required to correct coagulopathy [71–73]. In some centers TEG-based algorithms are used to diagnose DIC and to select the appropriate combination of blood components. DIC in antepartum women generally reverses rapidly after delivery and hence prompt delivery must be attempted under cover of blood component therapy [71–73].

Delivery of critically ill patients

Pharmacologic tocolysis is a controversial area even for healthy mothers, so its use in critically ill women is seldom indicated [42]. Priority should be given to stabilizing the mother. If maternal condition permits a short delay before effecting preterm delivery, administration of glucocorticoids for fetal lung maturity is a reasonable intervention [42]. Appropriate prophylaxis for infective endocarditis is initiated in women with congenital or valvular heart disease [48].

Intrapartum management

The important considerations in this period relate to timing, route and method of delivery. An accurate estimate of gestational age is very important. Several of the conditions listed in Box 23.7 are best managed by prompt delivery regardless of gestational age. A fundamental principle in critical care obstetrics is that the mother should be stabilized prior to intervening for fetal indications. A woman in the throes of an eclamptic seizure or comatose from diabetic ketoacidosis should not be subjected to emergency cesarean delivery for fetal bradycardia [50]. Often the abnormal fetal heart rate will respond to treatment of the maternal condition [50].

It is often difficult to decide on the appropriate route of delivery in critically ill pregnant women. Cesarean delivery is associated with increased risks of hemorrhage, infection, thromboembolism and anesthetic complications [74]. Hypotension may occur during cesarean delivery secondary to neuraxial anesthesia [34]. This can be reduced by fluid loading, ephedrine

---

Box 23.7 Conditions in which delivery by obstetric intervention improves maternal outcome

Early delivery improves maternal outcome	Severe pre-eclampsia with organ failure
	Eclampsia
	Acute fatty liver of pregnancy
	HELLP syndrome
	Placental abruption
	Status epilepticus
	Acute cardiac arrest ≥24 weeks gestation
	Severe chorioamnionitis
Operative vaginal delivery (forceps/ vacuum assisted) may improve maternal outcome*	Cardiac disease – NYHA Class III or IV
	Hypertensive crises
	Cerebrovascular disease, especially vascular malformations
	Myasthenia gravis
	Spinal cord injury

*Operative delivery shortens second stage of labor and reduces the effect of straining.

or phenylephrine [34]. Conversely, induction of labor with an unfavorable cervix requires time that may result in deterioration of maternal status. Selecting the route of delivery should therefore be individualized. Vaginal delivery is usually less difficult but obviously requires that the cervix be completely dilated. If shortening of the second stage of labor is indicated, the operator should select the instrument with which he or she is most comfortable [75]. Medical complications or drugs may either impair a woman's ability to push or relatively contraindicate active efforts to bear down [75]. This is not a contraindication to a vaginal delivery as mothers may have an assisted vaginal delivery even if heavily sedated and/or paralyzed. In these situations, forceps delivery has advantages over vacuum extraction, provided the operator has the requisite skills and there is no coagulopathy [75]. The decision to perform a cesarean delivery is usually based on obstetric indications and not medical ones. Regional anesthesia carries the risk of epidural hematomas if administered in the setting of thrombocytopenia and many anesthesiologists will not provide this technique to patients with platelet counts <50,000–75,000/µL. However, an absolute lower level of platelet count for acceptable regional anesthesia has not been determined. Individual assessment is warranted, and other factors (e.g. difficult airway) may influence the decision to use regional anesthesia [34].

Prevention of thromboembolic disease

Pregnant and postpartum women are at increased risk of developing venous thromboembolism. This risk is further increased by most critical illnesses, cesarean delivery, and immobility. Pregnant or postpartum women requiring critical care should receive thromboembolic prophylaxis. Routine use of thromboprophylaxis such as intermittent compression stockings and/or unfractionated/low molecular weight heparin is recommended in the critically ill obstetric patient unless she has a contraindication.

Prognosis and outcomes

Since organ dysfunction in many obstetric disorders reverses rapidly after delivery, the initial assessment may overestimate the risk of death [10,15,26]. Consequently, general prognostic scores like the APACHE II or SAPS II scores overestimate mortality in obstetric disorders; they perform relatively better in medical disorders in pregnancy [10,26].

A recent study comparing obstetric patients in the ICU of a publicly funded hospital in Mumbai, India, and a county hospital in Houston, Texas, highlighted preventable factors contributing to maternal mortality [16]. Patients were referred to the Indian ICU much later after onset of acute complications, resulting in high mortality. Significantly more American ICU patients were delivered by induction of labor (38.8% versus 27%) and

by cesarean section (78% versus 15%) than Indian ICU patients. This resulted in higher incidence of puerperal or postoperative sepsis in the American women, but a dramatic reduction in fetal (13% vs 51%) and maternal mortality (2.3% vs 25%). Thus, early referral of women with complicated pregnancies to large tertiary care centers with ICU facilities and timely intervention and delivery by skilled obstetricians and anesthetists are the keys to reducing maternal and perinatal mortality.

Conclusion

Critical illness may complicate even a low-risk pregnancy. Obstetricians must be familiar with the issues pertaining to care of pregnant women with multiple organ failure. Many obstetric disorders may mimic medical disorders: acute fatty liver of pregnancy mimics acute viral hepatitis, eclampsia mimics cerebral cortical venous thrombosis, pre-eclampsia mimics systemic lupus erythematosus and amniotic fluid embolism may mimic acute cardiogenic pulmonary edema. Once the correct diagnosis is made, the obstetrician and the intensivist must decide whether delivery will alter the natural history of the disease and improve maternal survival. If the maternal condition is expected to improve after delivery, then the decision to deliver vaginally or by cesarean section must be made. Meanwhile, hypovolemia, hypotension, respiratory failure and coagulopathy are treated while preparing for delivery. Timely delivery improves not only maternal outcome but fetal outcome too. Some maternal infections such as malaria, viral hepatitis, HIV and tuberculosis may be transmitted to the fetus. Appropriate steps must be taken to protect the newborn child against this. Finally, no efforts should be spared in the management of critically ill obstetric patients because their outcomes are often dramatically better than expected on the basis of the initial severity of illness [8,10,26].

References

1. Shaver SM, Shaver DC. Perioperative assessment of the obstetric patient undergoing abdominal surgery. J Perianesth Nurs 2005;20:160–6.
2. Yeomans ER, Gilstrap LC. Physiologic changes in pregnancy and their impact on critical care. Crit Care Med 2005;33(suppl): S256-S258.
3. Rizk NW, Kalassian KG, Gilligan T, Druzin MI, Daniel DL. Obstetric complications in pulmonary and critical care medicine. Chest 1996;110:791–809.
4. Chestnut AN. Physiology of normal pregnancy. Crit Care Clin 2004;20:609–15.
5. Catanzarite V, Cousins L. Respiratory failure in pregnancy. Immunol Allergy Clin North Am 2000;20:775–806.
6. Shapiro JM. Critical care of the obstetric patient. J Intens Care Med 2006;21:278–86.
7. Naylor DF, Olson MM. Critical care obstetrics and gynecology. Crit Care Clin 2003;19:127–49.
8. Karnad DR, Guntupalli KK. Critical illness and pregnancy: review of a global problem. Crit Care Clin 2004;20:555–76.

9. Ananth CV, Smulian JC. Epidemiology of critical illness and outcomes in pregnancy. In: Dildy GA, Belfort MA, Saade GR, Phelan JP, Hankins GDV, Clark SL (eds) Critical care obstetrics, 4th edn. Blackwell Scientific, Malden, MA, 2004: 3–12.

10. Karnad DR, Lapsia V, Krishnan A, Salvi VS. Prognostic factors in obstetric patients admitted to an Indian intensive care unit. Crit Care Med 2004;32:1294–9.

11. Vasquez DN, Elisa Estenssoro E, Canales HS, et al. Clinical characteristics and outcomes of obstetric patients requiring ICU admission. Chest 2007;131:718–24.

12. Zeeman GG, Wendel GD, Cunningham FG. A blueprint for obstetric care. Am J Obstet Gynecol 2003;188:532–6.

13. Mabie WC, Sibai BM. Treatment in an obstetric intensive care unit. Am J Obstet Gynecol 1990;162:1–4.

14. Maine D, Chavkin W. Maternal mortality: global similarities and differences. J Am Med Womens Assoc 2002;57:127–30.

15. Soubra SH, Guntupalli KK. Critical illness in pregnancy: an overview. Crit Care Med 2005;33(suppl):S248–S255.

16. Munnur U, Karnad DR, Bandi VDP, et al. Critically ill obstetric patients in an American and an Indian public hospital: comparison of case mix, organ dysfunction, intensive care requirements, and outcomes. Intens Care Med 2005;31:1087–94.

17. Graves CR. Organizing a critical care obstetric unit. In: Dildy GA, Belfort MA, Saade GR, Phelan JP, Hankins GDV, Clark SL (eds) Critical care obstetrics, 4th edn. Blackwell Scientific, Malden, MA, 2004: 13–18.

18. Task Force of the American College of Critical Care Medicine/Society of Critical Care Medicine. Guidelines for ICU admission, discharge and triage. Crit Care Med 1999;27:633–8.

19. Zeeman GG. Obstetric critical care: a blueprint for improved outcomes. Crit Care Med 2006;34(suppl):S208–S214.

20. Panchal S, Arria AM, Harris AP. Intensive care utilization during hospital admission for delivery. Anesthesiology 2000;92:1537–44.

21. Bouvier-Colle MH, Varnoux N, Salanave B, et al. Case-control study of risk factors for obstetric patients' admission to intensive care units. Eur J Obstet Gynecol Reprod Biol 1997;74:173–7.

22. Afessa B, Green B, Delke I, Koch K. Systemic inflammatory response syndrome, organ failure and outcome in critically ill obstetric patients treated in an ICU. Chest 2001;120:1271–7.

23. Budev MM, Arroliga AC, Emery S. Exacerbation of underlying pulmonary disease in pregnancy. Crit Care Med 2005;33(suppl):S313–S318.

24. Mattox KL, Goetzl L. Trauma in pregnancy. Crit Care Med 2005;33(suppl):S385–S389.

25. Stevens TA, Carroll MA, Promecene PA, Seibel M, Monga M. Utility of Acute Physiology, Age and Chronic Health Evauation (APACHE III) score in maternal admissions to the intensive care unit. Am J Obstet Gynecol 2006;194:e13–e15.

26. Harrison DA, Penny JA, Yentis SM, Fayek S, Brady AR. Case mix, outcome and activity for obstetric admissions to adult general critical care units: a secondary analysis of the ICNARC case mix program database. Crit Care 2005;9:S32–S37.

27. Karnad DR, Guntupalli KK. Neurologic disorders in pregnancy. Crit Care Med 2005;33(suppl):S362–S371.

28. Walters WAW, Ford JB, Sullivan EA, et al. Maternal deaths in Australia. Med J Aust 2002;176:413–14.

29. McKay DB, Josephson MA. Pregnancy in recipients of solid organs – effects on mother and child. N Engl J Med 2006;354:1281–93.

30. Barton JR, Sibai BM. HELLP and the liver diseases of preeclampsia. Clin Liver Dis 1999;1:31–48.

31. Munnur U, Suresh MS. Airway problems in pregnancy. Crit Care Clin 2004;20:617–42.

32. American Society of Anesthesiologists. Practice guidelines for management of the difficult airway: an updated report by the American Society of Anesthesiologists Task Force on Management of the Difficult Airway. Anesthesiology 2003;98:1269–77.

33. Munnur U, de Boisblanc B, Suresh MS. Airway problems in pregnancy. Crit Care Med 2005;33(suppl):S259–S268.

34. American Society of Anesthesiologists. Practice guidelines for obstetric anesthesia: an updated report by the American Society of Anesthesiologists Task Force on Obstetric Anesthesia. Anesthesiology 2007;106:843–63.

35. Fujitani S, Baldisseri MR. Hemodynamic assessment in a pregnant and peripartum patient. Crit Care Clin 2005;33(suppl):S354–S361.

36. Chichester M. When your patient is from the obstetric department: postpartum hemorrhage and massive transfusion. J Perianesth Nurs 2005;20:167–76.

37. Ganeshan A, Warakaulle DR, Uberoi R. Central venous access. Cardiovasc Intervent Radiol 2007;30:26–33.

38. Alamia V, Meyer BA. Peripartum hemorrhage. Obstet Gynecol Clin North Am 1999;26:385–98.

39. Beale RJ, Hollenberg SM, Vincent JL, Parillo JE. Vasopressor and inotropic support in septic shock: an evidence-based review. Crit Care Med 2004;32(suppl):S455–S465.

40. American Heart Association Guidelines for Cardiopulmonary Resuscitation and Emergency Cardiovascular Care. Cardiac arrest associated with pregnancy. Circulation 2005;112(suppl):IV-150–IV-153.

41. Luddington RJ. Thromboelastography/thromboelastometry. Clin Lab Haematol 2005;27:81–90.

42. Abbrescia K, Sheridan B. Complications of second and third trimester pregnancies. Emerg Med Clin North Am 2003;21 695–710.

43. Otero RM, Nguyen B, Huang DT, et al. Early goal-directed therapy in severe sepsis and septic shock revisited: concepts, controversies, and contemporary findings. Chest 2006;130:1579–95.

44. Cohen WR. Hemorrhagic shock in obstetrics. J Perinat Med 2006;34:263–71.

45. Vincent JL, Mendonca A, Cantraine F. Use of the SOFA score to assess the incidence of organ dysfunction/failure in intensive care units: results of a multicenter, prospective study. Crit Care Med 1998;26:1793–800.

46. Annane D, Bellissant E, Cavaillon JM. Septic shock. Lancet 2005;365:63–78.

47. Crochetière C. Obstetric emergencies. Anesthesiol Clin North Am 2003;21:111–25.

48. Martin SR, Foley MR. Intensive care in obstetrics: an evidence-based review. Am J Obstet Gynecol 2006;195:673–89.

49. Finfer S, Bellomo R, Boyce N, et al. A comparison of albumin and saline for fluid resuscitation in the intensive care unit. N Engl J Med 2004;350:2247–56.

50. Aagaard-Tillery KM, Belfort MA. Eclampsia: morbidity, mortality and management. Clin Obstet Gynecol 2005;48:12–23.

51. Sibai BM. Diagnosis, prevention and management of eclampsia. Obstet Gynecol 2005;105:402–10.

52. Vidaeff AC, Carroll MA, Ramin SA. Acute hypertensive emergencies in pregnancy. Crit Care Med 2005;33(suppl):S307–S312.

53. Bandi VD, Munnur U, Matthay MA. Acute lung injury and acute respiratory distress syndrome in pregnancy. Crit Care Clin 2004;20:577–607.

54. Jenkins TM, Troiano NH, Graves CR, Baird SM, Boehm FH. Mechanical ventilation in an obstetric population: characteristics and delivery rates. Am J Obstet Gynecol 2003;188:549–52.

55. Cole DE, Taylor TL, McCullough DM, Shoff CT, Derdak S. Acute respiratory distress syndrome in pregnancy. Crit Care Med 2005;33(suppl):S269–S278.

56. Worthley LIG. Oxygen therapy. In: Synopsis of intensive care medicine. Churchill Livingstone, Edinburgh, 1994: 387–92.

57. Gammill HS, Jeyabalan A. Acute renal failure in pregnancy. Crit Care Med 2005;33(suppl):S372–S384.

58. Drakeley AJ, Le Roux PA, Anthony J, Penny J. Acute renal failure complicating severe preeclampsia requiring admission to an obstetric intensive care unit. Am J Obstet Gynecol 2002;186:253–6.

59. Martin GS, Moss M, Wheeler AP, Mealer M, Morris JA, Bernard GR. A randomized, controlled trial of furosemide with or without albumin in hypoproteinemic patients with acute lung injury. Crit Care Med 2005;33:1681–7.

60. Naik V, Lohiya P, Lengade S, Chandran S, Karnad DR, Almeida AF. Obstetric acute renal failure revisited. Indian J Nephrol 2004;14:119–20.

61. Wolf JL. Liver disease in pregnancy. Med Clin North Am 1996;80:1167–87.

62. Steingrub JS. Pregnancy-associated severe liver dysfunction. Crit Care Clin 2004;20:763–76.

63. Jaiswal SP, Jain AK, Naik G, Soni N, Chitnis DS. Viral hepatitis during pregnancy. Int J Gynaecol Obstet 2001;72:103–8.

64. Dahiya M, Kumar A, Kar P, Gupta RK, Kumar A. Acute viral hepatitis in the third trimester of pregnancy. Indian J Gastroenterol 2005;24:128–9.

65. Han MK, Hyzy R. Advances in critical care management of hepatic failure and insufficiency. Crit Care Med 2006;34(suppl): S225–S231.

66. Sass DA, Shakil OA. Fulminant hepatic failure. Liver Transpl 2005;11:594–601.

67. Bhagwanjee S, Paruk F, Moodley J, Myckart DJJ. Intensive care unit morbidity and mortality from eclampsia: an evaluation of the Acute Physiology and Chronic Health Evaluation II score and the Glasgow Coma Scale score. Crit Care Med 2000;28:120–4.

68. Eclampsia Trial Collaborative Group. Which anticonvulsant for women with eclampsia? Evidence from the Collaborative Eclampsia Trial. Lancet 1995;345:1455–63.

69. Barrett C, Richens A. Epilepsy and pregnancy: report of an Epilepsy Research Foundation workshop. Epilepsy Res 2003;52:147–87.

70. Lowenstein DH, Allredge BK. Status epilepticus. N Engl J Med 1998;84:970–6.

71. Bick RL. Syndromes of disseminated intravascular coagulation in obstetrics, pregnancy and gynecology. Hematol Oncol Clin North Am 2000;14:999–1044.

72. Levi M. Current understanding of disseminated intravascular coagulation. Br J Haematol 2004;124:567–76.

73. Karnad DR, Vasani J Disseminated intravascular coagulation: a review with experience from an intensive care unit in India. J Postgrad Med 1992;38:186–93.

74. National Collaborating Centre for Women's and Children's Health. Caesarean section: clinical guidelines. RCOG Press, London, 2004.

75. Royal College of Obstetricians and Gynaecologists. Operative vaginal delivery. Guideline No 26. RCOG Press, London, 2005.

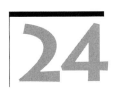

24 Embryologic and fetal development

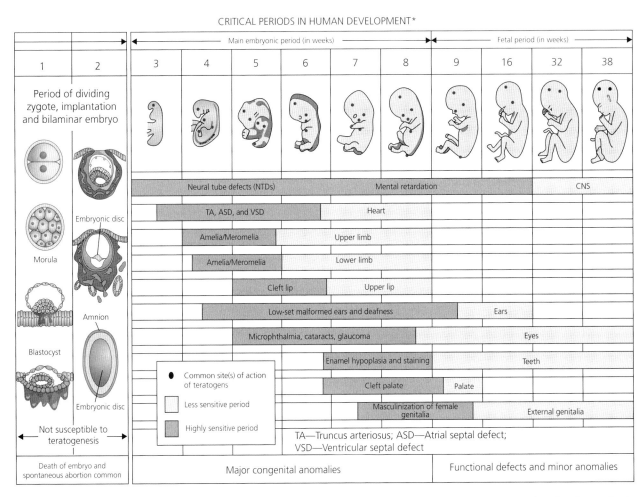

Figure 24.1 Reproduced with permission from Moore KL, Persaud TVN. *The Developing Human: Clinically Oriented Embryology*, 6th edn. WO Saunders: Philadelphia, 1998.
*Dark gray denotes highly sensitive periods when major birth defects may be produced.

de Swiet's Medical Disorders in Obstetric Practice, 5th edition.
Edited by R. O. Powrie, M. F. Greene, W. Camann. © 2010 Blackwell
Publishing.

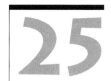

Global issues in maternal health

Rudiger Pittrof[1], *Moke Magoma*[1], *Véronique Filippi*[1]
with Medge D. Owen[2]

[1]Department of Epidemiology and Population Health, London School of Hygiene
and Tropical Medicine, London, UK
[2]Department of Anesthesia, Wake Forest University, Winston-Salem, NC, USA

Introduction

Too many women still die in pregnancy and childbirth in developing countries. The estimated number of maternal deaths has been stable for many years, with between 515,000 and 536,000 maternal deaths per year, most of which occur in developing countries [1,2]. The international community has recognized the gravity of the situation by endorsing the improvement of maternal health as the fifth of its eight millennium development goals (MDG) [3]. International efforts are increasing to meet the MDG-5 target of reducing maternal mortality by 75% from 1990 to 2015 but there are strong signs that this target might not be met [2]. There are many reasons for this, including a lack of political will, human and financial resources, as well as some biologic and demographic factors, such as the impact of the HIV epidemic on women and health systems, and the continuing population growth.

This chapter will review the levels and causes of maternal mortality and morbidity in the developing world, the role of some medical disorders, other reasons for the high levels of maternal deaths and what can be done to improve maternal health in developing countries. It will also consider global issues in obstetric anesthesia.

Levels and causes of maternal mortality and morbidity

Of the 536,000 maternal deaths estimated in 2007, 99% occurred in developing countries (see Figures 25.1 and 25.2). A further 9 million women have severe obstetric complications every year. The particularly high number of deaths in India (136,000) and Nigeria (37,000) can be attributed in part to the large populations of these countries. Another third

de Swiet's Medical Disorders in Obstetric Practice, 5th edition.
Edited by R. O. Powrie, M. F. Greene, W. Camann. © 2010 Blackwell
Publishing.

of all maternal deaths take place in 11 countries, including Pakistan, the Democratic Republic of the Congo, Ethiopia, Tanzania, Afghanistan, Bangladesh, Angola, China, Kenya, Indonesia and Uganda [4]. However, the risk of maternal death is highest in African countries and in Afghanistan. Women in Sierra Leone and Afghanistan have a lifetime risk of 1 in 6 of dying from a pregnancy, compared to 1 in 29,800 for women in Sweden [5] (see Table 25.1).

In poor countries, the causes of ill health and mortality in pregnancy can be difficult to establish because of the lack of diagnostic capability and vital registration. In addition, women may die at home or on the way to a provider and we have to rely on "verbal autopsies" to understand the reasons for their deaths. Available data indicate that the majority of deaths occur around the time of delivery and the most common causes are hemorrhage, infection, hypertensive disorders and obstructed labor (deaths associated with obstructed labor are classified separately even though obstructed labor usually causes death through infection, hemorrhage or uterine rupture) (Figure 25.3). Where diagnostic facilities exist, such as in South Africa, some causes of maternal mortality common in the "West," such as pulmonary embolism, appear to be comparatively rare [6]. In addition, many women still die because of unsafe abortions where abortions are illegal or costly to obtain [7]. Beyond these, there are also reasons related to the status of women and their financial and geographic accessibility to services.

The role of medical disorders in maternal mortality

Medical problems have a high prevalence in developing countries and are often detected in pregnancy, as this is often one of the rare occasions when women, including the poorest, use formal services. Nonfatal conditions can be highly prevalent (Table 25.2).

Indirect causes of maternal mortality such as anemia, malaria and HIV are increasingly recognized as important, particularly in Africa. Of these, maternal anemia is likely to be the most

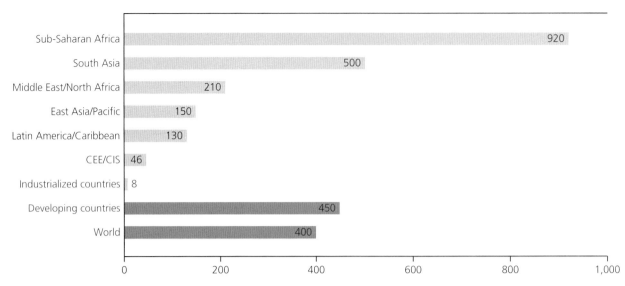

Figure 25.1 Maternal mortality ratios per 100,000 livebirths, by region, 2005. Reproduced with permission from World Health Organization, UNICEF, United Nations Population Fund and the World Bank, Maternal Mortality in 2005 (2007).

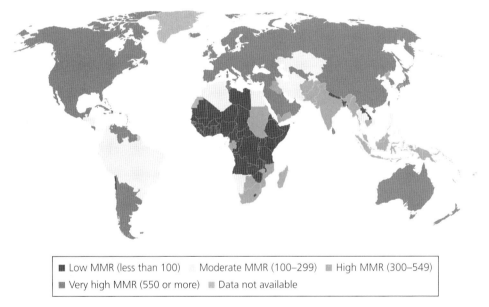

Figure 25.2 Maternal mortality ratios (MMR) per 100,000 livebirths, worldwide. Reproduced with permission from World Health Organization, UNICEF, Progress for Children: A Report Card on Maternal Mortality, Number 7, September 2008.

common medical problem. It usually results from nutritional deficiencies, intermittent (such as malaria) or chronic infections or hemoglobinopathies. Anemia is itself a cause of severe maternal morbidity [8] and can affect the case fatality rate of obstetric complications. Brabin *et al.* [9] estimated that the maternal mortality ratio for all-cause anemia was 40.8, 30.5 and 8.1 deaths per 100,000 livebirths for Africa, Asia and Latin America respectively.

In a hospital study of 251 maternal deaths in Zambia, 58% were caused by nonobstetric causes [10]. Of these, 30% were caused by malaria, 25% by tuberculosis and 22% by nonspecified chronic respiratory tract infections. While most studies, including those from Africa [6,11,12], continue to find that the majority of maternal deaths are caused by direct obstetric complications, a recent report from South Africa highlighted the importance of AIDS as the most common cause of maternal death in Durban [13]. In Malawi, maternal mortality level doubled between 1996 and 2000, reaching 1100 maternal deaths per 100,000 livebirths. Much of this is attributed to HIV/AIDS and its medical and social consequences.

Table 25.1 Lifetime risk of maternal death by region, 2005

Lifetime risk of maternal death	1 in:
Sub-Saharan Africa	22
Eastern/Southern Africa	29
West/Central Africa	17
Middle East/North Africa	140
South Asia	59
East Asia/Pacific	350
Latin America/Caribbean	280
CEE/CIS	1300
Industrialized countries	8000
Developing countries	76
Least developed countries	24
World	92

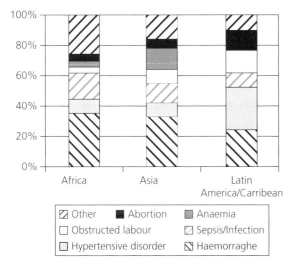

Figure 25.3 Causes of maternal mortality 1997–2002 [3].

In countries where malaria infection is common in pregnancy, such as in sub-Saharan Africa, one in four women has evidence of placental infection at delivery, and malaria-related maternal anemia, low birthweight, preterm delivery and infant and maternal mortality are prevalent [14]. Effective interventions, such as insecticide-treated bed nets and intermittent presumptive treatment, have the potential to reduce the risk of severe maternal anemia by 38%, low birthweights by 43% and perinatal mortality by 27% among women in their first and second pregnancies [14]. Multigravidae with HIV are also at increased risk from malaria [15] and malaria prevention may have to be aimed at all pregnant women in countries with a high HIV prevalence [4].

Reducing deaths from direct obstetric causes has been the focus of global initiatives such as Making Pregnancy Safer, with medical causes of ill health receiving less attention from the maternal health community. Integrating their management into routine obstetric services is important but requires careful attention, as they can create major disruption in service delivery and utilization. For example, well-resourced vertical HIV programs can attract the best staff away and undermine the ability of the routine services to provide skilled care [16]. Antenatal HIV screening programs often report a high loss to follow-up after HIV testing [17], and the fear of learning HIV results may contribute to poor uptake of intrapartum care for some of these women.

Current strategies to reduce maternal mortality

The provision of skilled birth attendants for all women in a health service setting and emergency obstetric care for those who need it are the two main strategies proposed for the reduction of maternal mortality (Box 25.1, Figure 25.4). Preventing unwanted pregnancies may also be able to avert around one-quarter of maternal deaths [3]. In addition to these, there are calls to reduce user fees and other financial or geographic barriers to enable access to obstetric services [18]. Countries which have successfully reduced maternal mortality are often middle-income countries. Lessons learnt from their success

Table 25.2 Selected examples of the frequency of chronic medical conditions in pregnancy

Condition	Country	Prevalence	Sample	Reference
Anaemia	Malawi	57%	Urban ANC	32
Intestinal worms	Indonesia	70%	Rural ANC	33
Schistosomiasis	Tanzania	63%	ANC	34
Iodine deficiency	Papua New Guinea	Pregnancy, 22%; lactation, 35%	Urban ANC	35
Maternal underweight	Bangladesh	52%	unclear	36
HIV	Botswana	37%	All mothers receiving ANC	37
Syphilis	Tanzania	7.3%	ANC	38
Trichomonas	Kenya	26%	Urban ANC	39
Gonorrhea		11%		
Domestic violence in pregnancy	Bangladesh, Brazil, Ethiopia, Namibia, Peru, Samoa, Tanzania, Thailand	4–28%	Population surveys	40

ANC, antenatal clinic.

Box 25.1 Definition of skilled birth attendants and emergency obstetric care

Skilled birth attendants: "an accredited health professional – such as a midwife, doctor or nurse – who has been educated and trained to proficiency in the skills needed to manage normal (uncomplicated) pregnancies, childbirth and the immediate postnatal period, and in the identification, management and referral of complications in women and newborns" [4]. Traditional birth attendants (TBA) – trained or not – are excluded from the category of skilled health-care workers.

Skilled birth attendance: refers to both the person and an enabling environment, including equipment, drugs and transportation for emergencies [41].

Emergency obstetric care: a minimal set of interventions which should be provided by hospitals to manage obstetric complications, including:
• Administration of parenteral oxytoxic drugs
• Administration of parenteral antibiotics
• Administration of parenteral sedatives/ anticonvulsants
• Performing manual removal of placenta
• Performing assisted vaginal delivery (vacuum extraction, forceps)
• Surgery (e.g. cesarean section, curettage, etc.)
• Blood transfusion

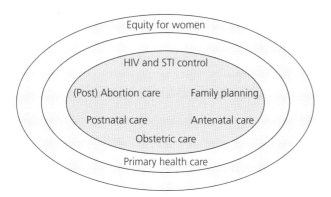

Figure 25.4 The main components of safe motherhood.

include the importance of increasing the professionalization of midwifery, improving access to skilled birth attendants and having an information system in place that monitors progress in maternal mortality [19].

The population growth momentum and migration of skilled staff away from rural areas and from poor countries, however, make it difficult to increase the proportion of deliveries attended by a skilled attendant. Between 1990 and 2005 the estimated proportion of deliveries attended by a skilled

attendant in poor countries only increased from 43% to 57% [3]. Because of skill shortage, new approaches to training, deploying and retaining health workers are required. Research from Mozambique suggests, for example, that it is safe and cost-effective to train nurses or medical assistants to conduct cesarean section [20].

Antenatal care

A successful safe motherhood program which reaches beyond obstetric causes of maternal deaths has the potential to achieve far more than maternal health. In particular, antenatal care can be used as a vehicle to improve the health of women more generally. Globally 71% of pregnant women receive antenatal care but only 63% then deliver with a skilled attendant [5] (Figure 25.5).

In industrialized countries, the scope of antenatal care is expanding to detect nonmedical risk factors for women's health (such as domestic violence). In poor countries, antenatal care has been much derided because of the low predictive value of its risk screening strategy for maternal mortality. The WHO promotes a new model of "focused antenatal care" including the identification of pre-existing conditions, the early detection of complications, health promotion and discussions on birth preparedness [21,22]. Many of the interventions on pre-existing conditions can be implemented in a standardized package. As HIV treatment becomes more accessible in poor countries, HIV testing and treatment during antenatal care may well be the most important means of improving health outcomes for many women, including after pregnancy.

Furthermore, while the scope of antenatal care to address direct obstetric problems is limited, antenatal care may present better value for money than is currently acknowledged,

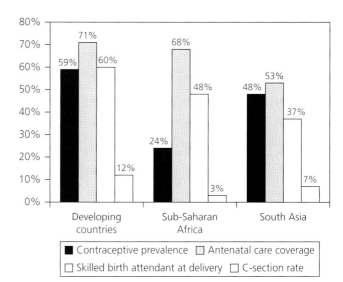

Figure 25.5 Use of reproductive health services in developing countries [5,42].

particularly when health outcomes in babies are taken into account [23].

- Estimates for the annual global incidence of congenital syphilis cases range from 713,600 to 1,575,000. Of these, 17–40% end in miscarriage or stillbirth, 12–20% in perinatal death, and 25–33% in the delivery of a premature or low birthweight infant [24]. Many of these adverse outcomes could be prevented through screening and treating or mass treatment in antenatal care.
- Antenatal tetanus toxoid vaccinations prevent maternal (30,000 deaths per year) and neonatal (215,000 deaths per year) deaths related to tetanus [25].
- In developing countries interventions to prevent congenital syphilis and maternal and neonatal tetanus can be extremely cost-effective [26] and may be more cost-effective than the provision of skilled intrapartum care [27].
- Other cost-effective interventions are calcium supplementation to prevent pre-eclampsia [28,29], intermittent presumptive treatment for malaria [29] and the detection and treatment of asymptomatic bacteriuria [29].

There are other promising interventions in pregnancy which require further evaluation. In randomized controlled trials, antibiotic mass treatment for sexually transmitted infections in antenatal care reduced low birthweight and preterm deliveries and early neonatal deaths in Uganda [30] while vitamin A or betacarotene supplementation before, during and after pregnancy reduced maternal mortality by 40% and 49% compared to placebo treatment in Nepal [31]. However, ongoing or recently terminated trials may be unable to replicate the findings from Nepal.

Conclusion

The reduction of maternal mortality is a key international development goal and the provision of skilled birth attendants and emergency care are rightly key strategies for achieving this goal. Medical conditions in pregnancy, however, can be extremely common. Even poor countries can have excellent uptake of antenatal care. Many medical conditions could be managed or prevented during the antenatal period even in a resource-restricted environment and should receive more attention by providers, planners and donors than at present. Where, for example, medical conditions such as neonatal tetanus or congenital syphilis are common, antenatal interventions to prevent these conditions will be a better use of limited resources than the provision of obstetric interventions such as intrapartum fetal monitoring.

Global issues in obstetric anesthesia

Anesthesia consistently ranks within the top ten leading causes of maternal mortality worldwide. In developed countries, the contribution of anesthesia to maternal mortality has fallen over the past two decades as anesthesia practices have become safer [43]. In developing countries it is estimated that anesthesia is responsible for 3–9% of hospital-based maternal deaths each year, [44–47] but reports vary widely [47] and in some cases, deaths due to anesthesia may be under-reported or unknown [44,47]. Considering the high number of maternal deaths in many countries, the impact of anesthesia is significant and many deaths are considered avoidable.

There are several factors that contribute to anesthesia-related maternal mortality. Emergency surgery is unavailable in many rural areas [48] and by the time a woman reaches a surgical center, conditions can be dire. Hypertensive crisis, hemorrhagic shock and sepsis are common preoperative problems that make anesthesia administration hazardous even for experienced practitioners [49]. Given these circumstances, it is not surprising that perioperative mortality in some countries is reported to be as high as 1–2%. [48,49] In addition, the numbers of trained anesthesiologists are inadequate [45,49,50]. In Ghana, for example, there are fewer than 20 anesthesiologists for over 22 million people. Anesthesia for cesarean section is frequently administered by junior medical officers, nurses or technicians with limited medical knowledge and inadequate equipment [44,47,50]. Most reported anesthesia-related maternal deaths occur during the administration of general anesthesia for cesarean section in both healthy and medically compromised patients [43–47,51]. The most common problems include gastric aspiration and/or hypoxemia related to difficult intubation or premature extubation and unrecognized esophageal intubation.

The most commonly used agents for the induction of general anesthesia are thiopental or ketamine followed by succinylcholine to facilitate tracheal intubation, not dissimilar from North American and European practices. The maintenance of anesthesia, however, differs greatly: ketamine, halothane or ether are most commonly used with or without muscle relaxants [49–51]. In very remote rural settings, anesthesia for cesarean section may be conducted with intravenous ketamine or facemask open drop ether as the sole anesthetic with spontaneous ventilation [49–52]. Practitioners of this method claim it is safer for untrained, unequipped anesthesia providers who should not attempt intubation or spinal anesthesia [49]. Ether produces slow change in the depth of anesthetic and can be administered in room air. The main disadvantages include delayed emergence, vomiting and flammability [53].

The airway complications that accompany general anesthesia could be minimized if regional anesthesia techniques were utilized for cesarean section [43–45,47,48,51]. Interestingly, even in countries with sufficient numbers of trained anesthesia providers or the availability of regional anesthesia, general anesthesia is still frequently preferred [44,46,51,54]. Reasons for this may include fear of regional anesthesia by patients, reluctance of surgeons to operate on "awake" patients and unfamiliarity of anesthesiologists with the regional techniques [50,54].

Efforts are underway by individuals and nongovernmental organizations (www.anaesthesiologists.org, www.oaa-anaes. ac.uk and www.kybeleworldwide.org) to train anesthesia providers in regional anesthetic techniques for cesarean section and labor analgesia.

Labor analgesia may seem unnecessary in countries with limited resources but it represents an index of healthcare quality and compassion. The provision of pain relief is now being considered as a basic human right although cultural and financial barriers impede its administration in many developing countries. Providing analgesia during labor could encourage patients to seek earlier hospital admission in urban settings and would promote multidisciplinary patient care with anesthesiologists outside the operating room. Earlier intervention by anesthesia providers could potentially improve patient outcome, especially in cases of hemorrhage or hypertensive crisis [48,51]. Finally, recent global initiatives that strive for greater availability of facility-based emergency obstetric services must also, by necessity, include a model of safe anesthesia care [45,48,51].

References

1. World Health Organization. Maternal mortality in 2000: estimates developed by WHO, UNICEF and UNFPA. WHO, Geneva. 2004.
2. Hill K, Thomas K, AbouZahr C, et al. Levels and trends in global and regional maternal mortality 1990 to 2005. Lancet 2007;370(9595):1311–19.
3. UN Millennium Goal Report, 2007. www.un.org/millenniumgoals/ www.un.org/millenniumgoals/pdf/mdg2007.pdf.
4. World Health Organization. Malaria and HIV interactions and implications: conclusions of a technical consultation convened by WHO, 23–24 June 2004. WHO, Geneva, 2004.
5. UNICEF 2007. The state of the world's children. www.unicef.org/sowc07/docs/sowc07.pdf.
6. Fawcus SR, van Coeverden de Groot HA, Isaacs S. A 50-year audit of maternal mortality in the Peninsula Maternal and Neonatal Service, Cape Town (1953–2002). Br J Obstet Gynecol 2005;112(9):1257–63.
7. Grimes, DA, Benson J, Singh S, et al. Unsafe abortion: the preventable epidemics. Lancet 2006;368(9550):1908–19.
8. Filippi V, Ronsmans C, Gouhou V, et al. Maternity wards or emergency obstetric rooms? Incidence of near-miss events in African hospitals. Acta Obstet Gynecol Scand 2005;84(1):11–16.
9. Brabin BJ, Hakimi M, Pelletier D. An analysis of anemia and pregnancy-related maternal mortality. J Nutr 2001;131(suppl 2):604S-15S.
10. Ahmed Y, Mwaba P, Chintu C, et al. A study of maternal mortality at the University Teaching Hospital. Int J Tuberc Lung Dis 1999;3:675–80.
11. Lema VM, Changole J, Kanyighe C, Malunga EV. Maternal mortality at the Queen Elizabeth Central Teaching Hospital, Blantyre, Malawi. East Afr Med J 2005;82(1):3–9.
12. Oyieke JB, Obore S, Kigondu CS. Millennium development goal 5: a review of maternal mortality at the Kenyatta National Hospital, Nairobi. East Afr Med J 2006;83(1):4–9.
13. Ramogale MR, Moodley J, Sebiloane MH. HIV-associated maternal mortality – primary causes of death at King Edward VIII Hospital, Durban. S Afr Med J 2007;97(5):363–6.
14. Desai M, ter Kuile FO, Nosten F, et al. Epidemiology and burden of malaria in pregnancy. Lancet Infect Dis 2007;7:93–104.
15. Van Eijk A, Ayisi JG, ter Kuile FO, et al. HIV increases the risk of malaria in women of all gravidities in Kisumu, Kenya. AIDS 2003;17:595–603.
16. England R. Are we spending too much on HIV? BMJ 2007;334:344.
17. Cartoux M, Msellati P, Meda N, et al. Attitude of pregnant women towards HIV testing in Abidjan, Cote d'Ivoire and Bobo-Dioulasso, Burkina Faso. AIDS 1998;12(17):2337–44.
18. Borghi J, Ensor T, Somanathan A, et al. Mobilising financial resources for maternal health. Lancet 2006;368(9545):1457–65.
19. Ronsmans C, Graham W. Maternal mortality: who, when, where and why. Lancet 2006;368(9542):1189–200.
20. Kruck M, Pereira C, Vaz F, Bergstrom S, Galea S. Economic evaluation of surgically trained assistant medical officers in performing major obstetric surgery in Mozambique. Br J Obstet Gynaecol 2007;114(10):1253–60.
21. World Health Organization, Antenatal Care Trial Research Group. WHO antenatal care randomized trial. Manual for implementation of the new model. WHO, Geneva, 2002.
22. Villar J, Ba'aqeel H, Piaggio G, et al. WHO antenatal care randomised trial for the evaluation of a new model of routine antenatal care. Lancet 2001;357:1551–64.
23. Graham WJ, Cairns J, Bhattacharya S, et al. Maternal and perinatal conditions. In: Alleyne G, Breman J, Claeson M, et al. (eds) Disease Control Priorities Project. World Bank and OUP, Oxford, 2006: 499–529.
24. World Health Organization. The global elimination of congenital syphilis. WHO, Geneva, 2007.
25. World Health Organization. Maternal and neonatal tetanus elimination by 2005. WHO, Geneva, 2000.
26. Schackman BR, Neukermans CP, Fontain SN, et al. Cost-effectiveness of rapid syphilis screening in prenatal HIV testing programs in Haiti. PLoS Med 2007;4(5):e183.
27. Adam T, Lim SS, Mehta S, et al. Cost effectiveness analysis of strategies for maternal and neonatal health in developing countries. BMJ 2005;331(7525):1107.
28. Hofmeyr GJ, Atallah AN, Duley L. Dietary calcium supplementation for prevention of pre-eclampsia and related problems: a systematic review and commentary. Br J Obstet Gynaecol 2007;114(8):933–43.
29. Darmstadt GL, Bhutta ZA, Cousens S, et al. Evidence-based, cost-effective interventions: how many newborn babies can we save? Lancet 2005;365(9463):977–88.
30. Gray RH, Wabwire-Mangen F, Kigozi G, et al. Randomized trial of presumptive sexually transmitted disease therapy during pregnancy in Rakai, Uganda. Am J Obstet Gynecol 2001;185(5):1209–17.
31. West K, Katz J, Khatry S, et al. Double blind, cluster randomised trial of low dose supplementation with vitamin A or beta carotene on mortality related to pregnancy in Nepal. BMJ 1999;318:570–5.
32. Van den Broek NR, Rogerson SJ, Mhango CG, et al. Anaemia in pregnancy in southern Malawi: prevalence and risk factors. Br J Obstet Gynaecol 2000;107(4):445–51.
33. Nurdia DS, Sumarni S, Suyoko, et al. Impact of intestinal helminth infection on anemia and iron status during pregnancy: a community based study in Indonesia. Southeast Asian J Trop Med Public Health 2001;32(1):14–22.

34. Ajanga A, Lwambo NJ, Blair L, *et al*. Schistosoma mansoni in pregnancy and associations with anaemia in northwest Tanzania. Trans R Soc Trop Med Hyg 2006;100(1):59–63.

35. Temple VJ, Haindapa B, Turare R, *et al*. Status of iodine nutrition in pregnant and lactating women in national capital district, Papua New Guinea. Asia Pac J Clin Nutr 2006;15(4):533–7.

36. UNICEF. Bangladesh – health and nutrition – women's health. www.unicef.org/bangladesh/health_nutrition_407.htm.

37. Centers for Disease Control and Prevention. Introduction of routine HIV testing in prenatal care – Botswana 2004. MMWR 2004;53(46):1083–6.

38. Swai RO, Somi GR, Matee MI, *et al*. Surveillance of HIV and syphilis infections among antenatal clinic attendees in Tanzania 2003/2004. BMC Public Health 2006;6:91.

39. Fonck K, Kidula N, Jaoko W. Validity of the vaginal discharge algorithm among pregnant and non-pregnant women in Nairobi, Kenya. Sex Transm Infect 2000;76(1):33–8.

40. World Health Organization. Multi-country study on women's health and domestic violence against women. WHO, Geneva, 2005.

41. Hussein J, Clapham S. Message in a bottle: sinking in a sea of safe motherhood concepts. Health Policy 2005;73(3):294–302.

42. Stanton C, Holtz S. Levels and trends in caesarean births in the developing world. Stud Family Plan 2006;37(1):41–8.

43. Hawkins JL. Anesthesia-related maternal mortality. Clin Obstet Gynecol 2003;46(3):679–87.

44. Enohumah KO, Imarengiaye CO. Factors associated with anesthesia-related maternal mortality in a tertiary hospital in Nigeria. Acta Anaesthesiol Scand 2006;50:206–10.

45. Rout C. Maternal mortality and anaesthesia in Africa: a South African perspective. Int J Obstet Anesth 2002;11:77–80.

46. Cetin M, Sumer H, Timuroglu T, Demirkoprulu N. Maternal mortality in the last decade at a university hospital in Turkey. Int J Obstet Anesth 2003;83:301–2.

47. McKenzie AG. Operative obstetric mortality at Harare Central Hospital 1992–94: an anaesthetic view. Int J Obstet Anesth 1998;7:237–41.

48. Clyburn P, Morris S, Hall J. Anaesthesia and safe motherhood. Anaesthesia 2007;62(1):21–5.

49. Fenton PM. Obstetric anesthesia in the developing world. In: Palmer CM, d'Angelo R, Paech MJ (eds) Handbook of obstetric anesthesia. BIOS, Oxford, 2002: 244–55.

50. Hodges SC, Mijumbi C, Okello M, McCormick BA, Walker IA, Wilson IH. Anaesthesia services in developing countries: defining the problems. Anaesthesia 2007;62:4–11.

51. Fenton PM, Whitty CJM, Reynolds F. Caesarean section in Malawi: prospective study of early maternal and perinatal mortality. BMJ 2003;327:1–5.

52. Maltby JR. Open drop ether anaesthesia for Caesarean section: a review of 420 cases in Nepal. Can Anaesth Soc J 1986;33(5):651–6.

53. Rahardjo E. The history of anesthesia: ether, the anesthetic from 19th to 21st century. International Congress Series 2002;1242:51–5.

54. Schnittger T. Regional anaesthesia in developing countries. Anaesthesia 2007;62(1):44–7.

26 Future health concerns for women who have had a complicated pregnancy

David J. Williams

UCL Institute for Women's Health, University College London and UCL Hospitals NHS Foundation Trust, London, UK

Introduction

During pregnancy, almost every organ of the mother's body has to work harder in order to meet the demands of the developing fetus [1]. Women with chronic disease struggle to fulfill these physiologic demands. As a consequence, pregnancy outcome can be compromised and long-term maternal health may be threatened.

Gestational syndromes generally develop in the second half of pregnancy when the physiologic burden is at its greatest. For example, the progressive insulin resistance of pregnancy acts as a stress test that transiently unmasks carbohydrate intolerance which we term "gestational diabetes mellitus" in women who are predisposed to type 2 diabetes. Childbirth leads to remission, but the disease returns in later life when the effects of aging and weight gain expose a persistent vulnerability to diabetes.

In this chapter, the consequences of an adverse pregnancy outcome on a woman's long-term health are discussed and recommendations are given that might prevent disease in later life.

Pre-eclampsia (see Chapter 6)

During healthy pregnancy the mother is propelled into an increasingly proatherogenic metabolic state [2,3]. Shortly after conception she develops a high cardiac output [4], hypercoagulability [5] and increased inflammatory activity [6]. After 20 weeks she develops insulin resistance [3,7] and hyperlipidemia [8]. Each of these gestational changes is more pronounced in women who later develop pre-eclampsia [3–8]. This must be at least partly due to the presence of subclinical classic cardiac risk factors in "healthy" women who go on to develop pre-eclampsia [9,10]. These women are more likely to be overweight, have higher lipid levels, higher blood pressure and insulin resistance and to have a thrombophilia, compared with women who go on to have a normotensive pregnancy [9–11].

Post partum, women who have had pre-eclampsia usually recover within 3 months of delivery, but are at an increased risk of developing cardiovascular disease in later life [12]. A systematic review and meta-analysis that included over 3.5 million women showed that women who had pre-eclampsia were more than twice as likely to develop future ischemic heart disease years after the index pregnancy compared with women who had a normotensive pregnancy (Table 26.1). A similar risk exists for future cerebrovascular accident [12].

Table 26.1 The relative risk of a woman developing future disease after pre-eclampsia

Pregnancy syndrome	Future disease	Relative risk (95% CI)
Pre-eclampsia	Chronic hypertension	3.70 (2.70–5.05)
Pre-eclampsia	Ischemic heart disease	2.16 (1.86–2.52)
Preterm pre-eclampsia	Ischemic heart disease	7.71 (4.40–13.52)
Pre-eclampsia	Cerebrovascular accident	1.81 (1.45–2.27)
Pre-eclampsia	Venous thromboembolism	1.79 (1.37–2.33)
Pre-eclampsia in 1st pregnancy only	Endstage renal disease	3.2 (2.2–4.9)
Pre-eclampsia in 1st and 2nd pregnancies	Endstage renal disease	6.4 (3.0–13.5)
Pre-eclampsia in 1st, 2nd and 3rd pregnancies	Endstage renal disease	15.5 (7.8–30.8)
Preterm labor	Fatal cardiovascular disease	1.8 (1.3–2.5)
Pre-eclampsia, fetal growth restriction and preterm labor	Fatal cardiovascular disease	7.0 (3.3–14.5)

de Swiet's Medical Disorders in Obstetric Practice, 5th edition.
Edited by R. O. Powrie, M. F. Greene, W. Camann. © 2010 Blackwell Publishing.

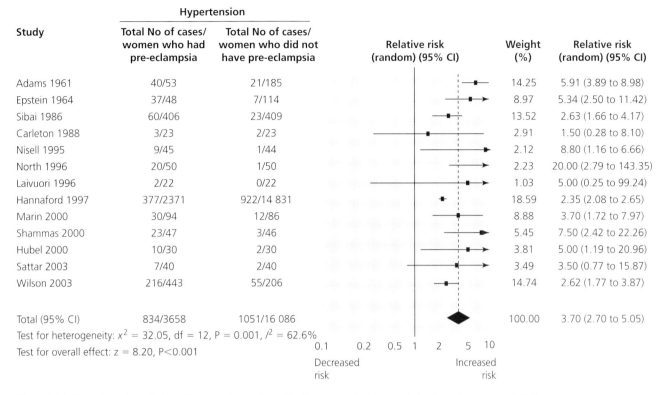

Study	Hypertension		Relative risk (random) (95% CI)	Weight (%)	Relative risk (random) (95% CI)
	Total No of cases/ women who had pre-eclampsia	Total No of cases/ women who did not have pre-eclampsia			
Adams 1961	40/53	21/185		14.25	5.91 (3.89 to 8.98)
Epstein 1964	37/48	7/114		8.97	5.34 (2.50 to 11.42)
Sibai 1986	60/406	23/409		13.52	2.63 (1.66 to 4.17)
Carleton 1988	3/23	2/23		2.91	1.50 (0.28 to 8.10)
Nisell 1995	9/45	1/44		2.12	8.80 (1.16 to 6.66)
North 1996	20/50	1/50		2.23	20.00 (2.79 to 143.35)
Laivuori 1996	2/22	0/22		1.03	5.00 (0.25 to 99.24)
Hannaford 1997	377/2371	922/14 831		18.59	2.35 (2.08 to 2.65)
Marin 2000	30/94	12/86		8.88	3.70 (1.72 to 7.97)
Shammas 2000	23/47	3/46		5.45	7.50 (2.42 to 22.26)
Hubel 2000	10/30	2/30		3.81	5.00 (1.19 to 20.96)
Sattar 2003	7/40	2/40		3.49	3.50 (0.77 to 15.87)
Wilson 2003	216/443	55/206		14.74	2.62 (1.77 to 3.87)
Total (95% CI)	834/3658	1051/16 086		100.00	3.70 (2.70 to 5.05)

Test for heterogeneity: $x^2 = 32.05$, df = 12, P = 0.001, $I^2 = 62.6\%$

Test for overall effect: z = 8.20, P<0.001

0.1 0.2 0.5 1 2 5 10

Decreased risk — Increased risk

Figure 26.1 Pre-eclampsia and risk of hypertension in later life. Reproduced with permission from Bellamy *et al.* [12].

These risks appear to be mediated through an even stronger future risk of chronic hypertension after pre-eclampsia (relative risk (RR) 3.70, 95% confidence interval (CI) 2.70–5.05) [12] (Figure 26.1).

Women who have preterm pre-eclampsia (before 37 weeks) have a particularly high RR of death from future cardiovascular disease (RR 8.12, 95% CI 4.31–15.33) and stroke (RR 5.08, 95% CI 2.09–12.35) [13], compared with women who had a normotensive pregnancy. Recurrent pre-eclampsia, which strongly suggests chronic renovascular disease in the mother, is associated with a particularly high risk of future hypertension and kidney disease in later life [14,15].

Fortunately, cardiovascular disease is rare in young women, but its prevalence increases with age. In the UK, 8.3% of women aged 50–59 years will have a cardiovascular event over the next 10 years [16]. If a woman in this age group had a pregnancy affected by pre-eclampsia, her calculated risk of having a cardiovascular event in the next 10 years could double to 17.8%. This pushes her towards a category of risk where therapeutic prophylaxis against cardiovascular disease is recommended with low-dose aspirin and HMG-CoA reductase inhibitors ("statins").

Conversely, women who have had a normotensive, term pregnancy appear to be in a privileged position with a lower than average risk of future cardiovascular disease compared with a general population [13,15].

Preterm birth and fetal growth restriction

Women who have had a pregnancy affected by preterm birth without pre-eclampsia are also at increased risk of death from future cardiovascular disease (RR 2.95, 95% CI 2.12–4.11) [17]. Similarly, a pregnancy complicated by fetal growth restriction identifies a woman as being at increased risk for future cardiovascular disease [17]. In one population, women who had a baby weighing less than 2500 g had an 11 times greater risk of dying from future ischemic heart disease (IHD) compared with those who had a baby weighing more than 3500 g [17]. These observations suggest that a different etiology may explain preterm pre-eclampsia, which is associated with low birthweight babies, compared with late pre-eclampsia, which is often associated with high birthweight babies [18]. Women who have a pregnancy complicated by all three of pre-eclampsia, preterm labor and fetal growth restriction (FGR) have the highest risk of cardiovascular disease in later life [13,17].

It is entirely possible that a woman who has had pregnancies complicated by FGR, preterm birth and/or pre-eclampsia has some combination of inherited and acquired risk factors for future cardiovascular disease that also caused her adverse pregnancy outcomes. It is therefore possible that such a woman would face the same long-term risk of cardiovascular disease even if she had never become pregnant and that the pregnancy complication only heralds but does not cause the later cardiovascular disease.

One epidemiologic study attempted to address this issue by comparing future cardiovascular risk according to classic risk factors for heart disease with or without a pregnancy affected by FGR or pre-eclampsia [19]. Women who had a pathologic pregnancy had a greater risk of ischemic heart disease compared with those who only had a classic risk factor for heart disease. It remains unclear whether this observation reflects an additional risk because of the pregnancy or that the pregnancy unmasks an as yet unknown additional risk factor for cardiovascular disease.

Furthermore, there is an association between an increasing number of healthy pregnancies and an increased risk of ischemic heart disease [20]. Parous women without pregnancy complications have a 1.95-fold (95% CI 1.03–3.7) higher cardiovascular disease prevalence than nulliparous women. Women who have had more than five pregnancies have the greatest risk of future cardiovascular disease [20]. Whether this reflects cumulative harm done due to the repeated physiologic strain of hemodynamic and metabolic changes of pregnancy or whether it follows weight retention after each pregnancy remains unclear.

Eclampsia

Eclampsia in a first pregnancy does not appear to be associated with the same increased risk of future hypertension as seen following pre-eclampsia [21–23]. The increased risk of future cardiovascular disease is, however, evident in multiparous women who develop eclampsia, or in primiparous women of black African origin. It is possible therefore that the pathology leading to isolated eclampsia is different from that which heralds the multiorgan syndrome of pre-eclampsia. Support for this suggestion follows the observation that women who have had eclampsia appear to be at greater risk of future epilepsy [24], in particular temporal lobe epilepsy, associated with hippocampal sclerosis. The hippocampus is supplied by the posterior circulation, which is most often compromised during eclampsia. Whether eclampsia unmasks a pre-existing vulnerability to hippocampal ischemia or causes it, is unclear.

When eclampsia occurs with pre-eclampsia, future maternal health is predicted by the gestation of onset of pre-eclampsia [25]. Women who had eclampsia before 30 weeks gestation were more than threefold more likely to develop chronic hypertension compared with those who had eclampsia after 37 weeks [25]. If the subsequent pregnancy was also complicated by pre-eclampsia then the incidence of chronic hypertension more than 7 years later has been estimated at 25%,

compared with only 2% for women who had a normotensive pregnancy following their eclamptic pregnancy [25].

The consistent findings that pre-eclampsia, preterm birth and intrauterine growth restriction (IUGR) are predictive of long-term maternal risk of cardiovascular disease provides an ideal opportunity for clinicians to initiate risk factor reduction in women whose pregnancies have been complicated by these conditions. Possibly helpful recommendations for these women (and for the other pregnancy complications listed below) are listed in Table 26.2. The potential importance of each of these interventions should be emphasized by the obstetrician to both the patient and the patient's medical primary care provider.

Pre-eclampsia and future kidney disease

Pre-eclampsia is more common in women with underlying renal disease, especially when associated with chronic hypertension [26]. Conversely, the prevalence of newly identified renal disease in women with pre-eclampsia depends on how hard and for how long you look.

More than 30 years ago, hypertensive pregnant women often had a postpartum renal biopsy. In one series, the classic renal histology of pre-eclampsia, glomerular endotheliosis, was associated with other renal disease in approximately 10% of primigravid pre-eclampsia and up to 30% of multiparous pre-eclampsia [15]. Currently, very few women who have had pre-eclampsia have a postpartum renal biopsy. It is more likely that persistent proteinuria will suggest underlying renal disease [27]. Microalbuminuria is also more common after pre-eclampsia, but also acts as a marker for cardiovascular disease, the major cause of morbidity in people with renal disease [28]. Women with proteinuria recognized during pregnancy should be followed up post partum, until either the proteinuria disappears or a diagnosis is made.

Given the strong association between pre-eclampsia and renal disease, it is no surprise that endstage renal disease (ESRD) is more common years after pre-eclampsia. This risk has been quantified from the combination of large Norwegian birth and renal registries [29]. If pre-eclampsia occurred only in the first pregnancy, the relative risk of future ESRD is 4.7 (95% CI 3.6–6.1) [29]. This risk of future ESRD increases progressively with two and three pregnancies affected by pre-eclampsia (see Table 26.1). If the pregnancy was also complicated by low birthweight and preterm labor, the relative risk of ESRD increases even further [29]. Prevention or delay in the development of renal disease will be helped by early identification and treatment of hypertension and may be helped by early identification of subsequent proteinuria (see Table 26.3).

Table 26.2 Possibly helpful interventions to decrease subsequent risk in mothers with pregnancy complications

Pregnancy complication that points to a future health risk	Future health risk	Possibly helpful advice, counselling or screening to reduce subsequent risk
Patients with pre-eclampsia prior to 37 weeks, recurrent pre-eclampsia or who have delivered pre-term or growth restricted infants	Cardiovascular disease (ischemic heart disease and stroke)	• Smoking cessation • Exercise for 20–30 minutes almost every day • Achieve and maintain ideal body weight • Undergo cholesterol screening 6 weeks postpartum and the subsequent appropriate treatment • Yearly blood pressure measurement and the subsequent appropriate treatment
	Renal disease	• Ensure that pre-eclampsia related protienuria completely resolves and if persistent, initiate appropriate investigations • Yearly blood pressure measurement and the subsequent appropriate treatment • Consider yearly urinalysis
Thromboembolic disease	Recurrent thromboembolism	• Consider screening patient for thrombophilia to help quantitate future risk • Smoking cessation • Achieve and maintain ideal body weight • Avoid estrogen containing medications • Employ frequent calf flexing and ambulation with prolonged road or plane trips • Consider thromboprophylaxis with any prolonged bed rest, surgery or a subsequent pregnancy • Educate patient as to signs and symptoms of acute VTE and encourage them to seek medical attention early if any of them occur at a subsequent date • Encourage the use of compression stockings early after the initial event to help reduce the risk and extent of this undesirable sequelae
Gestational diabetes	Type 2 diabetes	• Glucose tolerance test 6 weeks postpartum and a screening fasting glucose every 3 years • Exercise for 20–30 minutes almost every day • Achieve and maintain ideal body weight • Consider initiation of metformin if evidence of impaired glucose tolerance
Post-partum thyroiditis	Hypothyroidism	• Check thyroid peroxidise antibodies (anti-TPO) to assess risk of recurrence/subsequent hypothyroidism • Check TSH yearly • Check TSH prior to and/or early in the first trimester and 3–6 months after subsequent pregnancies • Patients who are known to have an elevated anti-TPO should have their TSH checked at three and six months postpartum
Peripartum cardiomyopathy	Persistent or worsening cardiac dysfunction	• Follow cardiac function with serial echocardiograms and optimize congestive heart failure therapy • Warn patient of risk of worsening with subsequent pregnancies
Postpartum depression	Recurrent depression	• Screen patient for depression yearly and with any presenting complaint potentially attributable to recurrent depression

anti-TPO, thyroid peroxidase antibodies; TSH, thyroid stimulating hormone; VTE, venous thromboembolism

Table 26.3 The relative risk of a woman developing future disease after gestational syndromes compared with women who had unaffected pregnancies

Gestational syndrome	Future maternal disease	Relative risk (95% CI)
Gestational diabetes mellitus	Type 2 diabetes mellitus	5.81 (4.77–7.08)
Gestational diabetes mellitus (gestational fasting glucose >6.05 mmol/L v <4.75 mmol/L)	Type 2 diabetes mellitus	21 (4.6–96)
Postpartum thyroiditis (with TPO antibodies)	Hypothyroidism	Approximately 50% will remain hypothyroid
Intrahepatic cholestasis of pregnancy	Hepatitits C	3.5 (1.6–7.6)
Intrahepatic cholestasis of pregnancy	Nonalcoholic liver cirrhosis	8.2 (1.9–35.5)
Intrahepatic cholestasis of pregnancy	Gallstones and cholecystitis	3.7 (3.2–4.2)
Intrahepatic cholestasis of pregnancy	Nonalcoholic pancreatitis	3.2 (1.7–5.7)
Peripartum cardiomyopathy	Chronic heart failure and cardiac transplantation	Relates to level of postpartum recovery
Postpartum depression	Psychiatric illness	30–75% of mothers hospitalized post partum have future psychiatric illness

This study reinforces the point that pre-eclampsia in multiparous women should alert the clinician to look carefully for underlying renal-vascular disease.

Pre-eclampsia and future cancer

Women who smoke have a lower incidence of pre-eclampsia [30]. This robust observation contradicts all other observations that cardiovascular risk factors predispose to pre-eclampsia. Initial observations even suggested that women who had pre-eclampsia were also protected from future cancer [13] because they were less likely to smoke. Further analysis shows that this does not appear to be true [12]. Furthermore, it remains the case that smoking increases the risk of pregnancy complications, including FGR, placental abruption, preterm rupture of membranes, placenta previa and ectopic pregnancy [30], which outweigh the benefit of a reduced risk of pre-eclampsia.

Pregnancy-induced hypertension

Women who had isolated pregnancy-induced hypertension have a similar risk of future chronic hypertension and cardiovascular disease as women who had term pre-eclampsia [12].

Thrombosis during pregnancy

(see Chapters 3 and 4)

Normal pregnancy is characterized by low-grade, chronic intravascular coagulation within both the maternal and uteroplacental circulation. As a consequence, the risk of deep venous thrombosis (DVT) is increased sixfold during pregnancy and for up to 6 weeks post partum [5]. Women who have an inherited thrombophilia may develop a DVT in combination with the hypercoagulable environment of healthy pregnancy [31]. Once treatment with anticoagulation is completed, a thrombophilia screen and family history of thrombosis will assess the woman's future risk of thrombosis. The recurrence risk of venous thromboembolism (VTE) is significant in all patients and particularly those with an associated thrombophilia. Patients who have had VTE in pregnancy should therefore be counseled as described in Table 26.3. Post-thrombotic syndrome with chronic venous congestion is also responsible for morbidity in later life and the use of compression stockings early after the initial event can help reduce the risk and extent of this undesirable sequela [5].

Thrombophilias have been associated with an increased risk of pre-eclampsia [32]. This observation is supported by studies that have followed up women who have had pre-eclampsia and who have been found to have twice the risk of future thrombosis as women who had a normotensive pregnancy [12] (see Figure 26.1).

Gestational diabetes mellitus

(see Chapter 11)

Most cases of gestational diabetes mellitus (GDM) emerge in the second half of pregnancy in women who either have pre-existing insulin resistance or who have limited capacity to increase insulin secretion in response to gestational insulin resistance [33]. As soon as the placenta is delivered, glucose homeostasis is restored to nonpregnant levels. This is a temporary situation. In time, either a further pregnancy will result in recurrent GDM or type 1 or usually type 2 diabetes mellitus will develop.

Depending on the severity of their insulin resistance, women who have had GDM have an approximately sixfold increased risk of developing type 2 diabetes mellitus within 5 years of the index pregnancy (Bellamy, personal communication) (Table 26.3). Over time, up to 80% of all women who have had GDM will develop type 2 diabetes [34] (Figure 26.2). It is therefore recommended that all women who have had GDM have an evaluation of their glucose tolerance 6 weeks post partum and a screening fasting glucose (or the more sensitive glucose tolerance test) every 3 years thereafter [33]. Despite this recommendation, few women who had GDM return for postpartum screening [35].

In order to stratify those at highest risk of long-term type 2 diabetes, a special effort should be made with women who have the highest fasting plasma glucose levels or who develop GDM earliest in pregnancy. In one study, a fasting glucose

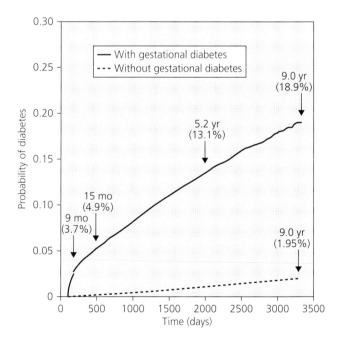

Figure 26.2 Cumulative incidence rate of diabetes mellitus, Reproduced with permission from Feig *et al.* [34].

above 6.71 mmol/L (121 mg/dL) during pregnancy was associated with a 36.7% rate of diabetes which is a 21-fold (95% CI 4.6–96) increased odds ratio of developing future diabetes mellitus, compared with women who had a maximum gestational fasting plasma glucose below 5.27 mmol/L (95 mg/dL) who had a 0.5% rate of developing diabetes [36]. In one study, a fasting glucose above 121 mg/dL during pregnancy was associated with a 37% risk of developing future diabetes mellitus, compared with a 0.5% risk for women who had a maximum gestational fasting plasma glucose below 95 mg/dL [36].

Further follow-up to encourage weight loss, a healthy diet and exercise, with regular assessment of blood glucose and blood pressure and timely intervention with disease-modifying drugs such as metformin is most likely to limit the emergence of morbidity associated with type 2 diabetes mellitus [37].

Gestational diabetes insipidus

During healthy pregnancy the placenta produces an enzyme, vasopressinase, which degrades vasopressin [38]. In response, the maternal posterior pituitary produces up to four times as much vasopressin in order to sustain water homeostasis [38]. During the third trimester, when the placenta is expressing the highest concentrations of vasopressinase, women who are unable to increase their pituitary output of vasopressin develop diabetes insipidus [39]. They have polyuria and polydipsia until the source of increased vasopressinase, the placenta, is removed. During the third trimester these women can be safely treated with 1-desamino-8-D-arginine vasopressin (DDAVP), which is resistant to placental vasopressinase and can be stopped immediately post partum. Although there are no long-term follow=up studies of these women, transient gestational diabetes insipidus almost always recurs in the third trimester of subsequent pregnancies [39]. Previously unrecognized subclinical hypothalamic or pituitary pathology is often responsible [40].

Thyroid disease (see Chapter 12)

Thyroid disease is common in young women. Hyperthyroidism affects 0.2% of pregnancies. Symptomatic hypothyroidism is present in 0.1–2% of the population, with the incidence of subclinical hypothyroidism being much higher [41]. Approximately 10% of all young women have antithyroid peroxidase (TPO) antibodies and they are even more prevalent (up to 25%) in euthyroid women who have a family history of thyroid disease [42]. Almost 50% of women with TPO antibodies develop postpartum thyroid dysfunction, which leads to more than 5% of all women developing the condition [41]. Almost half of all women who develop postpartum thyroid dysfunction and who have TPO antibodies will remain hypothyroid indefinitely [43].

Given the strong association between TPO antibodies and future thyroid disease, many advocate checking thyroid function at least once during (or preferably just before) a subsequent pregnancy and 6 weeks to 6 months post partum. Patients should also be screened subsequently for any symptoms consistent with the diagnosis of hypothyroidism.

Liver disease (see Chapter 9)

Healthy pregnancy is a cholestatic condition. As pregnancy progresses the liver metabolizes increasing concentrations of steroid hormones and secretes them into bile [44]. As a consequence, women with previously subclinical cholestatic disorders, including specific bile acid transporter defects [45], gallstones, hepatitis C or cholangitis, are at increased risk of developing symptomatic cholestasis when the concentration of steroid hormone overwhelms their limited ability to excrete metabolites into bile [45]. This usually develops in the third trimester and presents with pruritus and hepatic necrosis, raised alanine aminotransferase (ALT) and aspartate aminotransferase (AST) and raised serum bile acid concentrations. It is assumed that bile acids cause itching in areas where skin blood flow is greatest (i.e. palms and soles). The almost consistent recurrence of intrahepatic cholestasis of pregnancy in subsequent pregnancies further suggests an underlying maternal cholestatic disorder that is overwhelmed towards the end of each pregnancy. If liver function does not return to normal post partum, women with intrahepatic cholestasis of pregnancy should be investigated for subclinical hepatobiliary disease.

The long-term sequelae for women who have had obstetric cholestasis will relate to the underlying cholestatic defect. The most common conditions associated with obstetric cholestasis are hepatitis C and gallstones [46]. All women with cholestasis should likely be screened for hepatitis C and receive a right upper quadrant ultrasound if there are symptoms suggestive of biliary obstruction.

Acute fatty liver of pregnancy and pre-eclampsia/hemolysis, elevated liver enzymes and low platelets (HELLP) syndrome can lead to serious liver disease [47]. The long-term survival of women who have had hepatic failure in association with these conditions is good if they recover from the multisystem complications of the acute liver dysfunction [47].

Peripartum cardiomyopathy

(see Chapter 5)

Peripartum cardiomyopathy (PPCM) is an idiopathic form of heart failure that affects between 1:300 and 1:10,000 pregnancies depending on racial grouping and maternal phenotype [48]. Peripartum cardiomyopathy can be fatal or cause a mild reduction in left ventricular ejection fraction (LVEF) that recovers fully. In general, the amount of residual cardiac function after recovery from PPCM dictates maternal survival and cardiac function in a future pregnancy [49]. In women who make a good recovery (LVEF >50%) the hemodynamic demands of the next pregnancy lead to an average 20% fall in LVEF that usually recovers back to more than 50% post partum [49]. However, 20% of women who recovered well from PPCM and 44% of women who did not recover so well (LVEF <50%) have been shown to have a marked fall in LVEF during a first subsequent pregnancy. It is possible that this is due to recurrence of the idiopathic process that causes PPCM, but would more likely relate to the increased strain of another 9 months of pregnancy-related hemodynamic overload [49].

Women with PPCM who have LVEF below 50% are less likely to have complete recovery of cardiac function and more likely to worsen with a subsequent pregnancy [49] and women who recover from PPCM poorly, to a LVEF <25%, have a 57% risk of future cardiac transplantation [50]. In the absence of longer-term survival studies, it would seem likely that over time, women who recover from PPCM with the lowest LVEF have the worst prognosis. It is therefore critical that all women with PPCM be followed until complete resolution and receive optimal medical therapy for congestive heart failure to try to minimize the long-term risk.

Postpartum depression

(see Chapter 21)

Almost half of all women develop the "maternity blues." Approximately 10% of women develop nonpsychotic postnatal depression 4–6 weeks post partum and these women are at an increased risk of developing depression in later life. Less than 2 per 1000 women develop a severe postpartum psychiatric disorder, which is associated with a 70-fold increased risk of suicide in the first postnatal year [51]. A 23-year follow-up of 64 women who had been admitted to a psychiatric hospital within 6 months of childbirth revealed that 29% had recurrent puerperal psychiatric illness and 75% had further psychiatric illness, not related to pregnancy [52]. Postpartum depression therefore appears to unmask a life-long vulnerability to future psychiatric illness. Patients with a history of postpartum depression should likely be screened yearly for depression and with any presentation of symptoms that may be attributable to depression (e.g. fatigue, poor concentration). One widely used two-item screening tool involves asking the patient the following two questions: 1) During the past month, have you felt down, depressed or hopeless? 2) During the past month, have you felt little interest or pleasure in doing things? A yes answer to either of these questions is considered a positive screen and should trigger further evaluation.

Pregnancy in later life (see Chapter 28)

The menopause arrives at a time of life when the metabolic syndrome that leads to atherosclerosis is more advanced and aging will have diminished an organ's ability to accommodate the physiologic demands of pregnancy. Women in the developed world now often circumvent this timely and natural end to their fertility. There is an increasing tendency among some groups to delay pregnancy until later life, which exposes a woman to a physiologic challenge that would have optimally, from a medical standpoint, taken place up to 30 years earlier. The prevalence of pre-eclampsia, gestational diabetes and other complications is much greater in women over 40 years [53]. Despite this risk, increasing numbers of IVF practitioners are assisting women over 50 years old to become pregnant by oocyte donation. These women must be aware that they are at increased risk of pregnancy complications that may have a negative impact on their long-term health [54].

Conclusion

During pregnancy a transient metabolic syndrome develops, similar to that which predisposes to atherosclerosis. Women who develop pregnancy-induced hypertension, pre-eclampsia or gestational diabetes mellitus are at increased risk of developing cardiovascular disease and/or diabetes in later life. These women should be advised to adjust their lifestyle post partum by adjusting their diet and exercise routine and check their blood pressure and plasma glucose levels periodically so that early therapeutic intervention can minimize long-term morbidity. Other transient gestational syndromes result from the physiologic demands of pregnancy unmasking the limited reserves of a vulnerable organ system. At present, our knowledge of the long-term outcome for women who have had pregnancy-related syndromes is still incomplete. A past obstetric history may, however, prove useful in determining the origin and pathology of diseases in later life and allow intervention that may delay the development of maturity-onset conditions.

References

1. Williams DJ. Physiology of healthy pregnancy. In: Warrell DA, CoxTM, Firth JD (eds) Oxford textbook of medicine, 5th edn. Oxford University Press, Oxford, 2009.
2. Sattar N, Greer IA. Pregnancy complications and maternal cardiovascular risk: opportunities for intervention and screening. BMJ 2002;325:157–60.
3. Seely EW, Solomon CG. Insulin resistance and its potential role in pregnancy-induced hypertension. J Clin Endocrinol Metab 2003;88:2393–8.
4. Bosio PM, McKenna PJ, Conroy R, O'Herlihy C. Maternal central hemodynamics in hypertensive disorders of pregnancy. Obstet Gynecol 1999;94:978–84.

5. Greer IA. Thrombosis in pregnancy: maternal and fetal issues. Lancet 1999;10:1258–65.

6. Redman CW, Sacks GP, Sargent IL. Preeclampsia: an excessive maternal inflammatory response to pregnancy. Am J Obstet Gynecol 1999;180:499–506.

7. Kuhl C. Insulin secretion and insulin resistance in pregnancy and GDM: implications for diagnosis and management. Diabetes 1991;40:18–24.

8. Martin U, Davies C, Hayavi S, et al. Is normal pregnancy atherogenic? Clin Sci (Lond) 1999;96:421–5.

9. Magnussen EB, Vatten LJ, Lund-Nilsen TI, Salvesen KA, Davey Smith G, Romundstad PR. Prepregnancy cardiovascular risk factors as predictors of pre-eclampsia: population based cohort study. BMJ 2007;335:978.

10. Mello G, Parretti E, Marozio L, et al. Thrombophilia is significantly associated with severe preeclampsia: results of a large-scale, case controlled study. Hypertension 2005;46:1270–4.

11. Innes, KE, Wimsatt JH, McDuffie R. Relative glucose tolerance and subsequent development of hypertension in pregnancy. Obstet Gynecol 2001;97:905–10.

12. Bellamy L, Casas JP, Hingorani AD, Williams DJ. Pre-eclampsia and risk of cardiovascular disease and cancer in later life: a systematic review and meta-analysis. BMJ 2007;335:974–7.

13. Irgens HU, Reisaeter L, Irgens LM, Lie RT. Long term mortality of mothers and fathers after pre-eclampsia: population based cohort study. BMJ 2001;323:1213–17.

14. Sibai BM, el-Nazer A, Gonzalez-Ruiz A. Severe preeclampsia-eclampsia in young primigravid women: subsequent pregnancy outcome and remote prognosis. Am J Obstet Gynecol 1986;155:1011–16.

15. Fisher KA, Luger A, Spargo BH, Lindheimer MD. Hypertension in pregnancy: clinical-pathological correlations and remote prognosis. Medicine 1981;60:267–76.

16. National Institute of Health and Clinical Excellence. Statins for the prevention of cardiovascular events. Technology Appraisal 94. National Institute of Health and Clinical Excellence, London, 2006.

17. Smith GCS, Pell JP, Walsh D. Pregnancy complications and maternal risk of ischaemic heart disease: a retrospective cohort study of 129290 births Lancet 2001;357:1213–16.

18. Xiong X, Demianczuk NN, Buekens P, Saunders LD. Association of preeclampsia with high birth weight for gestational age. Am J Obstet Gynecol 2000;183:148–55.

19. Ray JG, Vermeulen MJ, Schull MJ, Redelmeier DA. Cardiovascular health after maternal placental syndromes (CHAMPS): population-based retrospective cohort study. Lancet 2005;366: 1797–803.

20. Catov JM, Newman AB, Sutton-Tyrrell K, et al. Parity and cardiovascular disease risk among older women: how do pregnancy complications mediate the association? Ann Epidemiol 2008;18: 873–9.

21. Chesley LC. Hypertension in pregnancy: definitions, familial factor, and remote prognosis. Kidney Int 1980;18:234–40.

22. Bryans CI Jr. The remote prognosis in toxaemia of pregnancy. Clin Obstet Gynecol 1966;9:973–90.

23. Marin R, Gorostidi M, Portal CG, et al. Long-term prognosis of hypertension in pregnancy. Hypertens Pregnancy 2000;19:199–209.

24. Lawn N, Laich E, Ho S, et al. Eclampsia, hippocampal sclerosis, and temporal lobe epilepsy. Accident or association? Neurology 2004;62:1352–6.

25. Sibai BM, Sarinoglu C, Mercer BM. Eclampsia. VII. Pregnancy outcome after eclampsia and long-term prognosis. Am J Obstet Gynecol 1992;166:1757–61.

26. Williams DJ, Davison JM. Chronic kidney disease in pregnancy. BMJ 2008;336: 211–15.

27. Reiter L, Brown MA, Whitworth JA. Hypertension in pregnancy: the incidence of underlying renal disease and essential hypertension. Am J Kid Dis 1994;24:883–7.

28. Romundstad S, Holmen J, Kvenild K, et al. Microalbuminuria and all-cause mortality in 2089 apparently healthy individuals: a 4.4 year follow-up study. The Nord-Trondelag Health Study (HUNT), Norway. Am J Kidney Dis 2003;42:466–73.

29. Vikse BE, Irgenss LM, Leivestad T, Skjaerven R, Iversen BM. Preeclampsia and the risk of end-stage renal disease. N Engl J Med 2008;359:800–9.

30. Castles A, Adams EK, Melvin CL, et al. Effects of smoking during pregnancy. Five meta-analyses. Am J Prev Med 1999;16:208–15.

31. Bowles L, Cohen H. Inherited thrombophilias and anticoagulation in pregnancy. Best Pract Res Clin Obstet Gynaecol 2003;17:471–89.

32. Walker ID. Prothrombotic genotypes and pre-eclampsia. Thromb Haemost 2002;87:777–8.

33. Kjos SL, Buchanan TA. Gestational diabetes mellitus. N Engl J Med 1999;341:1749–56.

34. Feig DS, Zinman B, Wang X, Hux JE. Risk of development of diabetes mellitus after diagnosis of gestational diabetes. CMAJ 2008;179:229–34.

35. Kim C, Tabaei BP, Bruke R, et al. Missed opportunities for type 2 diabetes mellitus screening with a history of gestational diabetes. Am J Public Health 2006;96:1643–8.

36. Schaefer-Graf UM, Buchanan TA, Xiang AH, et al. Clinical predictors for a high risk for the development of diabetes mellitus in the early puerperium in women with recent gestational diabetes mellitus. Am J Obstet Gynecol 2002;186:751–6.

37. Bentley-Lewis R, Levkoff S, Stuebe A, Seely EW. Gestational diabetes mellitus: postpartum opportunities for the diagnosis and prevention of type 2 diabetes mellitus. Nat Clin Pract Endocrinol Metab 2008;4:552–8.

38. Davison JM, Sheills EA, Barron WM, et al. Changes in the metabolic clearance of vasopressin and in plasma vasopressinase throughout human pregnancy. J Clin Invest 1989;83:1313–18.

39. Williams DJ, Metcalfe KA, Skingle L, et al. Pathophysiology of transient cranial diabetes insipidus during pregnancy. Clin Endocrinol (Oxf) 1993;38:595–600.

40. Monson JP, Williams DJ. Osmoregulatory adaptation in pregnancy and its disorders. J Endocrinol 1992;132:7–9.

41. Lazarus JH. Epidemiology and prevention of thyroid disease in pregnancy. Thyroid 2002;12:861–5.

42. Strieder TG, Prummel MF, Tijssen JG, et al. Risk factors for and prevalence of thyroid disorders in a cross-sectional study among healthy female relatives of patients with autoimmune thyroid disease. Clin Endocrinol (Oxf) 2003;59:396–401.

43. Premawardhana LD, Parkes AB, Ammari F, et al. Postpartum thyroiditis and long-term thyroid status: prognostic influence of thyroid peroxidase antibodies and ultrasound echogenicity. J Clin Endocrinol Metab 2000;85:71–5.

44. Elias E. URSO in obstetric cholestasis: not a bear market. Gut 1999;45:331–2.

45. Savander M, Ropponen A, Avela K, et al. Genetic evidence of heterogeneity in intrahepatic cholestasis of pregnancy. Gut 2003;52:1025–9.

46. Roppenen A, Sund R, Riikonen S, Ylikorkala O, Aittomaki K. Intrahepatic cholestasis of pregnancy as an indicator of liver and biliary diseases: a population based study. Hepatology 2006;43:723–8.

47. Rahman TM, Wendon J. Severe hepatic dysfunction in pregnancy. Q J Med 2002;95:343–57.

48. Sliwa K, Fett J, Elkayam U. Peripartum cardiomyopathy. Lancet 2006;368: 687–93.
49. Elkyam U, Tummala PP, Rao K, *et al.* Maternal and fetal outcomes of subsequent pregnancies in women with peripartum cardiomyopathy. N Engl J Med 2001;344:1567–71.
50. Habli M, O'Brien T, Nowack E, Khoury S, Barton JR, Sibai B. Peripartum cardiomyopathy: prognostic factors for long-term maternal outcome. Am J Obstet Gynecol 2008;199(4): 415 e1–5.
51. Appleby L, Mortensen PB, Faragher EB. Suicide and other causes of mortality after post-partum psychiatric admission. Br J Psychiatry 1998;173:209–11.
52. Robling SA, Paykel ES, Dunn VJ, *et al.* Long-term outcome of severe puerperal psychiatric illness: a 23 year follow-up study. Psychol Med 2000;30:1263–71.
53. Seoud MA, Nassar AH, Usta IM, *et al.* Impact of advanced maternal age on pregnancy outcome. Am J Perinatol 2002;19:1–8.
54. Paulson RJ, Boostanfar R, Saadat P, *et al.* Pregnancy in the sixth decade of life: obstetric outcomes in women of advanced reproductive age. JAMA 2002;288:2320–3.

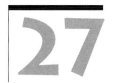

27 Special concerns for the obese patient

Hugh M. Ehrenberg[1] with Richard N. Wissler[2]

[1]Division of Maternal Fetal Medicine, Ohio State University Medical Center, Columbus, OH, USA

[2]Department of Anesthesiology, Obstetrics and Gynecology, University of Rochester, School of Medicine and Dentistry, Rochester, NY, USA

Introduction

Obesity continues to rise in prevalence around the globe and in the United States, now affects as many as 1 in 3 pregnancies delivered [1]. While the roots of the epidemic remain elusive, the consequences are becoming clearer. The medical implications of obesity outside pregnancy are well known, including hypertension and cardiovascular disease, joint disease, thromboembolism, dislipidemia and diabetes [2,3]. The ramifications of gravid obesity such as diabetes, hypertension and pre-eclampsia, fetal overgrowth and neonatal obesity, prolonged labor, cesarean delivery and surgical complications, are similarly far-reaching, with important implications for maternal health and fetal well-being [4,5]. The impact on the routine practice of prenatal care is significant, spanning from before conception through the postpartum period, leaving few obese patients unscathed. In the end, the challenges to the physician charged with caring for the obese gravida may be twofold. First, care must take into account the various increases in health risk to mother and child. Modifications in prenatal care and delivery may be dictated by maternal size at conception or excessive pregnancy weight gain. Second, pregnancy may also represent an opportunity for intervention, and an effort to break the cycle of obesity.

The obesity epidemic

The World Health Organization (WHO and National Institutes of Health (NIH) define "normal weight" by the Body Mass Index (BMI, calculated as weight in kg divided by the height in meters squared). Normal BMI is 18.5–24.9, overweight is BMI 25–29.9 and obesity is BMI ≥30 (Table 27.1). Obesity can be further characterized by BMI as class I (30–34.9), class II (35–39.9) and class III (≥40) [6].

Table 27.1 WHO body habitus categories

BMI	Category
<18.5	Underweight
18.5–24.9	Normal
25.0–29.9	Overweight
≥30.0	Obese

Table 27.2 Increase in adult obesity 1994–2000

	2000	1994–98
Obese	30.4%	22.9%
Overweight	64.5%	55.9%

The global epidemic of obesity continues to grow at an alarming rate, crossing boundaries of age, race and gender (Table 27.2). Indeed, it is now so common that it is replacing the more traditional public healthcare concerns including undernutrition and infectious disease as one of the most significant contributors to ill health [6].

The prevalence of adult obesity in the United States, defined as a BMI >30, rose to an alarming 30.5% in 2000, compared with 22.9% from 1994 to 1998. The proportion of the population meeting the definition of overweight (BMI >25) increased from 55.9% to 64.5% during the same period. Of particular concern is the rise of obesity among teens, with the prevalence of obesity in adolescents in the USA increasing by 11.3% between 1994 and 2000 [7]. The risk of increasing obesity is disproportionate among the races in the US and other countries, with the prevalence of obesity in the US increasing most among African American women [4].

Risks associated with obesity in pregnancy

Obesity appears to be associated with a wide range of increased risks to the mother and the pregnancy and a detailed

de Swiet's Medical Disorders in Obstetric Practice, 5th edition. Edited by R. O. Powrie, M. F. Greene, W. Camann. © 2010 Blackwell Publishing.

discussion of the literature on these risk associations is beyond the scope of this chapter. They are listed in Box 27.1 and discussed in detail in the associated references. What follows is a discussion of some of the more important known associations.

Obesity and the risk of cesarean delivery

Retrospective data describe the rate of cesarean delivery among overweight and obese women to be as high as 50% [4,9,10], applying to both the primary cesarean delivery [9] (Table 27.3) and the failure to successfully deliver vaginally after a previous cesarean [10] (Table 27.4). The etiology of this finding is likely to be multifactorial, including the influence of fetal macrosomia, maternal size, and other factors not yet described. There is no satisfactory single explanation as to the mechanism behind the failure to deliver vaginally in the obese. Chauhan *et al.* reported that 46% of obese women failing a trial of labor after cesarean to have an arrest disorder [11]. In a cohort studied by Edwards *et al.*, 39% of obese women were delivered by cesarean after labor dystocia, 29% due to nonreassuring fetal heart rate tracings, 10% due to malpresentation, and 8% secondary to failed induction [12].

In searching for the root cause of such findings, basic obstetrics relies on describing the *power* of contractions, the size and composition of the fetus (*passenger*), and the *pelvis*. The amount of power generated by the uterus in the obese and nonobese laboring woman is equivalent [13] and the degree of neonatal macrosomia alone cannot completely explain the elevated risk of cesareans in the obese [9]. The contribution of maternal pelvic fat to the failure of a trial of labor in the obese parturient has not yet been evaluated. Such a "soft tissue dystocia" may explain not only the increased rate of cesarean delivery, but also the prolongation of various stages of labor that has been described (Table 27.5) [14].

Box 27.1 Conditions seen with increased frequency in obese pregnant patients [57,58]

Preconception

- Subfertility

Antepartum

- Miscarriage
- Gestational diabetes
- Pre-eclampsia
- Congenital anomalies including orofacial, cardiac and neural tube defects
- Difficulty in obtaining detailed images with ultrasound
- Obstructive sleep apnea
- Fetal macrosomia

Intrapartum

- Prolonged labor
- Shoulder dystocia
- Difficulty with endotracheal intubation for general anesthesia
- Difficulty with placement of spinal or epidural catheter for regional anesthesia
- Special equipment needs (labor and OR beds, stretchers, wheelchairs)
- Cesarean delivery
- Post-term pregnancy

Postpartum

- Postpartum hemorrhage
- Wound infections and breakdown
- Endometritis
- Venous thromboembolism
- Increased weight in offspring
- Increased risk of childhood obesity
- Possible difficulty with breastfeeding

Table 27.3 Odds of cesarean with increasing maternal BMI

BMI (kg/m^2)	Odds ratio
<19.8	0.71 (0.4–1.24)
25.2–30	1.64 (1.09–2.47)
>30	2.5 (1.68–3.71)

Reproduced from Flegal *et al.* [8].

Table 27.4 Vaginal birth after cesarean (VBAC) success rates as affected by maternal body habitus

BMI (kg/m^2)	% VBAC	P value
<19.8	84.7%	0.04
19.8–25	70.5%	–
25–30	65.5%	0.35
>30	54.6%	0.003

Reproduced from Ehrenberg *et al.* [9].

Table 27.5 Perturbations of labor in nulliparous women as influenced by maternal weight at delivery

Weight (kg)	Rate of cervical dilation (cm/h)	Labor duration (h)	Cesarean rate (%)
	P = 0.01	P < 0.001	P < 0.001
<72	1.0	12	15
72–84.9	0.94	13	20
85–102.9	0.83	14	30
103–193	0.63	17	37

Reproduced from Buhimschi *et al.* [13].

Once the need for abdominal delivery has been declared, the risk of complications continues. Postoperative complications include wound infections and breakdown, endomyometritis, venous thromboembolism, febrile hospital stay and delayed return to productivity [15–18].

Skin incision choice

When a cesarean delivery is performed, the choice of skin incision may be important in reducing operative complications, though there is a paucity of data in this respect. In the past, without conclusive evidence supporting the use of either a Pfannenstiel or vertical skin incision, the selection of incision direction for cesarean delivery in the obese parturient has largely been one of operator choice. Each incision holds distinct theoretical benefits and risks to the patient, though these have not yet been adequately studied. Vertical skin incisions may offer improved exposure and ease of delivery with shorter operative times. They may be made through less fatty tissue and away from folds of skin, such that in the event of wound breakdown, better wound care would be feasible. For these reasons, predominant practice has been to perform a vertical skin incision on women perceived as extremely obese, and particularly those who may be more centrally obese. However, the vertical closure may be less secure, since it is acted upon by lateral forces and is more likely to be extended. Vertical incisions also may be at higher risk for breakdown and infection.

In a recent analysis, Wall *et al.* found the risk of postoperative complications requiring the reopening of the wound to be 12-fold higher in vertical skin incisions compared to the transverse Pfannenstiel. Unfortunately, the patients in the vertical incision group were also found to be significantly heavier than their Pfannenstiel counterparts [19]. Houston & Raynor, however, found no difference in postoperative morbidity based on incision type used in women >150% of ideal bodyweight undergoing cesarean delivery at term [15]. However, in this study again the vertically approached women were significantly heavier than those undergoing the more traditional transverse skin incisions (329 vs 246 lbs). These two studies represent the recent literature on the surgical approach to obese women undergoing cesarean delivery. Due to their retrospective design, it is possible that practice patterns had an influence on subject selection in each study. In the end, the factor most responsible for surgical morbidity with regard to incisional complications may be tissue depth at the site [17]. Interrupted closure of subcutaneous fat should therefore be considered as this appears to decrease the risk of wound rupture for incisions involving more than 2 cm of subcutaneous fat. They may work more by decreasing dead space than by increasing tensile strength but their use seems advisable in any case. Drains, however, do not appear to make a difference to the rate of wound infection or disruption.

In conclusion, these authors believe that for patients who appear to be less centrally obese, or whenever otherwise feasible, a Pfannenstiel incision remains preferable. These incisions are thought to be more secure, allowing for greater postoperative mobility, but are more difficult to manage intraoperatively for proper exposure. Transverse incisions, however, are commonly through more significant amounts of fatty tissue and may remain exposed to moist skinfolds postoperatively, predisposing to infection and wound breakdown.

Additional implications for management

Modifications in the management of a pregnancy affected by obesity should be considered in an effort to minimize both maternal and fetal risks. In the course of routine office-based prenatal care, fundal height measurements, used in the monitoring of fetal growth, are more difficult to obtain, and fetal heart tones can be difficult to auscultate early in pregnancy. Increased surveillance may be required to accomplish these otherwise routine tasks, including early ultrasound for pregnancy dating and more frequent scans during pregnancy for purposes of monitoring fetal growth.

Obesity may impart an independent small increase in the risk of fetal anomaly, particularly orofacial, cardiac and neural tube defects [20–26]. Preconception and antenatal folate supplementation is advised for obese patients but it is not clear if it is effective in decreasing this risk for these patients [27–29]. Co-morbid conditions such as diabetes also contribute to the increased risk of anomalies in the offspring of obese women. At the same time, maternal adipose tissue impedes the ability to satisfactorily image fetal anatomy, and may contribute to decreased sensitivity of ultrasound in anomaly screening[30–32]. Patients should be counseled as to the decreased sensitivity of ultrasound. It is possible that the decrease in sensitivity is responsible for a higher proportion of liveborn infants with anomalies. Increased frequency of screening and later scanning in the obese have each been attempted to increase the sensitivity, with mixed results [31,33,34].

Additional risks affecting pregnancy in the obese gravida include fetal overgrowth [35] and post-term pregnancy [36]. Late pregnancy ultrasounds will be helpful in predicting a macrosomic delivery, but error in overestimating fetal weight is common [37]. Prudence dictates careful consideration prior to induction of labor, attentive management of labor including invasive monitoring, which may be needed more often in this population due to difficulty in monitoring contractions. Physicians should be aware of the possible prolongation of the various stages of labor, particularly in the active and second stages, when evaluating laboring patients for the diagnosis of an arrest disorder. For those pregnancies delivering vaginally, shoulder dystocia is an unpredictable attendant risk. To avoid this complication, the ACOG has recommended cesarean delivery be offered to pregnancies affected by marcosomia >5000 g in the nondiabetic and >4200 g in the diabetic pregnancy [38] .

Obesity is a risk factor for venous thromboembolism. Early ambulation after delivery may reduce the risk of thrombosis, whether delivered vaginally or via cesarean. Although we lack evidence to guide recommendations in this area, consideration should be given to providing thromboprophylaxis to obese patients during their postpartum stay or even beyond it to day 5 postpartum (see Chapter 3). This can be provided in the form of either prophylactic-dose low molecular weight heparin, such as enoxaparin 40 mg once a day, or sequential compression devices. If sequential compression devices are to be effective, they should be continually on the patient throughout hospitalization and only removed for those periods when the patient is up walking.

Anesthesia

Obesity is a challenge to safe anesthesia care in the parturient and represents a significant risk factor for adverse anesthetic outcomes, including death [39]. The physiologic adaptations of pregnancy, combined with the pathophysiology of obesity, contribute to this phenomenon, especially in terms of pulmonary and cardiovascular function. For example, pregnant women have a more rapid decline in arterial oxygen saturation during apnea compared to nonpregnant women, and this is accentuated in obesity. The overall topic of anesthetic management in obese parturients has been reviewed by other authors [40–42].

In addition to the physiologic challenges of obesity, the obese body habitus provides technical challenges for either neuraxial or general anesthesia. The classic study of morbidly obese parturients by Hood & Dewan [43] documents greater difficulty with placement and maintenance of epidural analgesia/anesthesia, as well as increased difficulty with intubation during the induction of general anesthesia, compared to nonobese controls. The specific problems with obesity and neuraxial anesthesia include indistinct surface anatomy landmarks, a greater distance between lumbar skin and neuraxial target that accentuates the impact of small angle deflections of the block needle, and torsion on the epidural catheter from independent motion of the soft tissues of the trunk in relation to the bony vertebral column [44]. Ultrasound guidance for neuraxial block placement may be particularly useful in obese parturients to establish anatomic landmarks [45]. Technical challenges during lumbar epidural placement in obese patients increase the risk of unintended dural puncture, but the clinical impact is balanced by a lower incidence of headache after dural puncture in this population [46].

Prospective, randomized clinical data do not exist concerning the relative safety of neuraxial and general anesthesia for cesarean delivery. However, retrospective outcome data [47] and expert opinion [48] strongly support the use of neuraxial anesthesia for cesarean delivery, in the absence of contraindications. "Neuraxial techniques are preferred to general anesthesia for most (cesarean) deliveries … Early insertion of a spinal or epidural catheter (during labor) for obstetric … or anesthestic indications (e.g. anticipated difficult airway or obesity) should be considered to reduce the need for general anesthesia if an emergent procedure becomes necessary" [48]. Intubation is more difficult in nonobese patients during pregnancy [49] and also in obese versus normal weight nonpregnant patients [50]. The negative combination of obesity and pregnancy may be synergistic in terms of airway safety. The reasons include physical impairment of visualization during direct laryngoscopy, and difficult positive pressure mask ventilation if the initial intubation attempt fails. (The latter is the recommended step for maintenance of oxygenation during a difficult intubation in any patient [51].) Airway management challenges should be anticipated in all patients, but particularly in obese parturients. Minimizing the use of general anesthesia in these patients whenever possible is a prudent choice. It is unfortunate that obese parturients have a higher incidence of unplanned cesarean deliveries during labor [52], as well as emergency cesareans [53].

Equipment considerations for the safe peripartum care of obese parturients include operating room (OR) tables with appropriate weight load ratings (usually available on the manufacturer's website), OR table side extensions to stabilize wide patients, and longer neuraxial block needles. Obese patients can benefit from safe and comfortable waiting room chairs that lack restrictive side-arms.

Weight loss interventions

Attention has recently turned toward attempts at risk reduction for the obese pregnancy.

All healthcare providers should support public health initiatives to decrease the incidence of obesity in our society [5]. Primary care doctors and obstetricians should include discussion about pregnancy-related complications of obesity in their counseling of overweight women in the reproductive years.

A current area of interest is the modification of obesity-related risk in pregnancy by the limitation of gestational weight gain. Current Institute of Medicine recommendations for weight gain are only minimally restricted for those who conceive while obese (Table 27.6) [50]. Furthermore, recent evidence suggests that adherence to such guidelines is poor,

Table 27.6 Institute of Medicine gestational weight gain recommendations by pregravid BMI

BMI (kg/m^2)	Recommended weight gain (kg)
<18.5	28–40
18.5–24.9	25–35
25–29.9	15–25
≥30	11–20

with only 23% of obese women actually gaining the recommended amount of weight, and a full 46% gaining more than the recommended amount of weight during pregnancy [51]. In fact, patients adhering to these recommendations may remain at increased risk for obesity-related complications when compared to women who are more limited in their gestational weight gain [51]. While caloric restriction to the point of ketosis cannot yet be recommended due to a possible link to neural tube defects [52], limitation of carbohydrate intake, and aerobic exercise in an effort to limit weight gained in pregnancy may represent a point of intervention on behalf of affected pregnancies. Behavioral and diet changes instilled using pregnancy as a motivator may be carried forward into postpartum life, with positive influence on subsequent pregnancies and their outcomes.

An alternative strategy is to intervene in the first postpartum day(s) with several components including a practical weight loss program and a multidisciplinary meeting with the patient to emphasize weight loss as a long-term safety strategy [53]. Early referral for bariatric surgery may offer an exciting adjunct in the treatment of extreme obesity and when used with caution, may represent a means of reducing risk of adverse outcomes in subsequent pregnancies [54–56].

Conclusion

Obesity threatens to become one of the most far-reaching clinical challenges facing medicine in the new millennium. Gravid obesity represents part of this alarming trend, but also provides a unique opportunity to affect change in the course of two lives, and generations to come. Ongoing research is needed to assess the impact of intervention before pregnancy, during prenatal care, at delivery, into postpartum life, and between subsequent gestations.

References

1. Ogden C, Carroll M, Curtin L, Mcdowell M, Tabak C, Flegal K. Prevalence Of overweight and obesity in the United States, 1999–2004. JAMA 2006;295:1549–55.
2. Must A, Spadano J, Coakley E, Field A, Colditz G, Dietz W. The disease burden associated with overweight and obesity. JAMA 1999;282:1523–9.
3. Executive summary of the clinical guidelines on the identification, evaluation, and treatment of overweight and obesity in adults. Arch Intern Med 1998;158:1855–67.
4. Ehrenberg H, Dierker L, Milluzzi C, Mercer B. Prevalence of maternal obesity in an urban center. Am J Obstet Gynecol 2002;187:1189–93.
5. Reece E. Perspectives on obesity, pregnancy and birth outcomes in the United States: the scope of the problem. Am J Obstet Gynecol 2008;198:23–7.
6. Obesity: preventing and managing the global epidemic. Report of a WHO consultation. World Health Organ Tech Rep Ser 2000;894:I-Xii, 1–253.
7. Hedley A, Ogden C, Johnson C, Carroll M, Curtin L, Flegal K. Prevalence of overweight and obesity among US children, adolescents, and adults, 1999–2002. JAMA 2004;291:2847–50.
8. Flegal K, Ogden C, Carroll M. Prevalence and trends in overweight in Mexican-American adults and children. Nutr Rev 2004;62:S144–8.
9. Ehrenberg H, Durnwald C, Catalano P, Mercer B. The influence of obesity and diabetes on the risk of cesarean delivery. Am J Obstet Gynecol 2004;191:969–74.
10. Durnwald C, Ehrenberg H, Mercer B. The impact of maternal obesity and weight gain on vaginal birth after cesarean section success. Am J Obstet Gynecol 2004;191:954–7.
11. Chauhan S, Magann E, Carroll C, Barrilleaux P, Scardo J, Martin J Jr. Mode of delivery for the morbidly obese with prior cesarean delivery: vaginal versus repeat cesarean section. Am J Obstet Gynecol 2001;185:349–54.
12. Edwards R, Harnsberger D, Johnson I, Treloar R, Cruz A. Deciding on route of delivery for obese women with a prior cesarean delivery. Am J Obstet Gynecol 2003;189:385–9; discussion 389–90.
13. Buhimschi C, Buhimschi I, Malinow A, Weiner C. Intrauterine pressure during the second stage of labor in obese women. Obstet Gynecol 2004;103:225–30.
14. Nuthalapaty F, Rouse D, Owen J. The association of maternal weight with cesarean risk, labor duration, and cervical dilation rate during labor induction. Obstet Gynecol 2004;103:452–6.
15. Houston M, Raynor B. Postoperative morbidity in the morbidly obese parturient woman: supraumbilical and low transverse abdominal approaches. Am J Obstet Gynecol 2000;182:1033–5.
16. Vermillion S, Lamoutte C, Soper D, Verdeja A. Wound infection after cesarean: effect of subcutaneous tissue thickness. Obstet Gynecol 2000;95:923–6.
17. Grantcharov T, Rosenberg J. Vertical compared with transverse incisions in abdominal surgery. Eur J Surg 2001;167:260–7.
18. Myles T, Gooch J, Santolaya J. Obesity as an independent risk factor for infectious morbidity in patients who undergo cesarean delivery. Obstet Gynecol 2002;100:959–64.
19. Wall P, Deucy E, Glantz J, Pressman E. Vertical skin incisions and wound complications in the obese parturient. Obstet Gynecol 2003;102:952–6.
20. Ray J, Wyatt P, Vermeulen M, Meier C, Cole D. Greater maternal weight and the ongoing risk of neural tube defects after folic acid flour fortification. Obstet Gynecol 2005;105:261–5.
21. Shaw G, Velie E, Schaffer D. Risk of neural tube defect-affected pregnancies among obese women. JAMA 1996;275:1093–6.
22. Cedergren M, Kallen B. Maternal obesity and the risk for orofacial clefts in the offspring. Cleft Palate Craniofac J 2005;42:367–71.
23. Cedergren M, Kallen B. Maternal obesity and infant heart defects. Obes Res 2003;11:1065–71.
24. Mikhail L, Walker C, Mittendorf R. Association between maternal obesity and fetal cardiac malformations in African Americans. J Natl Med Assoc 2002;94:695–700.
25. Watkins M, Rasmussen S, Honein M, Botto L, Moore C. Maternal obesity and risk for birth defects. Pediatrics 2003;111:1152–8.
26. Haak M, Twisk J, van Vugt J. How successful is fetal echocardiographic examination in the first trimester of pregnancy? Ultrasound Obstet Gynecol 2002;20:9–13.
27. Hendler I, Blackwell S, Bujold E, et al. Suboptimal second-trimester ultrasonographic visualization of the fetal heart in obese women: should we repeat the examination? J Ultrasound Med 2005;24:1205–9; quiz 1210–1.

28. Hendler I, Blackwell S, Bujold E, et al. The impact of maternal obesity on midtrimester sonographic visualization of fetal cardiac and craniospinal structures. Int J Obes Relat Metab Disord 2004;28:1607–11.

29. Catanzarite V, Quirk J. Second-trimester ultrasonography: determinants of visualization of fetal anatomic structures. Am J Obstet Gynecol 1990;163:1191–5.

30. Lantz M, Chisholm C. The preferred timing of second-trimester obstetric sonography based on maternal Body Mass Index. J Ultrasound Med 2004;23:1019–22.

31. Ehrenberg H, Mercer B, Catalano P. The influence of obesity and diabetes on the prevalence of macrosomia. Am J Obstet Gynecol 2004;191:964–8.

32. Michlin R, Oettinger M, Odeh M, et al. Maternal obesity and pregnancy outcome. IMAJ 2000;2:10–13.

33. Field N, Langer O. The effects of maternal obesity on the accuracy of fetal weight estimation. Obstet Gynecol 1995;86:102–7.

34. ACOG Practice Bulletin. Clinical management guidelines for obstetrician-gynecologists. Obstet Gynecol 2002;100:1045–50.

35. Cooper G, McClure J. Anaesthesia chapter from Saving Mothers' Lives; Reviewing Maternal Deaths To Make Pregnancy Safer. Br J Anaesth 2008;100:17–22.

36. Saravanakumar K, Rao S, Cooper G. Obesity and obstetric anaesthesia. Anaesthesia 2006;61:36–48.

37. Mhyre J. Anesthetic management for the morbidly obese pregnant woman. Int Anesthesiol Clin 2007; 45:51–70.

38. Soens M, Birnbach D, Ranasinghe J, van Zundert A. Obstetric anesthesia for the obese and morbidly obese patient: an ounce of prevention is worth more than a pound of treatment. Acta Anaesthesiol Scand 2008;52:6–19.

39. Hood D, Dewan D. Anesthetic and obstetric outcome in morbidly obese parturients. Anesthesiology 1993; 79:1210–18.

40. Hamilton C, Riley E, Cohen S. Changes in the position of epidural catheters associated with patient movement. Anesthesiology 1997; 86:778–84.

41. Grau T, Leipold R, Conradi R, Martin E, Motsch J. Efficacy of ultrasound imaging in obstetric epidural anesthesia. J Clin Anesth 2002; 14:169–75.

42. Faure E, Moreno R, Thisted R. Incidence of postdural puncture headache in morbidly obese parturients. Reg Anesth 1994; 19:361–3.

43. Hawkins J, Koonin L, Palmer S, Gibbs C. Anesthesia-related deaths during obstetric delivery in the United States, 1979–1990. Anesthesiology 1997; 86:277 84.

44. American Society of Anesthesiologists. Practice guidelines for obstetric anesthesia. 2006. www.asahq.org.

45. Munnar U, de Boisblanc B, Suresh M. Airway problems in pregnancy. Crit Care Med 2005; 33(suppl):S259–68.

46. Juvin P, Lavaut E, Dupont H, Lefevre P, Demetriou M, Dumoulin J-L, Desmonts J-M. Difficult tracheal intubation is more common in obese than in lean patients. Anesth Analg 2003;97:595–600.

47. American Society of Anesthesiologists. Practice guidelines for management of the difficult airway. Anesthesiology 2003; 98:1269–77.

48. Sheerard A, Platt R, Vallerand D, Usher R, Zhang X, Kramer M. Maternal anthropometric risk factors for caesarean delivery before or after onset of labour. Br J Obstet Gynaecol 2007; 114:1088–96.

49. Bhattacharya S, Campbell D, Liston W, Bhattacharya S. Effect of Body Mass Index on pregnancy outcomes in nulliparous women delivering singleton babies. BMC Public Health 2007; 7:168.

50. Institute of Medicine (US). Weightgain during pregnancy. Re-examining the evidence. National Academies Press, Washington, DC, 1990.

51. Kiel D, Dodson E, Artal R, Boehmer T, Leet T. Gestational weight gain and pregnancy outcomes in obese women: how much is enough? Obstet Gynecol 2007;110:752–8.

52. Shaw G, Todoroff K, Carmichael S, Schaffer D, Selvin S. Lowered weight gain during pregnancy and risk of neural tube defects among offspring. Int J Epidemiol 2001;30:60–5.

53. Wissler R. Obesity in the parturient: an increasing burden. Int J Obstet Anesth 2008; 17:1–2.

54. Guelinckx I, Devleiger R, Vansant G. Reproductive outcome after bariatric surgery: a critical review. Hum Reprod Update 2009;15:189–201.

55. Wax JR, Cartin A, Wolff R, Lepich S, Pinette MG, Blackstone J. Pregnancy following gastric bypass for morbid obesity: effect of surgery-to-conception interval on maternal and neonatal outcomes. Obes Surg 2008;18:1517–21.

56. Patel JA, Patel NA, Thomas RL, Nelms JK, Colella JJ. Pregnancy outcomes after laparoscopic Roux-en-Y gastric bypass. Surg Obes Relat Dis 2008;4:39–45.

57. Sathy HK, Fleming A, Frey D, Barsoom M, Stapathy C, Khandalavala J. Maternal obesity and pregnancy. Postgrad Med 2008;120(3):E01–9.

58. Dixit A, Girling JC. Obesity and pregnancy. J Obstet Gynaecol 2008;29(10):14–23.

28 Special concerns for patients with advanced maternal age

Linda Heffner

Department of Obstetrics and Gynecology, Boston University School of Medicine, Boston, MA, USA

Introduction

Since Waters and Wagner introduced the term "elderly primigravida" in 1950 to describe pregnant women who have their first child after age 35 years [1], hundreds of articles have been written about the outcomes of pregnancies in older women. The field has been complicated by the introduction of the assisted reproductive technologies, notably egg donation, which have extended the childbearing years beyond their natural biologic limits at the same time that women lead healthier lifestyles that include regular exercise, balanced diets and no cigarettes. While the focus of this chapter will be on the care of healthy women without underlying medical problems who attempt pregnancies in the fourth and fifth decades of their lives, it is important to remember that advancing age carries with it increased risk of underlying medical disorders. The reader who cares for an older woman with a condition such as hypertension or diabetes is referred to that topic with the understanding that maternal age will be additive to the baseline risk in these pregnancies.

Preconception evaluation of older women considering pregnancy

In an ideal world, all women contemplating pregnancy would undergo preconception counseling. In the real world, the majority of pregnancies are unplanned; however, women who seek infertility services offer the medical practitioner the opportunity to assess and counsel about risk prior to conception. Currently, over half of the livebirths that occur with the use of assisted reproductive technologies in the United States are to mothers over the age of 35 years. Because all these women by necessity interact with the medical system, they have created the opportunity for a standardized approach to assessment and counseling.

de Swiet's Medical Disorders in Obstetric Practice, 5th edition.
Edited by R. O. Powrie, M. F. Greene, W. Camann. © 2010 Blackwell Publishing.

Because the likelihood of undiagnosed type 2 diabetes, hypertension, coronary artery disease, thyroid disease, cancer, and depression increases with age, it is important to take a directed personal and family medical history. Although we lack studies showing that these interventions will impact eventual outcome, it seems reasonable based on the recommendations for primary care that women over age 35 years who are obese or have strong family histories for diabetes, thyroid disease or coronary artery disease and all women age 45 and older should have a fasting blood sugar, thyroid-stimulating hormone (TSH) level and exertional exercise history. Women over the age of 50 should have a baseline mammogram and electrocardiogram (EKG) added to the above. Cigarette smoking, which has a strong age-dependent deleterious effect on pregnancy outcome, should be ascertained and aggressively addressed as should alcohol and prescription drug use.

Early pregnancy

While the strong relationship between maternal age and fecundity is well known, the equally strong association between maternal age and miscarriage is often overlooked (Figure 28.1). Women over the age of 40 years have, at best, a 50% chance of bearing a liveborn child after a spontaneous conception. It is wise to counsel caution for these women until the end of the first trimester when most miscarriages have occurred. Women who conceive using donor eggs have miscarriage rates that approximate the age of the donor and should be counseled accordingly.

Chromosomal abnormalities in the conceptuses of older women are probably the most widely recognized risk of delayed childbearing. The incidences of trisomies 13, 18 and 21 (Down's syndrome) and the sex chromosome abnormalities, except for XO (Turner's syndrome), all increase as maternal age increases. As with miscarriage, women whose pregnancy is conceived through egg donation carry the aneuploidy risk of the donor. Table 28.1 contains standard data used for counseling about the maternal age-associated risk of aneuploidy.

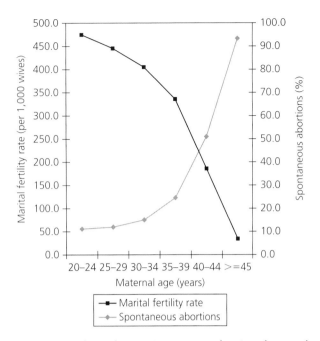

Figure 28.1 Fertility and miscarriage rates as a function of maternal age. Reproduced with permission from Heffner [2].

Table 28.1 Age-specific risks for chromosomal abnormalities in liveborn infants

Maternal age at delivery	Risk of Down's syndrome	Risk of any chromosomal abnormalities
20	1/1667	1/526
22	1/1429	1/500
24	1/1250	1/476
26	1/1176	1/476
27	1/1111	1/455
28	1/1053	1/435
29	1/1000	1/417
30	1/952	1/385
31	1/909	1/385
32	1/769	1/322
33	1/602	1/286
34	1/485	1/238
35	1/378	1/192
36	1/289	1/156
37	1/224	1/127
38	1/173	1/102
39	1/136	1/83
40	1/106	1/66
41	1/82	1/53
42	1/63	1/42
43	1/49	1/33
44	1/38	1/26
45	1/30	1/21
46	1/23	1/16
47	1/18	1/13
48	1/14	1/10
49	1/11	1/8

Data modified from the maternal age-specific rates derived by Hook *et al.* [3].

Historically, maternal age 35 years or older at the time of delivery has been an indication for genetic counseling and amniocentesis or chorionic villus sampling (CVS) for diagnosis of chromosomal abnormalities. Beginning with the introduction of universal second-trimester serum screening for aneuploidy in 1984, the practice of using age cutoffs to determine which women should be offered screening or diagnostic testing has been challenged. Practice has evolved toward a policy of offering universal noninvasive screening with counseling about the detection and false-positive rates, advantages, disadvantages and limitations of the tests along with the risks and benefits of both the noninvasive screening and invasive diagnostic procedures.

Three basic approaches to screening are currently available: first trimester, second trimester and a combination of first and second trimester. First-trimester options include an ultrasound measurement of the fluid collection at the back of the fetal neck, or "nuchal translucency," and assessment of the presence or absence of the nasal bone with or without a serum screen. Second-trimester serum screens include the triple panel of maternal serum markers and the quadruple screen, which adds inhibin A to the triple panel. Second-trimester ultrasound can detect ~50% of chromosomally abnormal fetuses; some experts advocate further adjusting the individual risk obtained from a serum screen by the ultrasound findings. The detection rates for each of the available tests are shown in Table 28.2. Which approach is offered to a given patient will depend on the gestational age at initiation

Table 28.2 Seven screening strategies and their associated Down's syndrome detection rates at a 5% false-positive rate

Screening strategy	Analytes	Down's syndrome detection rate (%)
Triple screen	MSAFP, HCG, estriol	69
Quadruple screen	MSAFP, HCG, estriol, inhibin-A	81
First-trimester screen	NT, PAPP-A, free beta-HCG	85
Integrated screen	NT, PAPP-A + quadruple screen (all results withheld until the second trimester)	95
Serum integrated screen	PAPP-A + quadruple screen	86
Stepwise sequential screen	First-trimester screen + quadruple screen with results given after each test	95
Contingent sequential screen	First-trimester screen with quadruple screen only for those with a "moderate" risk on first-trimester testing	93

MSAFP, maternal serum alpha-fetoprotein; NT, nuchal translucency; PAPP-A, pregnancy-associated plasma protein A.
Reproduced with permission from Reddy [4].

of prenatal care and the reliability or availability of specific tests such as nuchal lucency measurements and CVS.

Karyotyping of fetal material obtained by either CVS or amniocentesis is the only way a definitive diagnosis of aneuploidy can be made or excluded in the first or second trimester. Recent data indicate that the procedure-related loss rate for amniocentesis may be as low as 0.06%. In experienced hands, the procedure-related loss rate for CVS approaches 1%.

Advanced maternal age also appears to confer an additional 1% risk of congenital malformations not associated with aneuploidy. The odds ratio for cardiac defects was four times higher in the infants of women over age 40 when compared to women aged 20–24 years. Clubfoot and diaphragmatic hernias were also increased among the older mothers in the study population. Providers may want to consider fetal echocardiography in addition to an ultrasound fetal anatomic survey in their patients over age 40.

Late pregnancy

The incidence of gestational diabetes mellitus increases from a baseline of 2% to about 6% in the fifth decade, and in some populations as many as 8% of women over age 40 may enter pregnancy with undiagnosed type 2 diabetes. All women over the age of 35 years should be tested for gestational diabetes. Obese women, those with a strong family history of type 2 diabetes, and those with a prior history of gestational diabetes should be tested at the first prenatal visit. If testing is negative, it should be repeated in the late second trimester (24–26 menstrual weeks). Strategies for testing for diabetes in pregnancy are reviewed in Chapter 11 on diabetes. Strict glycemic control using diet, insulin and/or an insulin-sensitizing agent will reduce infant birthweight and the risk for hypoglycemia in the newborn period.

The incidence of the hypertensive complications of pregnancy is increased in older gravidas. Attention to any evidence of borderline or pre-existing mild hypertension is crucial. Baseline laboratory studies including a serum creatinine and urine microalbumin should be obtained if there is any concern.

Contrary to early data, more recent studies show that older mothers are at increased risk of premature birth. Contributing factors include the high incidence of multiple gestations seen with assisted reproductive technologies, notably egg donation, and the increased incidence of pre-eclampsia in older women.

Large population studies have consistently shown that the risk of stillbirth increases from a low of 4/1000 births at maternal age 25–29 years to >6/1000 after age 40. While a modest number of these intrauterine fetal deaths (IUFD) result from growth restriction or fetal aneuploidy, two conditions known to be associated with stillbirth, the majority of deaths are unexplained and occur between 36 and 41 weeks

of pregnancy. A recent decision analysis demonstrated that the use of weekly antepartum testing beginning at 37 weeks until delivery could reduce the risk of stillbirth by 75%, while only modestly increasing the cesarean delivery rate (11 additional cesareans for every IUFD averted) resulting from false-positive test results.

Management of labor and delivery

Labor and delivery in the older woman should be based on sound obstetric practice and not modified by age alone. That said, there is an increased risk for cesarean delivery in women over the age of 35 years. Clearly demonstrable reasons such as the increased incidence of placenta previa, multiple gestation and gestational diabetes account for some, but not all, of the increase.

Maternal mortality

Although difficult to discuss with patients, it must be acknowledged that maternal mortality does increase with advancing age. As compared to women 25–29 years of age, the risk of all-cause mortality is statistically significantly greater for women over 35 years of age, and continues to rise with advancing age beyond 35. This is true for white women regardless of parity, time of entry into prenatal care, and level of education. This risk is even greater for black women. However, it is fair to note that the overall absolute risk of maternal mortality for women greater than 35 years of age is relatively small (25 per 100,000 in the USA). The degree to which screening women greater than 35 years of age prior to pregnancy can reduce that risk is speculative.

References

1. Waters EG, Wagner HP. Pregnancy and labor experiences of elderly primigravidas. Am J Obstet Gynecol 1950;59:296–304.
2. Heffner LJ. Advanced maternal age: how old is too old? N Engl J Med 2004;351:1927–9.
3. Hook EB, Cross PK, Schreinemachers DM. Chromosomal abnormality rates at amniocentesis and in live-born infants. JAMA 1983;249:2034–8.
4. Reddy UM. The evolving prenatal screening scene. Obstet Gynecol 2007;110:2–4.

Further reading

American College of Obstetricians and Gynecologists. Screening for fetal chromosome abnormalities. ACOG Practice Bulletin 77. American College of Obstetricians and Gynecologists, Washington, DC, 2007.

Anderson A-MN, Wohlfahrt J, Christens P, Olsen J, Melbye M. Maternal age and fetal loss: population based register linkage study. BMJ 2000;320:1708–12.

Ball RH, Caughey AB, Malone FD, Nyberg DA, Comstock CH, Saade GR, *et al.* for the First and Second Trimester Evaluation of Risk (FASTER) Research Consortium. First- and second-trimester evaluation of risk for Down syndrome. Obstet Gynecol 2007;110:10–17.

Callaghan WM, Berg C. Pregnancy-related mortality among women aged 35 years and older, United States, 1991–1997. Obstet Gynecol 2003;102:1015–21.

Caughey AB, Hopkins LM, Norton ME. Chorionic villus sampling compared with amniocentesis and the difference in the rate of pregnancy loss. Obstet Gynecol 2006;108:612–16.

Cuckle H, Benn P, Wright D. Down syndrome screening in the first and/or second trimester: model predicted performance using meta-analysis parameters. Semin Perinatol 2005;29:252–7.

Eddleman KA, Malone FD, Sullivan L, Dukes K, Berkowitz RL, Kharbutli Y, *et al.* First- and Second-Trimester Evaluation of Risk (FASTER) Research Consortium. Pregnancy loss rates after midtrimester amniocentesis. Obstet Gynecol 2006;108:1067–72.

Fretts RC, Elkin EE, Meyers ER, Heffner LJ. Should older women have antepartum testing to prevent unexplained stillbirth? Obstet Gynecol 2004;104:56–64.

Hollier LM, Leveno KJ, Kelly MA, McIntire DD, Cunningham FG. Maternal age and malformations in singleton births. Obstet Gynecol 2000;96:701–6.

Hook EB. Rates of chromosomal abnormalities at different maternal ages. Obstet Gynecol 1981;58:282–5.

Malone F, Canick JA, Ball RH, Nyberg DA, Comstock CH, Buckowski R, *et al.* First- and Second-Trimester Evaluation of Risk (FASTER) Research Consortium. First-trimester or second-trimester screening, or both, for Down's syndrome. N Engl J Med 2005;353:2001–11.

Menken J, Trussell J, Larsen U. Age and fertility. Science 1986;233:1389–94.

Rosene-Montella K, Keely E, Laifer SA, Lee RV. Evaluation and management of infertility in women: the internists' role. Ann Intern Med 2000;132(12):973–81.

Salihu HM, Shumpert MN, Slay M, Kirby RS, Alexander GR. Childbearing beyond maternal age 50 and fetal outcomes in the United States. Obstet Gynecol 2003;102:1006–14.

29 Principles of obstetric anesthesia

Stephen Gatt[1] and William Camann[2]

[1]Division of Anaesthesia and Intensive Care, Prince of Wales and Sydney Children's
  Hospitals and Royal Hospital for Women, Randwick, New South Wales, Australia
[2]Department of Anesthesiology, Perioperative and Pain Medicine, Brigham
  and Women's Hospital, Boston, MA, USA

Introduction

This chapter will outline the basic principles of obstetric analgesia and anesthesia and deal with those borderline issues where the anesthesiologist interacts with the generalist obstetrician, maternal-fetal medicine specialist or medical specialist, or where the decisions of one group of clinicians impinge on another. The best clinical practice principles for a broad range of situations where joint management is necessary are reviewed.

Preanesthetic care

In all patients, but especially in those with significant maternal disease, a focused, directed history, past and recent history and chart review and physical examination prior to undertaking an anesthetic procedure reduce maternal, fetal and neonatal complications [1,2]. Particularly for those with concomitant medical problems, early referral to and consultation with the anesthesiologist is essential [2,3].

Principles of regional anesthesia for normal labor and delivery

Labor pain is caused mainly by uterine contractions, myometrial ischemia, and cervical stretching and distension, transmitted via the sympathetic (T10–L1) and somatic (S2–S4) afferent nerve pathways (Figure 29.1). These nerves project information to the autonomic, hormonal and somatosensory centers of the brain. Labor can also be viewed as an inflammatory process mediated by interleukins, tumor necrosis factor, nitric oxide, and prostaglandin E2 (PGE2).

Although the use of epidural analgesia for childbirth varies greatly throughout the world, approximately 60% of women in the USA and UK will choose epidural analgesia for pain relief during childbirth [4]. Labor pain is transmitted through lower thoracic, lumbar, and sacral nerve roots that are amenable to epidural blockade [5]. Epidural analgesia is achieved by placement of a catheter into the lumbar epidural space; this space surrounds the spinal column and allows analgesic medication to be administered directly to the appropriate afferent nerves. Solutions of a local anesthetic, an opioid or both can then be administered as intermittent boluses, a continuous infusion or a patient-controlled technique (PCEA). The technique of combined spinal-epidural (CSE) has gained popularity in recent years. With this, a single bolus of an opioid, or opioid and local anesthetic, is injected into the spinal space, in addition to the placement of an epidural catheter (Figure 29.2). The main advantage of CSE is extremely rapid onset of pain relief due to the rapid onset of the spinal component, with minimal motor blockade due to the extremely low dose of drug. The principal goal of labor analgesia is to produce sufficient pain relief without interference with motor function, to allow maximal participation from the mother during the expulsive phase of labor. The PCEA technique of epidural administration has become very popular, as it allows the patient to titrate to her particular desired level of analgesia, while minimizing side effects and providing maximal maternal satisfaction.

Regional anesthesia can cause hypotension, due to sympathetic block, as well as profound pain relief. The hypotension is usually more frequent during cesarean delivery, owing to the higher level of anesthetic block required, but can be a complication of labor analgesia as well. Common methods used to prevent hypotension include intravenous fluid administration, maintenance of lateral tilt position, and in some cases prophylaxis or treatment with a vasopressor, such as ephedrine, metaraminol or phenylephrine.

The Task Force on Obstetric Anesthesia of the American Society of Anesthesiologists has recently critically reviewed all available literature and produced guidelines with a view

de Swiet's Medical Disorders in Obstetric Practice, 5th edition.
Edited by R. O. Powrie, M. F. Greene, W. Camann. © 2010 Blackwell
Publishing.

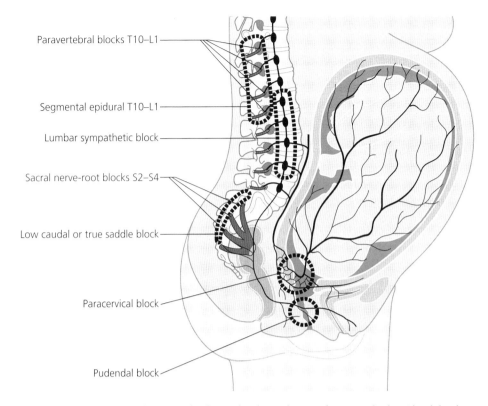

Paravertebral blocks T10–L1

Segmental epidural T10–L1

Lumbar sympathetic block

Sacral nerve-root blocks S2–S4

Low caudal or true saddle block

Paracervical block

Pudendal block

Figure 29.1 Innervation of the uterus, cervix and vagina. This figure also shows the site of paravertebral, epidural, lumbar sympathetic, sacral, caudal, paracervical and pudendal nerves blocks. Reproduced with permission from Eltzschig *et al.* [5].

to enhancing quality of anesthesia care, improving patient safety, reducing complications and increasing patient satisfaction [2]. These recommendations, as they apply to obstetric medicine, can be summarized as follows.

• No parturient should be denied pain relief in labor. The guidelines state that "Maternal request represents sufficient justification for pain relief."

• Epidural, spinal and combined spinal-epidural (CSE) anesthetic techniques can improve maternal and neonatal outcome. Parturients in early labor at less than 5 cm dilation can be safely offered neuraxial techniques without increasing their cesarean delivery or instrumental delivery risk compared to parenteral opioid analgesic techniques. Regional blocks do not increase risk to the fetus or neonate [6].

• In complicated parturients (e.g. twin gestation, pre-eclampsia, morbid obesity) early insertion of an epidural or spinal catheter reduces maternal complications.

• Neuraxial (epidural or spinal) catheter techniques are the best available modality for pain relief. They are efficacious, safe, flexible and versatile in the ability to offer good pain relief for a variety of clinical situations.

• Continuous infusion epidural local analgesia using local anesthetics with or without opioids, or spinal opioid with or without local anesthetic, provide better-quality analgesia than parenteral (IV or IM) opioid.

• Modern neuraxial analgesia does not increase the likelihood of cesarean delivery compared to parenteral opioid analgesia.

• The primary goal of neuraxial labor analgesia is to provide good sensory analgesia with a minimum amount of motor block. The lowest concentration of local anesthetic infusion that provides adequate maternal analgesia should be chosen. In most instances, this can usually be achieved with concentrations of 0.125% (or lower) of bupivacaine or ropivacaine.

• Compared to parenteral opioids, regional blocks do not significantly increase the duration of labor, decrease the incidence of vaginal delivery or increase the incidence of maternal, fetal or neonatal side effects.

• Addition of opioids to local anesthetics for both epidural and spinal techniques improves analgesia.

• For spinal analgesia, pencil point needles are better than cutting-bevel spinal needles in reducing the incidence of postdural puncture headache.

The trend towards using weaker local anesthetics (and combining them with opioids) for labor has brought major benefits – greater mobility, less motor blockade, fewer instrumental deliveries and less dystocia. All these techniques and agents aim at good pain relief coupled with retention of the maximum degree of control and the least interference with the pelvic muscles, the ability to push and to be ambulatory (or, at the very least, to be mobile). The optimal way to achieve these aims is either by using a CSE using opioid +/− a tiny dose of local anesthetic in the spinal component, or with an epidural with low-dose local anesthetic and opioid. Both methods have proven to be effective and safe [4–6].

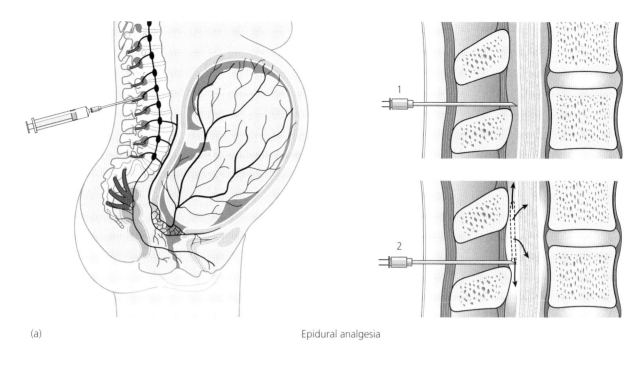

(a)   Epidural analgesia

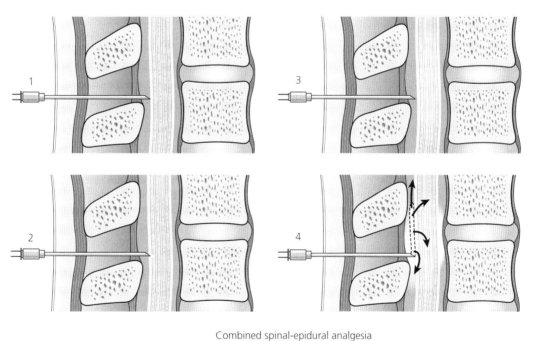

(b)   Combined spinal-epidural analgesia

Figure 29.2 (a) Epidural block showing site of needle insertion and location of tip of epidural needle and catheter. (b) Combined spinal epidural block showing (1) epidural needle placement, (2) spinal needle placement, (3) spinal needle removal, (4) epidural catheter placement. Reproduced with permission from Eltzschig *et al.* [5].

Principles of general anesthesia for cesarean delivery

In most situations, a regional anesthetic technique, albeit with some modifications tailored to the individual clinical situation, is preferable to general anesthesia and is often considerably safer for both mother and neonate. Nevertheless, there are situations, e.g. extreme urgency (due to rapid administration of general anesthesia), bleeding diathesis (due to possibility of epidural hematoma), generalized or local infection (due to possibility of epidural abscess), in which regional anesthesia may be absolutely or relatively contraindicated.

The standard, universal regimen for general anesthesia for cesarean delivery (CS) is used worldwide and is molded around a rapid-sequence induction, an anesthesia maintenance plan which is modified once the neonate is delivered and a course of action, the failed intubation algorithm [7–10], if intubation fails or proves difficult [11–15].

There are several reasons why the technique has gained such widespread acceptance.
• It allows anesthesiologists to secure the airway immediately under quasi-ideal intubating conditions.
• It has the lowest impact possible on the fetus such that the newborn is delivered with the lowest possible degree of depression.
• The technique is forgiving in that, if the intubation fails [16], there is a fair chance that the parturient will awake and breathe spontaneously before severe hypoxemia supervenes so that an alternative technique (e.g. laryngeal mask airway [16], spinal subarachnoid or epidural block) can then be tried.
• It virtually eliminates the incidence of maternal awareness.
• It provides maximum protection against pulmonary acid aspiration even in mothers with a full stomach.
• Anesthesia can be achieved within seconds so that delivery can start immediately, even in the most dire emergencies, and the distressed fetus can be delivered within minutes.
• General anesthesia (GA) can be achieved with relatively cheap and readily available medications and equipment.
• This GA sequence provides good surgical operating conditions.
The core of the rapid-sequence induction (RSI) technique consists of optimal preoxygenation, intravenous induction (using thiopental/thiopentone or propofol) followed by a rapid-acting neuromuscular block (usually succinylcholine) and endotracheal intubation under cricoid pressure, to prevent passive regurgitation of gastric contents. Anesthesia is then maintained using inhaled volatile agent (e.g. isoflurane, sevoflurane or desflurane). After delivery, the volatile concentration is reduced (as volatile inhalation agents can contribute to uterine atony) and an opioid (e.g. morphine, fentanyl, hydromorphone) and additional muscle relaxant, together with oxytocin and/or carbetocin, are administered.

Aspiration pneumonitis prophylaxis

Pulmonary aspiration of gastric contents has become an extremely rare event in modern obstetric anesthesia practice. While aspiration may occur during vaginal deliveries even in the absence of anesthesia, most cases will occur during, or immediately after, an emergency general anesthetic in a patient who has recently ingested a solid meal. In the past, this was attributed to a presumed delay in gastric emptying in laboring women and led to a general prohibition against any oral intake in women in labor. However, recent evidence indicates that gastric emptying of liquids is normal in normal pregnancy and labor [17–19]. Thus, the most recent guidelines for obstetric anesthesia by the American Society of Anesthesiologists support that a modest amount of oral clear liquids (water, carbonated beverages, sports drinks, fruit juice without pulp, clear tea, black coffee) administered up to 2 hours before induction of anesthesia in the uncomplicated patient does not increase maternal risk [2]. In those with additional risk factors for aspiration (e.g. obesity, diabetes, difficult airway), oral fluids may be restricted further, on a case-by-case basis. [2]. Fasting time for solids prior to elective surgery should be 6–8 hours depending on the type of food ingested (e.g. fat content) [2,19].

Timely administration of nonparticulate antacids (e.g. 30 mL of clear sodium citrate) and H2 receptor antagonists (e.g. ranitidine 150 mg) decreases gastric acidity and reduces peripartum maternal complications [2].

Principles of regional anesthesia for cesarean delivery

Cesarean delivery regional anesthesia can be achieved with spinal, epidural or CSE. The choice depends on many factors. Spinal anesthesia is quick, reliable, and simple, and provides excellent surgical anesthesia and operating conditions. However, spinal is associated with hypotension and a limited duration of action (generally 1–2 hours) although it is usually adequate for most cesarean deliveries. Epidural anesthesia is slower in onset and generally associated with less hypotension than spinal. The use of a catheter-based technique (versus a single-injection technique such as spinal) allows epidural anesthesia to be titrated and extended in the event of prolonged surgical operating times. However, epidural techniques can occasionally result in patchy anesthesia due to anatomic limitations. Moreover, epidural techniques require higher volumes of local anesthetic drugs, thus presenting the rare, but serious, possibility of local anesthetic toxicity if an intravascular injection occurs.

Pain relief following cesarean delivery

Women require less pain relief in the peripartum period than their age-matched, nonpregnant counterparts having equivalent surgery. Nevertheless, the postcesarean patient has had major surgery and will require significant analgesic support for a few days. This is especially true if there has been a poor obstetric outcome (e.g. infant with significant congenital anomaly), if there are postoperative complications (e.g. infection) or if the mother required additional surgery (e.g. cesarean hysterectomy).

Because there are so many anesthetic techniques available for cesarean delivery, it is unlikely that one formula for postoperative pain relief will be appropriate for all circumstances. Postoperative analgesia will depend on whether opioid has been placed in the subarachnoid or epidural space, whether an epidural catheter is *in situ* for analgesia top-up, on the temperament and estimated pain thresholds of the patient, and on the adjunct analgesic modalities available.

Most patients, at a minimum, will receive acetaminophen and/or a nonsteroidal analgesic (NSAID). Some will receive intraoperatively, after delivery of the baby, intravenous COX-2s (parecoxib) and acetaminophen. To this may be added:
• a recovery room morphine, pethidine (meperidine), tramadol or fentanyl pain protocol, and/or
• an intravenous patient-controlled opioid analgesia regimen (PCA), and/or
• intrathecal opioid, and/or
• epidural patient-controlled epidural boluses of opioid (PCEA), and/or
• epidural opioid boluses, and/or
• parenteral opioids.
The authors consider all of these interventions to be compatible with breastfeeding.

Ambulatory/mobile/walking epidurals and combined spinal-epidural for labor and delivery

In this context, "mobile" or "ambulatory" can mean walking, sitting out in a chair and/or toilet privileges, walking and/or sitting, sitting out of bed only, fully mobile in bed or even some motor impairment but not hugely incapacitating. Ambulatory/mobile/walking (M/A/W) epidurals can be achieved with low-dose epidural or a CSE using a tiny spinal dose followed by epidural bolus or infusion using very weak anesthetic solutions (preferably one with lowered motor blockade) + opioid combination [5]. It is not necessary to use the CSE technique in order to achieve a M/A/W epidural.

There has been no proven advantage in M/A/W epidurals and no substantial difference between CSE and low-dose epidural in improvements in:
• duration of labor
• instrumental delivery or cesarean rate

• fetal heart rate changes
• safety: hypotension, falls, respiratory depression, decreased muscle strength
• cardiovascular stability
• motor block
• side effects: urinary retention, deep vein thrombosis/venous thromboembolism (DVT/VTE), back pain, headache (postdural puncture headache), pruritus, ability to push in second stage.

Successful interdisciplinary team work

From the anesthesiologist's perspective, there are many clinical decisions made and treatments administered by the obstetric physician, which sometimes transfer one team's risk to another. In obstetrics, what sometimes seems like a reasonable treatment strategy to one group of clinicians can increase either the overall risk or the possibility of another complication.

This is confounded because the care of a pregnant and laboring woman is often shared by more than one clinician (obstetrician, anesthesiologist, physician, midwife, doula), each of whom may not have a complete understanding of the milieu in which the other works. Each group may be well aware of the risks within their specialty but not of those in another group.

For example, thrombosis management with potent, long-acting agents which are hard to reverse, in late pregnancy, in the milieu of high odds of postpartum hemorrhage, the need for major neuraxial pain relief in labor or of cesarean delivery or instrumental delivery, may pose a larger overall risk to the parturient than the risk of thrombosis. Furthermore, the risk of general anesthesia imposed by the administration of antithrombotics increases if the parturient has a "difficult airway" or is morbidly obese.

The only reliable way for each member of the team caring for a woman in labor to understand the perspective and concerns of the other team members is through early and continued open communication. No member of the team should be treated as simply a technician whose job is to serve the others. Making sure that anesthesiologists and nurses are brought in early to potentially concerning cases and creating an environment where all members of the care team are encouraged to speak their concerns and be heard is essential to the safety of laboring patients. Some key pointers for obstetricians and medical specialists looking to build collaborative working relationships with obstetric anesthesiologists are summarized in Box 29.1.

Urgent/emergency cesarean delivery

Good teamwork is particularly important when the possible need for an urgent caesarean delivery is identified. The call for an urgent cesarean delivery is associated with increased risk and morbidity. When justified, it can be

Box 29.1 Key aspects of successful collaboration between obstetricians, internists and anesthesiologists in the care of obstetric patients

1. Get anesthesiologists involved early if an obstetric patient is deemed to be at risk of respiratory failure.
2. Have multidisciplinary patient care conferences to create written delivery plans well in advance of the delivery date.
3. Most anesthesiologists are committed to offering regional anesthesia to patients in labor. Nonetheless, there are circumstances where the risk outweighs the benefits. Anesthesiologists should not be pressured unduly to place epidural or spinal catheters in situations not supported by the consensus statements of their professional societies
4. Endotracheal intubation of pregnant women is technically difficult and should generally be performed by the most experienced individual available.

life-saving but only when the term "urgency" is used judiciously. While speed is often of the essence when there is a nonreassuring fetal heart rate pattern, it is important to recognize that a degree of hazard is imposed by unnecessary haste. For example, rapidity of technique, especially in inexperienced hands, and inappropriately applied cricoid pressure may contribute to the increased incidence of difficult tracheal intubation or inadvertent esophageal intubation. Excessive emphasis on rapidity can also result in errors, and the ideal time until delivery should take into consideration both the benefits and risks of prioritization.

The "urgency" of "urgent CS" has been reviewed recently in the UK by Lucas *et al.* [20] such that we now have a working model for the categorization of the degree of speed of operation required of the anesthesiologist in certain circumstances. In this categorization schedule:

• category 1 = immediate threat to life of mother or fetus
• category 2 = maternal or fetal compromise, not immediately life threatening
• category 3 = needing early delivery but no maternal or fetal compromise
• category 4 = at a time to suit the mother and delivery team.

Implementation of this shared terminology on labor floors can help the interdisciplinary clinical team and related support staff triage safely and work together with a shared mental model of the circumstances. For category 1 cases, the management technique will generally involve immediate *in utero* resuscitation and expeditious cesarean delivery. *In utero* fetal resuscitation before induction of anesthesia in situations

where there are concerning fetal heart tracings consists of the following interventions.

• Turn oxytocin infusion off.
• Turn mother into left (or right) lateral position.
• Administer oxygen via facemask.
• Administer intravenous fluid.
• Consider administration of a vasopressor, either ephedrine (5–10 mg) or phenylephrine (40–80 μg).
• Consider administration of a tocolytic such as nitroglycerin 400 μg (sublingual or aerosol) or terbutaline 250 μg SC.

In most category 1 situations, the CS will be performed using general anesthesia with a rapid-induction sequence, unless an epidural catheter has already been placed. For other categories of cesarean deliveries, regional anesthesia may still be an option. Although an appropriate method to grade urgency, the "category 1–4" system is not yet common terminology in the USA.

Airway emergencies

Anesthesia-related maternal mortality in 2007 is low in the world's advanced economies, probably about 1.7 per million livebirths. Anesthesia accounts for only 3.2% of all maternal deaths. The percentage of general anesthesia deaths contributed by airway difficulties, however, is 49%. Obstetric anesthesiologists should be equipped with the tools to assess degree of risk and to prepare for the likelihood of intubation difficulty [21]. The incidence of failed intubation in obstetrics is 1 in 280 compared to 1 in 2330 in the general population. Airway assessment consists of history (congenital abnormality, faciomaxillary trauma, dental, cervical spine or faciomaxillary surgery, snoring), physical examination (obesity, receding mandible, short/thick neck, large breasts, over-riding upper teeth, protruding maxilla, short stature, large tongue, underslung jaw), specific airway testing (oropharyngeal class, Mallampati grade (Figure 29.3), incisor length, mandibular space and compliance, thyromental distance, atlanto-occipital extension, interincisor distance, Wilson risk sum, length and thickness of neck) and, in rare cases, radiologic tests (plain films, simulation laryngoscopy and X-ray laryngoscopy).

Personnel and equipment should be readily available in obstetric units to manage maternal airway emergencies. The anesthesiologist should be notified about and involved early with any pregnant patient with possible respiratory compromise. This allows an assessment of the patient's airway and preparation for the eventual possibility of the need for an emergency intubation.

The minimum monitoring equipment required should include a method to confirm endotracheal tube placement using expired carbon dioxide, and pulse oximetry. Airway equipment should include laryngoscope handles and blades of different designs, endotracheal tubes with bougies and stylets (to aid with difficult intubation), laryngeal mask airways

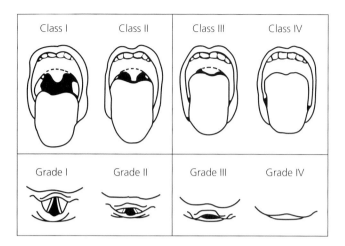

Figure 29.3 Classification of the airway (Mallampati score). Laryngeal view in the upper and lower panels respectively. Courtesy of Dr. R. Mallampati.

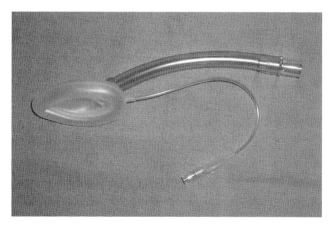

Figure 29.4 Laryngeal mask airway.

(LMA; Figure 29.4), a self-inflating bag and mask, and an oxygen source. Endotracheal tubes of different sizes, (5.5, 6.0. 6.5, 7.0 and 7.5) should be available, as well as a source of suction [2]. It is highly recommended that all obstetric units have ready access to these materials in a centrally stored, locked box or cart that is systematically and regularly reviewed.

Specialized devices for difficult airways (e.g. intubating LMA, fiberoptic intubation equipment, tracheostomy and cricothyroidotomy sets, light wands) and a predetermined failed intubation protocol algorithm should be available, and a failed intubation sequence should be pre-rehearsed [21–24].

Hemorrhagic emergencies (see also Chapter 2)

Obstetric units should have the resources to deal with massive hemorrhage. Pre-rehearsed emergency drills involving the entire team and occurring every 6–12 months have been shown to dramatically improve performance during emergencies. Equipment including large-bore intravenous cannulae, urinary catheters, massive transfusion devices, fluid warmers, blood pump infusion systems, forced air body warmers, automatic infusion devices and colloid and crystalloid solutions must be at hand.

Blood-banking facilities must also be readily available. A massive transfusion protocol which makes available red cells, fresh-frozen plasma, cryoprecipitate and platelets, as well as recombinant factor VIIa, has been useful in some special situations, such as catastrophic blood loss [25]. Oxytocics (oxytocin, methylergonovine), prostaglandins (prostaglandin F2-alpha 15-methyl, and misoprostol) and pressor agents should be readily available in obstetric units.

In those with severe pre-eclampsia, bleeding can be due to thrombocytopenia, abruptio placentae, disseminated intravascular coagulation, atonic uterus or the HELLP syndrome. The use of oxytocics to control postpartum bleeding in severe pre-eclampsia remains controversial, as methylergonovine can exacerbate hypertension. When massive bleeding occurs in severe pre-eclampsia, useful strategies may include misoprostol, recombinant factor VIIa and activation of a massive blood transfusion protocol [20]. More controversial is the use, in severe coagulopathy, of certain therapeutic agents (fibrinogen, aprotinin, antifibrinolytics, antithrombotics and, sometimes, heparins). The main controversy lies in when to administer them, in which order and to what endpoints. Likewise, blood products (platelets, fresh-frozen plasma, cryoprecipitate) must be used but the indications, endpoints and sequencing are more nebulous. In pre-eclampsia, both the best type of volume replacement and the optimum approach to volume replacement remain undetermined. In cases of massive postpartum hemorrhage, it is critical to maintain effective communication between the obstetrician and anesthesiologist as each attempts to provide their respective expertise to control of blood loss. Clear communication with blood bank personnel is also essential to maintain proper supply of blood products.

Other specific circumstances

Most of the major system-based chapters and some of the shorter "approach to" chapters include some practical advice from an obstetric anesthesiologist related to the specific diagnoses discussed in the chapter. Common questions about anesthetic management of pre-eclamptic patients and about regional anesthesia and thrombocytopenia or anticoagulation are addressed in this setting and the reader is encouraged to turn to the relevant chapters for this information.

Conclusion

Advances in obstetric anesthesia, in particular the use of regional anesthesia, have been of great benefit both for the comfort of women and for the management of medically complicated pregnancies. However, obstetric anesthesia also continues to represent a small but real potential source of risk, particularly in those medically complicated patients who may benefit the most from it. There are many situations in the interface between anesthesiologists and other clinicians (obstetricians, internists, midwives) where the optimal solution for the parturient's special condition is best achieved by prior consultation and consensus agreement between all team members.

References

1. Eagle KA and Task Force on Practice Guidelines. ACC/AHA guideline update for preoperative cardiovascular evaluation for noncardiac surgery – executive summary. Anesth Analg 2002;94:1052–64.

2. American Society of Anesthesiololgists Task Force on Obstetric Anesthesia. Practice guidelines for obstetric anesthesia: an updated report by the American Society of Anesthesiologists Task Force on Obstetric Anesthesia. Anesthesiology 2007;106(4):843–63.

3. American Society of Anesthesiologists Task Force on Preanesthesia Evaluation. Practice advisory for preanesthesia evaluation. Anesthesiology 2002;96:485–96.

4. Bucklin BA, Hawkins JL, Anderson JR, Ulrich JA. Obstetric Anesthesia Workforce Survey: twenty-year update. Anesthesiology 2005;103 645–53.

5. Eltzschig HK, Lieberman ES, Camann WR. Regional anesthesia and analgesia for labor and delivery. N Engl J Med 2003;348:319–32.

6. Analgesia and cesarean delivery rates. ACOG Committee Opinion #339, June 2006. Obstet Gynecol 2006;107:1487–8.

7. Thwaites AJ, Rice CP, Smith I. Rapid sequence induction: a questionnaire survey of its routine conduct and continued management during a failed intubation. Anaesthesia 1999;54:376–81.

8. Dean VS, Jurai SA, Naraynsingh GV, Serrao C. Failed intubation drill. Br J Anaesth 1997;78:231.

9. Nair A, Alderson JD. Failed intubation drill in obstetrics. Int J Obstet Anesth 2006;15:173.

10. Henderson J, Popat M, Latto I, Pierce AC. Difficult Airway Society guidelines for management of the unanticipated difficult intubation. Anaesthesia 2004;59:675–94.

11. Anserine JM, Bog CE, Carrie LE. Failed tracheal intubation at caesarean section and the laryngeal mask, Br J Anaesth 1992;68(1):116.

12. Duffy B. To paralyse a failed intubation or not? Anaesth Intens Care 1991;19(1):135–6.

13. Thind GS, Nagaraja SV. Airway management/failed intubation drill. Anaesthesia 2001;56(4):385.

14. Saravanakumar K, Copper GM. Failed intubation in obstetrics: has the incidence changed recently? Br J Anaesth 2005;94(5):690.

15. Russell R. Failed intubation in obstetrics: a self-fulfilling prophecy? Int J Obstet Anesth 2007;16:1–3.

16. Sharma B, Sahai C, Sood J, Kumra P. The ProSeal laryngeal mask airway in two failed obstetric tracheal intubation scenarios. Int J Obstet Anesth 2006;15:338–9.

17. Wong CA, McCarthy FJ, Fitzgerald PC, Raikoff, K, Avram MJ. Gastric emptying of water in obese pregnant women at term. Anesth Analg 2007;105:751–5.

18. Wong CA, Loffredi M, Ganchiff JN, Zhao J, Wang Z, Avram MJ. Gastric emptying of water in term pregnancy. Anesth Analg 2002;96:1395–400.

19. American Society of Anesthesiologists Task Force on Preoperative Fasting. Practice guidelines for preoperative fasting and the use of antacids to reduce the risk of pulmonary aspiration. Anesthesiology 1999;90:896–905.

20. Lucas DN, Yentis SM, Kinsella SM, et al. Urgency of caesarean section: a new classification. J R Soc Md 2000;93(7):346–50.

21. Gaiser RR, McGonigal ET, Litts P, Cheeck TG, Gutsche BB. Obstetricians' ability to assess the airway. Obstet Gynecol 1999;93:648–52.

22. Han TH, Brimacombe J, Lee EJ, Yang HS. The laryngeal mask airway is effective (and probably safe) in selected healthy parturients for elective Cesarean section: a prospective study of 1067 cases. Can J Anaesth 2001;48(11):1117–21.

23. Godley M, Reddy AR. Use of LMA for awake intubation for caesarean section. Can J Anaesth 1996;43(3):299–302.

24. Bailey SG, Kitching AJ. The laryngeal mask airway in failed obstetric tracheal intubation. Int J Obstet Anesth 2005;14(3):270–1.

25. Welsh A, McClintock C, Gatt S, Somerset D, Popham P, Ogle R. Guidelines for the use of recombinant activated factor VII in massive obstetric haemorrhage. Aust NZ J Obstet Gynaecol 2008;48:12–16.

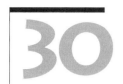

30

Prescribing in pregnancy: a practical approach

Sandra L. Kweder[1] and Raymond O. Powrie[2]

[1]Department of Medicine, Uniformed Services University, Bethesda, MD, USA
[2]Department of Medicine, Warren Alpert Medical School of Brown University, Women & Infants' Hospital of Rhode Island, Providence, RI, USA

Introduction

Deciding whether to prescribe a medication and which one to prescribe presents challenges in all areas of medical practice, but is especially difficult in caring for pregnant women. Information about pharmacologics and their risks in pregnancy, for both drugs and biologic therapeutics, is sparse at best. For the obstetrician caring for a patient who may need such treatment, the uncertainty this reality reveals is stark. Applying an organized, methodical approach to medical care in this setting is essential for clinicians and patients to make sound decisions for each unique situation. This chapter is intended to provide guidance to clinicians who are considering the need for pharmacologic intervention in a patient's care.

General approach

Start with the patient in mind

What is her condition and what are her concerns? It is remarkable how much patients have thought about the exact issues that their doctors think about, often long before and in different ways. Is she willing to consider pharmacologic treatment at all? What are her concerns about her condition? What is her need for certainty about the safety of a medication for her developing fetus? In today's environment, ask what she already knows about her condition and possible treatments. Chances are, she has already checked out internet sites and may even have already made a decision about what she thinks her options are. The patient must have a role in deciding whether to take a medicine and which one to take.

de Swiet's Medical Disorders in Obstetric Practice, 5th edition. Edited by R. O. Powrie, M. F. Greene, W. Camann. © 2010 Blackwell Publishing.

Ensure the diagnosis is correct

Pregnancy is not a time to treat empirically, so a confident diagnosis of the patient's problem is critical to selection of an appropriate therapy. It is surprising how often this is overlooked in the clinician's zeal to "do something." Patients who enter pregnancy with a chronic medical condition usually have had so much investigation that diagnostic testing, such as for rheumatoid arthritis, is not necessary. However, when the condition is of new onset or presents in a way that is different from manifestations the patient has previously experienced, determining the diagnosis is essential. Once a diagnosis is made, three major considerations merge in reaching a decision about treatment:
• how the pregnancy might affect the mother's condition or illness
• how the pathophysiology of the condition might affect the pregnancy or the fetus
• what the treatment options are.
A good rule to keep in mind is that at the end of pregnancy, a healthy baby is best assured by a healthy mother.

In general, conditions that will adversely affect the mother or the fetus, such as progressive acute or chronic medical conditions, should be considered as potentially detrimental to the developing fetus and likely to require treatment. Many self-limited, symptomatic illnesses (e.g. tension headaches, viral upper respiratory infections) can be managed with simple, nonpharmacologic treatments. However, there are also conditions that the pregnant woman may tolerate reasonably well but which still place fetal well-being at risk, such as some thyroid disease, asthma and some viral illnesses. Young women can have remarkable tolerance to substantial physiologic and immune alteration, while their developing fetus may not.

Will pregnancy affect the mother's medical condition?

Pregnancy itself can exacerbate some medical conditions, putting the pregnant woman at substantial risk. As stated above, the more healthy the mother, the greater the likelihood of a healthy fetus and infant. Conditions that worsen in pregnancy may place the mother at risk for morbidity and, in some cases, mortality. These are therefore likely to require pharmacologic intervention at some point. Examples include asthma, autoimmune conditions, congestive heart failure and cardiac arrhythmias. Unfortunately, for many such illnesses, it is not clear in advance which women will be adversely affected during pregnancy. For example, an uncomplicated first pregnancy in a woman with asthma is not necessarily reassurance that she will have a similar course in any subsequent pregnancy.

Will the medical condition affect the pregnancy and the fetus?

There are medical conditions that negatively affect pregnancy and fetal development, because of an effect on either maternal health or the fetus. These include some endocrine disorders, especially diabetes and thyroid disease, infections, and consequences of chronic conditions that manifest with episodic exacerbations. Examples of the latter include asthma and epilepsy, both of which can result in fetal hypoxia, even if the mother experiences no significant sequelae herself. Similarly, hypertension is usually asymptomatic in the mother, but its presence increases the risk of pre-eclampsia which may hamper fetal growth and development. Certain infections, even if mild in the mother, are well known to be associated with preterm labor.

It is not necessary to withhold medications from women who have self-limited conditions or those who have conditions that are not known to specifically adversely affect pregnancy. Here, understanding the patient's preferences and needs will guide whether or not to intervene with a medicine. For example, maternal migraine headaches are not likely to cause the fetus direct harm. They can, however, so substantially interfere with the woman's ability to carry out daily activities that she becomes depressed, sleep deprived and even poorly nourished – none of which are good for the fetus. Without a physician's willingness to consider prescribing an effective intervention, she may take matters into her own hands and use over-the-counter remedies she presumes are safe but which have their own risks (e.g. acetaminophen hepatotoxicity), to say nothing of herbal treatment and dietary supplements. Herbal-based or "natural" products are not necessarily safer than traditional medicine – they have simply not been tested.

Have a plan for drug treatment options

Whenever possible, it is prudent to have a plan for medical intervention should a patient with a medical illness worsen. Establishing such a plan well in advance is highly recommended – and it should be developed in partnership with the patient and any of her other healthcare providers, preferably before encountering an acute or emergency situation. A treatment plan can be simple, but should include the points in Box 30.1 including

---

Box 30.1 Developing a treatment plan

- Plan in the light, before the patient becomes ill
- Don't go it alone
  - Know the patient's concerns, worries, preferences about her illness and her pregnancy
  - Consult her other healthcare providers
- Write down potential risks and benefits of all possible treatments, including no medication
- Consider the dynamic physiology of gestation
  - Choose the right drug for the right trimester
- Write down criteria you will use to stop or change treatment. Don't keep it a secret – give the patient and other providers a copy

---

the diagnosis, what clinical changes will trigger starting pharmacologic treatment, and evidence that you and the patient have had frank discussions about her options and preferences.

Resources at the ready

With increasing emphasis on pharmacologics in medicine, choosing therapy can be difficult. Therapeutics in pregnancy has not kept pace with advances in the rest of the population, especially in understanding how medicines might affect fetal development. Some clinicians intentionally avoid newer medications, no matter how effective they may be, simply to allow their full safety profile to emerge over time as population experience grows. While a sound defensive practice, this may not always be in patients' best interest. Newer medicines are likely to be better characterized chemically, more pure in formulation and have up-to-date high-quality data regarding animal toxicology profiles.

Most nations with advanced economies have formal pregnancy safety categorization strategies to guide clinicians and their patients about the use of medications in pregnancy. One of the most widely referenced systems is the United States Food and Drug Administration (FDA) letter categories which are assigned at the time of US marketing approval. These letters are *not* a risk graded continuum, but instead are intended to reflect a balance of both the known risks and the quality of the information on which that risk assessment is based, on the one hand, and the potential benefits on the other hand (Box 30.2). Products with the same letter designation cannot be assumed to carry the same hazard. However, the letter designations are readily available when other sources of information may not be, and can be a useful general guide. A good rule of thumb when studying product labeling is to not stop with the letter. Read the full text accompanying it to understand the letter in its particular setting. Also, consider whether the information is up to date. If the drug is old (especially if there is no letter) and there are no human data about pregnancy in the label, it may be that there

Box 30.2 FDA pregnancy categories

Source

Found in most prescription medication package inserts/labeling and in *Physician's desk reference* published annually by Medical Economics Press.

Description

Well-known categories A, B, C, D, and X are a widely used resource for decisions about drug use in pregnancy.

Category A Controlled studies show no risk	Controlled studies in women fail to demonstrate a risk to the fetus in the first trimester, there is no evidence of a risk in later trimesters and therefore the possibility of fetal harm appears remote.
Category B No evidence of risk in humans	Either animal reproduction studies have not demonstrated a fetal risk but there are no controlled studies in pregnant women, or animal reproduction studies have shown an adverse effect (other than a decrease in fertility) that was not confirmed in controlled studies in women in the first trimester (and there is no evidence of a risk in later trimesters).
Category C Risk cannot be ruled out	Either studies in animals have revealed adverse effect on the fetus (teratogenic) or appropriate animal data are not available. Drugs should be given only if the potential benefit justifies the potential risk to the fetus.
Category D Positive evidence of risk	There is positive evidence of human fetal risk, but the benefits from use in pregnant women may be acceptable despite the risk (e.g. if the drug is needed in a life-threatening situation or for a serious disease for which safer drugs cannot be used or are ineffective). There will be an appropriate statement in the "warnings" section of the labeling.
Category X Contraindicated in pregnancy	Studies in animals or human beings have demonstrated fetal abnormalities or there is evidence of fetal risk based on human experience, or both, and the risk of the use of the drug in pregnant women clearly outweighs any possible benefit. The drug is contraindicated in women who are or may be pregnant.

are more up-to-date sources of information. In such cases, look to another source for additional information and guidance.

In Table 30.1, we have provided a few of the reference resources clinicians seem to value most in seeking information about individual drugs. The list is not complete but represents up-to-date, readily available sources, which were selected with the busy office-based clinician in mind. Several are texts or compendia in hard copy and others are available online. The hard-copy versions are increasingly being made available in forms that allow for downloading onto personal digital assistant devices (PDA). The online resources are updated often and may include information that is useful in counseling individual patients. Note that one reference is specific to drugs in nursing mothers, an important consideration as the patient transitions to the postpartum period.

Getting started

Having a sense of what treatment options to consider for a patient can be daunting. Every decision about the use of a

drug in pregnancy has to be made with the individual patient in mind, as was described earlier, making things even more daunting. The sources of information in Table 30.1 are best used once individual therapeutic options are being entertained. With that in mind, we have compiled Table 30.2 which includes commonly used medications for illnesses that are often diagnosed or managed by primary care physicians. It does not include medication recommendations for more complicated conditions such as epilepsy, bipolar affective disorder or conditions requiring immunosuppressive agents where details about the particular patient's condition and treatment history are critical to the decision-making process. It also does not include trade or brand names, because most of the drugs listed have more than one manufacturer and marketer. Finally, Table 30.2 is a general guide only, intended to get the busy office practitioner off to a start in thinking about commonly employed treatment options. It is not a drug safety table; for data on safety, you should refer to the sources listed in Table 30.1. Reference numbers in the table refer to ID numbers in PubMed (www.pubmed.gov).

Table 30.1 Some resources to assess medication safety in pregnancy

Publication	Authors	Publisher	Format
Drugs in pregnancy and lactation: a reference guide to fetal and neonatal risk	Briggs GS, Freeman RK, Yaffe SY	Solution Lippincott Williams & Wilkins; 8th edition 2008	Hardcover; 2144 pages
Teratogenic effects of drugs: a resource for clinicians (TERIS)	Friedman JM, Polifka JE.	Johns Hopkins University Press, 2nd edition 2000	Hardcover; 793 pages
Medication safety in pregnancy and breastfeeding: the evidence-based, A to Z clinician's pocket guide	Koren G	McGraw-Hill Professional, 1st edition 2006	Paperback; 312 pages
Medication safety in pregnancy and breastfeeding	Koren G	McGraw-Hill Professional, 1st edition 2007	Hardcover; 623 pages
Drugs for pregnant and lactating women	Weiner CP, Buhimschi C	Churchill Livingstone, 1st edition 2004	Hardcover; 1101 pages
Drugs during pregnancy and lactation	Schaefer C, Peters PWJ, Miller RK	Academic Press, 2nd edition 2007	Hardcover; 904 pages
Prescribing in pregnancy	Rubin PC, Ramsey M	BMJ Books, 4th edition 2008	Paperback; 256 pages
Catalog of teratogenic agents	Shepard TH, Lemire RJ	Johns Hopkins University Press, 12th edition 2007	Hardcover; 656 pages
Medications and mothers' milk: a manual of lactational pharmacology	Hale T	Pharmasoft Medical Publishing, 13th edition 2008	Paperback, 1172 pages
Online/computer databases			
REPRORISK: Thomson Reuters Micromedex Inc. Module (www.reprorisk.co.za)		Online database or diskette contains TERIS, REPROTOX, REPROTEXT and Shepard's Catalog of teratogenic agents	
TERIS: Information available at http://depts. washington.edu/terisweb/teris/		Online subscription or diskette	
Reprotox®: Thomson Reuters Micromedex Inc. Module www.REPROTOX.org		Online subscription or diskette; PDA version available	

Avoiding pitfalls

Just as every patient is unique, the considerations for every treatment course in every patient will be unique. Here are some suggestions for optimizing your patient's therapy.

• Do not start any medication unless it is clearly indicated. The urgent sense of needing to "do" something that often grips one upon seeing a patient who is seeking therapy is powerful.

• Do not discontinue any medication that successfully maintains the maternal condition unless there are clear indications to do so. In our experience, the reflex reaction of clinicians upon seeing a pregnant patient is to assume she should not be taking any medication. Taking no medicine is always an option, but in some cases is often a bigger threat to mother and fetus than any individual drug's risk. It is easy to be lulled into thinking a medication is not needed simply because the patient is doing well. If you are in doubt, seek a consultation with an expert in her condition.

• The physiology of pregnancy is dynamic: use principles of clinical pharmacology to make decisions about dosing. Do not assume that just giving a little bit of a drug is the best strategy. Doses that are or are likely to be subtherapeutic ensure no benefit, but never should be presumed to assure that risk is decreased. Drugs that are cleared renally are the most likely to require higher or more frequent dosing in pregnancy because

of increased rates of renal blood flow and, thus, glomerular filtration. Remember, these changes occur very early in gestation.

• Very few drugs are absolutely contraindicated in pregnancy. There are only a few dozen drugs that are known to be teratogenic, and these tend to be well known, such as isotretinoin and thalidomide. Unlike these examples, most others that have known teratogenic effects do so at much lower rates, such as warfarin, valproate and the ACE inhibitors.

• Fetal withdrawal syndromes require consideration in the third trimester. Drugs associated with withdrawal or withdrawal-like syndromes should be managed in anticipation of this. These include opiate analgesics, benzodiazepines, sympathomimetics, and some antidepressants, particularly serotonin reuptake inhibitors and their relatives.

• Pregnant women are susceptible to all the same adverse effects of drugs as those who are not pregnant. Complications of treatment unrelated to pregnancy are, in fact, far more likely than most teratogenic effects, but often forgotten in the intense focus on fetal risk. Know the possible adverse effects, educate your patient, and write it down – for you and for her. Remember that she may only leave the office remembering what you said about risk to the fetus.

• Encourage frank and open discussion. It is the only way you will learn what the patient is or is not doing with her medications, whether she is taking them, taking them occasionally,

Table 30.2 Suggested medications in pregnancy by indication

Condition or product type	Data suggest use justifiable when indicated	Data suggest use may be justifiable in unique circumstances	Data suggest rarely justifiable for indication listed	Useful review articles and comments
Acne	Topical erythromycin[B] Topical benzoyl peroxide[C] Topical clindamycin[B]	Oral erythromycin[B]	Tetracycline[D] Doxycycline[D] Topical tretinoin[C]	PMID: 2971690 PMID: 16487888
Analgesics	Acetaminophen[A] Codeine[C] Meperidine[C] Morphine[C]	All NSAID[B/C] (intermittent use of NSAID in the first two trimesters for anti-inflammatory purposes may be justifiable but repeated use after 28 weeks is to be avoided) ASA[D] (low-dose ASA <100 mg per day does appear to be safe in pregnancy)		These review articles detail issues surrounding the use of NSAID in pregnancy including case reports of constriction of the ductus arteriosus, renal dysfunction and hemostatic abnormalities in the fetus and neonate. Malformations associated with NSAID have not been reported, however. PMID: 16638921 PMID:16194696 PMID: 15013926
Antihistamines	Diphenhydramine[B] (but avoid in first trimester) Chlorpheniramine Dimenhydrinate[B] Loratidine[B] Cetirizine[B]	Fexofenadine[C]		These 2006 review articles systematically and critically review the literature on the treatment of allergic rhinitis in pregnancy. PMID: 16579874 PMID: 16443148
Anti-infectives	Erythromycin[B] base, ethyl succinate or stearate (not estolate) Penicillins[B] Cephalosporins[B] Azithromycin[B] Vancomycin[C] Nitrofurantoin[B] Metronidazole[B] (after first trimester) Isoniazid[C] Acyclovir[C] AZT[C] and other antiretrovirals except for efavirenz[D] (Sustiva)	Antifungals: (all [C] except amphotericin, nystatin, clotrimazole and terbinafine which are [B]) The following agents are commonly used in pregnancy but are best reserved for use when alternative agents are less effective: clarithromycin[C] aminoglycosides[D] trimethoprim[C] sulfonamides[C]	Tetracycline[D] Fluoroquinolones[C] despite very concerning animal data, increasing human data suggest flouroquinolones might warrant their placement in the "use may be justified in rare circumstances" category Erythomycin estolate[B] Efavirenz[D]	Two 1997 and one 2006 review article on the use of antimicrobials in pregnancy are: PMID: 9266582 PMID: 9067781 PMID: 16648419
Asthma	Beta agonists: albuterol[C] metaproterenol[C] salmeterol[C] pirbuterol[C] formeterol[C] Inhaled steroids: budesonide[B] beclomethasone[C] flunisolide[C] fluticasone[C] triamcinolone[C] Systemic steroids[C] ipratropium[B] cromolyn[B]	Zafirlukast[B] Montelukast[B] Omalizumab[B]		New national recommendations for the management of asthma in pregnancy were published in early 2005 and can be obtained through the NHLBI at www.nhlbi.nih.gov/health/prof/lung/asthma/astpreg.htm Most medications commonly used to treat asthma (aside from the leukotriene antagonists) have considerable clinical experience with their use in pregnancy that suggests their safety and particularly justifies their use to control asthma in pregnancy. PMID: 17363831 PMID: 17181448 PMID: 16946229 PMID: 16443145 See also Chapter 1. The use of steroids in pregnancy is discussed in Chapter 47.

(Continued on p. 638)

Table 30.2 (Continued)

Condition or product type	Data suggest use justifiable when indicated	Data suggest use may be justifiable in unique circumstances	Data suggest rarely justifiable for indication listed	Useful review articles and comments
Constipation	Bisacodyl[C] Docusate Glycerin Psyllium Sodium biphosphate Magnesium hydroxide Sorbitol Mineral oil			PMID: 17889809. See also Chapter 10
Cough	Guaifenesin[C] Dextromethorphan[C] Albuterol[C] Codeine[C]			This review article discusses the treatment of the common cold in pregnancy: PMID: 18474699
Depression	Amitriptyline[D] Nortriptyline[D] Fluoxetine[C] Sertraline[C]	Sertraline[C] Fluvoxamine[C] Escitalopram[C] Citalopram[C] Venlafaxine[C] Mirtazapine[C] Paroxetine[C] (increasingly data suggest this agent may fall into the category to the right because of a small risk of both teratogenicity and neonatal syndromes)		General review of behavioral health PMID: 18378767 Bipolar affective disorder PMID: 17764378 Depression PMID: 18760228 Anxiety PMID: 17955910 Schizophrenia PMID: 12553132 See Chapter 21.
Diabetes	Insulin (human, beef or pork, Lispro)	Glyburide[B] has a developing role in the management of gestational diabetes as an alternative to insulin with comparable outcomes. PMID:18622055 Metformin[B] Use of this agent in early pregnancies of women with PCO syndrome is increasing. PMID: 19084097	Chlorpropamide[C] Tolbutamide[D] Glipizide	PMID: 19104375 PMID: 18297574 PMID: 17596473 See also Chapter 11.
Diarrhea	Loperamide[B] Diphenoxylate/atropine			PMID: 12635420 PMID: 16673005
Dyspepsia	Ranitidine[B] Famotidine[B] Nazitidine[C] Cimetidine[B] Sulcrafate[C] Antacids[B] Al(OH)$_3$, Mg(OH)$_2$, CaCO$_3$	Omeprazole[B] Lansoprazole[C] Esomeprazole[B]	Misoprostol[X]	PMID: 12635419 PMID: 11430180 Despite placing proton pump inhibitors in the second category here, they are widely used in pregnancy and published data suggest they are not a mojor teratogenic risk in humans. We recommend their use if agents in the first column are ineffective in controlling symptoms.
Headache	Acetaminophen Codeine[C] Meperidine[C] Morphine[C] Metoclopramide[B] Caffeine[C]	All NSAID[B/C] (intermittent use of NSAID in the second trimester may be justifiable) Butalbital[C]	Sumatriptan[C] Noratriptan[C] Rizatriptan[C] Zolmatriptan[C] A growing literature about the use of these agents (particularly sumatriptan) in human pregnancies may	These review articles summarize the data about the treatment of migraine in pregnancy: PMID: 18583683 PMID: 18345969 PMID: 18332840

Table 30.2 (Continued)

Condition or product type	Data suggest use justifiable when indicated	Data suggest use may be justifiable in unique circumstances	Data suggest rarely justifiable for indication listed	Useful review articles and comments
	For prophylaxis: amitryptiline[B] nortiptyline[D] beta-blockers[B,C]		eventually support their use as a second-line agent in pregnancy. PMID 10649172 Ergotamine[X] (although unlikely to be a teratogen, this agent is concerning for its potent vasoconstrictive and uterotonic effects)	An effective role for nonpharmacologic management with biofeedback, physical therapy and relaxation is suggested in this small trial: PMID: 8682668 See also Chapter 35.
Hypertension	Labetalol[C] Methyldopa[B] Pindolol[B] Other beta-blockers: acebutalol[B] all others (may want to avoid atenolol because of an association with IUGR) nifedipine[C] hydralazine[C]	Calcium channel blockers other than nifedipine[C] Clonidine[C] Prazosin[C] Hydrochlorothiazide[B] Diazoxide[C]	ACE inhibitors[D] Accupril, perindopril, ramipril, captopril, benazepril, trandolapril, fosinopril, lisinopril, moexipril, enalapril Angiotensin II antagonists[D] Eprosartan, telmisartan, valsartan, candesartan, irbesartan, valsartan	PMID: 15805801 PMID:18259046 See also Chapter 5.
Immunosuppressive agents	These agents are discussed in disease-specific contexts in the chapters dealing with inflammatory bowel disease, rheumotologic disease and transplants (Chapters 10, 8 and 7)			
Nasal congestion	Oxymetazoline[C] Nasal steroids Nasal cromolyn[B] Nasal ipratropium[B]	Pseudoephedrine[C]		PMID: 16579874 PMID: 16443148
Nausea and vomiting	Metoclopramide[B] Prochloperazine[C] Dimenhydrinate[B] Promethazine[C] Doxylamine plus pyridoxine	Ondansetron[B]		PMID: 17967157 PMID: 18077743 PMID: 17889806 Although ondansetron is commonly used to treat nausea and vomiting in pregnancy, the published experience is limited and the authors view it as a second-line agent. See also Chapter 48.
Pruritus	Topical: moisturizing creams and lotions oatmeal cream or powder calamine lotion topical glucocorticoids[C] Systemic: hydroxyzine[C] chlorpheniramine[B] diphenhydramine[B]			PMID: 2289340 PMID: 10396430 PMID: 12031026
Thrombosis	Heparin (both low molecular weight and unfractionated)	Fibrinolytics such as streptokinase[C] and tPA *altepase*[C8]	Warfarin[X] (*coumadin*™) This agent is believed by some to have a role in the management of prosthetic heart valves after the first trimester as it may be associated with a lower risk of prosthetic valve thrombosis. PMID: 10647757	PMID: 1918847 PMID: 18987370 See also Chapters 3 and 46.

(Continued on p. 640)

Table 30.2 (Continued)

Condition or product type	Data suggest use justifiable when indicated	Data suggest use may be justifiable in unique circumstances	Data suggest rarely justifiable for indication listed	Useful review articles and comments
Vaccines	Diphtheria[C] Tetanus[C] Hepatitis A[C] Hepatitis B[C] Influenza[C] Immune globulin[C] Inactivated polio vaccine[C] Tuberculin test[C]		"Live vaccines": MMR sabin polio vaccine (oral) varicella	General PMID: 14719841 Influenza and pertussis PMID: 18677141 Pertussis, tetanus, diphtheria PMID: 18509304 For travelers PMID: 18760249 See also Chapter 17.

Letter designations are US FDA pregnancy categories from individual product package inserts.
References in the final column of this table are listed by their PubMed identification number. The citation and abstract can be obtained by going to www.pubmed.gov and entering this number into the search function.
NOTE: Every patient and circumstance are different and the literature on medication use in pregnancy is continually evolving. This table does not constitute specific therapeutic recommendations and the reader is referred to the resources in Table 30.1 as a guide to therapeutic decisions.

using alternative medicines or herbs, or some combination of these. Expect to review the same issues over at every visit.

Conclusion

Every obstetrician knows that pregnancy is a complicated time. Managing the patient who also has a medical problem, whether acute and short-lived or chronic, adds to this immensely. When pharmacologic intervention becomes part of the patient's management, this is often a step that adds more anxiety for the obstetrician than the patient herself. Using basic principles of good care, following those highlighted in this chapter and employing sound scientific resources in making decisions will go a long way toward a strong relationship between you and your patient and improve the likelihood of a good outcome for all.

Disclaimer

Dr Kweder is an official of the US Food and Drug Administration. The opinions and recommendations in this publication do not reflect the views or official policies of the FDA or the US government.

Further reading

Briggs GS, Freeman R, Yaffe S, Medication in pregnancy and lactation, 8th edn. Lippincott Williams and Wilkins, Philadelphia, 2008.
Buhimschi CS, Weiner CP. Medications in pregnancy and lactation: part 1 teratology. Obstet Gynecol 2009;113(1):166–88.
Buhimschi CS, Weiner CP. Medications in pregnancy and lactation: part 2 drugs with minimal or unknown human teratogenic effect. Obstet Gynecol 2009;113(2 pt1):417–32.
Friedman JM, Polifka JE. Teratogenic effects of drugs: a resource for clinicians (TERIS), 2nd edn. Johns Hopkins University Press, Baltimore, MD, 2000.
Hale T. Medications and mothers' milk: a manual of lactational pharmacology, 13th edn. Hale Publishing, Amarillo TX, 2008.
Koren G. Medication safety in pregnancy and breastfeeding. McGraw-Hill Professional, New York, 2007.
Rosene-Montella K, Keely E, Barbour LA, Lee RV. Medical care of the pregnant patient, 2nd edn. American College of Physicians/American Society of Internal Medicine, Philadelphia, 2008.
Rubin PC, Ramsey M. Prescribing in pregnancy, 4th edn. BMJ Books, London, 2008.
Schaefer C, Peters PWJ, Miller RK. Drugs during pregnancy and lactation, 2nd edn. Academic Press, London, 2007.
Shepard TH, Lamire RJ. Catalog of teratogenic agents, 12th edn. John Hopkins University Press, Baltimore, MD, 2007.
Weiner CP, Buhimschi CS. Drugs for pregnant and lactating women. Churchill Livingstone, Philadelphia, 2004.

31 Prescribing during lactation

Thomas W. Hale[1] and Teresa Baker[2]

[1]Department of Pediatrics, Texas Tech University of Medicine, Amarillo, TX, USA
[2]Department of Obstetrics and Gynecology, Texas Tech University of Medicine, Amarillo, TX, USA

Introduction

The rate of breastfeeding worldwide has continued to increase since the early 1970s. Now approximately 77% of American women opt to breastfeed their infants, at least initially. In many other countries, breastfeeding rates approach 95%. It has simply become clear to mothers around the globe that breastfeeding provides the best source of nutrition for their infant. Key benefits to the infant include perfect nutrition, enhanced neurocognitive development, stronger immune function, and significant reductions in infectious disease such as upper respiratory infections, otitis media, sudden infant death syndrome, and necrotizing enterocolitis [1–8].

Breastmilk is packed with large quantities of secretory IgA, interferons, antimicrobial proteins such as lactoferrin, lysozyme, and lipopolysaccharides. The presence of numerous growth factors (IgF-1), cytokines and gastric hormones (gastrin, motilin) enhances development of protective barriers in the gastrointestinal (GI) tract and stimulates elimination of meconium present during gestation.

While recent studies have suggested that the number of women who choose to breastfeed their infant is rising, the number of women who discontinue breastfeeding in order to take a medication is simply too high. Surveys of Western countries indicate that 90–99% of women who breastfeed will receive a medication during the first week post partum [9]. Another study of Scandinavian women suggests that in mothers who discontinue breastfeeding, the use of medications is a major reason and that 17–25% of breastfeeding women in this study had taken a medication during the prior 2 weeks [10]. The most frequently used drugs included analgesics, hypnotics, and methylergometrine [11].

Because so many women ingest medications during the early neonatal period, is it not surprising that one of the most common questions encountered by pediatricians and obstetricians is concerning the use of specific drugs during lactation. While in the past two decades we have developed extensive literature on the transfer of drugs into human milk, little of this information seems to have transferred to the practicing clinician. Too often, clinicians simply read the package insert, which always suggests discontinuing breastfeeding. Discontinuing breastfeeding is often the wrong decision and most mothers could easily continue to breastfeed and take the medication without risk to the infant.

In the past 20 years, we have developed a proficient understanding of the kinetics of drug entry into human milk. Most of the properties of drugs that facilitate transfer (molecular weight, pKa, lipophilicity) are known, but ultimately the degree of transfer of the medication must be determined in humans. Rodent studies have proven virtually worthless in comparison to human studies.

The following review covers a basic model for understanding how drugs enter milk, and numerous recommendations for drugs of choice for breastfeeding mothers.

The alveolar subunit

The parenchyma of the breast consists of approximately 10–15 ductal regions which ultimately drain toward the nipple. The alveolar unit (Figure 31.1) is lined with a specialized epithelial cell, formerly called the alveolar epithelial cell but now called the lactocyte. The entire alveolar unit is thoroughly perfused with capillaries and lymphatics and is innervated with small nerves. Closely juxtaposed to the basal membrane of the alveolus are numerous capillaries that serve as the primary source of nutrients, fats, and many other components (including drugs) needed for the production of human milk. Surrounding the alveolus like a basket is a specialized smooth muscle cell called the myoepithelial cell. This contains receptor sites for oxytocin. Upon the release of oxytocin from the pituitary, the let-down process occurs and forces milk down the ductal system toward the nipple.

Plasma cells from the lymphatics surround the entire alveolar unit and provide most of the immunoglobins present in milk. Each day, an infant receives 800–1200 mg of secretory IgA and smaller amounts of IgM and IgG. Millions of living cells also

de Swiet's Medical Disorders in Obstetric Practice, 5th edition.
Edited by R. O. Powrie, M. F. Greene, W. Camann. © 2010 Blackwell Publishing.

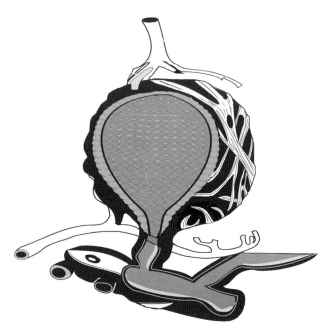

Figure 31.1 Typical mammary alveolus with secretory alveolar epithelium lining the lumen. Contractile myoepithelium cells are arrayed on the surface along with vascular supply. The alveolus empties into the mammary ductal system.

enter milk, including lymphocytes, T-cells, and macrophages, all of which function to prepare the infant gut for exposure to microbes.

Drug transfer into human milk

The ability of a medication to transfer into the milk compartment is largely determined by a few physicochemical properties, such as molecular weight, lipophilicity, plasma protein binding, and pKa. Maternal factors include the concentration of medication in the plasma compartment, with higher transfer at higher plasma levels (particularly C_{max}–the peak plasma concentration of a drug).

The transfer of drugs into human milk is usually facilitated by passive diffusion down a concentration gradient. In the breast tissue, only a few transport systems (for drugs) are known to exist. Thus, most drugs normally transfer from areas of high concentration (plasma) to areas of low concentration (milk) by passive diffusion between compartments. During the first few days post partum, drugs may transfer into milk at slightly higher concentrations due to the lack of a tight junctional system. The retrograde diffusion of drugs from the milk back into the plasma is well documented and is probably controlled by the same kinetic factors as entry (size, pKa, lipophilicity). As the maternal plasma level of medication increases, so does the transfer into milk. As the maternal plasma level of medication drops, most drugs diffuse out of the milk compartment and back into the maternal plasma for elimination. Few drugs

are actually trapped in milk but those that are include iodine, cimetidine and nitrofurantoin, among others.

The physicochemical factors most important include the following.
- *Molecular weight*: the lower the molecular weight, the more the drug enters the milk compartment. Drugs >800 daltons are virtually excluded from milk.
- *pKa*: drugs with a basic pKa may become highly ionized at the pH of milk (7.2) and thus become trapped in the milk compartment (e.g. barbiturates).
- *Protein binding*: as with any drug in any compartment, the more protein binding in the maternal plasma compartment, the less drug available for transfer into the milk compartment.
- *Lipid solubility*: lipid-soluble drugs diffuse more readily across cell membranes than water-soluble drugs. Lipid-soluble agents therefore will generally transfer more quickly and in greater amounts into breast milk than water-soluble agents.
- *Maternal C_{max}*: drugs that produce low levels in the plasma compartment produce even lower levels in the milk compartment. Thus topical or inhaled medications are ideal, as are those whose maternal plasma levels are miniscule.
- CNS active drugs invariably enter the milk compartment to some degree due to their ability to pass tight endothelial barriers. Thus expect milk levels from CNS active drugs (antidepressants, neuroleptics) to be higher.
- If the drug is poorly bio-available orally, expect uptake by the infant via milk to be negligible.

Bio-availability

For medications to produce systemic effects in the breastfeeding infant, they generally have to have some degree of oral bio-availability. The bio-availability of a medication generally refers to the amount of medication that is transluminally absorbed into the portal circulation and is able to pass the liver and enter the plasma compartment.

Because infants receive drugs via the mother's milk, oral bio-availability is of major importance in evaluating potential risks to the infant. Drugs that have poor bio-availability are ideal for breastfeeding mothers and their infants. Sumatriptan (15% bio-available) would be preferred over rizatriptan which is >45% bio-available. In some instances, however, the active medication may concentrate in the GI tract of the infant, causing problems (e.g. methotrexate, antibiotics). Diarrhea and thrush are a relatively uncommon (11%) but reported complication following the use of some antibiotics.

Calculating infant dose

Without exception, the most critical evaluation of drugs in breastfeeding mothers is calculating the estimated dose to the

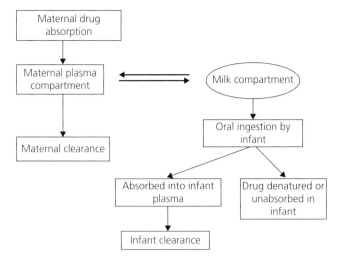

Figure 31.2 Compartmental representation of drug distribution and transfer into maternal plasma and the infant.

infant (D_{inf}) via milk. To do so, one must know the actual concentration of medication in the milk and the volume of milk transferred. While this is not always available for many drugs, we do have numerous studies providing the maximum concentration (C_{max}) or the average concentration (C_{av}) concentrations for various drugs. Many of the more recent studies now calculate the area under the curve (AUC) value for the medication. This methodology accurately estimates the average daily intake by the infant and is much more accurate than the C_{max} estimates.

Ultimately, the most clinically relevant method for determining the safety of the medication is to relate the weight-normalized dose received by the infant via milk. Termed the relative infant dose (RID), this value is generally expressed as a percentage of the mother's dose present in the mother's milk. It provides a standardized method of relating the infant's dose to the maternal dose. In full-term infants, many authors now recommend that a relative infant dose of <10% should be theoretically safe for most medications. While increasingly popular, the 10% level of concern is relative and each situation should be individually evaluated according to the overall toxicity of the medication, the oral bio-availability of the medication, and the ability of the infant to handle small amounts of the medication. Figure 31.2 provides a schematic of a step-wise approach to evaluate the relative risks of drugs in breastfeeding mothers.

Conclusion

All medications transfer into human milk to some degree. Fortunately, the amount transferred to the infant is often sub-clinical and the mother should almost always be advised to continue breastfeeding. Certain medications are obviously contraindicated, including anticancer agents, radio-active drugs, and those that specifically inhibit milk production,

Box 31.1 Lactation risk categories

L1 Safest

Drug which has been taken by a large number of breastfeeding mothers without any observed increase in adverse effects in the infant. Controlled studies in breastfeeding women fail to demonstrate a risk to the infant and the possibility of harm to the breastfeeding infant is remote or the product is not orally bio-available in an infant.

L2 Safer

Drug which has been studied in a limited number of breastfeeding women with either no increase in adverse effects in the infant and/or a demonstrated risk which is remote.

L3 Moderately safe

There are no controlled studies in breastfeeding women; however, the risk of untoward effects to a breastfed infant is possible or controlled studies show only minimal nonthreatening adverse effects. Drugs should be given only if the potential benefit justifies the potential risk to the infant.

L4 Possibly hazardous

There is positive evidence of risk to a breastfed infant or to breast milk production but the benefits from use in breastfeeding mothers may be acceptable despite the risk to the infant (e.g. if the drug is needed in a life-threatening situation or for a serious disease for which safer drugs cannot be used or are ineffective).

L5 Contraindicated

Studies in breastfeeding mothers have demonstrated that there is significant and documented risk to the infant based on human experience or it is a medication that has a high risk of causing significant damage to an infant. The risk of using the drug in breastfeeding women clearly outweighs any possible benefit from breastfeeding. The drug is contraindicated in women who are breastfeeding an infant.

Reproduced with permission from Hale [13].

but many are quite suitable for use in breastfeeding mothers (Box 31.1). Typical questions that need to be answered prior to using a medication are listed in Box 31.2.

However, in each case the clinician must first evaluate the relative risk to the infant by considering the absolute

Box 31.2 Questions to consider when prescribing to a breastfeeding mother

1. Is the medication really necessary? Avoid using medications where possible. Herbal drugs, high-dose vitamins, unusual supplements, etc. are simply not necessary; recommend avoiding the risk.

2. If the RID is less than 10%, most medications are quite safe to use. The RID of the vast majority of drugs is <1%.

3. How old is the infant? Older infants are able to handle small levels of medications quite adequately. With an unstable premature infant or a 1-week-old infant, be more cautious. After 6 months of age, the risk is negligible. After 1.5–2 years of breastfeeding, the risk is remote.

4. Is this drug safe or quite dangerous? Is it given to infants all the time (amoxicillin) or is it a toxic drug such as an anticancer or radio-active drug? More hazardous drugs may require periods of interruption before returning to breastfeeding.

5. Is this a drug for which we have breastfeeding information? Choose those drugs with good information available.

6. What volume of breast milk is the mother providing the infant? After 6 months the volume of milk starts to decline significantly. After 1 year the volume is often less than 100–200 mL/day or even less in many mothers. Low milk volumes mean low drug doses via milk.

7. Most drugs are quite safe in breastfeeding mothers while the risks of not breastfeeding and of using infant formulas are much higher for the infant.

or relative dose transferred via milk to the infant, but also the risk to the infant of not breastfeeding. Higher rates of GI syndromes, upper respiratory tract infection, and other diseases are now well documented in formula-fed infants. Other infant factors that must be included are the existence of prematurity, weakness, apnea, contraindicated medications or other factors that would reduce the ability of the infant to tolerate even low levels of maternal medications.

Often, the amount of medication delivered to the infant via milk is far less than 1% of the maternal dose, and the amount the infant actually absorbs orally is probably even less. In healthy, term infants, this amount is often easily tolerated without untoward effects. However, as the RID rises above 7–10% and the toxicity of the medication increases, the clinician should be more cautious in recommending breastfeeding.

In almost all situations, there are numerous medications that can be safely used for specific syndromes and should be carefully chosen with the breastfeeding mother in mind. This is not always difficult to do, as we now have hundreds of studies concerning medications and their use in breastfeeding mothers. Almost invariably, a more suitable drug can be chosen so that a mother can continue to breastfeed her infant. Some helpful resources for guiding clinicians with drug choices during lactation are listed in the references [12–22]. See also the Appendix at the end of this book, which reviews the lactation safety classification of most commonly used medications organized by clinical indication as an additional useful resource for clinicians prescribing to lactating women.

But most importantly, breast milk is the most beneficial nutrition a mother can give her infant. The immunologic and health benefits for both the mother and infant are now overwhelmingly documented in the literature. Interrupting breastfeeding for unsound reasoning, such as to take a relatively safe medication, should be avoided if at all possible.

References

1. Goldman AS, Hopkinson JM, Rassin DK. Benefits and risks of breastfeeding. Adv Pediatr 2007:54:275–304.
2. Cochi SL, Fleming DW, Hightower AW, Limpakarnjanarat K, Facklam RR, Smith JD, *et al*. Primary invasive Haemophilus influenzae type b disease: a population-based assessment of risk factors. J Pediatr 1986;108(6):887–96.
3. Ford RP, Taylor BJ, Mitchell EA, Enright SA, Stewart AW, Becroft DM, *et al*. Breastfeeding and the risk of sudden infant death syndrome. Int J Epidemiol 1993;22(5):885–90.
4. Goldman AS. The immune system of human milk: antimicrobial, antiinflammatory and immunomodulating properties. Pediatr Infect Dis J 1993;12(8):664–71.
5. Goldman AS, Chheda S, Keeney SE, Schmalstieg FC, Schanler RJ. Immunologic protection of the premature newborn by human milk. Semin Perinatol 1994;18(6):495–501.
6. Pisacane A, Graziano L, Mazzarella G, Scarpellino B, Zona G. Breast-feeding and urinary tract infection. J Pediatr 1992;120(1):87–9.
7. Turck D. Later effects of breastfeeding practice: the evidence Nestle Nutr Workshop Ser Pediatr Program 2007;60:31–9; discussion 39–42.
8. Depatrment of Health and Human Services Office on Women's Health. Benefits of breastfeeding. Nutr Clin Care 2003:6(3):125–31.
9. Bennett PN. Use of the monographs on drugs. In: Drugs and human lactation, 2nd edn. Elsevier, Amsterdam, 1996: 67–74.
10. Matheson I, Kristensen K, Lunde PK. Drug utilization in breast-feeding women. A survey in Oslo. Eur J Clin Pharmacol 1990;38(5):453–9.
11. Matheson I. Drugs taken by mothers in the puerperium. BMJ (Clin Res Ed) 1985;290(6481):1588–9.
12. Hale TW, Berens PD. Clinical therapy in breastfeeding patients, 2nd edn. Hale Publishing, Amarillo, TX, 2003.
13. Hale TW. Medications and mothers' milk, 13th edn. Hale Publishing, Amarillo, TX, 2008.
14. Buhimschi CS, Weiner CP. Medications in pregnancy and lactation: Part 2. Drugswith minimal or unknown human teratogenic effect. Obstet Gynecol 2009;113(2 Pt 1):417–32.

15. Buhimschi CS, Weiner CP. Medications in pregnancy and lactation: part 1. Teratology. Obstet Gynecol 2009;113(1): 166–88.

16. Berlin CM, Briggs GG. Drugs and chemicals in human milk. Semin Fetal Neonatal Med 2005;10(2):149–59.

17. Hale TW. Maternal medications during breastfeeding. Clin Obstet Gynecol 2004;47(3):696–711.

18. Koren G. Medication safety in pregnancy and breastfeeding. McGraw-Hill, New York, 2007.

19. Weiner CP, Buhimschi CS. Drugs for pregnant and lactating women. Churchill Livingstone, Philadelphia, 2004.

20. Schaefer C, Peters PWJ, Miller RK. Drugs during pregnancy and lactation, 2nd edn. Academic Press, London, 2007.

21. Rubin PC, Ramsey M. Prescribing in pregnancy, 4th edn. BMJ Books, London, 2008.

22. Briggs GS, Freeman R, Yaffe S. Medication in pregnancy and lactation, 8th edn. Lippincott Williams and Wilkins, Philadelphia, 2008.

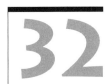

Diagnostic imaging in pregnancy

Sandra A. Lowe

Department of Medicine, Royal Hospital For Women and School of Women's and Children's Health, University of New South Wales, Sydney, Australia

Introduction

The pregnant woman is susceptible to the specific consequences and complications of pregnancy as well as the full array of medical events that may occur unrelated to the pregnancy. In many cases, some form of diagnostic imaging will be required to assess or manage these conditions. The selection and application of the most appropriate imaging modalities will often require a multidisciplinary approach involving obstetricans, maternal-fetal medicine specialists, internists, surgeons and radiologists. This must take into account the clinical situation as well as the risks and benefits of the various forms of diagnostic imaging: ultrasound, X-ray, computed tomography (CT), radionucleotide scanning or magnetic resonance imaging (MRI). Although this chapter focuses on what is known about the safety of various modalities of diagnostic imaging in pregnancy, it is worth emphasizing that both the available data and broad clinical experience suggest that more harm is likely to be caused to pregnant women and their fetuses by withholding diagnostic imaging than by its judicious application.

Absorbed dose

X-rays and gamma rays ionize tissue through the deposition of energy. This is the first step in a series of events that may subsequently lead to genetic and/or biologic effects Environmental exposures [1] (Table 32.1), diagnostic [2] imaging techniques including X-ray, fluoroscopy, angiography, mammography, positron emission tomography (PET), single photon emission computed tomography (SPECT), computed tomography (CT) and most nuclear medicine procedures involve exposure to ionizing radiation. Any adverse effects of ionizing radiation on the outcome of pregnancy are dependent on the fetal radiation dose, the timing of exposure and the form of administration.

de Swiet's Medical Disorders in Obstetric Practice, 5th edition.
Edited by R. O. Powrie, M. F. Greene, W. Camann. © 2010 Blackwell Publishing.

Radiation is measured in three distinct ways:
• the amount being given off or emitted by a radioactive material (measured in curie or becquerel)
• the amount deposited per unit of weight of human tissue (the "absorbed dose" measured in rad, milligray or gray)
• the biologic risk of the exposure (measured in rem or sievert). Absorbed dose and biologic risk are different depending on the type of radiation (alpha and beta particles, gamma rays and X-rays), and the particular tissue receiving the dose. This is because the different types of radiation have variable ability to transfer energy into the cells of the body.

Biologic risk of exposure, expressed as sieverts, is most often used when discussing radiation protection, particularly in environmental or occupational contexts. The radiation dose of interest in discussions about diagnostic imaging in pregnancy is the absorbed dose in grays or rads. (One Gy is equal to 1000 mGy is equal to 100 rad.) In assessing the potential effects of radiation in pregnancy, it is necessary to calculate both the maternal dose to a particular site as well as the estimated fetal absorbed dose. The remainder of this chapter will review what is known about the exposure risks to various common diagnostic imaging modalities.

Ultrasound and magnetic resonance imaging

Imaging techniques that do not involve electromagnetic radiation, i.e. ultrasound and MRI, are considered safe in pregnancy. The UK National Radiological Protection Board has recommended that "until further information becomes available, it is considered prudent to exclude pregnant women from NMR studies during the first 3 months of pregnancy. However, MR diagnostic procedures should be considered where the only reasonable alternative is an X-ray procedure" [4]. For MRI, gadolinium is used as a tracer to enhance imaging of vascular tissue or abnormal tissue. Gadolinium is teratogenic in high doses in animal studies, but a number of studies have evaluated the administration of gadolinium contrast material during human pregnancy and reported no obvious harmful effects. Administration of gadolinium

Table 32.1 Background/environmental radiation exposure

Environmental source	Exposure
Cosmic, gamma and radon	Varies from 1.8 mSv/yr in the UK and Australia to 7.8 mSv/yr in Finland
Occupational exposures in workplaces that involve radiation	Most safety laws limit radiation exposure during gestation to <20 mSv and <100 mSv/5years
Cosmic radiation with air travel	0.001–0.003 mSv/h on short-haul routes and up to 0.005 mSv/h on long haul
Nuclear accidents such as Chernobyl 1986	10–50 mSv over the subsequent 20 years (thyroid doses much higher) [3]

Table 32.2 Approximate fetal doses from common diagnostic procedures [7–10]

	Mean in mGy	Maximum in mGy
Conventional X-rays		
Abdomen	1.4 mGy (0.014 rad)	4.2 mGy (0.042 rad)
Chest	<0.01 (<0.0001 rad)	<0.01 (0.0001 rad)
Intravenous pyelogram	1.7 (0.017 rad)	10 (0.1 rad)
Lumbar spine	1.7 (0.17 rad)	10 (1 rad)
Pelvis	1.1 (0.11 rad)	4 (0.4 rad)
Skull	<0.01 (0.001 rad)	<0.01(0.01 rad)
Thoracic spine	<0.01 (0.001 rad)	<0.01 (0.001 rad)
DEXA posterior anterior spine	1.7 (0.17 rad)	4.9 (0.49 rad)
DEXA proximal femur	1.0 (0.1 rad)	2.7 (0.27 rad)
Fluoroscopic examinations		
Barium meal	1.1 (0.11 rad)	5.8 (0.58 rad)
Barium enema	6.8 (0.68 rad)	24 (2.4 rad)
ERCP	400 (40 rad)	1800 (180 rad)
Computed tomography		
Abdomen	8.0 (0.8 rad)	49 (4.9 rad)
Chest	0.06 (0.006 rad)	0.5 (0.05 rad)
Helical chest	<0.01 (0.001 rad)	0.13 (0.013 rad)
Head	<0.005 (0.0005 rad)	<0.005 (0.0005 rad)
Lumbar spine	2.4 (0.24 rad)	8.6 (0.86 rad)
Pelvis	25 (2.5 rad)	79 (7.9 rad)
Pelvimetry	0.2 (0.02 rad)	0.4 (0.04 rad)

DEXA, dual energy X-ray absorptiometry.

contrast material in the first trimester should therefore be avoided where possible. In practice, contrast material is of limited usefulness in most obstetric applications (with the exception of assessing placenta accreta) and would more likely be required for an extra-abdominal indication such as a suspected maternal brain tumor. In such a situation, the maternal benefits would probably outweigh the potential fetal risks. Both the American College of Radiology and the European Society of Urogenital Radiology have stated there is no requirement to cease breastfeeding following the administration of gadolinium to a lactating woman as excretion of gadolinium into breast milk is extremely limited.

Fetal absorbed radiation with X-rays and computed tomography

In estimating the absorbed dose to the fetus, a number of techniques have been used. Dosimetry surveys even within a particular country have been found to vary by a factor of up to 30 or more for the same examination. With fluoroscopy, e.g. for uterine artery embolization, endoscopic retrograde cholangiopancreatography (ERCP) or other procedures, additional factors such as location of the beam, duration of screening, magnification and conventional versus pulsed fluoroscopy will influence dose. Digital radiography techniques may reduce fetal absorbed dose considerably. In a study of X-ray pelvimetry, the use of digital radiography reduced fetal absorbed dose by 85% [5]. Estimations of fetal absorbed dose from CT examinations vary considerably, depending on the method used [6]. In addition to the radiation technique, site and dose administered, factors such as maternal thickness will influence the fetal absorbed dose following X-rays and CT scanning. Table 32.2 presents approximate fetal absorbed doses for a number of common radiologic procedures. Conventional X-ray examinations beyond the abdomen/pelvis are associated with a negligible fetal absorbed dose, related to scatter or leakage radiation. More direct examinations, particularly those with fluoroscopy such as barium enemas, are associated with a more significant fetal absorbed dose.

Fetal absorbed radiation with nuclear medicine imaging

In the case of nuclear medicine and PET studies, fetal absorbed dose will represent the cumulative effect of external irradiation from the maternal tissues as well as placental transfer and fetal uptake of radiopharmaceuticals (Table 32.3). The majority of radiopharmaceuticals are excreted in urine and irradiation from maternal bladder contents may be a more important source of fetal radiation. Hence, measures aimed at increasing the rate of urinary excretion may reduce the fetal absorbed dose significantly. Using smaller administered doses and longer imaging times can significantly reduce the fetal absorbed dose.

The special case of I^{131} and I^{123} requires specific mention. Radio-iodine crosses the placenta readily and the fetal thyroid begins to accumulate iodine from about 12 weeks after the last menstrual period. In early pregnancy, the major risk is from gamma radiation from the maternal bladder whilst after 12 weeks, the fetal thyroid dose is much greater than the fetal whole-body dose due to the avidity of the fetal thyroid for iodine. If therapeutic doses of radio-iodine are inadvertently given to a pregnant woman, there is a significant risk of fetal thyroid damage after 12 weeks gestation. If pregnancy is confirmed shortly after dose administration, maternal hydration

Table 32.3 Fetal whole-body dose from common radiopharmaceuticals in early pregnancy and at term. Dose includes maternal and fetal self-dose contributions [8,9,11,13]

		Administered activity (MBq)	Early pregnancy (mGy)	Late pregnancy (mGy)
^{99m}Tc	Bone scan	750	4.6–4.7 (0.46–0.47 rad)	1.8 (0.18 rad)
^{99m}Tc	Lung perfusion MAA	200	0.4–0.6 (0.04–0.06 rad)	0.8 (0.08 rad)
^{99m}Tc	Lung ventilation	40	0.1–0.3 (0.01–0.03 rad)	0.1 (0.01 rad)
^{99m}Tc	Thyroid scan	400	3.2–4.4 (0.32–0.44 rad)	3.7 (0.37 rad)
^{99m}Tc	Red blood cell	930	3.6–6.0 (0.36–0.6 rad)	2.5 (0.25 rad)
^{99m}Tc	Liver colloid	300	0.5–0.6 (0.05–0.06 rad)	1.1 (0.11 rad)
^{99m}Tc	Renal DTPA	750	5.9–9.0 (0.59–0.9 rad)	3.5 (0.35 rad)
^{67}Ga	Abcess/tumor	190	14–18 (1.4–1.8 rad)	25 (2.5 rad)
^{123}I	Thyroid therapy[a]	30	0.4–0.6 (0.04–0.06 rad)	0.3 (0.03 rad)
^{131}I	Thyroid therapy[a]	0.55	0.03–0.04 (0.003–0.004 rad)	0.15 (0.015 rad)
^{131}I	Metastases imaging[a]	40	2.0–2.9 (0.2–0.29 rad)	11.0 (1.1 rad)
^{51}Cr	Glomerular filtration estimation		Mean <0.01 (<0.001 rad)	Max. 0.01 (0.001 rad)
^{201}Tl	Thyroid, myocardium		Mean 3.7 (0.37 rad)	Max. 4.0 (0.4 rad)
^{18}F-FDG	Tumor localization	185–555	4–12 (0.4–1.2 rad)	3.1–9.4 (0.31–0.94 rad)

[a]Fetal thyroid doses are much higher than fetal whole-body dose.
DTPA, diethylenetriamine pentaacetic acid; FDG, fluorodeoxyglucose; MAA, macroaggregated albumin.

and frequent voiding should be encouraged and potassium iodide may be given as a thyroid-blocking agent. The total fetal absorbed dose is still likely to be <100 mGy (<10 rads).

Risks of radiation in pregnancy

Experimental assessments of radiation effects have identified a number of specific areas of potential concern:
- lethality
- teratogenicity
- intrauterine growth restriction
- mental retardation
- oncogenicity
- genetic damage
- sterility.

Radiation effects may be classified as either deterministic or stochastic. Cell killing leading to fetal death, gross malformation, developmental abnormalities or growth retardation is a *deterministic* event, i.e. there is a threshold dose below which no effect is seen and the higher the dose, the greater the effect. In comparison, malignancy and chromosomal abnormalities are *stochastic* effects, i.e. the absorbed dose influences the probability but not the severity of the effect.

Fetal effects of high-dose radiation

Excessive radiation doses to the fetus have been associated with all of the outcomes listed in Table 32.4. However, many of these data relate to massive radiation exposure in the experimental setting or from inadvertent exposure related to radiation therapy or nuclear events. The study of the radiation effects in Hiroshima and Nagasaki suggests an increase

in cancer in individuals heavily exposed to radiation *in utero* [14]. There was also an increased incidence of small head size and mental retardation which may have been a specific response to "fission neutron" exposure [15]. The Japanese bomb survivors and inhabitants of areas with high background radiation have shown no significant excess of known genetic disorders [8]. Reassuringly for the clinician, in most cases, a threshold dose exists below which these effects have not been demonstrated and the vast majority of diagnostic imaging procedures expose the fetus to a dose well below these thresholds.

More than 20 years since the nuclear accident at Chernobyl, there has been no detectable effect on fertility, numbers of stillbirths, adverse pregnancy outcomes or delivery complications in that period. A modest but steady increase in reported congenital malformations in both contaminated and uncontaminated areas of Belarus appears related to improved reporting and not to radiation exposure. The excessive thyroid radiation doses have led to a substantial and persistent increase in the rate of thyroid cancer in the areas affected by Chernobyl [3]. The most recent review by the International Commission for Radiation Protection states that with regard to fetal malformation, CNS damage and death, "a threshold of 100–200 mGy (10–20 rad) or higher" exists for all gestations [12]. This is well in excess of the fetal absorbed doses associated with most diagnostic imaging.

Radiation and genetic damage

The risk of developing genetic disease in all future generations after irradiation with a dose of 10 mGy has been estimated as between 0.012 and 0.099%. This compares with the risk of detecting chromosomal damage in a 35-year-old

Table 32.4 Estimated threshold and median radiation dose associated with adverse effects from radiation [8,12]

	Threshold in mGy (rad)	Median dose in mGy (rad)	Gestational sensitivity
Lethality	100 (10 rad)	1000 (100)	Preimplantation
Teratogenicity	100–200 (10–20 rad)	1000	First trimester
Mental retardation	300–900 (30–90 rad)	25 IQ points/1000	8–25 weeks
Growth impairment	250–500 (25–50 rad)	N/A	All
Cancer	No threshold	Excess absolute risk 0.006% (6 more cancers per 10,000 exposures of 1mGy or 0.1 rad when compared with background rates of exposure)	All, but greatest in first trimester
Genetic damage	Not available	1000	Not available
Sterility	Not available	1000	All

woman of 2.26% [8]. Although small changes in the rate of chromosomal damage are impossible to estimate, no radiation-induced transmissible gene mutations have ever been demonstrated unequivocally in humans.

Radiation and oncogenicity

A large number of epidemiologic studies have been performed to assess the possible effects of prenatal radiation on the incidence of malignant disease. All are flawed by problems such as retrospectivity, small study size, inadequate or inappropriate case and control selection, and variability in the determination of radiation exposure and measurement of outcome parameters. At least part of the increased risk associated with irradiation could be accounted for by the fact that mothers with a higher incidence of illness during pregnancy (a susceptibility which might be associated with an increased risk of tumor in their offspring) had a greater incidence of exposure to diagnostic radiation. In their most recent review, Wakeford & Little concluded "the reality of the statistical association between childhood cancer and antenatal X-ray exposure is not doubted but its explanation remains contentious" [16].

The largest study in this area remains the case–control study of Bithell & Stewart, now known as the Oxford Survey of Childhood Cancer (OSCC) [17]. Radiation exposure data both *in utero* and in childhood was obtained by patient recall although subsequent assessment of the medical records demonstrated the relative accuracy of this method. From this study, the relative risk for leukaemia prior to the age of 10 was 1.92 (95% confidence intervals 1.12–3.28) for women having abdominal radiation and 1.19 (0.63–2.16) for non-abdominal X-ray examinations. For all malignant disease the corresponding relative risks were 2.28 (1.31–3.97) and 1.15 (0.68–1.94). In 1962, McMahon reported a case–control study performed in the US using chart review to determine the radiation exposure *in utero* and reported similar findings [18].

Most of the studies in which a significant risk of oncogenicity was found failed to establish an association between the dose of radiation and the oncogenic effects. The exception was again the OSCC which interpolated a linear relationship between dose of radiation and excess risk of malignancy. At a dose of "one film," the estimated excess risk was approximately 0.3 (0.1–0.6), rising to 1.0 (0.5–3.0) with a dose of five films, an excess relative risk of 0.194 per film. The very crude measurement of dose based on numbers of films and the very large confidence intervals of these results must cast some doubt on their assumptions. In the large study by MacMahon, no significant association between radiation dose and cancer mortality was detected. However, there is some circumstantial evidence that improvement in radiographic techniques and reductions in radiation doses since the 1950s have been associated with a decreasing incidence of cancer deaths amongst children. However, these data do not indicate whether this association is causal. Against the proposition are the results from Hiroshima, the lack of specificity of the malignancies experienced and the data from a number of case–control and twin studies.

Dividing cells are more sensitive to injury from radiation than other cells and therefore it might be postulated that the rapidly growing fetus might be particularly susceptible to radiation, particularly in the first trimester. In general, the highest radiation exposures were in women in early pregnancy, before confirmation of the pregnancy. Although the studies of both MacMahon and Stewart suggest an increased risk at these times, the small numbers involved do not allow a statistically significant risk ratio to be determined. Court Brown *et al.* also noted that amongst the offspring of the 750 pregnant women identified as having been irradiated in the first trimester, there were no cases of leukemia with an average follow-up period of 6 years [19].

The increase in total malignancy associated with radiation is in contrast to the effects of postnatal radiation in which there has been a specific association with leukaemia. The excess risk per mGy is also much greater for *in utero* exposure, predominantly third trimester, than for child-hood exposure. In the studies by Bithell & Stewart [17] and MacMahon [18], there was no excess risk of leuke-mia (compared to other malignancies) although in another study such an increased risk was found [20]. Diamond *et al.* concluded that the relative risk of leukemia amongst white children was increased in fetuses exposed to radiation com-pared with nonexposed controls. This statement was based on an incidence of 10 cases of leukemia amongst approxi-mately 30,000 children: six cases in the exposed group and four in the control group. There was no excess of leuke-mia deaths amongst black children in the same study. They postulated that this may reflect either differences in the selection of subjects amongst the white group or possibly some difference in the susceptibility to radiation damage amongst white and black fetuses. Kaplan found a signifi-cantly increased risk of leukemia when radiation-exposed children were compared with their nonexposed siblings but not when compared with a control group derived from their playmates [21]. Harvey *et al.* reported the converse in a study of twins in which the relative risk ratio of solid cancers was greater than that for leukemia [22]. Hopton *et al.* identified two important diagnostic subgroups with a significantly high incidence of *in utero* radiation expo-sure: children dying of leukemia aged less than 2 years (RR 4.96; 1.39–17.7) and cases of the rare tumor histiocytosis X (RR 6.2; 1.89–19.99) [23]. This was not confirmed in the studies by Stewart or MacMahon. Stewart also noted an exceptional risk of teratoma in 12 women exposed to greater than "seven films."

Most cohort studies have failed to detect an association between radiation exposure *in utero* and malignancy. More recently, two European case–control studies with database ascertainment of cancer cases and comprising a total of 3289 case–control pairs have failed to demonstrate any association between recalled radiation exposure in pregnancy and risk of childhood malignancy [24,25]. This compares with 15,276 case–control pairs in the most recent OSCC.

In summary, although there are some inconsistencies in these studies, they do suggest that diagnostic imaging of the abdomen/pelvis (but not other sites) with fetal expo-sure is associated with a small but recognizable increased risk of malignancy, which is probably dose related. The UK National Radiological Protection Board has adopted an excess absolute risk coefficient for cancer incidence under 15 years of age following low-dose irradiation *in utero* of 0.006% per mGy compared with a risk of 0.0018% per mGy for a dose received just after birth. This assumes there is no threshold dose below which the risk is not increased (Table 32.5). However, in absolute terms, for an individual, this represents an additional one excess cancer death per 1700 children exposed *in utero* to 10 mGy dose [8]. The risk is equal in the second and third trimesters but may be greater in the first trimester than later in pregnancy.

Table 32.5 Probability of bearing healthy children as a function of radiation dose [28]

Dose to conceptus above natural background	Probability of NO malformation	Probability of NO cancer by age 19
0 mGy (0 rad)	97	99.7
1 mGy (0.1 rad)	97	99.7
5 mGy (0.5 rad)	97	99.7
10 mGy (1 rad)	97	99.6
50 mGy (5 rad)	97	99.4
100 mGy (10 rad)	97	99.1
>100 mGy (>10 rad)	Possible increased risk but may require doses >100 mGy (20 rad) to increase risk of malformation	Higher

Timing and fetal effects of radiation

During the preimplantation period (up to 2 weeks post con-ception), the embryo is most sensitive to the lethal effects of radiation but not to its teratogenic or growth-restricting effects. This means that the outcome after a significant expo-sure is either a normal conceptus or complete fetal resorption. The cells of the preimplantation stage are pluripotent; if a small number of cells are damaged, other cells multiply and take their place. However, if too many cells are dam-aged, the embryo does not survive [26]. In contrast, older studies have suggested somewhat surprisingly that low-dose radiation exposure *in utero* (estimated 10–50 mGy, i.e. 1–5 rad) has been associated with an increased fertility rate of 10–15% [12].

During organogenesis (weeks 3–15), the embryo is very sensitive to the teratogenic and growth-restricting effects of radiation. Because some limitations on growth can be "made up for" by the infant after birth, the most significant lasting effect in a liveborn infant exposed to significant radiation at this stage is malformation. In the second and third trimesters, the fetus is most sensitive to the growth-restricting effects of radiation, and malformations are unlikely. However, massive doses of radiation (500–1000 mGy) may have cell-depleting effects on the central nervous system, leading to microceph-aly and mental retardation. None of these adverse effects would be expected with the level of radiation associated with diagnostic imaging.

Iodinated contrast

A number of X-ray and CT procedures require the adminis-tration of contrast agents containing iodine. In radiocontrast media, the amount of inorganic iodine available to interfere with thyroid metabolism is about 0.1% of the dose adminis-tered. Nonionic contrast agents have been shown to cross the placenta and inhibit type II and III de-iodinases which can reduce intracellular tri-iodothyronine. In addition, depending on the dose of iodine, there is potential to blockade the fetal thyroid, in a manner similar to radio-iodine. The most recent European guidelines recommend that iodinated contrast agents be restricted to circumstances when radiographic examination is essential. Neonatal assessment should be performed within 1 week of delivery to assess for the small risk of fetal/neonatal hypothyroidism. Only very small amounts of iodinated contrast agent are excreted into the breast milk and even less is absorbed via the oral route. Hence, there is no requirement to cease breastfeeding following radiographic examinations involving the use of iodinated contrast agents.

Maternal risks from radiation in pregnancy

In the selection of the best diagnostic imaging modality during pregnancy, precedence is generally given to that technique which results in the minimum fetal dose. However, in certain situations, the maternal radiation risks will also need to be factored into the decision. CT pulmonary angiography (CTPA) is generally accepted as the recommended initial lung imaging modality for nonmassive pulmonary embolus. Ventilation-perfusion scanning may be considered as an alternative when the chest X-ray is normal and there is no intercurrent cardiac or pulmonary disease. This is often the case in pregnant or postpartum women with suspected pulmonary embolus. Numerous attempts have been made to compare the fetal radiation dose from CTPA versus ventilation-perfusion scanning for the detection of pulmonary embolus during pregnancy.

Most recent estimates indicate a fetal absorbed dose of <0.01 mGy (0.001 rad) for CTPA versus 0.12 mGy (0.012 rad) for low-dose perfusion scanning. Both these would be considered negligible doses and of no risk to the fetus [27]. However, the absorbed dose to the maternal breast was 10 mGy (1 rad) for CTPA and only 0.28 mGy (0.028 rad) from perfusion scanning. This can be reduced by the use of appropriate shielding. The risk of breast cancer is increased by radiation with an estimated additional risk of 18/million/mGy (180/million/rad). It is likely that the pregnant breast might be especially sensitive to such radiation, so the selection of the most appropriate imaging for the detection of pulmonary embolus needs to take into account the maternal as well as fetal risks. Magnetic resonance angiography (MRA) where available should also be considered as an alternative option in this setting.

Informed consent

For practical purposes, no specific counseling is required for women undergoing diagnostic imaging with a predicted fetal absorbed dose of less than 10 mGy. This includes all X-ray and CT scanning not involving the abdomen. For direct exposures or nuclear scanning with a potential exposure >10 mGy, women should be counseled on a risk/benefit basis. The specific risk appears to be childhood malignancy but, as described above, for each 10 mGy exposure, theoretical projections suggest a maximum risk of one additional cancer death per 1700 exposures. Balanced with this is the benefit of the imaging in terms of management of the maternal condition. Typical examples include ureteric obstruction requiring an IVP, trauma to the abdomen or malignancy. There are no diagnostic X-ray, CT or nuclear medicine procedures that can be considered a risk factor for genetic damage, congenital malformation or developmental effects based on current knowledge.

In general, the clinician ordering the imaging should be responsible for counseling the patient and obtaining informed consent in consultation with the radiologist or nuclear physician. The treating clinician must also take into account the total cumulative dose to the fetus if more than one procedure is undertaken. It is particularly important to liaise with the radiologist or nuclear physician to ensure that the most appropriate imaging is performed to obtain maximal information with minimal fetal absorbed dose. If possible, diagnostic imaging involving radiation should be delayed until after delivery if the information is not likely to alter immediate management. Alternatives such as ultrasound and MRI should be considered if appropriate.

References

1. www.epa.gov. United States Environmental Protection Agency.
2. Lowe SA. Diagnostic radiology in pregnancy: risks and reality. Aust NZ J Obstet Gynaecol 2004;44:191–6.
3. Bennett B, Repacholi M, Carr Z (eds). Health effects of the Chernobyl Accident and Special Health Care Programmes: report of the UN Chernobyl Forum Health Expert Group. World Health Organization, Geneva, 2006.
4. Saunders RD. Limits on patient and volunteer exposure during clinical magnetic resonance diagnostic procedures. Radiol Protect Bull 1991;125:20–4.
5. Claussen C, Kohler D, Christ F, et al. Pelvimetry by digital radiography and its dosimetry. J Perinat Med 1985;13(6):287–92.
6. Damilakis J, Perisinakis K, Voloudaki A, Gourtsoyiannin N. Estimation of fetal radiation dose from computed tomography scanning in late pregnancy. Invest Radiol 2000;35(9):527–33.
7. Damilakis J, Perisinakis K, Vrahoriti H, et al. Embryo/fetus radiation dose and risk from dual X-ray absorptiometry examinations. Osteoporos Int 2002;13(9):716–22.
8. Valentin J. Pregnancy and medical radiation. ICRP Publication 84. Ann ICRP 2000;30(1):1–43.
9. www.hpa.org.uk/radiation/publications/documents_of_nrpb/abstracts/absd4–4.htm#statement
10. Kahaleh M, Hartwell GD, Arseneau KO, et al. Safety and efficacy of ERCP in pregnancy. Gastrointest Endosc 2005;60(2):287–92.
11. Stabin MG. Proposed addendum to previously published fetal dose estimate tables for 18F-FDG. J Nucl Med 2004;45(4):634–5.
12. Valentin J. Biologic effects after prenatal irradiation (embryo and fetus). Ann ICRP 2003;33(1–2):1–206.

13. Steenvorde P, Pauwels EKJ, Harding LK, *et al*. Diagnostic nuclear medicine and risks for the fetus. Eur J Nucl Med 1998;25(2):193–9.
14. Yoshimoto Y, Kato H, Schull WJ. Risk of cancer among children exposed in utero to A-bomb radiations, 1950–84. Radiation Effects Research Foundation, Hiroshima, Japan. Lancet 1988;2(8612):665–9.
15. Miller RW, Blot WJ. Small head size after in utero exposure to atomic radiation. Lancet 1982;2:784–7.
16. Wakeford R, Little MP. Childhood cancer after low-level intrauterine exposure to radiation. J Radiol Prot 2002;22(3A):A123–7.
17. Bithell JF, Stewart AM. Prenatal irradiation and childhood malignancy. A review of British data from the Oxford survey. Br J Cancer 1975;31:271–87.
18. MacMahon B. Prenatal X-ray exposure and childhood cancer. J Natl Cancer Inst 1962;38:1173–91.
19. Court Brown WM, Doll R, Bradford Hill A. Incidence of leukaemia after exposure to diagnostic radiation in utero. BMJ 1960;2:1539–45.
20. Diamond EL, Schmerler H, Lilienfield AM. The relationship of intrauterine radiation to subsequent mortality and development of leukaemia in children. Am J Epidemiol 1973;97:283–313.
21. Kaplan HS. An evaluation of the somatic and genetic hazards of the medical uses of radiation. Am J Roentgenol 1958;80:696–705.
22. Harvey EB, Boice JD, Honeyman M, *et al*. Prenatal X-ray exposure and childhood cancer in twins. N Engl J Med 1985;312:541–6.
23. Hopton PA, McKinney PA, Cartwright RA, *et al*. X-rays in pregnancy and the risk of childhood cancer. Lancet 1985;2(8458):773.
24. Naumburg E, Bellocco R, Cnattingius S, *et al*. Intrauterine exposure to diagnostic X-rays and risk of childhood leukaemia subtypes. Radiat Res 2001;156(6):718–23.
25. Meinert R, Kaletsch U, Kaatsch P, *et al*. Associations between childhood cancer and ionising radiation: results of a population based case-control study in Germany. Cancer Epidemiol Biomarkers Prev 1999;8(9):793–9.
26. Brent RL. Saving lives and changing family histories: appropriate counseling of pregnant women and men and women of reproductive age, concerning the risk of diagnostic radiation exposures during and before pregnancy. Am J Obstet Gynecol 2009;200(1):4–24.
27. Cook JV, Kyriou J. Radiation from CT and perfusion scanning in pregnancy. BMJ 2005;331(7512):350.
28. Brent R, Mettler F, Wagner L, *et al*. International Commission on Radiological Protection Publication 84. www.icrp.org.

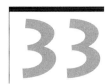

Contraception for women with medical disorders

Iris Tong and Raymond O. Powrie

Department of Medicine, Warren Alpert Medical School of Brown University, Women & Infants' Hospital of Rhode Island, Providence, RI, USA

Ideally, all women should have a reproductive life plan and all of their pregnancies should be intended and planned [1]. This is particularly true for women with medical problems in whom an unplanned pregnancy can have significant impact upon pregnancy outcome. Familiarity with the appropriate options for birth control in women with medical illness is therefore an integral part of their obstetric care.

Currently available options for contraception are listed in Table 33.1 along with their effectiveness in preventing pregnancy. While barrier methods, abstinence and the rhythm method can be used safely in the setting of any medical illness, these methods are less effective than hormonal methods and intrauterine devices. Their relative safety needs to be weighed carefully against the associated risks of an undesired pregnancy in a woman with significant medical disease. While tubal ligation and vasectomy are highly effective options for which the only medical risk is that of the procedure, their permanent nature makes them undesirable for many couples. It is the highly effective and reversible nature of hormonal contraception and intrauterine devices that makes these options so desirable for women with medical problems. However, both the clinician and the patient can be overwhelmed by the long list of cautionary statements and recommendations related to the use of these options in these same women. Table 33.2 is therefore provided to offer some helpful guidance to the clinician caring for women with medical illness during their reproductive years. It is based on the guidelines developed by the World Health Organization (WHO) in 2009.

It is worth noting that the WHO recommends no contraindication for the use of postcoital ("emergency") contraception in women with medical problems, including cardiovascular and thromboembolic disease. The short duration of exposure associated with single-dose hormonal therapy is unlikely to be of harm. In patients at risk for thromboembolic disease, it may be prudent, however, to favor progestin-only emergency contraceptive regimens over those that include estrogen. The efficacy of postcoital contraception and some various regimens is detailed in Table 33.1.

Table 33.1 Efficacy of various methods of contraception

Method	Women experiencing an unintended pregnancy within the first year of typical use (%)	Women experiencing an unintended pregnancy within the first year of perfect use (%)	Women continuing use at 1 year (%)
No method	85	85	–
Spermicides (foams, creams, gels, vaginal suppositories, vaginal film)	29	18	42
Withdrawal	27	4	43
Fertility awareness-based methods			
Fertility awareness-based methods overall	25	–	51
Standard days method (avoiding intercourse on cycle days 9–19)	–	5	–
Two day method (based on cervical mucus)	–	4	–
Ovulation method (based on cervical mucus)	–	3	–

(Continued on p. 654)

de Swiet's Medical Disorders in Obstetric Practice, 5th edition.
Edited by R. O. Powrie, M. F. Greene, W. Camann. © 2010 Blackwell Publishing.

Table 33.1 (Continued)

Method	Women experiencing an unintended pregnancy within the first year of typical use (%)	Women experiencing an unintended pregnancy within the first year of perfect use (%)	Women continuing use at 1 year (%)
Barrier methods			
Sponge in parous women	32	20	46
Sponge in nulliparous women	16	9	57
Diaphragm with spermicidal cream or jelly	16	6	57
Female condom without spermicides (Reality)	21	5	49
Male condom without spermicides (Reality)	15	2	53
Hormonal options			
Combined (estrogen and progestin) pill and progestin-only pill (COC/POP)	8	0.3	68
Evra® patch (transdermal norelgetromin/ethinyl estradiol) (P)	8	0.3	68
NuvaRing® (etonogestrel/ethinyl estradiol vaginal ring) (R)	8	0.3	68
Depo-Provera® (medroxyprogesterone acetate injectable suspension) (DMPA)	3	0.3	56
Implanon® (ethonogestrel implant) (ETG)	0.05	0.05	84
Intrauterine devices			
ParaGard® T (copper intrauterine device) (Cu-IUD)	0.8	0.6	78
Mirena® (levonorgestrel-releasing intrauterine system) (LNG-IUD)	0.2	0.2	80
Sterilization			
Female sterilization	0.5	0.5	100
Male sterilization	0.15	0.10	100
Other			
Lactational amenorrhea method (LAM)	LAM is a highly effective temporary method of contraception but to maintain effective protection against pregnancy, another method of contraception must be used as soon as menstruation resumes, the frequency or duration of breastfeeds is reduced, bottle feeds are introduced or the baby reaches 6 months of age		
Emergency contraceptive pills	Treatment initiated within 72 hours after unprotected intercourse reduces the risk of pregnancy by at least 75%, and treatment between 72 and 120 hours after unprotected intercourse still provides some protection against pregnancy		
	The treatment schedule is one dose of levonorgestrel 0.75 mg within 120 hours after unprotected intercourse, and a second dose 12 hours later. Plan B and Next choice (1 dose = 1 pill which contains levonorgestrel 0.75 mg) is the only dedicated product specifically marketed for emergency contraception. Both doses can be taken at the same time. A levonorgestrel 1.5 mg – tablet is also available and is marketed as Plan B One – Step		
	Combination estrogen and progesterone oral contraceptive pills can also be used for emergency contraception. The US Food and Drug Administration has in addition declared the following 22 brands of oral contraceptives to be safe and effective for emergency contraception: Ogestrel or Ovral (1 dose = 2 white pills), Levlen or Nordette (1 dose = 4 light-orange pills), Cryselle, Levora, Low-Ogestrel, Lo/Ovral or Quasence (1 dose = 4 white pills), Tri-Levlen or Triphasil (1 dose = 4 yellow pills), Jolessa, Portia, Seasonale or Trivora (1 dose = 4 pink pills), Seasonique (1 dose = 4 light-blue-green pills), Empresse (1 dose = 4 orange pills), Alesse, Lessina or Levlite (1 dose = 5 pink pills), Aviane (1 dose = 5 orange pills), and Lutera (1 dose = 5 white pills)		

Adapted from Trussell J. Contraceptive efficacy. In: Hatcher RA, Trussell J, Nelson AL, *et al.* (eds) Contraceptive technology, 19th edn. Ardent Media, New York, 2007.

Table 33.2 WHO recommendations for contraceptive use in women with medical problems

Condition	COC/P/R	CIC	POP	DMPA NET-EN	LNG/ETG Implants	Cu-IUD	LNG-IUD	Comments [1,2]
Thrombosis risk								
History of thromboembolic disease (TED)	4	4	2	2	2	1	2	COC have been associated with an increased risk of VTE [3]. COC/P/R should therefore be avoided in women with a history of VTE or hypercoagulable state. COC use, however, has a lower increase in risk of VTE (3–4-fold) [4] than pregnancy (5–6-fold) [5].
Acute TED	4	4	3	3	3	1	3	
TED presently on anticoagulants	4	4	2	2	2	1	2	The contraceptive patch has also been shown to be associated with a higher risk of VTE when compared with OCP containing levonorgestrel, a second-generation progestin [6]. Serum estrogen levels are 60% higher when using the contraceptive patch than when using an OCP containing
Family history of TED in first-degree relatives	2	2	1	1	1	1	1	
Major surgery with prolonged immobilization	4	4	2	2	2	1	2	35 μg of ethinyl estradiol. A recent case–control study conducted by the manufacturer of the patch demonstrated that the odds ratio of VTE was 1.9 (95% confidence interval 1.1–3.3) with the patch versus OCP containing levonorgestrel [7].
Major surgery without prolonged immobilization	2	2	1	1	1	1	1	
Minor surgery without immobilization	1	1	1	1	1	1	1	
Thrombogenic mutations	4	4	2	2	2	1	2	Copper IUD is recommended by the WHO for women with current VTE, a history of VTE or a hypercoagulable state. However, its use may increase vaginal bleeding which may be exacerbated in the setting of anticoagulation. POP are acceptable alternatives for women with a history of VTE or a hypercoagulable state. Women with hypercoagulable states who use COC have an even greater increased risk of VTE. COC users with the factor V Leiden mutation have a 10–30-fold increase in risk of VTE [8].
Varicose veins	1	1	1	1	1	1	1	
Superficial thrombophlebitis	2	2	1	1	1	1	1	
Obesity >30 kg/m² BMI >18 years	2	2	1	1	1	1	1	Several studies have provided evidence that POP and COC may be less effective in obese women, resulting in an average of 2–4 more
Obesity menarche to <18 years and >30 kg/m² BMI	2	2	1	DMPA 2 NET-EN 1	1	1	1	pregnancies per year in obese women on COC and POP than in women of normal weight [9]. Studies also suggest an increased risk of TED in obese women on COC as compared to lean women on COC [5].
Rheumatic disease								
SLE with positive or unknown antiphospholipid antibody status	4	4	3	3	3	1	3	COC, POP and the copper IUD do not appear to affect the course of SLE [10,11].
SLE with severe thrombocytopenia	2	2	2	3/2	2	3/2	2	Precautions related to antiphospholipid antibodies relate to the risk of thrombosis. Precautions related to thrombocytopenia relate to the risk of bleeding.
SLE on immunosuppressive treatment	2	2	2	2	2	2	2/1	Many clinicians are wary of placing IUD in women on immunosuppressive therapy but the WHO supports their use in this setting.
SLE with none of the above	2	2	2	2	2	1	2	Patients with rheumatologic conditions may also have cardiovascular disease and the additional concerns related to contraception in women with cardiac risk factors or disease should therefore also be considered.

(*Continued on p. 656*)

Table 33.2 (Continued)

Condition	COC/P/R	CIC	POP	DMPA NET-EN	LNG/ETG Implants	Cu-IUD	LNG-IUD	Comments [1,2]
Liver disease								
Acute or flaring viral hepatitis	3–4 /2	3/2	1	1	1	1	1	In the setting of severe acute hepatitis, COC/P/R are contraindicated.
Carrier viral hepatitis	1	1	1	1	1	1	1	
Chronic viral hepatitis	1	1	1	1	1	1	1	
Mild (compensated) cirrhosis	1	1	1	1	1	1	1	
Severe (decompensated) cirrhosis	4	3	3	3	3	1	3	
Benign focal nodular hyperplasia liver	2	2	2	2	2	1	2	
Benign hepatocellular adenoma	4	3	3	3	3	1	3	
Malignant hepatoma	4	3/4	3	3	3	1	3	
Gallbladder disease: symptomatic treated by cholecystectomy	2	2	2	2	2	1	2	
Gallbladder disease: symptomatic, medically treated	3	2	2	2	2	1	2	
Gallbladder disease: current	3	2	2	2	2	1	2	
Gallbladder disease: asymptomatic	2	2	2	2	2	1	2	
History of cholestasis related to pregnancy	2	2	1	1	1	1	1	
History of cholestasis related to combined oral contraceptives	3	2	2	2	2	1	2	
Infection and its treatment								
High risk of HIV	1	1	1	1	1	2	2	IUD do not appear to increase the risk of PID or viral shedding in HIV-positive women [12,13].
HIV infected	1	1	1	1	1	2	2	
HIV infected, clinically well on ARV therapy	1	1	1	1	1	2	2	COC/P/R/POP do not increase disease progression or risk of transmission.
AIDS	1	1	1	1	1	3/2	3/2	
Nucleoside reverse transcriptase inhibitors (NRTI)	1	1	1	DMPA 1 NET-EN 2	1	2–3/2	2–3/2	The concomitant use of hormonal contraception and some antiretroviral medications, however, may increase or decrease contraceptive steroid or antiretroviral efficacy.
Non-nucleoside reverse transcriptase inhibitors (NNRTI)	2	2	2	DMPA 1 NET-EN 2	2	2–3/2	2–3/2	
Ritonavir boosted protease inhibitors	3	3	3	DMPA 1 NET-EN 2	2	2–3/2	2–3/2	
Broad-spectrum antibiotics	1	1	1	1	1	1	1	

Condition	COC / P / R	POP	DMPA / NET-EN	Implant	Cu-IUD	LNG-IUD	Comments
Rifampicin or rifabutin therapy	3	3	DMPA 1 / NET-EN 2	2	1	1	
Antifungal therapy	1	1	1	1	1	1	
Antiparasitic therapy	1	1	1	1	1	1	
Schistosomiasis (uncomplicated)	1	1	1	1	1	1	
Schistosomiasis with hepatic fibrosis	1	1	1	1	1	1	
Nonpelvic tuberculosis	1	1	1	1	1	1	
Pelvic tuberculosis	1	1	1	1	4/3	4/3	
Malaria	1	1	1	1	1	1	
Neurologic illness							
Epilepsy	1	1	1	1	1	1	Epilepsy of itself is not a contraindication to any form of contraception but some anticonvulsants will affect contraceptive efficacy (see below).
Anticonvulsant therapy with phenytoin, carbamazapine, barbiturates, primidone, topiramate, oxcarbazepine	3	3	DMPA 1 / NET-EN 2	2	1	1	These anticonvulsants induce the cytochrome P450 system and enhance steroid metabolism by the liver, thereby reducing serum concentrations of estrogen and/or progesterone and making all hormonal forms of contraception less effective aside from DMPA [14,15]. Oral contraceptive pills have a 6% failure rate per year in this population [16]. Switching to an antiepileptic which does not induce the P450 system or to a nonhormonal form of contraception should be considered. Some women on these agents may still prefer hormonal methods despite their lower efficacy and these women should consider addition of a barrier method.
Anticonvulsant therapy with lamotrigine	3	1	1	1	1	1	Lamotrigine metabolism is significantly increased by COCs decreasing lamotrigine bio-availability without affecting contraceptive steroid concentrations.
Headaches (nonmigrainous)	1/2	1	1	1	1	1	
Migraine without aura age <35	2/3	1/2	2	2	1	2	Combination OCP use and migraine headaches are independently associated with an increased risk of stroke [5,17]. Multiple studies have demonstrated an increased risk of stroke in women with migraine headaches with aura, but not in women without aura [18,19].
Migraine without aura age >35	3/4	1/2	2	2	1	2	
Migraine with aura (at any age)	4	2/3	2/3	2/3	1	2/3	COC may be considered for women with migraine headaches who do not smoke, who do not have focal neurologic symptoms, and who are younger than 35 years of age given the low incidence of stroke among women with migraines. COC should be avoided in women with migraine headaches who smoke, have focal neurologic symptoms or are older than 35 years of age. POP can be used as they have not been associated with an increased risk of stroke [8].
Depression							
Depressive disorders	1	1	1	1	1	1	

(Continued on p. 658)

Table 33.2 (Continued)

Condition	COC/P/R	CIC	POP	DMPA NET-EN	LNG/ETG Implants	Cu-IUD	LNG-IUD	Comments [1,2]
Cardiovascular disease Multiple risk factors for arterial cardiovascular disease (such as older age, smoking, diabetes, and hypertension)	3/4	3/4	2	3	2	1	2	Both hypertension and COC use are associated with an increased risk of myocardial infarction and stroke [20–22]. However, the absolute risk of cardiovascular events among women of reproductive age with and without COC use is low. Therefore, when considering the use of COC, the risk of a cardiac event must be weighed against the risks and consequences of a pregnancy. COC should be avoided in women with poorly controlled hypertension, with established cardiovascular disease or with multiple cardiac risk factors. POP are good options in women who smoke as they have not been associated with vascular events [23]. COC can be used in women smokers who are <35 years old. COC should be avoided in women smokers who are >35 years old.
Hypertension history where blood pressure cannot be measured	3	3	2	2	2	1	2	DMPA and NET-EN have not been associated with increases in blood pressure [24] or with increased risk of cardiovascular events.
Well-controlled hypertension	3	3	1	2	1	1	1	COC can be considered in nonsmoking women with well-controlled hypertension who are less than 35 years of age. Small studies have demonstrated that COC use is associated with a slight increase in systolic [25] and diastolic blood pressures [26] of <10 mmHg. Therefore women using COC should have their blood pressure monitored.
Hypertension 140–159/90–99 mmHg	3	3	1	2	1	1	1	
Hypertension >160/100 mmHg	4	4	2	3	2	1	2	
Hypertension with known vascular disease	4	4	3	3	2	1	2	
History of high blood pressure in pregnancy but presently normal	2	2	1	1	1	1	1	
Current and history of ischemic heart disease	4	4	2/3	3	2/3	1	2/3	
Stroke	4	4	2/3	3	2/3	1	2	
Known hyperlipidemias	2/3	2/3	2	2	2	1	2	The estrogen component of COC decreases low-density lipoprotein (LDL) cholesterol and increases high-density lipoprotein (HDL) cholesterol and triglycerides. The progestin component attenuates the effects of estrogen. POP are appropriate options as they do not affect lipid levels. COC containing 35 mg or less of estrogen can be used in women with well-controlled hyperlipidemia given the low absolute risk of myocardial infarction in women of reproductive age. After initiating COC, fasting lipid panels should be monitored. COC should be avoided in women with poorly controlled hyperlipidemia, established cardiovascular disease or other cardiac risk factors.

Condition							Comments
Complicated valvular heart disease	4	4	1	1	2	2	
Uncomplicated valvular heart disease	2	2	1	1	1	1	
Breast cancer							
Undiagnosed breast mass	2	2	2	2	1	2	
Benign breast disease	1	1	1	1	1	1	
Family history of breast cancer	1	1	1	1	1	1	
Current breast cancer	4	4	4	4	1	4	
Past history of breast cancer with no evidence of current breast cancer for 5 years	3	3	3	3	1	3	
Endocrine							
History of gestational diabetes	1	1	1	1	1	1	Although data are limited, it does not appear that hormonal contraception, aside from high-dose COC, significantly affects glucose control. COC can worsen hyperlipidemia while POP may improve it.
Noninsulin-dependent diabetes with no vascular disease	2	2	2	2	1	2	
Insulin-dependent diabetes with no vascular disease	2	2	2	2	1	2	Restrictions related to contraceptive choices in diabetic women relate to vascular complications.
Diabetes with nephropathy/retinopathy/neuropathy	3/4	3/4	3	2	1	2	
Diabetes with vascular disease or diabetes of >20 years gestation	3/4	3/4	3	2	1	2	
Simple goiter	1	1	1	1	1	1	
Hyperthyroid	1	1	1	1	1	1	
Hypothyroid	1	1	1	1	1	1	
Hematology							
Thalassemias	1	1	1	1	2	2	
Sickle cell disease	2	2	2	2	1	2	
Iron deficiency anemia	1	1	1	1	2	2	

Adapted from World Health Organization. Medical eligibility criteria for contraceptive use, 4th edn. WHO, Geneva, 2009. http://www.who.int/reproductive-health/publications/mec/mec.pdf.

ARV, antiretroviral; BMI, Body Mass Index; COC/P/R, combined oral contraceptive pills/patch/vaginal ring; CIC, combined injectable contraceptives; POP, progestogen-only pills; DMPA, depot medroxyprogesterone injectable; NET-EN, norethisterone enanthate injectable; LNG/ETG, levonorgestrel (Jadelle®) and etonogestrel (Implanon®) implants; Cu-IUD, copper-bearing intrauterine device; LNG-IUD, levonorgestrel-releasing intrauterine device; OCP, oral contraceptive pill; PID, pelvic inflammatory disease; SLE, systemic lupus erythematosus; TED, thromboembolic disease; VTE, venous thromboembolism.

1, a condition for which there is no restriction for the use of the contraceptive method; 2, a condition in which the advantages of using the method generally outweigh the theoretical or proven risks; 3, a condition in which the theoretical or proven risks usually outweigh the advantage of using the method; 4, a condition which represents an unacceptable health risk if the contraceptive method is used.

When two numbers are seen in a cell on this table, the first number applies to the WHO rating for the *intiation* of the contraceptive method and the second refers to its *continuance* in patients already on that method.

References

1. CDC/ATSDR Preconception Care Work Group and the Select Panel on Preconception Care. Recommendations to improve preconception health and health care. MMWR 2006;55(RR06):1–23.

2. Teal SB, Ginosar DM. Contraception for women with chronic medical conditions. Obstet Gynecol Clin North Am 2007;34:113–26.

3. American College of Obstetricians and Gynecologists. ACOG practice bulletin no. 73: use of hormonal contraception in women with coexisting medical conditions. Clinical management guidelines for obstetrican-gynecologists. Obstet Gynecol 2006;107(6):1453–72.

4. Lidegaard O, Edstrom B, Kreiner S. Oral contraceptives and venous thromboembolism: a five-year national case-control study. Contraception 2000;65:187–96.

5. Sidney S, Petitti DB, Soff GA, et al. Venous thromboembolic disease in users of low-estrogen combined estrogen-progestin oral contraceptives. Contraception 2004;70:3–10.

6. Farmer RDT, Preston, TD. The risk of venous thromboembolism associated with low oestrogen oral contraceptives. Journal of Obstetrics & Gynaecology 1995; 15: 195–200.

7. Boston Collaborative Drug Surveillance Program. Postmarketing study of ORTHO EVRA® and levonorgestrel oral contraceptives containing hormonal contraceptives with 30 µg of EE in relation to non-fatal venous thromboembolism, ischemic stroke and myocardial infarction. http://www.clinicaltrials.gov/ct2/show/NCT00511784

8. Vandenbroucke JP, Koster T, Briet E, et al. Increased risk of venous thrombosis in oral-contraceptive users who are carriers of factor V Leiden mutation. Lancet 1994; 344: 1453–1457.

9. Holt VL, Scholes D, Wicklund KG, et al. Body mass index, weight, and oral contraceptive failure risk. Obstet Gynecol 2005;105(1):46–52.

10. Schwarz EB, Lohr PA. Oral contraceptives in women with systemic lupus erythematosus. N Engl J Med 2006;354(11):1203–4 [author reply: 1203–4].

11. Sanchez-Guerrero J, Uribe AG, Jimenez-Santana L, et al. A trial of contraceptive methods in women with systemic lupus erythematosus. N Engl J Med 2005;353(24):2539–49.

12. Richardson BA, Morrison CS, Sekadde-Kigondu C, et al. Effect of intrauterine device use on cervical shedding of HIV-1 DNA. AIDS 1999;13(15):2091–7.

13. Grimes DA. Intrauterine device and upper-genital-tract infection. Lancet 2000;356(9234):1013–9.

14. Mattson RH, Cramer JA, Darney PD, Naftolin F. Use of oral contraceptives by women with epilepsy. JAMA 1986; 256: 238–40.

15. Haukkamaa M. Contraception by Norplant subdermal capsules is not reliable in epileptic patients on anticonvulsant treatment. Contraception 1986; 33: 559–65.

16. Morrell MJ. Epilepsy in Women. American Family Physician 2002; 66: 1489 - 94.

17. Lidegaard O. Oral contraceptives, pregnancy and the risk of cerebral thromboembolism: the influence of diabetes, hypertension, migraine, and previous thrombotic disease. British Journal of Obstetrics and Gynaecology 1995; 102: 153–59.

18. Kurth T, Slomke MA, Kase CS, et al., Migraine, headache and the risk of stroke in women: a prospective study. Neurology 2005; 64: 1020–26.

19. Stang PE, Carson AP, Rose KM, et al. Headache, cerebrovascular symptoms, and stroke: the atherosclerosis risk in communities study. Neurology 2005; 64: 1573–77.

20. Khader YS, Rice J, Lefante J, Abueita O. Oral contraceptives use and the risk of myocardial infarction: a meta-analysis. Contraception 2003; 68:11–17.

21. Baillargeon JP, McClish DK, Essah PA, Nestler JE. Association between the current use of low-dose oral contraceptives and cardiovascular disease: a meta-analysis. Journal of Clinical Endocrinology and Metabolism 2005; (90): 3863 – 70.

22. Tanis BC, van den Bosch MA, Kemmeren JM, et al. Oral contraceptives and the risk of myocardial infarction. New England Journal of Medicine 2001; 345: 1787–93.

23. Hussain SF. Progestogen-only pills and high blood pressure: is there an association? A literature review. Contraception 2004; 69: 89–97.

24. Black HR, Leppert P, DeCherney A. The effect of medroxyprogesterone acetate on blood pressure. International Journal of Gynaecology and Obstetrics 1978; 17: 83–7.

25. Cardoso F, Polonia J, Santos A, et al. Low-dose oral contraceptives and 24-hour ambulatory blood pressure. International Journal of Gynaecology and Obstetrics 1997; 59: 237–43.

26. Narkiewicz K, Graniero GR, D'Este D, et al. Ambulatory blood pressure in mild hypertensive women taking oral contraceptives. A case-control study. American Journal of Hypertension 1995; 8: 249–53.

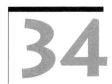

34 Effect of pregnancy on common laboratory tests

Michael P. Carson[1] and Elvis R. Pagan[2]

[1]UMDNJ-Robert Wood Johnson Medical School, Departments of Medicine and Obstetrics/Gynecology, Jersey Shore University Medical Centre, Neptune, NJ, USA
[2]Virginia Tech Carilion School of Medicine, Department of Medicine, Carilion Clinic, Roanoke, VA, USA

Test	Expected antepartum values during pregnancy (conventional units)	Expected antepartum values during pregnancy (SI units)	Comments	Evidence
Alimentary system				
Albumin	Decreased 3.2 g/dL (2.7–3.6)	Decreased 32 g/L (27–36)	Dilutional decrease during pregnancy.	Lockitch, G. Clinical biochemistry of pregnancy. Crit Rev Clin Lab Sci 1997;34(1):67–139. Pirani BB, Campbell DM, MacGillivray I. Plasma volume in normal first pregnancy. J Obstet Gynaecol Br Commonw. 1973;80(10):884–7.
Alkaline phosphatase	Increases with gestational age First and second trimester: 65 U/L (25–100) Third trimester: 140 U/L (125–250)	Increases with gestational age First and second trimester: 65 U/L (25–100) Third trimester: 140 U/L (125–250)	Increased due to the presence of placental alkaline phosphatase. The degree of elevation is not predictable. This cannot be used to differentiate hepatic parenchymal disease from cholestatic disease.	Kaplan MM. Alkaline phosphatase. Gastroenterology 1972;62(3):452–68.
Amylase/lipase	No change from nonpregnant	No change from nonpregnant		Lockitch, G (ed). Handbook of diagnostic biochemistry and hematology in normal pregnancy. CRC Press, Boca Raton, FL, 1993:537.
AST, ALT, bilirubin, GGT	No change from nonpregnant	No change from nonpregnant		Berg B, Petersohn L, Helm G, Tryding N. Reference values for serum components in pregnant women. Acta Obstet Gynecol Scand.1984;63(7):583–6.
Protein–total	Decreased 5.8 g/dL (5.1–6.5)	Decreased 58 g/L (51–65 g/L)	Dilutional decrease during pregnancy.	Lockitch G (ed) 1993: full reference above under amylase.

(Continued on p. 662)

de Swiet's Medical Disorders in Obstetric Practice, 5th edition.
Edited by R. O. Powrie, M. F. Greene, W. Camann. © 2010 Blackwell Publishing.

Test	Expected antepartum values during pregnancy (conventional units)	Expected antepartum values during pregnancy (SI units)	Comments	Evidence
Biochemistry				
Bicarbonate, serum (HCO$_3^-$)	Decreased 21 mEq /L18–25)	Decreased 21 mmol /L (18–25)	Compensation for normal respiratory alkalosis.	Lim VS, Katz AI, Lindheimer MD. Acid-base regulation in pregnancy. Am J Physiol 1976;231(6):1764–9.
Calcium	Total: Decreased 8.6 mg/dL (8–9.4)[δ] Ionized: Unchanged	Total: Decreased 2.2 mmol/L (2–2.4) Ionized: Unchanged	Decrease due to decreased protein bound calcium from physiologic hypoalbuminemia.	Pitkin RM. Calcium metabolism in pregnancy and the perinatal period: a review. Am J Obstet Gynecol 1985;151(1):99–107.
Ceruloplasmin	Increased 47 mg/dL (30–60)	Increased 470 mg/L (300–600)	Evaluation for Wilson's complicated due to the increase in this and copper with normal pregnancy.	Lockitch G 1997: full reference above under albumin.
Chloride	No change from nonpregnant	No change from nonpregnant		Lockitch G 1997: full reference above under albumin.
Copper	Increased 191 micrograms/dL (127–255)	Increased 30 micromol/L (20–40)	See above comment under Ceruloplasmin.	Lockitch G 1997: full reference above under albumin.
Drug levels	May decrease	May decrease	Dilutional decreases in serum protein levels can result in altered protein binding of medications. The total level of a protein bound medication such as phenytoin may decrease by 20%, but the free level may only decrease by 10%. Obtain free levels of medications when available.	
Glucose	Second and third trimester fasting 60 (55–65) mg/dL, 2 hrs postprandial 100 (95–105) mg/dL	Second and third trimester fasting 3.3 mmol/L (3–3.6) 2 h postprandial 5.5 mmol/L (5.3–5.8)		Parretti E, Mecacci F, Papini M, et al. Third trimester maternal glucose levels from diurnal profiles in nondiabetic pregnancies; correlation wih sonographic parameters of fetal growth. Diabetes Care 2001;24:1319–23
Magnesium	Slightly decreased 1.76 mg/dL (1.59–1.93)[δ]	Slightly decreased 0.72 mmol/L (0.65–0.79)		Bardicef M, Bardicef O, Sorokin Y, Altura BM, Altura BT, Cotton DB, Resnick LM. Extracellular and intracellular magnesium depletion in pregnancy and gestational diabetes. Am J Obstet Gynecol 1995;172(3):1009–13.
Partial pressure of carbon dioxide in arterial blood (PaCO2)	Decreased 31 mmHg (28–34)[δ]	Decreased 31 mmHg (28–34)[δ]	Hyperventilation due to progesterone effect on the respiratory center.	McAuliffe F, Kametas N, Krampl E, Ernsting J, Nicolaides K. Blood gases in pregnancy at sea level and at high altitude. Br J Obstet Gynecol 2001;108:980–5. Lim VS, et al, 1976: full reference above under bicarbonate.
Partial pressure of oxygen in arterial blood (PaO2)	Increased 99 mmHg (89–109) at sea level	Increased 99 mmHg (89–109) at sea level	Increased because of hyperventilation.	McAuliffe F, et al, 2001: full reference above under PaCO2.
Phosphorus	No change from nonpregnant	No change from nonpregnant		Pitkin RM, 1985: full reference above under calcium.

Test	Expected antepartum values during pregnancy (conventional units)	Expected antepartum values during pregnancy (SI units)	Comments	Evidence
Potassium	No change from nonpregnant	No change from nonpregnant		Lockitch G 1997: full reference above under albumin.
pH	Slightly increased 7.45 (7.43–7.47)[δ]	Slightly increased 7.45 (7.43–7.47)[δ]	Hyperventilation results in respiratory alkalosis, partially offset by compensatory renal excretion of bicarbonate.	McAuliffe F, et al, 2001: full reference above under PaCO2. Lim VS, et al, 1976: full reference above under bicarbonate.
Sodium	Decreased slightly, but in the normal range 135 mEq/L (132–140)	Decreased slightly, but in the normal range 135 mmol/L (132–140)	Osmotic threshold for thirst and antidiuretic hormone release (ADH) decreases in pregnancy resulting in increased free water retention and resultant decreased plasma osmolality.	Berg B, et al, 1984: full reference above under AST.
Uric acid	Decreased 3.0 mg/dL (1.7–4.2)	Decreased 178 micromol/L (101–250)	Due to increased renal plasma flow and increased vasopressin which decreases tubular reabsorption. Uric acid levels may return to pre-pregnancy values in the third trimester.	Lockitch G 1997: full reference above under albumin.
Zinc	Decreased 65 micrograms/dL (46–88)	Decreased 10 micromol/L (7–13.5)		Lockitch G 1997: full reference above under albumin.
Cardiac				
Brain natriuretic peptide (BNP)	May increase at term and postpartum. First and second trimester: 24 pg/mL (21–27)[δ] At term: 49 pg/mL (40–58)[δ] Postpartum: 116 pg/mL (99–133)[δ]	May increase at term and postpartum. First and second trimester: 24 ng/L (21–27) At term: 49 ng/L (40–58) Postpartum: 116 ng/L (99–133)	In conjunction with other clinical markers, BNP may be helpful in identifying antepartum patients with heart failure. There may be a modest increase in BNP at term and postpartum in normal pregnancies as well as in pregnancies complicated by pre-eclampsia.	Yoshimura T, Yoshimura M, Yasue H, Ito M, Okamura H, Mukoyama M, Nakao K. Plasma concentration of ANP and BNP during normal pregnancy and the postpartum period. J Endocrinol 1994;140:393–7.
Creatinine kinase-MB (CK-MB)	May be elevated after delivery	May be elevated after delivery	CK-MB makes up about 6% of the total CPK from the placenta and myometrium.	Chemnitz G, Nevermann L, Schmidt E, Schmidt FW, Lobers J. Creatinine kinase and CK isoenzymes during pregnancy and labor and in the cord blood. Clin Biochem. 1979;12(6):277–81.
Troponin I	No change from nonpregnant	No change from nonpregnant	Mild elevations have been documented in women who were classified as having gestational hypertension or pre-eclampsia.	Fleming SM, O'Gorman T, Finn J, Grimes H, Daly K, Morrison JJ. Cardiac troponin I in pre-eclamsia and gestational hypertension. Br J Obstet Gynaecol 2000;107:1417–20.
Endocrine Adrenal				
ACTH	Increases with gestational age. First trimester: 23 pg/mL (18.4–27.6)[δ] Third trimester: 59 pg/mL (43–75)[δ]	Increases with gestational age. First trimester: 23 ng/L (18.4–27.6)[δ] Third trimester: 59 ng/L (43–75)[δ]	Due to placental secretion of ACTH.	Carr BR, Parker CR Jr, Madden JD, MacDonald PC, Porter JC. Maternal plasma adrenocorticotropin and cortisol relationships throughout human pregnancy. Am J Obstet Gynecol 1981;139(4):416–22.

(Continued on p. 664)

Test	Expected antepartum values during pregnancy (conventional units)	Expected antepartum values during pregnancy (SI units)	Comments	Evidence
Aldosterone	Increases with gestational age. First trimester: 15 ng/dL (12–18)[δ] Second trimester: 52 ng/dL (45–69)[δ] Third trimester: 76 ng/dL (65–87)[δ]	Increases with gestational age. First trimester: 0.4 nmol/L (0.2–0.5)[δ] Second trimester: 1.4 nmol/L (1.2– 1.9)[δ] Third trimester: 2.1 nmol/L (1.8–2.4)[δ]	Will increase by 30–48% due to ACTH stimulation. Progesterone can counteract the potassium wasting seen in patients with true hyperaldosteronism (Conn's disease). Testing may need to be repeated after pregnancy.	Elsheikh A, Creatsas G, Mastorakos G, Milingos S, Loutradis D, Michalas S. The renin-aldosterone system during normal and hypertensive pregnancy. Arch Gynecol Obstet 2001;264:182–5. Suri D, Moran J, Hibbard JU, Kasza K, Weiss RE. Assessment of adrenal reserve in pregnancy: defining the normal response to the adrenocorticotropin stimulation test. J Clin Endocrinol Metab 2006;91(10):3866–72.
Catecholamines (urine and serum)	No change from nonpregnant	No change from nonpregnant	May increase with pre-eclampsia. Labetalol (a commonly used antihypertensive for pregnant patients) can cause false positive elevations.	Lindsay JR, Nieman LK. Adrenal disorders in pregnancy. Endocrinol Metab Clin North Am 2006;35:1–20.
Cortisol	Increases with gestational age. First trimester: No change from nonpregnant (9–14 micrograms/dL)[δ] Second trimester: 14.5 micrograms/dL (10.3–18.8)[δ] Third trimester: 35.3 micrograms/dL (26.2–44.2)[δ]	Increases with gestational age. First trimester: No change from nonpregnant 0.25–0.39 micromol/L[δ] Second trimester: 0.4 micromol/L (0.28–0.53)[δ] Third trimester: 0.99 micromol/L (0.73–1.24)[δ]	Evaluation for Cushing's syndrome may be difficult based on physiologic elevation of cortisol level. This could also result in inadequate suppression of cortisol with the dexamethasone suppression test.which is typically used to diagnose hypercortisolism.	Carr BR, et al, 1981: full reference above under ACTH. Suri D, et al, 2006: full reference above under aldosterone.
Free urine cortisol	Increases with gestational age. Second and third trimester levels may be up to three times greater than in nonpregnant patients	Increases with gestational age. Second and third trimester levels may be up to three times greater than in nonpregnant patients	In the second and third trimester 24–h urine cortisol does not reasonably predict patients who may have Cushing's syndrome; however, it is suggested if levels are greater than 3 times normal.	Lindsay JR, et al, 2005: full reference above under catecholamines.
Plasma renin activity	Increases with gestational age. First trimester: 8.3 ng/mL/h (4.2–12.4)[δ] Second trimester: 10.1 ng/mL/h (7.5–12.7)[δ] Third trimester: 15.7 ng/mL/h (10.5–20.9)[δ]	Increases with gestational age. First trimester: 8.3 micrograms/L/h (4.2–12.4)[δ] Second trimester: 10.1 micrograms/L/h (7.5–12.7)[δ] Third trimester: 15.7 micrograms/L/h (10.5–20.9)[δ]	Increased renin activity may occur due to decreased vascular resistance that is associated with pregnancy.	Elsheikh A, et al, 2001: full reference above under aldosterone.

Test	Expected antepartum values during pregnancy (conventional units)	Expected antepartum values during pregnancy (SI units)	Comments	Evidence
Bone metabolism				
Calcitonin	Studies vary. Some report no change, others that it increases.	Studies vary. Some report no change, others that it increases.	If calcitonin does increase, it may do so to counter the bone resorption effects of increased parathyroid hormone seen in pregnancy thereby protecting the maternal skeleton.	Pitkin R, 1985: full reference above under calcium. Pedersen EB, Johannesen P, Kristensen S, Rasmussen AB, Emmertsen K, Moller J, Lauritsen JG, Wohlert M. Calcium, parathyroid hormone and calcitonin in normal pregnancy and preeclampsia.Gynecol Obstet Invest 1984;18(3):156–64.
Intact parathyroid hormonne (iPTH)	No significant change	No significant change	Assay type may contribute to earlier varying reports of iPTH changes. Newer, more sensitive, assays suggest no significant changes with normal pregnancy.	Kovacs CS, Kronenberg HM. Maternal-fetal calcium and bone metabolism during pregnancy, puerperium and lactation. Endocrine Rev 1997;18 (6):832–72.
Vitamin D	1, 25–hydroxy-vitamin D (calcitriol): Increases with gestational age First trimester: 26 pg/mL (20–33)[δ] At term: 128 pg/mL (96–160)[δ] 25–hydoxy-vitamin D (calcidiol): No change	1,25-hydroxy-vitamin D (calcitriol): Increases with gestational age First trimester: 62.4 pmol/L (48–79)[δ] At term: 307 pmol/L (230–384)[δ] 25-hydoxy-vitamin D (calcidiol): No change	25-Hydroxy is the commonly ordered test. Increases in calcitriol may be related to increases in parathryoid hormone activity of pregnancy, but the hormonal activity is not necessarily maternal PTH.	Ardawi MS, Nasrat HA, BA'Aqueel HS. Calcium-regulating hormones and parathyroid hormone-related peptide in normal human pregnancy and postpartum: a longitudinal study. Eur J Endocrinol 1997;137(4):402–9.
Lipids				
Cholesterol HDL	Increases by 25%, peak second trimester	Increases with peak in second trimester	Because of the expected increases we generally avoid testing during pregnancy.	Piechota W, Staszewski A. Reference ranges of lipids and apolipoproteins in pregnancy. Eur J Obstet Gynecol Reprod Biol 1992 16;45(1):27–35. Lippi G, Albiero A, Montagnana M, Salvagno GL, Scevarolli S, Franchi M, Guidi GC. Lipid and lipoprotein profile in physiological pregnancy. Clin Lab 2007;53(3–4):173–7.
Cholesterol LDL	Increases by 36%, peak third trimester	Increases with peak in third trimester	Because of the expected increases we generally avoid testing during pregnancy.	Piechota W, Staszewski A, 1992: full reference above under HDL cholesterol.
Cholesterol total	Increases by 43%, peak third trimester (180–280 mg/dL)	Increases, with peak in third trimester (4.7–7.3 mmol/L)	Because of the expected increases we generally avoid testing during pregnancy.	Piechota W, Staszewski A, 1992: full reference above under HDL cholesterol.
Triglycerides	May increase 2.7 times, peak third trimester	Increases with peak in third trimester	Because of the expected increases we generally avoid testing during pregnancy.	Piechota W, Staszewski A, 1992: full reference above under HDL cholesterol.
Pituitary				
Antidiuretic hormone (ADH)	Increased	Increased	Osmotic threshold for ADH release is lowered in pregnancy.	Lindheimer MD, Barron WM, Davison JM. Osmoregulation of thirst and vasopressin release in pregnancy. Am J Physiol 1989; 257(26):159–69.

(*Continued on p. 666*)

Test	Expected antepartum values during pregnancy (conventional units)	Expected antepartum values during pregnancy (SI units)	Comments	Evidence
Follicle stimulating hormone (FSH), lutenizing hormone (LH)	Decreased	Decreased	Suppressed by estradiol and progesterone.	
Growth hormone	Decreased	Decreased	Replaced by placental-derived GH.	Mirlesse V, Frankenne F, Alsat E, Poncelet M, Hennen G, Evain-Brion D. Placental growth hormone levels in normal and pathological pregnancies. Pediatr Res 1993;34(4):439–42.
Prolactin	Increases throughout pregnancy. At term: 207 ng/mL (35–600)	Increases throughout pregnancy. At term: 207 micrograms/L (35–600)	Increased by estradiol in preparation for lactation.	Tyson JE, Hwang P, Guyda H, Friesen HG. Studies of prolactin secretion in human pregnancy. Am J Obstet Gynecol. 1972 1;113(1):14–20.
Thyroid				
Free Thyroxine Index	No change from nonpregnant (2–4.8)	No change from nonpregnant (2–4.8)	Multiply the total T4 by the T3RU (expressed as a percentage).	
T3 resin uptake (T3RU)	Decreased	Decreased	Decreased due to the increase of thyroid-binding globulin (TBG).	
Total thyroxine (TT4), total tri-iodothyronine (TT3)	Increased	Increased	TT4 and TT3 increase in pregnancy due to increased thyroid-binding globulin concentrations (TBG). Therefore free T4 or Free Thryoxine Index should be used to assess for thryoid disorders in pregnancy.	Soldin OP, 2006: full reference above under TSH.
Thyroid-stimulating hormone (TSH)	May be decreased in first trimester. First trimester: 0.89 uU/mL (0.24–2.99)	May be decreased in first trimester. First trimester: 0.89 mIU/L (0.24–2.99)	May be low in the first trimester since the structure of HCG is similar to TSH. Diagnosis of true hyperthyroidism during pregnancy should be associated with undetectable serum TSH, elevated free thyroxine levels and clinical features of the disease. Consider use of pregnancy specific ranges. See Chapter 12.	Soldin OP. Thyroid function in pregnancy and thyroid disease: trimester-specific reference intervals. Ther Drug Monit 2006;288–11.
Thyroxine, free (FT4)	No change from nonpregnant	No change from nonpregnant	Free T4 can be slightly elevated in the first trimester in normal pregnancies and in 40% of patients with hyperemesis gravidarum. Should normalize after the first trimester.	Lao TT, Chin RK, Chang AM. The outcome of hyperemetic pregnancies complicated by transient hyperthyroidism. Aust N Z J Obstet Gynaecol 1987;27(2):99–101.
Hematologic				
Ferritin	Decreases with gestational age. At term: 14 ng/mL (7–28)[φ]	Decreases with gestational age. At term: 14 micrograms/L (7–28)[φ]	Decrease partially related to dilutional effect of pregnancy. It is the most accurate measure of iron deficiency in pregnancy. Consider iron repletion if low (<15 micrograms/L). See comments under iron below.	Milman N, Agger AO, Nielson OJ. Iron status markers and serum erythropoietin in 120 mothers and newborn infants. Acta Obstet Gynecol Scand 1994;73:200–4.

Test	Expected antepartum values during pregnancy (conventional units)	Expected antepartum values during pregnancy (SI units)	Comments	Evidence
Folate	Decreased. Small decrease as pregnancy progresses. First trimester: 5.4 ng/mL (3.9–7.7) Third trimester: 4.1 ng/mL (3.0–6.0)	Decreased. Small decrease as pregnancy progresses. First trimester: 12.2 nmol/L (8.8–17.4) Third trimester: 9.3 nmol/L (6.7–13.6)	Folic acid dietary supplementation prior to pregnancy and through the first trimester has been demonstrated to reduce the incidences of both occurrence and recurrence of neural tube defects.	Makedos G, Papanicolaou A, Hitoglou A, Kalogiannidis I, Makedos A, Vrazioti V, Goutzioulis M. Homocysteine, folic acid and B12 serum levels in pregnancy complicated with preeclampsia. Arch Gynecol Obstet 2007;275(2):121–4.
Iron	Decreases with gestational age. First trimester: 106.5 micrograms/dL (82–131)[δ] Third trimester: 56 micrograms/dL (25–87)[δ]	Decreases with gestational age. First trimester: 32.6 micromol/L (14.7–23.4)[δ] Third trimester: 10 micromol/L (4.5–15.6)[δ]	Decrease is both dilutional and due to the increased metabolic needs of mother and fetus. This is partially offset by increased gastrointestinal iron absorption. See comment on ferritin above.	Kaneshige E. Serum ferritin as an assessment of iron stores and other hematologic parameters during pregnancy. Obstet Gynecol 1981;57:238–42.
Hemoglobin/ hematocrit	Decreased 12 g/dL (10–1 3.5)	Decreased 120 g/L (100–135)	Red cell mass increases but plasma volume increases to a greater extent resulting in dilutional anemia of pregnancy. Elevated hemoglobin/ hematocrit may be reflective of hemoconcentration or pre-eclampsia.	Chesley LC. Plasma and red cell volumes during pregnancy. Am J Obstet Gynecol 1972 1;112(3):440–50.
Lactate dehydrogenase (LDH)	Increases at term. At term: 550 U/L (350–650)	Increases at term. At term: 550 U/L (350–650)	LDH may increase at term and postpartum as the uterine myometrium has LDH activity.	Lockitch G, 1997: full reference above under albumin.
Platelets	No significant change fron nonpregnant	No significant change from nonpregnant	Gestational thrombocytopenia is a diagnosis of exclusion that complicates 5% of pregnancies. If low, rule out HIV, consider ITP and pre-eclampsia.	Burrow GN, Ferris TF (eds)1995: full reference above under C3.
TIBC/transferrin	Normal to increased	Normal to increased	Increased due to increased hepatic production and erythropoiesis of pregnancy. Iron deficiency should be diagnosed based on ferritin, TIBC, and iron levels.	Kaneshige E, 1981: full reference above under iron.
Transferrin saturation	Normal to decreased	Normal to decreased	Decreases due to increased TIBC (see above) and decreased iron levels. It should not be used as the sole determinant of iron deficiency.	Milman N, et al, 1994: full reference above under ferritin.
Vitamin B12	Decreases with gestational age. First trimester: 419 pg/mL (338–527)[δ] Third trimester: 270 pg/mL (243–297)[δ]	Decreases with gestational age. First trimester: 309 pmol/L (249–389)[δ] Third trimester: 199 pmol/L (179–219)[δ]		Van Wersch JWJ, Janssens Y, Zandvoort JA. Folic acid, vitamin B12, and homocysteine in smoking and non-smoking pregnant women. Eur J Obstet Gynecol Reprod Biol 2002;103:18–21.
White blood cell count	Increased $9 \times 10^3/mm^3$ (6–14)	Increased $9 \times 10^9/L$ (6–14)	There is a leukocytosis noted to occur with pregnancy. Further escalation in WBC may occur with delivery.	Burrow GN, Ferris TF (eds) 1995: full reference above under C3.

(Continued on p. 668)

Test	Expected antepartum values during pregnancy (conventional units)	Expected antepartum values during pregnancy (SI units)	Comments	Evidence
Hemostatic				
Antithrombin	No change from nonpregnant	No change from nonpregnant		Bremme KA, Haemostatic changes in pregnancy. Best Pract Res Clin Haematol 2003;16(2):153–68.
D-Dimer	Increases with gestational age. First trimester: 0.091 micrograms/mL (0.043–0.139) Third trimester: 0.198 micrograms/mL (0.08–0.316)	Increases with gestational age. First trimester: 0.091 mg/L (0.043–0.139) Third trimester: 0.198 mg/L (0.08–0.316)	The normal increase in pregnancy makes it difficult to interpret when assessing for the likelihood of a thrombotic event. It is reasonable to apply the negative predictive value for venous thrombosis to pregnant women, although trials are lacking.	Bremme KA, 2003: full reference above under antithrombin.
Factor levels	Factors VII, VIII, IX, X, XII: Increase Factor V: Unchanged Factor XI: Small decrease	Factors VII, VIII, IX, X, XII: Increase Factor V: Unchanged Factor XI: Small decrease	Most factor levels increase as pregnancy progresses. Patients with underlying factor deficiencies (vWD or VIII) may have fewer bleeding complications during pregnancy/and postpartum. Postpartum factor levels drop precipitously to pre-pregnancy levels and patients should be monitored closely during this period.	Bremme KA, 2003: full reference above under antithrombin.
Fibrinogen	Increased. First trimester: mean: 370 mg/dL (310–430)[δ] Third trimester: mean: 540 mg/dL (460–620)[δ]	Increased. First trimester: mean: 3.7 g/L (3.1–4.3)[δ] Third trimester: mean: 5.4 g/L (4.6–6.2)[δ]	Due to a decrease in fibrinolytic activity as defense against postpartum hemorrhage.	Bremme KA, 2003: full reference above under antithrombin.
Protein C	No change from nonpregnant	No change from nonpregnant		Bremme KA, 2003: full reference above under antithrombin.
Protein S activity	Decreased. Nonpregnant antigen or activity level usually greater than 60%. During pregnancy, 2nd and 3rd trimester median levels are about 50%. Although the normal range is not easily defined, it may be as low as 30%	Decreased	Diagnosis of protein S deficiency cannot be made with certainty in pregnancy.	Comp PC, Thurnau GR, Welsh J, Esmon CT. Functional and immunologic protein S levels are decreased during pregnancy. Blood 1986;68(4):881–5. Wickstrom K, Edelstan G, Lowbeer CH, Hansson LO, Siegbahns A. Reference intervals for plasma levels of fibronectin, von Willebrand factor, free protein S and antithrombin during third-trimester pregnancy. Scand J Clin Lab Invest 2004;64(1):31–40. Hojo S, Tsukimori K, Kinukawa N, Hattori S, Kang D, Hamasaki N, Wake N. Decreased maternal protein S activity is associated with fetal growth estriction. Thromb Res 2008;123(1):55–9.
PT, PTT	No change from nonpregnant	No change from nonpregnant		Burrow GN, Ferris TF (eds) 1995: full reference above under C3.

Test	Expected antepartum values during pregnancy (conventional units)	Expected antepartum values during pregnancy (SI units)	Comments	Evidence
Resistance to activated protein C (functional)	High risk for false positives	High risk for false positives	Increase in factor VIII levels can cause a "false-positive" resistance to APC that will not be found when testing is performed before or 6 weeks after pregnancy. Prevalence increases from 5% nonpregnant to 60% during pregnancy.	Walker MC, Garner PR, Keely EJ, Rock GA, Reis MD. Changes in activated protein C resistance during normal pregnancy. Am J Obstet Gynecol 1997;177(1):162–9
Von Willebrand factor (vWF)	Increased	Increased	Clinical significance is the same as described above for factor levels.	Bremme KA, 2003 full reference above under antithrombin.
Renal system				
Blood urea nitrogen (BUN)	Decreased 7 mg/dL (4–14)	Decreased 2.5 mmol/L (1.4–5)	Due to increased renal plasma flow and resultant increased glomerular filtration rate (GFR). Generally <14 mg/dL (5 mmol/L)	Burrow GN, Ferris TF (eds) 1995: full reference above under C3.
Creatinine clearance	Increased 150 cc/min (120–160)	Increased 2.5 mL/sec (2– 2.7)	50% higher than the nonpregnant value. Change usually seen by second trimester	Brown C, Saffan B, Howard C, Preedy J. The renal clearance of endogenous estrogens in late pregnancy. J Clin Invest. 1964;43:295–303.
Creatinine	Decreased 0.6 mg/dL (0.3–0.9)	Decreased 53 micromol/L (26–79)	Due to increased GFR. Generally <0.9 mg/dL (79 micromol/L)	Girling JC. Re-evaluation of plasma creatinine concentration in normal pregnancy. Obstet Gynaecol 2000;20(2):128–31.
24-Hour urine protein	Increased. Normal is <300 mg Mean 117 mg (47–260)	Increased. Normal is <300 mg Mean 117 mg (47–260)	Increased urinary protein excretion may be double of that of nonpregnant patients due to increased GFR and perhaps changes in glomerular permeability and/or altered tubular reabsorption of protein. When elevated consider pre-eclampsia or glomerular disease.	Higby K, Suiter CR, Phelps JY, Siler-Khodr T, Langer O. Normal values of urinary albumin and total protein excretion during pregnancy. Am J Obstet Gynecol 1994;171(4):984–9.
Rheumatologic				
Complement C3	Slightly increased 165 mg/dL(161–169)[δ]	Slightly increased 1.65 g/L (1.61–1.69)[δ]	May be 10 mg/dL lower in antiphospholipid antibody positive individuals. Levels do not change with pre-eclampsia.	Buyon JP, Cronstein BN, Morris M, Tanner M, Weissmann G. Serum complement values (C3 and C4) to differentiate between systemic lupus activity and pre-eclampsia. Am J Med 1986;81(2):194–200. Sugiura-Ogasawara M, Nozawa K, Nakanishi T, Hattori Y, Ozaki Y. Complement as a predictor of further miscarriage in couples with recurrent miscarriages. Hum Reprod 2006;21(10):2711–4. Burrow GN, Ferris TF (eds) Medical complications during pregnancy. W.B. Saunders. Philadephia, 1995.

(Continued on p. 670)

Test	Expected antepartum values during pregnancy (conventional units)	Expected antepartum values during pregnancy (SI units)	Comments	Evidence
Complement C4	Slightly increased 37 mg/dL (35–39)[δ]	Slightly increased 0.37 g/L (0.35–0.39)[δ]	May be 5 mg/dL lower in antiphospholipid antibody positive individuals. Levels do not change with pre-eclampsia.	Buyon JP, *et al*, 1986: full reference above under C3. Burrow GN, Ferris TF (eds) 1995: full reference above under C3.
Complement CH50	Increases with gestational age. Nonpregnant controls: 67.3 U/mL (64.1–70.6)[δ] First trimester: 71.0 U/mL (67.2–74.8)[δ] Second and third trimester: 81 U/mL (78.6–83.4)[δ]	Increases with gestational age. Nonpregnant controls: 67.3 U/mL (64.1–70.6)[δ] First trimester: 71.0 U/mL (67.2–74.8)[δ] Second and third trimester: 81 U/mL (78.6–83.4)[δ]		Jagadeesan V. Serum complement levels in normal pregnancy and pregnancy-induced hypertension. Int J Gynaecol Obstet 1988;26(3):389–91. Burrow GN, Ferris TF (eds) 1995: full reference above under C3.
C-reactive protein (CRP)	Increased in pregnancy and further elevated in labor 0.7 mg/dL (0.1–1.5)	Increased in pregnancy and further elevated in labor 7 mg/L (1–15)	Pregnancy is a relative inflammatory state that results in the elevation of acute phase reactants. Because of the normal increase we discourage ordering this test during pregnancy.	Watts DH, Krohn MA, Wener MH, Eschenbach DA. C-reactive protein in normal pregnancy. Obstet Gynecol 1991;77(2):176–80.
Sedimentation rate	Increased <20 weeks: 18 mm/h (6–46)[φ] >20 weeks: 30 mm/h (12–70)[φ]	Increased <20 weeks: 18 mm/h (6–46)[φ] >20 weeks: 30 mm/h (12–70)[φ]	Increased primarily due to the increase in fibrinogen. Because of the normal increase we discourage ordering this test during pregnancy.	Van Den Broek NR, Letsky EA. Pregnancy and the erythrocyte sedimentation rate. Br J Obstet Gynaecol 2001;108(11):1164–67.

Reference range includes mean followed by 95% CI in parenthesis unless otherwise stated.
[δ]indicates the interval in parenthesis +/– 1SD, [φ]indicates a median value.

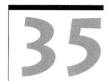

Approach to headaches in pregnancy

Jessica Illuzzi[1], Emma Barber[1] and Men-Jean Lee[2]

[1]Department of Obstetrics, Gynecology and Reproductive Sciences, Yale University School of Medicine, New Haven, CT, USA
[2]Department of Obstetrics, Gynecology and Reproductive Science, Mount Sinai School of Medicine, NY, USA

Introduction

Headache is a common symptom among pregnant women. Differentiating between benign, often chronic, headache syndromes and acute conditions signifying more serious pathophysiology is crucial. A careful history and physical exam can often aid the clinician in distinguishing between chronic and acute headache syndromes in pregnant women. Likewise, diagnostic imaging and the appropriate use of medical therapy need to be tailored to pregnancy, to avoid known teratogenic, uterotonic or otherwise potentially harmful agents.

In 2004, the International Headache Society (IHS) presented an updated classification system [1], which categorizes headaches as primary (tension and migraine) or secondary (tumor, trauma) (Box 35.1) and describes the typical signs and symptoms associated with each type (Table 35.1).

Box 35.1 IHS classification (2004)

Primary headaches

- Migraine with and without aura
- Tension-type
- Cluster
- Other
  - Stabbing
  - Cough
  - Orgasmic
  - Exertional

Secondary headaches

- Trauma
- Vascular disorders
  - Subarachnoid hemorrhage
  - Cerebral venous thrombosis
  - Vasculitis
  - Ischemic stroke
  - Vascular malformation
  - Arterial dissection
- Intracranial disorders
  - Idiopathic intracranial hypertension
  - Postdural puncture
  - Neoplasm
- Substance abuse or withdrawal
  - Alcohol
  - Caffeine
  - Cocaine
  - Medication overuse
- Infections
  - Meningitis
- Disorders of homeostasis
  - Pre-eclampsia
  - Hypoglycemia
- Disorders of cranial structures
  - Sinusitis
  - TMJ
- Psychiatric disorders
  - Somatization
  - Psychosis
- Neuralgias
  - Trigeminal neuralgia

Primary headaches

Chronic headache syndromes, classified as primary headaches by IHS, include tension, migraine, and cluster headaches. Melhado *et al.* interviewed a prospective cohort of 1101 pregnant women at three points during their pregnancies [2]; 93% reported a history of headache prior to pregnancy. Using the

de Swiet's Medical Disorders in Obstetric Practice, 5th edition. Edited by R. O. Powrie, M. F. Greene, W. Camann. © 2010 Blackwell Publishing.

Table 35.1 Characteristics of headaches in pregnancy

Headache type	Onset	Location	Character	Duration	Worsened by	Other symptoms	Course with pregnancy	Diagnosis
Tension type	Gradual	Bilateral	Constant, pressing/ tightening, mild/moderate	30 minutes to 7 days	–	Pericranial tenderness, minimal photophobia	No change	Symptomatology and history
Migraine	Progressive, may be preceded by aura	Unilateral, frontotemporal	Pulsating, moderate/severe	4–72 h	Exertion	Nausea, vomiting, photo/phonophobia	Majority improve	Requires at least 5 attacks to fulfill definition
Cluster	Sudden, up to 8 times per day	Unilateral, periorbital	Severe, constant	15–180 minutes	–	Ipsilateral tearing, sweating, congestion, edema, miosis, agitation	Rare	Symptomatology and history
Pre-eclampsia/ eclampsia	Gradual	Bilateral	Pulsating	Persists intermittently until delivery	Exertion	Scotomata, right upper quadrant and epigastric pain	Occurs during pregnancy after 20 weeks gestation and up to 7 days post partum	Typically blood pressure >140/90 on 2 instances 6 hrs apart and proteinuria >300mg/24hrs
Hypertensive crisis	Gradual	Bilateral	Pulsating	Resolves within 1 hour of normalization of blood pressure	Exertion	–	Increased incidence in women with chronic hypertension	Blood pressure >160/120
Cerebral venous thrombosis	Progressive	Diffuse	Severe	Weeks, until dissolution of thrombus by anticoagulation	–	Neurologic deficits, seizures, loss of consciousness, increased intracranial pressure	Increased incidence	MR or CT angiography
Subarachnoid hemorrhage	Abrupt	Unilateral	Incapacitating, worst ever	Days	Exertion	Nausea/vomiting, altered consciousness	Unchanged	CT, MRI, LP
Idiopathic intracranial hypertension	Progressive	Diffuse	Constant	Resolves within 72 h of normalization of ICP	Coughing, Valsalva	Papilledema, visual field defects	Unchanged	LP to measure ICP (>200mm H20)
Postdural puncture	Progressive within 5 days of dural puncture	Diffuse	Constant	1 week or 48 h after epidural blood patch	Upright position	Neck stiffness, tinnitus, hypacusia, photophobia, nausea	Associated with epidural and spinal analgesia	Symptomatology and history
Neoplasm	Progressive	Localized	Worse in morning	Indefinite, unless surgically resected	Cough or bending forward	Focal neurologic signs	Unchanged	CT, MRI
Caffeine withdrawal	Within 24 h of last caffeine intake	Bilateral	Pulsating	1 h if caffeine ingested, 7 days if not	–	–	Frequent in first trimester	Symptomatology and history
Meningitis	Progressive	Diffuse	Constant	Up to months after resolution of infection	–	Fever, stiff neck, nausea, photo/phonophobia	Unchanged	LP
Sinus headache	Gradual	Frontal, facial	Constant	7 days	–	Acute sinusitis	Unclear	CT, MRI

IHS headache classification system, 82.4% had a history of migraine or probable migraine with or without aura and 11.3% had tension-type headaches; 55% of women reported improvement in the first trimester, 60% in the second trimester, and 65% during the third trimester. Of the 7% of women who experienced a new or different headache during the pregnancy, 34.2% were classified as migraine, 2.6% as tension type, and 32.9% as headache secondary to hypertension. The remainder were characterized as secondary (e.g. sinusitis, neck or facial pain, withdrawal from caffeine or medication).

Migraine headache

Severe migraines affect approximately 17% of American women [3]. They are usually characterized as unilateral and pulsating and may be associated with photophobia, phonophobia, nausea, and exacerbation by physical activity [1]. Migraines are associated with fluctuations in estrogen levels and may actually improve during pregnancy when estrogen levels are higher and constant [4,5]. For this reason, migraines tend to recur during the postpartum period when estrogen levels fall, particularly in women with a history of menstrual-associated migraines. Of note, migraines are less frequent in breastfeeding women [6].

When migraines recur during pregnancy, treatment must consider the effect on the developing fetus. Box 35.2 reviews the components of many combination formulation medications used to treat headaches, and Box 35.3 provides the US Food and Drug Administration's pregnancy safety category for many of the agents used to treat headaches. Table 35.2 lists many of

Box 35.2 Components of common headache medications

- Excedrin ®   Acetaminophen, aspirin, caffeine
- Fioricet ®   Acetaminophen, butalbital, caffeine
- Fiorinal ®   Aspirin, butalbital, caffeine
- Vicodin ®   Acetaminophen, hydrocodone
- Darvocet ®   Acetaminophen, propoxyphene
- Midrin ®   Acetominophen, isometheptene, dichloralphenazone

Box 35.3 US FDA classification of medications used to treat headaches and associated conditions

NSAID and analgesics		Ergot alkaloids	
Acetaminophen	B	Ergotamine	X
Ibuprofen	B	**Beta-blockers**	
Naproxen	B	Propranolol	D
Aspirin	C/D	Timolol	D
Indometacin	B	Atenolol	D
Narcotics		Labetalol	B
Codeine	C	**Tricyclic antidepressants**	
Hydrocodone	C	Amitriptyline	C
Oxycodone	B	Nortriptyline	D
Propoxyphene	C	Doxepin	C
Meperidine	B	**Calcium channel blockers**	
Barbiturates		Nifedipine	C
Butalbital	C	Nimodipine	C
Serotonin agonists		Verapamil	C
Sumatriptan	C	**Anticonvulsants**	
Adjunctive medications		Valproic acid	D
Caffeine	B	**Corticosteroids**	
Metoclopramide	B	Prednisone	B
Prochlorperazine	C	Methylprednisolone	C
Promethazine	C	**Decongestants**	
Droperidol	C	Guaifenisen	C
Acetazolamide	C	Pseudoephedrine	C
Isometheptene	Unknown	**Anticoagulants**	
Dichloralphenazone	C/D	Heparin	C
		Warfarin	X

See Box 30.2 for a description of the FDA pregnancy classification system and meaning of each letter.

Table 35.2 Treatment options for migraines in pregnancy

Agent	US FDA category	Dose	Maximum total daily dose (rarely necessary, especially for headache prevention)	Comments
Acute therapies				
Acetominophen (paracetamol)	B	325–1000 mg PO up to every 4–6 hours	4000 mg/day	Can be helpful if used early on in migraine as "cocktail" of acetaminophen, metoclopramide and caffeine
Metoclopramide	B	10 mg PO up to every 6 hours		Can be helpful if used early on in migraine as "cocktail" of acetaminophen, metoclopramide and caffeine
Caffeine	B	40 mg PO up to every 4 hours (caffeine in 8 oz of coffee is 60–120 mg, black tea 45 mg and cola 21 mg)		Can be helpful if used early on in migraine as "cocktail" of acetaminophen, metoclopramide and caffeine
Magnesium	A	1 g IV		
Prochlorperazine	C	5–10 mg PO up to every 6–8 hours	40 mg/day	Useful for nausea associated with migraines and the treatment of them
Promethazine	C	12.5–25 mg PO/IV/IM every 4–6 hours		Useful for nausea associated with migraines and the treatment of them
Opioids	B/C	Varies with formulations		Avoid daily use which can cause rebound headaches and neonatal withdrawal syndromes
Ibuprofen	B	400–800g PO up to every 6–8 hours	3200 mg/day	Single dose, intermittent use only (if at all) after 20 weeks gestation
Butalbital	C	50–100 mg PO up to every 4 hours. Usually dispensed in a formulation combined with acetaminophen and/or caffeine		Avoid daily use which can cause rebound headaches and neonatal withdrawal syndromes
Sumatriptan	C	25–100 mg PO × 1, may repeat × 1 in 2 hours if ineffective 4–6 mg SC × 1, may repeat × 1 in 1 hour if ineffective		Safety data in pregnancy are still evolving. Best used as a third-line agent and infrequently at this point
Preventive therapies: used in patients with 3 or more migraines per month. Can take 4–6 weeks to have an effect				
Amitriptyline	C	25–150 mg PO daily at bedtime	300 mg	Start at 25 mg daily taken at bedtime. Main side effects are sleepiness, dry mouth and weight gain
Timolol	D	10–30 mg PO as daily or divided into twice daily dosing	30 mg	Start with 10 mg bid and adjust up. Discontinue if no effect in 6 weeks
Nortriptyline	D	25–150 mg PO daily at bedtime	150 mg	Start at 25 mg daily taken at bedtime. Main side effects are sleepiness, dry mouth and weight gain
Nifedipine	C	30–90 mg PO daily of a once a day formulation of this drug	90 mg	Aim to keep BP >100/60 or higher
Verapamil	C	120–480 mg PO daily of a once a day formulation of this drug	480 mg	Aim to keep BP >100/60 or higher
Trimagnesium dicitrate	A	600 mg PO daily	N/A	Main side effect is diarrhea

the agents that may be used to treat or prevent migraines in pregnancy that are reviewed in the following paragraphs.

Acetominophen is a first-line agent as it is considered safe for the mother and fetus. A dose of 1000 mg has been shown to be effective in reducing pain, photophobia, phonophobia, and is also effective in improving daily functioning [7]. Other medications may be given in combination with acetaminophen to potentiate its effect, such as metoclopramide (10 mg) or caffeine (either in beverages or as a tablet). Nonsteroidal anti-inflammatory drugs (NSAIDs), of which ibuprofen is the most studied, may also be used periodically in the first 20 weeks of gestation.

As gestation progresses, increasing consideration of potential risks versus benefits of the medication should occur because of potential effects of NSAIDs on platelet function, fetal renal function, and premature closure of the ductus arteriosus. If NSAIDs are utilized in the third trimester, many experts would caution against daily use and suggest regular testing of fetal well-being, including measurement of the amniotic fluid volume. The barbiturate butalbital is commonly used in conjunction with acetaminophen or caffeine in pregnancy but in our experience has a significant propensity for causing rebound headaches with frequent use as well as potential for withdrawal and neurodevelopmental issues in the neonate. We therefore recommend that, if used at all, this agent be used only infrequently. Lastly, narcotics, specifically opioids such as codeine, oxycodone, propoxyphene, and morphine, may be considered in refractory cases. Again, caution should be exercised in the prolonged use of any narcotic agents, due to the potential for rebound headaches and their addictive potential for both mother and fetus [8]. We see many patients with rebound headaches from daily use of butalbital or narcotics by well-meaning physicians and therefore instruct patients to try to never use narcotics to treat headaches for more than one day in a row or more than three times a month.

Nonsteroidal anti-inflammatory drugs, acetaminophen, and opioids all reduce pain associated with migraine; however, to abort a migraine as it is beginning, triptans (5-hydroxytryptophan (5-HT) agonists) can be used. These drugs include almotriptan, sumatriptan, rizatriptan, zolmitriptan and anratriptan. Currently, there is limited experience with triptan use during pregnancy, but for patients with symptoms refractory to first-line medications, sumatriptan use may be considered. Sumatriptan is an FDA category C drug and has not been associated with adverse pregnancy outcomes in humans; however, data are limited [9,10]. The sumatriptan registry has the largest number of cases with 7/183 pregnancies showing birth defects, which is consistent with the 2–4% background rate of congenital anomalies in the general population [11]. While some experts would not use these agents in pregnancy until further evidence is published, we believe that the data on sumatriptan suggest that this agent does have a role in second- or third-line treatment of headaches in pregnancy [12].

Another class of drugs used to abort migraines are the ergotamine derivatives. Ergot alkaloids (e.g. Cafergot®) have been helpful for nonpregnant patients but their role as potent vasoconstrictors precludes their use during pregnancy. These drugs are absolutely contraindicated in pregnancy (FDA category X) as they have been associated with increased uterine contractions resulting in abortion or decreased blood flow to the fetus leading to hypoxic sequelae [13].

For patients with a history of severe migraines or chronic, recurrent migraines >4 times per month, beta-blockers, calcium channel blockers and antidepressants can all be used prophylactically to reduce the onset of new migraines [14].

When appropriate, underlying conditions (i.e. hypertension, depression) should help guide the selection of which class of drugs is most appropriate.

Beta-blockers such as propranolol, 80–240 mg/d, and timolol, 20–30 mg/d, have been proven efficacious for the prevention of migraine [15]. Beta-blockers with intrinsic sympathomimetic activity (acebutolol, alprenolol, oxprenolol, pindolol) seem to be ineffective for the prevention of migraine [16]. The long-acting beta-blockers such as propranolol and atenolol are FDA class D due to the possible risk of intrauterine fetal growth restriction in the second and third trimesters. Beta-blockers also have the potential adverse effect of causing a beta-blockade in the fetus as well as the mother. Beta-blockade produces fetal hypoglycemia, bradycardia, hyperbilirubinemia, and can cause fetal growth restriction. However, these studies are largely among women with underlying hypertension, also a risk factor for growth restriction, and whether there truly is a cause for significant concern about the use of any beta-blocker in pregnancy is widely questioned [17]. In women refractory to conventional therapy, we support the use of prophylactic beta-blockers after discussing risks and benefits.

Tricyclic antidepressants, such as amitriptyline (US FDA Class C), nortriptyline (US FDA Class D), doxepin (US FDA Class C), are also effective for headache prophylaxis [16]. In the antidepressant class, amitriptyline, 30–150 mg/d, has been more frequently studied than other antidepressants and is the only one with consistent support for efficacy in migraine prevention. Nortriptyline is a metabolite of amitriptyline and therefore likely has similar efficacy (and toxicities). Occasional reports have associated the therapeutic use of amitriptyline with congenital malformations; however, the bulk of the evidence indicates it is safe during pregnancy [18]. Additionally, because of the extensive experience with tricyclic antidepressants, amitriptyline and nortriptyline are preferred over other antidepressants for use in pregnancy. In patients who are depressed with severe migraine, a tricyclic antidepressant may treat both conditions; however, the addition of a newer atypical antidepressant may be needed. The use of some tricyclics have been associated with neonatal withdrawal symptoms; however, no significant long-term effects have been attributed to their use [19].

Calcium channel blockers such as nifedipine, nimodipine, cyclandelate, and verapamil seem to have modest effects in preventing the onset of migraines [20]. Nifedipine is the most studied of these agents in pregnancy, and verapamil is perhaps the next best studied. These calcium channel blockers seem to be safe in pregnancy as long as the patient's blood pressure remains normal [21]. Magnesium may have some role both as an acute treatment for migraine (IV 1 g magnesium sulfate) and in prophylaxis (PO trimagnesium dicitrate 600 mg once daily [22]).

Anticonvulsants such as divalproex sodium and sodium valproate are efficacious in treating migraines in nonpregnant patients [23,24]. However, these drugs have been associated with an increased risk for congenital malformations, significant neurodevelopmental problems and fetal death and are therefore to be avoided in pregnant patients and in women who may become pregnant [25,26].

Both migraines themselves and the migraine drugs listed have the potential to cause nausea and vomiting. Prochlorperazine and promethazine (centrally acting dopaminergic antagonists) can be used relieve these symptoms. Prochlorperazine has been found to be safe during pregnancy [27,28], although it is currently not listed as compatible with breastfeeding by the American Academy of Pediatrics.

For intractable migraine, which is refractory to the above treatments, corticosteroids can be used. Both prednisone and methylprednisolone are metabolized by the placenta and, therefore, are associated with no significant risk of birth defects [29]. Dexametasone and betametasone, in contrast, are not metabolized in the placenta and remain metabolically active in the fetal bloodstream and tissues. Intravenous droperidol can also be used in refractory cases and is not associated with risk of birth defects or spontaneous abortions; however, it has been associated with maternal akathisia [30].

Tension headache

Tension headaches, characterized in Table 35.1, are common and typically less severe. They are often difficult to distinguish from migraines. However, tension headaches are usually bilateral and constant, while migraines are usually unilateral and associated with photophobia, phonophobia, nausea, and exacerbation by physical activity. They can be markers for domestic strife and should prompt screening for domestic violence and substance misuse although the vast majority of sufferers of tension headaches will have neither. Tension headaches often respond to over-the-counter medications, such as acetaminophen, ibuprofen or other NSAID with or without caffeine [31]. Similar precautions should be taken regarding the chronic use of these medications. For patients using analgesics daily, prophylactic therapy is indicated. Tricyclic antidepressants (amitriptyline, up to 100 mg/d) have shown the most success in prophylaxis [32]. Nonpharmacologic options such as biofeedback, stress therapy, psychotherapy, and relaxation therapy have all been reported to be effective for tension headaches, although the therapy may take months before producing a reduction in headache.

Cluster headache

Cluster headache is a devastating primary headache disorder that is characterized by autonomic symptoms [33]. It has a 3:1 male preponderance and is believed not to be affected by hormonal fluctuation. Cluster headaches have an unknown mechanism and are characterized by frequently recurring, short-lasting, extremely severe headache that can occur in bouts (clusters), typically of 6–12 weeks' duration once a year or 2 years and at the same time of year. It is typically one-sided,

periorbital, and occurs mostly at night. It can be associated with conjunctival erythema and tearing. The patient may experience rhinorrhea and ptosis on the affected side. This type of headache is rarely encountered in pregnant women. Several retrospective studies reported no apparent increase in cluster headaches in pregnancy in women with a previous history of cluster headaches [33,34]. Cluster headache during pregnancy may be difficult to treat, but may include corticosteroids, narcotics or calcium channel blockers such as verapamil. Ergot alkaloids and lithium may be used outside pregnancy. One novel therapy that may be considered during pregnancy in refractory cases is inhalation therapy with 100% oxygen. This has been found to be effective in about 70% of attacks [35].

Secondary headaches

Secondary headaches include those that are a symptom of an underlying process, such as trauma, neoplasm, vasculitis, and meningitis. Certain secondary headaches more commonly seen in pregnancy are described below.

Rebound headaches

Perhaps the most under-reported headache presenting in pregnancy is the rebound headache which may occur when a newly pregnant woman decides to immediately abstain from caffeine or other regularly used analgesic medications that contain caffeine or narcotics. While unnecessary medications should be avoided in pregnancy, tapering usage until cessation may be prudent. If a woman uses headache medications containing narcotics or caffeine more than 2 or 3 days per week, she may have a strong propensity to develop rebound headaches. Likewise, caffeine withdrawal headaches usually occur in the setting of daily caffeine intake greater than 200 mg for at least 2 weeks. If caffeine ingestion is stopped without a taper, headaches may ensue that last for about 1 week [1]. Caffeine consumption greater than 500 mg daily (equivalent to five 10 oz cups of coffee) has been linked to adverse outcomes, such as increased spontaneous abortion rates [36], so women may be encouraged to taper their caffeine consumption to lower levels (<100 mg) rather than abruptly ceasing caffeine consumption when pregnancy occurs.

Sinus headaches

Due to increase in vascularity and mucus production, pregnancy is associated with an increased susceptibility to sinus congestion [37]. Women who are prone to sinus congestion and sinusitis may note an increase in sinus headaches during pregnancy. They are typically periorbital or temporal and constant [1]. Treatment of a sinus headache should include acetaminophen and decongestants, as well as antibiotic therapy if there are signs and symptoms of bacterial sinusitis, such as fever and tenderness to palpation over sinuses on physical examination. Guaifenesin and pseudoephedrine (both FDA class C) may help to loosen mucus secretions and decrease mucus production, respectively, in order to relieve sinus pressure. The latter should be used with caution in women with underlying hypertension. Steroid nasal sprays, ipratropium nasal sprays and short-term use of oxymetazoline nasal sprays may have a role in patients with predominant nasal symptoms.

Pre-eclampsia/eclampsia

Pre-eclampsia should be considered in all women at greater than 20 weeks gestation who present with either new-onset headaches or a change in their previous headache pattern. A careful evaluation for hypertension, epigastric tenderness and laboratory testing of complete blood count, uric acid, aspartate aminotransferase (AST), creatinine and urinary protein is appropriate in these cases. The underlying pathophysiology of headache in pre-eclampsia is likely related to cerebral edema, increased cerebral perfusion pressure, and cerebral ischemia from vasospasm [38–40]. The headache associated with pre-eclampsia is often bilateral, throbbing and exacerbated by activity and worsening hypertension. Treatment, therefore, is aimed at controlling blood pressure and, if appropriate, promoting delivery; magnesium sulfate is used to prevent seizures. In a study by Chames et al., worsening headache was present in 87% of women who subsequently became eclamptic [41]. Likewise, worsening headache may also be a sign of rising blood pressure. Blood pressures above 160/110 are associated with a 14-fold increased risk of hemorrhagic stroke [42] and therefore should be controlled with appropriate antihypertensive therapy, such as labetalol or hydralazine.

Cerebral vascular hemorrhage

Cerebrovascular accidents remain the sixth leading cause of maternal mortality [43]. Subarachnoid hemorrhage is often noted to cause a sudden and severe headache ("thunderclap" headache or "the worst headache of one's life") accompanied by loss of consciousness and vomiting. These typically occur in the setting of an arteriovenous malformation or a saccular or berry aneurysm. The risk of rupture of these congenital defects appears to be constant and not affected by pregnancy itself [1]. However, diagnosis and therapy may be delayed in pregnancy, due to concerns about performing diagnostic imaging studies in pregnant women. Prompt therapy is potentially life saving and may prevent long-term neurologic injury, so work-up of a sudden and excruciating headache should not be delayed in pregnant women. Hemorrhagic stroke may occur either during pregnancy or during the postpartum period [44], at which time the risk of subarachnoid hemorrhage may actually be elevated [45].

Cerebral venous thrombosis

This ischemic stroke is rare, but potentially devastating to the pregnant woman. The hypercoagulable state of pregnancy in combination with a prothrombotic disorder, such as deficiencies in protein S, C or antithrombin or antiphospholipid syndrome, is often the setting in which cerebral venous thrombosis occurs. During pregnancy, the sagittal sinus is a common site of cerebral thrombosis [46]. Patients will present with a diffuse, severe, persistent headache and hypertension [1], which often leads healthcare providers to suspect pre-eclampsia. However, the presence of neurologic deficits, altered level of consciousness or headache not relieved by pharmacotherapy should raise suspicion of cerebral venous thrombosis; magnetic resonance imaging (MRI) with or without venography is usually required for diagnosis [47]. Therapy includes anticoagulation and possible thrombolysis or thrombectomy; anticoagulation is continued for at least 6 months.

Postdural puncture

Postdural puncture headaches are a significant cause of headache in the immediate (<72 h) postpartum period after the use of epidural or spinal analgesia during childbirth [48]. These headaches are characterized as "severe and searing like hot metal" in the frontal and occipital regions, radiating to the neck [49]. They are postural and worsened by the upright position. Fortunately, most are self-limited and respond to bedrest in a supine position, aggressive hydration, analgesics with or without narcotic, Occasionally, an epidural blood patch (EBP) (injection of the patient's own blood into the epidural space) is required to prevent further seepage of cerebrospinal fluid at the dural puncture site [1]. An EBP is almost always performed by an anesthesiologist and involves injection of fresh, autologous blood into the epidural space. Relief is almost immediate and the success rate is very high. Side effects can include transient back pain, repeat dural puncture or, rarely, infection. At one time, there was enthusiasm for caffeine in treating postdural puncture headaches (either orally caffeine 300 mg or as IV caffeine sodium benzoate 500 mg in 1 L of normal saline over 1 h) but this is approach is less effective than an EBP. As noted, the sudden decrease in estrogen levels and the sleep-deprived state after delivery may also trigger a migraine headache, so differentiating a postdural puncture headache from migraine and other diagnoses such as pre-eclampsia or cerebral venous thrombosis is important before proceeding to attempt epidural blood patch placement.

Idiopathic intracranial hypertension (pseudotumor cerebri)

This disorder is characterized by a generalized, progressive, nonpulsating headache, aggravated by Valsalva maneuvers. Papilledema is common and usually occurs concomitantly with visual changes such as diplopia. This type of headache most commonly occurs in young, obese women who may or may not be pregnant [1]. Diagnosis requires measurement of cerebrospinal fluid pressure by lumbar puncture. If elevated, cerebrospinal fluid production can be curtailed by the the the use of acetazolamide (500 mg twice daily) or by sequential lumbar punctures. Fortunately, intracranial hypertension seems to improve after delivery, and recurrence risks are only 10% in future pregnancies [50].

Evaluation

The most important tool in the evaluation of a pregnant patient with headache is obtaining a thorough history in order to establish whether the headache syndrome is chronic or acute in nature. The history should include information about the location, duration, severity, and frequency, as well as associated symptoms such as nausea, fever, congestion, numbness, weakness, and visual or other sensory disturbances. Danger signs of serious pathology that should prompt immediate cerebral imaging are reviewed in Box 35.4 and include sudden onset of a new and severe headache (e.g."the worst headache of my life") especially if accompanied by neurologic symptoms, change in mental status, speech abnormalities, seizure or fever [51,52]. History of recent trauma should also be determined.

In addition, the use of medications, caffeine consumption, and substance use should be thoroughly investigated. A complete medical and psychiatric history should be elicited, as well as a description of sleeping patterns, current life stressors, and occupational exposures to noxious stimuli. Patients with frequent or chronic headaches should be screened for depression, domestic violence and substance use.

Physical examination should include temperature, heart rate, blood pressure assessment (with an appropriate sized cuff), and a neurologic assessment of the cranial nerves, motor, sensory and cerebellar function, deep tendon reflexes, gait and Romberg tests. Additionally, the eyes, ears, nose, throat, and neck should be examined to assess for abnormities such as papilledema, meningismus, bruits or infection. Any asymmetry or focal abnormalities should trigger further evaluation, neurologic consultation, and imaging [52]. Box 35.5 summarizes the Cincinatti Stroke Scale, a sensitive screening test for stroke designed for prehospital care that may have applications to obstetric patients who report headache in ambulatory settings. Any positive finding on this screen requires emergency transport to a hospital with a stroke team readily available.

Diagnostic imaging should be pursued in patients with danger signs, worsening headache refractory to therapy or with focal or asymmetric neurologic findings. Noncontrast computed tomography (CT) is the first-line imaging study used in the acute setting to evaluate for intracranial hemorrhage as well as bony trauma. The sensitivity of noncontrast CT falls to 76% by 2 days after subarachnoid hemorrhage [53], so if this etiology is still suspected, lumbar puncture (looking for blood in the cerebrospinal fluid or the more specific finding of xanthochromia) should be performed. Magnetic resonance imaging is indicated to evaluate for cerebral venous thrombosis, vascular abnormalities, tumors, and infectious or inflammatory processes [54].

Both noncontrast head CT and MRI are considered safe in pregnancy and should be obtained when indicated in pregnant patients. Radiation exposure less than 5 rads has not been

---

Box 35.4 Features of headaches that may indicate a serious underlying cause

- Sudden onset
- New-onset headaches
- Severe ("worst headache of my life")
- Headaches increasing in frequency and severity
- Concomitant HIV/cancer
- Headache subsequent to head trauma
- Associated neurologic findings including sleepiness or change in mental status
- Association with fever
- Association with seizures

Box 35.5 Cincinnati stroke scale

1. Facial droop
   - Have the patient smile and assess for facial droop
     - Normal: both sides of face move equally
     - Abnormal: one side of face does not move
2. Arm drift
   - Have the patient hold both arms out and up with palms facing upwards
     - Normal: both arms move equally
     - Abnormal: one arm drifts compared with the other
3. Speech
   - Have the patient repeat a sentence
     - Normal: patient uses correct words with no slurring
     - Abnormal: slurred or inappropriate words of mute

If any of these three elements or any other neurologic findings are newly abnormal, the possibility of acute stroke is high and the patient should have urgent imaging and evaluation by a neurologist.

Reproduced with permission from Kothari RU, Pancioli A, Liu T, Brott T, Broderick J. Ann Emerg Med 1999;33(4):373–8.

associated with fetal loss or abnormalities. A typical head CT results in <0.05 rads of fetal radiation exposure, and an MRI does not use ionizing radiation [55]. If contrast is indicated, it should be noted that gadolinium (FDA class C) crosses the placenta and is excreted by the fetal kidneys, but no adverse effects have been documented. The decision to use gadolinium during MRI should therefore weigh the fetal exposure against the need to visualize with contrast (e.g. suspected maternal arteriovenous malformation prone to rupture). Magnetic resonance venograms and angiography can be performed without contrast as well [56].

References

1. International Headache Society. The international classification of headache disorders: 2nd edition. Cephalalgia 2004;24 (suppl 1):9–160.
2. Melhado EM, Maciel JA Jr, Guerreiro CA. Headache during gestation: evaluation of 1101 women. Can J Neurol Sci 2007;34(2):187–92.
3. Lipton RB, Scher AI, Kolodner K, Liberman J, Steiner TJ, Stewart WF. Migraine in the United States: epidemiology and patterns of health care use. *Neurology.* 2002;58(6):885–894.
4. Marcus DA. Interrelationships of neurochemicals, estrogen, and recurring headache. Pain 1995;62(2):129–39.
5. Melhado EM, Maciel JA Jr, Guerreiro CA. Headache during gestation: evaluation of 1101 women. Can J Neurol Sci 2007;34(2):187–92.
6. Sances G, Granella F, Nappi RE, *et al.* Course of migraine during pregnancy and postpartum: a prospective study. *Cephalalgia.* 2003;23(3):197–205.
7. Lipton RB, Stewart WF, Ryan RE, Jr., Saper J, Silberstein S, Sheftell F. Efficacy and safety of acetaminophen, aspirin, and caffeine in alleviating migraine headache pain: three double-blind, randomized, placebo-controlled trials.[see comment]. *Archives of Neurology.* 1998;55(2):210–217.
8. Mathew NT. Transformed migraine, analgesic rebound, and other chronic daily headaches. Neurol Clin 1997;15(1):167–86.
9. Olesen C, Steffensen FH, Sorensen HT, Nielsen GL, Olsen J. Pregnancy outcome following prescription for sumatriptan.[see comment]. *Headache.* 2000;40(1):20–24.
10. Hilaire ML, Cross LB, Eichner SF. Treatment of migraine headaches with sumatriptan in pregnancy. *Annals of Pharmacotherapy.* 2004;38(10):1726–1730.
11. Reiff-Eldridge R, Heffner CR, Ephross SA, Tennis PS, White AD, Andrews EB. Monitoring pregnancy outcomes after prenatal drug exposure through prospective pregnancy registries: a pharmaceutical company commitment. *American Journal of Obstetrics & Gynecology.* 2000;182(1 Pt 1):159–163.
12. Soldin OP, Dahlin J, O'Mara DM. Triptans in pregnancy. Ther Drug Monit 2008;30(1):5–9.
13. Raymond GV. Teratogen update: ergot and ergotamine. Teratology 1995;51(5):344–7.
14. Modi S, Lowder DM. Medications for migraine prophylaxis. Am Fam Physician 2006;73(1):72–8.
15. Pradalier A, Serratrice G, Collard M, *et al.* Long-acting propranolol in migraine prophylaxis: results of a double-blind, placebo-controlled study. *Cephalalgia.* Dec 1989;9(4):247–253.
16. Buchanan TM, Ramadan NM. Prophylactic pharmacotherapy for migraine headaches. Semin Neurol 2006;26(2):188–98.
17. Pruyn SC, Phelan JP, Buchanan JC. Long-term propranolol therapy in pregnancy: maternal and fetal outcome. Am J Obstet Gynecol 1979;135(4):485–9.
18. Kalra S, Born L, Sarkar M, Einarson A. The safety of antidepressant use in pregnancy. *Expert Opinion on Drug Safety.* 2005;4(2):273–284.
19. Ananth J. Side effects on fetus and infant of psychotropic drug use during pregnancy. Int Pharmacopsych 1976;11(4):246–60.
20. Magee LA, Schick B, Donnenfeld AE, *et al.* The safety of calcium channel blockers in human pregnancy: a prospective, multicenter cohort study. *American Journal of Obstetrics & Gynecology.* 1996;174(3):823–828.
21. Davis WB, *et al.* Analysis of the risks associated with calcium channel blockade: implications for the obstetrician-gynecologist. Obstet Gynecol Surv 1997;52(3):198–201.
22. Peikert A, Wilimzig C, Kohne-Voland R. Prophylaxis of migraine with oral magnesium: results from a prospective multi-center placeb0-controlled and double blind randomized trial. Cephalgia 1996;16(4):257–63.
23. Mathew NT, Saper JR, Silberstein SD, *et al.* Migraine prophylaxis with divalproex.[see comment]. *Archives of Neurology.* 1995;52(3):281–286.
24. Hering R, Kuritzky A. Sodium valproate in the prophylactic treatment of migraine: a double-blind study versus placebo. Cephalalgia 1992;12(2):81–4.
25. Samren EB, van Duijn CM, Koch S, *et al.* Maternal use of antiepileptic drugs and the risk of major congenital malformations: a joint European prospective study of human teratogenesis associated with maternal epilepsy.[see comment]. *Epilepsia.* 1997;38(9):981–990.
26. Kaneko S, Battino D, Andermann E, *et al.* Congenital malformations due to antiepileptic drugs. *Epilepsy Research.* 1999;33(2–3):145–158.
27. Slone D, Siskind V, Heinonen OP, Monson RR, Kaufman DW, Shapiro S. Antenatal exposure to the phenothiazines in relation to congenital malformations, perinatal mortality rate, birth weight, and intelligence quotient score. *Am J Obstet Gynecol.* Jul 1 1977;128(5):486–488.
28. Miklovich L, van den Berg BJ. An evaluation of the teratogenicity of certain antinauseant drugs. Am J Obstet Gynecol 1976;125(2):244–8.
29. Park-Wyllie L, Mazzotta P, Pastuszak A, *et al.* Birth defects after maternal exposure to corticosteroids: prospective cohort study and meta-analysis of epidemiological studies. *Teratology.* 2000;62(6):385–392.
30. Wang SJ, Silberstein SD, Young WB. Droperidol treatment of status migrainosus and refractory migraine. Headache 1997; 37(6):377–82.
31. Mathew NT. The prophylactic treatment of chronic daily headache. Headache 2006;46(10):1552–64.
32. Holroyd KA, O'Donnell FJ, Stensland M, Lipchik GL, Cordingley GE, Carlson BW. Management of chronic tension-type headache with tricyclic antidepressant medication, stress management therapy, and their combination: a randomized controlled trial.[see comment]. *JAMA.* 2001;285(17):2208–2215.
33. van Vliet JA, Favier I, Helmerhorst FM, Haan J, Ferrari MD. Cluster headache in women: relation with menstruation, use of oral contraceptives, pregnancy, and menopause. *J Neurol Neurosurg Psychiatry.* May 2006;77(5):690–692.
34. Ekbom K, Waldenlind E. Cluster headache in women: evidence of hypofertility(?) Headaches in relation to menstruation and pregnancy. Cephalalgia 1981;1(3):167–74.
35. Fogan L. Treatment of cluster headache. A double-blind comparison of oxygen v air inhalation. Arch Neurol 1985;42(4):362–3.

36. Cnattingius S, Signorello LB, Anneren G, *et al.* Caffeine intake and the risk of first-trimester spontaneous abortion. *N Engl J Med*. Dec 21 2000;343(25):1839–1845.

37. Ellegard EK. Pregnancy rhinitis. Immunol Allergy Clin North Am 2006;26(1):119–35, vii.

38. Belfort MA, Saade GR, Grunewald C, *et al.* Association of cerebral perfusion pressure with headache in women with pre-eclampsia. *Br J Obstet Gynaecol*. Aug 1999;106(8):814–821.

39. Schwartz RB, Jones KM, Kalina P, *et al.* Hypertensive encephalopathy: findings on CT, MR imaging, and SPECT imaging in 14 cases. *AJR Am J Roentgenol*. Aug 1992;159(2):379–383.

40. Cunningham FG, Twickler D. Cerebral edema complicating eclampsia. Am J Obstet Gynecol 2000;182(1 Pt 1):94–100.

41. Chames MC, Livingston JC, Ivester TS, Barton JR, Sibai BM. Late postpartum eclampsia: a preventable disease? *Am J Obstet Gynecol*. Jun 2002;186(6):1174–1177.

42. Zia E, Hedblad B, Pessah-Rasmussen H, Berglund G, Janzon L, Engstrom G. Blood pressure in relation to the incidence of cerebral infarction and intracerebral hemorrhage. Hypertensive hemorrhage: debated nomenclature is still relevant. *Stroke*. Oct 2007;38(10):2681–2685.

43. Berg CJ, Chang J, Callaghan WM, Whitehead SJ. Pregnancy-related mortality in the United States, 1991-1997. *Obstet Gynecol*. Feb 2003;101(2):289–296.

44. Stella CL, Jodicke CD, How HY, Harkness UF, Sibai BM. Postpartum headache: is your work-up complete? *Am J Obstet Gynecol*. Apr 2007;196(4):318 e311–317.

45. Kittner SJ, Stern BJ, Feeser BR, *et al.* Pregnancy and the risk of stroke. *N Engl J Med*. Sep 12 1996;335(11):768–774.

46. Roos KL, Pascuzzi RM, Kuharik MA, Shapiro AD, Manco-Johnson MJ. Postpartum intracranial venous thrombosis associated with dysfunctional protein C and deficiency of protein S. *Obstet Gynecol*. Sep 1990;76(3 Pt 2):492–494.

47. Appenzeller S, Zeller CB, Annichino-Bizzachi JM, *et al.* Cerebral venous thrombosis: influence of risk factors and imaging findings on prognosis. *Clin Neurol Neurosurg*. Aug 2005; 107(5):371–378.

48. Reynolds F. Dural puncture and headache. BMJ 1993; 306(6882):874–6.

49. Weir EC. The sharp end of the dural puncture. BMJ 2000; 320(7227):127.

50. Katz VL, Peterson R, Cefalo RC. Pseudotumor cerebri and pregnancy. Am J Perinatol 1989;6(4):442–5.

51. Edmeads J. Emergency management of headache. Headache 1988;28(10):675–9.

52. Lipton RB, Bigal ME, Steiner TJ, Silberstein SD, Olesen J. Classification of primary headaches. *Neurology*. Aug 10 2004;63(3):427–435.

53. Edlow JA, Caplan LR. Avoiding pitfalls in the diagnosis of subarachnoid hemorrhage. N Engl J Med 2000;342(1):29–36.

54. Martin SR, Foley MR. Approach to the pregnant patient with headache. Clin Obstet Gynecol 2005;48(1):2–11.

55. American College of Obstetricians and Gynecologists. Guidelines for diagnostic imaging during pregnancy. Int J Gynacol Obstet 1995;51(3):288–91.

56. Lin SP, Brown JJ. MR contrast agents: physical and pharmacologic basics. J Magn Reson Imaging 2007;25(5):884–99.

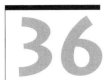

36 Approach to anemia in pregnancy

Dorothy Graham[1] and Jami Star[2]

[1]Obstetric Medicine, University of Western Australia and King Edward Memorial Hospital, Perth, Australia
[2]Department of Obstetrics and Gynecology, University of Massachusetts Medical School, University of Massachusetts Memorial Medical Center, Worcester, MA, USA

Introduction

Anemia is one of the most common medical disorders in pregnancy, with a 75% prevalence in some developing countries. Anemia is defined as a significant reduction in the hemoglobin level or the number of circulating red blood cells. This results in a decrease in the oxygen-carrying capacity of the blood. It is most common in the third trimester as iron reserves have often been depleted by then. Mild anemia is usually asymptomatic but more severe anemia may result in tiredness, light-headedness, palpitations or fainting.

Definition in pregnancy

Erythropoietin levels rise from early in pregnancy and by term are approximately double the level seen at initial booking. This results in an 18–25% increase in the red cell mass which meets the increased maternal oxygen requirements during pregnancy. The rise in red cell mass is even greater in multiple pregnancies. The plasma volume expands by 50% in pregnancy, however, and therefore, despite this increase in red cell mass, a physiologic fall in hemoglobin concentration is seen during pregnancy. The hemoglobin concentration reaches a nadir at about 20 weeks gestation and increases slowly from about 30 weeks until term. It is thought that the lower hematocrit may result in lower blood viscosity which aids placental perfusion and oxygenation of the fetus. The degree of plasma volume expansion is strongly associated with fetal size [1]. Maternal hemoconcentration (determined by an elevated hematocrit reflecting inadequate plasma volume expansion) is associated with premature labor, intrauterine growth restriction and pre-eclampsia.

The World Health Organization has recommended that hemoglobin levels during pregnancy should ideally be maintained at or above 11 g/dL (6.83 mmol/L) compared to 12 g/dL (7.44 mmol/L) in nonpregnant women. The US Centers for Disease Control and Prevention (CDC) considers anemia to be defined by a hemoglobin of <11g/dL in the first and third trimesters and <10.5 g/dL in the second trimester. Other investigators report that the lower limit of normal variation of hemoglobin levels is about 10 g/dL (6.2 mmol/L), with the nadir at around 25 or 26 weeks gestation [2,3]. While anemia is common in pregnancy, it is important to distinguish between physiologic anemia, which is harmless, and pathologic anemia, which may cause harm and/or represent a manifestation of an underlying disease.

Clinical consequences of anemia in pregnancy

Several investigators have found an association between iron deficiency anemia, detected early in pregnancy, and adverse pregnancy outcome. The data are most compelling for cases of severe maternal anemia (i.e. hemoglobin levels less than 6 g/dL) and include increased risks of preterm delivery, low birthweight and both perinatal and maternal mortality. While similar associations have been reported in some studies of women with less severe anemia, the data do not support a clear causal link. It is important to consider that it may be the factors causing the maternal anemia (i.e. infection, chronic illness, hereditary conditions and/or nutritional deficiencies) rather than the anemia *per se* that are responsible for pregnancy complications. Studies on the efficacy of iron supplementation to reduce the incidence of low birthweight and preterm delivery have been limited and inconclusive thus far, although there are no clear contraindications to routine supplementation in most pregnant women.

With respect to neonatal effects, there is increasing evidence that maternal iron deficiency may result in lower infant iron stores, an outcome which can be prevented by adequate maternal iron supplementation during pregnancy [4,5].

de Swiet's Medical Disorders in Obstetric Practice, 5th edition.
Edited by R. O. Powrie, M. F. Greene, W. Camann. © 2010 Blackwell Publishing.

Approach to anemia

Anemia identified on a screening complete blood count in pregnancy is most easily approached from a morphologic standpoint based on the volume of the red blood cells as measured by the mean cell volume (MCV). Table 36.1 classifies the common causes and the initial investigations of anemia by the associated MCV. Many of these etiologies are discussed in more detail in Chapter 2. Some details of the most common causes of iron deficiency anemia are listed in Box 36.1.

In some cases there may be several different populations of red cells with varying red blood cell volumes averaging out to cause a normal MCV. In this case the range distribution width (RDW) on the routine automated red cell indices should be elevated. This is often the case with thalassemia and can also be seen with a combination of abnormalities in one individual (e.g. co-existence of iron and folate deficiency).

It is also important when approaching anemia to confirm that the white blood cells and platelets are normal in number and morphology on the complete blood count. Abnormalities of more than one cell line suggest a different differential diagnosis in many cases that is beyond the scope of this chapter.

Table 36.1 Common causes and initial investigations of anemia

Mean cell volume	Possible etiologies	Initial investigations
Reduced (microcytic), i.e. <80 fL	Iron deficiency anemia (MCV usually only mildly decreased) Thalassemia (MCV may be dramatically decreased) Hemoglobinopathies Sideroblastic anemia (can be congenital or caused by lead or alcohol) Infrequently, anemia of chronic disease	Obtain a serum ferritin If ferritin is low, this is iron deficiency (see Box 36.1): – ask about and look for GI blood loss with three stools for occult blood or colonoscopy – undertake a trial of iron therapy If ferritin is normal: – obtain a hemoglobin electrophoresis – look for evidence of a chronic disease – have a peripheral smear evaluated for sideroblastic changes
Normal (normocytic), i.e. 80–100 fL	Anemia of chronic disease Acute blood loss Hypothyroidism Chronic kidney disease Bone marrow suppression Hemolysis (enzyme deficiencies, membranopathies, hemoglobinopathies, autoimmune or microangiopathic)	Obtain a reticulocyte count If reticulocyte count is greater than 3% of total RBC, suggestive of hemolysis or blood loss: – look for bleeding sources – obtain hemolysis studies (LDH, bilirubin, haptoglobin, peripheral smear) If reticulocyte count is <3%: – review for chronic disease and measure serum iron and ferritin (iron will be low but serum ferritin elevated with anemia of chronic disease) – measure TSH, creatinine and if all are normal consider bone marrow biopsy
Increased (macrocytic), i.e. >100 fL	B12 deficiency Folate deficiency Medications, e.g. zidovudine Alcohol Liver disease Reticulocytosis (e.g. from correction of iron deficiency, hemolytic anemia or after acute blood loss) Myelodysplastic/dyserythropoietic syndrome and aplastic anemia	Take medication, nutritional and alcohol history Check serum B12 levels and serum and red blood cell folate and reticulocyte count If reticulocyte count elevated, suggests reticuloytosis is causing increase in MCV and patient should be evaluated for acute blood loss or hemolysis (LDH, haptoglobin, bilirubin, and peripheral smear) If history and other testing not suggestive of an etiology, consider bone marrow biopsy

LDH, lactate dehydrogenase; MCV, mean cell volume; RBC, red blood cell; TSH, thyroid-stimulating hormone.

Box 36.1 Iron deficiency anemia

- Worldwide, iron deficiency anemia is the most common cause of anemia in pregnancy. Many women of childbearing age enter pregnancy with low iron stores (because of inadequate dietary intake, previous recent pregnancies or menorrhagia) and the red cell expansion in pregnancy requires iron. Maternal iron deficiency anemia without proper iron replacement will worsen in pregnancy as fetal iron requirements are met before maternal iron needs.

- Clinical symptoms of iron deficiency may include pica (particularly the eating of clay or dirt or pica for ice (pagophagia)). Signs of iron deficiency include glossitis (a swollen, smooth and/or discolored tongue), cheilitis (chapped lips), koilonychia (flattened or even concave nails also known as "spoon" nails).

- Outside pregnancy the earliest abnormality seen on the complete blood count in patients with iron deficiency anemia is a reduction in the red cell size as measured by the MCV. In pregnancy the increased numbers of circulating larger young erythrocytes may mean that the MCV may remain normal in the early stages of iron deficiency anemia [6].

- The first laboratory test to become abnormal with iron deficiency anemia is the serum ferritin. Low ferritin levels in pregnancy have been found to correlate with absent iron stores on bone marrow aspiration which is considered the "gold standard" method for assessment of iron stores but is invasive. However, ferritin levels may not reflect iron stores in inflammatory states where they act as an acute phase reactant and rise.

- Pregnant patients who are otherwise well and have a mild anemia with a decreased MCV on CBC are likely to have iron deficiency anemia. They should be asked about gastrointestinal blood loss, nutritional status and pregnancy history and menstrual blood loss. They should also have a confirmatory serum ferritin measured, and be given a trial of iron supplementation. While screening the stool for blood is likely warranted (and consideration of evaluation of the bowels for a bleeding source), this practice is in fact rarely done in obstetric practice unless the anemia is severe.

- In patients with iron deficiency anemia who are given adequate iron supplementation, an increase in hemoglobin concentration of 0.8 g/dL/week can be expected. If the hemoglobin concentration is not responding adequately to iron therapy in a patient with microcytic red blood cells and a low ferritin, an additional cause such as ongoing blood loss or an additional vitamin deficiency should be considered.

References

1. Gibson HM. Plasma volume and glomerular filtration rate in pregnancy and their relation to differences in fetal growth. J Obstet Gynaecol Br Commonw 1973;80(12):1067–74.
2. Garn SM, Ridella SA, Petzold AS, Falkner F. Maternal hematologic levels and pregnancy outcomes. Semin Perinatol 1981;5(2):155–62.
3. Murphy JF, O'Riordan J, Newcombe RG, Coles EC, Pearson JF. Relation of haemoglobin levels in first and second trimesters to outcome of pregnancy. Lancet 1986;1(8488):992–5.
4. Blot I, Tchernia G, Chenayer M, Hill C, Hajeri H, Leluc R. [Iron deficiency in the pregnant woman. Its repercussions on the newborn. The influence of systematic iron treatment (author's transl).] J Gynecol Obstet Biol Reprod (Paris) 1980;9(4):489–95.
5. Puolakka J, Jänne O, Vihko R. Evaluation by serum ferritin assay of the influence of maternal iron stores on the iron status of newborns and infants. Acta Obstet Gynecol Scand 1980;95(suppl):53–6.
6. Thompson WG. Comparison of tests for diagnosis of iron depletion in pregnancy. Am J Obstet Gynecol 1988;159(5):1132–4.

37 Approach to moderately elevated liver function tests in pregnancy not attributable to pre-eclampsia/HELLP syndrome

Margaret A. Miller

Department of Medicine, Warren Alpert Medical School of Brown University, Women & Infants' Hospital of Rhode Island, Providence, RI, USA

Introduction

A number of laboratory tests are available to test the health and function of the liver (Table 37.1). In this chapter, a review of the evaluation of elevated transaminase will be presented.

Transaminases include alanine aminotransferase (ALT) and aspartate aminotransferase (AST) and are markers of hepatocellular injury. The prevalence of elevated transaminases in the US has been found to be as high as 9.8% [1]. Comparing data from the National Health and Nutrition Examination Survey (NHANES) from 1988–1994 and 1999–2002, it appears that there has been a significant rise in the prevalence of elevated transaminases in the US [1]. It is likely that more sensitive assays account for at least some of this apparent rise, but the current prevalence of elevated transaminases is closely associated with risk factors for nonalcoholic fatty liver disease (NAFLD), suggesting that obesity and insulin resistance may be important predictors of chronic liver dysfunction.

While this is not the focus of this brief chapter, the differential diagnosis of elevated transaminases in pregnancy must always include pre-eclampsia/HELLP. In patients beyond 20 weeks gestation, it is important to look for other features of these conditions including hypertension, proteinuria, thrombocytopenia, hemolysis and elevated creatinine and maintain a high index of suspicion for these diagnoses which can be an important cause of both maternal and fetal morbidity and mortality (see Chapters 6 and 9).

Elevated transaminases are often encountered as an incidental finding in the pregnant woman. Common clinical scenarios include the pregnant patient who is less than 20 weeks gestation, is asymptomatic, and has mildly abnormal transaminases or the pregnant woman in the latter half of pregnancy who is screened for pre-eclampsia and has isolated elevation of transaminases with no other features of pre-eclampsia or HELLP. Although the clinician must maintain continued vigilance for the development of pre-eclampsia, it is important to investigate for other causes of elevated transaminases. This chapter will focus on the evaluation and etiology of nonobstetric causes of mild to moderate elevation of transaminases (less than five times normal) in the asymptomatic patient.

Table 37.1 Common liver chemistry tests

Liver test	Clinical implication of abnormality
Alanine aminotransferase (ALT)	Hepatocellular damage
Aspartate aminotransferase (AST)	Hepatocellular damage
Bilirubin	Cholestasis, impaired conjugation or biliary obstruction
Alkaline phosphatase	Cholestasis, infiltrative diseases or biliary obstruction
Prothrombin	Synthetic function
Albumin	Synthetic function
Gamma-glutamyltransferase (GGT)	Cholestasis or biliary obstruction
Bile acids	Cholestasis or biliary obstruction
Lactate dehydrogenase (LDH)	Hepatocellular damage, not specific for hepatic damage

Adapted from Green & Flamm [7].

de Swiet's Medical Disorders in Obstetric Practice, 5th edition.
Edited by R. O. Powrie, M. F. Greene, W. Camann. © 2010 Blackwell Publishing.

Diagnosis

The differential diagnosis of elevated transaminases is quite broad and includes many rare and unusual conditions.

Therefore, a stepwise approach to the evaluation of these laboratory abnormalities is often the most efficient and cost-effective. Once pre-eclampsia and HELLP syndrome have been ruled out, the evaluation should begin with a search for the most common causes of mild, asymptomatic elevated transaminases (Table 37.2). If the initial evaluation does not produce a diagnosis, then the next step is to test for the less common causes including rare liver disorders and nonhepatic causes of elevated transaminases.

In order to recognize the most common causes of mild asymptomatic elevated transaminases, the practitioner should be familiar with the clinical presentation and unique features of each condition.

Nonalcoholic fatty liver disease (NAFLD) is the most common cause of mild elevation of transaminases. In this condition fat accumulates in hepatocytes, causing inflammation. Risk factors include hyperlipidemia, obesity and diabetes, but this condition may occur in the absence of risk factors. There are no serologic tests for the diagnosis of NAFLD. Ultrasound of the liver may reveal a hyperechoic texture or a "bright liver" because of diffuse fatty infiltration [2]. These findings are suggestive but not confirmatory, and should not be used alone to make the diagnosis. Both computed tomography (CT) and magnetic resonance imaging (MRI) may also show a pattern suggestive of steatosis but are not sufficiently sensitive to detect inflammation or fibrosis [3]. A presumptive diagnosis is often made in a patient who presents with risk factors for NAFLD, asymptomatic mild elevation of transaminases, a negative evaluation for other causes of liver dysfunction and an imaging study that is suggestive of NAFLD. A liver biopsy is, however, required to confirm the diagnosis. The decision to perform a biopsy and the timing of the biopsy should be individualized and require consultation with a gastroenterologist. Effective treatment of NAFLD is generally directed at the primary metabolic disorder, including optimizing bodyweight and treating diabetes. Pathologic findings are indistinguishable from alcoholic hepatitis, but the prognosis is significantly different. NAFLD is generally considered to be a clinically stable disease but will progress to cirrhosis in approximately 3–10% of cases [4]. Alcoholic liver disease, on the other hand, is associated with a 30% rate of progression to cirrhosis.

Hepatitis C affects 2% of the US population [5]. Risk factors include a history of intravenous or intranasal drug use, blood transfusion, exposure to contaminated needles or sexual exposure. Screening assays for hepatitis C detect antibody to hepatitis C virus (HCV) and should be done as an initial step. The most commonly used test is an enzyme immunoassay (ELISA) that detects HCV proteins. Patients with positive results should have a confirmatory test. Most hepatologists are now using HCV ribonucleic acid (RNA) (viral load) to confirm the diagnosis. The radioimmunoblot (RIBA) test is still available in some labs, but is less useful. Like the ELISA, the RIBA is also

Table 37.2 Top five causes of mild, asymptomatic nonobstetric causes of elevation of liver enzymes once pre-eclampsia and HELLP syndrome have been ruled out

	Risk factors	Diagnosis
Nonalcoholic fatty liver disease (NAFLD)	Hyperlipidemia, obesity, and diabetes	No serologic tests. Ultrasound with diffuse fatty infiltration is suggestive. Biopsy needed to confirm diagnosis
Viral hepatitis	IV or intranasal drug use, blood transfusion, contaminated needles, sexual exposure	HbsAg, Hbs Ag, Hbc Ab ELISA for HCV Ab to screen HCV RNA to confirm
Medications	Female Common drugs include NSAID, antibiotics, statins, antiepileptic drugs and antituberculosis drugs	Medication history to screen Diagnosis confirmed if LFTs abnormalities resolve with discontinuation of drug
Hemochromatosis	Family history of hemochromatosis Symptoms include fatigue, abdominal pain, arthralgias Can cause congestive heart failure and diabetes	Iron saturation test (serum iron/TIBC) to screen Genetic testing or liver bipsy to confirm
Alcohol	Family history of alcoholism, depression	CAGE questionnaire to screen for problem drinking (2 questions answered positively suggests problem drinking) Have you ever felt you should *cut* down on your drinking? Have people *annoyed* you by criticizing your drinking? Have you ever felt bad or *guilty* about your drinking? Have you ever had a drink first thing in the morning to steady your nerves or get rid of a hangover (an "*eye-opener*")? AST:ALT ratio >2.0 is suggestive Liver biopsy needed to confirm

an antibody test, which has less sensitivity but better specificity than the ELISA. For this reason, it is most useful to test low-risk populations (blood donors with a positive HCV-Ab) where a high false-positive rate is likely. Eighty percent of patients infected with hepatitis C will develop chronic disease and of these, 20–30% will progress to cirrhosis [6]. Hepatitis C is the most common cause of chronic liver disease and the most common indication for liver transplantation in the US.

Hepatitis B is a common cause of mild liver enzyme abnormalities. The prevalence of the hepatitis B surface antigen carrier state is estimated to be 0.1–2% of the US population [7]. An estimated 1.2 million people are chronic carriers of hepatitis B in the US and are potential sources of infection to others. Risk factors are similar to hepatitis C, with the most common being multiple sexual partners, men having sex with men and injection drug use. Vertical transmission at birth or with sexual contact is significantly higher than with hepatitis C. Patients with abnormal transaminases should be screened for hepatitis B with the following tests:

• hepatitis B surface antigen (HbsAg)
• hepatitis B surface antibody (HbsAb)
• hepatitis B core antibody (HbcAb).

Patients with a positive surface antigen and a positive core antibody but negative surface antibody have chronic infection. Additional testing with hepatitis B virus (HBV) DNA (to confirm disease) and hepatitis B e antigen and e antibody (marker of infectivity) is indicated in these patients. A positive hepatitis B surface antibody (HbsAb) indicates immunity and another cause of elevated transaminases should be sought. For patients who acquire hepatitis B in adulthood, the rate of progression to chronic disease is significantly less than with hepatitis C. However, perinatally acquired hepatitis B is associated with a rate of progression from acute to chronic disease that approaches 90% [8].

Almost any medication can cause liver injury. Drug-induced liver injury is thought to cause more than 50% of the cases of acute liver failure in the US today [9]. Women account for a much higher percentage of cases of hepatic drug reactions than men [10]. A 2002 prospective study of liver failure at 17 tertiary care centers in the US found that 79% of cases of liver failure due to acetaminophen and 73% due to idiosyncratic drug reactions occurred in women [11]. Of note, this study also found that women accounted for 73% of all patients with liver failure from any cause. The reason for this female preponderance is not clear. Although it is possible that women are innately more susceptible to liver failure, an alternative explanation is that women take more medications and therefore have a higher risk.

Drug-induced liver injury generally presents with sudden, dramatic clinical findings and often leads to liver transplant. It is likely that mild degrees of liver injury due to medication are much more common, but significant under-reporting of these less dramatic cases makes it difficult to estimate a true incidence [10]. Common offenders include nonsteroidal anti-inflammatory drugs, antibiotics, statins, antiepileptic drugs, and antituberculosis drugs. In addition, herbal preparations and illicit drug use may also be the cause. Careful questioning about the use of over-the-counter drugs, herbs, supplements and illicit drugs (and other high-risk behavior patterns) is critical and should be a routine part of the medical history. Hepatotoxicity may occur at any time after initiating medications, but most often within 1–2 months. It is most likely that the hepatic injury due to medications is reversible once the medication is discontinued, but data on long-term effects of drug-induced hepatotoxicity are lacking.

Alcohol-induced liver injury can be difficult to diagnose because many patients conceal information about their drinking habits. An accurate history is essential and a validated questionnaire screening for alcoholism such as the four-question CAGE questionnaire is helpful (see Table 37.2) [12]. Although alcohol abuse is less common in pregnancy than in a primary care population, it is still a significant issue for many patients and must be considered in the differential diagnosis. The hallmark lab finding in alcoholic liver injury is an AST:ALT ratio greater than 2. It is estimated that 90% of patients with alcoholic liver injury will have an AST:ALT ratio >2 [13]. The higher the ratio, the more likely it is that alcohol is the cause. An elevated gamma-glutamyl transferase (GGT) alone is not specific for alcohol-induced liver injury, but when it is seen in the context of a high AST:ALT ratio, it is supportive of the diagnosis. It is important to note that the AST:ALT ratio may be elevated in an alcoholic pattern in other disease, especially nonalcoholic steatohepatitis and hepatitis C with cirrhosis. Pathologic lesions of alcoholic liver disease progress from hepatic steatosis to hepatitis to cirrhosis. If found early in the course of disease, alcohol-induced injury may be reversible.

Hemochromatosis is a common inherited disorder of iron overload that is often overlooked as a cause of mild liver enzyme abnormalities. In hereditary hemochromatosis, mutations in the genes that are involved in iron metabolism lead to an increased absorption of iron from the gastrointestinal tract. This condition is inherited in an autosomal dominant pattern with a homozygous frequency of 1:200 to 1:400. Clinical manifestations of disease are often not evident until after many years of iron accumulation. Women tend to present later in life because iron loss through menstruation partially balances the iron overload. Iron deposition in the liver, pancreas and heart causes a variety of symptoms including weakness, fatigue, abdominal pain and arthralgias. Hemochromatosis is characterized by congestive heart failure, diabetes mellitus and darkening of the skin. Patients should be screened with an iron saturation test (serum iron/TIBC), also called a transferrin saturation. Genetic testing or liver biopsy is necessary to confirm the diagnosis.

The majority of patients with mild, asymptomatic elevation of transaminases will be found to have one of the above causes. If the initial evaluation is negative, then a less common cause of the abnormality should be sought.

Elevations of transaminases are not always due to liver injury and nonhepatic causes should be considered. Muscle injury due to heavy exercise such as long distance running, inborn errors of muscle metabolism, myopathy or seizure may be a cause [14]. In this case, creatine phosphokinase (CPK) will usually be elevated as well. Thyroid disorders have been associated with elevated transaminases in several studies [15]. A number of reports have described elevated liver enzymes in patients with celiac disease which improve with gluten-free diet [16]. Screening tests for celiac disease include antigliadin antibodies, antiendomysial antibodies (EMA) and tissue transglutaminase (tTG). Other causes of elevated liver enzymes not related to primary liver disease include starvation due to anorexia nervosa or severe hyperemesis gravidarum and adrenal insufficiency [17,18].

Rare liver conditions may also be the cause of mild asymptomatic elevation of transaminases. Autoimmune hepatitis (AIH) is a condition found primarily in young to middle-aged women. Although this condition may cause fulminant hepatic failure, patients may also be asymptomatic or present with a variety of mild, nonspecific symptoms. A useful screening test for AIH is the serum protein electrophoresis (SPEP). More than 80% of patients with autoimmune hepatitis will have evidence of hypergammaglobulinemia on SPEP. Additional tests commonly ordered include antinuclear antibodies (ANA), anti-smooth muscle antibodies (SMA), and liver-kidney microsomal antibodies (LKMA).

Wilson's disease is a rare autosomal recessive condition that usually presents as liver disease and neurologic/psychiatric dysfunction in adolescents. It is caused by impaired secretion of copper into bile and results in excess copper in body tissues, especially in the liver. Hemolysis is common. Serum ceruloplasmin is low and urinary copper is high. Clinically, patients present with arthritis, Kayser–Fleischer rings (pathognomonic brownish corneal ring). A liver biopsy is required to confirm the diagnosis. Alpha-1-antitrypsin deficiency is inherited in an autosomal recessive pattern and causes a chronic hepatitis, eventually leading to cirrhosis. An alpha-1-antitrypsin level may be done to screen for this condition.

Evaluation of elevated transaminases

The evaluation of mild, asymptomatic elevation of transaminases not attributable to pre-eclampsia/HELLP syndrome is reviewed in Figure 37.1 and should begin with a thorough

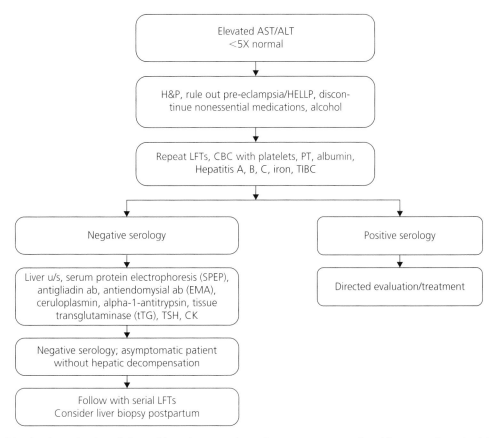

Figure 37.1 Algorithm for the evaluation of elevated hepatic transaminases in pregnancy not attributable to pre-eclampsia. Adapted from American Gastroenterological Association. Medical Position Statement: valuation of liver chemistry test. Gastroenterology 2002;123:136.

history and physical exam focused on identifying the top five causes (see Table 37.2). Patients should be advised to discontinue any nonessential medications and alcohol use. Repeat liver function tests should be ordered within a month to confirm the abnormality along with some further tests of liver function such as albumin and prothrombin time (PT). Screening for viral hepatitis and hemochromatosis is accomplished with the following set of labs: hepatitis A antibody, hepatitis B surface antigen, hepatitis B surface antibody and hepatitis B core antibody, hepatitis C antibody, serum iron and TIBC. Patients with positive findings on this initial work-up should have directed evaluation and treatment. If initial testing is negative, then the less common causes of elevated transaminases should be ruled out. A panel of tests including a liver ultrasound, ANA, antimitochondrial antibody (AMA), antigliadin antibody, antiendomysial antibody, ceruloplasmin, alpha-1-antitrypsin, and thyroid-stimulating hormone (TSH) will effectively rule out these conditions.

In many cases, patients will have a complete work-up that is negative and the provider is left with the question of what to do about mild liver enzyme abnormalities in an asymptomatic patient. Studies have found that liver biopsy in such patients may help to establish the diagnosis, but this infrequently changes the prebiopsy diagnosis and often does not affect treatment [19,20]. If this is the case, it is unlikely that the underlying condition will affect the outcome of the pregnancy; the majority of these cases will turn out to be NAFLD. If the patient is stable with no evidence of hepatic decompensation, it is acceptable to follow with monthly transaminases through the pregnancy. If liver enzyme levels remain stable, then liver biopsy may be deferred until after delivery. If liver enzymes continue to rise during the pregnancy, consultation with a gastroenterologist is warranted after ruling out pre-eclampsia.

Conclusion

It is estimated that abnormal elevations of liver enzymes may occur in nearly 10% of the asymptomatic population. Since liver chemistry tests are included in the panel of standard screening tests for pre-eclampsia, the obstetrician is often confronted with the patient with mild, asymptomatic elevation of transaminases without evidence of pre-eclampsia. In these cases, the differential diagnosis is quite broad, but is most commonly due to one of five leading causes. An informed approach to this evaluation will prevent missed opportunities to identify chronic liver dysfunction and to intervene in treatable or reversible cases.

References

1. Ioannou GN, Boyko EJ, Lee SP. The prevalence and predictors of elevated serum aminotransferase activity in the United States in 1999–2002. Am J Gastroenterol 2006;101:76–82.
2. Lonardo, A, Bellini, M, Tondelli, E, et al. Nonalcoholic steatohepatitis and the "bright liver syndrome": should a recently expanded clinical entity be further expanded? Am J Gastroenterol 1995;90:2072–4.
3. Rofsky, NM, Fleshaker, H. CT and MRI of diffuse liver disease. Semin Ultrasound CT MRI 1995;16:16.
4. Farrell GC, Larter CZ. Nonalcoholic fatty liver disease: from steatosis to cirrhosis. Hepatology 2006;43:S99–S112.
5. Armstrong, GL, Wasley, A, Simard, EP, et al. The prevalence of hepatitis C virus infection in the United States, 1999 through 2002. Ann Intern Med 2006;144:705.
6. Thomas DL, Seef LB. Natural history of hepatitis C. Clin Liver Dis 2005;9:383–98.
7. Green RM, Flamm S. AGA technical review on the evaluation of liver chemistry tests. Gastroenterology 2002;123:1367–84.
8. Stevens CE, Beasley RP, Tsui J, Lee WC. Vertical transmission of hepatitis B antigen in Taiwan. N Engl J Med 1975;292(15):771–4.
9. Lee WM. Drug-induced hepatoxicity. N Engl J Med 2003;349:474–85.
10. Sgro C, Clinard F, Ouazir K, et al. Incidence of drug-induced hepatic injuries: a French population-based study. Hepatology 2002;36(2):451–5.
11. Ostapowicz G, Fontana RJ, Schiodt FV, et al. Results of a prospective study of acute liver failure at 17 tertiary care centers in the United States. Ann Intern Med 2002;137:947–54.
12. Ewing JA. Detecting alcoholism. The CAGE Questionnaire. JAMA 1984;252(14):1905–7.
13. Cohen JA, Kaplan MM. SGOT/SGPT ratio – an indicator of alcoholic liver disease. Dig Dis Sci 1979;24(11):835–8.
14. Nathwani RA, Pais S, Reynolds TB, et al. Serum alanine aminotransferase in skeletal muscle disease. Hepatology 2005;41(2):380–2.
15. Bayraktar M, van Thiel DH. Abnormalities in measures of liver function and injury in thyroid disorders. Hepatogastroenterology 1997;44:1614–18.
16. Bardella MT, Vecchi M, Conte D, et al. Chronic unexplained hypertransaminasemia may be caused by occult celiac disease. Hepatology 1999;29(3):654–7.
17. Olson RG, Lindren A. Liver involvement in addison's disease. Am J Gastroenterol 1990;85:435.
18. Rivera-Nieves J, Kozaiwa K, Parrish CR, et al. Marked transaminase elevation in anorexia nervosa. Dig Dis Sci 2000;45:1959–63.
19. Sorti D, McGill DB, Thistle JL, et al. An assessment of the role of liver biopsies in asymptomatic patients with chronic liver test abnormalities. Am J Gastroenterol 2000;95(11):3206–10.
20. Skelly MM, James PD, Ryder SD. Findings on liver biopsy to investigate abnormal liver function tests in the absence of diagnostic serology. J Hepatol 2001;35(2):195–9.

38 Approach to shortness of breath in pregnancy

Ghada Bourjeily[1], *Hanan Khalil*[2] *and Michael J.Paglia*[3]

[1]Department of Medicine, Warren Alpert Medical School of Brown University, Women & Infants' Hospital of Rhode Island, Providence, RI, USA
[2]Department of Diagnostic Imaging, Warren Alpert Medical School of Brown University, Providence, RI, USA
[3]Department of Obstetrics and Gynecology, Warren Alpert Medical School of Brown University, Women & Infants' Hospital of Rhode Island, Providence, RI, USA

Introduction

Dyspnea is a common complaint in pregnancy. About half of gravidas, without any known history of cardiac or pulmonary disease, experience dyspnea at some point during their pregnancy. In most cases, dyspnea is related to the physiologic changes of pregnancy; however, given the fact that pregnancy is a stressor to the cardiovascular and the respiratory systems, breathing difficulties may indicate a decompensation of an underlying cardiac or pulmonary disorder.

Physiologic changes

In order to be able to differentiate between the various causes of breathlessness (Table 38.1), it is important to understand the normal physiologic changes that occur in the respiratory and the cardiovascular systems. Although respiratory rate in pregnancy remains unchanged at 10–18 breaths per minute, minute ventilation, a product of tidal volume and respiratory rate, is increased in pregnancy as a result of the rise in tidal volume [1–5]. Oxygen consumption also increases gradually in pregnancy starting in the first trimester.

Mechanical changes that occur in pregnancy include widening of the distal ribcage resulting in a larger anteroposterior chest wall diameter [6,7] and a rise in the diaphragm[8]. Respiratory and cardiovascular physiology are discussed in detail in Chapters 1 and 5 respectively.

History

A detailed history should be obtained from the pregnant patient complaining of dyspnea. It is important to understand what exactly a patient is describing as dyspnea. Some details of the description of dyspnea are discussed in Table 38.2.

Other clues that help differentiate different types of dyspnea include the timing of the symptoms and whether they are progressive. For instance, dyspnea that occurs at rest but does not affect the patient's ability to exercise is typical for dyspnea of pregnancy. On the other hand, symptoms that occur with exertion and progress to symptoms at rest are much more worrisome. This usually indicates the presence of an underlying cardiac or pulmonary pathology (see Table 38.2).

Timing and circumstances around the development of symptoms may also provide important pointers.

A certain degree of orthopnea is expected in late pregnancy because of diaphragmatic elevation. Progressive orthopnea and orthopnea associated with paroxysmal nocturnal dyspnea are more worrisome and may be suggestive of left ventricular dysfunction or diaphragmatic dysfunction/paralysis.

Associated symptoms may also help differentiate the various causes of dyspnea and are detailed in Table 38.2.

Physical examination

A thorough physical examination can provide vital clues as to the severity of symptoms and their etiology. Physical examination findings are detailed in Table 38.3.

Pulse oximetry is a simple test that may be performed in the outpatient or inpatient setting. It provides critical information with regard to the etiology and the severity of symptoms. Walking oximetry also helps differentiate between various etiologies of dyspnea. Desaturation with exertion

de Swiet's Medical Disorders in Obstetric Practice, 5th edition.
Edited by R. O. Powrie, M. F. Greene, W. Camann. © 2010 Blackwell Publishing.

Table 38.1 Causes of dyspnea

Type of dyspnea	Cause
Dyspnea of pregnancy	This is an isolated and common physiologic symptom. Dyspnea of pregnancy is usually not associated with any indicators of heart or lung disease and physical exam is usually normal. It is likely related to the awareness of hyperventilation.
Cardiac disease	This may be related to either underlying or new-onset cardiac disease. The presence of nonproductive cough, orthopnea, paroxysmal nocturnal dyspnea and limitation of usual activities are all suggestive of cardiac causes of dyspnea and should be asked about in all patients with dyspnea. Often cardiac causes of dyspnea will be associated with tachypnea and tachycardia on examination.
	Patients with structural heart disease predating the pregnancy such as *valvular disease* may develop symptoms during pregnancy, usually around the time that cardiac output and plasma volume are peaking.
	Cardiac disease that is related to the pregnancy such as *peripartum cardiomyopathy* occurs in the last month of pregnancy or within 5 months following delivery. Specific criteria are needed for the diagnosis of this condition and are discussed in more detail in Chapter 5.
	Coronary artery disease is an unusual cause in a young population but may occur more often in pregnant patients with underlying cardiovascular risk factors such as diabetes, hypertension and smoking. Although classically coronary artery disease presents with chest pain, in women the presentation is often atypical and may present with dyspnea as the primary symptom.
Pulmonary disease	Airway disease is likely the most common cause of nonphysiologic dyspnea in the outpatient population. *Asthma* is the most common chronic medical condition in pregnancy which frequently presents with dyspnea and chest tightness. Patients usually carry a diagnosis of asthma; however, new-onset bronchospastic events may certainly occur in pregnancy, especially in smokers. Other airway disorders include *upper airway infections*.
	Pulmonary vascular disease is another important cause of dyspnea. *Venous thromboembolism* (VTE) is much more common in pregnancy given venous stasis and the hypercoagulable state of pregnancy. VTE is the leading cause of mortality from nonobstetric causes. Clinical predictors have not been studied in pregnancy and the diagnosis of pulmonary embolism is more difficult in pregnancy than the general population.
	Amniotic fluid embolism is a rare but catastrophic complication of pregnancy. Risk factors for the development of this condition include prolonged labor, multiparity and advanced maternal age. This diagnosis should be considered in any woman in labor with an acute cardiorespiratory failure.
	Pulmonary arterial hypertension (PAH) is a rare disease. Idiopathic PAH occurs most commonly in the 3rd and 4th decades of life and more frequently in women. Thus, fertile women represent a subpopulation of patients that have the highest incidence of PAH regardless of whether or not they are pregnant. Pulmonary hypertension is associated with high mortality in pregnancy and patients with a prior diagnosis are usually advised against pregnancy.
	Parenchymal pulmonary disease may also result in dyspnea but is not a common occurence. Sarcoidosis is one of the more common causes since it has a predilection for young adults. The characteristic noncaseating granulomas can be found in almost any organ. Parenchymal disease may also be associated with autoimmune disorders. Other rare causes include lymphangioleiomyomatosis (LAM), a disorder characterized by proliferation of abnormal smooth muscle cells in the peribronchial, perivascular and perilymphatic areas leading to cystic lesions. Dyspnea in this case may be associated with pneumothoraces and chylous effusions. Women with LAM are advised to avoid pregnancy and contraceptive agents to avoid exacerbation of the disease or acceleration of death. Another rare disease characterized by dyspnea and cystic changes in the lung and which occurs in young adults is pulmonary Langerhans cell histiocytosis. Idiopathic pulmonary fibrosis is uncommon in women of childbearing age.
	More acute parenchymal disease include acute pulmonary edema which may be secondary to cardiogenic or noncardiogenic causes. *Cardiogenic pulmonary edema* result from conditions such as underlying valvular disease or cardiomyopathy. Pulmonary edema may also be related to tocolytics. *Noncardiogenic pulmonary edema* or acute lung injury/ARDS may be secondary to pre-eclampsia, pneumonia, aspiration, trauma, tocolytics or sepsis. This results in acute respiratory failure and usually requires admission to an intensive care unit for supportive care. This condition should be suspected in patients with acute dyspnea, severe hypoxemia, bilateral infiltrates on chest radiographs with a predisposing cause and without a history or findings consistent with cardiac disease.
	Pneumonia is the most common cause of fatal nonobstetric infection and a common cause for acute respiratory failure in pregnancy.
	Pleural disease may be a cause of dyspnea. *Pneumothoraces* may occur but are rare. Those may be primary or secondary to underlying lung disease.
	Pleural effusions may also occur and when large, they may be associated with dyspnea. Causes of pleural effusions are the same in pregnancy as in the nonpregnant population.
Neuromuscular or chest wall diseases	*Kyphoscoliosis* occurs in less than 1/1000 pregnancies. In severe cases, it may be associated with dyspnea related to the restrictive physiology. *Upper and lower motor neuron diseases* and diseases associated with *bulbar dysfunction* may cause complications in pregnancy and may be associated with dyspnea either because of respiratory muscle weakness or because of infections associated with bulbar dysfunction.

Table 38.2 History

Description of dyspnea	Likely diagnosis
Dyspnea described as the need to take a deep breath or the inability to get a deep enough breath. Onset is generally gradual and not acute. Patients often reports having to "catch their breath" while talking on the phone but the condition has no functional limitations	Dyspnea of pregnancy
Dyspnea with chest tightness or wheezing	Airway disease, asthma or cardiovascular disease
Dyspnea started on exertion and progressed to dyspnea on minimal exertion or at rest	Nonspecific but suggestive of pathology
Dyspnea following exposure to specific triggers	Reactive airway disease and asthma
Dyspnea on exertion that does not progress	Weight gain, possible deconditioning and anemia
Progressive orthopnea or orthopnea with paroxysmal nocturnal dyspnea	Left ventricular dysfunction or diaphragmatic dysfunction/paralysis
Timing of dyspnea	
Starts early pregnancy and gets better towards term	Dyspnea of pregnancy
Starts mid-term and progresses	Cardiac disease or asthma [22,23]
Following *in vitro* fertilization	Venous thromboembolic disease or pleural effusions
During labor and delivery	Aspiration pneumonitis, pulmonary embolism, pulmonary edema, amniotic fluid embolism or high-level epidural block
In association with the use of tocolytics or the presence of systemic infection or pre-eclampsia	Pulmonary edema
Associated symptoms	
Chest tightness	Airway or cardiac disease
Hemoptysis	Acute infections, pulmonary vascular disease, cardiac disease, tumors
Chest pain	Pulmonary vascular disease or cardiac disease
Cough	Airway disease or cardiac disease

Table 38.3 Physical examination

Signs	Implications
Tachypnea	This often neglected vital sign is critical to the evaluation and monitoring of patients with dyspnea. Elevations in respiratory rate are suggestive of underlying cardiac, pulmonary or neuromuscular disease
Tachycardia	Heart rate often elevated in setting of hypoxia and with cardiac or pulmonary causes of dyspnea
Paradoxic breathing, use of accessory muscles	Impending respiratory failure
Jugular venous distension	Normal pregnancy, fluid overload or ventricular dysfunction
Peripheral edema	Normal pregnancy or heart failure
Clubbing or cyanosis	Cardiac or pulmonary disease
Displaced left ventricular apex	Hypervolemia, cardiac disease with left ventricular hypertrophy or normal pregnancy
Persistent S2 splitting	Normal pregnancy or pulmonary hypertension
S3	Fluid overload
Soft systolic murmur	Likely a flow murmur (normal finding in pregnancy)
Loud systolic murmur	Valvular or congenital heart disease
Diastolic murmurs	Valvular heart disease
Basilar crackles	Common in normal pregnancy due to atelectasis but may suggest pneumonia, pulmonary edema or pulmonary fibrosis
Wheezing	Airway, pulmonary vascular disease or cardiac disease

usually suggests a diffusion problem that usually results from a parenchymal or vascular disorder. Nevertheless, normal oximetry, whether at rest or with exertion, does not rule out serious disorders. In a small study by Powrie *et al.* [9] in pregnant patients with documented pulmonary embolism, more than 50% had no evidence of hypoxemia on their arterial blood gases.

Diagnostic testing

Arterial blood gases

Arterial blood gases (ABG) help in the detection of hypercapnia, acid–base balance and the degree of hypoxemia. Patients presenting with an acute asthma attack, for instance,

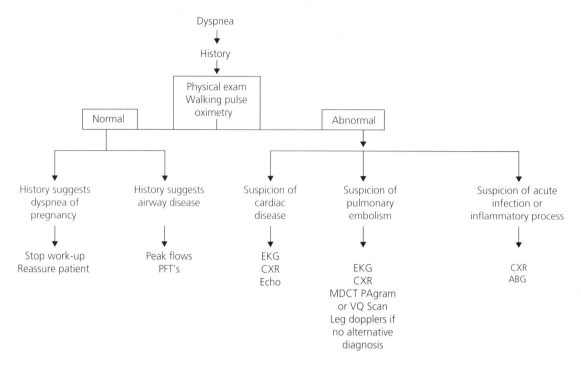

Figure 38.1 Diagnostic approach to dyspnea in pregnancy.

benefit from having an arterial blood gas checked, especially if their symptoms are not improving with initial therapy or in case their peak flows are persistently low. Patients with an acute asthma exacerbation usually hyperventilate and this normally results in hypocapnia and respiratory alkalosis. When the attack is severe, however, the respiratory dead space is increased and normocapnia or hypercapnia ensues. Normocapnia and hypercapnia are ominous signs of respiratory failure. On the other hand, patients with severe chronic lung disease may be hypercapnic at baseline.

Electrocardiogram

Electrocardiograms (EKG) are a quick noninvasive tool that gives the clinician essential information during the work-up of a patient with dyspnea. Arrhythmias may occasionally be diagnosed on an EKG. EKG also supplies evidence suggestive of chamber dilation or ischemia. It is important to keep in mind, though, that pregnancy may result in an axis shift – a leftward axis could be related to hypervolemia and chest wall changes that occur in pregnancy [10]. While heart rate increases by close to 20% in pregnancy, sinus tachycardia is not a normal finding in pregnancy. This increase is most prominent in the late stages of pregnancy. Premature complexes are also common in normal pregnancy. Nonspecific T wave and ST wave changes are not uncommon [10].

Chest radiographs

Chest radiographs (CXR) are an invaluable test in the evaluation of patients with dyspnea, in both the outpatient and the inpatient setting. Fetal exposure to radiation is minimal and is generally <0.001 rad (radiation absorbed dose) (1 rad is equal to 0.01 gray). Please refer to Table 38.4.

Echocardiography

Echocardiography (Echo) helps diagnose cardiac disorders such as right or left ventricular dysfunction, cardiomyopathy, valvular heart disease, congenital heart disorders and pulmonary hypertension. It is important to recognize that there are also changes on echocardiograms seen in a normal pregnancy. These include increased diastolic dimensions of the ventricles, slight increase in systolic function, left atrial dilation, small pericardial effusions and a mild degree of tricuspid regurgitation [11]. Pulmonary arterial pressures may therefore be overestimated by echocardiography. Therefore, a cardiologist experienced in reading this test should make the interpretation, when available.

Ventilation/perfusion scans

Ventilation/perfusion (VQ) scans help diagnose pulmonary embolism in pregnancy. Fetal radiation exposure has been

Table 38.4 Diagnostic tests

Test	Reason for performance
ABG	Obtain to evaluate degree of hypoxemia, presence or absence of hypercapnia (suggestive of hypoventilation) and acid–base status. Helps with management and decision for intubation as well as differentiating etiologies of dyspnea
ECG	Perform to rule out cardiac disease or pulmonary disease with secondary cardiac involvement. Can help detect rate, rhythm, ST or T wave changes that may suggest ongoing ischemic disease, axis deviation, right ventricular strain or left ventricular size/function
Chest radiograph	Helps rule out lung diseases such as pneumonia, pulmonary edema, aspiration pneumonitis, pleural disease or some secondary signs of pulmonary embolism. Chest radiographs also show heart size and help evaluate the mediastinum for widening or masses
VQ scan	Rules out acute pulmonary embolism or chronic thromboembolic disease in patients with pulmonary hypertension. A perfusion scan may be performed first to reduce the amount of radiation associated. If that is abnormal, a ventilation scan is performed and the result is based on the presence or absence of mismatched defects between the ventilation and the perfusion suggesting pulmonary embolism
CTPA	Rules out pulmonary embolism and helps with the evaluation of the pulmonary parenchyma. May offer an alternative diagnosis to pulmonary embolism and supply some prognostic clues in the case of massive pulmonary embolism. Radiation dose is likely less than VQ scans or even perfusion scans alone
CT chest (non-PE protocol)	Helps evaluate the mediastinum, the parenchyma and the airways. This is helpful in diagnosing lung or mediastinal masses or nodules as well as interstitial lung disease. Interstitial lung disease is better assessed with a high-resolution protocol performed with inspiratory and expiratory cuts, both in the supine and prone position in the nonpregnant patient. Prone positioning is usually quite challenging in patients in mid-to-late pregnancy
Pulmonary angiogram	Rarely used now with the advent of CTPA. Considered the gold standard in the diagnosis of pulmonary embolism in pregnancy for decades. The brachial approach is preferred in pregnancy to reduce the amount of fetal radiation exposure
Two-dimensional echocardiography	Helps diagnose cardiac disease including ventricular dysfunction as well as valvular function and pulmonary hypertension. Interpretation of the test should keep in mind the hemodynamic changes associated with normal pregnancy
Pulmonary function tests	Help diagnose obstructive lung disease such as asthma, assess response to bronchodilators and direct therapy. PFT also detect a restrictive physiology that may be associated with interstitial lung disease, neuromuscular or chest wall disease or body habitus and provide clues to differentiate between them

estimated to be around 0.02–0.06 rad for the perfusion scan and 0.03 rad for the ventilation scan [12] and is an acceptable amount of radiation in pregnancy, especially when the morbidity and mortality related to misdiagnosing pulmonary embolism are taken into account.

Perfusion scans are usually performed first. A normal perfusion scan usually obviates the need for a ventilation scan. Although VQ scans are associated with a high number of intermediate results [13] requiring further testing to rule out pulmonary embolism, the rate of intermediate scans is much lower in pregnancy (about 25% in one study) than in the nonpregnant population [14,15]. Another major disadvantage of a VQ scan is, however, the fact that it does not offer an alternative diagnosis. Although there are no data available to confirm the accuracy of VQ scans in pregnant patients (and the outcome data that have been published are retrospective only), we still recommend that until further data become available the test be used and interpreted in a similar manner in pregnancy as is presently done for the general population. It is important to keep in mind, however, that the predictive value of a VQ scan is likely lower in pregnancy than in the general population since the interpretation of the results depends highly on clinical pretest probability; the predictive

power of the clinical assessment or clinical decision tools has not been specifically studied in pregnancy.

Radiation exposure can be minimized by using a smaller dose of radioactive albumin, hydration and encouraging pregnant women to void frequently to avoid pooling of radioactive material in the bladder. Please refer to Chapter 32 for more discussion of imaging risks in pregnancy.

Computed tomography (CT) pulmonary angiography

Both single-detector CT scans and multiple generations of multidetector CT (MDCT) are now widely available and have replaced VQ scans at many centers as the initial diagnostic test for pulmonary embolism in nonpregnant patients. A major advantage of a CT pulmonary angiogram (CTPA) in the diagnosis of pulmonary embolism is the fact that it offers an alternative diagnosis and provides clues of the clot burden and even some prognostic information about the right ventricle. Multidetector CT scans are likely better at identifying small peripheral emboli than are single-detector scans but the clinical importance of this remains unclear. Breath-holding time is also much briefer for CTPA than it is for ventilation scans and can be as short as 5 seconds with 64-row multidetector scanners.

The accuracy of MDCT PA in the detection of pulmonary embolism in pregnancy has not been studied. One study has shown that out of 78 patients with negative CTPA that had leg Dopplers performed within 48 hours, two had evidence of DVT [16]. This study did not compare CT to another imaging procedure. In addition, there are currently no outcome studies available in this patient population. There are, however, ongoing retrospective and prospective outcome studies.

There are also some difficulties associated with the performance of CT angiograms in pregnancy. The increase in plasma volume and the cardiac output may affect the opacification of the vessels, leading to a suboptimal study. In the general population, the rate of inconclusive studies varies between 2% and 9% [17–19] but this rate is likely higher in pregnancy [20]. Given the previously described limitations of MDCT PA in pregnancy, we recommend adding bilateral leg Dopplers to those patients without any evidence of pulmonary emboli and no alternative pulmonary process to explain symptoms.

Fetal radiation exposure in CT angiograms in pregnancy has been shown to vary between 0.01 and 0.02 rad and was suggested to be even lower than that of VQ scans [21]. The risk of breast radiation exposure to young women persists from CT scans of the chest and is estimated to be around 2–5 rads.

Pulmonary function tests

Pulmonary function tests (PFT) can be performed without any risk in pregnancy. In patients with chronic lung disease, a baseline measurement of pulmonary function would be helpful in monitoring disease progression. PFT provide important information regarding flow rates, lung volumes and diffusion capacity. Patients with asthma typically have a reduction in their FEV_1/FVC ratio during an acute attack which usually normalizes between attacks. Peak expiratory flows are also reduced during attacks. Lung volumes may show evidence of restriction or hyperinflation (see Table 38.4). Diffusion capacity can be reduced in patients with restrictive lung disease or pulmonary vascular disease. Respiratory muscle strength can also be assessed during PFT and would help to rule out significant respiratory muscle weakness.

References

1. Cugell DW, Frank NR, Gaensler EA, et al. Pulmonary function in pregnancy. I. Serial observations in pregnant women. Am Rev Tuberc 1953;67:568–97.
2. Knuttgen HG, Emerson K Jr. Physiological response to pregnancy at rest and during exercise. J Appl Physiol 1974;36:549–53.
3. Liberatore SM, Pistelli R, Patalano F, Moneta E, Incalzi RA, Ciappi G. Respiratory function during pregnancy. Respiration 1984;46:145–50.
4. Rees GB, Broughton Pipkin F, Symonds EM, Patrick JM. A longitudinal study of respiratory changes in normal human pregnancy with cross-sectional data on subjects with pregnancy-induced hypertension. Am J Obstet Gynecol 1990;162:826–30.
5. Pernoll ML, Metcalfe J, Kovach PA, Wachtel R, Dunham MJ. Ventilation during rest and exercise in pregnancy and postpartum. Respir Physiol 1975;25:295–310.
6. Contreras G, Gutierrez M, Beroiza T, et al. Ventilatory drive and respiratory muscle function in pregnancy. Am Rev Respir Dis 1991;144:837–41.
7. Weinberger SE, Weiss ST, Cohen WR, et al. Pregnancy and the lung: state of the art. Am Rev Repsir Dis 1980;121:559–81.
8. Gilroy RJ, Mangura BT, Lavietes MH. Rib cage and abdominal volume displacements during breathing in pregnancy. Am Rev Respir Dis 1988;137:668–72.
9. Powrie RO, Larson L, Rosene-Montella K, Abarca M, Barbour L, Trujillo N. Alveolar-arterial oxygen gradient in acute pulmonary embolism in pregnancy. (Erratum appears in Am J Obstet Gynecol 1999;181(2):510.) Am J Obstet Gynecol 1998;178(2):394–6.
10. Carruth JE, Mirris SB, Brogan DR. The electrocardiogram in normal pregnancy. Am Heart J 1981;102:1075–8.
11. El-Khayam U, Gleicher N. Cardiac evaluation during pregnancy. In: Elkhayam U, Gleicher N (eds) Cardiac problems in pregnancy, 3rd edn. Wiley-Liss, New York, 1998.
12. Scarsbrook AF, Evans AL, Owen AR, Gleeson FV. Diagnosis of suspected venous thromboembolic disease in pregnancy. Clin Radiol 2006;61(1):1–12.
13. Anonymous. Value of the ventilation/perfusion scan in acute pulmonary embolism. Results of the prospective investigation of pulmonary embolism diagnosis (PIOPED). The PIOPED Investigators. JAMA 1990;263(20):2753–9.
14. Chan WS, Ray JG, Murray S, Coady GE, Coates G, Ginsberg JS. Suspected pulmonary embolism in pregnancy: clinical presentation, results of lung scanning, and subsequent maternal and pediatric outcomes. Arch Intern Med 2002;162(10):1170–5.
15. Yoo D, Lazarus E, Khalil H, Bourjeily G, Noto RB, Mayo-Smith WW. Diagnostic yield of ventilation perfusion (V/Q) scans in pregnancy: review of the findings in 315 consecutive pregnant patients from 1999 through 2006. Presented at RSNA Meeting, November 2007.
16. Bourjeily G, Khalil H, Habr F, Miller M, Rosene-Montella K. Multidetector-row computed tomography in the detection of pulmonary embolism in pregnancy. Chest 2007;132(4):500S.
17. Quiroz R, Kucher N, Zou K, et al. Clinical validity of a negative computed tomography scan in patients with suspected pulmonary embolism: a systematic review. JAMA 2005;293(16):2012–17.
18. Moores LK, Jackson WL, Shorr AF, Jackson JL. Metaanalysis: outcomes in patients with suspected pulmonary embolism managed with computed tomographic pulmonary angiography. Ann Intern Med 2004;141:866–74.
19. Stein PD, Fowler SE, Goodman LR, et al. for the PIOPED II investigators. Multidetector computed tomography for acute pulmonary embolism. N Engl J Med 2006;354(22):2317–27.
20. Khalil H, Bourjeily G, Lazarus E, Yoo D, Mayo-Smith W. Multidetector CT pulmonary angiograms in pregnant patients: the "limited, no central PE" – how limited? Presented at RSNA Meeting, November 2007.
21. Winer-Muram HT, Boone JM, Brown HL, Jennings SG, Mabie WC, Lombardo GT. Pulmonary embolism in pregnant patients: fetal radiation dose with helical CT. Radiology 2002;224(2):487–92.
22. Stenius-Aarniala B, Riikonen S, Teramo K. Asthma and pregnancy: a prospective study of 198 pregnancies. Thorax 1988;43:12–18.
23. Shatz M, Harden, Forsythe A, et al. The course of asthma during pregnancy, post-partum, and with successive pregnancies: a prospective analysis. J All Clin Immunol 1988;81:509–17.

39 Approach to hypertensive emergencies in pregnancy

Laura A. Magee[1,3], Peter von Dadelszen[2,3] with David Wlody[4]

[1]Department of Medicine, University of British Columbia, Vancouver, BC, Canada
[2]Department of Obstetrics and Gynecology, University of British Columbia, Vancouver, BC, Canada
[3]British Columbia Women's Hospital, Vancouver, BC, Canada
[4]Department of Anesthesiology, State University of New York Downstate Medical Center, Brooklyn, NY, USA

Introduction

Acute severe hypertension may occur in association with any of the hypertensive disorders of pregnancy (HDP). Persistent, severe hypertension must be treated. This is universally endorsed by all international guidelines for the management of HDP [1–3].

The purpose of treating persistent, severe hypertension is to decrease the risk of cerebrovascular, cardiovascular and renal events, although the absolute risk of any of these events is very low in young women. Although the treatment of severe hypertension will not alter the course of pre-eclampsia, which is not primarily a hypertensive disorder (Chapter 6), control of severe hypertension in this setting may help prevent the particularly undesirable complication of maternal hemorrhagic stroke.

What is severe hypertension?

• Severe hypertension is a systolic blood pressure (SBP) ≥160 mmHg or a diastolic blood pressure (DBP) ≥110 mmHg.
• Persistence of hypertension should be confirmed after at least 5–15 minutes of rest.
The definition of severe diastolic hypertension is quite consistently a DBP ≥110 mmHg. The definition of severe systolic hypertension varies between 160 and 170 mmHg or greater. Support for use of a SBP ≥160 mmHg is based on its

association with an increased risk of stroke in pregnancy [4]. We favor use of this more conservative threshold for treatment. Consideration of the patient's baseline blood pressure may also be important, as cerebral hemorrhage can occur at lower blood pressures, particularly if there has been a significant acute change from prior readings. A rise in systolic or diastolic blood pressure of >50 mmHg may be associated with stroke in pre-eclamptic patients even in the absence of severe hypertension [5].

These statements assume that proper BP measurement technique is being employed, including ensuring that the brachial artery is held at the level of the heart during measurement and that the appropriate cuff size is being used (see Chapter 5).

That severe hypertension should be *persistent* is an important clinical management point. By this we mean that the severe elevation of BP be confirmed by repeat measurement, in 5–15 minutes.

Treatment of severe hypertension is not without its risks, as discussed below.

How should patients with severe hypertension be assessed?

• Patients with severe hypertension should undergo a brief assessment by history, physical and laboratory evaluation for evidence of acute target organ damage. Key features of this assessment are reviewed in Box 39.1.
• Severe hypertension that is not clearly secondary to pre-eclampsia should prompt consideration of secondary causes of hypertension. Secondary cause of hypertension and some suggestive features of each etiology are reviewed in Table 42.1.

de Swiet's Medical Disorders in Obstetric Practice, 5th edition.
Edited by R. O. Powrie, M. F. Greene, W. Camann. © 2010 Blackwell Publishing.

1. Perform fundoscopy looking for papilledema and retinal hemorrhages.
2. Ask about chest pain. If chest pain is present:
   - obtain EKG and serial cardiac enzymes (troponin every 8 hours times three) if cardiac ischemia is suspected
   - screen for aortic dissection:
     - measure blood pressure in both arms to assess for significant discrepancies caused by disruption of proximal blood flow
     - listen to the patient's heart sounds for evidence of aortic regurgitation caused by aorta dissecting proximally into aortic valve (a blowing diastolic murmer is heard best over the the right upper sternal border in the 2nd intercostal space while the patient is leaning forward and has fully exhaled)
     - consider CT or MRI aorta if chest pain radiates to back or any abnormal findings on above screening.
3. Assess for persistent headache and any change in neurologic status. Strongly consider prompt neuroimaging and or neurologic consultation if any of the following are present: somnolence, confusion obtundation, visual complaints, slurred speech, facial asymmetry or inability to hold both arms steadily out in front.
4. Assess for renal injury by obtaining a serum creatinine and urinalysis.

How urgent is it to treat severe hypertension?

- Persistent, severe hypertension should be treated with an antihypertensive agent.
- Whether or not there is maternal end-organ dysfunction will determine whether there is a hypertensive "urgency" or "emergency."
- Blood pressure should be lowered to <160 mmHg systolic and <110 mmHg diastolic, but by no more than 25% over minutes to hours.

Persistent, severe hypertension should always be treated. This will usually be by administration of antihypertensive therapy. However, if other factors that may be contributing to the severe hypertension (such as pain) can be addressed (by epidural analgesia, for example), observation may be appropriate over minutes to an hour or so.

Hypertensive urgencies are those associated with severe hypertension but not end-organ dysfunction (such as pulmonary edema or eclampsia). Severe hypertension with end-organ dysfunction defines a hypertensive "emergency." Whether or not visual disturbances or headache should be defined as end-organ dysfunction is not clear, but many clinicians would regard them as such. In the setting of pregnancy and especially after 20 weeks gestation, hypertensive urgencies likely require hospitalization for treatment and monitoring. Urgencies may be treated with oral agents, which have peak drug effects in 1–2 hours (e.g. labetalol). Hypertensive emergencies should be treated with parenteral agents (and an arterial line) aimed at lowering mean arterial BP by no more than 25% over minutes to hours, and then further lowering BP to 160/100 mmHg over subsequent hours. Parenteral agents may also be preferable for women in active labor in whom gastric emptying may be delayed.

Which antihypertensive agents should be used to treat severe hypertension?

- The following are recommended as first-line drugs: labetalol, nifedipine short-acting capsules, nifedipine intermediate-acting tablets and hydralazine (the once-daily extended-release formulations of nifedipine do not have a role in the acute control of severe hypertension). Information about using the medications is reviewed in Table 39.1.
- $MgSO_4$ is not recommended as an antihypertensive agent.
- Nifedipine preparations and $MgSO_4$ can be used contemporaneously.

By meta-analysis of the relevant n = 21 trials (1085 women), parenteral hydralazine may be associated with more adverse effects than are other antihypertensives; these effects include maternal hypotension and cesarean section [6]. Labetalol was associated with more neonatal bradycardia which required intervention in one of six affected babies. Observational literature emphasizes that hypotension may result with any short-acting antihypertensive agent used in women with pre-eclampsia, who are intravascularly volume depleted.

In randomized controlled trials (RCT) for treatment of severe hypertension, labetalol was administered parenterally. However, in some jurisdictions, it has been given orally for hypertensive urgencies, with good effect [7].

Based on a 1999 survey of Canadian practitioners, obstetricians most frequently prescribe parenteral hydralazine and labetalol for severe hypertension [8]. However, 40% also described frequent use of $MgSO_4$ for this indication despite the evidence that magnesium has no sustained effect on blood pressure. The relevant (and observational) literature is limited, with reports of no [9] or transient decreases in BP at 30 minutes after 2–5 g of IV $MgSO_4$, with/without ongoing infusion, usually in the setting of pre-eclampsia [10–13].

Table 39.1 Dosing recommendations for treatment of acute, severe hypertension in pregnancy

Agent	Starting dose	Maximum dose
For severe hypertension		
Short-acting nifedipine (capsules) (begins to work in 20–30 minutes and lasts for 4–5 hours)	5–10 mg PO every 30 min	10 mg PO every 30 min, generally giving not more than a total dose of 40 mg
Intermediate-acting nifedipine (tablets)	10–20 mg PO every 45 min	20 mg PO every 45 min, generally not giving more than a total dose of 60 mg
Labetalol IV (begins to work in 5–10 minutes and lasts for 3–6 hours)	5–20 mg IV every 30 min or infusion of 1–2 mg/min*	80 mg IV every 30 min to a maximum of 240–300 mg/24 h
Hydralazine IV (begins to work in 5–20 minutes and lasts for 3–6 hours)	5–10 mg IV/IM every 30 min or infusion of 0.5–1.0 mg/h	10 mg IV/IM every 30 min. Doses as high as 40 mg IV have been given in nonpregnant patients. It is recommended to switch to PO as soon as possible
For mild-to-moderate hypertension		
Methyldopa PO	750 mg PO loading dose, then 250–500 mg PO bid	2000 mg/day in up to four doses
Labetalol PO	100–200 mg PO bid	1200 mg/day in up to four doses
Hydralazine PO	10 mg PO qid	200 mg/day in up to four doses
Long-acting nifedipine (XL) PO	20–30 mg PO daily	120 mg/day in one dose

The starting doses are lower than for nonpregnant subjects given the greater potential to cause maternal hypotension and its important consequences for the fetus.

*Labetalol infusions can be mixed as follows: labetalol comes in vials of 100 mg/20 mL. Put 5 vials (100 mL) of labetalol into 150 mL of IV fluid to get a solution of 2 mg/mL. Start at 15 mL/h (0.5 mg/min) and titrate up to as high as 60 mL/h (2 mg/min). Labetalol has a long half-life and may accumulate with prolonged infusion, so the infusion rate may need to be titrated down over time after BP control is established.

Reproduced with permission from Magee LA, Abdullah S. The safety of antihypertensives therapy in pregnancy. Expert Opin Drug Saf 2004;3:25–38.

Therefore, a sustained lowering of BP cannot be anticipated following a MgSO$_4$ bolus.

Nifedipine is available in a number of preparations. Those appropriate for treatment of severe hypertension include the short-acting capsules and the intermediate-release tablets [14]. Most authors of randomized trials did not specify whether nifedipine capsules were bitten prior to swallowing; biting may be associated with greater effects on BP. Although the 5 mg capsule may be used to decrease the risk of a precipitous fall in BP, there are no published studies comparing the 5 mg and 10 mg doses. The risk of neuromuscular blockade with contemporaneous use of nifedipine and MgSO$_4$ is <1%, based on a single-center, controlled study, and a complete data synthesis from the literature [15]; blockade is reversed with 10 g of IV calcium gluconate.

Nitroglycerine (glyceryl trinitrate) is primarily venodilatory. Theoretically, it may not be a good choice of antihypertensive in women with pre-eclampsia. However, no adverse clinical effects have been demonstrated in small studies [16,17]. For refractory hypertension, in an intensive care setting, consideration can be given to using sodium nitroprusside or diazoxide [18].

What other monitoring or treatment is advised?

• Fetal heart rate (FHR) monitoring is advised during treatment of severe hypertension.
• Plasma volume expansion is not recommended.

• Despite anecdotal suggestions to the contrary, antihypertensive agents have not been proven to have direct pharmacologic effects on FHR or pattern.
• Ongoing oral antihypertensive therapy should probably be initiated after severe hypertension has been treated.

Fetal heart rate monitoring is advised because of the potential for any short-acting antihypertensive agent to cause maternal hypotension, which may result in adverse maternal or fetal effects. Firstly, the maternal cerebrovasculature may lose its autoregulatory ability at the levels of BP being treated, particularly if the woman's BP has been, in the recent past, much lower (e.g. 100/60 mmHg). Secondly, the uteroplacental circulation is unable to autoregulate blood flow, so that maternal hypotension may precipitate a nonreassuring FHR pattern and iatrogenic delivery. Maternal hypotension is a particular risk among women with severe pre-eclampsia given their intravascular volume depletion [19].

Although volume expansion (with crystalloid or colloid) has been recommended for women who are responding to antihypertensive therapy with precipitous falls in BP, the small trials in the area have been designed primarily to examine maternal safety, and a RCT in severe pre-eclampsia demonstrated no maternal or perinatal benefits [20,21].

There is no evidence that antihypertensives alter FHR or pattern, although the quality of the evidence is poor [22].

Following treatment of severe hypertension, oral antihypertensive therapy should be started to maintain BP levels, unless there was a clear, modifiable precipitant (such as the pain of labor). BP peaks on days 3–6 after delivery, so oral antihypertensive therapy should be restarted after delivery, particularly in women with pre-eclampsia in whom postpartum hypertension is more common [23].

Anesthetic considerations

The great majority of parturients with severe hypertension will require some anesthetic intervention, either in the form of neuraxial analgesia for labor, or the provision of anesthesia for cesarean section. The presence of severe hypertension, as well as the associated manifestations of end-organ involvement, will have significant implications for the conduct of anesthesia.

Coagulation function

• While significant alterations in coagulation function may occur even in patients with mildly elevated blood pressure, as is common in the HELLP syndrome, it is especially important to evaluate patients with severe hypertension for the presence of coagulopathy.

• There is considerable controversy regarding the minimal acceptable platelet count for patients undergoing regional anesthesia. There is little evidence to support the commonly cited figure of 100,000 platelets/mm3. In the absence of clinically apparent bleeding and other contributing factors, such as concomitant anticoagulant treatment, most obstetric anesthesiologists will accept a platelet count as low as 75,000. The rate of decrease of the platelet count is probably more significant than the absolute number.

• It should be recognized that in patients with a relative contraindication to general anesthesia, such as a known difficult airway, the use of regional anesthesia may be appropriate at a level of thrombocytopenia that might be unacceptable in a patient without such a contraindication to general.

• Severe alterations of PT and PTT are unlikely in the absence of thrombocytopenia; therefore, a normal platelet count should serve as an adequate rapid screening tool.

Anesthetic responses in severe hypertension

• The hypertensive response to laryngoscopy and intubation can potentially lead to left ventricular failure, as well as hypertensive intracranial hemorrhage. Various agents can be used to attenuate this response, including intravenous opioids; this may be associated with newborn depression.

Monitoring

• Patients receiving rapidly-acting vasoactive drugs such as sodium nitroprusside should have their blood pressure monitored via an indwelling arterial catheter.

• CVP or PA catheter monitoring should be considered if severe hypertension is complicated by persistent oliguria, pulmonary edema, or pre-existing cardiac disorder but it's utility in these settings remains unproven.

References

1. Report of the National High Blood Pressure Education Program Working Group on High Blood Pressure in Pregnancy. Am J Obstet Gynecol 2000;183(1):S1–S22.
2. Brown MA, Hague WM, Higgins J, Lowe S, McCowan L, Oats J, et al. The detection, investigation and management of hypertension in pregnancy: executive summary. Aust NZ J Obstet Gynaecol 2000;40(2):133–8.
3. Magee LA, Helewa M, Rey E, Côté AM, Douglas J, Gibson P, Gruslin A, Lange I, Leduc L, Logan AG, Smith GN, STIRRHS Pre-eclampsia Scholars (Appendix 1), Cardew S, Firoz T, Moutquin J-M, von Dadelszen P. SOGC Guidelines: Diagnosis, evaluation and management of the hypertensive disorders of pregnancy. JOGC 2008;30(3):Suppl 1, S1-48.
4. Martin JN Jr, Thigpen BD, Moore RC, Rose CH, Cushman J, May W. Stroke and severe preeclampsia and eclampsia: a paradigm shift focusing on systolic blood pressure. Obstet Gynecol 2005;105(2):246–54.
5. Magee LA, Cham C, Waterman EJ, Ohlsson A, von Dadelszen P. Hydralazine for treatment of severe hypertension in pregnancy: meta-analysis. BMJ 2003;327(7421):955–60.
6. Tuffnell DJ, Jankowicz D, Lindow SW, Lyons G, Mason GC, Russell IF, et al. Outcomes of severe pre-eclampsia/eclampsia in Yorkshire 1999/2003. Br J Obstet Gynaecol 2005;112(7):875–80.
7. Caetano M, Ornstein M, von Dadelszen P, Hannah ME, Logan AG, Gruslin A, et al. A survey of Canadian practitioners regarding the management of the hypertensive disorders of pregnancy. Hypertens Pregn 2003;23(1):61–74.
8. Scardo JA, Hogg BB, Newman RB. Favorable hemodynamic effects of magnesium sulfate in preeclampsia. Am J Obstet Gynecol 1995;173(4):1249–53.
9. Cotton DB, Gonik B, Dorman KF. Cardiovascular alterations in severe pregnancy-induced hypertension: acute effects of intravenous magnesium sulfate. Am J Obstet Gynecol 1984;148(2):162–5.
10. Mroczek WJ, Lee WR, Davidov ME. Effect of magnesium sulfate on cardiovascular hemodynamics. Angiology 1977;28(10):720–4.
11. Pritchard JA. The use of the magnesium ion in the management of eclamptogenic toxemias. Surg Gynecol Obstet 1955;100(2):131–40.
12. Young BK, Weinstein HM. Effects of magnesium sulfate on toxemic patients in labor. Obstet Gynecol 1977;49(6):681–5.
13. Brown MA, Buddle ML, Farrell T, Davis GK. Efficacy and safety of nifedipine tablets for the acute treatment of severe hypertension in pregnancy. Am J Obstet Gynecol 2002;187(4):1046–50.
14. Magee LA, Miremadi S, Li J, Cheng C, Ensom MH, Carleton B, et al. Therapy with both magnesium sulfate and nifedipine does not increase the risk of serious magnesium-related maternal side effects in women with preeclampsia. Am J Obstet Gynecol 2005;193(1):153–63.
15. Cetin A, Yurtcu N, Guvenal T, Imir AG, Duran B, Cetin M. The effect of glyceryl trinitrate on hypertension in women with severe preeclampsia, HELLP syndrome, and eclampsia. Hypertens Pregn 2004;23(1):37–46.
16. Neri I, Valensise H, Facchinetti F, Menghini S, Romanini C, Volpe A. 24-hour ambulatory blood pressure monitoring: a comparison between transdermal glyceryl-trinitrate and oral nifedipine. Hypertens Pregn 1999;18:107–13.
17. Hennessy A, Thornton C, Makris A, Ogle R, Henderson-Smart D, Gillin A, et al. Parenteral intravenous optimal therapy trial – a RCT of hydralazine versus mini-bolus diazoxide for hyupertensive crises in the obstetric setting. Hypertens Pregn 2006;25:22.
18. Gallery ED, Hunyor SN, Gyory AZ. Plasma volume contraction: a significant factor in both pregnancy-associated hypertension (pre-eclampsia) and chronic hypertension in pregnancy. Q J Med 1979;48(192):593–602.

19. Ganzevoort W, Rep A, Bonsel GJ, Fetter WP, van Sonderen L, de Vries JI, *et al.* A randomised controlled trial comparing two temporising management strategies, one with and one without plasma volume expansion, for severe and early onset pre-eclampsia. Br J Obstet Gynaecol 2005;112(10):1358–68.

20. Magee LA, Ornstein MP, von Dadelszen P. Fortnightly review: management of hypertension in pregnancy. BMJ 1999;318 (7194):1332–6.

21. Waterman EJ, Magee LA, Lim KI, Skoll A, Rurak D, von Dadelszen P. Do commonly used oral antihypertensives alter fetal or neonatal heart rate characteristics? A systematic review. Hypertens Pregn 2004;23(2):155–69.

22. Sadeghi S, Magee LA. Treatment for postpartum hypertension (Protocol for a Cochrane Review). Cochrane Library 2003; (Issue 2).

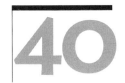

Approach to palpitations in pregnancy

Winnie W. Sia[1], Paul S. Gibson[2] and Rshmi Khurana[1]

[1]Departments of Medicine and Obstetrics and Gynecology, University of Alberta, Royal
Alexandra Hospital, Edmonton, Alberta, Canada
[2]Departments of Medicine and Obstetrics and Gynecology, University of Calgary,
Foothills Medical Centre, Calgary, Alberta, Canada

Introduction

Palpitations, defined as a subjective unpleasant awareness of heart beating, are a common symptom in pregnancy. Several physiologic alterations in pregnancy may exacerbate palpitations (Box 40.1). In addition, the increased awareness that a pregnant woman has of her body, concern about fetal well-being and more frequent contact with healthcare providers may make pregnant women more likely to report palpitations. Although most cases of palpitations in pregnant women will have a benign etiology, their benign nature should not be immediately assumed as palpitations may sometimes be a clue to a more serious underlying cause such as cardiac arrhythmia or thyrotoxicosis.

Sinus tachycardia, while not a normal finding in pregnancy, is a common finding that may present as palpitations. Sinus tachycardia can be a sign of conditions such as thyrotoxicosis, anemia, fever, pulmonary embolus, hypoglycemia, medications or illicit drug use. Obese pregnant women are more

likely to be tachycardic, presumably due to deconditioning [1]. Premature atrial or ventricular beats are also common during pregnancy [2]. Although most cases are of little clinical significance and do not warrant treatment in and of themselves, the ectopic beats may represent underlying cardiomyopathy, ischemia or electrolyte disturbances and these etiologies should be considered if the clinical picture suggests the possibility of these conditions. Notably, women with ectopic beats are more likely to sense the compensatory pause after the premature beat than the premature beat itself.

More serious rhythm disturbances may be unmasked during pregnancy because of the physiologic changes that occur to the cardiovascular system. Arrhythmias may present for the first time during pregnancy [3] or may represent a previously unrecognized problem that is now occurring more frequently [4]. These rhythms may be supraventricular (e.g. paroxysmal supraventricular tachycardia (PSVT), atrial fibrillation or flutter) tachycardia or, less commonly, ventricular tachycardia. These arrhythmias may be due to underlying causes such an accessory pathway (e.g. Wolff-Parkinson-White syndrome causing a PSVT), structural heart diseases (e.g. obstructive cardiomyopathy, peripartum cardiomyopathy, valvular heart disease), congestive heart failure or ischemic heart disease [5].

The challenge to healthcare providers is to distinguish benign causes of palpitations from serious ones. A targeted history, physical exam and several key investigations can help in this process. The following is an approach to assessing palpitations in pregnancy.

Box 40.1 Physiologic changes in pregnancy that increase the likelihood of palpitations

- Increased stroke volume and cardiac output
- Increased heart rate by an average of 15 beats/minute
- Increased ectopic beats (atrial and ventricular)
- Increased catecholamine levels in pregnancy
- Increased sensitivity of the heart to catecholamines (from effect of estrogen)
- Rotation of the heart closer to the chest wall such that the sensation of the heart beating is felt more readily

---

History

- Ask the patient to count her heart rate during an episode and have her attempt to tap out the rhythm with her fingers on a table. Ask about the *duration* and *frequency* of episodes and whether the rhythm is *irregular* or *regular*. Irregular heart beats of less than 5 minutes in duration that are unassociated with lightheadedness or underlying cardiac disease are very likely to be benign. Description of an irregular heartbeat

de Swiet's Medical Disorders in Obstetric Practice, 5th edition.
Edited by R. O. Powrie, M. F. Greene, W. Camann. © 2010 Blackwell
Publishing.

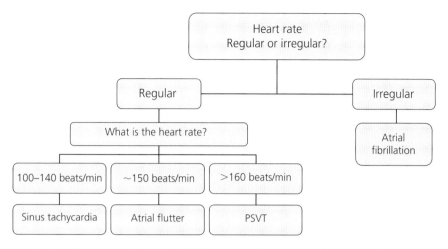

Figure 40.1 Likely diagnoses based on heart rate and rhythm. PSVT, paroxysmal supraventricular tachycardia. Note: palpitations with a slow heart rate may suggest atrioventricular block or sinus node disease.

Table 40.1 Suggestive diagnoses based on associated symptoms

Symptoms associated with palpitations	Suggestive diagnoses
Followed by syncope	Asystole or severe bradycardia following a tachyarrhythmia, or Stokes–Adams attack*
Presyncope (esp. history of myocardial infarction)	Ventricular tachycardia, rapid and unstable PSVT
Preceded by angina	Ischemic heart disease
Relieved by Valsalva maneuver (breath holding, etc.) or vagal maneuver	Paroxysmal supraventricular tachycardia
During mild exertion	Anemia, thyrotoxicosis, atrial fibrillation, heart failure or "deconditioning" (or being "out of shape")
On standing	Postural hypotension
Lump in the throat, tingling in hands and face	Tachycardia due to anxiety and/or hyperventilation

*Sudden loss of consciousness usually due to episodic intermittent high-grade atrioventricular block, or profound bradycardia.
PSVT, paroxysmal supraventricular tachycardia.

and/or duration of palpitations >5 minutes are more suggestive of a cardiac etiology [6]. Certain heart rates and rhythms may suggest specific diagnoses (Figure 40.1).

• Ask how the palpitations start and end – abruptly or gradually? When palpitations begin and end abruptly, they are often due to paroxysmal tachycardia (i.e. atrial or junctional), atrial flutter or atrial fibrillation. Alternatively, if the palpitations have a gradual onset and gradual cessation, it may suggest sinus tachycardia or an anxiety disorder as the cause.

• Ask about associated symptoms and events: the presence of syncope, chest pain or angina, anxiety or an exertional precipitant may suggest certain diagnoses (Table 40.1).

• Rule out diet and drug effects. See Box 40.2 for a list.

• Ask about any personal history of cardiac disease. The presence of an underlying cardiac condition such as valvular heart disease, ischemia or cardiomyopathy makes any complaint of palpitations far more likely to be due to an arrhythmia and

may also suggest a specific rhythm. Mitral valve disease puts patients at increased risk of atrial fibrillation. Cardiomyopathy increases the likelihood of ventricular tachycardia.

• Ask about family history, especially of arrhythmias, syncope and sudden death. Myotonic dystrophy and Duchenne muscular dystrophy can result in arrhythmias. Familial conduction system disorders, such as prolonged QT syndrome, can be a cause of unexplained sudden death in family members.

Physical examination

• Assess heart rate and rhythm (see Figure 40.1). Ask the patient to walk down the corridor to see whether that will unmask a poorly controlled ventricular response [7].

• Perform a precordial exam looking for a palpable murmur ("thrill") or parasternal heave ("lift") which likely reflects

Box 40.2 Drugs, diet and lifestyle factors which may exacerbate palpitations

Diet/lifestyle

- Excessive caffeine
- Heavy cigarette smoking

Medications

- Psychotropic drugs with antihistamines (i.e. tricyclic antidepressants) and monoamine-oxidase inhibitors (MAOI)
- Nasal decongestants containing sympathomimetic vasoconstrictors
- Cardiac medications such as nifedipine which may cause vasodilation and reflex tachycardia
- Asthma medications such as theophylline or excessive use of beta-2 agonists (e.g. sabutamol/albuterol)

Illicit drugs

- Cocaine
- Amphetamine

underlying structural cardiac abnormalities. The apical beat should be about the size of an American 25 cent coin and readily palpable in the fifth intercostal space along the midclavicular line. Its displacement can suggest an underlying ventricular dilation or hypertrophy.

• Look for jugular venous pulsation (JVP). It should be easily visible and biphasic (i.e. have a "flickering" quality) but not elevated in normal pregnancy. Normal JVP should be <4 cm above sternal angle. Elevated JVP may suggest congestive heart failure. A canon (or amplified) wave of the biphasic JVP wave may suggest atrial-ventricular dissociation as occurs with premature atrial contractions.

• Auscultate for heart sounds and murmurs. Loud systolic murmurs (>Grade 3), a harsh holosystolic murmur heard along the left sternal border that increases with Valsalva (suggestive of hypertrophic obstructive cardiomyopathy), diastolic murmurs, mid-systolic click (suggestive of mitral valve prolapse) should all be investigated with an echocardiogram.

• Examine for enlarged thyroid gland (i.e. goiter) and temperature to rule out fever.

Investigations

After a thorough history and physical examination, the extent of investigations depends on the clinical judgment of the care provider. Most patients should have a thyroid-stimulating hormone (TSH) (or a free T4 or free thyroxine index in the first trimester), hemoglobin, 12-lead electrocardiogram and electrolytes performed. As palpitations are usually intermittent, an EKG may not capture any abnormalities if the patient does not have symptoms at the time of the test. In this circumstance, a 24- or 48-hour Holter monitor (i.e. a simultaneously recorded ambulatory electrocardiogram while the patient keeps a diary of the time of any symptoms) or continuous loop event recorder (i.e. a transtelephonic transmission of electrocardiogram which the patient can carry with them for weeks) can be performed if arrhythmia is suspected. Ambulatory monitoring with Holter monitor or event recorder should be considered in patients whose history, physical examination and/or EKG suggest(s) an arrhythmic cause, and also in those with organic heart disease that increases the likelihood of serious arrhythmias. Continuous loop event recorder is more cost-effective than Holter monitor in the evaluation of palpitations and a 2-week monitoring duration will suffice for most patients [8,9]. The presence of the patient's typical palpitation symptoms with a normal recording on these tests is usually reassuring.

An echocardiogram can rule out structural heart disease when suspected, but is not essential in the setting of a normal clinical cardiac exam and normal EKG and no sinister symptoms. Cardiology consultation should be considered when noncardiac causes have been ruled out, and either an abnormality suggestive of arrhythmia is found or the patient has significant symptoms and testing is negative. If myocardial ischemia is suspected, troponin I and stress echocardiogram can be considered. For unexplained palpitations associated with syncope or uncaptured fast heart rate noted by medical personnel, consider referring to a cardiologist for electrophysiologic (EP) testing [10]. The treatment of arrhythmias in pregnancy is discussed elsewhere in this book.

Psychiatric disorders, such as generalized anxiety disorders and panic attacks, can cause palpitations but they should be considered as a diagnosis of exclusion made in conjunction with a behavioral health specialist. Many patients with an anxiety disorder also have arrhythmias [11].

Conclusion

The assessment of palpitations in pregnancy should begin with a targeted history and physical examination. Most patients should have basic investigations including a 12-lead electrocardiogram, TSH (with free T4 or free T4I in first trimester), hemoglobin and electrolytes. If arrhythmia is suspected, an event recorder or Holter monitor should be performed. Echocardiography may be performed to investigate suspected structural cardiac disease but is not routinely indicated. Referral to a cardiologist should be considered if an arrhythmia is detected or if there is a high clinical suspicion of arrhythmia despite negative investigations (such as recurrent symptoms associated with syncope).

Premature atrial or ventricular beats and sinus tachycardia are the most common cause of palpitations in pregnancy. In many cases, however, no diagnosis can be made despite appropriate testing. In such cases, if there are no sinister signs or symptoms, the pregnant woman should be reassured and be followed up closely.

References

1. Carson MP, Powrie RO, Rosene-Montella K. The effect of obesity and position on heart rate in pregnancy. J Matern Fetal Neonatal Med 2002;11(1):40–5.
2. Shotan A, Ostrzega E, Mehra A, Johnson J, Elkayam U. Incidence of arrhythmis in normal pregnancy and relation to palpitations, dizziness, and syncope. Am J Cardiol 1997;79(8):1061–4.
3. Brodsky M, Doria R, Allen B, Sato D, Thomas G, Sada M. New-onset ventricular tachycardia during pregnancy. Am Heart J 1992;123(4 Pt 1):933–41.
4. Silversides CK, Harris L, Haberer K, Sermer M, Colman JM, Siu SC. Recurrence rates of arrhythmias during pregnancy in women with previous tachyarrhythmia and impact on fetal and neonatal outcomes. Am J Cardiol 2006;97(8):1206–12.
5. Braunwald E (ed). Heart disease: a textbook of cardiovascular medicine. 5th edn. W.B. Saunders, Philadelphia, 1997.
6. Weber BE, Kapoor WN. Evaluation and outcomes of patients with palpitations. Am J Med 1996;100(2):138–48. Erratum in: Am J Med 1997;103(1):86.
7. Zimetbaum P, Josephson ME. Evaluation of patients with palpitations. N Engl J Med 1998;338(19):1369–73.
8. Fogel RI, Evans JJ, Prystowsky EN. Utility and cost of event recorders in the diagnosois of palpitations, presyncope, and syncope. Am J Cardiol 1997;79:207–8.
9. Zimetbaum PJ, Kim K, Josephson ME, Goldberger AL, Cohen DJ. Diagnostic yield and optimal duration of continuous-loop event monitoring for the diagnosis of palpitations. A cost-effectiveness analysis. Ann Intern Med 1998;128(11):890–5.
10. Blomstrom-Lundqvist C, Scheinman MM, Aliot EM, et al. ACC/AHA/ESC guidelines for the management of patients with supraventricular arrhythmias – executive summary: a report of the American College of Cardiology/American Heart Association Task Force on Practice Guidelines and the European Society of Cardiology Committee for Practice Guidelines (Writing Committee to Develop Guidelines for the Management of Patients With Supraventricular Arrhythmias). Circulation 2003;108:1871–909.
11. Lee RV, Rosene-Montella K, Barbour LA, Garner PR, Keely E (eds). Medical care of the pregnant patient. American College of Physicians, Philadelphia, 2000: 370–4.

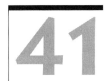

Approach to proteinuria identified remote from term

Margaret A. Miller

Department of Medicine, Warren Alpert Medical School of Brown University, Women & Infants' Hospital of Rhode Island, Providence, RI, USA

Introduction

Proteinuria is a common incidental finding. Routine screening for proteinuria in pregnancy is done primarily to screen for evidence of pre-eclampsia, but it is likely to lead to recognition of underlying renal disease in a number of cases. Patients who present with proteinuria prior to 20 weeks gestation or those who have proteinuria without other features of pre-eclampsia should be evaluated for underlying renal disease. A national survey found that the prevalence of chronic kidney disease (CKD) in a US adult population was 11% [1]. Among subjects of reproductive age, advanced (stage 3–5) kidney disease was rare; however, 13.7% of subjects aged 20–39 were found to have a mild reduction in glomerular filtration rate (GFR) consistent with stage 1 or 2 CKD. Therefore, even mild degrees of proteinuria should be thoroughly investigated. Pregnancy offers an opportunity to identify renal disease at an early stage when initiation of treatment may prevent progression of disease.

Physiology of proteinuria

The kidney handles three major types of protein: albumin, small molecular weight proteins such as peptide proteins and amino acids, and occasionally light chains derived from immunoglobulins. Albumin is the major protein in plasma and is important in maintaining Starling forces which regulate the circulating plasma volume. The healthy kidney has a number of mechanisms by which it conserves albumin. Blood enters the glomerulus through the afferent arteriole and is filtered across the glomerular capillary wall and the glomerular basement membrane. The glomerular basement membrane

(GBM) is the primary barrier to filtration of protein. The GBM is negatively charged and repels the negatively charged proteins including albumin. In addition to this charge barrier, the GBM also acts as a size barrier, preventing albumin and larger protein molecules from passing into the tubules. As a result, only a small percentage of the total albumin that enters the glomerulus is filtered into the renal tubules. Furthermore, 90% of the albumin that reaches the tubules is reabsorbed so that an even smaller amount is eventually excreted in the urine (<150 mg/24 h in a nonpregnant woman and <300 mg/24 h in a pregnant woman).

Types of proteinuria

There are three mechanisms which lead to proteinuria. Glomerular proteinuria results from the filtration of macromolecules, namely albumin, across the glomerular basement membrane. Defects in the GBM may lead to an alteration in the charge barrier, the size barrier or both. Glomerular proteinuria is a marker of glomerular disease that may result from primary renal disease or from systemic disease that affects the kidney. Tubular proteinuria is due to tubular or interstitial injury which impairs resorption of protein, resulting in increased excretion of small molecular weight proteins and small amounts of albumin. Overflow proteinuria is less common and is due to an excess production of small molecular weight protein which overwhelms the resorptive capacity of the tubules. The classic example of overflow proteinuria is the overproduction of light chains from immunoglobulins in multiple myeloma.

Measurement of proteinuria

A number of methods are available to measure urine protein. The urine dipstick is the most common screening test. This tests measures only albumin and will miss tubular or overflow proteinuria. The urine dipstick is a poor measure of the

de Swiet's Medical Disorders in Obstetric Practice, 5th edition. Edited by R. O. Powrie, M. F. Greene, W. Camann. © 2010 Blackwell Publishing.

severity of proteinuria. It measures albumin concentration and since concentration is dependent on volume, results may vary according to the patient's volume status. The 24- hour urine collection is the gold standard for quantifying urine. It measures all types of protein. Its primary disadvantage is a high degree of collection error such as missed samples or timing errors. For this reason, the National Kidney Foundation has recommended that, in the nonpregnant patient, a urine/protein creatinine ratio be the preferred method for measuring proteinuria [2]. When the urinary protein and the urinary creatinine are expressed in mg/dL, the ratio provides a correlation with the 24-hour urine that is easy to interpret. For example, a urine protein/creatinine ratio of 0.1 represents 100 mg of protein in a 24-hour urine; 0.2 would represent 200 mg, etc. A number of studies show significant correlation between the 24-hour urine collection and the urine protein/creatinine ratio in pregnancy [3,4]. However, there is no clear consensus on the best cut-off value to distinguish normal from abnormal levels of proteinuria. Still, other studies conclude that the urine protein/creatinine ratio is a poor predictor of significant proteinuria in women with suspected pre-eclampsia [5,6]. More studies are needed to clarify the role of the urine protein/creatinine ratio in pregnancy but in the absence of pre-eclampsia, it is reasonable to use this test to initiate the investigation of unexplained proteinuria.

Differential diagnosis of proteinuria

Proteinuria may be divided into two broad categories: benign and disease related. There are only two benign cause of proteinuria, while there are many disease-related causes (Box 41.1). Benign causes include transient and orthostatic proteinuria and are usually associated with low-range proteinuria, that is less than 1 g. The urinalysis and creatinine are normal in both of these conditions. Transient proteinuria occurs in 7% of women on a single exam [7]. It is most often triggered by some type of physiologic stress such as fever, heavy exercise, cold exposure or stress. The diagnosis is confirmed if a repeat urine dipstick is negative for protein once the physiologic stress is resolved. Orthostatic proteinuria is primarily a disease of children but it occurs in 2–5% of adolescents and can be seen in women in their 20s [8]. Orthostatic proteinuria is rare in women over the age of 30 years. In this condition, the patient excretes an abnormal amount of urine while in the upright position, but normal levels of protein while supine.

Disease-related proteinuria has many causes, both primary renal and systemic disease (see Box 41.1) There are a number of classification systems causing much confusion. A classification system based on clinical presentation seems to be the most clinically useful approach to the evaluation of disease-related proteinuria and will be presented here.

Box 41.1 Differential diagnosis of proteinuria

Benign causes

- Transient proteinuria
- Orthostatic proteinuria

Disease-related causes

- *Primary renal*
  - Tubulointerstitial disease
  - Minimal change disease
  - Membranous GN
  - Focal-segmental GN
  - IgA nephropathy
  - Membranoproliferative GN
  - Mesangioproliferative GN
- *Systemic*
  - Hypertension
  - Postinfectious GN (bacterial endocarditis, post-strep GN)
  - Vasculitic-immunologic
  - Multiple myeloma
  - Hereditary/metabolic
  - Diabetes
  - Systemic lupus erythematosus
  - Malignancy
  - Drugs
  - Infections
  - Obesity
  - Reflux nephropathy

Evaluation of proteinuria

The first step in the evaluation of proteinuria is to check the urinalysis and creatinine. An abnormal urinalysis or creatinine indicates disease-related proteinura and a work-up for benign causes is not necessary (Figure 41.1). If the urinalysis and creatinine are both normal, then benign causes may be considered. Patients should be questioned about physiologic stressors such as a recent febrile illness, heavy exercise, stress or cold exposure that may precipitate transient proteinuria. If present, then a repeat dipstick should be done once the condition resolves. A negative repeat dipstick confirms the diagnosis. No further work-up is needed and the patient may be reassured. If the patient is less than 30 years old, then a split urine collection may be done to rule out orthostatic proteinuria (Box 41.2).

If benign causes cannot be confirmed or if the patient has an abnormal creatinine or urinalysis, then the evaluation should move directly to the disease-related algorithm (Figure 41.2). The differential diagnosis may be narrowed initially based on the clinical presentation.

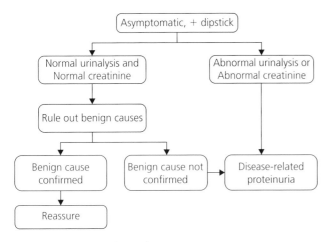

Figure 41.1 Initial work-up of asymptomatic proteinuria.

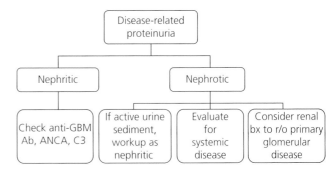

Figure 41.2 Disease-related proteinuria. Anti-GBM, antiglomerular basement membrane antibody; ANCA, antineutrophilic cytoplasmic antibodies; C3, a type of complement assay.

Box 41.2 Patient instructions for split urine collection

- You must collect *all* of your urine for 24 hours.
- The urine must be refrigerated during the process of collection.
- You will need two jugs and a funnel. Label the two jugs: (1) Daytime urine and (2) night-time urine.
- Start your collection in the morning;
- After waking, discard the first morning urine.
- For the rest of the day, collect *all* of the urine each time you void. Pour urine into the jug marked "Daytime" and keep jug in the refrigerator.
- In the evening, lie down 2 hours before you plan to sleep. Just before sleeping, void for the last time during the day and add this urine to the "Daytime" jug. By lying down for 2 hours before beginning the night-time collection, you will avoid contaminating the night-time collection with urine formed during the day when you were upright.
- The next morning (approximately 8 hours after you went to sleep) collect the first morning urine and add it to the "Night-time" urine jug.
- Return both jugs to the laboratory.
- Errors in collection are sometimes unavoidable. Please inform your provider if you think your sample is not complete (you missed some samples) as this can affect the results of the test.

Evaluation of proteinuria based on clinical presentation

Based on clinical presentation, it is possible to classify patients as having either nephritic or nephrotic renal disease.

Patients who do not clearly fall into one of these categories may in fact have early renal disease and warrant close monitoring throughout gestation.

Nephritic renal disease

Nephritis is primarily due to inflammation in the kidney and the hallmark finding is an "active" urine sediment. On microscopic exam of the urine, a number of abnormal cells such as red blood cells (RBC), white blood cells (WBC) or casts may be seen. The types of cells may provide a clue to the diagnosis (Table 41.1). By definition, nephritic proteinuria does not exceed 3.5 g/24h. The creatinine may be elevated on presentation, but is often normal. There are three distinct clinical syndromes associated with nephritis [9] (Table 41.2). Acute nephritic syndrome is characterized by sudden onset of acute renal failure and oliguria. Rapidly progressive glomerulonephritis (RPGN) is more subacute and may progress to renal failure over weeks to months. Chronic nephritis follows a more indolent course, with slow progression to renal impairment. Of note, any of the causes of nephritis may evolve into RPGN. For this reason, any patient with clinical evidence of nephritis should be referred to a nephrologist.

The differential diagnosis of nephritic syndrome includes a long list of both primary renal and systemic diseases. A few simple blood tests may help to significantly narrow this differential diagnosis and they include anti-GBM antibody, ANCA, and C3. The pattern of results will indicate the possible diagnosis (Table 41.3). Once the likely causes are narrowed, directed evaluation may be done.

Nephrotic renal disease

Nephrotic syndrome is defined as protein excretion that exceeds 3.5 g in 24 hours. The urine sediment is usually bland; that is, no RBC, WBC or casts are seen with the exception of oval fat bodies or casts. Creatinine may be normal at presentation.

Table 41.1 Urinalysis in proteinuria

Sediment	Clinical significance
Crystals	Most commonly of little diagnostic importance
Cells	
RBC	Transient hematuria in young women often not indicative of disease, may occur with urinary tract infection; persistent hematuria warrants evaluation
	Hematuria in women >50 years is more serious, malignancy should be ruled out
	Dysmorphic RBC suggest glomerular disease
WBC	Pyuria most commonly seen with infection
	Eosinophils associated with interstitial nephritis
	Lymphocytes may be seen with tubulointerstitial disease
Epithelial cells	The occasional epithelial cell is normal
	Large numbers of epithelial cells or epithelial cells in cast may indicate underlying renal disease
Casts	
Hyaline casts	Not indicative of disease
Red cell casts	Always abnormal.
	Diagnostic of glomerular disease or vasculitis
White cell casts	Seen most commonly with tubulointerstitial disease or acute pyelonephritis
Epithelial casts	Associated with acute tubular necrosis and acute glomerulonephritis
Fatty casts	Seen with nephrotic range proteinuria
Granular casts	May be seen in numerous disorders
	Multiple muddy brown granular casts are highly suggestive of acute tubular necrosis
Waxy casts	May indicate advanced renal failure
Broad casts	May indicate advanced renal failure

Table 41.2 Clinical presentation of disease-related proteinuria

	Clinical presentation	Urine sediment	Protein	Creatinine
Nephritic	• *Acute nephritic syndrome* characterized by sudden onset of ARF and oliguria • *RPGN* is more subacute. Can progress to renal failure over weeks to months • *Chronic nephritis*	Active (RBC, RBC casts, WBC)	<3.5 g/d	May be elevated
Nephrotic	• Key component is proteinuria • Hypertension, hypoalbuminemia, edema, hyperlipidemia and lipiduria are all secondary to protein loss	Bland (may see oval fat bodies)	>3.5 g/d	Usually normal at presentation

ARF, acute renal failure; RBC, red blood cells; RPGN, rapidly progressive glomerulonephritis; WBC, white blood cells.

Patients may also present with hypertension, edema, hypoalbuminemia, hyperlipidemia, and lipiduria (see Table 41.2).

The first step in the evaluation of a patient with nephrotic range proteinuria is to look for systemic disease that is associated with nephrotic renal disease (Table 41.4). Diabetes is the most common condition and patients should be screened for diabetes mellitus. Glomerular deposition disease such as multiple myeloma is uncommon in a population of reproductive age woman, but may be ruled out with a serum and urine protein electrophoresis. Drugs, such as nonsteroidal anti-inflammatories, gold, lithium, penicillamine and some antibiotics, may be common offenders so it is important to include a complete medication history, including over-the-counter medications, in the assesment. Nephrotic syndrome may be associated with malignancy, most commonly hematologic malignancies, and patients should be questioned about symptoms and a complete blood count (CBC) should be done. Obesity has been found to be an independent risk factor for proteinuria [10]. Reflux nephropathy may lead to nephrotic syndrome and a history of recurrent urinary tract

Table 41.3 Work-up for nephritic syndrome

	Anti-GBM AB	ANCA	C3	Diagnosis
Anti-GBM disease	+	−	Normal	Anti-GBM disease Goodpasture's (renal and lung disease)
Pauci-immune GN	−	+	Normal	Wegener's Microscopic PAN Renal-limited crescentic GN
Immune complex	−	−	Low	Primary glomerular disease (renal bx) Postinfectious GN (ASO, ADNAse) Bacterial endocarditis (echo, blood cx) Lupus (ANA, ds-DNA)
			Normal	Cryoglobulinemia (cryocrit, HCV) IgA nephropathy (hematuria after URI) Henoch–Schönlein purpura Fibrillary GN
Mimickers	−	−	Normal	Hypertension HUS/TTP Interstitial nephritis (WBC casts) Scleroderma crisis Atheroemboli

Anti GBM, antiglomerular basement membrane antibody; ANCA, antineutrophilic cytoplasmic antibodies; ANA, antinuclear antibody; ASO, antistreptolysis; C3, type of complement assay; Ds-DNA, double-stranded DNA; GN, glomerulonephritis; HCV, hepatitis C virus; HUS/TTP, hemolytic uremic syndrome/thrombotic thrombocytopenic purpura; PAN, polyarteritis nodosa; URI, upper respiratory infection.

Table 41.4 Work-up for nephrotic syndrome

Systemic disease	Clinical	Investigation
Diabetes	Accounts for 40% of ESRD	Check blood sugar
Glomerular deposition disease	Almost always due to multiple myeloma	SPEP, UPEP
Drugs	Common offenders include NSAIDS, gold therapy, penicillamine, IV heroin	Medication history
Malignancy	Most common with lymphoma/leukemia. Rarely seen with solid tumors	CBC; Usual cancer screening
Obesity	Morbid obesity is independent risk factor for renal disease	Check BMI
Reflux nephropathy	History of recurrent UTI	Voiding cystourethrogram

BMI, Body Mass Index; CBC, complete blood count; ESRD, endstage renal disease; NSAID, nonsteroidal anti-inflammatory drugs; SPEP, serum protein electrophoresis; UPEP, urine protein electrophoresis; UTI, urinary tract infection.

infection (UTI) should be sought. If there is no clear evidence of systemic disease, then it is most likely that the patient has a primary glomerulopathy which can only be confirmed by renal biopsy. Renal biopsies should be done in the pregnant woman for the same indications as a nonpregnant woman [11]. Indications would include proteinuria >2–3 g/24 h, evidence of progressive renal dysfunction (increasing creatinine) or renal disease with new onset of hypertension.

Occasionally patients present in early gestation with asymptomatic proteinuria that is less than 3.5 g, with a normal creatinine and normal urine sediment. Such patients do not meet criteria for either nephritis or nephrotic syndrome.

If transient and orthostatic proteinuria has been ruled out, such patients should be monitored closely for progression of disease throughout pregnancy. Little is known about the natural history of mild asymptomatic proteinuria in pregnancy. However, one study found that 29% of women with isolated asymptomatic proteinuria diagnosed before 20 weeks developed pre-eclampsia; 21 of 57 women who eventually underwent renal biopsy had evidence of renal disease [12]. A reasonable approach is to monitor the creatinine and 24-hour urine or urine protein/creatinine ratio every 4–6 weeks. Patients who develop more than 2 g of protein should be referred to a nephrologist for biopsy.

Conclusion

The evaluation of proteinuria in pregnancy that is discovered remote from term (<20 weeks gestation) should progress in a stepwise fashion. Testing should begin with a urinalysis and creatinine. If both are normal, benign causes of proteinuria may be considered. If either test is abnormal or benign cause cannot be confirmed, disease-related cause should be sought. Patients with <3.5 g protein on 24-hour urine, abnormal urine microscopy (nephritic syndrome), should be further evaluated with anti-GBM antibody, ANCA and C3. The pattern of results of these three tests will narrow the differential so that directed testing may proceed in a more efficient and cost-effective manner. Patients with >3.5 g protein in 24 hours (nephrotic syndrome) should be evaluated first for systemic disease associated with the nephrotic syndrome. If there is still no diagnosis, renal biopsy should be considered. Commonly, patients do not clearly fall into any of the above categories; that is, they have mild asymptomatic proteinuria with a normal creatinine and a normal urinalysis. Data from the Collaborative Perinatal Project suggest that, even in the absence of hypertension or pre-eclampsia, proteinuria is associated with an increased risk for fetal mortality (relative risk = 4). So all patients with proteinuria, regardless of severity, should be monitored closely for progression of renal disease, development of pre-eclampsia or other adverse pregnancy outcomes.

References

1. Coresh J, Astor B, Greene T. Prevalence of chronic kidney disease and decreased kidney function in the adult US population: third National Health And Nutrition Examination Survey. Am J Kidney Dis 2003:41(1);1–12.

2. National Kidney Foundation. K/DOQI clinical practice guidelines for chronic kidney disease: evaluation, classification and stratification. Am J Kidney Dis 2002;39:S1.

3. Neithardt A, Dooley S, Borensztajn J. Prediction of 24-hour protein excretion in pregnancy with a single voided urine protein-to-creatinine ratio. Am J Obstet Gynecol 2002;186:883–6.

4. Rodriguez-Thompson D, Lieberman E. Use of a random urinary protein-to-creatinine ratio for the diagnosis of significant proteinuria during pregnancy. Obstet Gynecol 2001;185:808–11.

5. Al RA, Baykal C, Karacay O, et al. Random urine protein-creatinine ratio to predict proteinuria in new-onset mild hypertension in late pregnancy. Obstet Gynecol 2004;104:367–71.

6. Durnwald C, Mercer B. A prospective comparison of total protein/creatinine ratio versus 24-hour urine protein in women with suspected preeclampsia. Am J Obstet Gynecol 200;189(3): 848–52.

7. Robinson RR. Isolated proteinuria in asymptomatic patients. Kidney Int 1980;18:395.

8. Springberg PD, Garrett LE JR, Thompson AL, et al. Fixed and reproducible orthostatic proteinuria: results of a 20-year follow-up study. Ann Intern Med 1982;97:516.

9. Chadban SJ, Atkins RC. Glomerulonephritis. Lancet 2005;365: 1797–806.

10. Kambham N, Markowitz GS, Valeri AM, et al. Obesity-related glomerulopathy: an emerging epidemic. Kidney Int 2001;59(4):1498–509.

11. Fuiano G, Massa G, Comi N, et al. Current indications for renal biopsy: a questionnaire based survey. Am J Kidney Dis 2000;35(3):448–57.

12. Stettler RW, Cunningham FG. Natural history of chronic proteinuria complicating pregnancy. Am J Obstet Gynecol 1992;167(5):1219–24.

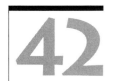

Approach to new-onset hypertension remote from term

Margaret A. Miller

Department of Medicine, Warren Alpert Medical School of Brown University,
Women & Infants' Hospital of Rhode Island, Providence, RI, USA

Introduction

Hypertension is the most common chronic medical problem encountered in pregnant women, with chronic essential hypertension estimated to complicate 1–5% of pregnancies [1]. While many women enter pregnancy with a diagnosis of chronic hypertension, others may present with elevated blood pressure (BP) for the first time in pregnancy. Hypertension that occurs remote from term, prior to 20 weeks gestation, is presumed to be chronic hypertension.

The Seventh Report of the Joint National Committee on Prevention, Detection, Evaluation and Treatment of High Blood Pressure provides a new classification of blood pressure for nonpregnant adults [2] (Box 42.1). A new category within this classification is that of "prehypertension" (BP 130– 139/80–89). It is estimated that individuals with blood pressure in this range are at twice the risk of developing chronic hypertension as those with normal values (BP <120/80) [3]. Furthermore, there is clear and consistent evidence that even mild hypertension is associated with a significantly increased risk of cardiovascular disease [4,5]. The new classification of prehypertension acknowledges this relationship and emphasizes the need for better education of providers and patients in order to prevent the development of hypertension. Pregnancy offers a unique opportunity to identify women with hypertension early in the course of disease and initiate prevention strategies.

Women with severe hypertension in early pregnancy are easily identified and require close monitoring as their risk of pregnancy complications may be greater [6]. However, identification of prehypertension or stage I hypertension in pregnant women may be more difficult and requires a working knowledge of the hemodynamic changes of pregnancy. In normal pregnancy, maternal blood pressure decreases in early

gestation due to a reduction in systemic vascular resistance and resistance to vasoconstricting hormones such as angiotensin II and norepinephrine. A mean decrease of 10–15 mmHg begins in the early weeks of pregnancy and reaches a nadir at 24–28 weeks. For this reason, it is very likely that a woman with prehypertension would present with normal BP values in early gestation. It is also for this reason that an elevated BP in early gestation, even if mild, should be interpreted as significant and warrants evaluation and close follow-up.

The approach to the patient with hypertension detected either prior to pregnancy or prior to 20 weeks gestation should include:
- screening for secondary or reversible causes
- evaluation for end-organ damage
- assessment of cardiovascular risk factors.

Screening for secondary causes of hypertension

Screening for secondary or reversible causes of hypertension is an essential part of the evaluation for all newly diagnosed hypertensive patients, including pregnant women. Although only 5–10% of chronic hypertension is due to a secondary or reversible cause, many of these conditions are associated with significant complications in pregnancy if left undetected. Secondary causes of hypertension are summarized in Table 42.1.

> ### Box 42.1 Classification of hypertension in non-pregnant individuals
>
> | | |
> |---|---|
> | Normal | <120/80 |
> | Prehypertension | 120–139/85–89 |
> | Hypertension: | |
> | Stage I | 140–159/90–99 |
> | Stage II | >160/100 |

de Swiet's Medical Disorders in Obstetric Practice, 5th edition.
Edited by R. O. Powrie, M. F. Greene, W. Camann. © 2010 Blackwell Publishing.

Table 42.1 Secondary causes of hypertension

	Symptoms	Signs other than hypertension	Screening test
Renal disease: renal artery stenosis, glomerular disease		Abdominal/flank bruit Hematuria, large palpable kidneys, edema	Screen all patients with a urinalysis and creatinine. Ultrasound or MR angiogram if renal artery stenosis is suspected
Drugs (OCP, NSAIDs, pseudoephedrine, steroids, alcohol, tobacco)	Usually asymptomatic	None	Medication/drug use history in all patients
Pheochromocytoma	Paroxysms of headache, sweating, palpitations	Tremor, weight loss, anxiety	If suspected, 24-h urine for metanephrines and catecholamines or serum catecholamines
Primary hyperaldosteronism	Usually asymptomatic	Abnormalities on exam are rare	Screen all patients with electrolytes (low K+, high Na is suggestive of hyperaldosteronism)
Hyperthyroidism	Anxiety, sweating, heat intolerance, palpitations, dyspnea, fatigue, weight loss	Tachycardia, weight loss, may have goiter, tremor, warm, moist skin, exophthalmos	Screen all patients with a TSH
Hyperparathyroidism	"Bones, stones, groans, moans" – painful bones, renal stones, abdominal pain and psychiatric symptoms	Nephrolithiaisis, polyuria, weight loss, bone pain, muscle weakness, apathy	Screen all patients with a calcium
Cushing's disease or syndrome	Emotional lability, muscle weakness, easy bruising	Moon facies, central obesity, striae, osteoporosis, diabetes, hirsutism	If suspected, review glucose and electrolytes and consider investigation with a 24-h urine cortisol
Sleep apnea	Excessive daytime sleepiness, snoring	Obesity, low-lying palate	If suspected, refer for sleep study
Coarctation of the aorta	Usually asymptomatic, may have headaches, exertional leg fatigue and pain, epistaxis	Prominent neck pulsations, delayed peripheral pulses, bruit over back	If suspected, check CXR (may have rib notching, "3 sign")

CXR, chest X-ray; MR, magnetic resonance; NSAID, nonsteroidal anti-inflammatory drugs; OCP, oral contraceptive pill; TSH, thyroid-stimulating hormone.

Renal artery stenosis is the most common secondary cause of hypertension in young patients. Although less common in mild to moderate hypertension, the incidence of renal artery stenosis in patients with acute, severe or refractory hypertension is 10–45% [7]. For unclear reasons, renovascular disease is less common in black patients. Renal function and urinalysis may appear normal. The optimal screening test is a matter of much debate as even the finding of a significant stenotic lesion on imaging studies may not, ultimately, be the cause of the hypertension [8]. In pregnancy, optimal initial screening tests include ultrasound and/or magnetic resonance (MR) angiogram. Stenosis of greater than 75% in one or both renal arteries or stenosis of 50% or greater with poststenotic dilation is suggestive of renovascular hypertension. Given that no test is sufficiently accurate to completely exclude the diagnosis, correlation with clinical history is important. Clinical clues to renal artery stenosis include a history of an acute elevation of blood pressure over a previously stable baseline, severe or refractory hypertension, severe hypertension with an otherwise unexplained atrophic kidney or an acute elevation

of creatinine after the initiation of an angiotensin-converting enzyme (ACE) inhibitor or angiotensin receptor-blocking drug. Patients with both a significant stenotic lesion and a typical clinical presentation should be referred to a nephrologist for further evaluation and treatment.

Chronic renal disease also causes hypertension and is associated with an increased risk of pregnancy complications [9]. Patients with early-stage disease may have no significant signs or symptoms on history and physical examination, but will generally have an abnormal urinalysis and/or creatinine.

Pheochromocytoma, although rare, can be a dangerous condition for the pregnant patient, particularly at the time of labor and delilvery [10]. The classic presentation includes paroxysmal hypertension, palpitations, headache and sweat ing, but many patients present with a less dramatic picture, leading to a delay in diagnosis. Although paroxysmal hypertension is often thought to be a typical feature of the disease, it occurs in only about 50% of cases; 5–15% of cases present with normal blood pressure and the rest have what appears to be essential hypertension [11]. A unique presentation of pheochromocytoma in pregnancy includes paradoxic supine hypertension with normal blood pressure in the sitting or erect position. This may occur as a result of compression of the adrenal tumor by the gravid uterus in the supine position. A 24-hour urine assessment for metanephrine and catecholamines or serum catecholamine levels is required to make the diagnosis. MR or computed tomography (CT) may be safely used to identify adrenal tumors if needed.

Other endocrine causes of hypertension include hyperaldosteronism and Cushing's disease. Primary hyperaldosteronism is an unusual cause of hypertension and is usually suggested by abnormal electrolytes (low potassium, high sodium). Patients with Cushing's disease are often infertile. This condition may be difficult to diagnose in pregnancy due to changes in steroid hormone levels. Patients with typical clinical features such as hypertension with central obesity, moon facies, striae, proximal muscle weakness and ecchymoses should be evaluated with the help of an internist or endocrinologist. Hyperthyroidism often presents with obvious physical symptoms and is easily diagnosed with thyroid function tests.

Obstructive sleep apnea as a cause of hypertension is often overlooked [12]. All hypertensive patients and their bed partners should be asked about symptoms of obstructive sleep apnea such as excessive daytime sleepiness, snoring or apneic episodes during sleep.

An extensive laboratory evaluation for secondary causes of hypertension is of little utility but all patients with newly diagnosed hypertension should have some basic labs and a directed evaluation to screen for secondary or reversible causes (Box 42.2). Secondary causes of hypertension should be suspected and further evaluation pursued in patients with onset of hypertension at an early age (<30 years), patients with severe (>180/110) or refractory (i.e. more than three medications are needed to control blood pressure) hypertension, patients with an acute elevation of blood pressure over a previously stable baseline, or patients who present with relevant signs and symptoms.

Box 42.2 Routine lab evaluation for all newly diagnosed hypertensive patients

- Electrolytes
- Urinalysis
- Creatinine
- Thyroid-stimulating hormone
- Hematocrit
- Calcium
- Fasting glucose
- Fasting lipid profile (may be difficult to interpret in pregnancy)
- Electrocardiogram

Evaluation for end-organ damage

The next step in the evaluation of hypertension is an assessment for end-organ damage. The risk of end-organ damage correlates with the duration and severity of blood pressure, as well as the presence or absence of other risk factors. The most common organs affected by hypertension include the heart, brain, kidney, eyes and peripheral vasculature. Cardiac conditions associated with hypertension include left ventricular hypertrophy, coronary artery disease or heart failure. Hypertension is also associated with an increased risk of transient ischemic attack or stroke, chronic kidney disease, retinopathy and peripheral vascular disease. Evaluation for end-organ damage is summarized in Table 42.2. If end-organ damage is identified, patients should be counseled that pregnancy may worsen these conditions.

Assessment of cardiovascular risk factors

Lastly, patients should be evaluated for cardiac risk factors. In general, any patient who is diagnosed with one cardiac risk factor should be screened for others [13]. Although lipid levels are often elevated in pregnancy, other cardiovascular risk factors can and should be assessed. Pregnant women are often highly motivated to optimize their health and frequent contact with the provider offers an ideal opportunity to address lifestyle changes to reduce long-term cardiovascular risk. Box 42.3 outlines the primary cardiac risk factors.

Table 42.2 Evaluation for end-organ damage

Organ	Screening test
Heart	Electrocardiogram for left ventricular hypertrophy
Kidney	Urinalysis, creatinine. If abnormal, do urine protein/creatinine ratio or 24-hour urine
Eyes	Fundoscopic exam to evaluate for retinopathy
Brain	Evaluate for signs or symptoms of ischemic brain injury
Peripheral vasculature	Evaluate for exertional leg pain, check peripheral pulses

---

Box 42.3 Primary cardiac risk factors

- Diabetes
- Hyperlipidemia
- Smoking
- Family history
- Peripheral vascular disease

Evaluation of hypertension

A thorough history and physical examination are critical parts of the evaluation of chronic hypertension. Clinicians should adopt a standard approach in all patients with newly diagnosed hypertension, including pregnant women. In addition, some laboratory testing should be done routinely in all patients with new hypertension. For those patients diagnosed prior to pregnancy, documentation of this assessment is important. The primary objective of the history, physical exam and lab testing is to evaluate for signs or symptoms of secondary causes of hypertension or end-organ damage from hypertension, and to assess for cardiovascular risk factors as outlined above.

History

Patients should be questioned about the following.
• Duration of hypertension and prior treatment.
• Family history of hypertension, cardiovascular disease or other conditions that may cause hypertension.
• Symptoms of secondary or reversible causes of hypertension (see Table 42.1).
• Symptoms of end-organ damage:
  • chest pain
  • dyspnea
  • exertional leg pain
  • decreased visual acuity
  • transient blindness or speech abnormality
  • unilateral loss of strength or sensation.
• Assessment of other cardiovascular risk factors:
  • family history of hypertension or cardiovascular disease
  • smoking status
  • personal history of hypertension, diabetes or hyperlipidemia
  • dietary habits (including salt intake and saturated fats)
  • exercise habits.

Physical examination

Proper blood pressure measurement is essential in the assessment and management of hypertension. The blood pressure should be measured with the patient in the seated position. The common practice of measuring blood pressure while the pregnant woman is lying on her left side may produce false low blood pressure readings and should be avoided. Inferior vena caval compression by the gravid uterus while supine may lead to a decrease in systolic pressure of more than 30% in some patients in the third trimester [14]. Patients should refrain from caffeine or tobacco intake in the 30 minutes prior to the exam. The arm should be fully extended and held at the level of the heart. Cuff size is extremely important in accurate blood pressure measurement. A cuff that is too large will falsely lower the blood pressure and one that is

too small will give a false high reading. Chronic hypertension is diagnosed if the blood pressure is greater than 140/90 on two separate readings done at least a week apart.

The rest of the physical exam is directed at evaluation for signs of secondary causes of end-organ damage of hypertension (see Tables 42.1 and 42.2).

Laboratory testing

Routine lab testing on all newly diagnosed hypertensive patients should include a complete blood count (CBC), electrolytes, creatinine, urinalysis, thyroid-stimulating hormone and calcium. An electrocardiogram should be done at the time of diagnosis and every year thereafter (see Box 42.2).

Conclusion

It is estimated that 24% of the adult population of the US has chronic hypertension [15]. Data from the Framingham Heart Study suggest that women who are normotensive at age 55 have a 90% lifetime risk for developing hypertension [16]. The prevalence of chronic hypertension in reproductive age women is estimated to be approximately 7% and as high as 10% in African American women [17]. Women with chronic hypertension have an increased risk of pregnancy complications including pre-eclampsia, intrauterine growth restriction and abruption. The obstetrician should be acutely aware of these potential complications and the need for close monitoring during gestation. The detection, evaluation and treatment of hypertension in pregnancy is, however, not only relevant to the pregnancy, but is essential in reducing long-term cardiovascular morbidity and mortality in women. A thoughtful and careful approach to the evaluation of hypertension in pregnancy provides an opportunity for the obstetrician to affect the health of their patients long after their reproductive years.

References

1. Magee L, Ornstein MP, von Dadelszen P. Management of hypertension in pregnancy. BMJ 1999;318:1332–6.
2. Chobanian AV, Bakris GL, Black HR, et al. The Seventh Report of the Joint National Committee on Prevention, Detection, Evaluation, and Treatment of High Blood Pressure. JAMA 2003;289(19):2560–72.
3. Vasan RS, Larson MG, Leip EP, et al. Assesment of frequency of progression to hypertension in nonhypertensive participants in the Framingham Heart Study. Lancet 2001;358: 1682–6.
4. Ogden LG, He J, Lydick E, et al. Long-term absolute benefit of lowering blood pressure in hypertensive patients according to the JNC VI risk stratification. Hypertension 2000;35:539–43.
5. Vasan RS, Larson MG, Leip EP, et al. Impact of high normal blood pressure on the risk of cardiovascular diseases. N Engl J Med 2001;345(18):1291–7.
6. Bagga R, Aggarwal N, Chopra V, et al. Pregnancy complicated by severe chronic hypertension: a 10-year analysis from a developing country. Hypertens Pregn 2007;26(2):139–49.

7. Mann SJ, Pickering TG. Detection of renovascular hypertension. State of the art: 1992. Ann Intern Med 1992;117:845.

8. Textor SC. Pitfalls in imaging for renal artery stenosis. Ann Intern Med 2004;141:730.

9. Fischer MJ, Lehnerz SD, Hebert JR, Parikh CR. Kidney disease is an independent risk factor for adverse fetal and maternal outcomes in pregnancy. Am J Kidney Dis 2004;43 415.

10. Grodski S, Jung C, Kertes P. Pheochromocytoma in pregnancy. Int Med J 2006;36:604–6.

11. Baguet JP, Hammer L, Mazzuco TL, *et al*. Circumstances of discovery of phaeochromocytoma: a retrospective study of 41 consecutive patients. Eur J Endocrinol 2004;150:681.

12. Nieto F, Young T, Lind B, *et al*. Association of sleep-disordered breathing, sleep apnea, and hypertension in a large community-based study: Sleep Heart Health Study. JAMA 2000;283:1829–36.

13. Padwal R, Straus SE, McAlister FA. Evidence based management of hypertension. Cardiovascular risk factors and their effects on the decision to treat hypertension: evidence based review. BMJ 2001;322:977.

14. Holmes F. Incidence of supine hypotension syndrome in late pregnancy. J Obstet Gynecol British Empire 1960;67:254–8.

15. Burt VL, Whelton P, Roccella EJ. Prevalence of hypertension in the US adult population: results from the third National Health And Nutrition Examination Survey, 1988–1991. Hypertension 1995;25(3):305–13.

16. Vasan RS, Beiser A, Seshadri S, *et al*. Residual lifetime risk for developing hypertension in middle-aged women and men. The Framingham Heart Study. JAMA 2002;287(8):1003–10.

17. Ihab H, Kotchen T. Trends in prevalence, awareness, treatment, and control of hypertension in the United States, 1988–2000. JAMA 2003;290(2):199–206.

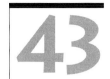

43 Approach to presyncope and syncope in pregnancy

Paul S. Gibson[1], Rshmi Khurana[2] and Winnie W. Sia[2]

[1]Departments of Medicine and Obstetrics and Gynecology, University of Calgary, Foothills Medical Centre, Calgary, Alberta, Canada
[2]Departments of Medicine and Obstetrics and Gynecology, University of Alberta, Royal Alexandra Hospital, Edmonton, Alberta, Canada

Introduction

Syncope is a common and important medical problem resulting from a transient reduction in cerebral blood flow to the parts of the brain that control consciousness. Individual episodes of syncope may lead to death or serious injury, and recurrent episodes of syncope or presyncope can be disabling.

Syncope and recurrent presyncope are common, and poorly understood, problems in pregnancy. Pregnant women have long been said to be "fainters" with little thought given to the underlying pathophysiology. Very little systematic research had been done to evaluate these symptoms among pregnant women. A postpartum survey identified a prevalence of syncope in pregnancy of 4.6% [1]. Furthermore, 28.2% of women reported at least one episode of presyncope during pregnancy, and 10.3% reported troublesome recurrent presyncope. These symptoms often have a dramatic effect on these women's quality of life.

Causes of syncope

The causes of syncope and recurrent presyncope are diverse (Table 43.1). Among nonpregnant patients presenting to an emergency room with syncope, the most common etiologies were neurally mediated (vasovagal), arrhythmia, seizures, orthostasis and situational syncope [1]. At least one-third of these patients did not have a definite cause of syncope identified despite appropriate investigations. During pregnancy, the differential diagnosis of syncope is relatively unchanged, although the physiologic changes of pregnancy make certain causes more likely.

Neurally mediated (also known as vasovagal or neurocardiogenic) syncope is the most common cause of syncope. It constitutes one-third of identified cases of syncope, and is the dominant etiology among patients without known heart disease [2]. The pathophysiology involves an initial reduction in venous return to the heart, triggering an aberrant reflex in susceptible individuals, which leads to sympathetic nervous system withdrawal and paradoxic peripheral venous dilation and/or bradycardia. These changes lead to hypotension, hypoperfusion of the brain and loss of consciousness [3].

Several physiologic changes predispose pregnant women to neurally mediated syncope. Elevated progesterone levels cause reduced venous tone and venous pooling in the upright posture, predisposing to orthostatic hypotension. Some pregnant women may be dehydrated due to severe nausea or hyperemesis gravidarum. The resulting reduced venous return to the heart, particularly with prolonged standing, may trigger a vasovagal episode in susceptible women. The increased cardiac contractility seen in pregnancy probably also contributes to the increased risk of neurally mediated syncope by enhanced stimulation of cardiac mechanoreceptors, which triggers the aberrant reflex.

In the latter part of pregnancy, the gravid uterus may compress the inferior vena cava (IVC) in the supine position, causing a temporary minor drop in cardiac output and blood pressure in most women. In susceptible individuals, however, this may precipitate the vasovagal reflex with accompanying profound hypotension and syncope. This is referred to as the "supine hypotension syndrome" [4,5]. IVC compression leading to syncope may even occur while sitting in some women [6]. Another period of enhanced risk for vasovagal episodes is during regional anesthesia for labour or cesarean delivery [7]. During these procedures, regional anesthetics may reduce neural tone of the peripheral vascular system, leading to venous pooling, reduced cardiac preload and triggering of the vasovagal reflex.

Other causes of syncope may also occur with increased frequency in pregnancy (see Table 43.1).

de Swiet's Medical Disorders in Obstetric Practice, 5th edition.
Edited by R. O. Powrie, M. F. Greene, W. Camann. © 2010 Blackwell Publishing.

Table 43.1 Causes of presyncope and syncope in pregnancy

Cause of presyncope or syncope	Investigations	Comments
Cardiac and circulatory causes		
Neurally mediated (vasovagal) syncope and presyncope (most common)	History Physical exam 12-lead EKG	Features that suggest vasovagal syncope include: gradual onset; accompanying nausea, hot flushes, diaphoresis, mild dyspnea and palpitations, visual graying; onset while sitting, standing or lying flat in late pregnancy; improvement with assumption of a lateral recumbent position; and absence of postevent confusion after syncope. Most women who experience vasovagal syncope do not suffer injury, as the onset of symptoms is gradual, and following resolution of the episode they feel exhausted
Situational syncope (cough syncope, micturition syncope, carotid sinus hypersensitivity, etc.)	History	Situational syncope is usually apparent on a careful history

Cardiac arrhythmias:
  bradyarrhythmias
  tachyarrhythmias (SVT, VT, WPW, long QT syndrome with torsades)
	EKG
	24- or 48-hour
	Holter monitor
	Event monitor
		Cardiac arrhythmias, particularly supraventricular [10] and ventricular tachycardia [11,12] , occur with increased frequency during pregnancy. While these arrhythmias more typically present with palpitations characterized as a rapid and regular heart beat, they may precipitate presyncope or syncope with rapid rates. Tachycardia-induced syncope is a particular risk in women with pre-existing cardiac conduction abnormalities such as pre-excitation [13] (e.g. WPW or Lown-Ganong-Levine syndromes) or long QT syndrome [14]. Bradycardia provoking syncope is rare in pregnancy but may be precipitated by medications such as beta-blockers or nondihydropyridine calcium channel blockers (such as verapamil and diltiazem)

Structural cardiac disease (aortic stenosis, atrial myxoma, cardiac tamponade, obstructive cardiomyopathy, massive pulmonary embolism)	History Physical exam Echocardiogram	A history or physical findings suggestive of cardiac disease would indicate a primary cardiac cause for syncope. Cardiac syncope is more likely to be sudden in onset, associated with severe palpitations of a fast regular heart beat and result in injury. Suspicious findings should be pursued with a detailed cardiac echo
Endocrine causes		
Hypoglycemia	Review diabetic monitoring record	Pregnant diabetics are at enhanced risk of hypoglycemia, which may progress to syncope or seizures if unrecognized or untreated
Hyperventilation	History	
Neurologic/psychiatric causes		
Seizures	Collateral history EEG MRI	A collateral history of convulsive activity, particularly with a history of epilepsy or neurologic disease, would support a diagnosis of seizure as the cause of syncope. This diagnosis would be supported by transient confusion following the episode, tongue biting or incontinence. Pregnant women with epilepsy may experience a worsening of their seizure disorder during pregnancy, most often due to either medication noncompliance or pregnancy-related changes in the pharmacokinetics of their anticonvulsant drug leading to subtherapeutic levels
TIA/CVA (rare)	History Physical exam CT/MRI brain	TIA and CVA are rare causes of syncope and will generally be associated with some focal neurologic deficit
Subclavian steal syndrome	History	Rapid or vigorous upper extremity movement may precipitate presyncope or syncope in susceptible individuals
Generalized anxiety disorders and panic attacks	History Psychiatric consultation	Among women with a history of psychiatric illness and/or atypical or inconsistent symptoms, a psychiatric etiology should be considered [15]

CT, computed tomography; CVA, cerebrovascular accident; EEG, electroencephalogram; EKG, electrocardiogram; MRI, magnetic resonance imaging; SVT, supraventricular tachycardia; TIA, transient ischemic attack; VT, ventricular tachycardia; WPW, Wolff-Parkinson-White syndrome.

Investigations

The approach to syncope in pregnancy begins with a complete history and physical examination. All patients with unexplained syncope or recurrent presyncope merit an initial 12-lead electrocardiogram (EKG). This study may identify an arrhythmia or evidence of underlying electrical or structural cardiac disease. Beyond the initial history, physical exam and EKG, the remaining work-up should be individualized according to the differential diagnosis that is suspected (Table 43.2). In women with a history compatible with vasovagal syncope and a reassuring physical examination and EKG, the clinician may move on to counseling and treatment.

Table 43.2 Investigations for presyncope and syncope in pregnancy

Investigation	Comments
Electrocardiography	Premature ventricular and supraventricular beats are common in pregnancy. Other changes reported in normal pregnancy include a small leftward shift of the QRS axis, small Q wave and inverted P wave in lead III (abolished by inspiration), ST segment and T wave changes in inferior and lateral leads and an increased R/S ratio in leads V1 and V2 [16]. In the setting of presyncope or syncope the EKG may reveal frequent PAC or PVC or occasionally capture a discrete episode of arrhythmia. It may also reveal evidence of pre-excitation (PR interval <120 msec with or without the slurred upstroke in the QRS complex referred to as a delta wave), QT prolongation (>440 msec after correction for rate) or other abnormalities suggesting underlying structural cardiac disease
Holter monitor	If arrhythmia is suspected and symptoms are occurring frequently, a 24–48 h Holter monitor may be very useful. It can identify an abnormal rhythm and may correlate symptoms with the cardiac rate and rhythm
Event monitor	Occasionally an event monitor may be necessary to obtain an accurate diagnosis, typically when arrhythmia is suspected but symptoms are infrequent and a Holter monitor is uninformative. The monitor is worn for days to weeks, with the ability to capture and transmit recordings of infrequent cardiac events
Echocardiography	Transthoracic or (rarely) transesophageal echocardiography utilizes sound waves to measure and record details of cardiac structures. Chamber sizes and aortic annulus increase in size by 5–15% throughout gestation and return to normal after delivery. Minor valvular regurgitation is common and small pericardial effusions are seen in up to 44% of women by the third trimester; they resolve by 6 weeks postpartum [17]. Major concerns that might be identified on echocardiogram that could be associated with syncope would include: severe aortic valve/outflow obstruction, severe mitral stenosis, myocardial dysfunction, cardiomyopathy and (rarely) atrial myxoma
Electroencephalogram	An EEG and/or neurologic consultation may be undertaken to pursue a possible seizure disorder
Psychiatric consultation	Formal psychiatric consultation may be helpful when evaluating women with a history of psychiatric illness and/or atypical or inconsistent symptoms
Diabetic glucometer recording	Diabetic women experiencing syncope should have a review of their control via review of their records or glucometer memory

EEG, electroencephalogram; EKG, electrocardiogram; PAC, premature atrial contraction; PVC, premature ventricular contraction.

Treatment of neurally mediated (vasovagal) presyncope and syncope (Box 43.1)

Upon diagnosis of recurrent neurally mediated syncope and presyncope, several effective treatment options are available. Initially, reassurance regarding the pathophysiology and generally benign nature of the condition may be very helpful to the woman. Specific instructions should be given to respond to further episodes by ceasing activity and changing position (preferably assuming a sitting or lateral decubitus position) until the symptoms resolve, thereby avoiding potential injury. Having the patient cross her legs with isometric muscle tensing in the upper limb (hand gripping) may also help postpone or prevent syncope in patients experiencing neurally mediated syncope [8]. Women should be advised to avoid prolonged standing and to keep a record of other potential precipitating/exacerbating factors [9]. Common precipitants include stress, fatigue, skipped meals, and hot or crowded environments. If symptoms persist, liberalization of salt intake along with generous fluid intake may be very effective in reducing the frequency and severity of the episodes [4]. The use of full-length graded compression stockings may also reduce venous pooling of blood and improve symptoms.

If the above measures are ineffective at preventing recurrent vasovagal syncope or presyncope, and a woman is finding her

Box 43.1 Management of neurocardiogenic presyncope and syncope

Reassurance

- Avoidance of precipitating and exacerbating factors, including:
  - prolonged standing
  - stress
  - fatigue
  - dehydration
  - skipped meals
  - hot or crowded environments
- Increased salt and fluid intake
- Compression stockings

Beta-blockers:

- Metoprolol: start at 25 mg PO bid
- Pindolol: start at 5 mg PO bid
- Propranolol: start at 40 mg PO bid

symptoms incapacitating, the use of pharmacologic therapy may be considered. Outside pregnancy there are multiple treatment options, including beta-blockers, alpha-agonists, selective serotonin reuptake inhibitors, fludrocortisone, disopyramide, scopolamine, and anticholinergic agents [18]. Many of these agents may not be routinely warranted for this indication in pregnancy, but beta-blockers have a record of safe use in pregnancy for a variety of conditions. Beta-blockers can help prevent neurally mediated presyncope and syncope by inhibiting the initiation of the vasovagal reflex at the level of the cardiac mechanoreceptors. Atenolol should be avoided due to its association with intrauterine growth restriction, but metoprolol (25 mg orally twice daily), pindolol (5 mg orally twice daily) or propranolol (40 mg orally twice daily) may be initiated and titrated gently upward to clinical effect. If effective, these agents should be continued throughout pregnancy and tapered off post partum.

Conclusion

Syncope and recurrent presyncope are common symptoms faced by pregnant women. While the etiology is usually benign, the symptoms may be incapacitating. Serious underlying causes should be excluded by a careful history, physical examination, EKG and other judiciously selected investigations. The majority of cases will prove to be due to the vasovagal mechanism. These women will benefit from reassurance, advice on safe behavior, generous sodium and fluid intake, use of graded compression stockings and occasionally specific pharmacotherapy with beta-blockers.

References

1. Gibson PS, Powrie R, Pipert J. Prevalence of syncope and recurrent presyncope during pregnancy. Obstet Gynecol 2001;97: S41–S42.
2. Fitzpatrick AP, Cooper P. Diagnosis and management of patients with blackouts. Heart 2006;92(4):559–68.
3. Soteriades ES, Evans JC, Larson MG, *et al.* Incidence and prognosis of syncope. N Engl J Med 2002;347(12):931–3.
4. Grubb BP. Clinical practice. Neurocardiogenic syncope. N Engl J Med 2005;352(10):1004–10.
5. Lanni SM, Tillinghast J, Silver HM. Hemodynamic changes and baroreflex gain in the supine hypotensive syndrome. Am J Obstet Gynecol 2002;187(6):1636–41.
6. Kinsella SM, Tuckey JP. Perioperative bradycardia and asystole: relationship to vasovagal syncope and the Bezold-Jarisch reflex. Br J Anaesth 2001;86(6):859–68.
7. Huang MH, Roeske WR, Hu H, Indik JH, Marcus FI. Postural position and neurocardiogenic syncope in late pregnancy. Am J Cardiol 2003; 92(10):1252–3.
8. Watkins EJ, Dresner M, Calow CE. Severe vasovagal attack during regional anaesthesia for caesarean section. Br J Anaesth 2000; 84(1):118–20.
9. Krediet CT, van Dijk N, Linzer M, van Lieshout JJ, Wieling W. Management of vasovagal syncope: controlling or aborting faints by leg crossing and muscle tensing. Circulation 2002;106(13):1684–9.
10. Chen-Scarabelli C, Scarabelli TM. Neurocardiogenic syncope. BMJ 2004;329(7461):336–41.
11. Silversides CK, Harris L, Haberer K, Sermer M, Colman JM, Siu SC. Recurrence rates of arrhythmias during pregnancy in women with previous tachyarrhythmia and impact on fetal and neonatal outcomes. Am J Cardiol 2006;97(8):1206–12.
12. Brodsky M, Doria R, Allen B, Sato D, Thomas G, Sada M. New-onset ventricular tachycardia during pregnancy. Am Heart J 1992;123(4 Pt 1):933–41.
13. Brodsky MA, Sato DA, Oster PD, Schmidt PL, Chesnie BM, Henry WL. Paroxysmal ventricular tachycardia with syncope during pregnancy. Am J Cardiol 1986;58(6):563–4.
14. Widerhorn J, Widerhorn AL, Rahimtoola SH, Elkayam U. WPW syndrome during pregnancy: increased incidence of supraventricular arrhythmias. Am Heart J 1992;123(3):796–8.
15. McCurdy CM Jr, Rutherford SE, Coddington CC. Syncope and sudden arrhythmic death complicating pregnancy. A case report of Romano-Ward syndrome. J Reprod Med 1993;38(3):233–4.
16. Kouakam C, Lacroix D, Klug D, Baux P, Marquie C, Kacet S. Prevalence and prognostic significance of psychiatric disorders in patients evaluated for recurrent unexplained syncope. Am J Cardiol 2002;89(5):530–5.
17. Elkayam U, Gleicher N (eds). Cardiac problems in pregnancy, 3rd edn. Wiley-Liss, New York, 1998: 26–27.
18. Lee RV, Rosene-Montella K, Barbour LA, Garner PR, Keely E (eds). Medical care of the pregnant patient. American College of Physicians, Washington, DC, 2000: 353.

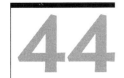

Approach to chest pain in pregnancy

Rshmi Khurana[1], Winnie W. Sia[1] and Paul S. Gibson[2]

[1]Departments of Medicine and Obstetrics and Gynecology, University of Alberta, Royal Alexandra Hospital, Edmonton, Alberta, Canada
[2]Departments of Medicine and Obstetrics and Gynecology, University of Calgary, Foothills Medical Centre, Calgary, Alberta, Canada

Introduction

Chest pain is a common symptom and can be challenging to evaluate. Most pregnant women who complain of chest pain will have a benign etiology. However, it is crucial to identify those who have serious or life-threatening conditions. Unfortunately, the literature on chest pain in pregnancy is sparse. Most of the algorithms developed to deal with chest pain in primary care populations are poorly applicable to pregnancy as they deal with an older male population and are targeted primarily towards excluding coronary artery disease, which is rare in pregnancy.

In evaluating a chest pain history, the mnemonic PQRST is useful (Box 44.1). Physical examination of the pregnant woman presenting with chest pain should include general appearance and level of distress, and full vitals (heart rate, temperature, blood pressure in both arms and respiratory rate). Assessment of oxygenation with a pulse oximeter is useful if available. Examination of the skin for jaundice, bruising, cyanosis or a vesicular rash may point to specific causes. Percussion and auscultation of the chest to pick up crackles, bronchial breath sounds, dullness, and absence of breath sounds may further help in determining the etiology of the chest pain. Cardiac exam should include examination for elevation of the jugular venous pressure, and auscultation to detect any murmurs, extra heart sounds or rubs. As upper abdominal pathology may also present with chest pain, examination of the abdomen should be performed. Palpation of the liver should be performed to check for tenderness and to elicit Murphy's sign. Epigastric or right upper quadrant tenderness may also be seen in pre-eclampsia/HELLP. Table 44.1 reviews several common and uncommon causes of chest pain in pregnancy and the initial investigations suggested.

Most of the usual investigations used to evaluate patients with chest pain can be employed during pregnancy. However, some may need to be excluded or modified due to concerns about fetal safety, and the interpretation of some may change slightly. Table 44.2 reviews some of the tests that may be useful in evaluating chest pain and any pregnancy considerations with them. Most patients with significant chest pain should have an electrocardiogram and chest X-ray performed if no other obvious cause is found. Fetal health should also be evaluated and considered when selecting maternal investigations, although in life-threatening situations, maternal health should be the primary factor in determining diagnostic and treatment decisions.

In summary, the pregnant woman with chest pain can pose a diagnostic challenge to her healthcare provider. Whether or not to evaluate for pulmonary embolus is a common clinical conundrum. If no other cause is apparent and the pain

Box 44.1 Chest pain history (PQRST)

P – precipitating and palliative features	Precipitating: exertion, palpation, eating fatty meal, emotion Palliative: rest, antacids
Q – quality of the pain	Dull, sharp, pressure, etc.
R – region of the pain and radiation	Region – epigastric, substernal Radiation – to back, shoulders, abdomen
S – severity of the pain	Rate 0–10 with 0 being no pain and 10 being worst pain imaginable
T – temporal quality of the pain	Onset of symptoms – sudden or gradual Duration – measured in seconds to hours

de Swiet's Medical Disorders in Obstetric Practice, 5th edition.
Edited by R. O. Powrie, M. F. Greene, W. Camann. © 2010 Blackwell Publishing.

Table 44.1 Causes of chest pain in pregnancy

Causes of chest pain	Investigations	Comments
Chest wall		
Breast	Consider ultrasound if fluctuant area of tenderness to rule out abscess	Breast tenderness is common during pregnancy and with breast engorgement post partum. Mastitis is common post partum, often caused by *Staphylococcus aureus*, and should be treated with antibiotics (breastfeeding can continue). Breast abscess can complicate mastitis and may require drainage
Musculoskeletal and costochondritis	None	Often is associated with chest wall tenderness, although tenderness over the sternum is common and should not be overinterpreted. Pain may be precipitated by movement of chest/arms. Costochondritis presents with diffuse pain that is reproduced by palpation of the upper costal cartilages without associated heat, erythema or swelling in the area. Treatment may include local heat or ice and acetaminophen. NSAIDs should be avoided
Shingles (herpes zoster)	If diagnosis unclear, viral culture of lesion	Severe, sharp pain assoiated with a vesicular rash in the distribution of a dermatome. Not a risk for fetus (unlike primary varicella infection). Treatment is symptomatic or could consider acyclovir/valacyclovir +/− prednisone for severe cases (shown to be beneficial only in patients >age 50)
Trauma		Examine skin for bruising. Elicit appropriate history. Ask specifically about domestic violence as women may not offer this history and it is common during pregnancy
Vascular		
Pulmonary embolism	Chest X-ray, V/Q scan or CT angiogram of the chest	1/1600 pregnancies. 5–6 times more common in pregnancy than nonpregnant. Pain often sudden in onset, pleuritic and associated with dyspnea. May have tachycardia and hemoptysis. Arterial blood gases and A-a gradient often normal. Risk is higher with caesarean section, obesity, prior history or thrombophilia or family history. Treatment is therapeutic anticoagulation with heparin or low molecular weight heparin. Warfarin can be used post partum while breastfeeding
Aortic dissection	Chest X-ray, MRI or CT chest, transesophageal echocardiogram	Rare but occurrence during pregnancy accounts for 50% of all dissections under age 40 [1]. Life-threatening disorder. More common in pregnancy likely due to increase in cardiac output and changes in connective tissue of blood vessels. Described as severe, sharp "tearing" pain, often radiating to back. Pain may be intermittent. Symptoms in territories supplied by branches from aorta (stroke, loss of pulses, myocardial ischemia, new aortic insufficiency murmur, etc.). Check for blood pressure difference in arms and pulse deficits. Predisposing factors include Marfan's or other collagen diseases, vasculitis (Takayasu's arteritis), crack cocaine use, Turner's syndrome, trauma, coarctation of aorta, bicuspid aortic valve and aortic valve replacement. Treatment should include admission to intensive care unit, control of hypertension. May require surgery for definitive treatment
Pulmonary		
Pneumonia	Chest X-ray, sputum culture. Consider nasopharyngeal swab for nucleic acid testing for respiratory viruses (including influenza)	Common, incidence in pregnancy same as in nonpregnant women. Often associated cough, fever, sputum production, dyspnea, leukocytosis. Similar pathogens to nonpregnant individuals, but may have more severe case. Also consider aspiration as pregnancy a risk factor. Decreased cell-mediated immunity may lead to more severe case of pneumonia if viral pathogen, particularly influenza. Treatment is supportive with appropriate antibacterials or antivirals
Pneumothorax	Chest X-ray	Pain usually of sudden onset, pleuritic and associated with dyspnea. Patient may have prior history of pneumothorax. Treatment is with needle or tube thoracostomy. May observe if small
Pneumomediastinum	Chest X-ray	Pain is intense and sharp. Can radiate from substernal area to shoulders. Rare, but has been reported with labor [2], likely secondary to rupture of alveolus with Valsalva maneuver. Chest pain is most common presentation, but other symptoms include dyspnea, cough, palpitations, dysphagia, dysphonia and neck swelling. Examine for subcutaneous emphysema. Treatment is usually supportive care only. May require mediastinotomy if tension pneumomediastinum

Table 44.1 (Continued)

Causes of chest pain	Investigations	Comments
Cardiac		
Myocardial ischemia/infarction [9]	EKG, troponin I, stress echocardiography, coronary angiography	Rare, but 3–4-fold higher risk in pregnancy compared to nonpregnant women. Acute myocardial infarction complicates about 1 in 10,000 pregnancies. Most cases in third trimester or post partum. Risks factors include advanced maternal age, hypertension, diabetes, smoking and thrombophilia. When angiography is performed, etiology can include atherosclerosis, but coronary artery dissection, thrombosis in normal arteries and vasospasm are more common than in nonpregnant individuals. Drugs implicated as risks include bromocriptine (to suppress lactation post partum), ergotamine and cocaine use. Management includes admission to coronary care unit and early coronary angiography
Pericarditis	EKG, echocardiogram. Consider ANA, viral studies	May have preceding viral infection or history of autoimmune disease. Pain can be at tip of shoulder, anterior chest or upper chest depending on area of pericardium involved. Often a pleuritic component to pain, which is usually relieved by sitting up and leaning forward. Listen for pericardial friction rub. Check for elevated jugular venous pressure and pulsus paradoxus to rule out cardiac tamponade
Gastrointestinal		
Gastroesophageal reflux disease (GERD) and esophageal spasm	None	GERD is common, especially late pregnancy. Incidence is 30–50%. Most common cause for chest pain in pregnancy. Progesterone causes relaxation of the lower esophageal sphincture, leading to exacerbation of GERD. Pain usually retrosternal and "burning." May be accompanied by nausea, vomiting, regurgitation or dysphagia. Pain often related to eating or supine position. Usually relieved with antacids or food intake. Esophageal spasm may present with squeezing pain that can mimic the pain of angina. Treatment includes lifestyle modification (avoid caffeine, eat small meals, avoid recumbent position after meals), antacid therapy, sucralfate, H2 blockers such as ranitidine, metoclopramide. Proton pump inhibitors may be used in refractory cases
Peptic ulcer disease	Endoscopy +/− biopsy	Usually epigastric or substernal pain that is relieved with antacids or milk. May have associated nausea or vomiting. If *H. pylori* diagnosed, consider eradication post partum
Esophageal rupture	Chest X-ray	Rare and usually occurs secondary to vomiting. May occur in patients with hyperemesis gravidarum. Pain is usually severe and retrosternal and preceded by retching and vomiting. May have odynophagia, tachypnea, dyspnea, cyanosis, fever and shock
Biliary tract disease (biliary colic, cholecystitis)	Liver enzymes, ultrasound of abdomen	Most often right upper quadrant abdominal pain, but can present as lower chest or epigastric. Pain usually occurs after eating fatty meal and may be colicky. Pain may also radiate to back and right shoulder area. Often associated nausea and vomiting. Pregnancy a risk factor for gallstones and biliary tract disease. Up to 10% of pregnant women will have gallstones or sludge, but only 0.16% will develop complications [3] (cholecystitis, choledocholithiasis or pancreatitis). Conservative management often successful; may require surgery if recurrent, severe disease or complication such as infection or pancreatitis. ERCP can also be performed for choledocholithiasis. Elective surgery safest in second trimester
Pancreatitis	Lipase, ultrasound abdomen	Incidence is 1 in 2000 deliveries. Pain is usually mid-epigastric, constant and often radiates to the back. Usually accompanied by nausea and vomiting. Most common cause in pregnancy is gallstone pancreatitis. Treatment is supportive
Other		
Effect of beta-adrenergic agonists (e.g. ritodrine, terbutaline) used as tocolytic	History of use, EKG	These drugs often used to stop preterm labor and chest pain is a common side effect [4,5]. Other side effects include palpitations, dyspnea, tremor, nausea. Complications include pulmonary edema, myocardial ischemia, and arrhythmias. Discontinuation of therapy usually resolves symptoms. Treatment may require diuretic if pulmonary edema develops
Pre-eclampsia/HELLP syndrome	Blood pressure, assessment of proteinuria, CBC, liver enzymes, creatinine, peripheral smear, uric acid	Pre-eclampsia occurs in 5% of pregnancies and HELLP occurs in 10–15% of patients with pre-eclampsia. Only occurs after 20 weeks gestation. Chest pain would be an uncommon presentation, but can occur. Epigastric or right upper quadrant pain more common (from liver capsule distension). Rarely, myocardial ischemia may occur with severe pre-eclampsia [6]. Delivery is the definitive treatment

(Continued on p. 722)

Table 44.1 (Continued)

Causes of chest pain	Investigations	Comments
Acute fatty liver of pregnancy (AFLP)	Liver enzymes, CBC, INR, PTT, fibrinogen, creatinine, bilirubin, glucose, ammonia	Occurs in 1 in 16,000 deliveries after 20 weeks, but usually in third trimester. Usual symptoms are nausea, vomiting, epigastric pain, jaundice. 50% of patients also have signs of pre-eclampsia. Cardinal feature is evidence of liver synthetic dysfunction (coagulopathy, elevated ammonia levels, hypoglycemia). Acute renal failure often a feature. May be difficult to distinguish between AFLP and HELLP syndrome. Definitive treatment for both is delivery
Ovarian hyperstimulation syndrome (OHSS)	History of pharmacologic ovarian stimulation, chest x-ray, abdominal ultrasound	OHSS [7] has become a recognized entity with the increased use of assisted reproductive technology. Patients have enlarged ovaries, increased vascular permeability leading to ascites, pleural effusions, hemoconcentration and are at higher risk for thrombosis. Chest pain may occur in this condition from a large pleural effusion or from pulmonary embolism. Patients present with abdominal distension, cough, and dyspnea. Treatment involves supportive care, thoracocentesis and paracentesis for symptomatic relief of pleural effusions and ascites
Sickle cell crisis	History of sickle cell disease	Increased risk of acute chest syndrome during pregnancy in patients with sickle cell disease. Treatment includes hydration and analgesics (often opioids)
Pheochromocytoma	Measurement of urinary metanephrines and catecholamines	Rare, but life-threatening, especially if undiagnosed in pregnancy. Classic presentation is sweating, tachycardia, episodic headache and hypertension; chest pain less common presentation, but reported in pregnancy. Diagnosis more likely if family history of Multiple endocrine neoplasia (MEN) II syndrome. Methyldopa can interfere with assay for urinary metanephrines test. Treatment includes adequate alpha-adrenergic blockade followed with beta-blockade (beta-blockade prior to alpha-blockade can trigger hypertensive crisis). Definitive treatment with surgery
Anxiety/panic disorder	Need to rule out organic disease	Diagnosis of exclusion. Hyperventilation can occasionally cause nonspecific ST and T wave abnormalities

ANA, antinuclear antibody; CBC, complete blood count; EKG, electrocardiogram; ERCP, endoscopic retrograde cholangiopancreatography; INR, international normalized ratio; NSAID, nonsteroidal anti-inflammatory drugs; PTT, partial thromboplastin time.

Table 44.2 Investigations for chest pain in pregnancy

Investigations	Comments
Chest X-ray	May provide a diagnosis such as in pneumothorax or pneumonia. May be useful in excluding other causes of chest pain if suspect pulmonary embolism. Radiation dose to the fetus from a maternal PA and lateral chest X-ray with appropriate shielding is <0.001 rads [8], well below the maximum 5 rads total exposure that is considered safe in pregnancy. Chest X-ray findings generally remain unchanged in pregnancy, but may demonstrate slight cardiomegaly with a horizontal position of the heart and straightening of the left heart border (due to diaphragmatic elevation), increased lung markings suggesting elevated pulmonary venous pressure, and increased breast shadows. Post partum, small pleural effusions may be present [9]
Electrocardiography (EKG)	Useful when considering the diagnosis of myocardial ischemia or pericarditis. Typical findings of acute MI are peaked T waves followed by ST elevation in the leads recording the involved myocardium and finally development of Q waves. A new left bundle branch block may also be seen with acute MI. Patients may also have non-ST elevation MI and EKG can be normal in 20% of patients with acute MI. Premature ventricular and supraventricular beats more common in pregnancy. Other changes reported in normal pregnancy include a small shift of the QRS axis to the left, small Q wave and inverted P wave in lead III (abolished by inspiration), ST segment and T wave changes in inferior and lateral leads and an increased R/S ratio in leads V1 and V2 [10]. Transient EKG changes suggestive of ischemia can occur in healthy women undergoing cesarean section, usually in leads I, aVL and V5. These changes should be correlated with clinical presentation and biochemical markers to ensure that they are not due to myocardial ischemia. Most of these EKG changes are minor, but if confusion about their significance, consider consultation with an internist or cardiologist
Cardiac enzymes	Cardiac troponin I has been shown to be reliable and useful when investigating pregnant women for myocardial ischemia [11]. Caution needs to be exercised when using creatine kinase (CK) and CK-MB to diagnose myocardial ischemia peripartum as it can be elevated with normal labor and after caesarean section [12]
Arterial blood gases	Normal pCO_2 in pregnancy is 28–32 mmHg due to physiologic hyperventilation from stimulation of the respiratory center by progesterone. Normal range for pO_2 in pregnancy at sea level is 95–105 mmHg. The arterial-alveolar (A-a) gradient remains normal in normal pregnancy, and often remains normal even in the setting of documented pulmonary embolism [13]

Table 44.2 (Continued)

Investigations	Comments
Ventilation/perfusion (V/Q) scan	When available, this is probably the test of choice when pulmonary embolism is being considered in pregnancy and the patient's chest X-ray is normal. A normal perfusion scan by itself effectively rules out pulmonary embolism, making the ventilation scan unnecessary and thereby limiting further radiation exposure. However, even when both a ventilation scan and perfusion scan are done, the radiation dose to the fetus is still acceptable at 0.02–0.05 rads
Computed tomography (CT) pulmonary angiography of the chest	An alternative to rule out pulmonary embolism when chest X-ray abnormal, when patient cannot co-operate with a prolonged test and when V/Q not available or indeterminate. CT pulmonary angiography may miss smaller peripheral emboli, however. Therefore many experts would recommend also obtaining bilateral leg Doppler compression ultrasounds when there is no evidence of pulmonary emboli on CT but there exists no alternative pulmonary process to explain the patient's symptoms. Radiation dose to the fetus from CT pulmonary angiography is less than 0.02 rads (1 rad is equivalent to 0.01 gray). CT may confer a higher maternal radiation dose to the breasts, and some experts fear it may increase maternal cancer risk later in life [14]. Theoretical risk of thyroid dysfunction in the fetus with exposure to iodinated contrast *in utero*; suggest that thyroid function be tested in first week of life but this is not recommended by all experts
Echocardiography	No risk to fetus. May be useful in diagnosis of aortic dissection, pericarditis, and suspected ischemia. Chamber sizes and aortic annulus increase in size by 5–15% throughout gestation and return to normal after delivery. Small pericardial effusions are seen in up to 44% of women by the third trimester; they resolve by 6 weeks post partum [15]
Pre-eclampsia labs	Hemoglobin, platelets, creatinine, uric acid, AST, ALT, and assessment of proteinuria (urine dipstick, 24-hour urine for protein or random urine protein to creatinine ratio) should be ordered in patients suspected of having pre-eclampsia

ALT, alanine transaminase; AST, aspartate transaminase.

is suggestive, a computed tomography scan or ventilation/perfusion scan should be performed as pulmonary embolus is one of the leading medical causes of maternal mortality. Although most pregnant women will have a benign etiology for their chest pain, such as musculoskeletal discomfort or gastroesophageal reflux, they are at risk for some very serious causes that must be excluded. A detailed history, physical exam and a few targeted investigations will usually provide information to provide a diagnosis and rule out the other more serious etiologies.

References

1. Ray P, Murphy GJ, Shutt LE. Recognition and management of maternal cardiac disease in pregnancy. Br J Anaesth 2004;93:428–39.
2. Seidl JJ, Brotzman GL. Pneumomediastinum and subcutaneous emphysema following vaginal delivery. Case report and review of the literature. J Fam Pract 1994;39(2):178–80.
3. Swisher SG, Schmit PJ, Hunt KK, *et al.* Biliary disease during pregnancy. Am J Surg 1994;168(6):576–9.
4. Perry KG, Morrison JC, Rust OA, Sullivan CA, Martin RW, Naef RW. Incidence of adverse cardiopulmonary effects with low-dose continuous terbutaline infusion. Am J Obstet Gynecol 1995;173:1273–7.
5. Canadian Preterm Labor Investigators Group. Treatment of preterm labor with the beta-adrenergic agonist ritodrine. N Engl J Med 1992;327:308–12.
6. Nabatian S, Quinn P, Brookfield L, Lakier J. Acute coronary syndrome and preeclampsia. Obstet Gynecol 2005;106(5 Pt 2):1204–6.
7. Delvigne A, Rozenberg S. Review of clinical course and treatment of ovarian hyperstimulation syndrome (OHSS). Hum Reprod Update 2003;9(1):77–96.
8. Lee RV, Rosene-Montella K, Barbour LA, Garner PR, Keely E (eds). Medical care of the pregnant patient. American College of Physicians, Washington, DC, 2000: 110–15.
9. Elkayam U, Gleicher N (eds). Cardiac problems in pregnancy, 3rd edn. Wiley-Liss, New York, 1998: 80.
10. Elkayam U, Gleicher N (eds). Cardiac problems in pregnancy, 3rd edn. Wiley-Liss, New York, 1998: 26–7.
11. Koscica KL, Bebbington M, Bernstein PS. Are maternal serum troponin I levels affected by vaginal or cesarean delivery? Am J Perinatol 2004;21(1):31–4.
12. Abramov Y, Abramov D, Abrahamov A, Durst R, Schenker J. Elevation of serum creatine phosphokinase and its MB isoenzyme during normal labor and early puerperium. Acta Obstet Gynecol Scand 1996;75(3):255–60.
13. Powrie RO, Larson L, Rosene-Montella K, Abarca M, Barbour L, Trujillo N. Alveolar-arterial oxygen gradient in acute pulmonary embolism in pregnancy. Am J Obstet Gynecol 1998;178(2):394–6.
14. Matthews S. Short communication: imaging pulmonary embolism in pregnancy: what is the most appropriate imaging protocol? Br J Radiol 2006;79(941):441–4.
15. Lee RV, Rosene-Montella K, Barbour LA, Garner PR, Keely E (editors). Medical care of the pregnant patient. American College of Physicians, Washington, DC, 2000: 353.

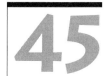

New-onset seizures in pregnancy

Laura A. Magee[1–4], Anne-Marie Côté[5] and Peter von Dadelszen[2–4]

[1]Department of Medicine, University of British Columbia, Vancouver, BC, Canada
[2]Department of Obstetrics and Gynecology, University of British Columbia, Vancouver, BC, Canada
[3]Centre for Applied Health Research and Evaluation, Child and Family Research Institute, University of British Columbia, Vancouver, BC, Canada
[4]Department of Health Care and Epidemiology, University of British Columbia, Vancouver, BC, Canada
[5]Department of Medicine, Université de Sherbrooke, Sherbrooke, Quebec, Canada

Physiologic changes

Eclampsia and epilepsy are the leading causes of seizures in pregnancy. Eclampsia is a pregnancy-induced condition, caused by the endothelial cell dysfunction of pre-eclampsia. Many physiologic changes in pregnancy may increase seizure risk for other women, particularly those with epilepsy. Chronic respiratory alkalosis, stress, anxiety, and sleep deprivation may lower the seizure threshold. For women taking antiepileptic drug (AED) therapy, nausea and vomiting may decrease drug absorption. Increases in maternal weight, plasma estrogens, and total body water may decrease AED levels through expansion of volume of distribution, decreased protein binding, and increased AED clearance [1–3]. Most important of all is maternal noncompliance with AED therapy, which occurs in up to two-thirds of women with epilepsy [4] and is responsible for 20% of status epilepticus [5].

General introduction

Evaluation and investigation of the pregnant woman with a seizure should follow the same general principles as for any adult, with attention paid to the diagnostic possibility of eclampsia.

Diagnosis

Epidemiology

A seizure in pregnancy is most likely to be secondary to epilepsy or eclampsia, which occur in 30–60/10,000 [1,6,7] and 5/10,000 pregnancies [8].

de Swiet's Medical Disorders in Obstetric Practice, 5th edition. Edited by R. O. Powrie, M. F. Greene, W. Camann. © 2010 Blackwell Publishing.

Etiology/pathophysiology

Epilepsy results from a genetically or acquired brain disorder. Eclampsia is associated with vasomotor instability, hypercoagulability, and inflammation of pre-eclampsia. Other causes of seizures may be structural or metabolic.

General course in pregnancy

Increased seizure frequency occurs in 15–30% of pregnant women with epilepsy [1,9,10] but status epilepticus is no more frequent and is rare (<1%) [2]. Among women with epilepsy, seizure frequency has not been associated with seizure type, duration of epilepsy or seizure frequency in a previous pregnancy [1].

Clinical presentation

Signs and symptoms

A seizure is a sudden change in behavior as a result of excessive neuronal activation in the cerebral cortex. Status epilepticus is a single unremitting seizure or frequent recurrent seizures without interictal recovery of consciousness lasting for at least 30 minutes; however, status should be assumed if a woman has seized for 10 minutes [11,12]. Eclamptic seizures are indistinguishable (clinically or by electroencephalogram (EEG) criteria) from other types of generalized tonic-clonic seizures, but there are some unique features (Box 45.1).

Diagnosis

A detailed description should be sought of the pre-"seizure" period, "seizure" itself, and post-"seizure" period in order to guide the differential diagnosis (Box 45.2). Specific points to verify include: signs or symptoms of pre-eclampsia; noncompliance with AED in women with epilepsy; history of childhood seizures; illicit, prescription and over-the-counter drug use; and intrapartum anesthesia (if relevant). The physical exam should be focused on "ABCs" of assessment, establishing

Box 45.1 Characteristics of eclampsia

Timing

- By definition, occurs after 20 weeks gestation, but presentations before 20 weeks have been reported rarely
- Women may seize antepartum (38%, and usually at preterm gestational ages), intrapartum (18%) or post partum (44%, usually within 48 hours of delivery, although reports exist of eclamptic seizures occurring as late as 14 days post partum)
- The majority (75%) of eclamptic seizures that occur during labor and in the postpartum period are observed in women who deliver at term

Symptoms and signs

- Self-limited, generalized tonic-clonic event that lasts less than 3–4 minutes
- May occur in the absence of antecedent pre-eclampsia, significant hypertension or maternal symptoms; prior to their first eclamptic convulsion, 40% of women do not have both hypertension and proteinuria (i.e. the traditional definition of pre-eclampsia) and 40% are asymptomatic

Box 45.2 Causes of a seizure in pregnancy

Pregnancy-induced causes

- Eclampsia
- Complications of regional anesthesia†

Other causes of seizure*

- Epileptic seizure (recurrent or *de novo*)
- CNS infection
- Metabolic:
  - hypoglycemia
  - extreme hyperglycemia
  - hyponatremia
  - hypocalcemia
  - uremia
  - hepatic encephalopathy
- Tumor/mass (e.g. AVM, cerebral meningioma)*
- AED withdrawal or overdose
- Illicit stimulant drug use
- Alcohol or drug withdrawal
- Trauma (e.g. subdural hematoma)
- Hemorrhage (e.g. subarachnoid or intracerebral hemorrhage)*
- Thromboembolism (e.g. cerebral sinus thrombosis)*
- Psychogenic nonepileptic seizures ("pseudo-seizures")

AED, antiepileptic drugs; AVM, arteriovenous malformation; CNS, central nervous system; SAH, subarachnoid hemorrhage.
†For example, bacterial or aseptic meningitis, "high" spinal anesthesia or intravascular injection of local anesthetic.
*Causes more likely to occur or worsen in pregnancy.

maternal and fetal well-being, ruling out complications (e.g. aspiration) and ascertaining the cause of the suspected seizure. Assessment of fetal heart rate (FHR) and pattern must also be included.

Laboratory evaluation and diagnostic testing

Basic investigations are the same as for the nonpregnant patient (Table 45.1). These detailed investigations and neurology consultation may be useful in any case of eclampsia but are definitely indicated for:

- a first seizure that occurs without the other characteristic features of eclampsia (i.e. hypertension, proteinuria or end-organ complications), even in the presence of another clear identifiable precipitant (e.g. hypoglycemia) [13,14]
- a seizure that has focal onset, is of a nongeneralized nature or is associated with focal neurologic findings, sustained obtundation or loss of consciousness
- recurrent/persistent eclamptic seizures
- a seizure in a patient with known epilepsy that is not consistent with their usual pattern or has no clear precipitant.

Detailed investigations may consist of one/more of the following.

- **Either computed tomography or magnetic resonance imaging, both of which are acceptable.** Computed tomography (CT) of the head is abnormal in approximately one-third of women with typical eclampsia. Typical changes are hypodensities in the cerebral cortex and subcortical white matter, usually localized to the posterior parietal and occipital areas, but also in the watershed area between the anterior, middle and posterior cerebral arteries [15]. Magnetic resonance imaging (MRI) demonstrates similar changes (characterized by high signal intensity on T2-weighted scans), but in a higher proportion (i.e. 46%) of women with eclampsia.

Magnetic resonance imaging is preferable if there is a strong suspicion of a posterior fossa lesion or cerebral venous thrombosis, a clinical stroke (particularly if the CT head is

Table 45.1 Investigations for a woman with a seizure in pregnancy

Investigation	Remarks
Needed in all women	
Bloodwork	"Pre-eclampsia laboratory markers": CBC, creatinine, uric acid, AST, ALT, LDH, bilirubin Other biochemistry: electrolytes, glucose, calcium, magnesium Toxicology screen
Urinalysis	Urinary protein quantification
May be needed depending on history and physical exam	
Neuroimaging	CT scan or MRI of head
EEG	Without, and possibly with, sleep deprivation
Lumbar puncture*	Opening pressure, minimal CSF parameters†: cell count, glucose, protein, gram stain and culture
ECG +/− Holter monitor	Rule out arrhythmia
Echocardiogram	Rule out valvular heart disease

*After excluding increased intracranial pressure.
† Other tests should be guided by clinical situation (e.g. cryptococcal antigen in a woman with known HIV).
ALT, alanine transaminase; AST, aspartate transaminase; CBC, complete blood count; CSF, cerebrospinal fluid; ECG, electrocardiogram; EEG, electroencephalogram; LDH, lactate dehydrogenase.

normal) or no obvious cause of a seizure and the brain CT is normal. Neither CT nor MRI is associated with significant fetal radiation exposure and neither has been associated with adverse fetal effects [16]. The choice of technique will depend in part on local availability.

- **EEG, which may be useful to predict seizure recurrence.** Outside pregnancy, a normal EEG, in the presence of a normal physical exam, reduces the risk of seizure recurrence in the subsequent year by almost two-thirds, from 33% to 12% in all patients [17]. The yield of EEG is highest when performed within 24 hours of the seizure, and when performed after sleep deprivation.
- **Lumbar puncture.** This is indicated if there is suspicion of an infectious process or a subarachnoid hemorrhage that has been missed on neuroimaging. First, neuroimaging or fundoscopy (if local access to neuroimaging access is limited) should be performed to rule out causes of increased intracranial pressure. Cerebral spinal fluid (CSF) should be sent for cell count, gram stain, culture, glucose and total protein. If meningitis is perceived as a possible cause, then antibiotic therapy should be initiated while awaiting the CSF results. Interpretation of the CSF laboratory studies is not altered by pregnancy. A prolonged seizure or status epilepticus may occasionally cause CSF pleocytosis [14].

Differential diagnosis

The differential diagnosis of a seizure in pregnancy is large, and includes specific pregnancy-induced causes and/or those that can occur in either nonpregnant or pregnant women (see Box 45.2). Consideration should be given to a "seizure mimicker" including: syncope, excessive daytime sleepiness, transient ischemic attack (TIA) and psychogenic nonepileptic seizure (PNES), also known as pseudoseizures. Typically, PNES is characterized by seizures that only occur in the presence of others and are often associated with some emotional precipitant. Common suggestive features of pseudoseizures include side-to-side shaking of the head, bilateral asynchronous movements (e.g. bicycling), weeping, stuttering, and arching of the back. Even when characteristic features exist, the diagnosis of pseudoseizure should be generally made in conjunction with a neurologist after the usual investigations for a seizure have been completed.

Management

Of the acute episode

Treatment of seizures in pregnancy includes the same supportive and therapeutic measures taken in the nonpregnant patient (i.e. the "ABCs"). The following are of particular importance.
- Left lateral decubitus positioning to avoid aspiration and supine hypotension.
- Adequate ventilation as pregnant women become hypoxemic more quickly.
- Investigations, including rapid maternal electrocardiogram (EKG) and glucometer testing (to exclude hypoglycemia). Venous blood should be drawn for laboratory investigations (see Table 45.1).
- Fetal heart rate assessment as the following have been associated with in-hospital generalized seizures: prolonged bradycardia (i.e. up to 30 min), decreased short-term FHR variability, and late decelerations in FHR [1,6,18,19]. These changes may occur in the absence of maternal hypoxemia or hypotension, possibly as a result of a seizure-related increase in sympathetic tone. There are no reliable data to indicate when to perform an emergency cesarean section for fetal indications.
- The assumption that a seizure in pregnancy is eclampsia until proven otherwise. This is true even in a woman with known epilepsy.

For eclampsia, the treatment of choice is $MgSO_4$ (4 g IV over 5–10 min) which halves the recurrence risk (to 5%) and is superior to both phenytoin and diazepam [20–22]. Benzodiazepines (lorazepam or diazepam) are not usually needed as the eclamptic seizures are generally short-lived but they may be used for prolonged seizures. They should not be administered once the seizure has finished as they are inferior to magnesium in this context. Recurrent seizures are treated with a further 2–4 g IV $MgSO_4$. Doses should be adjusted according to clinical response (e.g. a decrease in deep tendon reflexes), and lowered in renal failure. Eclampsia is "pre-eclampsia in the brain" so attention must be paid to other end-organ complications (e.g. renal failure). MgSO$_4$ and nifedipine may be used together, as the risk (if any) of neuromuscular blockade is <1%, and can be reversed with calcium gluconate 10 g IV [24].

If seizures do not remit or they recur, then one should treat as for other causes of seizures/status, in addition to proceeding with further investigations and consulting with intensive care and neurology.

- Noneclamptic seizures should be terminated by benzodiazepines. Lorazepam (0.1 mg/kg) is the benzodiazepine of choice because of its short half-life [24]. Diazepam (10 mg IV over 2 min, maximum 20 mg) is an alternative and is available as a rectal gel. Phenytoin (20 mg/kg IV administered no more rapidly than 50 mg/min) or the more expensive but more rapidly administered phenytoin pro-drug fosphenytoin is indicated when benzodiazepines fail or when a long-acting drug is needed (e.g. in preparation for transport).

- If after 10 minutes, the seizure has not remitted, or seizures are recurring, a higher level of care is needed. The following should be initiated: intubation, detailed investigations (as discussed above), and urgent consultation by neurology and intensive care.

Antenatal aftermath

Delivery is indicated for eclampsia. These women should receive an additional 24 hours of MgSO$_4$ therapy post partum [20].

For women with established epilepsy, consideration should be given to increasing the dose of AED (or restarting AED if previously stopped), unless there were clear modifiable precipitants that can be treated/eliminated. For women for whom the presumptive diagnosis is new-onset primary epilepsy, AED therapy will likely be initiated but this decision should be made in conjunction with a neurologist. For women with other causes of seizure, the primary cause should be treated. If structural, then the risk of seizure recurrence is much higher, and in nonpregnant women, AED therapy would be prescribed. However, the wisdom of AED administration will be guided by the gestational age, fetal risks of the proposed AED therapy, and the cause of the seizure.

All women with a seizure in pregnancy should be prohibited from driving or participating in activities that could result in personal injury. All physicians should be aware of local regulations in relation to their obligation to report these women to driving licensing authorities.

Therapeutic drug monitoring of AED levels may be useful. Monitoring of AED levels has practical limitations, is controversial, and has not been proven to improve seizure control and/or identify serum drug levels that are associated with lower fetal risk [25]. However, if AED levels

Table 45.2 Changes in AED levels with other medication

Drugs which may decrease AED levels	Drugs which may increase AED levels	AED may decrease levels of these drugs
Antacids	Erythroymycin	Corticosteroids*
St John's wort	Omeprazole	Benzodiazepines
Folic acid*	Psychoactive medication (e.g. fluoxetine, tricyclic antidepressants, sertraline)	Tricyclic antidepressants

*Guidelines for the administration of either folic acid or antenatal corticosteroids (for acceleration of fetal pulmonary maturity) do not advise any dose increase in women on hepatic enzyme-inducing AED. AED, antiepileptic drugs.

are performed (usually monthly), then it must be noted that pregnancy is associated with a decrease in total serum AED levels (but possibly, an increase in free AED fraction) [26]. Therapeutic drug monitoring may also be useful if women are taking other drugs that inhibit or induce hepatic enzymes that metabolize AED (Table 45.2) [28]. Note that AED may themselves interfere with the metabolism of other drugs.

Vitamin K supplementation of the mother on AED should be considered. Early hemorrhagic disease of the newborn (EHDN) manifests in the first 24 hours of life and has been associated with use of enzyme-inducing AED, although the risk is probably <1% [1,28]. Presumably, cytochrome P450 enzyme induction in the maternal and fetal liver leads to rapid consumption of vitamin K. Normal maternal coagulation parameters cannot be used to predict elevated fetal prothrombin and partial thromboplastin times [1]. The American Academy of Neurology states that there is no evidence for or against the standard recommendation that women on AEDs receive vitamin K supplementation (10–20 mg/day vitamin K, orally) during the last month of pregnancy to avoid EHDN [1,2,6]. Vitamin K tablets are not widely available.

Labor and delivery

Delivery should take place in an obstetric unit with facilities for maternal and neonatal resuscitation and a multidisciplinary plan should be established [1,16]. Cesarean section should be reserved for obstetric indications, including inadequate maternal co-operation because of impaired awareness [2].

During labor and delivery and the immediate postpartum period, the risk of seizure is <5% in the woman with epilepsy [2]. AED should be continued. Orally administered AED may not be adequately absorbed, because of delayed gastric emptying. If women are nauseated, AED may be held altogether because many are not available (e.g. carbamazepine) or widely available (e.g. valproic acid) in parenteral form, and extended-release preparations cannot be crushed and given

Table 45.3 Postpartum management

	Issue	Action
Postpartum eclampsia	Eclampsia may occur up to 14 days post partum	For a seizure within 14 days post partum, BP and urinalysis, in addition to "pre-eclampsia bloodwork" should be done
AED monitoring	AED clearance falls and levels rise post partum	AED tapering should be initiated, and women should be aware of symptoms of AED toxicity
Infant safety advice (for all women bar those with eclampsia)	Infant injury may occur in association with a maternal seizure, although the absolute risk is low [2]	Common seizure triggers should be avoided Bathing should be done by sponge bath or in the presence of another adult Feeding and changing of the infant should also be done on the floor Carrying the child should be minimized by stocking supplies on each floor of the house A stroller with a "dead's man" arm can also be used indoors for transportation of the infant Access to stairs and the outdoors should be secured to prevent wandering of walking siblings
Lactation	There is some passage of AED into breast milk (as there is for almost all medications)	Women taking AEDs should be encouraged to breastfeed given the well-known benefits [2,4] When breastfeeding is stopped, the infant should be weaned slowly (over weeks) given the potential for withdrawal symptoms
Contraception	Many AED induce hepatic enzymes and warrant higher doses of estrogen in OCP	Both barrier methods and OCP are available and acceptable methods of contraception [4] Carbamazepine, phenytoin, phenobarbital, primidone, ethosuximide, topiramate and felbamate [2] mandate OCP with higher doses of estrogen Valproate and newer AED (including vigabatrin, gabapentin, lamotrigine and tiagabine) do not induce hepatic enzymes, and women using these medications can receive standard low-dose 35 μg ethinyl estradiol OCP [2] Breakthrough bleeding mandates an increase in ethinyl estradiol dosage (to 75–100μg) and temporary use of additional methods of birth control (e.g. condoms) [2] Medroxyprogesterone injections appear to be effective [2] but levonorgestrel implants are contraindicated due to an unacceptably elevated failure rate [2]
Subsequent pregnancy	Planning, as 50% of pregnancies are unplanned	For women with epilepsy, the experience in one pregnancy does not necessarily predict the experience in the next For women with eclampsia, the risk of recurrent pre-eclampsia is 10–50% Folic acid supplementation should be started preconception to decrease the risk of NTD. Although unproven, most authors recommend higher doses of folic acid (i.e. 4–5 mg/d), particularly for women taking valproic acid or carbamazepine who have a higher risk of NTD (i.e. 1–2% and approximately 1%, respectively) [3,4]

AED, antiepileptic drugs; BP, blood pressure; NTD, neural tube defects; OCP, oral contraceptive pills.

through a nasogastric tube [16]. Meperidine, used at some centers for analgesia in labor, lowers the seizure threshold through an active metabolite with a long half-life; morphine is therefore preferable for control of pain. Labor is associated with hyperventilation, pain, emotional stress, and sleep deprivation, all of which are known precipitants of seizures [2]; an early epidural may be very helpful.

Postnatal aftermath

Several issues require attention following delivery, to optimize management in the postpartum period, between pregnancies, and in future pregnancies (Table 45.3). Advice relates mainly to the women with seizures unrelated to eclampsia, all of whom need neurologic follow-up. The website epilepsynse.org.uk has excellent information for patients.

Conclusion

A new seizure in pregnancy has a broad differential diagnosis. Epilepsy and eclampsia are the most common causes, but it

may be difficult to differentiate between them. Because of the serious maternal and fetal complications associated with pre-eclampsia, eclampsia should always be considered until proven otherwise. $MgSO_4$ is the pharmacologic treatment of choice for eclampsia and delivery is the definitive treatment. Monitoring must be initiated for other end-organ complications of pre-eclampsia. For all but eclampsia, recurrence in the peripartum period must be actively avoided by continuing AED therapy (if prescribed) throughout labor and delivery, and avoiding sleep deprivation and pain. Women should be encouraged to breastfeed, and recommendations about infant safety should be provided.

References

1. Yerby MS. Pregnancy and epilepsy. Epilepsia 1991;32(suppl 6): S51–S59.
2. Delgado-Escueta AV, Janz D. Consensus guidelines: preconception counseling, management, and care of the pregnant woman with epilepsy. Neurology 1992;42(4 suppl 5):149–60.
3. Pschirrer ER. Seizure disorders in pregnancy. Obstet Gynecol Clin North Am 2004;31(2):373–84, vii.

4. Williams J, Myson V, Steward S, Jones G, Wilson JF, Kerr MP, *et al*. Self-discontinuation of antiepileptic medication in pregnancy: detection by hair analysis. Epilepsia 2002;43(8):824–31.

5. Britton JW. Antiepileptic drug withdrawal: literature review. Mayo Clin Proc 2002;77(12):1378–88.

6. Quality Standards Subcommittee of the American Academy of Neurology. Practice parameter: management issues for women with epilepsy (summary statement). Report of the Quality Standards Subcommittee of the American Academy of Neurology. Neurology 1998;51(4):944–8.

7. Fairgrieve SD, Jackson M, Jonas P, Walshaw D, White K, Montgomery TL, *et al*. Population based, prospective study of the care of women with epilepsy in pregnancy. BMJ 2000; 321(7262):674–5.

8. Douglas KA, Redman CW. Eclampsia in the United Kingdom. BMJ 1994;309(6966):1395–400.

9. Tomson T, Lindbom U, Ekqvist B, Sundqvist A. Epilepsy and pregnancy: a prospective study of seizure control in relation to free and total plasma concentrations of carbamazepine and phenytoin. Epilepsia 1994;35(1):122–30.

10. Pennell PB. EURAP outcomes for seizure control during pregnancy: useful and encouraging data. Epilepsy Curr 2006;6(6):186–8.

11. Bone RC. Treating convulsive status epilepticus. Nursing 1994;24(10):32F, 32H.

12. Willmore LJ. Epilepsy emergencies: the first seizure and status epilepticus. Neurology 1998;51(5 suppl 4):S34-S38.

13. Blume WT. Diagnosis and management of epilepsy. CMAJ 2003; 168(4):441–8.

14. Moore-Sledge CM. Evaluation and management of first seizures in adults. Am Fam Physician 1997;56(4):1113–20.

15. Dahmus MA, Barton JR, Sibai BM. Cerebral imaging in eclampsia: magnetic resonance imaging versus computed tomography. Am J Obstet Gynecol 1992;167(4 Pt 1):935–41.

16. Crawford P, Appleton R, Betts T, Duncan J, Guthrie E, Morrow J. Best practice guidelines for the management of women with epilepsy. The Women with Epilepsy Guidelines Development Group. Seizure 1999;8(4):201–17.

17. Van Donselaar CA, Geerts AT, Schimsheimer RJ. Idiopathic first seizure in adult life: who should be treated? BMJ 1991; 302(6777):620–3.

18. Paul RH, Koh KS, Bernstein SG. Changes in fetal heart rate-uterine contraction patterns associated with eclampsia. Am J Obstet Gynecol 1978;130(2):165–9.

19. Teramo K, Hiilesmaa V, Bardy A, Saarikoski S. Fetal heart rate during a maternal grand mal epileptic seizure. J Perinat Med 1979;7(1):3–6.

20. Collaborative Eclampsia Trial Investigators. Which anticonvulsant for women with eclampsia? Evidence from the Collaborative Eclampsia Trial. Lancet 1995;345(8963):1455–63.

21. Duley L, Henderson-Smart D. Magnesium sulphate versus phenytoin for eclampsia. Cochrane Database of Systematic Reviews, 2003;4:CD000128.

22. Duley L, Henderson-Smart D. Magnesium sulphate versus diazepam for eclampsia. Cochrane Database of Systematic Reviews, 2003;4:CD000127.

23. Magee LA, Miremadi S, Li J, Cheng C, Ensom MH, Carleton B, *et al*. Therapy with both magnesium sulfate and nifedipine does not increase the risk of serious magnesium-related maternal side effects in women with preeclampsia. Am J Obstet Gynecol 2005;193(1):153–63.

24. Rey E, Treluyer JM, Pons G. Pharmacokinetic optimization of benzodiazepine therapy for acute seizures. Focus on delivery routes. Clin Pharmacokinet 1999;36(6):409–24.

25. Adab N. Therapeutic monitoring of antiepileptic drugs during pregnancy and in the postpartum period: is it useful? CNS Drugs 2006;20(10):791–800.

26. Nulman I, Laslo D, Koren G. Treatment of epilepsy in pregnancy. Drugs 1999;57(4):535–44.

27. Patsalos PN, Froscher W, Pisani F, van Rijn CM. The importance of drug interactions in epilepsy therapy. Epilepsia 2002;43(4):365–85.

28. Kaaja E, Kaaja R, Matila R, Hiilesmaa V. Enzyme-inducing antiepileptic drugs in pregnancy and the risk of bleeding in the neonate. Neurology 2002;58(4):549–53.

Further reading

www.aan.com

Collaborative Eclampsia Trial Investigators. Which anticonvulsant for women with eclampsia? Evidence from the Collaborative Eclampsia Trial. Lancet 1995;345(8963):1455–63.

Douglas KA, Redman CW. Eclampsia in the United Kingdom. BMJ 1994;309(6966):1395–400.

Pennell PB. EURAP outcomes for seizure control during pregnancy: useful and encouraging data. Epilepsy Curr 2006;6(6):186–8.

Zupanc ML. Antiepileptic drugs and hormonal contraceptives in adolescent women with epilepsy. Neurology 2006;66(6 suppl 3):S37–S45.

Approach to prosthetic heart valves in pregnancy

Wee Shian Chan[1], Mark C. Walker[2] and Marc A. Rodger[2,3]

[1]Department of Medicine, University of Toronto, Sunnybrooke and Women's Health Sciences Center, Toronto, Canada

[2]Ottawa Health Research Institute and Department of Obstetrics and Gynecology, University of Ottawa, Ontario, Canada

[3]Division of Hematology, The Ottawa Hospital, University of Ottawa, Ottawa, Ontario, Canada

Introduction

Prosthetic heart valves have been used since the 1950s for the replacement of both congenital and acquired valvular heart disease; more than 60,000 valve replacement procedures are performed in the United States annually [1]. There are two primary types of prosthetic valves: mechanical heart valves (MHV) and bioprosthetic heart valves (BPV). The former is primarily composed of metal or carbon alloys, the latter is derived from bovine or porcine tissue mounted on a metal support or preserved human valves [1].

The major differences between MHV and BPV are durability and thrombogenicity. Mechanical heart valves are highly durable, lasting 20–30 years whereas up to 30% of BPV will fail in 10–15 years [1]. MHV are more thrombogenic and require ongoing anticoagulation throughout the lifespan of the valve; with adequate anticoagulation, the risk of valve thrombosis with MHV is decreased from 12–22% per patient-year to 0.1–5.7% per patient-year [1,2]. The thrombogenicity of MHV is dependent on valve type: the newer generation bileaflet-tilting disks are less thrombogenic than the older generation single-tilting or caged-ball types [1]. Thrombogenicity is also influenced by valve position (mitral greater than aortic), adequacy of anticoagulation therapy and number of prosthetic heart valves [2].

In comparison to MHV, the risk of valve thrombosis is low with BPV and anticoagulation is not usually required after the initial 3 months following valve replacement, at which point aspirin is recommended [1,2].

Regardless of valve type, patients with prosthetic heart valves (MHV or BPV) may have an increased risk of thromboembolic complications (TEC). If atrial fibrillation, left ventricular

dysfunction and previous history of TEC are present in these patients, ongoing antithrombotic agents should independently be considered [2].

Based on the durability of MHV and the fact that anticoagulation therapy may be less well tolerated in the older patients, younger patients (<40 years), such as women of childbearing age, tend to be implanted with MHV, while BPV are used in older individuals [1].

Anticoagulation therapy for patients with MHV in the nonpregnant population

Vitamin K antagonists (VKA), like warfarin, are the mainstay anticoagulant for thromboprophylaxis in patients with MHV [1,2]. For most newer generation MHV (i.e. excluding the caged-ball valves) in the aortic position, a target international normalized ratio (INR) of 2.0–3.0 is recommended while for valves in the mitral position, an INR of 2.5–3.5 is recommended [2]. In patients with concurrent risk factors (such as atrial fibrillation, low ejection fraction, previous TEC, myocardial infarction, left atrial enlargement or endocardial damage), an INR target of 2.5–3.5 and addition of low-dose aspirin (75–100 mg/day) should be considered [2].

For bridging anticoagulation, i.e. in situations where therapeutic anticoagulation with VKA has not yet been achieved or during short periods in which interruption of VKA therapy is required (such as invasive procedures), both intravenous unfractionated heparin (UFH) or full-dose low molecular weight heparin (LMWH) have been used successfully, with minimal risks of TEC during the period of VKA interruption [3,4]. However, the risk of major bleeding in the postprocedure phase is significant with full-dose LMWH or IV heparin and major bleeding can result in interruption of anticoagulation with subsequent TEC. In a multicenter cohort study of 224 patients treated with full-dose LMWH, the postoperative

de Swiet's Medical Disorders in Obstetric Practice, 5th edition.
Edited by R. O. Powrie, M. F. Greene, W. Camann. © 2010 Blackwell Publishing.

TEC rate was 3.1% and 75% of these occurred in patients who had anticoagulation held due to bleeding [4].

Bacterial endocarditis prophylaxis

Patients with prosthetic heart valves have an increased lifetime risk of developing infective endocarditis (IE) (400 per 100,000 patient-years); antibiotic prophylaxis is recommended for MHV patients who undergo:
• dental procedures involving the manipulation of gingival tissue, periapical region of teeth or perforation of the oral mucosa
• procedures on the respiratory tract
• procedures on infected skin, skin structures or musculoskeletal tissue [5].
Antibiotic prophylaxis is no longer recommended in BPV patients undergoing these procedures unless they have had previous IE, congenital heart disease or cardiac transplant [5].

In previous guidelines, antibiotic prophylaxis could be considered in patients with BPV or MHV undergoing vaginal delivery or cesarean section; however, more recent guidelines do not advocate the use of antibiotic prophylaxis solely for the purpose of preventing bacterial endocarditis for these procedures [5,6] (see also Chapter 5).

Management of valve thrombosis

Valve thrombosis is an infrequent but potentially life-threatening complication in patients with MHV. The presentation of valve thrombosis may be sudden death, acute pulmonary edema, embolic accidents, onset of shortness of breath or heart failure. Currently the best diagnostic studies for the detection of MHV thrombosis are transesophageal echocardiogram or fluoroscopy [6,7]. If valve thrombosis is suspected, a consultation with a cardiologist and/or cardiovascular thoracic surgeon is recommended. Depending on the degree of valve thrombosis, right- or left-sided valve thrombosis and patient factors (e.g. NYHA class symptoms, reviewed in Chapter 5), valve thrombus could be managed medically with intravenous heparin therapy (small clot burden and minimal symptoms) or thrombolysis (right-sided lesions with NYHA class III or IV symptoms or large clot burden), or surgically with valve replacement (left-sided lesions with NYHA class III or IV symptoms or large clot burden) [6].

There is little in the literature to guide the management of valve thrombosis during pregnancy. Case studies of the use of both thrombolytic therapy and surgery in pregnant women with MHV thrombosis have been reported [8,9] but with some complications [10]. In these latter situations, the risks and benefits of these procedures must be weighed carefully against the risk of maternal morbidity and mortality associated with valve thrombosis.

Pregnant women with prosthetic heart valves

Bioprosthetic heart valves

Young patients (16–40 years) implanted with BPV undergo structural valve deterioration in 50% at 10 years, and 90% at 15 years [6,11].

Pregnant women with BPV avoid the need for anticoagulation and the problems associated with the need for VKA therapy (see below), so the pregnancy outcomes, from the fetal point of view, in these patients are mostly favorable [5]. However, in these patients, the risk of structural valve deterioration during pregnancy and shortly after (within 1 year) is high, at about 28% [5]. This rate of valve deterioration is, however, similar to other age-matched patients who do not undertake pregnancy [12–14]. For patients with BPV who require valve reoperation, the mortality rate, although decreasing over the past 20 years, is still significant at 3.5–11.1% [15].

The presentation of valve deterioration in patients with BPV is often the gradual onset of dyspnea and symptoms of heart failure. These symptoms often mimic the normal symptoms associated with physiologic changes with pregnancy [1] so careful auscultation and regular functional assessment with echocardiography may be required.

Mechanical heart valves

Anticoagulation therapy

The major challenge with managing women with MHV during pregnancy is that VKA, which are highly effective in preventing valve thrombosis and TEC in the nonpregnant MHV population [6], are associated with adverse effects on the pregnancy and developing fetus [16]. The use of either UFH or LMWH, which are both "safe" for the developing fetus, is associated with an apparent higher risk of valve thrombosis than VKA and even maternal death [16]. In addition, there are no large clinical trials comparing anticoagulation therapies in pregnant women with MHV to dictate appropriate choice; recommendations are largely based on cohort studies, case series and expert opinion. In this section, an overview of the reported pregnancy experiences in women with MHV with the respective anticoagulant therapy will be presented, as well as the fetal and maternal risks associated with each regimen.

Vitamin K antagonists

Coumarin derivatives (or VKA such as warfarin) depresses synthesis of vitamin K-dependent clotting factors (factors II, VII, IX, and X) by blocking reduction of the epoxide form of vitamin K. Because of their low molecular weight, coumarins cross the placenta, achieving clinically significant levels in the fetus [17]. Fetal exposure to coumarin derivatives leads to congenital anomalies, presumably through inhibition of vitamin K-dependent proteins in bone and brain. A specific pattern of congenital anomalies known as coumarin embryopathy is recognized in children exposed *in utero* to coumarin derivatives between 6 and 12 weeks of pregnancy [18]. These anomalies consist of nasal hypoplasia (depressed nasal bridge and underdeveloped or absent nasal septum) and chondrodysplasia punctata (radiographic epiphyseal and vertebral stippling). This stippling resolves after the growth plates calcify but it may lead to limb and digit hypoplasia [18]. Beyond the first trimester of pregnancy, coumarin exposure, likely through fetal anticoagulation, has also been associated with central nervous system abnormalities such as intraventricular hemorrhages, microcephaly, hydrocephalus, cerebellar and cerebral atrophy, eye and vision abnormalities (optic atrophy, cataracts, blindness, microphthalmia) seizures, and growth and mental retardation [17,18].

Beyond these CNS side effects diagnosed at birth, recent prospective studies evaluating neurodevelopmental outcomes in children exposed to coumarin *in utero* have revealed the presence of neurodevelopmental abnormalities [19]. In a pooled analysis of studies [16], the risk of congenital fetal abnormalities associated with the use of coumarin throughout pregnancy was 6.4%, the risk of spontaneous losses was 24.8%, and the overall fetal wastage associated with coumarin use throughout pregnancy was significant at 33.6%. In a multicenter prospective cohort study based in European teratology information services, 666 VKA-exposed pregnancies were compared to a nonexposed group (n = 1094), Schaefer demonstrated that with first-trimester coumarin exposure, the absolute risk of major birth defects (defined as serious medical, surgical or cosmetic consequences) was 4.8% compared to 1.4% in controls (relative risk (RR) 3.9, 95% confidence interval (CI) 1.9–8.0); the risk of coumarin embryopathy was low (0.6%) (with no cases with exposure <8 weeks after LMP). However, the rate of miscarriage was higher in the exposed (42%) compared to the nonexposed group (14%) [20].

Despite its adverse effects on the fetus and pregnancy, coumarin derivatives are unquestionably an effective thromboprophylaxis agent in pregnant women with MHV. Pregnant women who are given coumarin derivatives throughout pregnancy have a 3.9% risk of TEC; this risk is doubled even if coumarin derivatives are replaced only for a few weeks, in the first trimester, with adjusted-dose UFH [16].

Unfractionated heparin and low molecular weight heparin

Low molecular weight heparin, like UFH, does not cross the placenta and is safe for use during pregnancy [21,22]. For many reasons, LMWH has supplanted UFH as the anticoagulant of choice during pregnancy, particularly for the treatment of venous thromboembolic disease [23].

Several large reviews of LMWH use in pregnant women have been published confirming the safety of LMWH exposure to the developing fetus [24,25]. The advantage of LMWH over UFH is clear: LMWH are associated with a low risk of heparin-induced thrombocytopenia (<1 in a 1000) [24,26,27], low risk of osteoporosis at 0.04% (95% CI 0–0.2%) and low risk of bleeding at 1.98% (95% CI 1.5–2.5%) [24]. However, like UFH, LMWH use can result in erythematous cutaneous plaques at injection sites (1.8%, 95% CI 1.3–2.4%) [24].

Although safe and effective for the management of venous thromboembolic disease in pregnancy, UFH use, even in adjusted doses, in pregnant women with MHV has been associated with high rates of valve thrombosis (25%) [16]. LMWH, with its better bio-availablility and ease of dosing, appeared to offer clinicians an alternative therapy to UFH. Unfortunately, in the last decade, multiple case reports and case series have reported on the failure of LMWH therapy [28]. In a review, the use of LMWH in pregnant women with MHV was associated with a rate of valve thrombosis of 8.8% (95% CI 2.5–14.8), while the frequency of overall thromboembolic complications was 12.4% (95% CI 5.2–19.5%) [28]. The concern with LMWH use was heightened further after a small clinical trial was discontinued prematurely, because two of the seven women treated with LMWH (versus warfarin) developed valve thrombosis resulting in maternal deaths [23]. However, in both patients, subtherapeutic antifactor Xa levels were recorded in the weeks prior to these events [3]. This study also resulted in manufacturers' labeling changes and warnings against the use of LMWH for this specific cohort of patients.

The failure of LMWH in preventing valve thrombosis in pregnant women as compared to its success as bridging anticoagulant therapy in nonpregnant patients [2,3] may relate in part to the unforgiving nature of the medication's short half-life that makes single missed doses far more dangerous than missed doses of warfarin. It may also relate to the altered pharmacokinetics of LMWH in pregnancy and/or the hypercoagulable state of pregnancy. When LMWH is used for the treatment of venous thromboembolism (VTE) in pregnant patients, it is usually administered based on the patient's weight. However, as the pregnancy progresses, it remains unclear if dose adjustment is needed based on changes in the patient's weight, volume of distribution or renal excretion rate [29]. Several prospective cohort studies which followed antifactor Xa levels 3–4 hours post injection (therapeutic LMWH for acute VTE) have yielded conflicting results (target peak 0.5–1.0 IU/mL) but most suggest that dose increases are necessary as pregnancy progresses [23]. It is also unknown if anti-Xa levels correlate with efficacy of treatment in any setting. However, pharmacokinetic studies conducted in women on low doses of LMWH suggest that twice-daily dosing may be superior to once-daily dosing in pregnancy [30].

Extrapolating the results of these small pharmacokinetic studies in pregnant women with VTE and studies from nonpregnant patients, experts have recommended that for pregnant women with MHV, LMWH should be administered as a twice-daily dose to keep a 4-hour postinjection antifactor Xa level of at least 1.0–1.2 U/mL [23] and some have even advocated higher targets of up to 1.5 U/mL [3].

Antiplatelet agents

Low-dose aspirin (<100 mg/day) is safe for use in pregnancy [31]. The indications for adding aspirin to pregnant women with MHV would be similar to those for nonpregnant patients (i.e. concurrent risk factors such as atrial fibrillation, low ejection fraction, previous TEC, etc.) [2,5]. Some centers advocate the addition of aspirin in all pregnant women with MHV when they are treated with LMWH. The increased risk of hemorrhage, conferred by the addition of aspirin, in pregnant women has, however, not been evaluated but would no doubt be higher.

Approach to pregnant women with mechanical heart valves (Table 46.1) [32]

Shared decision making is crucial with the very important question of anticoagulant choice in pregnant women with MHV. These women need to be carefully and thoughtfully informed about the potential risks of fetal events and maternal complications with the available options (as detailed above). That is, mothers should make informed decisions and be well aware of the trade-off between maternal and fetal safety with approaches maximizing VKA use (increased maternal safety but increased fetal risk) and with approaches maximizing heparin/LMWH use (decreased maternal safety and decreased (if any) fetal risk). In patients at high risk (and some would argue in all patients), the addition of aspirin should be considered whenever LMWH is used.

Pre-pregnancy counseling

Women with MHV should initially undergo a careful structural and functional evaluation of the heart by a cardiologist, in addition to an evaluation of the choice of anticoagulant regimen prior to pregnancy. Assessment of the underlying cardiac function and underlying reason for valve replacement would ensure that high-risk cardiac lesions (e.g. poor functional class or cyanosis, left heart obstruction) can be identified and the patient counseled appropriately regarding the risks of pregnancy [33].

With respect to the management of anticoagulation prior to conception, one of two approaches could be considered:
• a switch from VKA to twice-daily full therapeutic LMWH can be made, with close monitoring of anti-Xa levels (peak levels, drawn 3–4 hours after injection of 1.0–1.5 IU/mL and trough levels maintained above 0.5)
• continue on VKA until pregnancy is confirmed (at its soonest) with a serum blood test, and then a switch to LMWH can be made.

Our preference is the latter given the apparent higher risk of valve thrombosis with LMWH than VKA and the lack

Table 46.1 Management of anticoagulation in women with mechanical heart valves during pregnancy

Period	Pre-pregnancy	Pregnancy				Peripartum	Postpartum
		0–6 weeks	6–12 weeks	12–32/34 weeks	34 weeks–term (planned induction)		
Anticoagulation	a) **VKA** b) LMWH c) UFH	a) **VKA** b) LMWH c) UFH	a) **VKA** b) **LMWH** c) UFH	a) **VKA** b) LMWH c) UFH	a) LMWH b) UFH	Discontinue LMWH or UFH 24 hours prior to induction. Consider IV UFH (especially in high-risk women) until active labor	Resume VKA with bridging LMWH or UFH therapy
Antiplatelet (ASA <100 mg daily)	ASA	ASA	**ASA**	ASA	ASA. Consider discontinuing 1 week prior to planned induction*		ASA

LMWH: twice-daily full therapeutic low molecular weight heparin with close monitoring of anti-Xa levels (peak levels, drawn 3–4 hours after injection of 1.0–1.5 IU/mL and trough levels maintained above 0.5); UFH: subcutaneous unfractionated heparin twice a day (mid-interval activated partial thromboplastin time at least twice control or preferably attain an anti-Xa heparin level 0.35–0.70 IU/mL) [3,23].
VKA, vitamin K antagonists.
Bold – option preferred by authors.
*While there is no evidence of an increased risk of peripartum bleeding or complications of regional anesthesia in patients on <100 mg of ASA at the time of delivery, some experts (including the authors but not the editors) hold ASA for 1 week prior to planned delivery.

of evidence for adverse embryonic events with VKA if they are discontinued prior to 6 weeks gestation. Furthermore, it may take some couples over a year to conceive, exposing these women to an extended period at higher risk of valve thrombosis with LMWH than with VKA. We advise on the liberal use of pregnancy tests while these women are trying to conceive to ensure that VKA are discontinued as early as possible in pregnancy.

Occasionally LMWH is not available and it is necessary to use UFH. In this case, UFH should be administered subcutaneously two or three times a day with monitoring by mid-interval activated partial thromboplastin time at least twice control or preferably with anti-Xa assays to attain an anti-Xa heparin level 0.35–0.70 IU/mL [3,6,23].

Antepartum

Once pregnancy is confirmed, exposure to coumarins should be avoided from 6 to 12 gestational weeks. During this period, a switch to twice-daily full therapeutic LMWH should be considered with close monitoring (at least weekly) of anti-Xa levels (peak levels, drawn 3–4 hours after injection of 1.0–1.5 IU/mL and trough levels maintained above 0.5) [3,6,23].

Beyond 12 weeks, the choice of anticoagulation therapy could be one of two regimens: continue therapeutic twice-daily LMWH with anti-Xa monitoring as above, or switch to VKA (INR 2.0–3.5, dependent on valve type) [3,6,23]. If LMWH is not available then UFH can be substituted as discussed above.

If coumarins are to be used after 12 weeks, a switch to heparin or LMWH (dosing and monitoring as above) should then be made at 34–36 weeks, when delivery is imminent, to avoid fetal anticoagulation at the time of delivery.

Peripartum

For patients receiving therapeutic LMWH or UFH to prevent TEC of MHV, induction of labor at term would be ideal to maximize access to neuraxial anagelsia and minimize bleeding complications. Both subcutaneous LMWH and UFH should be discontinued 24 hours prior to planned induction (i.e. last dose administered 24 hours earlier) [3,6,23].

In patients at high risk of thrombosis, defined as those with MHV and any risk factors (atrial fibrillation, previous thromboembolism, LV dysfunction, hypercoagulable conditions, older-generation thrombogenic valves), intravenous UFH could be used throughout the period of labor induction and discontinued at the first sign of active labor. Intravenous UFH has a half-life of 1.5 hours and its effects should resolve by 4 hours after cessation of the drip. In some centers this is the preferred approach in all patients.

Patients who present unexpectedly in labor or requiring urgent delivery while on therapeutic LMWH, UFH or

warfarin may need a reversal of these agents to proceed with delivery, especially if a cesaren delivery is planned. Vitamin K with or without fresh-frozen plasma may be used to reverse warfarin therapy (see Chapter 3 for details of administration and dosing). Protamine will fully reverse UFH and partially reverse LMWH and is an option for these patients (see Chapters 3 and 4 for details of administration and dosing). Both strategies are best approached in consultation with cardiology and hematology.

Postpartum

In the postpartum period, VKA can be started the same day as delivery, given that it usually takes 2–5 days of treatment before a therapeutic INR level is achieved. Administration of bridging LMWH or UFH anticoagulation should only be started once it is considered safe from the neuraxial procedure point of view (typically not until 2 hours after the epidural or spinal catheter has been removed; see Chapter 4, section on obstetric anesthesia and anticoagulation) and when postpartum hemorrhage is not a concern (i.e. usually 12–24 hours postpartum). Although LMWH is not completely reversible with protomaine, it is less likely to cause bleeding than IV UFH (and the associated necessary UFH boluses) and therefore LMWH would be our preferred agent in this setting. Clinicians should be reassured that the daily risk of major hemorrhage with full therapeutic heparin/LMWH (>1%) clearly exceeds the risk of valve thrombosis (<0.1%) in the first 24 hours postpartum with comparable case fatality rates. Furthermore, as discussed above, major bleeding also frequently leads to withholding anticoagulants for days and exposure to heightened risk of thrombosis [4].

Some centers, concerned about the possibility of bleeding, delay the introduction of warfarin and use LMWH exclusively for 2–14 days in postpartum patients. There is no supporting evidence to demonstrate improved outcomes for such an approach. This approach may be a reasonable one as long as LMWH compliance and careful antifactor Xa monitoring are achieved throughout this period.

Unfractionated heparin, LMHW and VKA are all compatible with breastfeeding.

References

1. Vongpatanasin W, Hillis LD, Lange RA. Prosthetic heart valves. N Engl J Med 1996;335(6):407–16.
2. Salem DN, Stein PD, Al Ahmad A, Bussey HI, Horstkotte D, Miller N, et al. Antithrombotic therapy in valvular heart disease – native and prosthetic: the Seventh ACCP Conference on Antithrombotic and Thrombolytic Therapy. Chest 2004;126 (3 suppl):457S–482S.
3. Seshadri N, Goldhaber SZ, Elkayam U, Grimm RA, Groce JB, III, Heit JA, et al. The clinical challenge of bridging anticoagulation with low-molecular-weight heparin in patients with mechanical prosthetic heart valves: an evidence-based comparative review

focusing on anticoagulation options in pregnant and nonpregnant patients. Am Heart J 2005;150:27–34.

4. Kovacs MJ, Kearon C, Rodger MA, Anderson DR, Turpie AGG, Bates SM, et al. Single-arm study of bridging therapy with low-molecular-weight heparin for patients at risk of arterial embolism who require temporary interruption of warfarin. Circulation 2004;110:1658–63.

5. Wilson W, Taubert KA, Gewitz M, Lockhart PB, Baddour LM, Levison M, et al. Prevention of infective endocarditis. Guidelines From the American Heart Association. A Guideline From the American Heart Association Rheumatic Fever, Endocarditis, and Kawasaki Disease Committee, Council on Cardiovascular Disease in the Young, and the Council on Clinical Cardiology, Council on Cardiovascular Surgery and Anesthesia, and the Quality of Care and Outcomes Research Interdisciplinary Working Group. Circulation 2007;116(15):1736–54.

6. Bonow RO, Carabello BA, Kanu C, de Leon AC Jr, Faxon DP, Freed MD, et al. ACC/AHA 2006 guidelines for the management of patients with valvular heart disease: a report of the American College of Cardiology/American Heart Association Task Force on Practice Guidelines (Writing Committee to Revise the 1998 Guidelines for the Management of Patients With Valvular Heart Disease): developed in collaboration with the Society of Cardiovascular Anesthesiologists: endorsed by the Society for Cardiovascular Angiography and Interventions and the Society of Thoracic Surgeons. Circulation 2006;114(5):e84–231.

7. Gueret P, Vignon P, Fournier P, Chabernaud JM, Gomez M, LaCroix P, et al. Transesophageal echocardiography for the diagnosis and management of nonobstructive thrombosis of mechanical mitral valve prosthesis. Circulation 1995;91(1):103–10.

8. Nassar AH, Abdallah ME, Moukarbel GV, Usta IM, Gharzuddine WS. Sequential use of thrombolytic agents for thrombosed mitral valve prosthesis during pregnancy. J Perinat Med 2003 31(3):257–60.

9. Alessandrini F, Lapenna E, Nasso G, de Bonis M, Possati GF. Successful thrombectomy for thrombosis of aortic composite valve graft in pregnancy. Ann Thorac Surg 2003;75(4):1317–18.

10. Usta IM, Abdallah M, El Hajj M, Nassar AH. Massive subchorionic hematomas following thrombolytic therapy in pregnancy. Obstet Gynecol 2004;103(5 Pt 2):1079–82.

11. Hung L, Rahimtoola SH. Prosthetic heart valves and pregnancy. Circulation 2003;107(9):1240–6.

12. Avila WS, Rossi EG, Grinberg M, Ramires JA. Influence of pregnancy after bioprosthetic valve replacement in young women: a prospective five-year study. J Heart Valve Dis 2002;11(6):864–9.

13. El SF, Hassan W, Latroche B, Helaly S, Hegazy H, Shahid M, et al. Pregnancy has no effect on the rate of structural deterioration of bioprosthetic valves: long-term 18-year follow up results. J Heart Valve Dis 2005;14(4):481–5.

14. North RA, Sadler L, Stewart AW, McCowan LM, Kerr AR, White HD. Long-term survival and valve-related complications in young women with cardiac valve replacements. Circulation 1999;99(20):2669–76.

15. Jamieson WR, Burr LH, Miyagishima RT, Janusz MT, Fradet GJ, Lichtenstein SV, et al. Reoperation for bioprosthetic mitral structural failure: risk assessment. Circulation 2003;108 (suppl 1):II98–102.

16. Chan WS, Anand SS, Ginsberg JS. Anticoagulation of pregnant women with mechanical heart valves. Arch Intern Med 2000;160:191–6.

17. Hall JG, Pauli RM, Wilson KM. Maternal and fetal sequelae of anticoagulation during pregnancy. Am J Med 1980;68(1):122–40.

18. van Driel D, Wesseling J, Sauer PJ, Touwen BC, van der Veer E, Heymans HS. Teratogen update: fetal effects after in utero exposure to coumarins overview of cases, follow-up findings, and pathogenesis. Teratology 2002;66(3):127–40.

19. Ansell JE, Hirsh J, Poller L, Bussey H, Jacobson A, Hylek E. The pharmacology and management of the vitamin K antagonists: the Seventh ACCP Conference on Antithrombotic and Thrombolytic Therapy. Chest 2004;126(3 suppl):204S–233S.

20. Schaefer C, Hannemann D, Meister R, Elefant E, Paulus W, Vial T, et al. Vitamin K antagonists and pregnancy outcome. A multi-centre prospective study. Thromb Haemost 2006;95(6):949–57.

21. Forestier F, Sole Y, Aiach M, Alhenc GM, Daffos F. Absence of transplacental passage of fragmin (Kabi) during the second and the third trimesters of pregnancy. Thromb Haemost 1992;67(1):180–1.

22. Forestier F, Daffos F, Rainaut M, Toulemonde F. Low molecular weight heparin (CY 216) does not cross the placenta during the third trimester of pregnancy. Thromb Haemost 1987;57(2):234.

23. Bates SM, Greer IA, Hirsh J, Ginsberg JS. Use of antithrombotic agents during pregnancy: the Seventh ACCP Conference on Antithrombotic and Thrombolytic Therapy. Chest 2004;126 (3 suppl):627S–644S.

24. Greer IA, Nelson-Piercy C. Low-molecular-weight heparins for thromboprophylaxis and treatment of venous thromboembolism in pregnancy: a systematic review of safety and efficacy. Blood 2005;106:401–7.

25. Sanson BJ, Lensing AW, Prins MH, Ginsberg JS, Barkagan ZS, Lavenne-Pardonge E, et al. Safety of low-molecular-weight heparin in pregnancy: a systematic review. Thromb Haemost 1999;81:668–72.

26. Huhle G, Geberth M, Hoffmann U, Heene DL, Harenberg J. Management of heparin-associated thrombocytopenia in pregnancy with subcutaneous r-hirudin. Gynecol Obstet Invest 2000;49(1):67–9.

27. Lepercq J, Conard J, Borel-Derlon A, Darmon JY, Boudignat O, Francoual C, et al. Venous thromboembolism during pregnancy: a retrospective study of enoxaparin safety in 624 pregnancies. Br J Obstet Gynaecol 2001;108:1134–40.

28. Oran B, Lee-Parritz A, Ansell J. Low molecular weight heparin for the prophylaxis of thromboembolism in women with prosthetic mechanical heart valves during pregnancy. Thromb Haemost 2004;92(4):747–51.

29. Crowther MA, Spitzer K, Julian J, Ginsberg JS, Johnston M, Crowther R, et al. Pharmacokinetic profile of a low-molecular weight heparin (Reviparin) in pregnant patients: a prospective cohort study. Thromb Res 2000;98:133–8.

30. Casele HL, Laifer SA, Woelkers DA, Venkataramanan R. Changes in the pharmacokinetics of the low-molecular-weight heparin enoxaparin sodium during pregnancy. Am J Obstet Gynecol 1999;181(5 Pt 1):1113–17.

31. Duley L, Henderson-Smart D, Knight M, King J. Antiplatelet drugs for prevention of pre-eclampsia and its consequences: systematic review. BMJ 2001;322:329–33.

32. Bates SM, Greer IA, Pabinger I, Sofaer S, Hirsh J, American College of Chest Physicians. Venous thromboembolism, thrombophilia, antithrombotic therapy, and pregnancy: American College of Chest Physicians evidence-based clinical practice guidelines (8th Edition). Chest 2008;133(6 suppl):844S–886S.

33. Siu SC, Sermer M, Colman JM, Alvarez AN, Mercier LA, Morton BC, et al. Prospective multicenter study of pregnancy outcomes in women with heart disease. Circulation 2001;104(5):515–21.

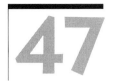

Approach to the use of glucocorticoids in pregnancy for nonobstetric indications

Kenneth K. Chen and Raymond O. Powrie

Department of Medicine, Warren Alpert Medical School of Brown University, Women & Infants' Hospital of Rhode Island, Providence, RI, USA

Introduction

Glucocorticoids are essential for life and have a wide spectrum of effects on many organ systems. Physiologically, endogenous glucocorticoid levels rise in response to a threat in homeostatic balance. In humans, the primary glucocorticoid is cortisol. The major role of the hypothalamic-pituitary-adrenal (HPA) axis is to control the synthesis and secretion of cortisol from the adrenal cortex. Glucocorticoids in turn regulate their own release through the action of a negative feedback system. The adrenal cortex secretes cortisol in a pulsatile fashion and exhibits a diurnal circadian rhythm, with cortisol levels peaking early in the morning and reaching a nadir at midnight.

Clinical administration of synthetic glucocorticoids has widespread application for a variety of medical conditions including autoimmune disease, allergic conditions, asthma, inflammatory bowel disease, and enhancement of fetal lung maturation, as in the case of threatened preterm delivery. In each case, the administration of glucocorticoids can result in both desirable (i.e. immune suppression) and undesirable effects (summarized in Table 47.1) and clinicians are well advised to always consider both the risks and benefits of their use and have a clear goal in mind when these agents are prescribed. The situation becomes even more complicated in pregnancy when clinicians must also consider all the potential risks and benefits to the embryo or fetus [1,2].

The most commonly used synthetic glucocorticoids are prednisone, methylprednisolone, triamcinolone, dexamethasone and betamethasone. Their relative potencies and degree of mineralocorticoid effect are listed in Table 47.2. Hydrocortisone is a natural metabolic intermediary of cortisol with predominantly glucocorticoid effects though it has some mineralocorticoid effects as well. Therefore, it is often used to treat patients with primary adrenal insufficiency as these patients require replacement with an agent with both effects. Prednisone, methylprednisolone, triamcinolone, dexamethasone and betamethasone were designed to have higher glucocorticoid potency, reduced mineralocorticoid effects and a longer duration of action. The latter two cross the placenta much more than prednisone and so they tend to be used in situations where it is necessary for the fetus to receive glucocorticoids (dexamethasone in reducing the incidence of female virilization in congenital adrenal hyperplasia and betamethasone in enhancing fetal lung maturation of preterm neonates). Prednisone tends to be the most common synthetic glucocorticoid used in pregnant women with chronic medical conditions as placental transfer is much less compared to the others.

Safety of glucocorticoids in pregnancy

Systemic

The concerns surrounding the use of glucocorticoids in pregnancy began more than 50 years ago following the publication of various studies which showed that large doses of glucocorticoids administered to pregnant rabbits, mice and rats during organogenesis lead to a higher incidence of cleft palate in the exposed offspring [3–6]. This was followed by the publication of two case reports of neonates with isolated cleft palate after pregnancy exposure to cortisone [7,8]. However, several subsequent case reports in which pregnant women were treated with prednisone throughout the first trimester [9–17] for various medical conditions (including renal transplantation, Hodgkin's disease, steroid-dependent asthma and systemic lupus erythematosus) did not reveal a consistent pattern of embryopathy. The increased incidence of low birthweight, miscarriages and stillbirths that is noted in some studies is difficult to discriminate from the effects of the underlying maternal conditions for which the glucocorticoids were being administered.

Two large prospective cohort studies published over the past decade have shown that there is, firstly, no risk of major

de Swiet's Medical Disorders in Obstetric Practice, 5th edition.
Edited by R. O. Powrie, M. F. Greene, W. Camann. © 2010 Blackwell Publishing.

congenital anomalies with first-trimester use of glucocorticoids and, secondly, either only a very small (odds ratio of 3.35; 95% confidence interval (CI) 1.97–5.69) [18] or no increased rate [19] of cleft lip or palate. Although the latter prospective study was only powered to detect a risk of 2.5-fold or greater, a pooling of the prospective data from these two studies describes a total of 499 pregnancies exposed to glucocorticoids with no cases of cleft lip or palate in any of

the exposed offspring. It seems safe to say that glucocorticoids at therapeutic doses do not represent a major teratogenic risk in humans. Given the serious nature of the conditions treated with glucocorticoids and the fact that fetal well-being is dependent on maternal well-being, it would be difficult to envisage a situation where it would be justifiable to cease or withhold these agents during pregnancy on the basis of concerns about their teratogenic risk. This concept has made it much easier for clinicians to consider using glucocorticoids to treat a wide range of conditions, including hyperemesis gravidarum or migraines, which may be refractory to conventional treatments in early pregnancy.

Whilst systemic glucocorticoids are not significant teratogens, long-term use of the equivalent of 30 mg of prednisone per day has been shown in several studies to increase the risk of premature preterm rupture of membranes and this is consistent with the authors' experience [20–22]. However, this again needs to be interpreted in the context of the very serious maternal and fetal implications of untreated inflammatory conditions such as asthma, systemic lupus erythematosus and inflammatory bowel disease.

Studies examining the effects of high-dose betamethasone given repeatedly to women with preterm labor do suggest an increased risk of intrauterine growth restriction [23–25] despite the marked advantage they confer to premature infants with respect to decreasing the risk of neonatal respiratory distress syndrome, intraventricular hemorrhage and necrotizing enterocolitis. Concern also exists about the long-term neurodevelopmental effects of high-dose steroids on premature infants [26,27] but it should be remembered that these concerns refer to supraphysiologic doses of glucocorticoids administered with the intention of getting most of the medication to the fetus and the applicability of these data to the use of prednisone in pregnancy is doubtful. Numerous other studies, in any case, have found that there are no significant differences

Table 47.1 Possible side effects of exogenous glucocorticoid use

Affected system	Possible side effect
Behavioral	Euphoria, psychosis, depression, akathisia, insomnia
Blood	Leukocytosis (typically increased mature neutrophils with a mild lymphopenia)
Bone	Osteoporosis, avascular necrosis
Cardiovascular	Hypertension, premature coronary artery disease, hyperlipidemia
Endocrine	Hyperglycemia, secondary adrenal insufficiency from suppression of the HPA axis
Eye	Glaucoma, cataracts
Gastrointestinal	Gastritis, peptic ulcer disease, steatohepatitis, pancreatitis
Gynecologic	Amenorrhea
Immunologic	Increased risk of both typical and opportunistic infections including reactivation of herpes zoster and tuberculosis
Muscle	Myopathy
Neurologic	Pseudotumor cerebri
Obstetric	Intrauterine growth restriction
Renal	Hypokalemia, fluid retention
Skin and soft tissue	Skin thinning, purpura, alopecia, hypertrichosis, hirsutism, striae, moon facies, centripetal obesity and buffalo hump

Table 47.2 Approximate equivalent doses of commonly used corticosteroids

Corticosteroid	Mineralocorticoid effect	Approximate equivalent dose with respect to glucocorticoid effect	Fetal exposure
Betamethasone	−	0.75	Crosses placenta readily so often used for fetal benefits
Dexamethasone	−	0.75	Crosses placenta readily (used in congenital adrenal hyperplasia)
Methylprednisolone	−	4	Form of prednisolone so fetal exposure similar to prednisolone
Triamcinolone	−	4	Topical glucocorticoid
Prednisolone	−	5	Metabolized by the placenta (11-beta-HSD1 enzyme) so minimal fetal exposure
Prednisone	−	5	Prodrug of prednisolone (converted in liver) so fetal exposure similar to prednisolone
Hydrocortisone	+	25	Natural metabolic intermediary of cortisol, crosses placenta to a limited degree

in neurocognitive development of infants who were exposed to antenatal high-dose glucocorticoid therapy [28–31].

Glucocorticoids can cause insulin resistance and may unmask some impaired glucose tolerance in women at risk. Consideration of early or additional screening for gestational diabetes may be warranted in women receiving glucocorticoids in pregnancy, particularly if they have additional risk factors for gestational diabetes mellitus. It should be noted that betamethasone administered up to 7 days prior to a glucose challenge test or a formal glucose tolerance test may cause a spurious elevation in the result [32].

Topical

Patients and clinicians have also expressed concerns about the effects of topical steroids used on the skin, nasopharynx, airways and rectal mucosa for conditions such as eczema, allergic rhinitis, asthma and ulcerative colitis. Systemic absorption of these agents does occur to some degree and varies with the medication, its formulation, the condition being treated, thickness of exposed skin (scalp and feet absorbing much less than the face or genitals) and whether an occlusive dressing is used. The large number of preparations available on the market also makes it difficult to develop meaningful pregnancy safety data for any one of them.

Among the topical steroids, the best studied is budesonide. A review published in 2005 showed that regular maternal exposure to oral inhaled budesonide for chronic asthma during pregnancy is not associated with an increased risk of congenital malformations (including cleft palate) or other adverse fetal outcomes [33–37]. However, there is also extensive clinical experience with the use of inhaled beclomethasone, triamcinolone, fluticasone and systemic hydrocortisone for the treatment of asthma in pregnant women. Given the favorable data about systemic steroids and the limited systemic absorption of the topical agents, use of the most commonly available topical steroids is likely justifiable in pregnancy but budesonide might be considered the preferred agent, with hydrocortisone, beclomethasone, triamcinolone and fluticasone all being reasonable alternatives.

Breastfeeding

More than 50% of all American women now breastfeed their infants upon discharge from hospital. Although there are limited studies describing the use of systemic steroids during lactation, the molecular weights of these are low enough that excretion in the breast milk should be expected. Prednisolone (and presumably the closely related agent methylprednisolone) and prednisone have all been shown to be detectable in breast milk [38] but the American Academy of Pediatrics considers them to be entirely compatible with breastfeeding [38–40].

Use of stress-dose glucocorticoids at time of labor and delivery

As outlined above, there are an increasing number of women who require daily or frequent usage of glucocorticoids during their pregnancy for treatment of their chronic medical ailments.

Historically, the concept of "stress-dose steroids" arose in the early 1950s following the case report of the death of a patient who developed perioperative secondary adrenal insufficiency as a consequence of preoperative withdrawal from glucocorticoid therapy [41]. It is well documented that long-term use of glucocorticoids for chronic autoimmune or inflammatory diseases suppresses the HPA axis. In normal patients, severe illness, trauma, stress and surgery are accompanied by activation of the HPA axis. Patients with HPA axis suppression from long-term glucocorticoid therapy may be unable to produce this physiologic response to stress.

The first set of recommendations regarding the appropriate dosage of "stress-dose steroids" came about as part of another case report of perioperative secondary adrenal insufficiency due to the cessation of glucocorticoids preoperatively [42]. Without any scientific basis, it was recommended that the dose of glucocorticoids be quadrupled routinely around the time of surgery. However, it was also recognized that supraphysiologic doses of glucocorticoids lead to adverse clinical consequences, such as reduced tissue repair rates, glucose tolerance, and increased susceptibility to infection [43].

Fortunately, knowledge of adrenal cortical responses to physical stressors has been much refined over the past 30 years and as a consequence, perioperative glucocorticoid management can now be prescribed in a much more rational fashion [43]. Axelrod's 1976 dictum [44] that "anyone who has received a glucocorticoid in doses equivalent to 20 mg of prednisone per day for more than a week should be suspected of having HPA suppression until proven otherwise" has stood the test of time. Kehlet did much work in the mid-1970s looking at the normal cortisol secretion rate in response to surgery and he concluded that adults secrete 75–150 mg per day in response to major surgery and 50 mg per day during minor procedures [45]. No one has been able to show that exceeding this amount of glucocorticoid administration in the peripartum or perioperative period is ever beneficial [43].

There has also been much progress in recent years in predicting which patients are most at risk for HPA axis suppression. It is generally held now that although Axelrod's dictum remains physiologically true, current recommendations recognize three groups of patients with respect to the need for stress-dose steroids that are reviewed below and summarized in Table 47.3.

The first group are patients for whom HPA suppression is very unlikely and therefore stress-dose steroids for these patients are inappropriate. These include patients who have received any dose of glucocorticoids for less than 3 weeks over the past year and patients on 5 mg or less of prednisone per day.

Table 47.3 Who warrants stress-dose steroids

HPA axis status	Characteristics of patients' steroid exposure	Recommendation
HPA axis suppression unlikely	Equivalent of <5 mg prednisone per day for any length of time Alternate-day steroids for any duration Any dose of steroids for <3 weeks	No need for stress-dose steroids
HPA axis suppression likely	Equivalent of 20 mg prednisone per day for more than 3 weeks in the past year Cushingoid appearance	Give stress-dose steroids appropriate for stress level (see Table 47.4)
HPA axis suppression unknown	Patient received 5–20 mg of prednisone for more than 3 weeks in the past year	Give stress-dose steroids appropriate for stress level (see Table 47.4) OR Perform ACTH stimulation test (see Box 47.1) and give stress-dose steroids only if patient fails to show an adequate response
Documented HPA axis suppression	Documented adrenal insufficiency or HPA axis suppression on formal testing (see Box 47.1)	Give stress-dose steroids appropriate for stress level (see Table 47.4)

Box 47.1 How to test the HPA axis by the Cosyntropin (tetracosactide) test

1. Draw baseline serum cortisol on patient.
2. Administer synthetic ACTH (Cosyntropin) 250 μg preferably IV (but IM acceptable).
3. Draw serum cortisol at 30 minutes and 60 minutes after dose of Cosyntropin-tetracosactide given.

Interpretation: a normal healthy response outside pregnancy is indicated by a basal cortisol level >250 nmol/L (9.0 μg/dL) and/or 30-minute peak cortisol level >600 nmol/L (21.6 μg/dL).

In pregnancy, cortisol levels are increased compared with the nonpregnant state due to increased corticosteroid-binding globulin (CBG) levels. Furthermore, cortisol levels increase gradually towards term. Therefore, cortisol values below the above ranges are definitely suggestive of adrenal insufficiency. However, these ranges are not validated in pregnancy and values above this range may therefore still represent HPA axis suppression. The lack of clarity over "normal values" in pregnancy for an ACTH stimulation test justifies the administration of stress-dose steroids empirically in the peripartum period and delaying the formal testing of the HPA axis until the postpartum period.

The exception to this rule would be if the patient is cushingoid in appearance even on this dosage of glucocorticoids and therefore has clinical evidence of adrenocorticol excess.

The second group are patients for whom HPA axis suppression is so likely that stress-dose steroids should always be given. This group includes any patient who has received more than 20 mg of prednisone (or equivalent) for more than 3 weeks in the past year or patients who are on glucocorticoids at any dose and who are cushingoid in appearance.

The third and definitely the most challenging group are those patients who fall in between the previous two groups. Patients who are on more than 5 mg and less than 20 mg per day of prednisone (or its equivalent) for more than 3 weeks in the past year fall into this gray zone. For these patients, two theoretical options exist. The first option is to test their HPA axis by administering a synthetic analog of adrenocorticotropin hormone (ACTH) and testing the adrenal response to this pituitary hormone. An overview to this test is reviewed in Box 47.1. The second option is to presume HPA axis suppression in these patients and administer stress-dose steroids. This is our routine clinical practice based on the following reasoning:
• a normal response to ACTH suggests but does not guarantee a fully functional HPA axis
• postpartum adrenal insufficiency may be hard to distinguish from some of the normal postpartum symptoms and (especially in the era of early postpartum discharges) may easily be missed

• we find the logistics of doing and interpreting an ACTH stimulation test during pregnancy challenging, given that this test is very uncommonly performed at obstetric centers and no validated pregnancy reference ranges are available (see Box 47.1).

If stress-dose steroids are not given to patients who may be at risk of HPA axis suppression, it is advisable to monitor the patient very closely for signs of adrenal insufficiency (anorexia, nausea, vomiting, weakness, hypotension, hyponatremia and/or hyperkalemia) in the postpartum period.

Once the decision is made to give stress-dose steroids, how much should be given? The current consensus is that the amount should be based on the magnitude of the stress and the known glucocorticoid production rate associated with it. Unfortunately, this area has not been studied very much since the mid-1990s and all the available data focus on the nonobstetric surgical patient [43,46,47] and our recommendations are based solely on extrapolation from these limited data and our own experience (Table 47.4).

For minor surgical stress (e.g. dilation & curettage and it is our opinion that a normal vaginal delivery fits into this category), the daily cortisol secretion rate and static plasma cortisol measurements [48,49] suggest that the glucocorticoid target is about 25 mg of hydrocortisone equivalent.

Table 47.4 What dose of stress-dose steroids to give

Physiologic stress level	Representative surgeries	Recommended glucocorticoid protocol
Minor surgical stress	Dilation and curettage Vaginal delivery	Hydrocortisone 25 mg IV prior to surgery and then resume previous dose
Moderate surgical stress	Cesarean delivery	Hydrocortisone 50–75 mg IV prior to delivery and then 25 mg every 8 hours for 1–2 days and then resume previous dose
Major surgical stress	Emergency cesarean hysterectomy	Hydrocortisone 100–150 mg IV intraoperatively and then 50 mg every 8 hours for 2–3 days and then resume previous dose

For moderate surgical stress (e.g. cesarean section), cortisol production rates suggest that the glucocorticoid target is about 50–75 mg per day of hydrocortisone equivalent for 1–2 days.

Finally, for major surgical stress (e.g. an emergency cesarean hysterectomy in the setting of major hemorrhage), the glucocorticoid target should be 100–150 mg of hydrocortisone equivalent per day for 2–3 days.

Lastly, it should be noted that a patient who is receiving a maintenance dose of glucocorticoid therapy that exceeds the estimated stress requirements will not need more glucocorticoid coverage during the stress period. After uncomplicated major surgery, plasma cortisol concentrations decrease rapidly. The circulating cortisol concentration is normal by 24–48 hours after surgical stress in most patients [50]. A postoperative increase in cortisol secretion is presumptive evidence for a continued or new stressor (e.g. fever, peritonitis, etc.). In the case of postoperative complications, the patient should continue to receive glucocorticoid administration consistent with the postoperative stress response.

References

1. Sloboda DM, Challis JRG, Moss TJM, Newnham JP. Synthetic glucocorticoids: antenatal administration and long-term implications. Curr Pharmaceuti Des 2005;11(11):1459–72.
2. Newnham JP, Moss TJM, Nitsos I, Sloboda DM. Antenatal corticosteroids: the good, the bad and the unknown. Curr Opin Obstet Gynaecol 2002;14:607–12.
3. Baxter H, Fraser FC. Production of congenital defects in offspring of female mice treated with cortisone. McGill Med J 1950;19:245–9.
4. Fainstat T. Cortisone induced congenital cleft palate in rabbits. Endocrinology 1954;55:502–8.
5. Pinsky L, DiGeorge AM. Cleft palate in the mouse: a teratogenic index of glucocorticoid potency. Science 1965;147:402–3.
6. Walker B. Induction of cleft palate in rats with anti-inflammatory drugs. Teratology 1971;4:39–42.
7. Harris JWS, Ross IP. Cortisone therapy in early pregnancy: relation to cleft palate. Lancet 1956;1:1045–17.
8. Doig RK, Coltman O. Cleft palate following cortisone therapy in early pregnancy. Lancet 1956;2:730.
9. Sinykin MB, Kaplan H. Leukaemia in pregnancy. Am J Obstet Gynecol 1962;83:220–34.
10. Morris WI. Pregnancy in rheumatoid arthritis and systemic lupus erythematosus. Aust NZ J Obstet Gynaecol 1969;9:136–44.
11. Nolan GH, Sweet RL, Laros RK, Roure CA. Renal cadaver transplantation followed by successful pregnancies. Obstet Gynecol 1974;43(5):732–9.
12. Cote CJ, Meuwissen HJ, Pickering R. Effects on the neonate of prednisone and azathioprine administered to the mother during pregnancy. J Pediatr 1974;85:324–8.
13. Schatz M, Patterson R, Zeitz S, Rourke J, Melam H. Corticosteroid therapy for the pregnant asthmatic patient. JAMA 1975;233:804–7.
14. Tozman ECS, Urowitz MB, Gladman DD. Systemic lupus erythematosus and pregnancy. J Rheumatol 1980;7:624–32.
15. Schilsky RL, Sherins RJ, Hubbard SM, Wesley MN, Young RC, DeVita VT. Long-term follow-up of ovarian function in women treated with MOPP chemotherapy for Hodgkin's disease. Am J Med 1981;71:552.
16. Mogadam M, Dobbins WO, Korelitz BI, Ahmed SW. Pregnancy in inflammatory bowel disease: effect of sulfasalazine and corticosteroids on foetal outcome. Gastroenterology 1981;80:72–6.
17. Coulam CB, Zincke H, Sterioff S. Pregnancy after renal transplantation: estrogen secretion. Transplantation 1982;33:556.
18. Park-Wyllie L, Mazzota P, Pastuszak A, et al. Birth defects after maternal exposure to corticosteroids: prospective cohort study and meta-analysis of epidemiological studies. Teratology 2000;62:385–92.
19. Gur C, Diav-Citrin O, Shechtman S, Arnon J, Ornoy A. Pregnancy outcome after first trimester exposure to corticosteroids: a prospective controlled study. Reprod Toxicol 2004;18:93–101.
20. Cowchock S. Prevention of fetal death in the antiphospholipid antibody syndrome. Lupus 1996;5(5):467–72.
21. Lockshin MD, Sammaritano LR. Corticosteroids during pregnancy. Scand J Rheumatol Scandinavian 1998;107:136–8.
22. Silver RM, Branch DW. Immunologic disorders. In: Creasy RK, Resnik R (eds) Maternal fetal medicine. WB Saunders, Philadelphia, 1999.
23. French NP, Hagan R, Evans S, et al. Repeated antenatal corticosteroids: size at birth and subsequent development. Am J Obstet Gynecol 1999;180:114–21.
24. Thorp JA, Jones PG, Knox E, Clark RH. Does antenatal corticosteroid therapy affect birthweight and head circumference? Obstet Gynecol 2002;99:101–8.
25. Banks BA, Cnaan A, Morgan MA, et al. Multiple courses of antenatal corticosteroids and outcome of premature neonates. Am J Obstet Gynecol 1999;181:709–17.
26. French NP, Hagan R, Evans SF, Mullan A, Newnham JP. Repeated antenatal corticosteroids: effects on cerebral palsy and childhood behaviour. Am J Obstet Gynecol 2004;190:588–95.
27. Jackson JR, Kleeman S, Doerzbacher M, Lambers DS. The effect of glucocorticosteroid administration on foetal movements and biophysical profile scores in normal pregnancies. J Maternal Fetal Neonat Med 2003;13(1):50–3.
28. Doyle LW, Ford GW, Rickards AL, Kelly EA, Davis NM, Callanan C, et al. Antenatal corticosteroids and outcome at 14 years of age in children with birth weight less than 1501 grams. Paediatrics 2000;106(1):E2.
29. Dessens AB, Haas HS, Koppe JG. Twenty-year follow-up of antenatal corticosteroid treatment. Paediatrics 2000;105(6):E77.
30. Hasbargen U, Reber D, Versmold H, Schulze A. Growth and development of children to 4 years of age after repeated antenatal steroid administration. Eur J Paediatr 2001;160:552–5.

31. Hirvikoski T, Nordenstrom A, Lindholm T, Lindblad F, Ritzen EM, Lajic S. Long-term follow-up of prenatally treated children at risk for congenital adrenal hyperplasia: does dexamethasone cause behavioural problems? Eur J Endocrinol 2008;159:309–16.

32. Mathiesen ER, Christensen AB, Hellmuth E, et al. Insulin doses during glucocorticoid treatment for foetal lung maturation in diabetic pregnancy: test of an algorithm. Acta Obstet Gynaecol Scand 2002;81:835.

33. Gluck PA, Gluck JC. A review of pregnancy outcomes after exposure to orally inhaled or intranasal budesonide. Curr Med Res Opin 2005;21(7):1075–84.

34. Norjavaara E, de Verdier MG. Normal pregnancy outcomes in a population-based study including 2968 pregnant women exposed to budesonide. J Allergy Clin Immunol 2003;111:736–42.

35. Kallen B, Rydhstroem H, Aberg A. Congenital malformations after the use of inhaled budesonide in early pregnancy. Obstet Gynecol 1999;93:392–5.

36. Silverman M, Sheffer A, Diaz P, et al. Prospective pregnancy outcome data in patients with newly diagnosed, mild persistent asthma treated with once-daily budesonide: 5-year results from the START study. Am J Respir Crit Care Med 2004;169:A91.

37. Namazy J, Schatz M, Long L, et al. Use of inhaled steroids by pregnant asthmatic women does not reduce intrauterine growth. J Allergy Clin Immunol 2004;113:427–32.

38. Briggs GG, Freeman RK, Yaffe SJ. Drugs in pregnancy and lactation, 6th edn. Lippincott Williams and Wilkins, Philadelphia, 2002.

39. Coustan DR, Mochizuki TK. Handbook for prescribing medications during pregnancy, 3rd edn. Lippincott-Raven, Philadelphia, 1998.

40. Larimore WL, Petrie KA. Drug use during pregnancy and lactation. Primary Care 2000;27(1):35–53.

41. Fraser CG, Preuss FS, Bigford WD. Adrenal atrophy and irreversible shock associated with cortisone therapy. JAMA 1952;149:1542–3.

42. Lewis L, Robinson RF, Yee J, et al. Fatal adrenal cortical insufficiency precipitated by surgery during prolonged continuous cortisone infusion. Ann Intern Med 1953;39:116–25.

43. Salem M, Tainsh RE, Bromberg J, Loriaux DL, Chernow B. Perioperative glucocorticoid coverage – a reassessment 42 years after emergence of a problem. Ann Surg 1994;219(4):416–25.

44. Axelrod L. Glucocorticoid therapy. Medicine 1976;55:39–63.

45. Kehlet H. Clinical course and hypothalamic-pituitary-adrenocortical function in glucocorticoid-treated surgical patients. FADL's Forlag, Copenhagen, 1976.

46. Glowniak JV, Loriaux DL. A double-blind study of perioperative steroid requirements in secondary adrenal insufficiency. Surgery 1997;121(2):123–9.

47. Bromberg JS, Alfrey EJ, Barker CF, et al. Adrenal suppression and steroid supplementation in renal transplant recipients. Transplantation 1991;51(2):385–95.

48. Udelsman R, Ramp J, Gallucci WT, et al. Adaptation during surgical stress – a re-evaluation of the role of glucocorticoids. J Clin Invest 1986;44:1377–81.

49. Udelsman R, Goldstein DS, Loriaux DL, Chrousos GP. Catecholamine–glucocorticoid interactions during surgical stress. J Surg Res 1987;43:539–45.

50. Chernow B, Alexander HR, Thompson WR, et al. The hormonal responses to surgical stress. Arch Intern Med 1987;147:1273–8.

Approach to hyperemesis gravidarum

Sumona Saha[1], *Catherine Williamson*[2], *Niharika Mehta*[1],
Edward K.S. Chien[3] *and Silvia Degli Esposti*[1]

[1]Department of Medicine, Warren Alpert Medical School of Brown University, Women &
Infants' Hospital of Rhode Island, Providence, RI, USA
[2]Institute of Reproductive and Developmental Biology, Imperial College London, London, UK
[3]Department of Obstetrics and Gynecology, Warren Alpert Medical School of Brown
University, Women & Infants' Hospital of Rhode Island, Providence, RI, USA

Background and epidemiology

Hyperemesis gravidarum (HG) is a condition of severe nausea
and vomiting during pregnancy leading to fluid, electrolyte
and acid–base imbalance, nutritional deficiency and weight
loss [1]. Ketonuria and weight loss of greater than 5% pre-
pregnancy bodyweight, which cannot be attributed to other
causes, distinguishes HG from the more common nausea and
vomiting of pregnancy [2]. Although the prognosis is generally favorable, severe, untreated disease may lead to significant maternal and fetal morbidity.

While up to 50% of all pregnant patients will experience
some nausea and vomiting of pregnancy (NVP), HG occurs in
only 0.3–2% of all pregnancies [3]. The incidence appears to
vary with ethnicity [4]. Symptoms usually begin at 4–5 weeks
gestation and improve by 14–16 weeks. However, in up to
20% of patients, symptoms persist throughout pregnancy [5].

Hyperemesis gravidarum places a significant financial burden on the healthcare system and on society in general by
leading to time loss from work, frequent hospitalizations and
frequent visits to healthcare professionals. A study from 2002
estimated the cost of treating a single patient with HG in the
United States could be as high as $17,000 [6].

Reported risk factors include personal or family history of
hyperemesis, female sex of the offspring, multiple gestation, gestational trophoblastic disease, trisomy 21, hydrops fetalis and
Helicobacter pylori (*H. pylori*) infection [7,8]. Maternal age
greater than 30 and cigarette smoking may be protective [9].

Pathophysiology

The exact etiology of HG is unknown. Whether HG is an
extreme form of gestational vomiting or a distinct entity has

also not been determined. Many possible causes have been
investigated including hormonal changes, thyroid dysfunction, gastrointestinal tract dysmotility, *H. pylori* infection and
psychologic factors.

The pregnancy-related hormones, specifically human chorionic gonadotropin (HCG) and estrogen, have been suggested
to be the stimulus for nausea and vomiting of pregnancy [10].
It is well recognized that the peak symptoms of HG occur
during periods of peak HCG concentration.

States of high estrogen concentration such as low parity
and high maternal Body Mass Index have also been associated with higher incidence of HG [11]. Estrogen is thought
to contribute to HG by slowing gastric intestinal transit
time and gastric emptying. Among the estrogens, estradiol
has been found in some studies to correlate with nausea
and vomiting of pregnancy and higher rates of HG, whereas
estriol has not [12,13]. It is unlikely that estrogens are the
sole cause of HG, especially considering that estrogen levels
peak in the third trimester of pregnancy while HG tends to
improve during late pregnancy [1].

Nonpregnancy-related hormones implicated in the pathogenesis of HG include the thyroid hormones (thyroid-stimulating
hormone (TSH), free tri-iodothyronine (FT3), and free thyroxine (FT4)) and leptin. Abnormal results on thyroid function tests are common in HG, occurring in two-thirds of
women [14]. "Biochemical thyrotoxicosis" characterized by
suppressed TSH and slightly elevated FT4 may be seen due to
the mild thyroid-stimulating activity of HCG. Despite these
laboratory abnormalities, women with HG are generally
euthyroid with no history of prior thyroid diseases, absent
goiter and negative antithyroid antibodies [7]. Treatment is
generally not necessary as the thyroid function tests normalize
in most patients by 18 weeks [15].

Recently, a relationship between the hormone leptin and
HG has been proposed. Increased serum leptin levels during pregnancy, possibly the result of increased total fat mass
and placental production have been found to be significantly

de Swiet's Medical Disorders in Obstetric Practice, 5th edition.
Edited by R. O. Powrie, M. F. Greene, W. Camann. © 2010 Blackwell
Publishing.

higher in patients with HG when compared to healthy pregnant controls [16,17].

The role of the gram-negative spiral bacterium *H. pylori* in HG remains controversial. Several studies have found *H. pylori* seropositivity to be significantly associated with HG [8,18], whereas others could not determine any relationship between the two conditions [19]. In the single study which used endoscopy with gastric mucosal biopsies to identify active *H. pylori* infection, 95% of women with HG were positive for *H. pylori* infection compared with 50% of healthy pregnant controls [20]. A small case series of the effect of treatment of *H. pylori* infection in patients with HG reported dramatic improvement in symptoms after eradication [21]. Currently, there are no guidelines regarding whom or how to check for *H. pylori* infection in pregnancy; however, in severe cases of HG, *H. pylori* infection should be considered a contributing cause and should be treated.

Early studies proposed that HG may be a psychosomatic illness [1]. Recent studies, however, have not found definite psychogenic causes of HG [22,23]. It is likely that sociocultural factors rather than scientific evidence have led to the labeling of HG as a psychologically based condition and that psychologic disturbances are the result rather than the cause of HG [24].

Clinical presentation

Hyperemesis gravidarum presents in the first trimester of pregnancy, usually starting at 4–5 weeks gestation. In addition to severe nausea and vomiting, patients may report ptyalism, spitting and retching. Patients may also complain of gastroesophageal reflux symptoms such as retrosternal discomfort and heartburn. The initial evaluation of patients with HG is reviewed in Box 48.1. A pregnancy unique quantification of emesis and nausea (PUQE) score that is calculated using the number of hours of nausea per day, number of episodes of emesis per day and number of episodes of retching per day can be used to track the severity of symptoms [25] (Box 48.2).

On physical exam, patients may have evidence of volume depletion with dry mucous membranes, tachycardia and postural hypotension. Weight loss of greater than 5% of prepregnancy bodyweight or inadequate weight gain are viewed by many experts to be the features that distinguish HG from nausea and vomiting of pregnancy. Severely affected patients may have muscle wasting and weakness.

Laboratory studies that are useful in diagnosing and managing patients with HG include urinalysis to assess for specific gravity, ketonuria and infection. Electrolytes and renal function should also be assessed to evaluate for hyponatremia, hypokalemia, and metabolic alkalosis from severe dehydration. Complete blood count testing may reveal an elevated hemoglobin due to hemoconcentration and volume depletion. Prealbumin (plasma transthyretin) levels may be

---

Box 48.1 Initial approach to hyperemesis gravidarum

History and physical exam

- Assess duration and severity of symptoms
- Assess for weight loss
- Assess for dehydration
- Elicit presence of other symptoms (e.g. fever, abdominal pain, etc.)
- Calculate PUQE score

Laboratory studies

- Urinalysis
- Electrolytes
- Liver function tests
- TSH and free T4
- Serum lipase
- Prealbumin

Imaging

- Consider abdominal ultrasound
- Consider obstetric ultrasound

Endoscopy

- EsophagoGastroDuodenoscopy (EGD) if nausea is accompanied by hematemesis, odynophagia and dysphagia

---

Box 48.2 Motherisk-PUQE score system

1. In the last 12 hours, for how long have you felt nauseated or sick to your stomach?
   a. Not at all (1 point)
   b. 1 hour or less (2 points)
   c. 2–3 hours (3 points)
   d. 4–6 hours (4 points)
   e. More than 6 hours (5 points)
2. In the last 13 hours have you vomited or thrown up?
   a. I did not throw up (1 point)
   b. 1–2 times (2 points)
   c. 3–4 times (3 points)
   d. 5–6 times (4 points)
   e. 7 or more times (5 points)
3. In the past 12 hours how often have you had retching or dry heaves without bringing anything up?
   a. At no time (1 point)
   b. 1–2 times (2 points)
   c. 3–4 times (3 points)

d. 5–6 times (4 points)

e. 7 or more times (5 points)

Calculate total score and categorize patient's symptoms as follows: 1–3 no symptoms; 4–6 mild; 7–12 moderate symptoms; >13 severe.

Adapted from Koren G, Baskovic R, Hard M, *et al.* Motherisk-PUQE (pregnancy unique quantification of emesis and nausea) scoring system for nausea and vomiting of pregnancy. Am J Obstet Gynecol 2002;186:S228–31.

---

low, reflecting poor protein nutrition status in the mother and possibly predicting lower fetal birthweights [26].

Liver function tests may be abnormal in up to 50% of hospitalized patients [27]. Mild hyperbilirubinemia (bilirubin <4 mg/dL) and/or a rise in alkaline phosphatase to twice the upper limit of normal may be seen [28]. A moderate transaminitis is the most common liver function test abnormality, with alanine aminotransferase (ALT) levels generally greater than aspartate aminotranferase (AST) levels. The transaminase elevation is usually 2–3 times the upper limit of normal; however, levels greater than 1000 U/mL have been reported [29]. The abnormal liver tests are likely related to starvation and resolve promptly upon resolution of the vomiting.

Hyperamylasemia is common in HG. One study found elevated amylase levels in 24% of patients with HG [30]. This is likely due to excessive salivary gland production of amylase rather than pancreatic secretion and a result rather than a cause of HG [1].

Thyroid stimulating hormone levels may be low in HG, as mentioned above, due to cross-reaction between the alpha-subunit of HCG with the TSH receptor. In the majority of cases, this biochemical thyrotoxicosis is not clinically relevant as patients are euthyroid. Thyroid hormone levels generally normalize without treatment by 18 weeks gestation. In cases where it is hard to exclude thyrotoxicosis, thyroid autoantibodies (TSH receptor antibodies suggestive of Graves' disease and thyroid peroxidase and thyroglobulin antibodies most commonly seen in Hashimoto's thyroiditis) may be of value. In HG the raised liver transaminases and abnormal thyroid function tests should improve as the disease resolves and if they do not, further investigation should be undertaken to exclude other liver disease or hyperthyroidism.

Diagnosis

Hyperemesis gravidarum is a clinical diagnosis based on symptoms and the exclusion of other conditions. No clear delineation exists between HG and nausea and vomiting of pregnancy which may complicate making the diagnosis. No specific testing is needed to diagnose HG; however, ultrasound of the abdomen and/or obstetric ultrasound may be helpful to exclude other causes such as gallbladder disease, hydatidiform mole and multiple gestation. The differential diagnosis is reviewed in Table 48.1 and includes nausea and vomiting of pregnancy, acute thyroiditis, eating disorders, viral gastroenteritis, biliary tract disease, pancreatitis, hepatitis, gastroesophageal reflux disease and less commonly, intracerebral neoplasm and Addison's disease.

Table 48.1 Differential diagnosis of hyperemesis gravidarum

System	Diagnosis	Investigation/initial assessment
Genitourinary	Urinary tract infection	Mid-stream urine specimen for culture
	Uremia	Urinalysis, electrolytes, BUN and creatinine
	Molar pregnancy	Ultrasound of the uterus
Gastrointestinal	Gastritis/peptic ulceration	*Helicobacter pylori* antibodies
	Gastroesophageal reflux and ulcerative esophagitis	Endoscopy or empirical proton pump inhibitor therapy
	Pancreatitis	Amylase, blood glucose, calcium
	Bowel obstruction	Plain supine abdominal X-ray
Endocrine	Addison's disease	Urinalysis and electrolytes, early morning cortisol, a cosyntropin (a synthetic peptide with similar activity to ACTH that is known as tetracosactrin in the UK) stimulation test
	Hyperthyroidism	Surveillance for symptoms and signs of hyperthyroidism, thyroid function tests, thyroid autoantibodies (especially TSH receptor antibodies)
	Diabetic ketoacidosis	Blood glucose, urinary dipstick for ketones, glucose tolerance test
	Renal tubular acidosis	Urinalysis (with urinary pH), electrolytes, BUN and creatinine
CNS	Intracranial tumor	Neurologic examination, brain imaging
	Vestibular disease	History (vertigo should be a prominent feature) and neurologic examination (sudden movements of the head may precipitate symptoms and nystagmus)
Respiratory	Asthma	Chest examination, peak expiratory flow rate (asthma can be associated with vomiting especially if there are large amounts of swallowed respiratory secretions)

Complications

Mild-to-moderate nausea and vomiting of pregnancy is not associated with adverse fetal outcomes and may, in fact, be associated with reduced risks for miscarriage, preterm delivery and stillbirth [31]. In contrast, severe, refractory HG has been associated with adverse maternal and fetal outcomes. In a study of more than 150,000 singleton pregnancies, infants born to women with hyperemesis and low pregnancy weight gain (less than 7 kg) were more likely to be low birthweight, born before 37 weeks of gestation and have a 5-minute Apgar score of less than 7 [3]. If the mother develops Wernicke's encephalopathy the fetal outcome is worse; of 45 cases in the published literature, only 44% were reported as having been born alive [32].

Common maternal complications include weight loss, dehydration, micronutrient deficiency, and muscle weakness. More severe, albeit rare, complications of intractable vomiting or retching that have been reported include Mallory–Weiss tears (tears of the lower esophageal mucosa with subsequent gastrointestinal bleeding), esophageal perforation, retinal hemorrhage and spontaneous pneumomediastinum with or without subcutaneous emphysema [7]. Central pontine myelinolysis and Wernicke's encephalopathy with or without Korsakoff's psychosis are catastrophic but preventable complications of HG. Central pontine myelinolysis is seen in cases of HG where severe hyponatremia is corrected too rapidly. It is a symmetric destruction of myelin at the center of the basal pons. It can cause pyramidal tract signs, spastic quadraparesis, pseudobulbar palsy and impaired consciousness. Wernicke's encephalopathy is seen in cases of HG with untreated thiamine deficiency, especially if these patients are given glucose or fed before thiamine has been replaced. A review of 45 reported cases established that the most common presenting symptoms are ocular signs (diplopia, sixth nerve palsy or nystagmus, 82%), confusion (71%) and ataxia (69%) [32]. If untreated, Wernicke's encephalopathy may lead to Korsakoff's psychosis (amnesia, impaired ability to learn) or death. Lastly, severe depression with elective termination of pregnancy has also been reported in association with HG [33].

Management

Given the potential for adverse outcomes, HG should be aggressively treated with the goals of maintaining fluid and electrolyte balance, maintaining adequate caloric intake and controlling symptoms. Patients able to maintain some oral intake benefit from nutritional counseling. Women are advised to eat several small meals throughout the day and to avoid an empty stomach as this may precipitate nausea. Avoiding offensive odors, separating solids and liquids and eating high-carbohydrate foods may also be helpful [34].

Complementary therapies such as acupressure, hypnosis, and herbal remedies have been variably effective in treating nausea and vomiting of pregnancy [35]. Recently, tactile massage [36] and acupressure have been found to be effective in HG [37]; other literature suggests that hypnosis as an adjunctive therapy may also be helpful [38]. Regarding herbal therapy, ginger was found to be more effective than placebo in a randomized controlled trial for treatment of HG [39]. And in a retrospective Canadian study, medicinal cannabis obtained through a compassion society was found to be over 90% effective in treating nausea and vomiting of pregnancy [40].

Pharmacologic therapy with antiemetics and antireflux medications constitute first-line treatment for outpatients who fail dietary changes. An evidence-based algorithm for the treatment of nausea and vomiting of pregnancy is detailed below (Figure 48.1). Although there is often anxiety and reluctance to prescribe antiemetics in pregnancy, extensive data show lack of teratogenesis and good fetal safety for many of these medications [41,42]. Patients may, however, not tolerate oral therapy and a trial of treatment with rectal, sublingual or intravenous formulations should be attempted in these cases.

Promethazine (12.5–25 mg PO/4 h), the phenothiazines (chlorpromazine 10–25 mg PO/6 h and prochlorperazine 5–10 mg PO or 2.5–10 IV/6 h), the dopamine antagonist metoclopramide (10 mg PO or IV/6 h), and pyridoxine (vitamin B6 typically as 10–25 mg PO three to four times daily) by itself or in combination with doxylamine (where available; typically given as 10–12.5 mg PO three or four times a day) are often used as first-line therapy for nausea and vomiting of pregnancy [43]. In patients who fail or cannot tolerate these medications due to severe side effects (e.g. extreme sedation and extrapyramidal symptoms in the case of the phenothiazines or extrapyramidal symptoms in the case of metoclopramide), treatment with newer antiemetics such as ondansetron can be considered.

A 5-hydroxytryptamine (5-HT) receptor antagonist, ondansetron is widely used for the treatment of postoperative and chemotherapy-induced nausea and vomiting [44]. Its safety in pregnancy was suggested in a recent study which showed no significant increase in the number of miscarriages, major malformations or birthweight between infants exposed to ondansetron and unexposed controls [45]. It is categorized as a category B drug ("No evidence of risk in humans") in the US Food and Drug Administration (FDA) Pregnancy Risk Classification (see Chapter 30 on prescribing in pregnancy). A pilot study of 30 pregnant women with hyperemesis did not find any benefit of ondansetron 10 mg given intravenously every 8 hours as needed over promethazine 50 mg given intravenously every 8 hours in terms of nausea, weight gain, days of hospitalization or total doses of medicine [46]. However, the entry criteria for this study were not stringent and so the reproducibility of its findings remains in question. Both case reports and widespread clinical experience support the superior efficacy

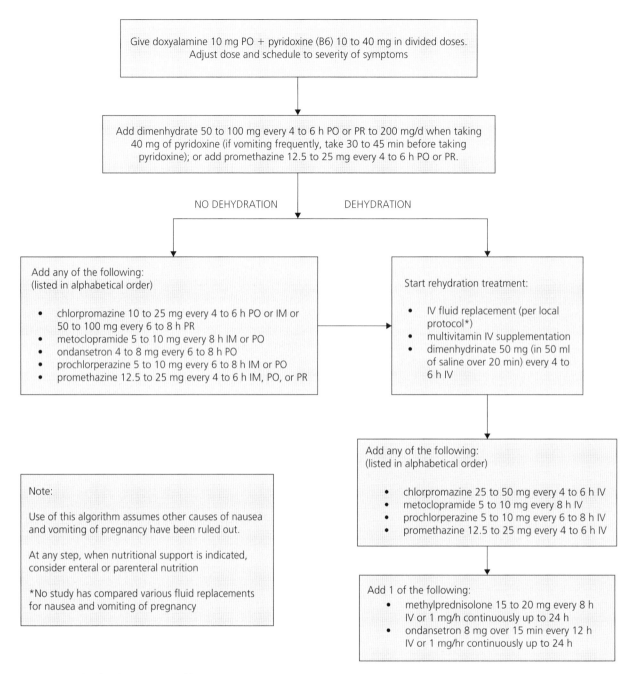

Figure 48.1 Algorithm for the treatment of hyperemesis gravidarum. From Levichek Z, Atanackovic G, Oepkes D, *et al*. Motherisk Update. Nausea and vomiting of pregnancy: evidence-based treatment algorithm. Can Fam Physician 2002;48:267–8,277.

of ondansetron 8 mg every 8 hours for the treatment of HG and its better tolerability over older antiemetics [47,48].

5-HT4 receptor antagonists (cisapride) may also be used as an alternative to standard treatment of hyperemesis but cisapride is no longer marketed in the US because of its association with cardiac arrhythmia.

Oral and intravenous corticosteroids have been used for refractory cases of HG with variable results. One randomized placebo-controlled trial of 25 women with HG found an

increased sense of well-being, improved appetite and increased weight gain in women treated with steroids compared with placebo, although no statistically significant improvement in actual nausea and vomiting was seen [49]. In another study 40 women with hyperemesis were randomized to receive either oral methylprednisolone (16 mg three times a day for 3 days and then tapered over 2 weeks) or oral promethazine (25 mg three times a day for 2 weeks). There was a similar response to both drugs after 2 days, but no woman who received methylprednisolone was readmitted within 2 weeks of discharge while five women who received promethazine were readmitted with hyperemesis [50]. Other randomized controlled trials, however, have reported less optimistic results with the same rates of rehospitalization found in women treated with steroids compared with conventional therapy [51]. Direct comparison of these studies is limited, however, by differences in the type of corticosteroid used and differences in the doses and durations of steroid use. If corticosteroids are used for longer than 4 weeks to treat HG, they should be reduced gradually because of the possibility of adrenal suppression and stress-dose steroids should be considered for labor and delivery (see Chapter 47). A cosyntropin (a synthetic peptide with similar activity as ACTH known as tetracosactrin in the UK) stimulation test should be considered before corticosteroids are stopped.

Patients who are ketotic and not able to maintain hydration by oral intake require intravenous hydration. Normal saline (NaCl 0.9%, 150 mmol/L Na), lactated Ringer's solution (130 mmol/L Na) or Hartmann's solution (NaCl 0.6%; 131 mmol/L Na) are preferred since fluids containing dextrose may precipitate Wernicke's encephalopathy if given before thiamine. In addition, these three solutions are more effective at preventing or correcting hyponatremia than fluids containing dextrose [52]. Hypertonic saline is never required and may precipitate central pontine myelinosis by the overly rapid correction of serum sodium levels.

Potassium supplements should be added to the intravenous fluid replacement therapy as required. Thiamine should be given to prevent Wernicke's encephalopathy, as a daily dose of either 50–150 mg orally or 100 mg diluted in 100 mL normal saline as an intravenous infusion.

Intravenous hydration is often started during hospitalization. In severely affected patients, this may need to be continued after discharge [53]. Patients may be treated with fluid boluses or with continuous fluid infusions at home via peripheral IV, midline catheters or peripherally inserted central catheters (PICC).

In addition to hydration, patients with refractory HG may also require nutritional support. Both parenteral and enteral nutrition have been described in HG. Total parenteral nutrition (TPN) given via central catheters or PICC lines requires close supervision and monitoring. Hyperglycemia and abnormal liver function tests due to cholestatic liver disease are common complications of TPN. Other serious complications of parenteral nutrition in pregnancy, reported to be as high as 50% in one study, are sepsis, pneumothorax, and thrombosis [54]. Immunosuppression and the hypercoagulable state associated with pregnancy dramatically increase the risks of indwelling catheters in the pregnant population and reduce the safety of TPN. Other disadvantages to parenteral nutrition are its attendant care and expense.

Enteral feeding in HG has been described via nasoenteric tubes [55], percutaneous gastrostomy (PEG) [56] and jejunostomy [57,58]. Although relatively easy and safe to place, nasoenteric tube use in clinical practice has been limited by tube dislodgment, occlusion and poor patient tolerance. Altered anatomy in pregnancy poses risks with respect to PEG placement although in small case series both feeding gastrostomy and jejunostomy have been reported to be safe and efficacious in the treatment of HG.

Patients who are hospitalized with HG should be considered for thromboprophylaxis with either heparin or intermittent compression stockings. Immobilization, dehydration and pregnancy may predispose these patients to thromboembolism.

Women who have had HG in a previous pregnancy have a 20-fold increased risk of developing it in a subsequent pregnancy compared to women with previous uncomplicated pregnancies [58]. The risk is slightly lower with a different partner. It is important to exclude associated conditions (Figure 48.1) and to optimize their management. For example, "triple therapy" (typically a proton pump inhibitor, amoxicillin and clarithromycin) can be used for *Helicobacter pylori* infection before conception and women with thyroid dysfunction can have their treatment optimized.

References

1. Verberg MFG, Gillott DJ, Al-Fardan N, *et al*. Hyperemesis gravidarum, a literature review. Human Reprod Update 2005;11:527–39.
2. Goodwin TM. Hyperemesis gravidarum. Clin Obstet Gynecol 1998;41:597–605.
3. Dodds, L, Fell DB, Joseph KS, *et al*. Outcomes of pregnancies complicated by hyperemesis gravidarum. Obset Gynecol 2006;107:285–92.
4. Bashiri A, Neumann L, Maymon E, *et al*. Hyperemesis gravidarum: epidemiologic features, complications and outcome. Eur J Obstet Gynecol Reprod Biol 1995;63:138–8.
5. Kelly CK, Degli-Esposti S. Hyperemesis gravidarum. In: McGarry K, Tong IL (eds) 5-Minute clinical consult companion to women's health. Lippincott, Williams and Wilkins, Philadelphia, 2007:238–40.
6. Attard CL, Kholi MA, Coleman S, *et al*. The burden of illness of severe nausea and vomiting of pregnancy in the United States. Am J Obstet Gynecol 2002;186:S220–7.
7. Kuscu NK, Koyuncu F. Hyperemesis gravidarum: current concepts and management. Postgrad Med J 2002;78:76–9.
8. Frigo P, Lang C, Reisenberger K, *et al*. Hyperemesis gravidarum assoicated with Helicobacter pylori seropositivity. Obstet Gynecol 1998;91:615–17.
9. Fell DB, Dodds L, Joseph KS, *et al*. Risk factors for hyperemesis gravidarum requiring hospital admission during pregnancy. Obstet Gynecol 2006;107:277–84.
10. Goodwin TM. Nausea and vomiting of pregnancy: an obstetric syndrome. Am J Obstet Gynecol 2002;186:S184–9.
11. Depue RH, Bernstein L, Ross RK, *et al*. Hyperemesis gravidarum in relation to estradiol levels, pregnancy outcome, and other maternal factors: a seroepidemiologic study. Am J Obstet Gynecol 1987;156:1137–41.
12. Goodwin TM, Montoro M, Mestman JH, *et al*. The role of chorionic gonadotropin in transient hyperthyroidism of hyperemesis gravidarum. J Clin Endocrinol Metab 1992;75:1333–7.
13. Lagiou P, Tamimi R, Mucci LA, *et al*. Nausea and vomiting in pregnancy in relation to prolactin, estrogens, and progesterone: a prospective study. Obstet Gynecol 2003;101:639–44.

14. Goowin TM, Montero M, Mestman JH. Transient hyperthyroidism and hyperemesis gravidarum: clinical aspects. Am J Obstet Gynecol 1992;167:638–52.

15. Caffrey TJ. Transient hyperthyroidism of hyperemesis gravidarum: a sheep in wolf's clothing. J Am Board Fam Pract 200;13:35–8.

16. Aka N, Atalay S, Sayharman S, et al. Leptin and leptin receptor levels in pregnant women with hyperemesis gravidarum. Aust NZ J Obstet Gynecol 2006;46: 274–7.

17. Demir B, Erel CT, Haberal A. Adjusted leptin level (ALL) is a predictor for hyperemesis gravidarum. Eur J Obstet Gynecol Reprod Biol 2006;124:193–6.

18. Kocak I, Akcan Y, Ustun C, et al. Helicobacter pylori seropositivity in patients with hyperemesis gravidarum. Int J Gynecol Obstet 1999;66:251–4.

19. Karadeniz RS, Ozdegirmenci O, Altay MM, et al. Helicobacter pylori seropositivity and stool antigen in patients with hyperemesis gravidarum. Infect Dis Obstet Gynecol 2006;2:1–3.

20. Bagis T, Gurmurdulu Y, Kayaselcuk F, et al. Endoscopy in hyperemesis gravidarum and Helicobacter pylori infection. Int J Gynaecol Obstet 2002;79:105–9.

21. Jacoby EB, Porter KB. Helicobacter pylori infection and persistent hyperemesis gravidarum. Am J Perinatol 1999;16:85–8.

22. Simpson SW, Goodwin TM, Robins SB, et al. Psychological factors and hyperemesis gravidarum. J Womens Health Gend Based Med 2001;10:471–7.

23. Munch S. Women's experiences with a pregnancy complication: causal explanations of hyperemesis gravidarum. Soc Work Health Care 2002;36:519–24.

24. Munch S. Chicken or the egg? The biological-psychological controversy surrounding hyperemesis gravidarum. Soc Sci Med 2002;55:1267–8.

25. Koren G, Piwko C, Ahn E, et al. Validation studies of the Pregnancy Unique Quantification of Emesis (PUQE) scores. J Obstet Gynaecol 2005;25:241–4.

26. Jain SK, Shah M, Ransonet L, et al. Maternal and neonatal plasma transthyretin (prealbumin) concentrations and birth weight of newborn infants. Biol Neonate 1995;68:10–14.

27. Wallstedt A, Riely CA, Shaver D, et al. Prevalence and characteristics of liver dysfunction in hyperemesis gravidarum. Clin Res 1990;38:970A.

28. Knox TA, Olans LB. Liver disease in pregnancy. N Engl J Med 1996;335:569–76.

29. Conchillo JM, Pijnenborg JMA, Peeters P, et al. Liver enzyme elevation induced by hyperemesis gravidarum: aetiology, diagnosis and treatment. Neth J Med 2002;60:374–8.

30. Robertson C, Miller H. Hyperamylasemia in bulimia nervosa and hyperemesis gravidarum. Int J Eat Disord 1999;26:223–7.

31. Flaxmann SM, Sherman PW. Morning sickness: a mechanism for protecting mother and embryo. Q Rev Biol 2000;75:113–48.

32. Selitsky T, Chandra P, Schiavello HJ. Wernicke's encephalopathy with hyperemesis and ketoacidosis. Obstet Gynecol 2006; 107:486–90.

33. Mazzotta P, Stewart DE, Koren G, et al. Factors associated with elective termination of pregnancy among Canadian and American women with nausea and vomiting of pregnancy. J Psychosom Obstet Gynaecol 2001;22:7–12.

34. Kaiser LL, Allen L. Position of the American Dietetic Association: nutrition and lifestyle for a healthy pregnancy outcome. J Am Diet Assoc 2002;102:1479–90.

35. Jewell D, Young G. Interventions for nausea and vomiting in early pregnancy. Cochrane Database of Systematic Reviews, 2003;4:CD000145.

36. Agren A, Berg M. Tactile massage and severe nausea and vomiting during pregnancy- women's experiences. Scand J Caring Sci 2006;20:169–76.

37. Neri I, Allais G, Schiapparelli P. Acupuncture versus pharmacological approach to reduce hyperemesis gravidarum discomfort. Minerva Ginecol 2005;57:471–5.

38. Simon EP, Shwartz J. Medical hypnosis for hyperemesis gravidarum. Birth 1999;26(4):248–54.

39. Fischer-Rasmussen W, Kjaser SK, Dahl C, et al. Ginger treatment of hyperemesis gravidarum. Eur J Obstet Gynecol Reprod Biol 1991;38:19–24.

40. Westfall RE, Janssen PA, Lucas P, et al. Survey of medicinal cannabis use among childbearing women: patterns of its use in pregnancy and retroactive self-assessment of its efficacy against 'morning sickness'. Complement Ther Clin Pract 2006;12:27–33.

41. Milkovich L, van den Berg BJ. An evaluation of the teratogenicity of certain antinauseant drugs. Am J Obstet Gynecol 1976;125:244–8.

42. Seto A, Einarson T, Koren G. Pregnancy outcome following first trimester exposure to antihistamines – a meta-analysis. Am J Perinatol 1997;14:119–24.

43. Bsat FA, Hoffman DE, Seubert DE. Comparison of three outpatient regimens in the management of nausea and vomiting in pregnancy. J Perinatol 2003;23(7):531–5.

44. Rubenstein EB, Slusher BS, Rojas C, et al. New approaches to chemotherapy-induced nausea and vomiting: from neuropharmacology to clinical investigations.Cancer J 2006;12:341–7.

45. Einarson A, Malatepe C, Navioz Y. The safety of ondansetron for nausea and vomiting of pregnancy: a prospective comparative study. Br J Obstet Gynecol 2004;111:940–3.

46. Sullivan CA, Johnson CA, Roach H. A pilot study of intravenous ondansetron for hyperemesis gravidarum. Am J Obstet Gynecol 1996;174:1565–18.

47. Tincello DJ, Johnstone MJ. Treatment of hyperemesis gravidarum with the 5-HT3 antagonist ondansetron (Zofran). Postgrad Med J 1996;72:688–9.

48. Siu SS, Yip SK, Cheung CW. Treatment of intractable hyperemesis gravidarum by ondansetron. Eur J Obstet Gynecol Reprod Biol 2002;105:73–4.

49. Nelson-Piercy C, Fayers P, de Swiet M. Randomised, double-blind, placebo-controlled trial of corticosteroids for the treatment of hyperemesis gravidarum. Br J Obstet Gynaecol 2001;108(1):9–15.

50. Safari HR, Fassett MJ, Souter IC, Alsulyman OM, Goodwin TM. The efficacy of methylprednisolone in the treatment of hyperemesis gravidarum: a randomized, double-blind, controlled study. Am J Obstet Gynecol 1998;179: 921–4.

51. Yost N, McIntire D, Winans F, et al. A randomized, placebo-controlled trial of corticosteroids for hyperemesis due to pregnancy. Obstet Gynecol 2003;102:1250–4.

52. Nelson-Piercy C. Treatment of nausea and vomiting in pregnancy. When should it be treated and what can be safely taken? Drug Safety 1998;19:155–64.

53. Cowan MJ. Hyperemesis gravidarum: implications for home care and infusion therapies. J Intraven Nurs 1996;19:46–58.

54. Russo-Stieglitz KE, Levine AB, Wagner BA, et al. Pregnancy outcome in patients requiring parenteral nutrition. J Matern Fetal Med 1999;8:164–7.

55. Vaisman N, Kaider R, Levin I, et al. Nasojejunal feeding in hyperemesis gravidarum–a preliminary study. Clin Nutr 2004;23:53–7.

56. Serrano P, Velloso A, Garcia-Luna PP, et al. Enteral nutrition by percutaneous endoscopic gastrojejunostomy in severe hyperemesis gravidarum: a report of two cases. Clin Nutr 1998;17:135–9.

57. Erick M. Nutrition via jejunostomy in refractory hyperemesis gravidarum: a case report. J Am Dietet Assoc 1997;97:1154–6.

58. Trogstad LIS, Stoltenberg C, Magnus P, Skaerven R, Irgens LM. Recurrence risk in hyperemesis gravidarum. Br J Obstet Gynaecol 2005;112:1641–5.

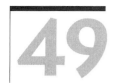

Approach to fetal assessment, optimization of neonatal outcome, mode of delivery and timing for nonobstetric readers

Michael Peek[1], George J. Mangos[2] and Mark A. Brown[2]

[1]Department of Obstetrics and Gynaecology, University of Sydney and Nepean Hospital, Sydney, Australia
[2]Department of Renal Medicine, St George Hospital and University of New South Wales, Sydney, Australia

Introduction

While this book is written recognizing that our main audience is the practicing obstetrician, we realize that there will be many nonobstetric readers who would benefit from some clarification of how fetuses are assessed *in utero* in women with medical problems and what factors influence mode and timing of delivery. A detailed discussion of this material is beyond the scope of this book and the purpose of the following is to provide some very general background to these topics for readers who are not obstetricians.

Assessment of fetal well-being *in utero*

The assessment of fetal well-being is an imprecise science and is carried out in a number of ways:
- fetal growth assessment
- amniotic fluid volume assessment
- nonstress tests (NST), contraction stress tests (CST) (both also known as cardiotocography (CTG))
- biophysical profile
- fetal Doppler velocimetry
- maternal Doppler velocimetry.

Each of these modalities is briefly summarized below. While all of these modalities are commonly used in clinical practice,

the evidence for their impact upon pregnancy outcome remains unclear.

Fetal growth

Maternal medical disorders such as hypertension, hypoxia, and chronic renal disease can affect placental function and lead to intrauterine growth restriction (IUGR). The greater and earlier the onset of the IUGR, the greater the risk of perinatal morbidity and mortality [1]. Fundal height (the height of the uterus as measured from the pubic bone) is a screening test for appropriate fetal growth but has limited sensitivity and specificity. Ultrasound is currently the most useful method of determining fetal growth. Clinical determination of fetal growth such as fundal height can be misleading and should always be backed up by ultrasound. In cases where there is high risk of IUGR, serial ultrasound examinations to assess fetal growth should be carried out every 2–4 weeks depending upon the severity of the problem. The routine growth parameters used are biparietal diameter, head circumference, abdominal circumference and femur length. Due to wide normal ranges for these measurements, particularly at later gestations, and the errors of measurement, growth is best assessed by ultrasound examinations carried out 2–4 weeks apart. The classic picture of IUGR related to maternal medical disease is asymmetric IUGR where the abdominal measurements are more decreased than the fetal head and femur measurements. In severe early-onset IUGR, all parameters are often decreased.

Amniotic fluid volume

It is well documented that amniotic fluid volume correlates well with perinatal outcome and is very helpful in identifying

de Swiet's Medical Disorders in Obstetric Practice, 5th edition.
Edited by R. O. Powrie, M. F. Greene, W. Camann. © 2010 Blackwell Publishing.

those babies that are small due to uteroplacental insufficiency from those that are constitutionally small. It has been demonstrated in animal models that fetuses subject to chronic hypoxia redirect blood flow from less vital organs (such as the kidneys) to more critical organs (such as the brain). This diversion of blood flow from the kidneys leads to reduced fetal urine production and thus to a decreased amniotic fluid volume or oligohydramnios.

Amniotic fluid volume is usually measured in one of two ways. The first is the maximum vertical pocket of amniotic fluid as measured by ultrasound. Normal values fall between 2 cm and 8 cm, with oligohydramnios being present when the value is less than 2 cm. The Amniotic Fluid Index (AFI) is the second ultrasound method of assessing amniotic fluid volume. With this method, the maximum vertical pocket in each of the four quadrants is measured and then the values are summed. In general, the normal range is between 5 and 24, but gestational age-related ranges have been developed [2].

Nonstress tests and contraction stress test (also known as cardiotocography)

The measurement of fetal heart rate and its relationship to fetal activity (NST) or uterine contractions (CST) are the most commonly used methods in assessing fetal well-being [3], despite lack of convincing data on the overall benefits of such testing. Although used extensively antenatally, it is the mainstay of intrapartum fetal monitoring. It is beyond the scope of this chapter to cover all aspects of CTG interpretation. Many authorities have published guidelines for the use and interpretation of CTG, including the American College of Obstetricians and Gynecologists and the Royal College of Obstetricians and Gynaecologists [1,4].

Fetal heart rate is measured either externally by a Doppler ultrasound transducer placed on the maternal abdomen or internally by an electrode (fetal scalp electrode) affixed to the fetus. Maternal contractions are measured by an external tocodynamometer attached to the maternal abdomen or an intrauterine pressure catheter. A number of fetal heart rate parameters including baseline rate, heart rate variability, and accelerations and decelerations are measured when assessing a CTG record. In general, a reactive NST as assessed by these parameters is very predictive of a nonhypoxic, noncompromised fetus. On the other hand, a nonreactive NST pattern is not highly predictive of a compromised fetus and should be interpreted in association with the clinical situation (such as pre-eclampsia, antepartum hemorrhage) and should be used as a screening test for further investigation. Either an unsatisfactory or a nonreactive NST provides no reassurance of fetal well-being and usually warrants further investigation by a CST (administering oxytocin and assessing the fetal heart rate response to uterine contractions) or ultrasound (a biophysical

profile –see below). Similarly, a nonreassuring CTG in labor requires further evaluation, including the possibility of the collection of a fetal scalp blood sample for assessment of pH. If, for example, the scalp pH is less than 7.20, delivery should be expedited. There are also very sinister CTG patterns (such as prolonged decelerations) that require immediate delivery without other testing.

Biophysical profile

The biophysical profile (BPP) combines an assessment of fetal NST and ultrasound assessments of amniotic fluid volume, fetal tone, fetal breathing and spontaneous fetal movement in an attempt to improve upon the specificity and sensitivity of NST and amniotic fluid levels alone. The BPP is often used as an alternative test to monitor fetal well-being in pregnancies at increased risk of fetal loss or as a follow-up test for patients who have an abnormal NST [5].

Fetal Doppler velocimetry

Doppler flow velocity waveforms in a number of fetal vessels have been used to assess fetal health: umbilical artery, middle cerebral artery, the ductus arteriosus and the umbilical vein. They are each discussed below.

Umbilical arteries

Umbilical arteries are the most commonly studied [4,6]. In normal pregnancy umbilical artery resistance falls progressively throughout pregnancy as the number of small placental vessels increases. As placental function deteriorates, there can be an increase in resistance to flow through the umbilical arteries. This resistance can be assessed by Doppler ultrasound. As placental function deteriorates, forward flow in diastole is at first reduced, then can be absent and may even be reversed in serious dysfunction. The time course of this progression can vary and depends upon a number of factors, including gestational age, the type and severity of the cause of the dysfunction. Nevertheless, the appearance of absent end-diastolic flow is usually an indication that delivery may be indicated soon, depending upon both fetal and maternal factors such as gestational age and severity of maternal disease. Preparation for delivery will include further fetal assessment (for example, cardiotocography), consideration of administration of maternal corticosteroids to help mature the fetal lungs and transfer to a hospital with appropriate neonatal care. The development of reversed end-diastolic flow is usually an indication for delivery as there is a high risk of fetal hypoxia, acidosis and death. The interpretation of these findings can be difficult and advice should be sought from an experienced perinatologist.

Middle cerebral arteries

As uteroplacental insufficiency worsens, the fetus redirects more of its circulation to vital organs such as the brain. This is represented by an increase in diastolic velocity in the middle cerebral artery (MCA) signal. MCA velocimetry is useful in distinguishing between fetuses that are small because of placental compromise and those that are constitutionally small [7,8]. High-flow velocities are also seen with fetal anemia of any cause [9].

Fetal venous Dopplers

The fetal venous system can also be investigated. The two main vessels that are used clinically are the ductus venosus and the umbilical vein. Abnormal velocimetry in these vessels can be due to cardiac failure secondary to a large increase in afterload as seen in placental insufficiency. These changes usually occur late in the disease process and are often seen as an indication for delivery.

Maternal Doppler velocimetry

The maternal uterine artery is probably the most commonly measured maternal vessel in obstetrics. While it does not provide immediate information regarding fetal well-being, it does help in identifying those pregnancies at high risk of developing pre-eclampsia or growth restriction [10]. This is particularly helpful in distinguishing fetuses that are small for nonpathologic reasons from those that are growth restricted due to placental dysfunction. Normally there is a progressive reduction in resistance and increased flow with gestation in the uterine arteries. In pregnancies affected by abnormal placentation, there can be persistence of the high-resistance patterns, including diastolic notching.

Indications for and frequency of fetal assessment

It is important to emphasize that antepartum assessment of fetal well-being is intended only to prevent fetal demise, and reassuring fetal assessments do not rule out all fetal pathology, including pathology that may become obvious only later in life such as neurodevelopmental disability. In general, fetal assessment by one or more of the above means is not initiated until after 32–34 weeks but testing can be started as early as 26–28 weeks gestation. The specific gestational age at which periodic assessments of fetal well-being are initiated will be determined by the clinician's assessment of the magnitude of the risk of fetal demise and the gestational age at which it might begin. The frequency of testing also varies considerably by indication and center; growth and amniotic fluid assessments are typically carried out every 2–4 weeks in women suspected to be at risk for

a growth-restricted fetus. The frequency of NST may vary from episodic based on some acute concern to daily, with patients deemed to be at high risk of fetal demise typically being tested once or twice weekly.

Optimization of fetal outcome

There are no proven treatments for growth restriction due to uteroplacental insufficiency or any other cause. The mainstay of management is timely diagnosis and delivery when it is considered that the risks (to both mother and fetus) of delivery are less than the risks of remaining undelivered. This is often a difficult and individual decision requiring consultation from a number of specialties (including obstetrics, neonatology and obstetric medicine). In coming to a decision, there are a number of issues to be considered to optimize fetal outcome:
- gestational age
- administration of antenatal glucocorticoids
- delivery in an appropriate center
- intrapartum and postpartum management.

Each of these issues is briefly discussed below.

Gestational age

Decisions are often difficult to make at the threshold of viability (23–25 weeks gestation). Gestational age is the most important determinant of outcome, but fetal gender, receipt of antenatal glucocorticoids and being a member of a multiple gestation also affect neonatal survival. It is essential that up-to-date neonatal morbidity and mortality outcome data are used in counseling so that an informed decision can be made [11]. The outcome data vary from country to country but the approximate survival rates increase from 30% at 23 weeks to 65% at 25 weeks to 95% at 30 weeks gestation. Babies born less than 30 weeks gestation have significant risks of long-term morbidity, including chronic lung disease and cerebral palsy.

Antenatal corticosteroids

The most common problem faced by preterm babies is respiratory distress syndrome. Surfactant produced by type II pneumocytes is required to reduce surface tension and help expand alveoli, leading to adequate gas exchange. Maternally administered antenatal corticosteroids have been shown to reduce respiratory distress syndrome by 50% when given between 24 and 34 weeks gestation [12]. With this, there are also reductions in necrotizing enterocolitis, chronic lung disease and mortality. For best effect, the corticosteroids need to be administered at least 24 hours prior to delivery. Two standard regimens are betamethasone 12 mg q24 h × 2 doses and dexamethasone sol6 mg q12h × 4 doses. There is some controversy over the length of effect of steroids and whether the dose needs to be repeated as there have been concerns about the possibility of adverse fetal effects of repeated doses of steroids [13,14].

Delivery in an appropriate center

Outcome data suggest that there is less neonatal morbidity and mortality if babies are born in hospitals where there is appropriate neonatal care rather than being transferred after delivery. *Ex utero* transfer carries the risks of hypothermia and cardiorespiratory instability. Thus if preterm delivery is likely, transfer of the mother to an appropriate unit prior to delivery should be considered.

Intrapartum and postpartum management

Regardless of the method of delivery, the intrapartum care needs to be carried out by obstetrical and midwifery staff familiar with high-risk intrapartum care with access to specialists from other disciplines. Infrastructure needs to be in place to be able to carry out emergency deliveries in a timely fashion. Referral centers equipped to look after women with major medical problems such as chronic renal disease should be able to have a decision-to-delivery time within 30 minutes for emergency cesarean sections.

Women with medical problems and particularly those who undergo operative or preterm delivery often have difficulties with postnatal issues such as care of the newborn and breastfeeding. Access to lactational consultants and experienced midwives is often required.

Mode of delivery

The method of delivery, either vaginal or by cesarean section, in women with medical illness is normally determined by fetal or obstetric concerns (such as previous cesarean section, prematurity, presentation or previous poor obstetric history) rather than medical ones. Even women under critical care can have successful vaginal deliveries if they receive excellent pain control and an assisted second stage. Vaginal deliveries are generally better tolerated in medically compromised women than is a cesarean delivery.

Timing of delivery

In women with stable medical disease and no evidence of fetal compromise, pregnancies can normally be continued to term and spontaneous labor awaited. In other cases where there is a significant deterioration in either maternal or fetal health, intervention to bring about delivery may be indicated. Delivery for maternal or fetal indications should be considered if continued pregnancy places the mother or fetus at an ongoing risk that will be reduced by delivery. With the exception of some cases of cancer requiring toxic chemotherapy or radiation therapy to a field that would include the fetus, delivery simply to make medical care of the mother "less complicated" is not generally justifiable. Again, the mode of delivery should be determined by obstetric and fetal issues with a careful consideration of the length of time needed for and the likelihood of a successful induction of labor. On occasion, a patient's delivery plan is so complicated that there is justification to induce labor or plan a cesarean delivery to increase the likelihood of having the right team in place at the time of delivery.

Neonatal outcomes overall are best when women deliver after 39 weeks gestation. The earlier an infant is delivered prior to term, the higher the risk of neonatal morbidity and mortality. Deliveries prior to 23–24 weeks gestation rarely survive. When counseling parents on the outcomes of such pregnancies and possible need for delivery, input from neonatologists with up-to-date local or national data can be of great help, as discussed above.

References

1. Royal College of Obstetricians and Gynaecologists. Evidence-based clinical guideline number 8: the use of electronic fetal monitoring. Clinical Effectiveness Support Unit, Royal College of Obstetrcians and Gynaecologists, London, 2001. www.rcog.org.uk.
2. Nabhan AF, Abdelmoula YA. Amniotic Fluid Index versus single deepest vertical pocket as a screening test for preventing adverse pregnancy outcome. Cochrane Database of Systematic Reviews, 2008;3:CD006593.
3. Banta DH, Thacker SB. Historical controversy in health technology assessment: the case of electronic fetal monitoring. Obstet Gynecol Surv 2001;56(11):707–19.
4. American College of Obstetricians and Gynecologists. Antepartum fetal surveillance. ACOG practice bulletin #9. American College of Obstetricians and Gynecologists, Washington, DC, 1999.
5. Lalor JG, Fawole B, Alfirevic Z, Devane D. Biophysical profile for fetal assessment in high risk pregnancies. Cochrane Database of Systematic Reviews, 2008;1:CD000038.
6. Westergaard HB, Langhoff-Roos J, Lingman G, *et al*. Critical appraisal of the use of umbilical artery Doppler ultrasound in high-risk pregnancies: use of meta-analyses in evidence-based obstetrics. Ultrasound Obstet Gynecol 2001;17(6):466–76.
7. Van den Wijngaard JAGW, Groenenberg IAL, Wladimiroff JW, *et al*. Cerebral Doppler ultrasound of the human fetus. Br J Obstet Gynaecol 1989;96:845–9.
8. Sherer DM. Prenatal ultrasonographic assessment of the middle cerebral artery: a review. Obstet Gynecol Surv 1997;52(7):444–55.
9. Mari G, Deter RL, Carpenter RL, *et al*. Noninvasive diagnosis by Doppler ultrasonography of fetal anemia due to maternal red-cell alloimmunization. Collaborative Group for Doppler Assessment of the Blood Velocity in Anemic Fetuses. N Engl J Med 2000;342(1):9–14.

10. Bewley S, Cooper D, Campbell S. Doppler investigation of uteroplacental blood flow resistance in the second trimester: a screening study for pre-eclampsia and intrauterine growth retardation. Br J Obstet Gynaecol 1991:98:871–9.

11. Tyson JE, Parikh NA, Langer J, Green C, Higgins RD, National Institute of Child Health and Human Development Neonatal Research Network. Intensive care for extreme prematurity – moving beyond gestational age. N Engl J Med. 2008;358(16):1672–81.

12. Roberts D, Dalziel S. Antenatal corticosteroids for accelerating fetal lung maturation for women at risk of preterm birth. Cochrane Database of Systematic Reviews, 2006;3:CD004454.

13. Crowther CA, Doyle LW, Haslam RR, Hiller JE, Harding JE, Robinson JS, ACTORDS Study Group. Outcomes at 2 years of age after repeat doses of antenatal corticosteroids. N Engl J Med 2007;357(12):1179–89.

14. Wapner RJ, Sorokin Y, Mele L, *et al.*, National Institute of Child Health and Human Development Maternal-Fetal Medicine Units Network. Long-term outcomes after repeat doses of antenatal corticosteroids. N Engl J Med 2007;357(12):1190–8.

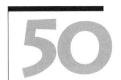

Promoting safe care for women with medical problems during pregnancy

Raymond O. Powrie[1], James A. O'Brien[2] with Kue Chung Choi[3]

[1]Department of Medicine, Warren Alpert Medical School of Brown University, Women & Infants' Hospital of Rhode Island, Providence, RI, USA
[2]Department of Obstetrics and Gynecology, Warren Alpert Medical School of Brown University, Women & Infants' Hospital of Rhode Island, Providence, RI, USA
[3]Department of Anesthesiology, Women & Infants' Hospital of Rhode Island, Providence, RI, USA

Introduction

In the past decade there has been a dramatic increase in our understanding of the important contribution of medical errors as a cause of morbidity and mortality. National attention in the United States was brought to this issue in 1999 with the publication of the Institute of Medicine's Report *To err is human: building a safer health system* [1]. This report summarized data that presented medical errors as the eighth leading cause of death in the US, being responsible for between 48,000 and 98,000 deaths per year – more deaths than are attributable each year to motor vehicle accidents, breast cancer or HIV infection. Similar reports have been published in many other Western countries before and since 1999 suggesting that this problem is not unique to the US healthcare system [2,3]. Nor does this problem appear unique to medical or surgical patients. A 4-year review of maternal mortality in North Carolina in the US found that 40% of deaths were potentially preventable by improvements in care [4]. The United Kingdom's excellent Confidential Enquiry into Maternal and Child Health (CEMACH), which reviews all maternal deaths in the UK, identified some degree of substandard care in 64% of deaths directly attributable to a pregnancy complication and in 40% of those patients for whom pregnancy was considered to be at least a contributing factor in their death [5].

After a dramatic progressive drop in the maternal mortality rate over the first three-quarters of the past century in both the US and the UK, little progress has since been made in either country. In recent data from both the UK and US, medical illness, rather than obstetric causes, appears to be a key contributor in a manner that was not true in the past.

In 1952, a little under half of the maternal mortality in the UK was attributable to medical causes while in the year 2000, this portion had risen to 81%. Delayed childbearing, advances in reproductive technologies, and better medical care of women with chronic medical illness have all likely contributed to an increase in the number of pregnant women with medical problems. However, the change in relative proportion of deaths due to obstetric versus medical causes may also suggest the possibility that the progress in obstetric and anesthetic care seen in the past century has not been matched by medical care during pregnancy.

For the majority of obstetric patients, medical care follows a similar successful course down a well-worn path. Since serious medical complications are relatively rare, obstetricians, internists, anesthesiologists, and nurses are unable to gain day-to-day clinical experience that helps promote excellence in the management of serious medical complications during pregnancy. The obstetric population is one that is often highly resilient to less than optimal care; however, the stakes remain very high for the patient and her partner, her infant, and caregivers. What can be done to minimize the risk to women with medical illness in pregnancy? Application of safety principles from other industries and areas of healthcare offers our present best hope of adequately addressing errors in the care of obstetric patients with medical disorders. These principles are listed in Box 50.1 and discussed below.

> **Box 50.1** Four principles for increasing the medical safety of pregnant women
>
> - Promoting a safe culture
> - Identifying those at risk
> - Intervening early
> - Preparing for emergencies

de Swiet's Medical Disorders in Obstetric Practice, 5th edition.
Edited by R. O. Powrie, M. F. Greene, W. Camann. © 2010 Blackwell Publishing.

Increasing the medical safety of pregnant women

Safety culture

Of the four safety principles listed in Box 50.1, a "safety culture" is the least quantifiable but perhaps the most important. A culture of safety can be broadly defined as one that makes it more likely that the caregivers will do the right thing and less likely that they will do the wrong one. It has many contributing elements and factors, but four features listed in Box 50.2 are crucial and discussed below.

Standardizing care

Although many physicians pride themselves on the art of medicine and their unique and distinct approach to care, these variations in practice, although perhaps important to medical progress, come at a price to patient safety. Variations in practice over matters unlikely to affect clinical outcomes increase the likelihood of error by asking other providers, pharmacists, nurses, and midwives to "learn" a wide variety of practices, making it more likely that an error due to variance will occur. Safe hospital cultures are ones in which standardized guidelines and protocols of care are developed and disseminated and in which compliance with them is audited and promoted. Although the best justification for such protocols will be evidence based, standardization has merit from a safety perspective even in the absence of knowing the single best way to do something. In the best safety cultures, variation from accepted protocols is open to inquiry by and discussion with any member of the care team to ensure the variation is understood and carefully applied.

Promoting vigilance

In many cases of poor maternal outcome, early signs of maternal deterioration are missed, responded to inadequately and/or communicated poorly. There may even be a failure to obtain complete or accurate vital signs, or for abnormalities to be communicated to the patient's provider. There may be a failure on the provider's part to make a complete assessment of the patient and/or to clearly communicate a plan

---

Box 50.2 Elements of a safe culture

- Standardizing care according to accepted protocols
- Promoting vigilance
- Promoting transparency
- Promoting teamwork

---

to the patient and nurse. Defining the vital signs that require the obstetrician be notified, and delineating what the expected response to such calls should be can help prevent unnecessary delays in assessment and treatment that can contribute to poor outcomes. Ensuring that providers who have made an assessment share their conclusions and plan with other members of the care team is critical to creating a shared mental model of the next steps for patient care.

Transparency

Difficult medical outcomes or near misses in pregnant patients are thankfully relatively rare, so it is important that institutions learn as much as possible from the events in order to prevent similar events from reoccurring in the future. The UK CEMACH report in 2007 perhaps says this best: "Every maternal death and serious untoward incident should be critically reviewed and the lessons learnt actively disseminated to all clinical staff, risk managers, and administrators ... The precise educational actions taken as a result must be recorded, audited, and regularly reported to the Board by the clinical governance lead." Each unanticipated serious adverse outcome should trigger a prompt interdisciplinary review of all elements of care with a focus not on whether the outcome could have been different but on how could the care could have been better. The review should also focus less on attributing blame and more on how systems can be designed or improved to minimize the risk of error [6]. Open discussion is critical but the discussion must be followed by unambiguous action plans with clearly defined responsible individuals and deadlines. The lessons learned should be widely disseminated to all clinical staff and administrators and the interventions recorded, audited, and regularly reported to an oversight committee. Talking openly about potential and actual mistakes may be difficult, but can be very powerful in helping to create change. US Supreme Court Justice Louis Brandeis put this well when he said that "Sunlight is said to be the best of disinfectants; electric lights the most efficient policeman" [7].

Teamwork

Few areas of medical practice require an assembly of individuals with such a diverse set of skills and expertise as the care of medically complex obstetric patients. Often this assembly must occur in circumstances that are unanticipated, highly emotionally charged, and in a context where time is of the essence. Forging multidisciplinary teams that proactively work to design care plans which prevent adverse maternal outcomes is critical and can help different specialties to work together. Each specific serious medical problem in pregnancy is infrequent enough that no one specialty group should consider itself expert enough to provide exceptional care to these patients in isolation. The triumvirate of maternal-fetal medicine/obstetrician, medical subspecialist/obstetric internist and obstetric anesthesia/anesthesiologist that is represented by the authorship of each chapter of this book is an approach that is well worth pursuing.

Many hospitals, aware of the challenges of fostering teamwork in medical practice, have invested in "team training" based on experience from the aviation industry aimed at preventing errors through a team approach. The goal of such training is to create a culture that empowers every member of the care team (including those traditionally considered junior or subordinate) to "speak up" if they have concerns that the patient's care is less than it could be and encourages senior members of the team to address all such inquiries constructively (and never dismissively or derisively). "Speaking up" should be done in a manner that is not alarming to the patient. This often requires practice and the adoption of phrases such as "Can we update?" or "I need to clarify something with you" which are understood by all team members to trigger a review of the situation outside the patient's room. "Speaking up" should also be done in a manner that is constructive and specific. Rather than ask "Why are you giving methergine IV?" a more effective alternative might be "I realize the patient is bleeding, but she is a smoker with chronic hypertension and diabetes. IV Methergine can cause coronary artery spasm and myocardial ischemia. Can you help me understand why we are considering IV methergine in this circumstance?" Similarly important to "speaking up" in fostering a safe team environment is standardizing the format and content for all hands-off communications to ensure that both the provider who is being relieved and the provider who is doing the relieving share a similar understanding of the patient's status and the plan of care.

Identifying those at risk

Prenatal care in the rich nations of the world is a highly developed system intended to identify those mothers at increased risk and subsequently intervene at the appropriate time on behalf of both mother and fetus. For many obstetric issues the recommended screening and intervention are fairly standardized and practiced. However, development of standardized approaches to screening and the recommended interventions for many medical issues during pregnancy (such as the need for thromboembolic disease prophylaxis) remain highly variable. Similarly, compliance with screening for substance abuse, seat belt use, domestic violence, and depression is also variable despite our knowledge that these issues contribute significantly to many maternal deaths. Safe medical practice in obstetrics should include standard approaches to screening for medical illness and social ills regularly and the auditing of compliance with both screening recommendations and the clinician's knowledge of how to access effective interventions for patients identified to be at risk.

Some institutions have adopted policies where inpatients are color coded based on shared definitions of their potential risk in the hope of increasing situational awareness and vigilance among providers. With such an approach, it is important to include consideration of obesity, employment status, immigration status, language barriers, race, and ethnicity as each of these factors may place the mother at increased risk.

Intervening early

This element of safety has much in common with the above discussed cultural element of promoting vigilance. Conditions such as sepsis, cerebral hemorrhage from preeclampsia, and pulmonary edema in pregnancy are very often preceded by a period of subtle but progressive deterioration. In cases of sepsis, failure to respond to rising pulse and respiratory rate can be a problem. In cases of intracerebral hemorrhage, delayed response to marked increase in hypertension prior to the stroke is often seen. Early intervention is greatly facilitated by educating all staff about the early signs and symptoms of our most severe complications and defining triggers that will uniformly lead to contacting (and a standardized assessment by) a clinician. Two examples from the Women and Infants Hospital of Rhode Island of such protocols are found in Boxes 50.3 and 50.4. In addition to such disease-specific protocol-driven early interventions, many hospitals, including our own, have

---

Box 50.3 Early identification of sepsis

If patient has a suspected infection with any two of the following, call a physician to assess patient and consider sepsis investigation:

- systolic blood pressure <90, mean arterial pressure <65, heart rate >110 beats per minute, white blood cell count >12,000, <4000 or >10% bands, temperature >38 or <36.

Physician to consider: increasing frequency of vital signs, complete blood count, electrolytes, AST, glucose, lactic acid, urine output monitoring, and large-bore intravenous access.
Quality auditing

- Was serum lactate ordered on patient who met criteria for sepsis investigation?
- Were blood and urine cultures obtained prior to antibiotic administration?
- Were antibiotics administered within 3 hours of admission to the emergency room or within 1 hour of presentation on an inpatient unit in patients with sepsis?

Box 50.4 Early intervention for severe hypertension

Patients with BP >160 systolic or >105 diastolic need the blood pressure reported to the physician and the physician to perform a bedside assessment of the patient.

- Measurement must be done using proper patient positioning and an appropriately sized cuff. If two blood pressures more than 10 minutes apart remain in this range, antihypertensive therapy should be administered.
  Quality auditing
- Was patient assessed promptly with BP >160 systolic or >105 diastolic?
- How long before antihypertensive therapy was administered?
- Was protocol followed for each subsequent elevation in blood pressure in this patient?

Box 50.5 Measures of hospital preparedness for cardiac disease in pregnancy

- Pulse and respiratory rate are always part of the assessment of patients with possible cardiac complaints in both hospital and ambulatory settings.
- Patients with chest pain or who have a syncopal episode should have their pulse and blood pressure measured, and be placed on a cardiac monitor immediately.
- A standardized approach to patients with chest pain is defined and complied with (patient on a monitor, placed on oxygen, serum troponin is obtained, EKG is obtained and read by trained personnel).
- All patients with known cardiac disease have a written standardized multidisciplinary delivery plan in place that has been disseminated to all team members in advance of admission to hospital for delivery.
- All members of the cardiac arrest team know how to get to the labor room in less than 5 minutes.
- All birth attendants for cardiac patients have up-to-date certification in basic and advanced cardiac resuscitation.
- Hospital has regular drills reviewing response to cardiac arrest in obstetric units.

developed a rapid response team of nurses and physicians who are called to provide a second set of eyes on a patient any time a trigger is reached (e.g. respiratory rate >24 or <8/minute, pulse >120/minute or<40/minute). This additional assessment by an experienced team is then relayed to the attending physician.

Being prepared

Even in the setting of all the above safety practices, certain medical diagnoses and emergencies, while infrequent in obstetrics, remain unavoidable. Many potentially harmful errors can be avoided by anticipating these challenges and developing clear standardized simple approaches to facilitate the initial response to these complications. Preparedness for cardiac disease in pregnancy, stroke, seizures, airway difficulties, cardiac resuscitation, massive hemorrhage, and the accommodation of the morbidly obese patient are essential quality hallmarks of an obstetric center that aims to care competently for women with medical problems in pregnancy. Such preparedness can come in many forms and some examples of how it might be measured as it applies to cardiac disease in pregnancy are offered in Box 50.5.

Most essential to this preparedness is the development of multidisciplinary delivery plans for patients with medical problems that include all relevant expertise working on a clear plan that is appropriate for the environment in which the mother will receive care. Maternal-fetal medicine, nursing, anesthesia, neonatology, obstetric medicine (where available), medical specialists, and any other relevant specialty should confer together to design a joint pregnancy management plan

that extends through the postpartum period. This plan needs to acknowledge the limits of obstetric nursing in caring for complex medical problems and the limits of intensive care nursing in caring for obstetric patients. A clear nursing and physician education plan needs to be put in place to facilitate competency and confidence. An educational briefing should ideally occur again on the day of admission for delivery. The plan should be as explicit as possible and anticipate and prevent potential causes of delays should an emergency arise (e.g. the plan for a patient with a potential ventricular arrhythmia in labor is less helpful if it says only "give amiodarone for ventricular tachycardia" and more helpful if it defines for the covering physician and nurse what ventricular tachycardia looks like on the monitor and offers some specific practical details as to how amiodarone is dosed, drawn up, administered and followed for toxicity). A clear list of who should be contacted (and how) when the mother is at risk is also important. In many situations the combination of a critical care and an obstetric nurse at the bedside may be advisable. Once the plan has been agreed upon, it should be disseminated in advance to all team members, with updates made if the patient's status changes. The use of an electronic medical record is particularly helpful in this regard.

Finally, practice drills are also important in preparedness. In addition to the standard cardiac arrest drills, obstetric centers would do well to incorporate regular drills on obstetric hemorrhage, difficult airways, and eclampsia.

Conclusion

This textbook has focused in the past 49 chapters on providing specific expert guidance for the care of a wide range of medical disorders in pregnancy. However, obstetric patients with medical illness may suffer preventable harm even under the care of the most knowledgeable of physicians if active attention is not given to the underlying culture, systems, and care models in which this knowledge is applied. Care should be standardized as much as is sensibly possible, and it should be characterized by teamwork that promotes readiness, early identification of, and intervention for any change in patient status [8].

References

1. Kohn LT, Corrigan J, Donaldson MS (eds). To err is human: building a safer health system. Washington, DC: Committee of Quality of Health Care in America, Institute of Medicine, 2000.
2. Baker G, Norton P, Flintoft V, et al. The Canadian Adverse Events Study: the incidence of adverse events among hospital patients in Canada. Can Med Assoc J 2004;170(11):1678–86.
3. O'Hagan J, MacKinnon NJ, Persaud D, Etchegary H. Self-reported medical errors in seven countries: implications for Canada. Healthcare Quart 2009;12(suppl):55–61.
4. Berg CJ, Harper MA, Atkinson SM, et al. Preventability of pregnancy-related deaths: results of a state-wide review. Obstet Gynecol 2005;106(6):1228–34.
5. CEMACH. Saving mothers' lives 2003–5. London: CEMACH, 2007.
6. American College of Obstetricians and Gynecologists. Patient safety in obstetrics and gynecology. Obstet Gynecol 2009;114(6):1424–7.
7. Brandeis LD. Other people's money and how the bankers use it. Whitefish, MT: Kessinger Publishing, 2009.
8. Gosman GG, Baldisseri MR, Stein KL, et al. Introduction of an obstetric-specific medical emergency team for obstetric crises: implementation and experience. Am J Obstet Gynecol 2008;198:367.

Appendix: Medications and their relative risk to breastfeeding infants

Syndrome or condition	Drugs justified when indicated	Lactation risk category: comments for use in breastfeeding*	RID %**
Acne	Adapalene (topical)	L3; Most unabsorbed topically	
	Benzoyl peroxide (topical)	L1; Unabsorbed, safe	
	Clindamycin topical	L2 ; See antibiotics below	
	Doxycycline	See antibiotics below	
	Isotretinoin (systemic)	L5; Unsafe, do not use	
	Metronidazole (topical)	L3; Compatible. See antibiotics below	
	Tetracyclines (topical)	L2; Topically, compatible. See antibiotics below. Absorption limited	
	Tretinoin topical	L3; Topically, compatible	
Addison's	Hydrocortisone	L2; Compatible. Steroid transfer to milk is negligible	
Attention deficit hyperactivity disorder (ADHD/ADD)	Atomoxetine	L4; No data available	
	Dextroamphetamine	L3; Caution recommended	1.8–6.9
	Methylphenidate	L3; Compatible but some caution recommended	0.2– 0.4
Alcohol use	Ethanol	L3; Compatible at low doses. Recommend 2 hours wait for each drink	16.0
Alcohol withdrawal	Chlordiazepoxide	L3; Probably compatible at low doses. No data however	
	Chlorpromazine	L3; Probably compatible but some risk of apnea. Caution	0.25
	Diazepam	L3; Probably compatible but some sedation reported with chronic use. Acute use is compatible	2.8–7.1
	Disulfiram	L5; Contraindicated	
	Lorazepam	L3; Compatible. Observe for sedation	2.9
	Thiamine	L1; Compatible. Milk levels proportional to intake	
Allergic rhinitis	Cetirizine	L2; Compatible	
	Clemastine	L4; Caution, sedation and irritability reported	5.2
	Desloratadine	L2; Compatible	0.03
	Diphenhydramine	L2; Compatible. Observed for sedation	0.7–1.4
	Fexofenadine	L2; Compatible	0.7
	Loratadine	L1; Compatible	0.29
	Nasal steroids	L3; Compatible. Systemic absorption minimal	
	Pseudoephedrine	L3; Caution. Milk production reduced	4.7
Analgesics	Codeine	L3; Compatible. Limit dose due to sedative effects	8.0
	Diclofenac	L2; Compatible	
	Fentanyl	L2; Compatible. Limit dose due to sedative effects	2.2–5.0
	Gabapentin	L3; Compatible. No adverse events noted	6.5
	Hydrocodone	L3; Compatible. Observe for sedation	
	Hydromorphone	L3; Compatible. Limit dose due to sedative effects	
	Ibuprofen	L1; Compatible. Ideal analgesic	0.65
	Ketorolac	L2; Compatible. Milk levels negligible	0.2
	Meperidine	L2; Compatible but not ideal. Observe for prolonged sedation	1.4–13.9
	Methadone	L3; Compatible	1.9–6.5
	Morphine	L3; Compatible but observe for sedation	9.1–34.9
	Naloxone	L3; Compatible. Poor oral absorption	

(Continued on page. 760)

de Swiet's Medical Disorders in Obstetric Practice, 5th edition.
Edited by R. O. Powrie, M. F. Greene, W. Camann. © 2010
Blackwell Publishing.

Syndrome or condition	Drugs justified when indicated	Lactation risk category: comments for use in breastfeeding*	RID %**
	Naproxen	L3; Compatible. Avoid prolonged use. Watery diarrhea reported	3.3
	Oxycodone	L3; Compatible but observe for sedation	3.5
	Propoxyphene	L2; Compatible	
Anesthesia	Alfentanil	L2; Compatible. Observe for sedation	0.4
	Bupivacaine	L2; Compatible	0.9
	Butorphanol	L2; Compatible	0.1–0.5
	Fentanyl	See analgesics	
	Halothane	L2; Compatible. Trace levels in milk	
	Lidocaine	L2; Compatible	0.5–3.1
	Meperidine	See analgesics	
	Midazolam	L2; Compatible. Cleared rapidly	0.63
	Morphine	L3; Compatible but observe for sedation	
	Nalbuphine	See analgesics	
	Naloxone	See analgesics	
	Nitrous oxide	L3; Compatible. Cleared almost instantly	
	Propofol	L2; Compatible. Cleared rapidly. Milk levels negligible	4.4
	Remifentanil	L3; Compatible. Brief half-life. Milk levels unknown	
	Ropivacaine	L2; Compatible	
	Sevoflurane	L3; Compatible. Brief half-life	
	Sufentanil	See fentanyl	
	Thiopental	L3; Compatible. Rapid distribution out of plasma. Milk levels minimal	2.6
	Tramadol	L2; Compatible. Minimal levels in milk	2.88
Antibiotics	Ampicillin	L1; Safe. Milk levels minimal	0.2–1.5
	Azithromycin	L2; Compatible. Observer for infant diarrhea and thrush	5.88
	Clarithromycin	L1; Compatible. Observer for infant diarrhea and thrush	2.1
	Cephalosporins	L1; Compatible. Observer for infant diarrhea and thrush	
	Chloramphenicol	L4; Avoid if possible. Milk levels low	3.2–8.5
	Clindamycin	L2; Compatible but observe infant for diarrhea	1.0–7.3
	Doxycycline	L3; Compatible. Do not use more than 3 weeks	4.2–13.3
	Gentamicin	L2; Compatible. Poor oral absorption from milk	2.0
	Erythromycin	L2; Compatible, but increased risk of pyloric stenosis in infants <13 days old	2.0
	Metronidazole	L2; Moderate transfer. No reported complications. May impose bitter taste to milk. Stop breastfeeding for 12–24h after 2 gram STAT dose	12.6–13.5
	Nitrofurantoin	L2; Compatible. Avoid in infants with G6PD or jaundice	6.8
	Penicillins	L1; Compatible. Observe for diarrhea or thrush	
	Ciprofloxacin	L3; Compatible. One case of pseudomembranous colitis reported. Ofloxacin or Levofloxacin may be preferred	2.1–6.34
	Sulfonamides	L2; Compatible. Avoid in infants with G6PD and hyperbilirubinemia	
	Tetracyclines	L2; Compatible but limit treatment to less than 3–4 weeks	0.6
	Vancomycin	L1; Compatible. Minimal oral bioavailability	6.7
Antihistamines	H-1 blockers		
	Diphenhydramine	L2; Compatible. Observe for sedation	0.7–1.4
	Chlorpheniramine	L3; Probably compatible. Observe for sedation	
	Brompheniramine	L3; Probably compatible. Observe for sedation	
	Loratadine	L1; Compatible	0.29
	Desloratadine	L2; Compatible	0.03
	Cetirizine	L2; Compatible	
	Fexofenadine	L2; Compatible	0.7
	Promethazine	L2; Probably compatible. Do not use with apneic infants	
	H-2 blockers		
	Cimetidine	L2; Compatible, but dose high	9.8–32.6
	Famotidine	L1; Compatible	1.9
	Nizatidine	L2; Compatible	0.5
	Ranitidine	L2; Compatible	1.3–4.6
Anxiety disorders	Diazepam	L3; Probably compatible. Observe for sedation, lethargy	2.7–7.1
	Buspirone	L3; Probably compatible. Limited data	
	SSRIs	See antidepressants	
	Tricyclics	See antidepressants	
	Zolpidem	L3; Probably compatible. Observe for sedation	4.7–19.1

Syndrome or condition	Drugs justified when indicated	Lactation risk category: comments for use in breastfeeding*	RID %**
Appetite suppressants	Dextroamphetamine	L3; Probably compatible but observed for anorexia and excitement	1.8–6.9
	Phentermine	L4; No data. Caution	
	Sibutramine	L4; No data. Caution	
Asthma	Albuterol/Salbutamol	L1; Safe	
	Beclomethasone	L2; Safe. Unabsorbed	
	Budesonide (oral)	L3; Safe. Unabsorbed orally	
	Cromolyn	L1; Safe	
	Fluticasone and salmeterol	L3; Probably safe. Virtually unabsorbed	
	Formoterol	L3; Probably safe. Maternal levels low	
	Ipratropium	L2; Safe	
	Methylprednisolone	L2; Probably safe. Avoid supratherapeutic or chronic doses	
	Montelukast	L3; Probably safe	
	Prednisone- Prednisolone	L2; Safe. Avoid supratherapeutic doses over prolonged periods	1.8–5.3
	Salmeterol	L2; Safe	
	Triamcinolone	L3; Probably safe. Avoid supratherapeutic doses over prolonged periods	
	Zileuton	L3; Probably safe but no data	
Atopic dermatitis Eczema	Corticosteroids	See asthma	
	Diphenhydramine	L2; Compatible. Observed for sedation	0.7–1.4
	Doxepin	See antidepressants	
	Pimecrolimus	L2; Minimal transcutaneous absorption	
	Hydroxyzine	L1; Safe, but observe for sedation	
	Tacrolimus	L3; Probably safe	0.1–0.5
Atrophic vaginitis	Estrogens (topical)	L3; Probably safe but may reduce milk production. Avoid any form of estrogen	
	Estradiol (vaginal)		
Bipolar affective disorder	Carbamazepine	L2; Probably safe	3.8–5.9
	Haloperidol	L2; Probably safe but observe for sedation	2.1–12.0
	Lamotrigine	L3; Probably safe but observe for sedation. Infant plasma levels drop over time	9.2–22.8
	Lithium	L3; Hazardous. Plasma levels in infants are approximately 40% of maternal plasma	12.0–30.1
	Olanzapine	L2; Probably safe. Observe for sedation	1.2
	Quetiapine	L2; Probably safe. Observe for sedation	0.07–0.1
	Risperidone	L3; Probably safe. Observe for sedation	2.8–9.1
	Topiramate	L3: Probably safe. Observe for sedation	24.5
	Valproic acid	L2; Safe. Possibly monitor liver function periodically	1.4–1.7
Breast cancer	Chemotherapeutic agents	See Hale's Medications and Mothers' Milk 2006, Appendix A	
Candidiasis	Betaconazole	L3; Probably safe	
	Boric acid	L3; Probably safe vaginally. Do not apply to nipples	
	Clotrimazole	L1; Safe but contact dermatitis reported when used on nipples	
	Fluconazole	L2; Safe	16.4–21.5
	Gentian violet	L3; Safe. Do not use more than 5 days due to mucositis	
	Miconazole	L2; Safe, preferred topical azole	
	Nystatin	L1; Safe but has offensive taste. Moderate to poor efficacy	
	Tetrazole	L3; Probably safe but no data	
Cardiac arrhythmia	Adenosine	L1; Safe, brief half-life	
	Amiodarone	L5; Chronic use contraindicated. Brief use (2–3 days) probably safe after 24–48 hour interruption	43.1
	Atropine	L3; Probably safe, but no data	
	Bicarbonate	Safe	
	Calcium gluconate	Safe	
	Digoxin	L2; Safe. Undetectable in infant plasma	2.7–2.8
	Diltiazem	L3; Probably safe but use nifedipine instead	
	Lidocaine	L2; Probably safe if doses are not massive	0.5–3.1
	Magnesium sulfate	L1; Safe, virtually excluded from milk	0.17
	Procainamide	L3; Probably safe but some caution recommended. Others preferred	5.3

(Continued on page. 762)

Syndrome or condition	Drugs justified when indicated	Lactation risk category: comments for use in breastfeeding*	RID %**
Cardiomyopathy/ congestive heart failure/cardiac resuscitation	ACE inhibitors	L2-L3; Probably safe. Avoid use in mothers with premature infants. Captopril, enalapril preferred	
	Digoxin	L2; Safe. Undetectable in infant plasma	2.7–2.8
	Diuretics-furosemide	L3; Probably safe. Limited oral absorption in infants	
	Dopamine	L2; Safe. Brief half life	
	Epinephrine	L1; Safe. Brief half life	
	Heparin	L1; Safe. Limited transport to milk and unabsorbed orally in infant	
	Hydralazine	L2; Safe	1.2
	LMW heparins	L3; Probably safe. Limited transport to milk. Unabsorbed orally	
	Vasopressin	L3; Safe	
	Warfarin	L2; Safe. Virtually excluded from milk. None detected in infant	
Chemicals	Hair dyes	L1; Safe. Limited transcutaneous absorption	
	Cleaning solutions	L1; Safe. Limited transcutaneous absorption	
	Nail polish	L1; Safe. Limited transcutaneous absorption	
	House paints (lead)	L5; Breastfeeding is contraindicated in mothers with high plasma lead levels	
	Asbestos	L5; Contraindicated	
	Mercury	L5; Mercury largely transferred in utero, limited via milk. No problem with mercury dental fillings	
	Pesticides	L5; Caution with some	
	Carbon monoxide	L5; Contraindicated in direct exposure. However, does not transfer into milk	
	Embalming fluids	L3; Probably safe in breastfeeding mother exposed to OSHA-safe environment	
Cholestasis	Cholestyramine	L1; Safe. Unabsorbed	
	Dexamethasone	L3; Probably safe for short duration	
	Diphenhydramine	L2; Compatible. Observe for sedation	0.7–1.4
	Hydroxyzine	L1; Safe, but observe for sedation	
	Ursodeoxycholic acid	L3; Probably safe. Only trace levels in maternal plasma	
Cytomegalovirus	Foscarnet	L4; Potentially hazardous. Milk levels may be excessive with significant toxicity	
	Ganciclovir	L4; Potentially toxic although oral absorption is only 5%	
Coagulation defects	Aminocaproic acid	L4; Possible bleeding but largely unknown	
	Aspirin	L3; Compatible. Safe in small doses (82mg/day), potentially hazardous in high daily doses	2.5–10.8
	Corticosteroids	See individual agents. Mostly compatible over brief intervals	
	Dalteparin	L2; Probably compatible but no data. Insignificant oral absorption	
	DDAVP	L2 Compatible, unabsorbed orally	
	Enoxaparin	L3; Compatible, unabsorbed orally	
	Factor VIII	L1; Compatible, unabsorbed orally	
	Heparin	L1; Compatible, absorption unlikely	
	Tinzaparin	L3; Compatible, unabsorbed	
Congential adrenal hyperplasia	Glucocorticoids	See individual agents. Mostly compatible over brief intervals	
	Fludrocortisone	L3: Probably compatible but no data are available	
Conjunctivitis	Bacitracin	L3; Safe, unabsorbed	
	Ciprofloxacin drops	L3; Safe in eyedrops. Limited absorption	2.1–6.3
	Gentamicin drops	L2; Compatible, limited milk levels and milk levels	2.0
	Polysporin	L3; Safe, largely unabsorbed	
	Sulfacetamide drops	L2; Safe, largely unabsorbed. Caution in hyperbilirubinemic infant	
Constipation	Bisacodyl	L2; Safe, gastric absorption limited	
	Bulking agents	L1; Safe, unabsorbed	
	Castor oil	L3; Moderately safe but some caution advised	
	Colace	L1; Safe, unabsorbed orally	
	Lactulose	L3; Probably safe but no data. Observe for diarrhea	
	Magnesium sulfate	L1; Safe, virtually excluded from milk	0.17
	Psyllium	L1; Safe, unabsorbed	
	Senna	L3; Probably safe. Observe for diarrhea	
	Sorbitol	L3; Probably safe. No data	

Syndrome or condition	Drugs justified when indicated	Lactation risk category: comments for use in breastfeeding*	RID %**
Contraception	Estrogen-progesterone	L3; Compatible but may suppress milk production. Avoid estrogens. especially before breastfeeding is well established	
	IUD-copper	L1; Compatible	
	IUD-progesterone	L1; Compatible	
	Levonorgestrel	L2; Safe	
	Medroxyprogesterone	L1; Safe, avoid early postnatally in some women	
	Etonogestrel/ethyinyl estradiol vaginal ring	L3; Compatible but avoid due to estrogen content. May suppress milk production	
	Emergency contraception	L2; Safe	
	Progestin-only	L3; Safe in most women	
	Prog-estrogen patch	L3; Compatible, but avoid estrogens if possible	
	Spermicide	L1; Safe	
Depression – postpartum	Amitriptyline	L2; Probably safe	1.9–2.8
	Bupropion	L3; Probably safe. Transfer into milk is low. Do not use in infants subject to seizure disorders	0.2–1.98
	Citalopram	L2; Probably safe. Some somnolence reported	3.5–3.6
	Doxepin	L5; Contraindicated. Significant hypotonia and sedation	1.2–3.0
	Duloxetine	L3; Probably safe. Limited data. Use venlafaxine instead	0.14
	Escitalopram	L2; Probably safe. Limited transport to infant	5.18–7.97
	Fluoxetine	L2; Probably safe. Extensively used with minimal problems	6.8
	Mirtazapine	L3; Probably safe. Minimal transfer to infant	1.6–6.3
	Paroxetine	L2; Probably safe. Minimal transfer to infant	1.2–2.8
	Sertraline	L2; Safe. Extensively used with high degree of safety. Limited transfer to infant. Preferred SSRI	0.4–2.2
	Venlafaxine	L3; Probably safe	6.8–8.1
Diabetes insipidus	Chlorpropamide	L3; Probably safe but some risk of hypoglycemia in infant	10.5
	Desmopressin	L2; Safe. No transfer to milk. Oral absorption minimal	0.07
	Thiazide diuretic	L2; Safe	
	Vasopressin	L3; Safe. No data but would be unabsorbed orally	
Diabetes mellitus	Glitazones		
	Rosiglitazone	L3; Probably safe. No data	
	Pioglitazone	L3; Probably safe. No data	
	Sulfonylureas		
	Glyburide	L2; Probably safe. Milk levels were undetectable	
	Glipizide	L3; Probably safe. Milk levels were undetectable	
	Biguanides		
	Metformin	L1; Safe	0.28–0.65
	Insulin	L1; Safe. Unabsorbed orally	
	Glucagon	L3; Probably safe. Unabsorbed orally	
Diuretics	Furosemide	L3; Probably safe. Limited oral absorption in infants	
	HCTZ	L3; Safe	0.15
	Spironolactone	L2; Probably safe	4.3
	Triamterene	L3; Probably safe but other better alternatives are suggested	
Eclampsia	Magnesium sulfate	L1; Safe, virtually excluded from milk	0.17
Endometriosis	Combination OCP	L3; Compatible, but avoid estrogens. May suppress milk supply	
	Danazol	L5; Contraindicated. May suppress prolactin production or milk production	
	Leuprolide	L5; Contraindicated. May suppress prolactin production or milk production	
	Progesterone	L3; Safe in most women. May suppress milk production in rare individual. Oral absorption nil	
Engorgement of breasts	Cabergoline	L4; Contraindicated due to suppression of prolactin production. May be used in hyperprolactinemia	
Fungal infections (Tinea)- cutaneous	Butenafine	L3; Probably safe. Minimal transcutaneous absorption	
	Ciclopirox cream	L3; Probably safe. Minimal transcutaneous absorption	
	Griseofulvin	L2; Probably safe but no data	
	Imidazoles	L3; Probably safe. Minimal transcutaneous absorption	
	Ketoconazole	L2; Safe	0.3
	Naftifine cream	L3; Probably safe but no data. Some absorbed transcutaneously (6%). Avoid if possible	

(Continued on page. 764)

Syndrome or condition	Drugs justified when indicated	Lactation risk category: comments for use in breastfeeding*	RID %**
Gastroenteritis	Bismuth subsalicylate	L3; Probably safe. Poorly absorbed from maternal GI	
	Diphenoxylate	L3; Probably safe but no data	
	Granisetron	L3; Probably safe	
	Loperamide	L2; Safe, limited oral absorption	0.03
	Metoclopramide	L2; Safe. Maternal depression after prolonged exposure. No reported complications in infants	4.7–14.3
	Ondansetron	L2; Safe	
	Promethazine	L2; Probably compatible. Do not use with apneic infants	
Gastroesophageal reflux disease (GERD) and peptic ulcer disease	Cimetidine	L2; Compatible. Observe for sedation	9.8–32.6
	Famotidine	L1; Compatible	1.9
	Lansoprazole	L3; Compatible. Unstable in GI tract	
	Esomeprazole	L2; Compatible. Unstable in GI tract	
	Omeprazole	L2; Compatible. Unstable in GI tract	1.05
	Rabeprazole	L3; Compatible. Unstable in GI tract	
	Ranitidine	L2; Compatible	1.3–4.6
	Sucralfate	L2; Safe, unabsorbed orally	
Heart valves and SBE prophylaxis	Ampicillin	L1; Compatible	0.2–1.5
	Coumadin	L2; Compatible	
	Gentamicin	L2; Compatible. Poor oral absorption from milk	2.0
	Heparin	L1; Safe. Limited transport to milk and unabsorbed orally in infant	
	Dalteparin	L2; Compatible. Insignificant oral absorption	
	Enoxaparin	L3; Probably compatible but no data. Insignificant oral absorption	
	Vancomycin	L1; Compatible. Minimal oral bioavailability	6.7
	Warfarin	L2; Safe. Virtually excluded from milk. None detected in infant	
Hemorrhage	Albumin	L1; Safe	
	Dobutamine	L2; Safe, unabsorbed orally	
	Dopamine	L2; Safe, unabsorbed orally	
	Epinephrine	L1; Safe. Brief half-life. Unabsorbed orally	
	Aminocaproic acid	L4; Possible bleeding but largely unknown	
Hepatitis A	Infection	Safe for breastfeeding	
	Hepatitis A vaccine	L2: Safe	
Hepatitis B	HB infection	Contraindicated. OK following injection of HBIG and vaccination	
	HB immune globulin	L2;Safe	
	Hepatitis B vaccine	L2;Safe	
Hepatitis C	HC infection	L2; Safe	
	Peginterferon	L3; Probably safe but no data	
	Ribavirin	L4; Probably contraindicated for chronic use	
	Amantadine	L3; Moderately safe. May suppress prolactin production. Long-term effects unknown	
Herbal remedies	Black cohosh	L4; Possibly hazardous. May suppress prolactin secretion	
	Blessed thistle	L3; Probably safe but unknown for sure. Commonly used to stimulate milk production	
	Blue cohosh	L5; Absolutely contraindicated. Myocardial toxicant	
	Echinacea	L3; Probably safe. Immune stimulant, but effect on lactation is unknown	
	Fenugreek	L3; Safe. May stimulate milk production but largely undocumented. Apparently quite safe	
	Garlic	L3; Probably safe but limited data	
	Ginkgo biloba	L3; Probably safe but limited data	
	Ginseng	L3; Probably safe but limited data	
	Kava Kava	L5; Contraindicated	
	St. John's Wort	L2; Safe. Levels in milk negligible. May have numerous drug-drug interactions. Caution	
HIV		L5; Contraindicated in the USA and other developed nations	
Human papilloma virus	Podophyllin	L5; Contraindicated. Milk levels are unreported but toxicity is high. Pump and discard milk for 24 hours	
	Topical 5-fluorouracil	L5; Contraindicated in mothers receiving IV therapy. Withhold breastfeeding 24 hours. OK following topical or intraocular therapy	
	Trichloroacetic acid	L3; Probably safe. Unabsorbed topically	

Syndrome or condition	Drugs justified when indicated	Lactation risk category: comments for use in breastfeeding*	RID %**
Herpes simplex virus 1 or 2	Acyclovir	L2; Safe	1.1–1.5
	Famciclovir	L2; Safe	
	Valacyclovir	L1; Safe. Precursor of acyclovir	4.7
Hypercholesterolemia	Cholestyramine	L1; Safe, unabsorbed	
	Clofibrate	L3; Probably safe but not recommended in breastfeeding mothers	
	Gemfibrozil	L3; Probably safe but not recommended in breastfeeding mothers	
	Niacin	L3; Probably safe. Avoid however due to high doses required	
	HMG-CoA reductase inhibitors (statins)	L3; Probably safe but not recommended in breastfeeding mothers. Avoid during lactation	
Hypertension	Beta blockers		
	Atenolol	L3; Probably safe but not recommended. Observe for hypotonia and weakness	6.6
	Labetalol	L2; Probably safe	0.2–0.6
	Metoprolol	L3; Probably safe. Preferred beta blocker	1.4
	Propranolol	L2; Safe in moderate to low doses	0.3–0.5
	Calcium channel blockers		
	Amlodipine	L3; Probably safe	
	Diltiazem	L3; Probably safe	
	Felodipine	L3; Probably safe, but no data	
	Nifedipine	L2; Safe. Preferred	2.3–3.4
	Verapamil	L2; Safe	0.15–0.2
	Angiotensin converting enzyme inhibitors and angiotensin receptor blockers		
	Benazepril	L2; Safe but avoid use in mothers with premature infants	0.00006
	Captopril	L2; Safe but avoid use in mothers with premature infants	
	Enalapril	L2; Safe but avoid use in mothers with premature infants	0.175–0.178
	Losartan	L3; Probably safe. No data	
	Diuretics		
	Furosemide	L3; Probably safe. Limited oral absorption in infants	
	HCTZ	L3; Safe. Thrombocytopenia reported but rare	0.16
	Nitrates		
	Isosorbide dinitrate	L3; Avoid if possible. Data limited on all nitrates	
	Nitroglycerin	L4; Avoid if possible. Data limited on all nitrates	
	Na nitroprusside	L4; Avoid if possible. No data	
	Hydralazine	L2; Safe	1.2
	Methyldopa	L2; Safe	0.1–0.3
	Spironolactone	L2; Safe	4.3
Hyperthyroidism	Iodides	L4; Unsafe. Concentrated in milk. May suppress infant thyroid	High
	Lithium	L3; Hazardous. Plasma levels in infants are approximately 40% of maternal plasma	12.5–30.1
	Methimazole	L3; Probably safe	2.3
	Propranolol	L2; Safe in moderate to low doses	0.3–0.5
	Propylthiouracil	L2; Safe	1.83–1.84
Hypothyroidism	Levothyroxine	L1; Safe. Does not transfer into milk	
	Armour thyroid	L1; Safe. Does not transfer into milk	
Inflammatory bowel disease (Crohn's ulcerative colitis)	Azathioprine	L3; Probably safe. Some caution recommended	0.06–0.26
	Ciprofloxacin	See antibiotics	
	Infliximab	L2; Probably safe. Milk levels low to undetectable. Not absorbed orally	
	Mesalamine	L3; Probably safe. Limited oral absorption in several cases	0.1–8.75
	Methylprednisolone	L2; Safe in moderate to low acute doses. Avoid prolonged and high doses	
	Metronidazole	See antibiotics	
	Prednisolone	L2; Safe in moderate to low acute doses. Avoid prolonged and high doses	1.8–5.3
	Sulfasalazine	L3; Probably safe. Transfer minimal	0.3–1.1
Influenza	Amantadine	L3; Moderately safe. May suppress prolactin production. Long-term effects unknown	
	Oseltamivir	L2; Probably safe but no data	
	Ribavirin	L4; Probably contraindicated for chronic use	0.5

(*Continued on page. 766*)

Syndrome or condition	Drugs justified when indicated	Lactation risk category: comments for use in breastfeeding*	RID %**
	Rimantadine	L3; Probably safe. Used in infants. No data. Caution	
	Zanamivir	L3; Probably safe. Limited systemic absorption in mother. Poor oral bioavailability	
Iron deficiency anemia	Erythropoietin	L3; Probably safe but no data. Unabsorbed orally	
	Ferrous gluconate	L2; Safe. Ferrous salts enter milk poorly	
	Ferrous sulfate	L2; Safe. Ferrous salts enter milk poorly	
	IM iron	L2; Safe. Ferrous salts enter milk poorly	
	Vitamin C	L1; Safe. Levels in milk limited	
Irritable bowel syndrome	Alosetron	L3; Probably safe but no data. Maternal plasma levels minimal	
	Dicyclomine	L4; Possibly hazardous	6.9
	SSRIs	See antidepressants	
	Tegaserod	L3; Probably safe but no data. Limited oral absorption. Some caution recommended	
Lyme disease	Ampicillin	L1; Safe. Milk levels minimal	0.2–1.5
	Cefuroxime	L2; Safe. Bitter taste	0.6–2.03
	Doxycycline	L3; Compatible. Do not use more than 3 weeks	4.2–13.3
Malaria	Chloroquine	L2; Probably safe. Much less than pediatric dose administered	0.6–2.3
	Doxycycline	L3; Compatible. Do not use more than 3 weeks	4.2–13.3
	Mefloquine	L2; Safe. Milk levels low. Dose via milk insufficient to protect infant from malaria. Infant requires own dosage	0.13–0.2
	Pyrimethamine	L3; Unsafe. Strong folic acid antagonist. Avoid	45.8
	Quinine sulfate	L2; Safe. Trace levels in milk	0.7–1.3
	Sulfadoxine	L3; Probably safe but no data. Caution	
	Tetracycline	L2; Compatible but limit treatment to less than 3–4 weeks	0.6
Mastitis or breast abscess	Ciprofloxacin	See antibiotics	
	Dicloxacillin	See antibiotics	
	Erythromycin	See antibiotics	
Migraine headache	Amitriptyline	L2; Probably safe	1.9–2.8
	Aspirin	L3; Compatible. Safe in small doses (82mg/day), potentially hazardous in high daily doses	2.5–10.8
	Atenolol	L3; Probably safe but not recommended. Observe for hypotonia and weakness	6.6
	Butalbital	L3; Probably safe. Limited data	
	Caffeine	L2; Safe but observe for excitement and insomnia	6–25.9
	Codeine	L3; Probably safe. Limit dose due to sedative effects especially in those rare individuals who metabolize this drug differently than others	8.1
	Ergotamines	L4; Contraindicated. Suppress prolactin release	
	Fioricet	L3; Probably safe	
	Meperidine	L2; Probably safe. Levels in milk limited but sedation is possible. Avoid in neonate due to sedation and poor feeding	1.4–13.9
	Midrin	L3; Probably safe but no data on any drug in this product. Avoid if possible	
	Promethazine	L2; Probably compatible. Do not use with apneic infants	
	Propranolol	L2; Safe in moderate to low doses	0.28–0.5
	Sumatriptan	L3; Probably safe. Preferred tryptan. Good data on this product. Avoid other tryptans due to lack of data	3.5–15.3
Multiple sclerosis	Alpha interferon	L2; Probably safe. Milk levels low to undetectable	
	Beta interferons	L3; Probably safe. Milk levels when determined will be low	
	Amitriptyline	L2; Probably safe	1.5
	Azathioprine	L3; Probably safe. Some caution recommended	0.06–0.26
	Baclofen	L2; Probably safe but may suppress prolactin production. Caution	6.9
	Carbamazepine	L2; Probably safe	3.8–5.9
	Corticosteroids	L2; Probably safe. Avoid high doses over prolonged periods	
	Cyclophosphamide	L5; Contraindicated. Transfer to milk suspected. One case of infantile neutropenia reported	
	Cyclosporine	L3; Probably safe but caution recommended. Several cases reported of safe use. One case of high infantile dose	0.4–3.0
	Phenytoin	L2; Safe. Numerous cases reported but measuring neonatal plasma initially recommended	0.6–7.7

Syndrome or condition	Drugs justified when indicated	Lactation risk category: comments for use in breastfeeding*	RID %**
Polycystic ovary syndrome	Clomiphene	L3; Probably safe but avoid using early postnatally. May suppress lactation	
	Metformin	L1; Safe. Minimal transfer to milk	
	Oral contraceptives	L3; Probably safe but avoid estrogen-containing forms	
	Progestins	L3; Probably safe but observe for changes in milk production	
	Spironolactone	L2; Probably safe	4.3
Prolactinoma	Bromocriptine	L5; Contraindicated. Suppresses prolactin production	
	Cabergoline	L4; Contraindicated. Suppresses prolactin production. May be used in lactation if lower doses carefully administered	
Pseudotumor cerebri	Acetazolamide	L2; Safe. Plasma levels in infant reportedly very low	2.2
	Dexamethasone	L3; Probably safe if used acutely, in moderate to low doses	
	Furosemide	L3; Probably safe. Limited oral absorption in infants	
Psoriasis	Anthralin (topical)	L3; Probably safe but do not use on areola or nipple	
	Calcipotriene (topical)	L3; Probably safe. Transcutaneous absorption limited	
	Corticosteroids (topical)	L2; Probably safe. Avoid high doses over prolonged periods	
	Pimecrolimus (topical)	L2; Safe. Limited transcutaneous absorption. Used in pediatric patients	
	Tacrolimus (topical)	L3; Probably safe. Transfer to milk is limited	
	Tar ointments (topical)	L3; Probably safe but do not use on areola or nipple	
Pulmonary HTN	Epoprostenol (prostacyclin)	L3; Probably safe. Rapidly metabolized (3–5 minutes)	
	Nifedipine	L2; Safe. Preferred	2.3–3.4
	Sildenafil	L3; Probably safe. Milk levels are likely low due to large molecular weight. Observe for priapism	
PUPPS	Hydroxyzine	L1; Safe	
	Bile salt chelator	L1; Unabsorbed. See cholestyramine	
	Corticosteroids	L2; Safe in moderate to low acute doses. Avoid prolonged high doses	
	Diphenhydramine	L2; Compatible. Observe for sedation	0.7–1.4
	Topical steroids	L2; Safe. Use low to medium potency steroids only	
Radiography	X-ray	L1; Safe	
	CT − contrast	All CT and Gadolinium contrast agents are considered safe by the American College of Radiology for use in breastfeeding women	
	CT + contrast		
	MRI − contrast		
	MRI + contrast		
	Fluoroscopy	L1; Safe	
	Nuclear scans	L4; Generally unsafe but check radiation tables in Hale's reference	
Radioisotopic procedures	^{131}I	L4; Contraindicated. Highly dangerous to breastfeeding infant. Stop breastfeeding until radioactive counts at background (<40 days)	
	^{123}I	L4; Contraindicated. Interrupt breastfeeding until radioactive counts at background (generally a few days)	
	^{99}mTc	L4; Potentially hazardous. Withhold breastfeeding for 0–48 hours. Brief half-life (6 hours). Check Hale*	
Renal failure or renal transplants	Antihypertensives	See hypertension	
	Azathioprine	L3; Probably safe. Some caution recommended	0.06–0.26
	Cyclosporine	L3; Probably safe but caution recommended. Several cases reported of safe use. One case of high infantile dose	0.4–3.0
	Prednisone	L2; Safe in even higher to moderate doses. Avoid high and prolonged doses	1.8–5.3
Rheumatologic conditions including rheumatoid arthritis and SLE	Adalimumab	L3; Probably safe	
	Anakinra	L3; Probably safe	
	Azathioprine	L3; Probably safe. Some caution recommended	0.06–0.26
	Corticosteroids	L2; Safe in even moderate to higher doses. Avoid high and prolonged doses	
	Cyclophosphamide	L5; Contraindicated. Transfer to milk suspected. One case of infantile neutropenia reported	
	Diclofenac	L2; Safe. Observe for GI symptoms	
	Etanercept	L3; Probably safe	
	Gold	L5; Contraindicated	0.6–2.8
	Hydroxychloroquine	L2; Probably safe. About 1 mg/liter of milk. Consult with ophthalmologist may be advised	2.88–2.89
	Indomethacin	L3; Probably safe. Some caution due to one case report of seizures, but no reported problems in large study of 16 patients	1.2

(Continued on page. 768)

Syndrome or condition	Drugs justified when indicated	Lactation risk category: comments for use in breastfeeding*	RID %**
	Infliximab	L2; probably safe. Large molecule unlikely to enter breast milk and not orally bioavailable	
	Leflunomide	L4; Possibly hazardous	
	Methotrexate	L3; Probably safe but only for acute use at low doses. L5 for chronic use or high doses. Milk levels are low	0.12
	NSAIDs	L2; Probably safe. Ibuprofen, celecoxib, and diclofenac preferred	
	Penicillamine	L4; Possibly hazardous	
	Salicylates	L3; Probably safe but only at low doses. Risk of Reye syndrome	
	Sulfasalazine	L3; Probably safe. Several studies suggest it is safe to use	0.3–1.1
	Sulindac	L3; Probably safe but no data. Use ibuprofen, diclofenac, celecoxib, or naproxen instead	
Scabies	Lindane	L4; Possibly hazardous. Do not use. Levels in milk possibly high	
	Permethrin cream	L2; Safe	
	Ivermectin	L3; Probably safe. Milk levels low. Limited transfer to infant	1.3
Schizophrenia and psychosis	Haloperidol	L2; Probably safe. Milk levels low. Observed for sedation	2.1–12
	Olanzapine	L2; Probably safe. Milk levels low	1.2
	Quetiapine	L2; Probably safe. Milk levels low	0.07–0.1
	Risperidone	L3; Probably safe. Milk levels low. None detected in infant plasmas	2.8–9.1
Seizure disorder	Carbamazepine	L2; Probably safe	3.8–5.9
	Ethosuximide	L4; Possibly hazardous. Milk levels high. Avoid	31.5
	Felbamate	L4; Possibly hazardous	
	Gabapentin	L2; Probably safe but detectable in infant plasma at low levels	6.59
	Lamotrigine	L3; Probably safe but observe for sedation. Infant plasma levels drop over time	9.2–22.8
	Levetiracetam	L3; Probably safe	3.36–7.8
	Phenobarbital	L3; Probably safe but infant plasma levels range from 30–40% of maternal levels	24.0
	Phenytoin	L2; Safe. Numerous cases reported but measuring neonatal plasma at least initially is recommended	0.6–7.7
	Topiramate	L3; Probably safe. Observe for sedation	24.5
	Valproic acid	L2; Probably safe. Milk levels average 1.4 mg/L. May need to monitor infant liver function initially	1.4–1.7
Sexually transmitted diseases	Azithromycin	L2; Compatible. Observe infant for diarrhea and thrush	5.88
	Cefixime	L2; Safe. Undetectable in milk. Absorbed poorly	
	Ceftriaxone	L1; Safe. Milk levels low. Unabsorbed orally. Observe for diarrhea	4.1–4.2
	Ciprofloxacin	L3; Compatible	2.1–6.3
	Doxycycline	L3; Compatible. Do not use for more than three weeks	4.2–13.3
	Levofloxacin	L3; Safe but no data. Milk levels should be low, similar to ofloxacin (3.1%)	10.5–17.2
Sleep disorders	Eszopiclone	L3; Probably safe, but studies incomplete	
	Zaleplon	L2; Probably safe. Levels in milk averaged 14 ug/liter	1.5
	Zolpidem	L3; Probably safe. Once case of sedation has been reported	4.7–19.1
	Temazepam	L3; Probably safe. Levels in infant undetectable	
	Melatonin	L3; Probably safe. No reports of somnolence in infants	
	Valerian	L3; Probably safe but data on this herbal remedy is limited. Some caution is recommended	
Smoking cessation	Bupropion	L3; Probably safe. Transfer into milk is low. Do not use in infants subject to seizure disorders	0.2–1.98
	Varenicline	L4; Probably safe but no data yet. Blocks nicotine receptor. Few side effects	
	Nicotine patches/gum	L2; Probably safe. Highest patch equivalent to 1 pack/day smoker. Start with mid level patch if possible	
Stroke- ischemic	Aspirin	L3; Compatible. Safe in small doses (82 mg/day), potentially hazardous in high daily doses	2.52–10.8
	Clopidogrel	L3; Probably safe. Irreversibly inhibits platelet function. Some caution is recommended	
	Coumadin (warfarin)	L2; Safe. Virtually excluded from milk. None detected in infant	
	Heparin	L1; Safe. Limited transport to milk and unabsorbed orally in infant	
	LMW heparins	L3; Probably compatible but no data. Insignificant oral absorption	
	Streptokinase	L2; Probably safe. Would not enter milk nor be orally bioavailable to infant	
	TPA	L2; Probably safe. Would not enter milk nor be orally bioavailable to infant	

Syndrome or condition	Drugs justified when indicated	Lactation risk category: comments for use in breastfeeding*	RID %**
Tuberculosis	Ethambutol	L2; Safe. Milk levels are reported to be 1.4 mg/liter	1.5
	Isoniazid	L3; Probably safe but monitor infant for liver function	1.2–18
	Pyrazinamide	L3; Probably safe	1.5
	Pyridoxine	L2; Safe, but avoid high doses (600 mg)	
	Rifampin	L2; Safe. Depending on dose, milk levels are moderate. No reported complications	5.3–11.5
Toxoplasmosis	Pyrimethamine	L3; Probably safe although relative infant dose is high. May produce clinical range for infant	45.8
	Sulfadiazine	L3; Probably safe. Do not use in infant with hyperbilirubinemia	
	Trisulfapyrimidines	L3; Probably safe. Do not use in infant with hyperbilirubinemia	
URI	Dextromethorphan	L1; Safe	
	Diphenhydramine	See antihistamines	
	Guaifenesin	See antihistamines	
	Pseudoephedrine	L3; Caution. Milk production may be reduced	4.7
	See antibiotics		
	See asthma		
Vaccines	HPV (Gardasil)	At this time, all vaccines are cleared by the CDC for use in breastfeeding mothers. Yellow fever should be avoided unless the infant is significantly subject to exposure in high endemic areas	
	Hepatitis A		
	Hepatitis B		
	Influenza		
	Yellow fever		
	MMR		
	Diphtheria-tetanus		
	Varicella		
	Pneumococcal		
	Meningococcal		
	Polio		
	Rabies		
	Typhoid		
	Tuberculin-PPD		
	BCG		

* Data and references derived, with permission, from Hale's *Medication and Mothers' Milk*, 14th edition. Hale Publishing, Amarillo, Texas, 2010.
** Relative infant dose (RID): calculated by dividing the infant's dose via milk (in mg/kg/day) by the mother's dose (in mg/kg/day). Many experts would submit that a RID of <10% is unlikely to be of concern to an infant's wellbeing.

BCG, bacillus Calmette-Guerin; CDC, Centers for Disease Control; CT, computed tomography; DDAVP, desmopressin; G6PD, glucose-6- phosphate dehydrogenase; HCTZ, hydrochlorothiazide; HIV, human immunodeficiency virus; HPV, human papilloma virus; HSV, herpes simples virus; HTN, hypertension; IM, intramuscular; IUD, intrauterine device; LMWH, low molecular weight heparin; MMR, mumps measles rubella; MRI, magnetic resonance imaging; NSAIDs, nonsteroidal anti-inflammatory drugs; OCP, oral contraceptive pill; OSHA, United States' Government's Occupational Safety and Health Administration; PPD, tuberculin skin test; PUPPS, pruritic urticarial papules and plaques of pregnancy; SLE, systemic lupus erythematosus; SSRIs, selective serotonin reuptake inhibitors; tPA, tissue plasminogen activator; URI, upper respiratory tract infection.

Index